Myles Textbook for
Midwives

Myles Textbook for **Midwives**

17THedition

Edited by

Jayne E **Marshall** FRCM, PFHEA, PhD, MA, PGCEA, ADM, RM, RGN

Foundation Professor of Midwifery / Lead Midwife for Education,
School of Allied Health Professions, College of Life Sciences,
George Davies Centre, University of Leicester, Leicester, UK

Maureen D **Raynor** MA PGCEA ADM RMN RN RM

Senior Lecturer in Midwifery, De Montfort University, Faculty of Health
and Life Sciences, Leicester School of Nursing and Midwifery, Division
of Maternal and Child Health, Leicester, UK

Foreword by
Professor Jacqueline Dunkley-Bent OBE

ELSEVIER

Edinburgh London New York Oxford Philadelphia St Louis Sydney 2020

First edition 1953
Second edition 1956
Third edition 1958
Fourth edition 1961
Fifth edition 1964
Sixth edition 1968
Seventh edition 1971
Eighth edition 1975

Ninth edition 1981
Tenth edition 1985
Eleventh edition 1989
Twelfth edition 1993
Thirteenth edition 1999
Fourteenth edition 2003
Fifteenth edition 2009
Sixteenth edition 2014

Notices

ISBN: 978-0-7020-7642-8
IE ISBN: 978-0-7020-7643-5

Content Strategist: Alison Taylor and Poppy Garraway
Content Development Specialist: Veronika Watkins
Content Coordinator: Susan Jansons
Project Manager: Anne Collett and Louisa Talbott
Design: Amy Buxton

Printed in India

Last digit is the print number: 9 8 7 6 5 4

Working together
to grow libraries in
developing countries

www.elsevier.com • www.bookaid.org

CONTENTS

CONTRIBUTORS

Kirsten Allen, BMBS, MMedSci
Obstetrics and Gynaecology,
Nottingham University Hospitals NHS Trust,
Nottingham, UK

Michelle Anderson, RM, BSc(Hons), Psy, BSc, PGCert (Med Sim)
Research Midwife
The Royal Free London NHS Foundation Trust
London, UK

Julia Austin, PGDip, BA(Hons), RM, RGN
Consultant Midwife
Public Health Research and Quality Standards/
    Professional Midwifery Advocate
University Hospitals of Leicester NHS Trust
Womens' and Childrens' Directorate
Leicester Royal Infirmary, Leicester, UK
Honorary Senior Lecturer, University of Leicester
Leicester, UK

Jenny Bailey, MMedSci/Clinical education, BN, DANS
Former Assistant Professor Midwifery (RGN, RM),
    Division of Midwifery,
University of Nottingham
Nottingham, UK

Helen Baston, BA(Hons), MMedSci, PhD, PGDipEd, ADM, RN, RM
Consultant Midwife Public Health
Sheffield Teaching Hospitals NHS Foundations Trust
UK;
Honorary Researcher/Lecturer
University of Sheffield
Honorary Lecturer Sheffield Hallam University
UK

Cecily Begley, RGN, RM, RNT, FFNRCSI, MSc, MA, PhD, FTCD
Professor of Nursing and Midwifery
School of Nursing and Midwifery
Trinity College Dublin
Dublin, Ireland

Jenny Brewster, MEd (open), BSc(Hons) Health Studies, RM
Senior Lecturer in Midwifery, CNMH
University of West London
Brentford, UK

Angela Brown, BNurs, BMid, MBA, PhD
Lecturer in Midwifery
School of Nursing and Midwifery
University of South Australia
Adelaide, Australia

Terri Coates, MSc, RN, RM, ADM, Dip Ed
Freelance Midwifery Advisor (Television and Film),
    London UK,
PhD Student: Media and communication
Bournemouth University
Bournemouth, UK

Sarah Coombes, BSc(Hons)
Trustee, Beat SCAD
Derbyshire, UK

Helen Crafter, RM, ADM, PGCEA, MSc Health Education
(Retired) Formerly College of Nursing
Midwifery and Healthcare
University of West London
Brentford
Middlesex, UK

Joanne Dickens, BSc, PgCert, RM
Bereavement Specialist Midwife/PhD Student
SAPPHIRE (Social Science Applied to Healthcare
    Improvement Research)/The Infant Mortality and
    Morbidity Studies (TIMMS)
Department of Health Sciences
College of Life Sciences
George Davies Centre
University of Leicester
Leicester, UK

Rowena Doughty, PhD, MSc, BA (Hons), ADM, RM, RN
Lead Midwife for Education
Leicester School of Nursing and Midwifery
De Montfort University
Leicester
Leicestershire, UK

Soo Downe OBE, PhD, MSc, RM, BA(Hons)
Professor of Midwifery Studies
Brook Building
University of Central Lancaster
Preston, Lancashire, UK

Clare Gordon, MSc Public Health Practice, BSc(Hons) Midwifery
Senior Lecturer in Midwifery
College of Nursing
Midwifery and Healthcare
University of West London
London, UK

Kerry Green, BSc(Hons) Midwifery
Health and Life Sciences
De Montfort University
Leicester, UK

Richard Hayman, MBBS FRCOG DM
Consultant, Obstetrics and Gynaecology
Gloucestershire Hospitals NHS Foundation Trust
Gloucester, UK

Jenny Hendley, PhD, MSc, PG Cert, BSc, RM, RGN
Senior Midwifery Lecturer
School of Health Sciences
University of Brighton
Brighton, East Sussex, UK

Karen Jackson, MPhil, BSc(Hons), ADM, RM, RN
Former Assistant Professor in Midwifery/PhD student
Division of Midwifery
University of Nottingham
Nottingham, Nottinghamshire, UK

Amar Jawad,
Consultant Obstetric Anaesthetist
Chesterfield Royal Hospital
Derbyshire, UK

Lucy Kean, BM BCh, DM FRCOG
Obstetrics and Gynaecology
Nottingham University Hospitals NHS Trust,
Nottingham, UK

Michael RB Keighley
Emeritus Professor of Surgery
President of the MASIC Foundation

Joy Kemp, RGN, RM, CTCM&H, MSc, PGCLT (HE), FHEA
Global Professional Advisor
The Royal College of Midwives,
London, UK

Michelle Knight, PGCEA, BSc, RM
Consultant Midwife
Epsom and St Helier Hospital NHS Trust
Carshalton, Surrey, UK

Joan G Lalor
Professor of Midwifery
School of Nursing and Midwifery
Trinity College Dublin, Ireland

Alison Ledward, PhD, MPhil, MSc, RM, RGN, BA
Freelance writer
School of Allied Health Professions
College of Life Sciences
George Davies Centre
University of Leicester
Leicester, UK

Jayne E Marshall, FRCM, PFHEA, PhD, MA, PGCEA, ADM, RM, RGN
Foundation Professor of Midwifery/Lead Midwife for
    Education
School of Allied Health Professions
College of Life Sciences
George Davies Centre
University of Leicester
Leicester, UK

Amy Mason
Writer and Comedian

Carol McCormick
Consultant Midwife (retired)
Nottingham, UK

John McIntyre, MBChB DM FRCPCH
Consultant Neonatologist
Derbyshire Children's Hospital
Derby, UK

**Helen McIntyre, SFHEA, DHSci, MSc, BSc(Hons)
PGDE, RM, RGN**
Associate Professor of Midwifery
School of Allied Health Professions
College of Life Sciences
George Davies Centre
University of Leicester
Leicester, UK

**Moira McLean, RGN, RM, ADM, PGCEA, PG Dip,
PMA**
Senior Lecturer Midwifery
Leicester School Nursing and Midwifery
De Montfort University
Leicester, UK

Aarti Mistry, MBChB, MRCPCH
Clinical Research Fellow
School of Medicine
University of Nottingham
Nottingham, UK

Sylvia Murphy Tighe
Lecturer/ Course Director BSc Midwifery
Dept of Nursing and Midwifery
University of Limerick

Irene Murray, BSc(Hons) Midwifery
Lecturer (Midwifery)
Department of Nursing and Midwifery
University of the Highlands and Islands
Old Perth Road, Inverness, Highland, UK

Mary L Nolan, PhD, MA, BA(Hons)
Nursing and Midwifery
University of Worcester
Worcester, UK

**Shalini Ojha, PhD, Diploma (Med Ed), MD,
MRCPCH, MBBS**
Clinical Associate Professor
School of Medicine
University of Nottingham
Nottingham, UK

Kathleen O'Reilly, MBChB, MA, MRCPCH
Consultant Neonatologist
Neonatal Medicine
Royal Hospital for Children
Glasgow, UK

Jean Rankin, PhD, MMedical Science, BSc(Hons)
Professor
Health, Nursing and Midwifery
University of the West of Scotland
Paisley, UK

Hazel Ransome, RM BSc(Hons), PGCLTHE
Senior Lecturer Midwifery
Department of Midwifery
Faculty of Health Social Care and Education
Kingston University
London, UK

**Maureen D Raynor, MA, PGCEA, ADM, RMN, RN,
RM**
Senior Lecturer in Midwifery
De Montfort University
Faculty of Health and Life Sciences
Leicester School of Nursing and Midwifery
Division of Maternal and Child Health
Leicester, UK

Mary J Renfrew, BSc, RN, RM, PhD, FRSE
Professor of Mother and Infant Research Unit
School of Nursing and Health Sciences
University of Dundee
Dundee UK

Mary Ross-Davie, BA(Hons), MA, RM, PhD, FHEA
Royal College of Midwives Director for Scotland
Edinburgh, UK

Lindsey Ryan BSc, RM
Lead Midwife for Clinical Education
Chesterfield Royal Hospital Foundation Trust
Derbyshire, UK

Judith Simpson, MRCPCH
Consultant Neonatologist
Neonatal Intensive Care Unit
Royal Hospital for Children
Glasgow, UK

Gill Skene, MA Eng
Scottish Representative
The Birth Trauma Association (BTA)
Maternal and Mental Health Scotland
Change Agent
Edinburgh, UK

Liz Snapes, MSc, PGCE(Ed), BSc(Hons), RM
Senior Lecturer Midwifery
Faculty of Health Education, Medicine and Social Care
Anglia Ruskin University
Cambridge, UK

Mary Steen, RGN, RM, BHSc, PGCRM, PGDipHE, MCGI, PhD
Professor of Midwifery
School of Nursing and Midwifery
University of South Australia
Adelaide, Australia

Abdul H Sultan, MB, ChB, MD, FRCOG
Consultant Obstetrician and UroGynaecologist
Obstetrics and Gynaecology
Croydon University Hospital
Croydon, Surrey, UK

Ranee Thakar, MD, MRCOG
Obstetrics and Gynaecology
Croydon University Hospital
Croydon, Surrey, UK

Liana Tsilika, BMedSci, BMBS, MRCPCH
Paediatric Registrar
Neonatal Intensive Care
Nottingham University Hospitals
Nottingham, UK

Helen Turier, RGN (retired)
Head of Family & Professional Support
Family & Professional Support
Twins Trust, Aldershot, UK

Pete Wallroth
Founder & CEO Mummy's Star (reg charity: 1152808 & SC046449)
Hadfield
Derbyshire, UK

Sherry Whibley, BSc, RGN
The University of Greenwich
London, UK

Mark Williams
Campaigner and Author
Father's Reaching Out

I am deeply humbled and honoured to write the foreword for this incredible text book. As the Chief Midwifery Officer for the NHS in England, I am passionate about the unique and significant contribution that midwives make to the maternity experiences of women, babies and their families. Globally midwives work tirelessly to provide the best maternity care for women and babies that women seldom forget. The old adage that a woman never forgets her midwife is a reality and I am keen that the memory is a positive one! The knowledge gained from the content of this textbook will provide an opportunity for student midwives and midwives to be the best that they can be.

Since the publication of the sixteenth edition of *Myles Textbook for Midwives* in 2014, the needs of childbearing women, babies and their families have continued to shape the provision of maternity care and the role of the midwife in contemporary society. More women in the United Kingdom are having babies when they are older, are of a greater weight and present with more underlying health conditions than ever before.

The proportion of mothers aged 35 years or older at the time of birth in England and Wales has increased year on year from 19.9% in 2010 to 23.4% in 2018, which continues a long-term increasing trend since the 1970s. More than half of women (50.4%) with a recorded BMI at booking were overweight or obese (up from 47.3% in 2015/16).[1] Inequalities in health outcomes continue to persist and perinatal mental health continues to drive the development of timely and appropriate short- and long-term healthcare.

Health care policy in the UK has kept pace with these changes and since the 2016 publication of *Better Births*,[2] the report of the national maternity review, the NHS

in England and system partners have collectively come together to implement its vision, for safer and more personalised care across England and deliver the national ambition to half the rates of stillbirths, neonatal mortality, maternal mortality and brain injury by 2025. I am mindful that healthcare policy and its focus on maternity care is not universal, but the knowledge espoused in this textbook will undoubtedly support midwives worldwide to improve this care.

The midwife plays a significant and pivotal role in improving health outcomes, ensuring that care is personalised and safe. This contribution is usually unique and involves the development of a special relationship between the woman and midwife and sometimes the family too, if they are present. This relationship develops and flourishes if the same midwife provides antenatal, intrapartum and postnatal care and is associated with improved experiences and health outcomes. I am reassured that the seventeenth edition of the *Myles Textbook for Midwives* provides the depth and breadth of knowledge to support a student midwife and the continuing professional development of a qualified midwife, to deliver personal and safe maternity care.

The content of the chapters in this addition of *Myles* has kept pace with the everchanging needs of maternity care and the varied and sometimes complex needs and circumstances of women, babies and their families. This edition provides the reader with knowledge and the associated practical application for the development of firm foundations, from which further learning, and development can take place, particularly as midwives frequently traverse the fine line between the intrepid joy of new life and the hurt and despair associated with loss and a life unlived.

I am heartened to see the logical progression and flow of the chapters, that takes the reader on a journey of discovery, but more importantly a journey that builds a comprehensive picture of the childbirth continuum and the midwife's role.

Section one provides the context of midwifery practice with an appropriate focus on professionalism, a much-needed chapter within a societal context where social media and the digital maternity platform grows

[1]National Maternity and Perinatal Audit: https://maternityaudit.org.uk/pages/cr2019km

[2]National Health Service (NHS) England (2016) National Maternity Review. Better Births: Improving outcomes of maternity services in England: A Five Year Forward View for maternity care, London, NHS England: https://www.england.nhs.uk/wp-content/uploads/2016/02/national-maternity-review-report.pdf

and develops at pace, to support women of childbearing age to be knowledgeable and empowered to make decisions about their reproductive health.

Chapter five skilfully describes the hormonal cycles, fertilization and early development that educates and or reminds the reader of the midwife's role in the knowledge required to educate women and their families in the basic principles of genomics and the significance of appropriate sign posting for specialist support where this is available. The benefits of understanding the aetiology and pathophysiology of medical and obstetric conditions is an essential and significant part of a midwife's role and I am inspired by the depth and breadth of information in Chapter 26 that supports the preparation of the midwife, with knowledge to recognise the acutely unwell woman, maternal collapse and resuscitation needs.

Generally, the depth of physiology and its application to maternity care and the midwife's role is exceptional in this edition of *Myles* and reflects the contribution of multidisciplinary authors that adds to the authenticity and credibility of the content. I am confident that the foundational principles describe in this text book will provide the reader with the firm foundations required for learners to practise safely and qualified midwives to refresh their knowledge.

Reflecting on my experiences of knowledge acquisition and how I learn best, I am mindful that reading a text book in the absence of reflecting on what I have read and applying knowledge gained to practice, reduces the depth of my learning and limits my desire to read wider. I appreciate that this is not the experience of every learner, but I am absolutely delighted to applaud the authors of this edition of *Myles Textbook for Midwives*, for the extraordinary lengths they have gone to ensure that chapters conclude with reflective activities for self-assessment. I encourage readers to undertake these activities that promise to assist with knowledge acquisition and learning, remembering always that your presence is evidence that your midwifery purpose is necessary!

Professor Jacqueline Dunkley-Bent, OBE
Chief Midwifery Officer
National Maternity Safety Champion
NHS England and NHS Improvement, London, UK

PREFACE

It is a great privilege to have been approached a second time by Elsevier to undertake the editorship of the seventeenth edition of *Myles Textbook for Midwives*. It is nearly 70 years since the Scottish midwife Margaret Myles wrote the first edition and this book remains highly regarded as a seminal text for student midwives and practising midwives alike throughout the world, with adaptation to the African context and a recent translation into Korean.

Over the ensuing decades, many changes have taken place in the education and training of future midwives alongside increasing demands and complexities associated with the health and wellbeing of childbearing women, their babies and families within a global context. Furthermore the development of evidence-based practice and advances in technology have also contributed to major reviews of how undergraduate curricula are delivered to ensure that today's graduate midwives are able to rise to the many challenges of the multifaceted role of the 21st century midwife, ensuring they are fit for practice and purpose. The seventeenth edition has been developed with these issues in mind, as we both would expect midwives to provide safe and competent care that is tailored to the individual needs of childbearing women, their babies and families with a professional and compassionate attitude.

The content and format of this edition of *Myles Textbook for Midwives* has been further developed and enhanced in response to the collated views regarding the format and contents of the sixteenth edition that have been received from students and midwives from around the world. While we acknowledge that midwifery practice should always be informed by the best possible up-to-date evidence, we also appreciate that since some research studies are still ongoing or just emerging, it is impossible to expect any new text to contain the most contemporary research and systematic reviews on every single topic relating to midwifery practice. Consequently, this edition provides the reader with comprehensive reference lists, details of annotated further reading and links to appropriate websites.

The online multiple-choice questions have been updated, revised with additions made to reflect the focus of the chapters in this edition as readers appreciate their use in aiding self-assessment of learning. New to this edition are reflective questions at the end of each chapter for the reader to utilise as a means of self-assessment of the content and as a revision aid as well as for lecturers to explore issues with their students within the learning environment.

There has been some revision in the ordering of chapters to replicate the childbirth continuum and improve the logical progression. Throughout its history, *Myles Textbook for Midwives* has always included clear and comprehensive illustrations to complement the text and, as with the sixteenth edition, full colour has been used throughout this text and in response to feedback, new diagrams and contemporary images have been added where appropriate.

We are grateful that a number of chapter authors have continued their contribution to successive editions of this seminal text and we also welcome the invaluable contributions from new authors who have passion and enthusiasm to impart their knowledge and experience in specific subject areas. It is vital to retain the ethos of the text being a textbook for midwives that is written by midwives with the appropriate expertise. Our role as editors as well as midwifery educationalists is to encourage and nurture new authors who have the potential to publish their work as well as continue the legacy of Margaret Myles. Furthermore, the text continues to reflect the eclectic nature of maternity and neonatal care and consequently some of the chapters have been written in collaboration with members of the multiprofessional team. This highlights the importance of health professionals working and learning together in order to enhance the quality of care women and their families receive. This is essential whenever complications develop in the physiological process throughout the childbirth continuum. In all clinical situations, the presence of the midwife is integral and the role is significant in ensuring the woman always receives the additional care required from the most appropriate health professional at the most appropriate time.

Where appropriate, case studies of personal experiences from childbearing women and some partners/fathers have been included to add depth to the contents of the chapter. Such contributions are invaluable to learning and, as editors we are indebted to these women and the fathers/partners who have unreservedly had to relive their childbirth experiences, often being a difficult and life changing event.

Since the sixteenth edition was published in 2014, there have been significant changes within the global context of midwifery education and practice that this text has aimed to capture. This includes the introduction of the Sustainable Development Goals, the *Lancet* series Global Framework for Quality Maternal and Newborn Care (presented in a new Chapter 8: Designing and implementing high quality midwifery care), employer-led supervision, the introduction of the Nursing and Midwifery Council's *Realising Professionalism: Standards for Education and Practice Framework*, safeguarding of vulnerable individuals and professional revalidation/continuing professional development (Chapter 2) that are fundamental to every midwife practising in the 21st century. We acknowledge that medicalization and consequential effect of a risk culture in the maternity services have eroded some aspects of the midwife's role over time. It is our aim to continue challenging midwives into becoming critical thinkers, compassionate leaders and effective change agents who have the confidence to empower women into making choices appropriate for them and their personal situation.

Recognizing that midwives increasingly care for women with complex healthcare needs within a multicultural society and take on specialist or extended roles, significant chapters have been added to make the text more contemporary. Chapter 12 explores the midwife's role in supporting women who have concealed their pregnancy; Chapter 18 examines the challenges that midwives face when women present with tocophobia (fear of childbirth) and Chapter 26 guides the reader through the principles of caring for the critically ill mother, including maternal resuscitation. This is a pivotal chapter given the increasing number of women presenting with co-morbidities and other complexities that may arise during pregnancy, labour and postpartum. Recognizing that not all pregnancies result in healthy babies, Chapter 38 explores end-of-life care provided to babies with life-limiting conditions within the context of legal and ethical issues and the dilemmas that families and healthcare professionals may face in such situations.

It is a great honour that the Foreword to the text has been written by Professor Jacqueline Dunkley-Bent, the first Chief Midwifery Officer for England. Her appointment to this role is pivotal in the history of midwifery in the United Kingdom in terms of strengthening midwifery leadership and recognizing the uniqueness of our profession and the importance of the role that midwives play in the lives of childbearing women, their babies and families.

We hope that this new edition of *Myles Textbook for Midwives* will continue to provide midwives with the foundation of the physiological theory and underpinning care principles to inform their clinical practice and support appropriate decision-making in partnership with childbearing women and members of the multiprofessional team. However, we recognize that knowledge is unlimited and that this text alone cannot provide everything midwives should know when fulfilling their multi-faceted roles. Nonetheless, it can afford the means to stimulate further enquiry and zest for continuing professional development.

Jayne E Marshall
Leicester (University of Leicester)
Maureen D Raynor
Leicester (De Montfort University)
2020

ACKNOWLEDGEMENT

As editors of the seventeenth edition of *Myles Textbook for Midwives,* we are indebted to the many authors of earlier editions of this seminal midwifery text whose work has provided the foundations from which this current volume has evolved. From the sixteenth edition, these contributors include the following chapter authors:

Susan Brydon
Margie Davies
Carole England
Angie Godfrey
Claire Greig
Sally inch
Rosemary Mander

Margaret R. Oates
Annie Rimmer
S Elizabeth Robson
Amanda Sullivan
Mary Vance
Stephen P. Wardle
Julie Wray

During the development of our second experience of editing *Myles Textbook for Midwives*, the production team at Elsevier has continued to be invaluable in providing the support and guidance to us, in the updating of the textbook in order that it remains a contemporary and internationally renowned resource for midwives, student midwives and other allied healthcare professionals. In addition, we wish to acknowledge the support of friends, family and colleagues that has enabled us to accomplish the task alongside our academic work commitments.

The Midwife in Context

1

The Midwife in Contemporary Midwifery Practice

Maureen D. Raynor, Joy Kemp, Michelle Anderson

CHAPTER CONTENTS

Midwives are global citizens who require a broad toolkit of skills and knowledge in order to work collaboratively with women as equal partners in their care, and across professional boundaries with key members of the multidisciplinary team (MDT). Contemporary midwifery education and practice are driven by key global initiatives such as the United Nations' Sustainable Development Goals (SDGs) and the International Confederation of Midwives' international definition of the midwife (UN 2015a,b; ICM 2017).

THE CHAPTER AIMS TO

- explore the midwife in context, taking a number of influential social and global issues into consideration especially the midwife as a global citizen with due consideration of the UN Sustainable Development Goals, the European (EU) Directives and International Confederation of Midwives Education Standards
- explore the emotional context of midwifery
- explore the concept of family in contemporary society
- explore working with women from socially disadvantaged groups
- explore research and the midwife.

GLOBAL HEALTH: THE CONTRIBUTION OF MIDWIVES

Midwives as Global Citizens

It is important that midwives have an understanding of the global context of midwifery as today's health professionals must be global citizens who are culturally congruent, able to provide effective care to multicultural communities with diverse needs (Academy of Medical Royal Colleges, AMROC 2016; Flying Start NHS 2018; West et al. 2017). Additionally, there is much that can be learned from international engagement, which can enrich and strengthen health services at home (DH 2014; THET 2017; Royal College of Physicians and Surgeons Glasgow, RCPSG 2017).

THE STATE OF THE WORLD: BETTER CONNECTED AND YET MORE UNEQUAL THAN EVER

Globalization means that the world is more connected than ever before; countries are becoming increasingly interdependent through greater economic integration, communication and technology, cultural dissemination and travel; this has the effect of making the world seem smaller (Labonté 2018). McLuhan and Fiore (1968) first described this connected world as a 'global village'. However, despite the world's greater connectedness, there is also growing inequity between and within nations and women, and children are often disproportionately disadvantaged.

Gender inequalities manifest themselves in every dimension of sustainable development (UN Women 2018). One person out of every nine in the world is under-nourished and women are often the first to go hungry; failure to reduce hunger is associated with increasing conflict and violence. While hunger grows, obesity is also rising which increases the risk of non communicable diseases such as diabetes and hypertension (FAO et al. 2018). Provision of clean water and sanitation is also inequitable; in households without water, responsibility for water collection mainly falls to women and girls with adverse implications for their health and safety (UN Women 2018). There are 844 million people globally without access to water and this is directly linked to 289,000 child deaths per year. Additionally, one in three people do not have access to a toilet (WHO/UNICEF 2017; WASH Watch 2017).

Gender discrimination and violence against women and girls remains pervasive across the world. One in five women and girls have experienced physical and/or sexual violence by an intimate partner within the last 12 months, yet 49 countries have no laws that specifically protect women from such violence (UN Women 2018). The number of people living in extreme poverty has fallen but this decline has slowed and rates remain stubbornly high in low-income countries and those affected by conflict and political upheaval (World Bank 2018). The effects of climate change are also experienced inequitably; women commonly face higher risks and greater burdens from the impact of climate change in situations of poverty, and the majority of the world's poor are women (United Nations Climate Change, UNCC 2019). Conflict is a major contributor to humanitarian need and there is a complex dynamic between poverty, environmental vulnerability and fragility that continues to affect significant numbers of poor people (Development Initiatives 2018). An estimated 136 million people in 20 countries require protection and humanitarian assistance each year; this figure comprises a total of 34 million women of reproductive age including 5 million pregnant women (UNFPA 2018).

At least half of the world's population does not have full coverage of essential health services and the need to pay for health care can push families into extreme poverty. 'Universal Health Coverage' is an ambition shared by all countries within the United Nations (UN), which aims to ensure all people have access to quality health services without suffering financial hardship as a result of paying for health care (World Health Organization, WHO 2018a).

Although the global maternal mortality ratio nearly halved between 1990 and 2015 (Koblinsky et al. 2016), approximately 830 women still die every day from preventable causes related to pregnancy and childbirth. Additionally, there are an estimated 7000 newborn deaths per day and 2.6 million stillbirths per year (UNICEF 2018; Lawn et al. 2016). More than 92% of all maternal and newborn deaths occur in 73 low- and middle-income countries; however, only 42% of the world's medical, midwifery and nursing personnel are available in these countries (UNFPA 2014). Moreover, poor-quality and inaccessible care exist even in high- and middle-income countries (Lancet 2014; WHO 2018b; Koblinsky et al. 2016). A total of 214 million women and girls around the world, most of them in poor and vulnerable communities, have an unmet need for contraception, contributing to 25 million unsafe abortions each year (Starrs et al. 2018; International Federation of Gynecology and Obstetrics, FIGO 2018). In recent years there has also been a sharp rise in inappropriate and harmful obstetric intervention in childbirth with a global epidemic of caesarean sections (Lancet 2018). All of this means that for many women around the world they receive 'too little, too late' or 'too much too soon' (Lancet 2016).

TABLE 1.1	Core Components of a Right to Health
Availability	Refers to the need for a sufficient quantity of functioning public health and healthcare facilities, goods and services, as well as programmes for all
Accessibility	Requires that health facilities, goods and services must be non-discriminatory in terms of physical accessibility, economical accessibility (affordability) and information accessibility
Acceptability	Health care must respect medical ethics, be culturally appropriate and sensitive to gender and the specific needs of diverse people groups
Quality	Services should be safe, effective, people-centred, timely, equitable, integrated and efficient. Quality is a key component of universal health coverage and includes the experience as well as the perception of health care

WHO (World Health Organization). (2017) Human rights and health. Available at: www.who.int/news-room/fact-sheets/detail/human-rights-and-health.

TABLE 1.2	The Seven Rights of Childbearing Women
1.	Freedom from harm and ill-treatment
2.	Right to information, informed consent and refusal and respect for choices and preferences, including the right to companionship of choice wherever possible
3.	Confidentiality, privacy
4.	Dignity, respect
5.	Equality, freedom from discrimination, equitable care
6.	Right to timely health care and to the highest attainable level of health
7.	Liberty, autonomy, self-determination and freedom from coercion

White Ribbon Alliance. (2011) Respectful maternity care: the universal rights of childbearing women. Available at: www.whiteribbonalliance.org/wp-content/uploads/2017/11/Final_RMC_Charter.pdf.

THE RIGHT TO HEALTH AND RESPECTFUL MATERNITY CARE

Global health factors are focused on improving health and achieving health equity for all people worldwide (Squires 2018). Every human being has a right to the highest achievable standard of health without distinction of race, religion, political belief, economic or social condition (WHO 2017). Table 1.1 highlights the (WHO 2017) core components of a right to health.

The right to health encompasses the right to sexual and reproductive health and to respectful maternity care. Sexual and reproductive health rights also cut across other human rights, such as the right to privacy, the right to education and the prohibition of discrimination (United Nations Human Rights Officer of the High Commissioner, OHCRH 2019). Sexual and reproductive health are fundamental for women's full participation in society (Zuccala and Horton 2018). Sexual and reproductive health rights are important, not only for

individuals' wellbeing and development, but for sustainable development (Starrs et al. 2018). However, progress towards the achievement of these rights has been slow for complex reasons.

Respectful maternity care is a concept that is based on respect for women's basic human rights and advocates for women to be free from disrespectful and abusive treatment at the hands of maternity care providers (Manning and Schaaf 2018). Table 1.2 details the seven rights of childbearing women charter from the White Ribbon Alliance (2011).

Health workers also have personal, employment and professional rights, including safe and decent working environments and freedom from all kinds of discrimination, coercion and violence (WHO 2016a). However, the recent global survey of 2470 midwives from 93 countries (WHO 2016b) found widespread experiences of: disrespect; subordination and gender discrimination; harassment; social isolation and lack of safe accommodation; salaries insufficient to meet basic needs; and a lack of

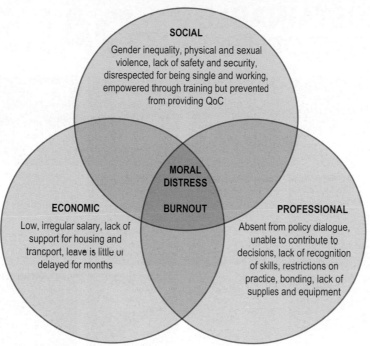

Fig. 1.1 Barriers to the provision of quality care by midwifery personnel. (Reproduced with permission from the World Health Organization 2016. Midwives voices, midwives realities: finding from a global consultation on providing quality midwifery care. Available at: www.who.int/maternal_child_adolescent/documents/midwives-voices-realities/en.)

opportunity for professional and leadership development. These experiences can lead to moral distress and burnout. Fig. 1.1 highlights the barriers to midwives being able to provide quality care (WHO 2016a).

MIDWIVES AND THE SUSTAINABLE DEVELOPMENT GOALS

In 2015, the 193 member states of the UN unanimously adopted the 17 sustainable development goals (SDGs), aiming to transform the world over the next 15 years. The SDGs built on the foundation of the Millennium Development Goals, which galvanized unprecedented efforts to meet the needs of the world's poorest (UN 2015a). Goal 3 relates to health, with the aim of ensuring good health and wellbeing for all. Within this goal there are subgoals relating to maternal and newborn health: to reduce the global maternal mortality ratio to fewer than 70 maternal deaths per 100,000 live births; reducing neonatal mortality to at least as low as 12 per 1000 live births; and ensuring universal access to sexual and reproductive healthcare services. The SDGs set ambitious targets for universal health coverage of essential health services by 2030 (UN 2015b). Fig. 1.2 sets out the UN SDGs.

Ultimately, sustainable development rests on the autonomy and empowerment of women and their health and wellbeing (Zuccala and Horton 2018). Midwives are central to achieving the SDGs. High quality midwifery care saves lives and midwives have the competence to meet 87% of women and their newborn service needs and to avert two-thirds of maternal and newborn mortality (Lancet 2014; UNFPA 2014; International Confederation of Midwives, ICM 2014a). No woman or newborn should face a greater risk of preventable death because of where they live or who they are; however, there is a global shortage of 17.4 million healthcare workers including 350,000 midwives (WHO 2015, 2016b; ICM 2014b). Investment in midwives is a key priority for the WHO (2016c). UNFPA (2014) suggests that investing in midwives could yield a 16-fold return on investment in terms of lives saved and costs of caesarean sections avoided, and is a 'best buy' in primary health care. It also frees other health carers to focus on other health needs.

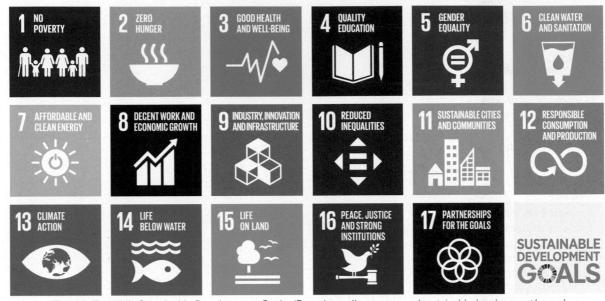

Fig. 1.2 The UN's Sustainable Development Goals. (From https:// www.un.org/sustainabledevelopment/news/ communications-material.) The content of this publication has not been approved by the United Nations and does not reflect the views of the United Nations or its officials or Member States.

The All Party Parliamentary Group on Global Health (2016) suggests that investing in nurses and midwives will have a triple impact: better health, greater gender equality and stronger economies.

THE DEFINITION AND SCOPE OF A MIDWIFE

The international definition of a midwife is provided by the International Confederations of Midwives (ICM 2017a) as delineated in Box 1.1.

Midwives are the primary (but not the only) providers of midwifery care (Renfrew et al. 2014). The ICM (2017a) International Definition of a Midwife, Global Standards for Midwifery Education (ICM 2013) and the Global Competencies (ICM 2019) provide a benchmark upon which individual regions or countries set their own frameworks for midwifery education and regulation. Table 1.3 details the ICM (2019) essential competencies for midwifery practice.

The provision of high quality midwifery should not be limited by politics or borders. However, even in high-income countries such as within Europe, maternity services and outcomes for women and their babies varies enormously (Euro-Peristat 2018).

In European law, midwives are governed by European Directive 2005/36/EC and Modernized Directive 2013/55/EU, which relate to the recognition of professional qualifications in practice. These directives strengthen midwifery education by setting minimum standards; they also allow midwives to move across borders and to practice their occupation or provide services abroad, provided they register with the relevant regulatory body in the host country. WHO (2015b) recommends that all midwives in the European region are educated to a minimum of degree level. In the UK, the Nursing and Midwifery Council regulates midwives and produces standards for midwifery education and competence, based on the ICM's international standards. Table 1.4 broadly outlines the global midwifery education standards (ICM 2013), which set benchmarks for the preparation of a midwife based on global norms. They are based on the values of trust in the midwifery education process, continuous quality improvement

---

BOX 1.1 The International Definition of a Midwife

A person who has successfully completed a midwifery education programme that is based on the ICM Essential Competencies for Basic Midwifery Practice and the framework of the ICM Global Standards for Midwifery Education and is recognized in the country where it is located; who has acquired the requisite qualifications to be registered and/or legally licensed to practice midwifery and use the title 'midwife'; and who demonstrates competency in the practice of midwifery.

(ICM 2017a)

Midwifery is defined as:

Skilled, knowledgeable and compassionate care for childbearing women, newborn infants and families across the continuum throughout pre-pregnancy, pregnancy, birth, postpartum and the early weeks of life. Core characteristics include optimising normal biological, psychological, social and cultural processes of reproduction and early life, timely prevention and management of complications, consultation with and referral to other services, respecting women's individual circumstances and views, and working in partnership with women to strengthen women's own capabilities to care for themselves and their families.

(Renfrew et al. 2014)

---

for midwifery education programmes, maintaining integrity through fair and honest education, fostering life-long learning and promoting autonomy for the midwifery profession.

Looking to the future, global midwifery education standards will need to prepare midwives for caring for women in conflict and crisis and make recommendations about adequate water and sanitation provision for student midwives and educators. Within Europe, the Erasmus programme provides opportunity to gain an international perspective by exchange programmes between students from different universities in different countries (European Commission 2018; UCAS 2018).

STRENGTHENING GLOBAL MIDWIFERY TOWARDS 2030

The evidence for midwives' contribution to global health is stronger than ever and the global momentum generated by SDGs provides a unique opportunity for advocacy aimed at strengthening midwifery and investing in midwives. The State of the World's Midwifery Report (UNFPA 2014) suggests a 'Midwifery 2030 Pathway' for all countries and any health systems designed to ensure provision of woman-centred sexual, reproductive, maternal, newborn and adolescent health care, through strengthening 10 key foundations. These include universal access to high quality midwifery care, a well-trained, regulated and managed midwifery workforce, supportive and accountable governments and strong professional midwives associations (ten Hoope-Bender et al. 2016).

The 2030 agenda compels midwives to have a strong voice, positioning themselves to help achieve high quality universal health coverage for all. However, although midwives can articulate solutions for achieving high quality maternity care, their voices are not always heard (WHO 2016a). Coming together in a professional midwives association gives midwives a stronger voice by combining their efforts, thoughts and ideas and giving credibility and power to the midwifery profession. The ICM promotes twinning between professional midwives associations for mutual strengthening (Survive & Thrive 2016; ICM 2014b, 2018). An example of this is the twinning initiative between the Royal College of Midwives (RCM) and the Bangladesh Midwifery Society; this project aims to strengthen midwifery both in Bangladesh and in the UK. (Further information about the RCM Twinning project can be accessed at: www.rcm.org.uk).

As well as partnering with other midwives, it is also important that midwives work in partnership with women to advocate for investment in midwifery; midwifery is a profession that is based upon a partnership between women and midwives aiming to promote health outcomes (ICM 2017b). Collaboration and partnership is also required with other health professionals, with other sectors and across geographical boundaries; improvements in global health can only be achieved through working together (Squires 2018). Within regions such as Europe, there is benefit in sharing success stories and learning from each other through collaborative working (Euro-Peristat 2018).

Achieving the vision for midwifery 2030 also requires political will and support from governments and policy-makers for each of the three pillars of midwifery: education, regulation and association development. Additionally, the provision of enabling practice environments for midwives with sufficient workforce and resources is vital, along with effective referral services to higher level facilities where necessary (UNFPA 2014).

TABLE 1.3	**Essential Competencies for Midwifery Practice**	
1. General competencies	1a.	Assume responsibility for own decisions and actions as an autonomous practitioner
	1b.	Assume responsibility for self-care and self-development as a midwife
	1c.	Appropriately delegate aspects of care and provide supervision
	1d.	Use research to inform practice
	1e.	Uphold fundamental human rights of individuals when providing midwifery care
	1f.	Adhere to jurisdictional laws, regulatory requirements, and codes of conduct for midwifery practice
	1g.	Facilitate women to make individual choices about care
	1h.	Demonstrate effective interpersonal communication with women and families, health-care teams and community groups
	1i.	Facilitate normal birth processes in institutional and community settings, including women's homes
	1j.	Assess the health status, screen for health risks and promote general health and wellbeing of women and infants
	1k.	Prevent and treat common health problems related to reproduction and early life
	1l.	Recognize conditions outside the midwifery scope of practice and refer appropriately
	1m.	Care for women who experience physical and sexual violence and abuse
2. Competencies specific to pre-pregnancy and antenatal care	2a.	Provide pre-pregnancy care
	2b.	Determine the health status of the woman
	2c.	Assess fetal wellbeing
	2d.	Monitor the progression of pregnancy
	2e.	Promote and support health behaviours that improve wellbeing
	2f.	Provide anticipatory guidance related to pregnancy, birth, breastfeeding, parenthood and change in the family
	2g.	Detect, manage and refer women with complicated pregnancies
	2h.	Assist the woman and her family to plan for an appropriate place of birth
	2i.	Provide care to women with unintended or mistimed pregnancy
3. Competencies specific to care during labour and birth	3a.	Promote physiological labour and birth
	3b.	Manage a safe spontaneous vaginal birth and prevent complications
	3c.	Provide care of the newborn immediately after birth
4. Competencies specific to the ongoing care of women and newborns	4a.	Provide postnatal care for the healthy woman
	4b.	Provide care to the healthy newborn infant
	4c.	Promote and support breastfeeding
	4d.	Detect and treat or refer postnatal complications in the woman
	4e.	Detect and manage health problems in the newborn infant
	4f.	Provide family planning services

Adapted from ICM (International Confederation of Midwives). (2019) Essential competencies for midwifery practice: 2019 update. Available at: www.internationalmidwives.org/our-work/policy-and-practice/essential-competencies-for-midwifery-practice.html.

It is important to involve professional midwives' associations in policy and planning for the midwifery workforce (Lopez et al. 2015). The quality of midwifery education is directly linked to the quality of midwifery care provision; students will only learn to provide high quality care when they are mentored by skilled midwives in a well-resourced and managed clinical learning environment (Kemp et al. 2018). Investment is required in career pathways and professional development for midwives including opportunities for leadership development. Exploring

TABLE 1.4   ICM (2013) Midwifery Education Standards

I. Organization and Administration	I.1.	The host institution/agency/branch of government supports the philosophy, aims and objectives of the midwifery education programme
	I.2.	The host institution helps to ensure that financial and public/policy support for the midwifery education programme are sufficient to prepare competent midwives
	I.3.	The midwifery school/programme has a designated budget and budget control that meets programme needs
	I.4.	The midwifery faculty is self-governing and responsible for developing and leading the policies and curriculum of the midwifery education programme
	I.5.	The head of the midwifery programme is a qualified midwife teacher with experience in management/administration
	I.6.	The midwifery programme takes into account national and international policies and standards to meet maternity workforce needs.
II. Midwifery Faculty (Teachers)	II.2.	The midwife teacher:
	II.2.a.	has formal preparation in midwifery
	II.2.b.	demonstrates competency in midwifery practise, generally accomplished with two (2) years full scope practise
	II.2.c.	holds a current license/registration or other form of legal recognition to practise midwifery
	II.2.d.	has formal preparation for teaching, or undertakes such preparation as a condition of continuing to hold the position
	II.2.e.	maintains competence in midwifery practise and education
	II.3.	The midwife clinical preceptor/clinical teacher:
	II.3.a.	is qualified according to the ICM Definition of a midwife
	II.3.b.	demonstrates competency in midwifery practise, generally accomplished with two (2) years full scope practise
	II.3.c.	maintains competency in midwifery practise and clinical education
	II.3.d.	holds a current license/registration or other form of legal recognition to practise midwifery
	II.3.e.	has formal preparation for clinical teaching or undertakes such preparation
	II.4.	Individuals from other disciplines who teach in the midwifery programme are competent
	II.5.	Midwife teachers provide education, support and supervision of individuals who teach students in practical learning sites
	II.6.	Midwife teachers and midwife clinical preceptors/clinical teachers work together to support (facilitate), directly observe and evaluate students' practical learning
	II.7.	The ratio of students to teachers and clinical preceptors/clinical teachers in the classroom and practical sites is determined by the midwifery programme and the requirements of regulatory authorities
	II.8.	The effectiveness of midwifery faculty members is assessed on a regular basis following an established process.
III. Student body	III.1.	The midwifery programme has clearly written admission policies that are accessible to potential applicants. These policies include:
	III.1.a.	entry requirements, including minimum requirement of completion of secondary education

Continued

TABLE 1.4   ICM (2013) Midwifery Education Standards—cont'd

	III.1.b.	a transparent recruitment process
	III.1.c.	selection process and criteria for acceptance
	III.1.d.	mechanisms for taking account of prior learning
	III.2.	Eligible midwifery candidates are admitted without prejudice or discrimination (e.g. gender, age, national origin, religion)
	III.3.	Eligible midwifery candidates are admitted in-keeping with national healthcare policies and maternity workforce plans
	III.4.	The midwifery programme has clearly written student policies that include:
	III.4.a.	expectations of students in classroom and practical areas
	III.4.b.	statements about students' rights and responsibilities and an established process for addressing student appeals and/or grievances
	III.4.c.	mechanisms for students to provide feedback and ongoing evaluation of the midwifery curriculum, midwifery faculty and the midwifery programme
	III.4.d.	requirements for successful completion of the midwifery programme
	III.5.	Mechanisms exist for the student's active participation in midwifery programme governance and committees
	III.6.	Students have sufficient midwifery practical experience in a variety of settings to attain, at a minimum, the current ICM Essential Competencies for Basic Midwifery Practice
	III.7.	Students provide midwifery care primarily under the supervision of a midwife teacher or midwifery clinical preceptor/clinical teacher.
IV. Curriculum	IV.1.	The philosophy of the midwifery education programme is consistent with the ICM Philosophy and model of care
	IV.2.	The purpose of the midwifery education programme is to produce a competent midwife who:
	IV.2.a.	has attained/demonstrated, at a minimum, the current ICM Essential Competencies for Basic Midwifery Practice
	IV.2.b.	meets the criteria of the ICM Definition of a Midwife and regulatory body standards leading to licensure or registration as a midwife
	IV.2.c.	is eligible to apply for advanced education
	IV.2.d.	is a knowledgeable, autonomous practitioner who adheres to the ICM International Code of Ethics for Midwives, standards of the profession and established scope of practise within the jurisdiction where legally recognized
	IV.3.	The sequence and content of the midwifery curriculum enables the student to acquire essential competencies for midwifery practise in accord with ICM core documents
	IV.4.	The midwifery curriculum includes both theory and practise elements with a minimum of 40% theory and a minimum of 50% practise
	IV 4.a.	Minimum length of a direct-entry midwifery education programme is three (3) years
	IV4.b.	Minimum length of a post-nursing/healthcare provider (post-registration) midwifery education programme is eighteen (18) months
	IV.5.	The midwifery programme uses evidence-based approaches to teaching and learning that promote adult learning and competency-based education

TABLE 1.4			ICM (2013) Midwifery Education Standards—cont'd
		IV.6.	The midwifery programme offers opportunities for multidisciplinary content and learning experiences that complement the midwifery content.
V.	Resources, facilities and services	V.1.	The midwifery programme implements written policies that address student and teacher safety and wellbeing in teaching and learning environments
		V.2.	The midwifery programme has sufficient teaching and learning resources to meet programme needs
		V.3.	The midwifery programme has adequate human resources to support both classroom/theoretical and practical learning
		V.4.	The midwifery programme has access to sufficient midwifery practical experiences in a variety of settings to meet the learning needs of each student
		V.5.	Selection criteria for appropriate midwifery practical learning sites are clearly written and implemented.
VI.	Assessment strategies	VI.1.	The Midwifery faculty uses valid and reliable formative and summative evaluation/assessment methods to measure student performance and progress in learning related to:
		VI.1.a.	knowledge
		VI.1.b.	behaviours
		VI.1.c.	practise skills
		VI.1.d.	critical thinking and decision-making
		VI.1.e.	interpersonal relationships/communication skills
		VI.2.	The means and criteria for assessment/evaluation of midwifery student performance and progression, including identification of learning difficulties, are written and shared with students
		VI.3.	Midwifery faculty conducts regular reviews of the curriculum as a part of quality improvement, including input from students, programme graduates, midwife practitioners, clients of midwives and other stakeholders
		VI.4.	Midwifery faculty conducts ongoing review of practical learning sites and their suitability for student learning/experience in relation to expected learning outcomes
		VI.5.	Periodic external review of programme effectiveness takes place.

ICM (International Confederation of Midwives). (2013) Global standards for midwifery education. Available at: www.internationalmidwives.org/assets/files/general-files/2018/04/icm-standards-guidelines_ammended2013.pdf.

different ways of organizing midwifery care, such as midwifery social enterprises, may provide models for women's empowerment and health systems' strengthening (Institute of Medicine of the National Academies, INMA 2015).

Lastly, midwives and others must continue to fund and engage in research, adding to the growing body of evidence for the effectiveness of midwifery as a high quality and cost-effective solution to women and newborn's global health. Powell-Kennedy et al. (2018) suggest three interconnected areas for this research: first, evaluating the effectiveness of midwifery care; second, identifying and describing which aspects of care optimize or disturb physiological processes in the childbearing continuum; and third, determining which indicators, measures and benchmarks are valuable in assessing quality maternal and newborn care.

THE EMOTIONAL CONTEXT OF MIDWIFERY

Much of midwifery work is emotionally demanding, an understanding by midwives of why this is so, and exploration of ways to manage feelings can only benefit women and midwives. How midwives 'feel' about their work and the women they care for is important. It has significant implications for communication and inter-personal relationships with not only women and families but also colleagues. It also has much wider implications for the quality of maternity services in general.

By its very nature, midwifery work involves a range of emotions. Activities that midwives perform in their day-to-day role are rarely dull, spanning a vast spectrum. What may appear routine and mundane acts to midwives are often far from ordinary experiences for women – the recipients of maternity care. While birth is often construed as a highly charged emotional event, it may be less obvious to appreciate why a routine antenatal 'booking' history or postnatal visit can generate emotions.

What is 'Emotion Work'?

Emotional labour can be defined as the work that is undertaken to manage feelings so that they are appropriate for a particular situation (Hunter and Deery 2009). This is done in accordance with 'feeling rules', social norms regarding which emotions it is considered appropriate to feel and to display.

Sources of Emotion Work in Midwifery Practice

It is suggested that there are various sources of emotion work in midwifery (Hunter and Deery 2009), which can be grouped into three key themes:
1. Midwife–woman relationships
2. Collegial relationships
3. The organization of maternity care.
It is important to note that these themes are often intertwined, for example, the organization of maternity care impacts on both midwife–woman relationships and on collegial relationships.

Midwife–Woman Relationships

The quality of the midwife–mother relationship is vital to ensure quality of care as it combines all the essential threads of the midwifery service. Equally, a trusting relationship between the woman and midwife is fundamental (Hunter and Deery 2009; Dahlberg and Aune 2013; Drach-Zahavy et al. 2016).

Pregnancy and birth are not always joyful experiences (see Chapter 30), for example midwives work with women who: may have concealed their pregnancy (see Chapter 12); have unplanned or unwanted pregnancies; who are in unhappy or abusive relationships; who are fearful of pregnancy and childbirth (see Chapter 18) or encounter pregnancies where fetal malformations or antenatal problems are detected (see Chapter 13). In these cases, midwives need to support women and their partners with great sensitivity and emotional awareness. This requires excellent communication and interpersonal skills to establish trust (Lewis et al. 2017). Relationships between midwives and women may vary considerably in their quality, level of intimacy and sense of personal connection. Some relationships may be intense and short-lived (e.g. when a midwife and woman meet on the labour suite or birth centre for the first time); intense and long-lived (e.g. when a midwife provides continuity of care throughout pregnancy, birth and the postnatal period via models of care such as caseholding). They may also be relatively superficial, whether the contact is short-lived or longer-standing. There is evidence that a key issue in midwife–woman relationships is the level of 'reciprocity' that is experienced (McCourt and Stevens 2009; Lewis et al. 2017). Reciprocity is defined as the mutual exchange of something between two individuals or groups of people when each person or group gives or allows something to the other (Collins English Dictionary 2019). When relationships are experienced as 'reciprocal' or 'balanced', the midwife and woman are in a harmonious situation. Both are able to give to the other and to receive what is given, such as when the midwife can give support and advice, the woman is happy to accept this and in return affirm the value of the midwife's care. Achieving a partnership with the women therefore requires reciprocity.

At times, relationships may become unbalanced, and in these situations emotion work is needed by the midwife. For example, a woman may be hostile to the information provided by the midwife, or alternatively, she may expect more in terms of personal friendship than the midwife feels it is appropriate or feasible to offer. Some midwives working in continuity of care schemes have expressed concerns about 'getting the balance right' in their relationships with women, so that they can offer authentic support without overstepping personal boundaries and becoming burnt out (McCourt and Stevens 2009). However, establishing and maintaining reciprocal relationships can also prove challenging.

Women want care from a midwife that is not only kind but is also attentive, intelligent and supportive. The woman also wants a midwife who is competent in her clinical skills to make the woman feel safe (Care Quality Commission, CQC 2018). Women's views of their maternity care experience are important. In England, a study by the CQC (2018) suggests that women are marginally more positive about their experiences of maternity care within the NHS than in 2015. The survey received 18,400 responses from women who gave birth in February 2017, across 130 NHS Trusts.

The fifth survey of its kind showed 59% of women reporting that they received help from members of staff within a reasonable amount of time after giving birth, a 5% increase in comparison to the last survey that was conducted in 2015. However, the majority of women (88%) felt they were 'always' spoken to in a way they could understand during labour and birth, and a high number 'definitely' felt they had confidence and trust in the staff caring for them (82%). Disappointingly, there were fewer improvements compared with the previous year. Postnatal care continues to remain less of a positive experience for women when compared with other aspects of their maternity journey. Information sharing and communication are the key areas where improvements are needed. Of equal concern is the fact that 15% of women reflected they are still not being offered choices about aspects of their care.

Collegial Relationships

Relationships between midwives and their colleagues, both within midwifery and the wider multidisciplinary (MDT) and multiagency teams are also key sources of emotion work. Much of the existing evidence attests to relationships between midwifery colleagues, which may be positive or negative experiences. Some reports investigating poor maternal and neonatal outcomes and avoidable harm, identified that a number of cases involved an element of substandard care, where poor communication, ineffective team work and interpersonal skills are common themes cited as particular areas of concern (RCOG 2017; Knight et al. 2019). Non-technical skills known as human factors (see Chapter 26) are essential within the MDT and collegiate relationship

and effective communication are at the nexus of a strong MDT. This is where a positive work culture is fostered, collaborative working and shared decision-making are realized and where the safety of mother and baby are the core business of maternity care.

Undermining behaviour on the other hand in the form of bullying and harassment has no place in the workforce. There are a myriad of definitions for bullying and harassment but for simplicity, the definitions employed by Illing et al. (2013) are adopted for use within the chapter.

- **Bullying** may be intimidating, malicious, offensive or insulting behaviour, or an abuse or misuse of power through means that undermine, humiliate, denigrate or injure the recipient.
- **Harassment** is unwanted conduct related to a relevant protected characteristic, which has the purpose or effect of violating an individual's dignity or creating an environment for that individual that is not only hostile but is intimidating, degrading, humiliating or offensive.

The sinister and covert nature of bullying and harassment can often make it challenging to recognize, in that they may not be blatantly obvious to others, making it all very insidious. Nonetheless, in the UK, much work has been done around undermining and bullying behaviour within healthcare institutions relating to definitions, occurrence, causes, consequences, prevention and management. Illing et al. (2013) provide an illuminating report about the issue, and the RCOG and RCM have produced a toolkit to address this challenge within the maternity services. (The toolkit can be accessed at: www.rcog.org.uk/underminingtoolkit.)

The Organization of Maternity Care

Globally, the way in which maternity care is organized may also be a source of emotion work for midwives. The fragmented, task-orientated nature of much hospital-based maternity care creates emotionally difficult situations for midwives as it reduces opportunities for establishing meaningful relationships with women and colleagues, and for doing 'real midwifery'.

Midwives working in community-based practice, continuity of care schemes or in birth centre settings are more emotionally satisfied in their work (Sandall et al. 2016). Although there is the potential for continuity of care schemes to increase emotion work as a result of altered boundaries in the midwife–woman relationship, there is also evidence to suggest that when these schemes are organized and managed effectively, they provide emotional rewards for women and midwives (NHS England 2016; Sandall et al. 2016).

Better Births

NHS England's (2016) National Maternity Review 'Better Births' transformative report considered how maternity services needed to change to meet the needs of the population and set out a clear vision for safe and efficient models of maternity care, including safer care, joined up across disciplines, reflecting women's choices and offering continuity of care along the pathway. This report is now driving much of the changes to the organization of maternity care in the UK (see Chapter 8). Globally, the midwifery framework by Renfrew et al. (2014) in the *Lancet* midwifery series focuses minds on providing models of care that are holistic and assure quality.

THE FAMILY IN SOCIETY

It is outside the scope of the chapter to explore all subgroups relating to the family. It can only offer a broad perspective of the modern family with some working examples to provide context. The family in contemporary society is part of social change that transforms with the modern trends in that given society. In other words, family function in any given society will be structured according to the overall changes that occur in all aspects of social life. Sixty years ago in Western societies, the so-called 'nuclear' family – a married couple with 2.5 children, was the norm. Transformation to family structures has meant that there are more diverse types of families today than ever before. A variety of families now exists within developed and developing countries, e.g. cohabiting couples, same sex couples, single parent families, childless families, etc. The main changes are a result of a variety of reasons, as postulated in Box 1.2.

Providing woman-centred care is a complex issue, particularly in a diverse society where individual's and families' health needs are not homogeneous and one size does not fit all. Listening and responding to women's views and respecting their ethnic, cultural, social, religious and family backgrounds is critical to developing a responsive midwifery service. Persistent concerns have been expressed about the poor neonatal and maternal health outcomes among disadvantaged and socially excluded groups (Marmot 2010; Knight et al. 2019),

---

> ### BOX 1.2   Some Possible Reasons for Changes to Traditional Family Structure
>
> - Couples marry later in life
> - More permissive society means that many couples choose to shun the patriarchal structure of marriage and choose to cohabit
> - Fewer couples choose to marry
> - Many women are now more career-oriented and the main 'bread winner', i.e. earner in households
> - Better equality and opportunity in education and work for women; many now opt to pursue and fulfil their ambition of career/success rather than marry and have children
> - Higher divorce rates
> - Changes to partnerships (i.e. more same sex couples, more cohabitation, more people living alone, childless couples)
> - Changes to children and families (i.e. higher rates of births outside marriage, women choosing to have fewer children, divorce rates and re-marriage, resulting in more step families/step children)
> - Increased incidence of lone parent families (this could be due to a host of different reasons, e.g. individuals choosing to parent alone, relationship break down, divorce, death of a parent, displaced people seeking asylum/refugee status, etc.).
>
>   Figures from the Office of National Statistics (ONS 2017) reveal the following trend:
> - In 2017, there were 19.0 million families in the UK – increased by 15% from 16.6 million in 1996.
> - There were 12.9 million married or civil partner couple families in the UK in 2017. This remains the most common type of family.
> - The second largest family type was the cohabiting couple family at 3.3 million families, followed by 2.8 million lone parent families.

suggesting not all groups in society enjoy equal access to maternity services.

Women from Disadvantaged Groups

There is strong evidence that disadvantaged groups have poorer health and poorer access to health care, with clear links between inequality in social life and inequality in health, demonstrating that inequality exists in both mortality and morbidity (Marmot 2010; Knight et al. 2019). WHO (2008) states that 'social justice is a matter of life or death' and refers to the social determinants of health as conditions in which people are born, live, develop, work and age. This includes the healthcare system, which paradoxically is formulated and influenced by the distribution of wealth, power and resources at all levels. The social determinants of health therefore are largely responsible for health inequalities, i.e. the unfair and avoidable differences in health status seen within and between countries The development of a society, be that wealthy or impoverished, can be judged by the quality of its population's health, the justice meted out to health distribution across the social spectrum and the degree of protection provided from disadvantage as a result of ill-health (WHO 2008).

Women from Black, Asian and Minority Ethnic Groups (BAME)

Maternal and infant health inequalities between and within developed and developing countries is well documented (WHO 2015c; Jones et al. 2017; Alkema et al. 2016). Concerns have also been expressed with the way in which access to services, lifestyle choices, sociocultural factors, ethnicity and globalization of the market economy continue to generate differences in health outcomes for different groups, especially those who are more likely to be marginalized due to unconscious bias and institutional racism (Jones et al. 2017; WHO 2015c, 2018c).

There are health disparities in maternal and infant birth outcomes of BAME women giving birth in the UK compared with white women (Garcia et al. 2015; Aquino et al. 2015). Knight et al.'s (2019) report on the confidential enquiries into maternal deaths in the UK raised some sobering issues, highlighting the almost five-fold higher mortality rate among black women compared with white women for the triennium 2015–2017. Much work is therefore needed to identify and address the underlying causes of this difference.

To improve maternal health for women from a BAME background, barriers that limit access to quality maternal health services must be identified and addressed at all levels of the health system (WHO 2018c). The World Health Organization (WHO 2015c) recommendation on supporting 'culturally-appropriate' maternity care services to improve maternal and newborn health is welcomed. The UN (2015) and WHO (2018c) states that between 2016 and 2030, as part of the SDGs target, the goal is to reduce the burden of global maternal mortality ratio to <70 per 100,000 live births. To help achieve this vision, skilled, well-informed and culturally

congruent midwives are central to the provision of safe and effective maternity care (Aquino et al. 2015; Garcia et al. 2015).

Teenage Parents

Data from Public Health England (PHE 2016) reflect that over recent decades, the under-18 conception rate has more than halved, to the lowest level since 1960s. This is the result of a concerted long-term evidence-based teenage pregnancy strategy, delivered with concerted effort by local government and their health partners. Teenage parents are no different from any other parent group; most manage extremely well with appropriate social support and these families want only the best for their children (PHE 2016). It is important to acknowledge that some young mothers and fathers do achieve a successful outcome to their pregnancy and parenting with appropriate social support via Family Nurse Partnership (FNP) (Olds 2002). Nonetheless, it is widely understood that there is a strong association between teenage pregnancy resulting in early parenthood and poor educational achievement coupled with wider health inequalities and social deprivation, e.g. poor physical and mental health, social isolation, poverty plus wider-related factors (Public Health England, PHE 2016). It should also be recognized that morbidity and mortality among babies born to these mothers is increased and that the mothers show a higher risk of developing complications, such as hypertensive disorders and intrapartum complications (PHE 2016; Knight et al. 2019). Many young teenage mothers tend to present late for antenatal care and are disproportionately likely to have some risk factors associated with poor antenatal health (e.g. poverty and smoking). Moreover, there is a growing recognition that socioeconomic disadvantage can be both a cause and effect of teenage parenthood. This affects the life chances not only for teenage parents but also the next generation of children. There are a variety of risk factors for early pregnancy affecting some young people entering parenthood that make them particularly vulnerable.

According to PHE (2016) these include:
- family poverty
- poor educational attainment due to persistent truancy from school by age 14
- slower than expected attainment between ages 11 and 14
- being looked after or being a care leaver.

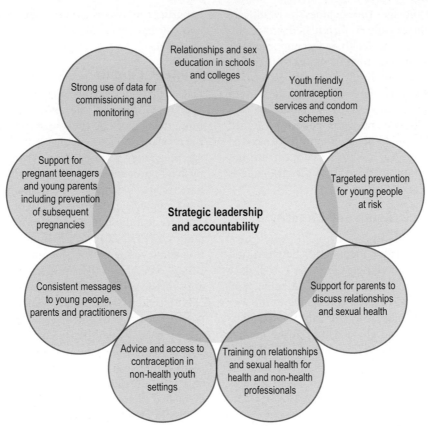

Fig. 1.3 Factors for the prevention of teenage pregnancies. (Adapted from PHE (2016), PHE Crown copyright 2019. This information (excluding logos) may be used free of charge in any format or medium, under the terms of the Open Government Licence v3.0.).

Furthermore, PHE (2016) identified that the above risk factors are reflected in the cohort of young parents in the FNP trial participants:

- 46% had been suspended, expelled or excluded from school
- 48% were not in education, employment or training at the time of recruitment.

Consequent to the above, some young parents will have missed out on the protective factors of:

- high quality sex and relationships education
- emotional wellbeing and resilience
- positive parenting role models and having a trusted adult in their life.

For a minority, these vulnerabilities may make parenting very challenging.

However, as mentioned previously, with appropriate support, young teenage parents can make an effective transition to parenthood. They can be assisted to develop good parenting and life skills to prevent a potential downward spiral and break the cycle of social deprivation and health inequalities by early intervention schemes such as FNP developed by Olds (2002). Fig. 1.3 identifies the factors highlighted by PHE (2016) for the prevention of teenage pregnancies.

Migrant Families

War, civil unrest and the fear of torture or persecution have resulted in many displaced populations worldwide. The number of families who are migrants and refugees throughout the world has continued to increase at a pace, with particular concerns for migrant and refugee women who are pregnant (ICM 2017c). The ICM (2017c:1) draws midwives attention to its International Code of Ethics (ICM 2014c) to convey the importance of midwives to *respect the basic Human Rights of all people and to value cultural diversity'*. The ICM (2017c:1) aptly and poignantly states that:

> The health and well-being of migrant and refugee women may have been damaged in their country of origin or during their journey and may expose them to reproductive health risks, including sexual violence, unwanted pregnancies and exposure to sexually transmitted diseases.

Javaweera (2016) identifies specific vulnerable categories of migrant women as being:

- asylum seekers
- refugees or those refused asylum seekers
- other undocumented migrant women
- women with no recourse to public funds that are supported by the local authority
- trafficked women
- some Roma women
- women with limited fluency in English
- migrants from the European Union (EU) with no health insurance card.

Midwives need to be aware of the complex needs of this group of vulnerable women who, in addition to the problems described above, have often experienced traumatic events in their home country, may be isolated from their family and friends and face uncertainty regarding their future domicile. Negative stereotypes and prejudice are damaging and can only lead to insensitive and ineffective care.

Women from Travelling Families

Travelling families are not a homogeneous group. Travellers may belong to a distinct social group such as the Romanies; their origins may lie in the UK or elsewhere such as Ireland or Eastern Europe, or they may be part of the social grouping loosely termed 'New Age' travellers or part of the Showman's Guild travelling community. As with all social groups, their cultural background will influence their beliefs about and experience of health and childbearing.

A common factor, which may apply to all, is the likelihood of prejudice and marginalization. Midwives need to examine their own beliefs and values in order to develop their knowledge to address the needs of travelling families with respect, plus provide a caring and non-judgemental service. An informed approach to lifestyle interpretation may stop the midwife identifying the woman as an 'antenatal defaulter' with the negative connotations that accompany that label. Moving on may be through choice related to lifestyle, but equally it may be the result of eviction from unofficial sites.

Some health authorities have designated services for travelling families that contribute to uptake and continuity of care. These carers understand the culture and are aware of specific health needs; they can also access appropriate resources, for example a general practitioner (GP) who is receptive to travellers' needs. A trusting relationship is important to people who are frequently subjected to discrimination. Handheld records contribute to continuity of care and communication between care providers, but the maternity service also needs to address communication challenges for individuals who do not have a postal address or who have low levels of literacy.

Homelessness

Homelessness is a complex concept; it knows no boundaries, no borders and no colour. It does not discriminate and is an issue that can affect anyone. This vulnerable population comprises a human kaleidoscope of people where health disparities are heightened. The homeless population constitute a heterogeneous community characterized by multiple comorbidities that make them more vulnerable:

- alcohol and drug dependence
- mental disorders illness
- infections, e.g. tuberculosis and HIV
- premature death.

Homeless individuals are often excluded from mainstream society; homelessness may arise for many reasons but the following risk factors may be implicated:

- those experiencing disputes and relationship breakdown
- those with learning difficulties and no/low educational attainment or unemployment
- alcohol or drug misuse
- mental health problems
- those in debt or lacking a social support network
- young teenagers who run away from home
- those subjected to domestic abuse/violence
- those who define themselves as LGBT – a number of adolescents become homeless after leaving home because of conflicts with parents regarding sexual orientation
- refugees or those seeking asylum
- individuals having contact with the criminal justice system.

Homelessness drives many to despair, as the daily struggle for safety, food, shelter, clothing and the bare necessities of daily living drives health to the bottom of the list in order of priorities. This in turn, exacerbates morbidity, complicates treatment and elevates mortality. Hirani and Richter (2019) attest that homelessness is a significant challenge to health care globally, with estimates of up to 100 million people worldwide who are homeless at any given time. Of particular concern, homeless women may have comorbidities and other vulnerability factors such as mental illness, poor nutritional status, substance misuse problems and infectious disease such as HIV, hepatitis B and C and tuberculosis (Rimawi et al. 2014).

A significant number of women who died in the UK had multiple and complex health problems or other vulnerability factors (Knight et al. 2019). Domestic and sexual violence is the leading cause of homelessness for women and families. Homeless women are far more likely to experience violence compared with women who are not homeless because of a lack of personal security when living outdoors or in shelters (Hirani and Richter 2019). Tackling vulnerability factors and complex physical and psychosocial health needs requires the midwife to develop cultural competence, which is held as a key strategy to reducing disparities and promoting health equity.

The Midwife Researcher: an Introduction

A midwife's work is consistently based on the knowledge gained from evidence. Midwives use this knowledge to provide high standards of care to women and families. It enables them to advocate for women and empowers midwives to keep developing knowledge and skills, both clinically and academically. It is an interesting question therefore, to think a little deeper about where this evidence comes from. Research, or perhaps more aptly put, the birth of all evidence, is becoming increasingly visible in the clinical environment globally. In the UK for example, this is largely due to the National Institute for Health Research (NIHR), which was set up in 2006 and is the overarching entity for all publicly funded research in the National Health Service (NHS). Among other initiatives, the NIHR setup local Clinical Research Networks (CRNs) to support the delivery of research across the NHS in England (NIHR 2018). There are 15 local CRNs in England, which tend to be divided by region. In 2016/17 the overall Clinical Research Network recruited over 665,000 people into clinical research studies (NIHR 2018).

International Confederation of Harmonization Good Clinical Practice

The ICH GCP is an international ethical and scientific quality standard for designing, conducting, recording and reporting trials that involve the participation of human subjects. Compliance with this standard ensures that the rights and safety of trial participants are protected. The basic principles of GCP originated from the World Medical Association's (WMA 2013) Declaration of Helsinki and aims to ensure that not only are trial participants protected but also that the data and reported results are credible and accurate. GCP was developed in response to historical tragedies such as the thalidomide scandal.

Any research study carried out in the NHS must meet the standards of ICH GCP (2016). The key principles of the ICH GCP (2016) are highlighted in Box 1.3

The Birth of Regulatory Frameworks

The conduct of research trials has not always been ethically sound. A number of experiments have been conducted over the last century, which led to dire consequences requiring the need for standards and regulatory frameworks ensuring the safety of all participants.

The Nuremberg Code was developed to serve as a foundation for ethical clinical research since its publication 60 years ago (Ghooi 2011). The Nuremberg Code was developed in response to a series of inhumane experiments which were conducted, mostly in concentration camps, on Jewish prisoners (Smith and Master 2014). These experiments included the study of the human body's resistance to low pressure, hypothermia, malaria, mustard gas, typhus and poison (Smith and Master 2014). During the Nuremberg trials (1945–46) the international military tribunal charged 23 Nazi doctors and scientists with war crimes and crimes against humanity; many were convicted and some sentenced to death (Smith and Master 2014). The Nuremberg Code is considered the historical basis for research ethics.

The Declaration of Helsinki was originally published in 1964 by the World Medical Association primarily to set international ethical principles for research involving human participants (Morris 2013). Once again, a number of studies preceding the declaration had involved

BOX 1.3 The Principles of ICH GCP E6 (2016)

Guideline to which all Clinical Trials should be Conducted

- Clinical trials should be conducted in accordance with the ethical principles that have their origin in the Declaration of Helsinki, and that are consistent with GCP and the applicable regulatory requirements.
- Before a trial is initiated, foreseeable risks and inconveniences are weighed against the anticipated benefit for the individual trail subject and society. A trial should be initiated and continued only if the anticipated benefits justify the risks.
- The rights, safety and wellbeing of the trial subjects are the most important considerations and should prevail over the interests of science and society.
- The available non-clinical and clinical information on an investigational product should be adequate to support the proposed clinical trial.
- Clinical trials should be scientifically sound and described in a clear detailed protocol.
- A trial should be conducted in compliance with the protocol that has received prior institutional review board (IRB)/Independent ethics committee (IEC) approval or favourable opinion.
- The medical care given to, and medical decisions made on behalf of subjects, should always be the responsibility of a qualified physician or, when appropriate, of a qualified dentist.
- Each individual involved in conducting a trial should be qualified by education, training and experience to perform his or her respective task(s).
- Freely given informed consent should be obtained from every subject prior to clinical trial participation.
- All clinical trial information should be recorded, handled and stored in a way that allows its accurate reporting, interpretation and verification.
- The confidentiality of records that could identify subjects should be protected, respecting the privacy and confidentiality rules in accordance with the applicable regulatory requirement(s).
- Investigational products should be manufactured, handled and stored in accordance with applicable good manufacturing practice (GMP). They should be used in accordance with the approval protocol.
- Systems with procedures that assure the quality of every aspect of the trial should be implemented.

CASE STUDY 1.1 Diethylstilboestrol

Diethylstilboestrol (DES) is a synthetic oestrogen. It was produced in London in 1938 and was prescribed from 1945 to 1971 to prevent miscarriages (Mastroianni et al. 1994). Early studies conducted at Harvard University found that DES was effective against a variety of pregnancy complications (Mastroianni et al. 1994). These studies were heavily criticized because they were conducted without the use of controls. However, despite this criticism, DES was approved by the Food and Drug Administration (FDA) federal agency in 1947 as a new drug application for the purpose of preventing miscarriages (Mastroianni et al. 1994).

Controlled studies on DES were carried out in the 1950s and the findings were very different. At the University of Chicago, every pregnant woman was enrolled into a clinical trial at the University's Lying-In Hospital. One half of the women were randomized to receive DES and the other half to receive a placebo. None of the women were told that they were part of the study and none of the women were told which drug they were taking (Mastroianni et al. 1994). This study found that twice as many of the mothers who had been given DES had miscarriages or smaller birth weight babies. Despite these studies, DES continued to be marketed as a drug to prevent miscarriage.

What are the ethical problems with this piece of research and how, now, might this piece of research be conducted differently?

the use of human subjects without consent, and would now be considered unethical and unacceptable within the scientific community.

The Declaration of Helsinki (WMA 2013) statement consists of the following general principles:

- risks
- burdens and benefits
- vulnerable groups and individuals
- scientific requirements and research protocols
- research ethic committees
- privacy and confidentiality
- informed consent
- use of placebo
- post-trial provision
- research registration
- public dissemination of results and unproven interventions in clinical practice.

Read Case Study 1.1 and then reflect on the WMA (2013) Declaration of Helsinki general principles.

CASE STUDY 1.2   **Thalidomide**

Thalidomide was used in the 1950s and 1960s to prevent morning sickness in pregnant women. It was first licensed in the UK in 1958 and was widely prescribed to pregnant women suffering with morning sickness.

During the time of thalidomide, the regulatory standards that are in place today were not present. Many of the medications taken by women during pregnancy had not been through robust clinical trials to investigate whether they would cause potential harm to the fetus. It soon became apparent that babies born to mothers who had taken thalidomide suffered severe teratogenic side-effects such as phocomelia (seal-like limbs in the fetus). Because of this, US senate hearings followed, and in 1962, the Kefauver Amendment to the Food, Drug and Cosmetic Act were passed into law to ensure drug efficacy and greater drug safety (Ray et al. 2016). For the first time, drug manufacturers were required to prove the effectiveness of their products to the FDA before marketing (Ray et al. 2016).

The consequences of unethical research can have extreme negative effects for participants. Between 1966 and 1971 seven cases of clear-cell adenocarcinoma (CCA), an extremely rare cancer, especially in young women, were found in teenage girls whose mothers had taken diethylstilboestrol (DES) a synthetic oestrogen during pregnancy. That same year, the agency responsible for food and drug administration (FDA) banned the use of DES as a preventer against miscarriage, but by that time it was estimated that 1.5 million babies had been exposed to DES *in utero* (Mastroianni et al. 1994).

Case Study 1.2 highlights the harm that can be wreaked on the lives of women and their families when untested drugs such as thalidomide are implemented without the regulatory standards and checks that now exist in contemporary practice around research on human subjects.

The Role of the Research Midwife

Globally, midwives play a pivotal role in the development of research; for example in the UK many NHS Trusts now employ research midwives to help coordinate the delivery of clinical studies within the maternity unit. Research midwives work within their local CRN to help support the delivery of local research. This research falls under the umbrella term of 'Reproductive Health and Childbirth' and is one of 30 specialties within the

Clinical Research Networks. Other specialties include mental health, diabetes and injuries as well as emergencies (NIHR 2018).

The research midwife's job is important and diverse. Many research midwives are involved in the selection, setup and recruitment of clinical trials. Very often they will coordinate the study establish the process and play a large part in recruiting participants to research studies. The research midwife is often the core person in a trial on site (Luyben et al. 2013). Midwives are also integral to any multidisciplinary research team, as they are in a unique and privileged position to understand the needs of pregnant women, and as midwifery education advances many midwives are now equipped with the necessary skills required for research (Rowland and Jones 2013).

The research midwife has a duty to work within the regulatory frameworks of clinical research. There are research governance frameworks to guide good practice in the field of research. In the UK for example, the NHS Health Research Authority (HRA 2018) Research Governance Framework for Health and Social Care guidelines provide a structure for the governance of research in health and social care. This framework applies to everybody involved in clinical and non-clinical research (Fig. 1.4).

This policy framework not only sets out good practice in the management and conduct of health and social care research, but also the legal requirements and other standards (Health Research Authority, HRA 2017). It is primarily used to ensure the safety of participants and sets out operational procedures that should be followed by institutions conducting research (HRA 2017).

Box 1.4 identifies the statement of principles that serves as a benchmark for good practice that the management and conduct of all health and social care research in the UK are expected to meet.

In addition to the principles outlined in Box 1.4, the key values in Box 1.5 apply to interventional research only, i.e. where a change in treatment, care or other services is made for the purpose of research.

Frontline Research

The research midwife does not work in isolation, and with any research study or clinical trial individuals who are part of the Site Team have duties and responsibilities (Fig. 1.5).

A good proportion of the research midwives' time is spent on recruiting eligible participants for studies. All studies will have an inclusion and exclusion criteria

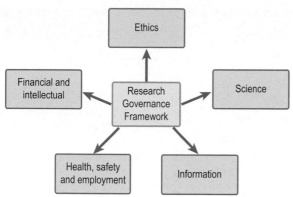

Fig. 1.4 The five domains of the Research Governance Framework for Health & Social Care. (From NHS Health Research Authority 2018.)

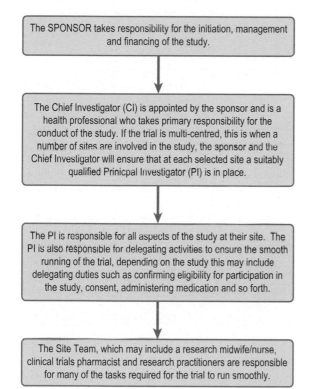

Fig. 1.5 Structure of responsibility for research study/clinical trial.

and it is important that this is followed when identifying potential participants for research studies. In some research studies/trials, eligibility has to be confirmed by a medical professional, in which case, the research midwife would refer onto the doctor designated to confirm eligibility for the study/trial. All information about the conduct of a trial can be found in the trial protocol, and this will outline the process for identifying participants.

Informed Consent

Informed consent is just as important in research as it is in routine clinical care. ICH-GCP states that informed consent is a process by which the subject voluntarily confirms his or her willingness to participate in a particular trial, after having been informed of all aspects of the trial that are relevant to the subject's decision to participate. Informed consent is documented by means of a written signed and dated 'Informed Consent Form' (ICH GCP 2016). Where research midwives/nurse are involved in the consent procedure it creates a bond of trust between the participant and the research midwife/nurse (Ray et al. 2016). This is because the research midwife is often the primary point of contact for the participant.

The safety of participants in any trial is of the upmost importance and respecting their decision of whether or not to participate in a research study is paramount. Everybody involved with the consenting process should be familiar with the study protocol, have knowledge of all available treatment options, have the time for a full discussion with the participant and be sensitive to the circumstances of the participants (NIHR 2018). A potential participant should never feel coerced into taking part in a research study and regardless of whether or not the individual chooses to participate clinical care should never be affected.

Read Case Study 1.3 and then answer the related questions.

Understanding the Basic Principles of Research

Understanding basic research principles are crucial in all aspects of health care. Whether this is to critique a research paper, or collate the latest evidence in healthcare practice. Research evidence is applied by midwives in day-to-day practice by gathering the best available evidence and applying it to health care and medicine. It is, quite broadly, the systematic investigation with the aim of advancing existing knowledge (Ray et al. 2016). Even if midwives do not choose to follow a research career path, a basic understanding of the principles of research helps inform all areas of midwifery practice and help to safeguard women and babies from harm. Integrating and normalizing research within clinical teams fosters a culture of research activeness, which benefits midwives and the very women for whom they care.

BOX 1.4   HRA (2017) Statement of Principles, Research Governance Framework for Health and Social Care

Principle 1: *Safety*
The safety and wellbeing of the individual prevails over the interests of science and society.

Principle 2: *Competence*
All the people involved in managing and conducting a research project are qualified by education, training and experience, or otherwise competent under the supervision of a suitably qualified person, to perform their tasks.

Principle 3: *Scientific and Ethical Conduct*
Research projects are scientifically sound and guided by ethical principles in all their aspects.

Principle 4: *The Woman as a Recipient of Care*
Service users and the public are involved in the design, management, conduct and dissemination of research, unless otherwise justified.

Principle 5: *Integrity*
Quality and transparency research is designed, reviewed, managed and undertaken in a way that ensures integrity, quality and transparency.

Principle 6: *Protocol*
The design and procedure of the research are clearly described and justified in a research proposal or protocol, where applicable conforming to a standard template and/or specified contents.

Principle 7: *Legality*
The researchers and sponsor familiarize themselves with relevant legislation and guidance in respect of managing and conducting the research.

Principle 8: *Benefits and Risks*
Before the research project is started, any anticipated benefit for the individual participant and other present and future recipients of the health or social care in question is weighed against the foreseeable risks and inconveniences once they have been mitigated.

Principle 9: *Approval*
A research project is started only if a research ethics committee and any other relevant approval body have favourably reviewed the research proposal or protocol and related information, where their review is expected or required.

Principle 10: *Information about the Research*
In order to avoid waste, information about research projects (other than those for educational purposes) is made publicly available before they start (unless a deferral is agreed by or on behalf of the research ethics committee).

Principle 11: *Accessible Findings*
Other than research for educational purposes and early phase trials, the findings, whether positive or negative, are made accessible, with adequate consent and privacy safeguards, in a timely manner after they have finished, in compliance with any applicable regulatory standards, i.e. legal requirements or expectations of regulators. In addition, where appropriate, information about the findings of the research is available, in a suitable format and timely manner, to those who took part in it, unless otherwise justified.

Principle 12: *Choice*
Research participants are afforded respect and autonomy, taking account of their capacity to understand. Where there is a difference between the research and the standard practice that they might otherwise experience, research participants are given information to understand the distinction and make a choice, unless a research ethics committee agrees otherwise. Where participants' explicit consent is sought, it is voluntary and informed. Where consent is refused or withdrawn, this is done without reprisal. A formal, structured risk assessment is only expected where identified as essential. The risk:benefit ratio will normally be sufficiently described and considered as part of review processes such as research ethics committee review, i.e. the HRA, the Administration of Radioactive Substances Advisory Committee (ARSAC), the Human Fertilisation and Embryology Authority (HFEA) or the Medicines and Healthcare products Regulatory Agency (MHRA). Either directly, or indirectly through the involvement of data or tissue that could identify them.

Principle 13: *Insurance and Indemnity*
Adequate provision is made for insurance or indemnity to cover liabilities, which may arise in relation to the design, management and conduct of the research project.

Principle 14: *Respect for Privacy*
All information collected for or as part of the research project is recorded, handled and stored appropriately and in such a way and for such time that it can be accurately reported, interpreted and verified, while the confidentiality

---

BOX 1.4 HRA (2017) Statement of Principles, Research Governance Framework for Health and Social Care—cont'd

of individual research participants remains appropriately protected. Data and tissue collections are managed in a transparent way that demonstrates commitment to their appropriate use for research and appropriate protection of privacy.

Principle 15: *Compliance*
Sanctions for non-compliance with these principles may include appropriate and proportionate administrative, contractual or legal measures by funders, employers, relevant professional and statutory regulators, and other bodies.

HRA (Health Research Authority) (2017) UK Policy for Health and Social Care Research. Available at: www.hra.nhs.uk/planning-and-improving-research/policies-standards-legislation/uk-policy-framework-health-social-care-research.

BOX 1.5 HRA (2017) Statement of Principles, Research Governance Framework for Health and Social Care. (Note: for use ONLY in Interventional Research)

Principle 16: *Justified Intervention*
The intended deviation from normal treatment, care or other services is adequately supported by the available information (including evidence from previous research).

Principle 17: *Ongoing Provision of Treatment*
The research proposal or protocol and the participant information sheet explain the special arrangements, if any, after the research intervention period has ended (e.g. continuing or changing the treatment, care or other services that were introduced for the purposes of the research).

Principle 18: *Integrity of the Care Record*
All information about treatment, care or other services provided as part of the research project and their outcomes is recorded, handled and stored appropriately and

in such a way and for such time that it can be understood, where relevant, by others involved in the participant's care and accurately reported, interpreted and verified, while the confidentiality of records of the participants remains protected.

Principle 19: *Duty of Care*
The duty of care owed by health and social care providers continues to apply when their patients and service users take part in research. A relevant health or social care professional retains responsibility for the treatment, care or other services given to patients and service users as research participants and for decisions about their treatment, care or other services. If an unmanageable conflict arises between research and patient interests, the duty to the participant as a patient prevails.

HRA (Health Research Authority). (2017) Statement of Principles, Research Governance Framework for Health and Social Care.

CASE STUDY 1.3 Mrs Jones

A maternity unit is involved in a study investigating the effects of a new medication to prevent postpartum haemorrhage. Mrs Jones is a primigravida and attends maternity triage contracting 3 in 10 min; she is 40+^{1} weeks' gestation. On examination, the cervix is 4 cm and she is diagnosed in established labour. She has a history of anxiety and presented to maternity triage 1 week previously with reduced fetal movements. The midwife looking after her thinks she might be eligible for the clinical trial and

asks the research midwife if she would like to discuss the study with the woman. When the research midwife enters the room the woman is using entonox and appears to be finding the contractions difficult to cope with.

1. *Do you think it is an appropriate time to discuss a research study investigating postpartum haemorrhage with the woman?*
2. *When might be a good time to give information on the study?*

REFLECTIVE ACTIVITY FOR SELF-ASSESSMENT

1. What contribution can midwives make to global health?
2. What are the key aims of the United Nations sustainable development goals?
3. Discuss this statement: 'Transformation to family structures has meant that there are more diverse types of families today than ever before'.
4. What are the basic research principles?

REFERENCES

AOMRC (Academy of Medical Royal Colleges). (2016). Global health capabilities for UK health professionals. Available at: www.aomrc.org.uk/wp-content/uploads/2016/08/Global_Health_Capabilities_100816–2.pdf.

Alkema, L., Chou, D., Hogan, D., et al. (2016). Global, regional, and national levels and trends in maternal mortality between 1990 and 2015, with scenario-based projections to 2030: A systematic analysis by the UN Maternal Mortality Estimation Inter-Agency Group. *Lancet, 387*(10017), 462–474.

All Party Parliamentary Group on Global Health. (2016). Triple impact: How developing nursing will improve health, promote gender equality and support economic growth. Available at: www.appg-globalhealth.org.uk.

Aquino, M. R., Edge, D., & Smith, D. M. (2015). Pregnancy as an ideal time for intervention to address the complex needs of black and minority ethnic women: Views of British midwives. *Midwifery, 31*(3), 373–379.

CQC (Care Quality Commission). (2018). Available at: 2018 survey of women's experiences of maternity care. Available at: www.cqc.org.uk/sites/default/files/20190424_mat18_statisticalrelease.pdf.

Collins English Dictionary. (2019). Online. Available at: www.collinsdictionary.com/dictionary/english.

Dahlberg, U., & Aune, I. (2013). The woman's birth experience—The effect of interpersonal relationships and continuity of care. *Midwifery, 29*(4), 407–415.

DH (Department of Health. (2014). Engaging in global health: The framework for voluntary engagement in global health by the UK health sector. Available at: www.gov.uk/government/publications/supporting-international-volunteering-in-the-health-and-care-sector.

Development Initiatives. (2018). Global humanitarian assistance report 2018. Available at: http://devinit.org/post/global-humanitarian-assistance-report-2018/#.

Drach-Zahavy, A., Buchnic, R., & Granot, M. (2016). Antecedents and consequences of emotional work in midwifery: A prospective field study. *International Journal of Nursing Studies, 60*, 168–178.

European Commission. (2018). Erasmus+ – Opportunities – Studying ABROAD. Available at: https://ec.europa.eu/programmes/erasmus-plus/opportunities/individuals/students/studying-abroad_en.

European Parliament and the Council of the European Union. (2005). Directive 2005/36/EC of the European Parliament and of the Council of 7 September 2005 on the recognition of professional qualifications. Available at: https://eur-lex.europa.eu/legal-content/EN/TXT/?uri=celex%3A32005L0036.

European Parliament and the Council of the European Union. (2013). Directive 2013/55/EU of the European Parliament and of the Council of 20 November 2013 amending Directive 2005/36/EC on the recognition of professional qualifications and Regulation (EU) No 1024/2012 on administrative cooperation through the Internal Market Information System ('the IMI Regulation'). Available at: www.education.ie/en/The-Education-System/Qualifications-Recognition/EU-Directive-2013-55-EU.pdf.

Euro-Peristat. (2018). *European perinatal health report: Core indicators of the health and care of pregnant women and babies in Europe in 2015*. Available at: www.europeristat.com.

FAO, IFAD, UNICEF, WFP, WHO. (2018). The State of Food Security and Nutrition in the World 2018. Building climate resilience for food security and nutrition. Rome, FAO. Licence: CC BY-NC-SA 3.0 IGO. Available at: www.fao.org/family-farming/detail/en/c/1152381.

FIGO (International Federation of Gynecology and Obstetrics). (2018). The global unmet need for modern contraceptives. Available at: www.figo.org/news/global-unmet-need-modern-contraceptives-0016065.

Flying Start NHS. (2018). Cultural competence. Available at: https://learn.nes.nhs.scot/735/flying-start-nhs.

Garcia, R., Ali, N., Papadopoulos, C., et al. (2015). Specific antenatal interventions for Black, Asian and Minority Ethnic (BAME) pregnant women at high risk of poor birth outcomes in the United Kingdom: A scoping review. *BMC Pregnancy and Childbirth, 15*, 226.

Ghooi, R. B. (2011). The Nuremberg Code – A critique. *Ethics, 2*(2), 72–76.

HRA (Health Research Authority). (2017). UK Policy for Health & Social Care Research. Available at: www.hra.nhs.uk/planning-and-improving-research/policies-standards-legislation/uk-policy-framework-health-social-care-research.

HRA (Health Research Authority). (2018). UK policy framework for health and social care research. Available at: www.hra.nhs.uk/planning-and-improving-research/policies-standards-legislation/uk-policy-framework-health-social-care-research.

Hirani, S. A. A., & Richter, S. (2019). Maternal and child health during forced displacement. *Journal of Nursing Scholarship*, 51(3), 252–261.

Hunter, B., & Deery, R. (Eds.). (2009). *Emotions in midwifery and reproduction*. Basingstoke: Palgrave Macmillan.

INMA (Institute of Medicine of the National Academies). (2015). Empowering women and strengthening health systems and services through investing in nursing and midwifery enterprise. Available at: www.nap.edu/read/19005/chapter/1.

ICH GCP (International Confederation of Harmonization Good Clinical Practice). (2016). Integrated addendum to ICH E6 (R1): Guideline for good clinical practice E6 (R2). Current Step 4 Version. Available at: www.ich.org/filcadmin/Public_Web_Site/ICH_Products/Guidelines/Efficacy/E6/E6_R2__Step_4_2016_1109.pdf.

ICM (International Confederation of Midwives). (2013). Global standards for midwifery education. Available at: www.internationalmidwives.org/assets/files/general-files/2018/04/icm-standards-guidelines_ammended2013.pdf.

ICM (International Confederation of Midwives). (2014a). Position statement: The midwife is the first choice health professional for childbearing women. Available at: www.internationalmidwives.org/assets/files/statement files/2018/04/the-midwife-is-the-first-choice-eng.pdf.

ICM (International Confederation of Midwives) (2014b). Why and how to create a midwives association. Available at: www.internationalmidwives.org/our-members/create-a-national-association.html.

ICM (International Confederation of Midwives). (2014c). International Code of Ethics for Midwives. Hague/Netherlands: ICM. Available at: www.internationalmidwives.org.

ICM (International Confederation of Midwives). (2017a). Core document: International definition of a midwife. Available at: www.internationalmidwives.org/assets/files/definitions-files/2018/06/eng-definition_of_the_midwife-2017.pdf.

ICM (International Confederation of Midwives). (2017b). Position statement: Partnership between women and midwives. Available at: www.internationalmidwives.org/assets/files/statement-files/2018/04/eng-partnership-between-women-and-midwives1.pdf.

ICM (International Confederation of Midwives). (2017c). Position statement migrant and refugee women and their families. Available at: www.internationalmidwives.org/assets/files/statement-files/2018/04/eng-migrant_refugee_women.pdf.

ICM (International Confederation of Midwives). (2018). Our work. Available at: www.internationalmidwives.org/our-work.

ICM (International Confederation of Midwives). (2019). Essential competencies for midwifery practice: 2019 update. Available at: www.internationalmidwives.org/our-work/policy-and-practice/essential-competencies-for-midwifery-practice.html.

Illing, J. C., Carter, M., Thompson, N. J., et al. (2013). *Evidence synthesis on the occurrence, causes, consequences, prevention and management of bullying and harassing behaviours to inform decision making in the NHS. Final report*. Durham: NIHR Service Delivery and Organisation programme.

Javaweera, H. (2016). *Commissioning health services for vulnerable migrant women in England evidence on policies and practices*. London: Women's Health Consortium.

Jones, E., Lattof, A. R., & Coast, E. (2017). Interventions to provide culturally appropriate maternity care services: Factors affecting implementation. *BMC Pregnancy and Childbirth*, 17(267), 1–10.

Kemp, J., Shaw, E., Nanjego, S., & Mondeh, K. (2018). Improving student midwives practice learning in Uganda through action research: The MOMENTUM project. *International Practice Development Journal*, 8(1), 7.

Knight M, Bunch K, Tuffnell D, et al. (Eds) (2019); on behalf of MBRRACE-UK. Saving Lives, Improving Mothers' Care – Lessons learned to inform maternity care from the UK and Ireland Confidential Enquiries into Maternal Deaths and Morbidity 2015–17. Oxford: National Perinatal Epidemiology Unit, University of Oxford.

Koblinsky, M., Moyer, C., Calvert, C., et al. (2016). Quality maternity care for every woman, everywhere: A call to action. *Lancet*, 388(10057), 2307–2320.

Labonté, R. (2018). Reprising the globalization dimensions of international health. *Globalization and Health*, 14(1), 49.

Lancet. (2014). Midwifery Series: Executive Summary. Available at: www.thelancet.com/series/midwifery.

Lancet. (2016). Maternal Health Series. Available at: www.maternalhealthseries.org.

Lancet. (2018). Stemming the global caesarean section epidemic. Editorial 392:1279. Available at: www.thelancet.com/pdfs/journals/lancet/PIIS0140–6736(18)32394–8.pdf.

Lawn, J., Blencowe, H., Waiswa, P., et al. (2016). Stillbirths: Rates, risk factors and potential for progress towards 2030. *Lancet*, 387(10018), 587–603.

Lewis, M., Jones, A., & Hunter, B. (2017). Women's experience of trust within the midwife–mother relationship. *International Journal of Childbirth*, 7(1), 50–52.

Lopez, S., Titulaer, P., Bokosi, M., et al. (2015). The involvement of midwives associations in policy and planning about the midwifery workforce: A global survey. *Midwifery*, 31, 1096–1103.

Luyben, A. G., Wijnen, H. A., Oblasser, C., et al. (2013). The current state of midwifery and development of midwifery research in four European countries. *Midwifery, 29*(5), 417–424.

Manning, A., & Schaaf, M. (2018). Respectful maternity care and human resources for health. Available at: www.whiteribbonalliance.org/wp-content/uploads/2018/04/6422_RMC-Maternity-Care-Resources-PPG_English.pdf.

Marmot, M. (2010). *Fair society, health lives: Strategic review of health inequalities in England post-2010.* London: The Marmot Review.

Mastroianni, A. C., Faden, R., & Federman, D. (1994). *Women and health research: Ethical and legal issues of including women in clinical studies* (Vol. I). Washington, DC: National Academies Press.

McCourt, C., & Stevens, T. (2009). Relationship and reciprocity in caseload midwifery. In B. Hunter, & R. Deery (Eds.), *Emotions in midwifery and reproduction* (pp. 17–35). Basingstoke: Palgrave Macmillan.

McLuhan, M., & Fiore, Q. (1968). *War and peace in the global village* (pp. 7). New York: Bantam Books

Powell-Kennedy, H., Cheyney, M., Dahlen, H., et al. (2018). Asking different questions: A call to action for research to improve the quality of care for every woman, every child. *Midwifery, 65,* 16–17.

Morris, K. (2013). Revising the Declaration of Helsinki. World Report. *Lancet, 381*(9881), 1889–1890.

NHS England. (2016). National maternity review: Better births – improving outcomes of maternity services in England, a five year forward view for maternity care. Available at: www.england.nhs.uk/wp-content/uploads/2016/02/national-maternity-review-report.pdf.

NIHR (National Institute for Health Research). (2018). Annual Report 2016/17: Improving the Health and Wealth of the Nation through Research. Available at: www.nihr.ac.uk/about-us/documents/NIHR%20ANNUAL%20REPORT%201617%-20FINAL.pdf.

ONS (Office of National Statistics). (2017). Families and Households: 2017.Trends in living arrangements including families (with and without dependent children), people living alone and people in shared accommodation, broken down by size and type of household. Available at: www.ons.gov.uk/peoplepopulationandcommunity/birthsdeathsandmarriages/families/bulletins/familiesandhouseholds/2017.

Olds, L. D. (2002). Prenatal and infancy home visiting by nurses: From randomized trials to community replication. *Prevention Science, 3*(3), 153–172.

PHE (Public Health England). (2016). (updated 2019). *A framework for supporting teenage mothers and young fathers.* London: PHE.

Ray, S., Fitzpatrick, S., Golubic, R., & Fisher, S. (2016). *Oxford handbook of clinical and healthcare research.* Oxford: Oxford University Press.

Smith, E., & Master, Z. (2014). Ethical practice of research involving humans. Reference module in biomedical sciences. Available at: www.sciencedirect.com/science/article/pii/B9780128012383001781.

Renfrew, M., McFadden, A., Bastos, M., et al. (2014). Midwifery and quality care: Findings from a new evidence-informed framework for maternal and newborn care. *Lancet, 384*(9948), 1129–1145.

Rimawi, B. H., Mirdamadi, M., & John, J. F. (2014). Infections and homelessness: Risks of increased infectious diseases in displaced women. *World Medical & Health Policy, 6,* 2.

Rowland, L., & Jones, C. (2013). Research midwives: Importance and practicalities. *British Journal of Midwifery, 21*(1), 60–64.

RCOG (Royal College of Obstetricians and Gynaecologists). (2017). *Each baby counts: 2015 full report.* London: RCOG.

RCPSG (Royal College of Physicians and Surgeons of Glasgow). (2017). Global citizenship in the Scottish health service: The value of international volunteering. Available at: https://rcpsg.ac.uk/college/influencing-healthcare/policy/global-citizenship.

Sandall, J., Soltani, H., Gates, S., et al. (2016). Midwife-led continuity models versus other models of care for childbearing women. *Cochrane Database of Systematic Reviews,* (4), CD004667.

Squires, N. (2018). Global Health – what it means and why Public Health England works globally. Available at: https://publichealthmatters.blog.gov.uk/2018/09/04/global-health-what-it-means-and-why-phe-works-globally.

Starrs, A., Ezeh, A., Barker, G., et al. (2018). Accelerate progress—sexual and reproductive health and rights for all: Report of the guttmacher–lancet commission. *Lancet, 391*(10140), 2642–2692.

Survive & Thrive. (2016). The professional association strengthening project Module 4: Functions of a professional association. Available at: www.strongprofassoc.org.

ten Hoope-Bender, P., Lopes, S., Nove, A., et al. (2016). Midwifery 2030: A woman's pathway to health. What does this mean? *Midwifery, 32,* 1–6.

THET. (2017). In our mutual interest. Available at: www.thet.org/resources/thet-in-our-mutual-interest.

UCAS. (2018). What is Erasmus? Available at: www.ucas.com/undergraduate/what-and-where-study/studying-overseas/what-erasmus.

UNICEF. (2018). Neonatal mortality. Available at: https://data.unicef.org/topic/child-survival/neonatal-mortality.

UN (United Nations). (2015a). Millennium Development Goals and beyond 2015. Available at: www.un.org/millenniumgoals.

UN (United Nations). (2015b). About the sustainable development goals. Available at: www.un.org/sustainabledevelopment/sustainable-development-goals.

UNCC (United Nations Climate Change). (2019). Introduction to gender and climate change. Available at: https://unfccc.int/topics/gender/the-big-picture/introduction-to-gender-and-climate-change.

OHCRH (United Nations Human Rights Officer of the High Commissioner). (2019). Sexual and reproductive health rights. Available at: www.ohchr.org/en/issues/women/wrgs/pages/healthrights.aspx.

UNFPA. (2014). State of the world's midwifery: A universal pathway, a woman's right to health. Available at: www.unfpa.org/sowmy.

UNFPA. (2018). Humanitarian Action: 2018 Overview. Available at: www.unfpa.org/sites/default/files/pub-pdf/UNFPA_HumanitAction_18_20180124_ONLINE.pdf.

UN Women. (2018). *UN Women Annual Report 2017–2018.* Available at: www.annualreport.unwomen.org.

WASHWatch. (2017). Wash: A global issue. Available at: https://washwatch.org/en/about/about-wash.

West, M., Eckert, R., Collins, B., et al. (2017). *Caring to change: How compassionate leadership can stimulate innovation in health care.* London: The King's Fund.

White Ribbon Alliance. (2011). Respectful maternity care: The universal rights of childbearing women. Available at: www.whiteribbonalliance.org/wp-content/uploads/2017/11/Final_RMC_Charter.pdf.

WHO (World Health Organization). (2008). *Commission on social determinants of health. Closing the gap in a generation: Health equity through action on the social determinants of health.* Geneva: WHO.

WHO (World Health Organization). (2015a). *Survive, thrive, transform: The global strategy for women's, children's and adolescents' health 2016–2030.* Available at: www.who.int/life-course/publications/global-strategy-2016–2030/en.

WHO (World Health Organization). (2015b). European strategic directions for strengthening nursing and midwifery towards Health 2020 goals. Available at: www.euro.who.int/en/health-topics/Health-systems/nursing-and-midwifery/publications/2015/european-strategic-directions-for-strengthening-nursing-and-midwifery-towards-health-2020-goals.

WHO (World Health Organization). (2015c). *Recommendations on health promotion interventions for maternal and newborn health.* Geneva: WHO.

WHO (World Health Organization). (2016a). Midwives voices, midwives realities: Finding from a global consultation on providing quality midwifery care. Available at: www.who.int/maternal_child_adolescent/documents/midwives-voices-realities/en.

WHO (World Health Organization). (2016b). *Global strategic directions for strengthening nursing and midwifery 2016–2020.* Available at: www.who.int/hrh/nursing_midwifery/global-strategy-midwifery-2016–2020/en.

WHO (World Health Organization). (2016c). *Global strategy on human resources for health: Workforce 2030.* Available at: www.who.int/hrh/resources/pub_globstrathrh-2030/en.

WHO (World Health Organization). (2017). Human rights and health. Available at: www.who.int/news-room/fact-sheets/detail/human-rights-and-health.

WHO (World Health Organization). (2018a). Universal health coverage (UHC) fact sheet. Available at: www.who.int/news-room/fact-sheets/detail/universal-health-coverage-(uhc.

WHO (World Health Organization). (2018b). Maternal mortality fact sheet. Available at: www.who.int/news-room/fact-sheets/detail/maternal-mortality.

WHO (World Health Organization). (2018c). Maternal mortality fact sheet. Available at: www.who.int/news-room/fact-sheets/detail/maternal-mortality.

WHO/UNICEF. (2017). *Progress on drinking water, sanitation and hygiene 2017.* Available at: https://washdata.org/sites/default/files/documents/reports/2018-01/JMP-2017-report-final.pdf.

WMA (World Medical Association). (2013). WMA Declaration of Helsinki Ethical Principles for Medical Research Involving Human Participants. Available at: www.wma.net/what-we-do/medical-ethics.

World Bank. (2018). Poverty and shared prosperity 2018: Piecing together the poverty puzzle. Available at: www.worldbank.org/en/publication/poverty-and-shared-prosperity.

Zuccala, E., & Horton, R. (2018). Addressing the unfinished agenda on sexual and reproductive health and rights in the SDG era. *Lancet, 391*(10140), 2581–2583.

ANNOTATED FURTHER READING

Alkema, L., Chou, D., Hogan, D., et al. (2016). Global, regional, and national levels and trends in maternal mortality between 1990 and 2015, with scenario-based projections to 2030: A systematic analysis by the UN Maternal Mortality Estimation Inter-Agency Group. *Lancet, 387*(10017), 462–474.

This study provides a comprehensive analysis of global maternal mortality trends based on the latest data from 171 countries.

Daniel, J. N. (2019). Disabled mothering? Outlawed, overlooked and severely prohibited: Interrogating ableism in motherhood. *Social Inclusion, 7*(1), 114–123.

This article provides a feminist perspective of how disabled women are excluded from the ideology of motherhood and the discrimination and marginalization mothers who are disabled encounter. This is a thought provoking read given that the chapter was unable to address the issue of disability due to work constraints.

Royal College of Midwives. (2016). (Update due 2019) Health inequalities and the social determinants of health. Available at: www.ilearn.rcm.org.uk.

This is an e-learning module that contains one short video and three soundbites. It explores social determinants of health in the UK and globally alongside its causes.

USEFUL WEBSITES

Care Quality Commission: www.cqc.org.uk
International Confederation of Midwives: www.internationalmidwives.org
United Nations: www.un.org
White Ribbon Alliance: www.whiteribbonalliance.org
Women's Health and Equality Consortium: www.whec.org.uk
World Bank: www.worldbank.org
World Health Organization: www.who.int

Professional Issues Concerning the Midwife and Midwifery Practice

Jayne E. Marshall, Julia Austin

CHAPTER CONTENTS

This chapter provides an overview of the key frameworks governing the midwifery profession and underpinning the professional practice of the midwife. Included is a resume of the regulation of midwifery and the demise of statutory supervision of midwifery along with the separate Midwives rules. It emphasizes how employer-led models of supervision are vital elements of leadership and clinical governance that support the provision of high quality maternity services and standards of midwifery practice. The concept of resilience is introduced to enable readers to contemplate their personal contribution in creating an environment that is conducive to protecting the wellbeing of themselves and colleagues within the workplace. The chapter also addresses the mandatory triennial revalidation process and the importance of continuing professional development in order for midwives to demonstrate they have maintained professional proficiency. Having knowledge of these various frameworks is essential to every midwife so they are able to function effectively as autonomous, accountable practitioners and provide care to all childbearing women, their babies and families that follows legal and ethical principles and is also contemporary, safe, compassionate and of a high quality.

THE CHAPTER AIMS TO

- identify the purpose of regulation of healthcare professionals in protecting public safety
- explain the role and functions of the regulatory body governing midwifery practice within the UK: namely the Nursing and Midwifery Council
- review the legal framework midwives should work within to maximize safety and minimize risk to women, their babies and families
- raise awareness of ethical frameworks and principles in supporting midwifery practice and empowering childbearing women

- compare the various models of employer-led supervision and their function in supporting professional leadership and the delivery of high quality midwifery care
- introduce the concept of resilience as a key component in developing a workplace that is compassionate and conducive to the wellbeing of all individuals
- affirm the value of continuing professional development and its contribution to the mandatory triennial revalidation

STATUTORY MIDWIFERY REGULATION

The statutory regulation of a profession provides structure and boundaries within a legal framework that can be understood and interpreted by both the professionals themselves and the public they serve and consequently, can be viewed as the basis of a contract of trust between the public and the profession. Regulation of midwifery should therefore play a key role in helping to improve women's experiences of the maternity services and preventing harm from occurring in midwifery practice.

It is essential that women and their families can be assured they are safe and are being cared for by competent and skilled midwives who are effectively educated and knowledgeable in contemporary midwifery practice. Consequently, midwifery regulation should *not* be viewed as an abstract concept but from how it is perceived in ordinary everyday healthcare terms, that is: *supporting the standard of care that women want* or *what midwives would want for themselves and their families*.

'**Midwife**' is a title protected in statute in the UK, which means that no-one can call themselves a midwife or practise

as a midwife unless they are registered on the Nursing and Midwifery Council's (NMC) Register. This registration must be *active*, in that the midwife has met the triennial revalidation requirements to remain on the Register (NMC 2019a). There are just under 37,000 midwives on the NMC Midwives Register with an increase of 1000 midwives from the preceding year's statistics (NMC 2019b).

PROFESSIONAL REGULATION FROM AN INTERNATIONAL PERSPECTIVE

The goal of the International Confederation of Midwives (ICM 2011) *Global Standards for Midwifery Regulation* is to promote regulatory mechanisms that protect the public (women and families) by ensuring that safe and competent midwives provide high standards of care to every woman and baby, within the global context. The six key functions, as shown in Box 2.1, enable this to be achieved.

The ICM (2011) founding values and principles include recognition that:

- Regulation is a mechanism by which the social contract between the midwifery profession and society

BOX 2.1 Purpose of Regulation

The safety of the public is achieved through:
- Setting the scope of practice
- Pre-registration education
- Registration
- Relicensing and continuing competence
- Complaints and discipline
- Code of conduct and ethics

Adapted from the International Confederation of Midwives. (2011) Global standards for midwifery regulation. The Hague: ICM. Available at: www.internationalmidwives.org/assets/files/general-files/2018/04/global-standards-for-midwifery-regulation-eng.pdf.

is expressed. Society grants the midwifery profession authority and autonomy to regulate itself. In return, society expects the midwifery profession to act responsibly, ensure high standards of midwifery care and maintain the trust of the public.

- Each woman has the right to receive care in childbirth from an educated and competent midwife authorized to practise midwifery.
- Midwives are autonomous practitioners, that is, they practise in their own right and are responsible and accountable for their own clinical decision-making.
- The midwife's scope of practice describes the circumstances the midwife must practise in collaboration with other health professionals, such as doctors.
- Midwifery is a profession that is autonomous, separate and distinct from nursing and medicine. What sets midwives apart from nurses and doctors is that **only** midwives can exercise the full scope of midwifery practice and provide all the competencies within the scope.
- Wherever a registered/qualified midwife with a midwifery practising certificate works with pregnant women during the childbirth continuum, no matter what the setting, they are practising midwifery. Therefore when a midwife holds dual registration/qualification as a nurse, they cannot practise simultaneously as a midwife and a nurse. In a maternity setting, a registered/qualified midwife always practises midwifery.

The ICM (2011) further asserts that the following principles of good regulation provide a benchmark against which regulatory processes can be assessed:

- **NECESSITY:** is the regulation necessary? Are current rules and structures that govern this area still valid? Is the legislation purposeful?

- **EFFECTIVENESS:** is the regulation properly targeted? Can it be properly enforced and complied with? Is it flexible and enabling?
- **FLEXIBILITY:** is the legislation sufficiently flexible to be enabling rather than too prescriptive?
- **PROPORTIONALITY:** do the advantages outweigh the disadvantages? Can the same goal be achieved better in another way?
- **TRANSPARENCY:** is the regulation clear and accessible to all? Have stakeholders been involved in the development?
- **ACCOUNTABILITY:** is it clear who is responsible to whom and for what? Is there an effective appeals process?
- **CONSISTENCY:** will the regulation give rise to anomalies and inconsistencies, given the other regulations already in place for this area? Are best practice principles being applied?

Self-regulation of midwifery does not exist in all countries and consequently, regulations for midwifery education or practice are set by the national government or by another professional group who may be perceived as senior/superior. In many high-income countries, midwifery regulatory frameworks, in the main, reflect the ICM (2011) global standards, but with the exception that regulation is rarely midwifery specific, indicating the regulator's governance does not lie predominantly with **midwives** at Board level.

In Europe, midwifery is mostly regulated within an autonomous nursing and midwifery regulatory body, such as in the UK, or through a shared responsibility between a ministry and a midwifery or a nursing and midwifery regulatory body (Nursing and Midwifery Council, NMC 2009). Currently, France is the only country where midwifery is regulated by an autonomous midwifery regulatory body. In Denmark and Norway, the regulatory authority for all health professionals lies with the Board of Health.

The African Health Profession Regulatory Collaborative for Nurses and Midwives was established following the publication of the 'global standards' (ICM 2011) in order to convene a group of leaders from 14 countries spanning east, central and southern Africa who had responsibility for regulation. The aim of this Collaborative is to increase the regulatory capacity of health professional organizations with the consequential impact of improving the regulation and professional standards within each African region. Support is provided from the Collaborative for between four and five countries each year to implement locally created regulation improvement projects. However, despite efforts to improve midwifery education and strengthen the midwifery profession through association, many low- to middle-income countries in Africa and other parts of the world have limited or non-existent regulatory processes. As a result, there continues to be a call for more work to be done in the development of legislation for midwifery regulation in these countries (UNFPA/ICM/WHO 2014; Castro Lopes et al. 2016).

Although midwifery is regulated in the USA, the legal status, definitions, regulations and scope of practice differ considerably across member states. In recent years, efforts have been made by the US Midwifery Education, Regulation and Association collective (USMERA) to achieve common goals that align with the ICM (2011) global standards for strengthening midwifery. In comparison, in New Zealand, there is a separate Midwifery Council, whereas in Australia, midwifery is regulated by a Nursing and Midwifery Board that has separate standards and code of conduct for nurses and midwives.

Self-Regulation in the United Kingdom

In the UK, midwives are members of a self-regulating profession. This is a real privilege, in that the standards for midwifery education and practice are set by midwives themselves. Self-regulating professions have regulatory bodies that are funded by their own professionals. In the case of midwives and nurses, their initial and subsequent retaining/renewal of registration fee payments is the sole funding that pays for all functions of the NMC.

It is acknowledged that the midwifery profession, as other health professions in the UK, is affected to varying degrees by national regulations that are set by others who are not part of the profession: for example, legislation for safeguarding vulnerable children or adults (Safeguarding Vulnerable Groups Act 2006; Department of Health, DH 2014; Her Majesty's Government, HM Government 2018a); medicines legislation (Human Medicines (Amendment) Regulations 2019); Health and Safety in the Workplace Regulations (Health and Safety at Work Act 1974). All midwives are bound by these national laws in the same way as others. However, during the late 1990s, power was devolved away from

the UK Parliament based in Westminster (England) to the other three nations, enabling them to establish their own parliaments or assemblies: the Scottish Parliament, the National Assembly of Wales and the Northern Ireland Assembly. Consequently, each governing body is able to determine their own legislative framework to guide health and social care practice, albeit these are usually based on very similar principles.

Protection of the public cannot be achieved by the regulatory body alone and thus it involves a combination of statutory regulation, personal self-regulation, efficient employment practices and effective collaborative working with professional and educational organizations. It can, however, be difficult for individuals to act ethically and escalate concerns about practices within their employing organizations. It is here, where the regulator and regulation can support the midwife by offering appropriate guidance. The NMC can also work actively with other service regulators such as the Care Quality Commission (CQC) in England, Healthcare Improvement Scotland (HIS), the Regulation and Quality Improvement Authority in Northern Ireland (RQIA) and Healthcare Inspectorate Wales (HIW), to ensure early action is taken to prevent unnecessary harm to women, their babies and families.

The Professional Standards Authority for Health and Social Care (PSA) was established in 2003 (originally known as the Council for Healthcare Regulatory Excellence, CHRE) to oversee the nine health professions' regulators that are identified in Fig. 2.1. As an independent body, the PSA has the legal powers to monitor the performance of the regulators, holding them to account and subsequently providing annual reports to the UK Parliament on their performance. The PSA also conducts audits, reviews and investigations and can appeal fitness to practise decisions in the courts if it considers the sanctions applied by the regulators are inadequate to safeguard the public.

STATUTORY MIDWIFERY PROFESSIONAL REGULATION

Historical Context

While it is appreciated that the governments in Austria, Norway and Sweden had established the legislation that governed the practice of midwifery as early as 1801, it was not until a century later, in 1902, that the

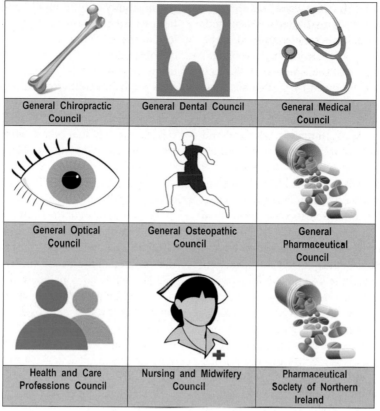

Fig. 2.1 Nine Regulatory Bodies in the UK.

first Midwives Act sanctioned the establishment of a statutory body: the Central Midwives Board (CMB) in England and Wales, followed by the Midwives (Scotland) Act 1915 and the Midwives (Ireland) Act 1918. In the UK, the drive for the legislation to regulate healthcare professionals so as to ensure the public receive quality care, arose from the profession itself, rather than political or public pressure. Professional self-regulation was developed in recognition of specialist skills and to ensure that only those individuals meeting such standards set by their peers gained professional status. The Pharmacy Act of 1852 was the first legislation in the UK to regulate health professionals (pharmacists and druggists) and establish the Pharmaceutical Society of Great Britain, which was followed by the Medical Act of 1858, which created the General Medical Council to regulate doctors in the UK.

The first Midwives Act in 1902 was promoted by individual members of Parliament through Private Members' Bills in the House of Lords and by others who supported midwife registration, rather than being initiated by the government of the time. All three Acts of the UK prescribed the constitution and function of the CMBs in each of the four countries and laid down their statutory powers, which included:

- maintaining a register of qualified midwives
- framing rules to regulate, supervise and restrict, within due limits the practice of midwives to keep the public safe
- arranging for the training of midwives and the conduct of examinations
- setting up professional conduct proceedings with the power to remove from the register any midwife found guilty of misconduct.

A series of further Acts of Parliament in 1926, 1934, 1936 and 1950 amended this initial legislation and were consolidated in the Midwives Act 1951 and Midwives (Scotland) Act 1951. However, all midwifery statutory bodies in the UK were dominated by doctors who had long opposed the regulation of midwives, unlike other professional regulatory bodies that were mainly constructed of members of the occupation to be regulated. There was no requirement for even one midwife to be included on the Council of any CMB, which remained the case until the dissolution of the CMBs in 1983.

The Midwives Act was followed by the Nurses Registration Act in 1919, which established the General Nursing Council (GNC) for England and Wales, followed by the establishment of councils in Scotland and Ireland. The two professions were regulated separately until the Nurses, Midwives and Health Visitors Act 1979 established the framework of the United Kingdom Central Council for Nursing, Midwifery and Health Visiting (UKCC) in 1983. National Boards were established in England, Scotland, Northern Ireland and Wales to approve and monitor pre- and post-registration education and practice as well as be responsible for the supervision of midwives. This was the first time that midwives had been amalgamated in law with other professional groups as, up to this point, midwifery had remained independent of any nursing infrastructure. After much campaigning by the midwifery profession, in particular, the Royal College of Midwives (RCM) and the Association of Radical Midwives (ARM) who feared that the UKCC register and Council would be dominated by nurses and that midwives would lose control of their profession, a special clause was inserted into the Act and put into legislation the requirement for a statutory midwifery committee. The scope of the Midwifery Committee was for it to be consulted on all midwifery matters and to formulate the rules for the practice and supervision of midwives.

The main underlying principles of the Nurses, Midwives and Health Visitors Act of 1979 were the protection of the public and self-regulation by the three professions. This was achieved by the majority of members of the Council being elected by the three professions from the four countries of the UK. However, this created a dichotomy – between the public and professional interest – that has been central to the development of the regulation of the professions and has played a key part in recent reforms of midwifery regulation in the UK.

A decade later, an external review of the Nurses, Midwives and Health Visitors Act 1979 was commissioned by the DH, which resulted in a smaller, directly elected central council with smaller national boards. Regional Health Authorities (RHA) were assigned the responsibility of funding nursing and midwifery education, whilst the national boards retained responsibility for course validation and accreditation. This in essence established the *purchaser–provider model*, where hospitals were expected to contract with education providers for a requisite number of training places for nurses and midwives to fulfil their local workforce planning. These arrangements and the new streamlined structure of the UKCC and national boards were incorporated into the 1992 Nurses, Midwives and Health Visitors Act. Further consolidation of the 1979 and 1992 Acts incorporating all the reforms, resulted in the 1997 Nurses, Midwives and Health Visitors Act.

Further reform of the health professions was included in the Health Act 1999 that repealed the Nurses, Midwives and Health Visitors Act 1997 following a review of the function of the UKCC undertaken by JM Consulting in 1998, who had concluded that more effective regulation required the balancing of the interests of the professions with those of employers, service-users, educators and others. In tandem with the emergence of patient and women-centred care in the 1990s, professional self-regulation gave way to professional regulation in the public interest.

It was against this background that primary legislation was replaced with a Statutory Instrument by Order, which meant a departure from the normal practice of parliamentary procedure experienced during the previous century, involving professional scrutiny through all the earlier stages, including the publication of Green and White Papers. Section 62 (9) of the Health Act 1999 set out the Order for the establishment of the Nursing and Midwifery Council (NMC), which commenced operating in 2002. The Order encompassed the main recommendations made by JM Consulting (1998) and strengthened the accountability of the professions to the public in general and in particular, around fitness to practise.

The NMC took over the quality assurance functions of the UKCC and the four national boards, although some of the functions of the national boards in Scotland, Northern Ireland and Wales are provided by NHS Education for Scotland (NES), the Northern Ireland Practice and Education Council for Nursing and Midwifery (NIPEC) and Healthcare Inspectorate Wales. This development reunited standards for education with standards for practice and supervision of midwives on a UK basis. However, the creation of this UK-wide regulatory body, the NMC, was contrary to the trend of Parliamentary devolution that had occurred in the late 1990s.

Midwifery Regulatory Reform

Public trust in the health professions' abilities and willingness to call those they regulated to account had failed in the late 1990s. In particular, two inquiries into failings within the NHS, the Bristol Royal Infirmary Inquiry (Kennedy 2001); and the Shipman Inquiry (Smith 2004) revealed a club culture among doctors, in which they placed their own professional loyalties and relationships before the safety of patients. The recommendations from the two inquiries concerned the regulation of healthcare professionals, including their education and training, assessment of competence, registration, continuing professional development (CPD) and revalidation. The government commissioned a further two reports (Donaldson 2006; DH 2006), which led to the publication of the white paper: 'Trust, assurance and safety: the regulation of health professionals in the 21st century' (DH 2007). This led to the introduction of the Health and Social Care Act 2012, resulting in significant reforms to the governance arrangements of all health profession regulators, moving from elected professional dominated boards to appointed boards consisting of equal representation of professionals and lay people. These reforms also improved the fitness to practise procedures and sanctions as well as advocated that all health professions adopt a form of periodic revalidation.

The Mid Staffordshire NHS Foundation Trust Public Inquiry (Francis 2013) and the University Hospitals of Morecambe Bay NHS Foundation Trust Investigation (Kirkup 2015) identified that the actions, motivation, responsibility and accountability of individual health professionals are important in upholding the standards of the profession and contributing to patient safety culture. Walshe (2003, 2009) however, claim that advocates of patient safety science see all, or most errors as being products of the system or organization of care. Such a sentiment was also supported in the Berwick report (National Advisory Group on the Safety of Patients in England 2013) who affirmed that a safer NHS depends far more on major cultural change than a new regulatory regime of rules, standards and control strategies.

The Parliamentary and Health Service Ombudsman (PHSO) in England, investigating the failures in maternity and neonatal care that occurred from January 2004 to June 2013 at Furness General Hospital (that later became the University Hospitals of Morecambe Bay NHS Foundation Trust), expressed concerns of the additional tier of regulation, which applied to midwives, namely the *statutory supervision of midwives* (PHSO 2013). The structural flaw permitting the local investigation of midwives by midwives, was viewed as leading to potential muddling of the supervisory and regulatory roles of midwives and the possibility of a perceived conflict of interest. As a result, the report recommended two principles for the future model of midwifery regulation that:

• midwifery supervision and regulation should be separated
• the NMC should be in direct control of regulatory activity (PHSO 2013).

Further consideration of the report by the PSA (2014) concluded that:

• there was a lack of evidence to suggest that the risks posed by contemporary midwifery practice required an additional tier of regulation
• the imposition of regulatory sanctions or prohibitions by one midwife on another without lay scrutiny is not in line with good regulatory practice.

As a consequence, the NMC commissioned an independent review of midwifery regulation by the King's Fund with the aim of recommending a future model that would be fit for public protection, be fair and proportionate and would give the NMC sufficient regulatory control to be accountable for its outcomes. The recommendation from the King's Fund was to remove the additional layer of regulation for midwives, that the NMC should restrict its role to the core functions of regulation and that the governments of the four UK countries, should consider other ways to ensure that the functions of supervision and professional development are provided by other organizations in the health system (Baird et al. 2015). A decision was subsequently made by the NMC to seek a change in its legislation to remove the additional tier of regulation, which included the supervision of midwives as a statutory function. Following consultation and debates in Parliament (House of Lords Hansard 2017), the Nursing and Midwifery (Amendment) Order 2017 was passed. However, these changes would be more far-reaching than just the removal of the supervision of midwives from statute as Gillman and Lloyd (2015) outlined. The changes included the removal of the *Midwifery* section of the Nursing and Midwifery Order 2001 (Section 60), which provided the legislation for:

- the Midwifery Committee
- rules defining midwifery practice
- local supervision of midwives.

In addition, Part V of the 2001 Order relating to certain fitness to practise functions of the NMC relating to both midwives and nurses, was also amended.

The NMC stated that the changes would **not** affect:

- the separate registration of midwives
- direct entry to the register as a midwife
- the protected title of a midwife
- the protected function of midwives attending a woman in childbirth or
- separate competencies and pre-registration education standards for midwives (NMC 2017a).

The statutory supervision of midwives consequently has been replaced by an *employer led model of clinical supervision* based on the principles set out by the DH (2016) and are explored in more detail later in the chapter.

Statutory Instruments

The Nursing and Midwifery Order 2001: SI 2002 No. 253 (*The Order*)

The Nursing and Midwifery Order 2001 (*The Order*) is the main legislation that established the NMC and was made under Section 60 of the Health Act 1999. The Order, which sets out what the Council is required to do (*shall*) and provides permissive powers for things that it can choose to do (*may*), is therefore classed as *secondary legislation*. A series of orders made by the Privy Council and Rules made by the Council sit *underneath* The Order. The numbered paragraphs within The Order are referred to as Articles.

There are 10 parts to The Order that outlined the establishment of the Nursing and Midwifery Council, its role and function, which include:

- Part III: Registration that resulted in three parts of the Register:
  - Nurses
  - Midwives
  - Specialist Community Public Health Nurses: namely health visitors, school nurses, occupational health nurses, health promotion nurses and sexual health nurses.
- Part IV: Education and Training
- Part V: *Fitness to Practise*
- Part VI: Appeals

- Part VII: EEA *provisions*
- Part VIII: Midwifery specific Articles that established the following:
  - Article 41: The Midwifery Committee
  - Article 42: Rules specific to midwifery practice
  - Article 43: Regulation of the LSA and supervisors of midwives
- Part IX: *Offences* that include
  - Article 45: Attendance by unqualified persons at childbirth.

To change how the NMC operates in the main, requires legislative changes and since its existence, The Order has been subject to a number of amendments, which are detailed in Box 2.2: the most significant to the midwifery profession being The Nursing and Midwifery (Amendment) Order 2017: SI 2017 No. 321. This SI **removed** provisions relating to the Midwifery Committee, the local supervision of midwifery and the Midwives Rules (NMC 2012).

THE NURSING AND MIDWIFERY COUNCIL

Being the UK-wide regulator for nurses and midwives and for nursing associates in England, the role of the Nursing and Midwifery Council (NMC) is to ensure these professionals have the knowledge and skills to deliver consistent, quality care that keeps people safe. It is accountable to the Privy Council, the Department of Health and the Professional Standards Authority. The NMC is governed by a Council whose role is to ensure that the NMC complies with all relevant legislation governing nursing and midwifery practice, the main legislation being the Nursing and Midwifery Order 2001 (The Order) and adheres to the Charities Act 2011 ultimately holding the Chief Executive and Registrar to account.

Being registered with the Charity Commission in England and Wales and the Office of the Scottish Charity Regulator, the NMC should use all funds received from its registrants purely for the benefit of the public, i.e. in the regulation of nursing and midwifery, ensuring that better and safer care is always at the heart of its function. The Council is committed to openness and transparency and holds meetings in public at least six times a year to which anyone is welcome to attend.

Membership

Standing Orders made by the Council under Article 12 Schedule 1 of The Order establish the fundamental

BOX 2.2 Notable Amendments to the Nursing and Midwifery Order

SI 2001 No. 253 and Subsequent Rules

Statutory Instrument (SI)	Title
SI 2008 No. 1485	**The Nursing and Midwifery (Amendment) Order 2008** *This Statutory Order related to improving the governance arrangements of the NMC in order to maintain and improve public confidence.* *This included changes to the membership of the NMC from being mostly an elected committee to becoming fully appointed. This also applied to the composition of the Midwifery Committee.*
SI 2014 No. 3272	**The Nursing and Midwifery (Amendment) Order 2014** *This Statutory Order introduced powers to the NMC to enable it to carry out its fitness to practise and registration functions more effectively and efficiently by improving consistency in decision-making and reducing the time it takes to deal with cases. The amendment clarified the law regarding the sanctions that could be imposed by a Practice Committee, as well as introduced amendments to the composition of a Registration Appeal Panel.*
SI 2015 No. 52	**The Nursing and Midwifery Council (Fitness to Practise) (Education, Registration and Registration Appeals) (Amendment) Rules Order of Council 2015** *This Statutory Instrument relates to amending the Fitness to Practise Rules and the Registration Rules as a result of the Nursing and Midwifery (Amendment) Order 2014 (see above). These rules were to improve the NMC's fitness to practise procedure and enhance public protection.* *Rules relating to indemnity arrangements as defined in the Indemnity Order (SI 2014 No. 1887) were also incorporated in this amendment. These rules enable the NMC Registrar to request information for the purposes of determining the eligibility of an individual's registration, application for admission or renewal of registration, that they have or will have appropriate cover under an indemnity arrangement.*
SI 2015 No. 1923	**The Nursing and Midwifery Council (Fitness to Practise) (Education, Registration and Registration Appeals) (Amendment No. 2) Rules Order of Council 2015** *This Statutory Instrument relates to further amending the Fitness to Practise Rules and the Registration Rules as a result of the Knowledge of English Order 2015 (SI 2015 No. 806). The rules set out the details pertaining to registrants demonstrating competence in the English Language for safe practice as a midwife or nurse.*
SI 2017 No. 321	**The Nursing and Midwifery (Amendment) Order 2017** *This Statutory Instrument removed provisions relating to the Midwifery Committee, local supervision of midwifery and the Midwives Rules (NMC 2012).* *Part V of The Order was amended in respect of further updating fitness to practise processes for nurses and midwives to ensure they are efficient and proportionate. This included replacing the Conduct and Competence Committee and the Health Committee with a single Fitness to Practise Committee.*
SI 2017 No. 703	**The Nursing and Midwifery Order (Legal Assessors) (Amendment) and the Nursing and Midwifery Council (Fitness to Practise) (Amendment) Rules Order of Council 2017** *This Statutory Instrument related to amending the NMC Fitness to Practise Rules as a result of the Nursing and Midwifery (Amendment) Order 2017 (see above).*
SI 2018 No. 838	**The Nursing and Midwifery (Amendment) Order 2018** *The Order was amended to include provisions relating to the regulation of nursing associates (England only) and to make consequential amendments in that regard to other secondary legislation.*

procedures by which the Council and its committees conduct their business. This involves appointing the Chair of the Council and its members. The NMC Council comprises of 12 members who are appointed by the Appointments Board of the Privy Council: six of whom are lay people and six are registrants. The Council must include at least one member from each of the four UK countries who lives or works wholly or mainly in that country. Each registrant member is from either a nursing or midwifery background with the lay members selected for their expertise in various areas and strategic experience. These members also sit on various Committees within the framework of the NMC.

Committees

Changes to the number of Statutory Committees occurred following the introduction of the Nursing and Midwifery (Amendment) Order 2017 on 31 March 2017. The significant amendments contained within the Statutory Instrument (SI) removed the Midwifery section from The Order, resulting in the abolition of the Midwifery Committee. In addition, the amendments in Part V of The Order that led to the replacement of the Conduct and Competence Committee and the Health Committee with Practice Committees. There are a number of Discretionary Committees that the Council may establish as it considers appropriate in connection with the discharge of its functions and delegate any of its functions to them other than the power to make rules. The Discretionary Committees include the Audit Committee, the Remuneration Committee, the Appointments Board, the Council Budget Scrutiny Group and the Investment Committee.

Statutory committees

The Practice Committees. The functions of the practice committees are stipulated in The Order and are not subject to delegation. They comprise of the Investigating Committee and the Fitness to Practise Committee, of which Fitness to Practise Panels are convened. The Practice Committees consider cases where a nurse, midwife or nursing associate's fitness to practise is alleged to be impaired. To reflect the NMC's accountability, fitness to practise hearings are usually held in public, however, the Investigating Committee meet in private to consider all the supporting evidence in a case. Both committees are made up of nurses, midwives and lay people who are from outside these professions.

Discretionary Committees (established by the Council under Article 3 (12) of The Order 2001)

The Audit Committee. The remit of this committee is to support the Council and management by reviewing the comprehensiveness and reliability of assurances on governance through internal and external auditing (including the National Audit Office), risk management, the control environment and the integrity of financial statements and the annual report.

The Remuneration Committee. The responsibility of this Committee is to ensure that there are appropriate systems in place for remuneration, rewards and succession planning at the NMC. This includes approving and overseeing the process for the recruitment and selection of the Chief Executive and Registrar, Chair and Council members, including appraisal.

The Appointments Board. This Board was established to assist the Council in connection with any function or process relating to the appointment of Panel Members and Legal Assessors. The Appointments Board should consist of up to five Partner Members, one of whom will be the Chair of the Board, selected and appointed in accordance with the Standing Orders. Part of the Board's remit is approving the code of conduct for Panel Members.

The Council Budget Scrutiny Group. This is a short-term group established from time to time by the Council, that operates during the budget setting process. The Group is appointed by the Chair of Council and additionally comprise at least the Chairs or members of the Audit and Remuneration Committees. Its remit is to provide scrutiny in relation to budget development and advice to the Chief Executive. In addition, the Budget Scrutiny Group provides assurance to the Council that appropriate analysis and consideration has been undertaken in the construction of the financial plans and budgets and makes any recommendations in the context of the NMC financial strategy.

The Investment Committee. The Council is responsible for determining the investment strategy, risk appetite and target returns on the advice of the Committee. The remit of this committee is to oversee implementation of the Council's investment strategy, determine the allocation and movement of funds and monitor the Council's investment portfolio. The Chair of the Council determines the membership of the Committee and its Chair from among the Council members. Membership will comprise at least three Council members and include at least one lay and one registrant member.

Suitably qualified independent members with extensive investment expertise may be co-opted or appointed to the Committee with the consent of the Chair of Council. Decision-making and implementation of the investment strategy is delegated to the Investment Committee.

Functions of the NMC

The powers of the NMC are specified within The Order and its subsequent amendments and, as was the case with the CMB and UKCC, its primary function is to establish and improve standards of midwifery and nursing care in order to keep the public safe by:

1. Establishing and maintaining a Register of all qualified nurses, midwives, specialist community public health nurses in the UK and nursing associates in England
2. Setting standards for the education and practice of all nurses, midwives, specialist community public health nurses and nursing associates to ensure they have the right skills and qualities at the point of registration which continue to develop throughout their professional careers
3. Regulating fitness to practise, conduct and performance through rules and codes.

Where a registrant does not meet the standards for skills, education and behaviour, the NMC has the power to remove them from the Register permanently or for a set period of time. It also has a statutory function to inform and educate registrants and to inform the public about its work. The three functions are examined in more detail in the following sections.

1. Establishing and maintaining the Register

The Privy Council determines the division of parts of the professional register and as a result of The Nursing and Midwifery (Amendment) Order 2018 (SI 2018 No. 838), there are currently four parts to the Register:

1. Nurses
2. Midwives
3. Specialist Community Public Health Nurses
4. Nursing Associates

The Council determines the initial registration fee, coordinates the registration process, including determining the status of the applicant's good health and good character and they have indemnity arrangements in place. In addition, the NMC's function is to coordinate the triennial renewal to the Register and the collection of the annual registration retention fee.

Under the Nursing and Midwifery Council (Fitness to Practise) (Education, Registration and Registration Appeals) (Amendment No. 2) Rules Order of Council 2015 (SI 2015 No. 1925), any midwife or nurse from outside the UK seeking registration with the NMC are subject to assessment of their competence in the English language and comparable qualifications and level of clinical proficiency.

2. Setting standards for education and practice (midwifery)

As part of its statutory function, the NMC is required to establish the pre-registration standards of education and training, including the requirements for good health and good character, leading to the award of midwifery qualifications. The standards also comply with the minimum EU law pertaining to standards for the training of midwives Directive 2005/36/EC of the European Parliament on the recognition of professional qualifications (amended by Directive 2013/55/EU) (see Chapter 1).

The NMC has developed a radical education and training strategy: Realizing Professionalism: standards for education and training, based on *The Code* (NMC 2018a), that affects pre-registration education and training provision across the UK. This strategy is expected to be fully implemented across all Approved Education Institutions (AEIs) and practice learning partners by 2021 through a staged approach. It consists of three parts, which should all be read in conjunction with each other:

- Part 1 – *Standards framework for nursing and midwifery education* (NMC 2018b): the NMC need to be assured that the AEI and practice partners can fulfil the institutional requirements to support the theoretical and practice components of the education programme.
- Part 2 – *Standards for student supervision and assessment* (NMC 2018c): define the changes to the role that clinicians (practice supervisors and practice assessors) and academics (academic assessors) play in supporting the learning and assessment of students in practice.
- Part 3 – *Programme standards*: one for each programme that the AEI provides: for midwifery this consists of the *Standards for pre-registration midwifery programmes* (NMC 2019c) and the *Standards of proficiency for midwives* (NMC 2019d).

The standards are all outcome-focused and compliance with all three sets of standards is required for an education institution to be approved and offer NMC approved programmes. This is part of the NMC quality assurance mechanism.

The NMC sets the proficiencies for students to achieve the standards, which are divided into six domains:

Domain 1: Being an accountable, autonomous, professional midwife

Domain 2: Safe and effective midwifery care: promoting and providing continuity of care and carer

Domain 3: Universal care for all women and newborn infants

Domain 4: Additional care for women and newborn infants with complications

Domain 5: Promoting excellence: the midwife as colleague, scholar and leader

Domain 6: The midwife as skilled practitioner (NMC 2019d).

These standards meet and exceed the ICM (2019) *Essential Competencies for Midwifery Practice*, incorporate Directive 2005/36/EC (amended 2013/55/EU) and the UNICEF Baby Friendly Initiative (BFI) Standards (UNICEF-UK 2019). The length of the programme is set at a minimum of 4600 h, or 3000 h for registered (adult) nurses (shortened programme), with an EQUAL balance of 50% theory and 50% practice, however there is no specified time limit to complete a midwifery programme and as a result, this is determined locally at AEI level. The minimum academic level is degree. Upon successful completion of the midwifery programme, the lead midwife for education at the AEI is responsible to sign the declaration of health and character of each student midwife. To stay on the register, midwives must keep their knowledge and skills up-to-date and demonstrate this through undertaking a process of revalidation very 3 years (NMC 2019a).

The Lead Midwife for Education. The NMC requires each AEI to appoint a lead midwife for education (LME), who is suitably qualified and experienced to lead and advise on all matters relating to midwifery education. This may include contributing to the development, delivery, quality assurance and evaluation of their programmes and providing midwifery input at strategic and operational levels within their AEI. Furthermore, to strengthen and support sustainable midwifery leadership in education, the RCM (2019) endorses the seniority and authority of the lead midwife for education, is

essential to be able to exercise strategic influence over all AEI business that impacts on the delivery of midwifery education.

The lead midwife for education and their designated midwife substitute must be a midwife who has active registration with the NMC. The AEI should inform the NMC Council of the name of the LME. A national network of LMEs that meets with the NMC twice per year ensures the standards and quality of midwifery education programmes across the UK remains high. The requirements of the LME are set out in Rule 6 (i)(a)(ii) and Rule 6 (3) of the Nursing and Midwifery Council (Education, Registration and Registration Appeals) Rules 2004 (SI 2004 No. 1767) that mandate the LME as being:

- responsible for midwifery education in the AEI
- accountable for signing declarations of health and character for applicants applying for admission to the register on or within six months of completing a pre-registration midwifery programme or for applicants applying for readmission to the register following a return to practise programme
- accountable for signing declarations of health and character for applicants who have successfully completed an adaptation programme in the UK.

It is imperative that the NMC Registrar is totally assured that an applicant is capable of safe and effective practice as a midwife for them to be admitted to the professional Register. If the LME cannot be assured of a student's health and character, they must NOT sign the supporting declaration. As a consequence the student CANNOT be recommended for admission to the midwives' part of the register.

3. Regulating fitness to practise, conduct and performance

This function is supported by the NMC rules, standards and guidance that are set out by the Practise Committees. The NMC has developed a number of key principles for fitness to practise that accord with NMC legislation and case law and which are consistent with the fitness to practise process that delivers the desired regulatory outcomes. These principles are summarized in Box 2.3 and are designed to inform those involved in the process, whether they are registrants, service-users, members of the public, employers or decision-makers.

There are two types of allegation where the NMC have statutory powers to undertake investigations: **fraudulent or incorrect entry** to the professional register or **allegations about the fitness to practise** of nurses

BOX 2.3 **The NMC Principles of Fitness to Practise**

These 12 principles are used to ensure consistency and transparency when making decisions about the fitness to practise of a nurse or midwife:

1. A person-centred approach to fitness to practise.
2. Fitness to practise is about managing the risk that a nurse or midwife poses to patients or members of the public in the future. It isn't about punishing people for past events.
3. We can best protect patients and members of the public by making final fitness to practise decisions swiftly and publishing the results openly.
4. Employers should act first to deal with concerns about a nurse or a midwife's practice, unless the risk to patients or the public is so serious that we need to take immediate action.
5. We always take regulatory action when there is risk to patient safety that is not being effectively managed by an employer.
6. We take account of the context in which the nurse or midwife was practising when deciding whether there is a risk to patient safety that requires us to take regulatory action.
7. We may not need to take regulatory action for a clinical mistake, even where there has been a serious harm to a patient or service-user, if there is no longer a risk to patient safety and the nurse or midwife has been open about what went wrong and can demonstrate that they have learned from it.
8. Deliberately covering up when things go wrong seriously undermines patient safety and damages public trust in the professions. Restrictive regulatory action is likely to be required in such cases.
9. In cases about clinical practice, taking action solely to maintain public confidence or uphold standards is only likely to be needed if the regulatory concern can't be remedied.
10. In cases that aren't about clinical practice, taking action to maintain public confidence or uphold standards is only likely to be needed if the concerns raise fundamental questions about the trustworthiness of a nurse or midwife as a professional.
11. Some regulatory concerns, particularly if they raise fundamental concerns about the nurse or midwife's professionalism, can't be remedied and require restrictive regulatory action.
12. Hearings best protect patients and members of the public by resolving central aspects of a case that we and the nurse or midwife don't agree on.

or midwives. Such allegations of fitness to practise can be based on:

- misconduct
- lack of competence
- criminal convictions and cautions
- health
- not having the necessary knowledge of English
- determinations by other health or social care organizations
- a finding by any other health or social care regulator or licensing body that fitness to practise is impaired.

Case Examiners and the Investigating Committee

When a referral about a registrant's fitness to practise has been made to the NMC, the details are initially screened to assess if there is any immediate risk to the safety of the public by nature of the allegation that determines there is a definite case to answer. Otherwise, a pair of case examiners will be assigned to the case to review and arrive at a joint decision as to whether there is a case to answer. One case examiner in the pairing is always a registered nurse or midwife and the other is a lay person who is neither registered as a nurse nor a midwife. The case examiners can decide that there is:

- no case to answer and close the case with no further action
- no case to answer and close the case with advice given to the nurse or midwife to remind them of their responsibilities
- a case to answer and issue a warning, which will be published for a period of 12 months
- a case to answer and recommend undertakings, which will comprise of restrictive and rehabilitative measures, setting out a clear plan back to safe and effective practice; these undertakings will be published for as long as they are in place
- a case to answer and refer the matter to the fitness to practise committee.

If the two case examiners are unable to reach a decision, the case would be referred to the panel of the *Investigating Committee*. Case examiners do not consider allegations of fraudulent or incorrect entries to the register as these are considered directly by the Investigating Committee. Any interested parties may request that the decisions made by the case examiners are reviewed by the Registrar.

Should the case examiners believe there to be a risk to the public, they may request that the case is considered for an *interim order application hearing*, which are usually made at the beginning of the case process, however, they can be made at any time should new information become available. Such an order temporarily suspends or restricts the registrant while their case is being investigated. Interim order cases may include cases of lack of competence, poor clinical practice, serious convictions or imprisonment and serious mental illness. Panels of any of the Practice Committees can decide to hold an interim orders hearing to which the nurse, midwife or nursing associate is invited to attend. *The Panel* can then impose the following:

- An interim suspension order: registration is suspended preventing the registrant from working during the investigation of the case
- An interim conditions of practice order: the panel imposes conditions on the registrant who can continue working in practice subject to defined conditions.

The Panel can only impose an interim order if it finds it is necessary to protect the public; it is in the public interest or in the registrant's interest. The investigation continues while the interim order is in effect. Interim orders can be imposed for up to 18 months, but must be reviewed after 6 months or earlier, should any new information become available. At an interim review hearing, the panel can continue, replace, vary the order or revoke it.

Fitness to Practise Committee

Panel meetings are held in public reflecting the NMC's public accountability and transparency. However, parts of the hearing may be held in private to protect the anonymity of the individual or if confidential medical evidence may need to be shared in cases where the registrant's fitness to practise may be impaired by reason of health issues. When deciding on whether a registrant's fitness to practise is impaired. Panels consider the standards expected of a registrant ordinarily working at that level of practise, not for the highest possible level of practice. Even if there has been a breach of a standard set out in *The Code* (NMC 2018a), it does not automatically follow that a registrant's fitness to practise is impaired. That is a judgement for the Panel to make, having considered any evidence regarding what has happened since the breach or failures occurred.

A range of sanctions is available and the Panel uses the Council's *sanctions* guidance to determine the one that is most appropriate for the particular case. The Panel must first consider whether, taking account of all the

circumstances of the case, it is appropriate to take no further action. If the Panel decides this option is not appropriate, the following sanctions are available (considering them in order from a 'caution order' to a 'striking off order'):

- to issue a *caution* for a specified period of between 1 and 5 years
- to impose *conditions of practice* for a specified period of up to 3 years
- to *suspend* the registrant's registration for up to 1 year
- to strike off the registrant from the Register.

A striking off order cannot be imposed if the registrant's fitness to practise is impaired, due to: their health, lack of competence or not having the necessary knowledge of English, until they have been on either a suspension order or subject to a conditions of practise order for a continuous period of 2 years.

Appeals

A registrant can appeal against a final substantive order hearing to the court: The High Court in England and Wales, the High Court Justice in Northern Ireland and the Court of Session in Scotland. In the case of an order to amend the register where an entry has been incorrectly made or fraudulently procured, the appeal is made to the County Court. The appeal has to be made within 28 days commencing from the day after the date on the letter informing the registrant of the outcome of the hearing, unless the court decides there are exceptional circumstances to extend the time period.

Consensual panel determination

Consensual panel determination enables a case to be resolved by agreement or consent. This arrangement reduces the length of hearings and the need for witnesses to attend hearings, enabling the NMC to concentrate their resources on cases where there are significant matters in dispute. Should a registrant indicate that they wish to resolve their case by consent, they must accept the facts of the allegation and that their fitness to practise is impaired. The NMC would then agree what the level of sanction is with the registrant, a statement of case is drawn up and signed by the NMC and registrant. The Fitness to Practise Panel would then consider the case and make the final decision about the outcome.

Voluntary removal from the Register

A registrant who is subject to fitness to practise proceedings and who does not intend to continue practising, can apply to be removed from the register by way of *voluntary removal*. This would then conclude the proceedings without the need for a full public hearing. Voluntary removal supports the NMC's aim to reach the outcome that best protects the public at the earliest opportunity. It is only appropriate in circumstances when it is not in the public interest to hold such a hearing, and the public and patients will be best protected by the registrant's immediate removal from the register.

Voluntary removal from the Register is only allowed if:

- the registrant accepts the details of the regulatory concern
- the registrant provides evidence that they do not intend to continue practising.

All voluntary removal applications are considered by the Registrar/Assistant Registrar. If the application is successful, the registrant is asked to sign a voluntary removal declaration form confirming their intention not to apply for readmission to the Register sooner than 5 years from the date of the removal decision. The register is adjusted with 'voluntarily removed' displayed against the registrant's name. If the voluntary removal decision is made before a final hearing, the NMC do not publish any other details about the case. Details of the regulatory concerns however, may be shared indefinitely with potential employers and other enquirers on request, with the only exception to this being relating solely to a registrant's health.

Restoration to the Register following a striking off order

A registrant's name is removed from the NMC Register for 5 years, during which time they are not allowed to work as a nurse, midwife or nursing associate in the UK. The application process to be restored to the Register can be made 5 years after the striking off order was made, as this is not done automatically. Only one application is considered in any 12-month period. A panel of the Fitness to Practise Committee will consider the application for restoration in light of the applicant satisfying the *fit and proper person test* and the other requirements for restoration. A restoration hearing however, is not an opportunity for the applicant to appeal the original striking-off order, reassess the finding of fact or the decision of the panel at the initial hearing. The powers of the Committee can:

- grant the application for restoration

- grant the application subject to the applicant completing a return to practise course
- grant the application and impose a conditions of practise order
- grant the application subject to the applicant completing a return to practise course **and** impose a condition of practise order
- refuse the application.

Promoting Professionalism

In the UK, the four Chief Nursing Officers launched a framework (Fig. 2.2) around enabling professionalism in midwifery and nursing that is supported by the NMC (2017b). Professionalism is determined by the autonomous evidenced-based decision-making by members of an occupation who share the same values and sphere of practise and is vital to delivering safe and high quality care to childbearing women, their babies and families. The framework embraces *The Code* (NMC 2018a) through the attributes or prerequisites of midwifery and nursing practice:

- **Accountable** (practise effectively)
- **A leader** (promoting professionalism and trust)
- **An advocate** (prioritizing people)
- **Competent** (preserving safety).

It is acknowledged that organizational and environmental factors are crucial in supporting and enabling professional practise and behaviours. NMC (2017b) define an environment that promotes professionalism as one that:

- recognizes and encourages midwifery leadership
- encourages autonomous innovative practice
- enables positive inter-professional collaboration
- enables practice learning and development
- provides appropriate resources.

It is becoming increasingly challenging for midwives where maternity services are under-resourced and societal health and social care needs are becoming more complex and demanding. Employers need to provide the systems and conditions for midwives to continually develop and practise safe care. The framework of enabling professionalism (NMC 2017b) explores how various strategies can support and promote professional practice and behaviour within the workplace, as well as identifying the ways in which the individual midwife should uphold their professional practise, such as raising concerns when issues arise that could compromise safety, quality and experience.

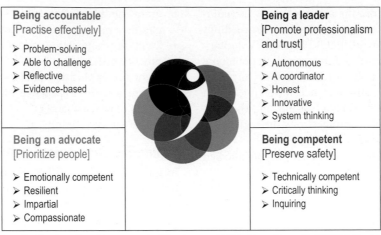

Being accountable
[Practise effectively]

> Problem-solving
> Able to challenge
> Reflective
> Evidence-based

Being a leader
[Promote professionalism and trust]

> Autonomous
> A coordinator
> Honest
> Innovative
> System thinking

Being an advocate
[Prioritize people]

> Emotionally competent
> Resilient
> Impartial
> Compassionate

Being competent
[Preserve safety]

> Technically competent
> Critically thinking
> Inquiring

Fig. 2.2 Enabling Professionalism Framework. (Nursing and Midwifery Council. (2017b) Enabling professionalism in nursing and midwifery practice. London: NMC. Available at: www.nmc.org.uk/globalassets/sitedocuments/other-publications/enabling-professionalism.pdf.)

Responsibility and Accountability

Although midwives practise in a wide range of settings, they are all unified by underlying values and *responsibilities*. Each midwife has a *personal responsibility* for their own practise by being aware of their personal strengths and limitations and is therefore required to continually develop their knowledge and skills to maintain proficiency. Self-regulation and professional freedom are based on the assumption that each professional can be trusted to work without supervision and, where necessary, take action against colleagues should their practise not be up to the appropriate standards. Furthermore, midwives share a *collective responsibility* in how women and their families are treated and cared for. This means that each midwife should highlight instances where individual practices or where the systems or processes within organizations providing maternity services, are compromising safe and appropriate care to women and their babies.

Accountability is more than having responsibility, although the concepts are used interchangeably, and means that midwives are answerable for their actions and omissions, regardless of advice or directions by another professional. To be accountable, a midwife is required to have the ability, responsibility and authority for their actions (Bergman 1981).

Each registrant is:

- professionally accountable for their actions and omissions to the NMC
- legally accountable to the law and
- contractually accountable to their employer.

They must always act in the best interests of the individuals to whom they are providing care. In the case of midwives, this would be the childbearing woman, her baby and family. There may be occasions when midwives have difficulty appreciating their own accountability, especially when carrying out the instructions of medical staff, but it is clear from *The Code* (NMC 2018a) that registrants' accountability cannot be delegated to, or borne by, others.

LEGAL ISSUES AND THE MIDWIFE

Contemporary midwifery practice is characterized by increasing complexities in respect of the health needs of childbearing women, their babies and families as well as increasing uncertainties about what is right and wrong. Midwives can find themselves faced with dilemmas and have to make decisions where there may not be evidence of any robust clinical evidence. It is therefore important each midwife is fully aware of the legislation and legal framework in which they should practise as accountable practitioners within the context of normal midwifery, for which they have been duly trained and have the appropriate expertise.

Legislation

The Nursing and Midwifery Order 2001 (SI 2002 No. 253) is the statutory legislation that currently governs the midwifery profession and endorsed the formation of the regulatory body, the NMC.

BOX 2.4 Equality Duty: Protected Characteristics

In terms of providing healthcare services, service providers cannot discriminate against individuals or groups and must consider the three facets of Equality Duty in relation to:
- age
- disability
- gender reassignment
- marriage or civil partnership
- pregnancy and maternity
- race
- religion, faith or belief
- sex
- sexual orientation.

Adapted from The Equality Act 2010, Section 149.

Primary legislation is enshrined in Acts of Parliament, which have been debated in the House of Commons and House of Lords before receiving Royal Assent. Such legislation is expected to last at least a couple of decades before being revised. With the pressure on Parliamentary time, Acts of Parliament are frequently designed as *enabling legislation* in that they provide a framework from which statutory rules may be derived: known as *secondary* or *subordinate legislation*. All secondary legislation is published in Statutory Instruments (SI), such as *The Order*.

Statutory rules/secondary legislation can in theory be implemented or amended much more quickly, as it is the Privy Council who lays the rules before the House of Commons for formal and generally automatic approval, rather than is the case for primary legislation that requires endorsement by the Secretary of State. However, this may still take several weeks or months to occur.

The Equality Act 2010 and the Human Rights Act 1998

The Equality Act 2010 consolidated UK law in relation to forms of discrimination such as race, disability and gender, by simplifying and strengthening the existing anti-discrimination legislation and provides clear guidance about individual rights and responsibilities through the identification of nine protected characteristics, as shown in Box 2.4. Discrimination, harassment and victimization in relation to any of these characteristics within employment, education and the provision of public services are unlawful. As a consequence, all public sector organizations are required to embed *due regard* within their decision-making processes in order to eliminate unlawful discrimination, victimization and harassment, promote equality of opportunity and facilitate good relations between groups of individuals. The Equality and Human Rights Commission (2016) affirm that the way in which employers act, design and deliver services, and how they develop policy to ensure the aims of *equality duty* are met, is essential to upholding the conventions of the Equality Act 2010.

There is provision within the Equality Act 2010, to assist individuals who share a protected characteristic and experience disadvantages, or suffer as a result of past or present discrimination. Section 158 of the Act enables service providers to take *positive action* to improve equality outcomes: this may include the favourable treatment of members of a group who share a protected characteristic. However, to be lawful, the action taken must always meet the conditions of the Act and the test of proportionality. This means that the disadvantages of a particular group are recognized and appropriate action is taken to enable or encourage persons who share the protected characteristic to overcome or minimize that disadvantage (Equality Act 2010: Section 158.1; Law Society 2012).

The European Convention for the Protection of Human Rights and Fundamental Freedoms (1951) set out to protect basic human rights and the UK was the first signatory to the Convention. The Convention is enforced through the European Court of Human Rights in Strasbourg. The **Human Rights Act** was passed in 1998 and came into force on 2 October 2000, since then most of the articles of the convention have been directly enforceable in the UK courts in relation to public authorities and organizations, such as the National Health Service (NHS). It is important that midwives are aware of, and encouraged to work within, the boundaries of this Act. Of particular significance to midwives and those working in health care are the following Articles of the Act:
- *Article 2: The right to life* (e.g. continuing treatment of the life of a severely disabled baby).
- *Article 3: The right not to be tortured or subjected to inhumane or degrading treatment* (e.g. chaining a pregnant prisoner to a bed during labour would contravene this Article).

- *Article 5: The right to liberty and security* (e.g. safe and competent care during childbirth).
- *Article 6: The right to a fair trial* (e.g. civil hearings and tribunals as well as criminal proceedings).
- *Article 8: The right to respect privacy and family life and to physical integrity* (e.g. supports a woman's right to give birth at home).
- *Article 12: The right to marry* (e.g. found a family, including fertility and assisted fertility).
- *Article 14: The right not to be discriminated against* (e.g. women with a disability, from a different ethnic/cultural background).

One benefit of this Act is that it has placed the public at the centre of health care. The individual's experience has become an important measure of quality and effectiveness in health care and as a consequence of this Act, the NHS complaints system has been reviewed. Midwives should be aware that when someone has a right to something, there is usually a corresponding duty on someone else to facilitate that right (Beauchamp and Childress 2019). It could be said that women have a *right to safe and competent care during childbirth*, fitting in with Article 5. It would therefore follow that as midwives are educated to provide midwifery care, they have an obligation that the care is both *safe and competent*. Similarly, the UK Government via the NMC has an obligation in regulating its practitioners to ensure they practise safely and competently through *The Order* and its subsequent amendments, rules and standards.

Legal Frameworks: Rules and Standards

Each midwife must meet the Standards of Proficiency for Midwives (NMC 2019d), which stipulate the knowledge, understanding and skills that all midwives must demonstrate to be eligible to enter the UK NMC professional register. These also comply with Article 42 of the European Union Directive on professional qualifications (2013/35/EU) and the ICM Global Standards for Midwifery Education (ICM 2013). The standards of proficiency (NMC 2019d) and *The Code* (NMC 2018a) are significant to midwives when considering their scope of practice, which may change depending on the nature of their roles and the learning they have acquired. *The Code* (NMC 2018a) specifies that midwives must not practise outside of their knowledge, skills or competence. It is therefore important that maternity service providers are aware of this professional duty when

they deploy midwives. Through the mandatory process of triennial professional revalidation (NMC 2019a), the midwife is able to demonstrate they are maintaining their knowledge, skills and competence alongside upholding the values and behaviours contained within *The Code* (NMC 2018a).

The Code: Professional standards of practice and behaviour for nurses, midwives and nursing associates

The Code (NMC 2018a) provides the registrant with the foundation of good nursing and midwifery practice and is a vital mechanism in safeguarding the health and wellbeing of the public, being central to the NMC's statutory duty to protect the public. It highlights the professional standards of practice and behaviour that each registrant must clearly demonstrate in order to meet public trust and is structured around four themes, identified in Box 2.5.

The values and principles set out in *The Code* apply to **all** registrants, regardless of their area of practice: be it in direct care provision, leadership, education or research. However, the values and principles are not negotiable or discretionary. *The Code* reaffirms the registrant's personal accountability for their actions and omissions and being able to justify their decisions. Furthermore, the registrant's actions should always be lawful, whether these relate to their professional or personal life. When joining the Register, each registrant commits to upholding these standards. Such commitment to professional standards is fundamental to being part of a profession. Those registrants who fail to uphold *The Code* may be subject to a fitness to practise allegation and in serious cases, this can include suspension from practice and/or removal from the professional Register.

The Professional Duty of Candour

All healthcare professionals have a 'duty of candour': that is a professional responsibility to be honest with those in their care when things go wrong. This is described as the *professional duty of candour*. Guidance was jointly developed by the GMC and NMC in 2015, following the Kirkup (2015) Inquiry into the failings at the University Hospitals of Morecambe Bay and the subsequent recommendations, which forms part of a joint statement from eight regulators of healthcare professionals in the

BOX 2.5 The Code (NMC 2018a)

Prioritize people	You put the interests of people using or needing nursing or midwifery services first. You make their care and safety your main concern and make sure that their dignity is preserved and their needs are recognized, assessed and responded to. You make sure that those receiving care are treated with respect, that their rights are upheld and that any discriminatory attitudes and behaviours towards those receiving care are challenged.
Practise effectively	You assess need and deliver or advise on treatment, or give help (including preventative or rehabilitative care) without too much delay, to the best of your abilities, on the basis of best available evidence. You communicate effectively keeping clear and accurate records and sharing skills, knowledge and experience where appropriate. You reflect and act on any feedback you receive to improve your practice.
Preserve safety	You make sure that patient and public safety is not affected. You work within the limits of your professional 'duty of candour' and raising concerns immediately whenever you come across situations that put patients or public safety at risk. You take the necessary action to deal with any concerns where appropriate.
Promote professionalism and trust	You uphold the reputation of your profession at all times. You should display a personal commitment to the standards of practice and behaviour set out in *The Code*. You should be a model of integrity and leadership for others to aspire to. This should lead to trust and confidence in the professions from patients, people receiving care, other health and care professionals and the public.

UK (GMC/NMC 2015). The guidance is divided into two parts:

- The duty to be open and honest with women and their families or those close to them if something goes wrong. This includes apologizing.
- The duty to be open and honest within their employing organization and to encourage a learning culture by reporting adverse incidents that lead to harm, as well as near misses.

This may include the midwife taking part in reviews and investigations when requested as well as being open and honest with the NMC, raising concerns where appropriate and not stopping others from raising concerns.

Raising and escalating concerns

Midwives also have a professional responsibility to put women, babies and families in their care first and to act to protect them if it is considered they may be at risk. It is important that midwives know how to raise concerns appropriately using the broad principles in the NMC (2019e) guidance along with *The Code* (NMC 2018a); specifically paragraphs 16 and 17. In addition, local

whistleblowing policies issued by the employer and clinical governance and risk management procedures will assist the midwife to report incidents early or any near misses. It is also important that midwives have a good working knowledge of their local authority's safeguarding practices.

Professional bodies and trade unions can assist in offering support and guidance to midwives who have concerns about any part of their work, including anxieties about care provision. These bodies can also raise matters formally with the midwife's organization on the midwife's behalf, as well as access other forums within the organization that may help. Raising a concern can often seem isolating and intimidating, so having such support can assist midwives to meet their professional standards with more confidence.

Raising and escalating concerns also applies to student midwives who should always seek the support from their practice supervisor, practice assessor, personal tutor, lecturer, etc., immediately, whenever they feel that a colleague or anyone else is placing another individual at risk of harm. To a student, raising a concern can appear daunting so seeking support from their university, professional body or trade union is essential to help guide them in the local process.

Record-Keeping

Paragraph 10 of *The Code* (NMC 2018a) addresses the responsibilities of the midwife in respect of keeping clear and accurate records relevant to their practice. This includes understanding and complying with the provision in law that cover the creation, maintenance, handling storage, retention and sharing of the personal details of women and babies in their care, as defined in the EU General Data Protection Regulations (GDPR 2018). Most midwives will need to meet the policy requirements of an employer/maternity service provider. Those who work outside of such a structure, such as independent midwives should take advice about their legal obligations relating to record-keeping to be compliant with legal requirements.

All records relating to the care of a woman and baby should be clear, concise, legible (if written) and of a high standard and retained securely for 25 years, including work diaries. Claims can arise up to 25–30 years after a baby's birth and, if the documentation is lost, or the records difficult to comprehend, it is difficult for the case to be successfully defended.

Conscientious Objection by Midwives

Paragraph 4.4 of *The Code* (NMC 2018a) clearly states that if a midwife (or student midwife) has a conscientious objection to a particular procedure, such as termination of pregnancy, they must inform colleagues, their manager and the person receiving care. As a consequence, the midwife must also arrange for a suitably qualified colleague to take over the responsibility for that person's care. As the law on conscientious objection varies by country of practice, it is the midwife's responsibility to always ensure they fully understand the legislation in the country where they are practising.

Guidance on Using Social Media Responsibly

With the growth in information technology and social media, there is an associated challenge in the increasing risk this poses to healthcare professionals regarding the safety and privacy of personal information. In upholding *The Code* (NMC 2018a), midwives and student midwives should always exercise extra care when using social media, blogs and other online platforms,

being mindful of the detail they share with others via such media. The NMC has issued specific guidance for the responsible use of social media in line with *The Code* paragraph 20.10 (NMC 2018a) that sets out the principles for professional behaviour and public protection in that conduct online should be judged in the same way as conduct in the real world (NMC 2019f).

It is important to remember that sharing particular characteristics, locations or details about an individual may mean that they are identifiable, even if they are not specifically named. The consequences of improper action or unprofessional behaviour through social media or other information sharing websites or applications could put a midwife's registration at risk or could jeopardize a student midwife from ultimately being eligible to join the professional Register.

Triennial Professional Revalidation

The process of revalidation in the UK has been effective since April 2016. Professional revalidation is a process which all midwives and nurses must complete every 3 years in order to maintain their registration with the NMC (2019a). It embraces the principles of *The Code* (NMC 2018a) as the guide for registrants to reflect upon and demonstrate that their practice is up-to-date, safe and effective. Failure to comply with the triennial revalidation requirement will result in a midwife or nurse being removed from the Register.

The NMC (2019a) requirements for revalidation include:

- 450 practice hours (or 900 practice hours if renewing as both a nurse or midwife)
- 35 h of Continuing Professional Development (CPD) including 20 h of participatory learning
- Five pieces of practice-related feedback
- Five written reflective accounts
- Reflective discussion with a fellow NMC registrant
- Health and character declaration
- Professional indemnity arrangement
- Confirmation.

The revalidation process does not assess a registrant's fitness to practise, as its purpose is to ensure midwives and nurses are conversant with *The Code* (NMC 2018a) and ultimately raise professional standards. It is also worth noting that revalidation is for **all** midwives, not just those working in clinical practice. Those midwives who are in leadership, education and research roles are legitimately practising midwifery in their respective fields and are also registered with and regulated by the NMC. In these situations, peer review with a fellow registrant, rather than clinical supervision is the more appropriate means for them to meet the requirements of revalidation. The midwife is expected to maintain a portfolio of evidence, which should be discussed with the confirmer who may be the midwife's line manager or another registrant from any of the professional statutory regulatory bodies (but not a friend). On the NMC website are templates that can be used to format the portfolio, such as a CPD log, a reflective account form, a feedback log and a practice hours log.

As there is some degree of self-certification in the revalidation process, the midwife is therefore required to provide an honest account of their activities in practice. Failure to do so would place the midwife's registration at risk. A measure of scrutiny by the NMC is made on a small number of registrant's portfolios of evidence to ensure quality and consistency across the UK.

Professional revalidation and student midwives

All nurses registered in the adult field who are undertaking a shortened pre-registration midwifery education programme are responsible for ensuring they pay their annual retention fee to maintain their registration with the NMC during their studies. For a proportion of these student midwives, their triennial revalidation may also fall within this time. It is therefore important that the student midwife is supported to complete the process successfully by their personal tutor/academic assessor and practice supervisor/practice assessor (any of whom could act as the student's registrant confirmer). However, at this stage, the evidence should only reflect **nursing** activities, as this is the part of the register on which the student midwife is registered and for which they will be undertaking the revalidation process.

Standards for Medicines Management

Medicines management and prescribing in the UK are governed by a complex framework of legislation, policy and standards, of which the NMC standards are only one part. However, the Human Medicines Regulations 2012 and Human Medicines Regulations (Amendment) 2019 have attempted to simplify medicines legislation, while maintaining effective safeguards for public health. The regulations replaced the majority of the Medicines Act 1968, repealing most of the obsolete law in the process to ensure the legislation is fit for purpose.

> **BOX 2.6 Categories of Medicines in Midwifery Practice**
>
> - General Sales List Medicines (GSL)*
> - Pharmacy Medicines (P)*
> - Prescription Only Medicines (POM)**
> - Controlled Drugs**
> - Patient Specific Direction (PSD)
> - Patient Group Direction (PGD)
> Midwives' Exemptions (Schedule 17 of Human Medicines Regulations 2012)

*All medicines in accordance with the midwife's scope of practice; **specified medicines.

At the point of registration, all midwives will have been deemed safe and competent by the AEI in medicines management in accordance with the Human Medicines Regulations 2012. The Regulations set out the rules for prescription, supply and administration of medicines by midwives with reference to patient-specific directions (PSD); patient-group direction (PGD); and midwives' exemptions (Box 2.6). Midwives can supply all general sale list medicines (GSL) and pharmacy medicines (P) in accordance with their scope of practice. Medicines not included in midwives' exemptions (which include GSL, P and specified prescription-only medicines, POM), require a prescription signed by a doctor, dentist or pharmacist. Schedule 17 of the Human Medicines Regulations 2012 lists the midwives exemptions (e.g. diclofenac, diamorphine and Anti-D immunoglobulin), from restrictions on supply and administration of prescription-only medicines, meaning that midwives can legally supply and administer certain POMs on their own professional licence. The Secretary of State for Health and Social Care can amend the list of medicines in the exemptions by exercise of the powers conferred within the European Communities Act 1972 Section 2 (2) in relation to medicinal products. Midwives are able to prescribe medicines within the scope of their role and qualifications, should they have completed an NMC approved independent and supplementary prescribing programme; the qualification of which must be recorded in the NMC's Register.

Midwives who supervise and assess student midwives in clinical practice, must be familiar with the law in relation to the supply of medicines, including midwives' exemptions, in order to safely support student midwives who may administer medicines to women in their care. Furthermore, in accordance with Part 3 of Schedule 17 of the Human Medicines Regulations 2012, student midwives may administer the medicines included within the midwives' exemptions (except controlled drugs) under the direct supervision of a midwife. Student midwives are not permitted to administer controlled drugs using midwives' exemptions, including diamorphine, morphine and pethidine hydrochloride. They may participate in the checking and preparation of controlled drugs under the direct supervision of a midwife. Student midwives may administer prescribed drugs parenterally (including controlled drugs) if prescribed by a doctor or an appropriate practitioner according to their direction. This must be under the direct supervision of a midwife. For the purposes of all medicines administration, registered nurses undertaking midwifery training should always act in the capacity of a student midwife.

In *The Code* (NMC 2018a), paragraph 18 specifically refers to medicines management, namely advising on, prescribing, supplying, dispensing or administering medicines. Such activities should always be within the limits of the midwife's training and proficiency, the law, NMC guidance and being conversant with national and local policies, guidance and regulations to maximize safety of the public. A useful source in providing information about medicines legislation and regulation in the UK that midwives can access is the Medicines Healthcare Products Regulatory Agency (MHRA). The NMC has also published guidance for those registrants who have undertaken further training to become a midwife or nurse prescriber.

Litigation

This is the term used for the process of taking a case through the courts, where a claimant brings a charge against a defendant to seek some form of redress: i.e. an *adversarial* process. In healthcare terms, this may be as a consequence of the claimant experiencing an *act of trespass* to their person by the defendant or suffering harm from the defendant's actions/omissions that could be proven as *negligence*. The *National Health Service (NHS) Resolution* predominantly handles negligence claims on behalf of the members of its indemnity schemes, namely NHS organizations and independent sector providers of health care in England. A similar organization exists in Scotland, namely the *Clinical Negligence and Other Risks Indemnity Scheme (CNORIS)* and in Wales, the *Welsh Risk Pool*.

Consent

The concept of consent is complex and this section is intended as only a brief introduction. It is important the midwife or doctor obtains consent from a childbearing woman before undertaking any procedure to avoid any future allegations of *trespass to the person* that may be made against them. **Obtaining consent is therefore the legal defence to trespass to the person.**

The law on Informed Consent has moved away from considering the actions of the reasonable doctor by a responsible body of medical opinion, based on the Bolam standard (*Bolam v. Friern Hospital Management Committee* 1957) following the case of *Montgomery v. Lanarkshire Health Board* [2015], to that of the reasonable person/patient standard. This means an individual should be given as much information about the risks of treatment and consent to treatment as any *reasonable person* could be expected to understand in order for them to autonomously determine the decision about their care and subsequent treatment. This implies that the person is mentally competent (is legally an adult: 18 years or over) or is not mentally incapacitated in any way. However, there are very few instances in contemporary practice (if any) where a healthcare professional ultimately makes the decision as to the extent of information that should be disclosed. This is due in part to the ease at which service-users can access information about their health situations through the advances in modern information technology.

The purpose and significance or potential complication of any procedure or treatment should also be discussed with the childbearing woman by the midwife or doctor. Where possible, the woman should be given time to consider her options before making a decision. This should be done voluntarily and without any duress or undue influence from health professionals, family or friends for it to be *valid*. Only the woman can give consent for treatment or intervention and although it is desirable for the partner or other relatives to be in agreement, ultimately the woman's views are the only ones that should be taken into consideration (DH 2009).

Incapacity may be temporary, for example as a result of shock, pain, fatigue, confusion or panic induced by fear. However, it would not usually be reasonable to consider that a woman in labour, experiencing the pain of contractions, would be so affected that she lacked capacity. If a healthcare professional fears that a woman's decision-making (capacity) is impaired, they should seek assistance in assessing capacity, which is usually provided by the courts. If a woman requires emergency treatment to save her life, and she is unable to give consent due to being unconscious, treatment can be carried out if it is in her best interests and according to the reasonable standard of the profession (Mental Capacity Act 2005). Once the woman has recovered, the reasons why treatment was necessary must be fully explained to her.

In the case of minors (children under 16 years), it is important to carefully assess whether there is evidence that they have sufficient understanding in order to give valid consent, i.e. considered to be *Gillick competent* (*Gillick v. West Norfolk and Wisbech AHA* 1985). Although Gillick competence was originally intended to decide whether a child under 16 years can receive contraception without parental knowledge it has, since 1986, had wider applications in health provision and is also referred to as *Fraser competence* (DH 2009). It is also advisable that the child's parents or other accompanying adults/guardians are kept informed of any clinical decisions that are made. Where there is a conflict of opinion regarding consent between child and parent, the health professional should always act in the child's best interest which in some instances may involve the courts determining whether it is lawful to treat the child (DH 2009).

It is good practice that the health professional who is to perform the procedure should be the one to obtain the woman's consent. Such details of the discussion and decision should be clearly documented in the woman's records for colleagues to see that consent has been duly obtained or declined.

Consent can be *implied*, *verbal* or *written*. It is a common misconception that written consent is more valid than verbal consent, when in fact written consent merely serves as evidence of consent. If appropriate information has not been provided, the woman feels that she is under duress or undue influence or she does not have capacity, then a signature on a form will make the consent *invalid*. It is advised that written consent for significant interventions such as surgery should always be obtained (DH 2009) but for many procedures such as vaginal examination or phlebotomy, verbal consent is sufficient. In an absolute emergency, it may be more appropriate to take witnessed verbal consent for caesarean section.

Although the law protects the rights of the woman, the fetus does **not** have any rights until it is born, in UK law. A mentally competent woman cannot be legally forced to have a caesarean section because of risks to the fetus. However, while accepting the law and respecting the woman's right to refuse such an intervention that may further endanger the life of the fetus, such a situation will be very uncomfortable for any midwife or obstetrician to sit back and allow a fetus to die. Cases such as this can be referred to court for an emergency application to determine whether the intervention can proceed lawfully.

Negligence

It is recognized that the most significant claims in obstetrics arise from birth trauma resulting in cerebral palsy. These are usually based on the allegation that there was negligence on the part of the health professionals involved in the intrapartum care and management, resulting in fetal asphyxia and consequently, neurological damage to the baby.

The Congenital Disabilities (Civil Liability) Act 1976 enables a child who is born disabled as a result of negligence prior to birth, to claim compensation from the person(s) responsible for the negligent act. A mother can only be sued for negligence to her unborn baby if this occurred through dangerous driving. In such cases, the child would sue the mother's insurance company. There has been an amendment to the Act so that children who have suffered damage during *in vitro* fertilization (IVF) treatment may also obtain compensation. As with all medicolegal cases, for the claimant to be successful, the following need to be proved:

- the health professional owed the woman a *duty of care*
- there was a *breach of duty of care* to the woman by the health professional such that the standard of care afforded to her was *below the standard that she could reasonably have expected*
- the harm/injury sustained was *caused by the breach of duty* and
- damages or other losses such as psychiatric injury (post-traumatic stress disorder/nervous shock, anxiety disorder or adjustment disorder), financial loss (loss of earnings) and future healthcare provision, recognized by the courts as being subject to compensation, have resulted from that harm.

In many cases where a baby suffers neurological damage and develops cerebral palsy, although it may be accepted that the care was substandard, proving **causation** is more difficult, i.e. whether the substandard care actually resulted in the disability. The situation is complicated by the fact that only a small percentage of babies born with significant neurological damage acquire their disability as a result of events that took place during labour and birth. However, parents will seek to assign the damage to issues of management during the intrapartum period when the health and wellbeing of some babies may have already been chronically compromised before this time. Experts are therefore required to assess the case on behalf of the claimant (the woman or mother on behalf of the baby) and the defendant (usually the provider of maternity services) to consider the issues of causation. This may mean that many medicolegal expert opinions are obtained from neonatologists, paediatric neurologists and obstetricians before finally reaching a conclusion.

The **burden of proof of negligence** falls on the claimant to prove that on the *balance of probabilities*, it is more likely than not that the defendant was negligent in order for them to be awarded any compensation by the courts. In cases of negligence, compensation is determined by agreeing the *liability* and the amount (*quantum*). However, if as a result of negligence the baby has died, then the parents can only recover bereavement costs. Where a fetus dies there is no bereavement costs, as the unborn child does not have any legal rights in the UK.

Vicarious Liability

In the event of an *employed* midwife being negligent, it would be usual for her employer to be sued. The doctrine of vicarious liability exists to ensure that any innocent victim obtains compensation for injuries caused by an employee. Under this doctrine, the employer is responsible for compensation payable for the harm. For vicarious liability to be established, the following elements however, **must** exist:

- there *must* be negligence: a duty of care has been breached and as a reasonably foreseeable consequence has caused harm/other failure by the employee
- the negligent act, omission or failure *must* have been by an employee
- the negligent employee *must* have been acting in the course of their employment.

It is worth noting that even where the employer is held to be vicariously liable, the midwife who is responsible for harm, such as death of a woman or baby, could be found guilty of manslaughter for their gross negligence which led to the death, could lose their job following

disciplinary action and be removed from the Professional Register following NMC Fitness to Practise proceedings.

The doctrine of vicarious liability does not necessarily deprive the employer of their rights against the negligent employee. If a midwife has been negligent then they are in breach of their contract of employment that requires them to take all reasonable care and skill. This breach gives the employer a right to be indemnified against the negligent midwife.

The Health Care and Associated Professions (Indemnity Arrangements) Order 2014 (referred to as 'The Indemnity Order SI 2014 No. 1887') specifies that **all** healthcare professionals, including midwives and nurses, are expected to have indemnity arrangements in place as *a condition of their registration*. This was included in the Nursing and Midwifery Council (Fitness to Practise) (Education, Registration and Registration Appeals) (Amendment) Rules Order of Council 2015. The Clinical Negligence Scheme for Trusts (CNST) fulfils this requirement, so each midwife should be covered via their employer's membership to CNST.

In the case of independent midwives who are self-employed, they have no vicarious liability or indemnity by an employer and are *personally liable* for the health and safety of themselves and others and thus to continue practising, must secure their own personal indemnity insurance cover according to the *Indemnity Order 2014*. However, due to the increase in compensation paid out to maternity cases and subsequent rising costs of insurance premiums, many independent midwives are no longer able to function alone. They have either established social enterprise schemes where they commission care from maternity care providers with whom they negotiate professional indemnity insurance cover, or have returned to employment in the NHS.

SAFEGUARDING AND THE ROLE OF THE MIDWIFE

Every midwife and student midwife has a professional duty to always put the interest of individuals within their care first and act to protect them if it is considered they may be at risk (NMC 2018a). This includes taking all reasonable steps to protect individuals who are vulnerable or at risk from harm, neglect or abuse and being fully aware of the laws relating to the disclosure of information should it be deemed appropriate to share details with others (NMC 2018a). Essentially, safeguarding means that the midwife has a responsibility to ensure the mental and physical health and wellbeing of all childbearing women and their babies in their care is paramount, including there being no risk of exposure to any type of abuse or neglect.

Where vulnerable individuals may be at risk from harm, the principle of confidentiality is important in order to build relationships of trust and enable concerns and fears to be shared. The right to confidentiality in these situations however, is not absolute. It is vital to safeguard and promote the health and welfare of children, young people and vulnerable adults that appropriate information is shared with the *right people* at the *right time*: the tenets of good safeguarding practice. One of the factors identified in many of the safeguarding serious case reviews has been the failure of professionals to record, share and understand the significance of pieces of information that may have prevented serious harm or death of a vulnerable individual (HM Government 2018a). The tenets of sharing information according to HM Government (2018a) can be seen in Box 2.7.

The Law Relating to Safeguarding the Child

The Articles contained within the United Nations (UN) Convention on the Rights of the Child 1989 specify the requirement that all children should live in a safe environment, be protected from harm and have access to the highest attainable standard of health. Midwives should be familiar with the national legislation relating to children within the country in which they practise. For those working within Europe, this also includes promoting the rights contained in the European Convention for the Protection of Human Rights and Fundamental Freedoms, which have been integrated into the national legal framework across the UK. However, this does not fully apply to the integration of the articles of the UN Convention on the Rights of the Child 1989 within UK law. Each UK nation is responsible for its own policies and laws around education, health and social welfare, which cover most aspects of safeguarding and child protection. The Children Act 1989 (England and Wales), the Children (Scotland) Act 1995 and the Children (Northern Ireland) Order 1995 established the framework for the protection and care of children and young people, providing clear principles to guide decision-making in

---

BOX 2.7   Seven Golden Rules to Sharing Information in Health and Social Care Settings

1. **The General Data Protection Regulations Act 2018 and Human Rights Law are not barriers to justified information sharing,** but provide a framework to ensure that personal information about living individuals is shared appropriately.

2. **Be open and honest with the individual** (and/or their family where appropriate) from the outset about why, what, how and with whom information will, or could be shared, and seek their agreement, unless it is unsafe or inappropriate to do so.

3. **Seek advice** from other practitioners if there is any doubt about sharing the information concerned, without disclosing the identity of the individual where possible.

4. **Share with informed consent** where appropriate and, where possible, respect the wishes of those who do not consent to share confidential information. **Information may still be shared without consent if there is good reason to do so, such as where safety may be at risk.** Judgement needs to be based on the facts

of the case. When sharing or requesting personal information from someone, be certain of the basis upon which you are doing so. Where you have consent, be mindful that an individual might not expect information to be shared.

5. **Consider safety and wellbeing.** Base information sharing decisions on considerations of the safety and wellbeing of the individual and others who may be affected by their actions.

6. **Necessary, proportionate, relevant, adequate, accurate, timely and secure.** Ensure it is necessary for the purpose for which it is being shared, is shared only with those individuals who need to have it, is accurate and up-to-date, is shared in a timely fashion and is shared securely.

7. **Keep a record of the decision and the reasons for it** – whether it is to share information or not. If a decision is made to share details, what exactly has been shared, with whom and for what purpose, should be clearly recorded.

Adapted from HM Government. (2018a) Information sharing advice for practitioners providing safeguarding services to children, young people, parents and carers. London: DfE. Available at: https://assets.publishing.service.gov.uk/government/uploads/system/uploads/attachment_data/file/721581/Information_sharing_advice_practitioners_safeguarding_services.pdf.

relation to their care within the four UK nations; however, subsequent legislation has developed to ensure the interests of the child always remain paramount and inter-agency working is strengthened. In Section 11 of The Children Act 2004, it is mandated that health organizations have a duty to cooperate with social services under Section 27 of the Children Act 1989. These duties are an explicit part of NHS employment contracts, with the Chief Executives having the responsibility to ensure there are arrangements in place in their organizations that reflect the importance of safeguarding and promoting the wellbeing of children.

The safeguarding of babies and children is everyone's responsibility, however within UK law, the fetus does not possess the legal rights of a child, until the moment of birth when they become a separate independent individual. This means that the fetus cannot be a party to an action for damages suffered before birth. Although safeguarding can be a challenging role for the midwife, they are well placed to recognize socially vulnerable women and families, including children requiring protection, identifying risks early and raising concerns in a timely and well planned way. This may include teenage parents, care-leavers, asylum seekers and refugees, those with a history of mental health or learning difficulties and others who may misuse substances (including alcohol) and are likely to experience abuse as well as families with a history of previous removal of a child. In such situations, the midwife is a source of information and support, working closely with appropriate health and social care services. It is important to recognize that child maltreatment can also occur in families with no known risk factors.

All NHS Trusts should have a designated safeguarding lead and where there is maternity services provision, a named midwife with responsibility for safeguarding is a statutory requirement (NHS England and NHS Improvement 2015). These midwives oversee safeguarding cases, providing support, knowledge and clinical supervision for midwives, where appropriate. Pre-birth protocols may be found in the protective procedures of Local Safeguarding Children Boards (LSCB) that set out the shared agency responsibility in the protection of children within every Local Authority.

During contact with a woman, the midwife may identify concerns about the safety of the baby once it is born. There is then a duty for the midwife to escalate that concern according to local safeguarding operating procedures, which every midwife should be familiar with. Initially, this would involve a discussion with the line manager or the safeguarding specialist (depending on their knowledge and experience) and a referral made to the local social care services. Any member of the public can make a direct referral to social care if they believe a child is at risk. Under Section 47 of the Children Act 1989, social care would then undertake an assessment of the family's situation, seeking opinion of healthcare professionals such as specialist community public health nurses (SCPHN)/health visitors, midwives, community support workers, General Practitioners (GPs), police officers, etc., involved in the care and support of the family in question (HM Government 2018b). This is to ascertain if any measures need to be put into place to protect the unborn baby and any other children in the family. A child protection conference may then be organized by social care where all professionals involved in the care of the family are invited to discuss the case with family members. This may occur before the birth of the baby and the timing of which needs careful consideration, bearing in mind the need for early action to allow time to plan for the birth. A pre-birth conference should always be convened where there is a need to consider if a multiagency child protection plan is required in England, or the child should be added to a child protection register in Northern Ireland, Scotland and Wales (HM Government 2018b). Box 2.8 highlights the situations where a pre-birth conference should be held to determine the subsequent protection of the baby and promotion of their wellbeing following birth.

These meetings may be particularly difficult for any health and social care professional, especially if the parents are present. However, each professional should always base their opinion on their code of practice and duty of care, in that the safety of the newborn baby and/or other children in the family should be paramount (NMC 2018a). If a decision is made that the child requires protection, social care will work with the team looking after the family to devise a multiagency *child protection plan* to meet the needs of the child or add them to a *child protection register*. Furthermore, the midwife may fear the relationship with the family may be in jeopardy following the outcome of the *child protection conference*, but must always be mindful of their professional and legal obligation to share information to other agencies where they may have safeguarding concerns. A midwife in such a situation

BOX 2.8   Child Protection: Pre-Birth Conference Criteria and Considerations

A pre-birth conference should be held where:

- A pre-birth assessment gives rise to concerns that an unborn child may be at risk of significant harm
- A previous child has died or has been removed from parent(s) as a result of significant harm
- A child is to be born into a family or household that already has children who are subjects of a child protection plan or on a child protection register.
- An adult or child who is a risk to children resides in the household or is known to be a regular visitor.

Other risk factors to be considered are:

- The impact of parental risk factors such as mental ill health, learning difficulties, substance misuse and domestic abuse and violence
- A mother under 18 years of age about whom there are concerns regarding her ability to self-care and/or care for the child.

TABLE 2.1   Types of Abuse

Domestic abuse	Physical abuse
Emotional/psychological	Neglect
Sexual abuse	Female genital mutilation
Human trafficking/modern slavery	Child exploitation/grooming

should seek specific safeguarding advice from their employer to support them, as well as from a clinical supervisor or professional midwifery advocate (PMA) (NHS 2017).

On occasions, social care may decide that following the joint case conference it would not be safe for a baby to remain with the mother/parents when it is born. Social care will seek a court order to remove the baby to a place of safety, which can only be applied for when the baby is born; known as an *Emergency Protection Order* (EPO). This will often occur within the postnatal ward and midwives will be supporting the safety of the baby and comfort to the parents. Although this is a very difficult and sad time for all concerned, midwives must always remember that the safety of the baby is paramount and parents will be represented in court where a judge will decide the course of action.

Types of Abuse

There are many different types of abuse, which are identified in Table 2.1.

Domestic violence and abuse

Domestic violence and abuse is any incident or pattern of incidents of controlling, coercive or threatening behaviour, violence or abuse between those aged 16 years or over who are or have been, intimate partners or family members regardless of gender or sexuality (Strickland and Allen 2018). This can encompass but is not limited to the following:

- Psychological abuse
- Physical abuse
- Sexual abuse
- Financial abuse
- Emotional abuse.

Strickland and Allen (2018) define *controlling behaviour* as being a range of acts designed to make an individual subordinate and/or dependent on another. This is done by isolating them from sources of support; exploiting their resources and capacities for personal gain; depriving them of the means needed for independence; resistance and escape; and regulating their everyday behaviour. In comparison, *coercive behaviour* is characterized by an act or a pattern of acts of assault, threats, humiliation or other abuse from a person that is used to harm, punish or frighten their victim.

Demographically, the abused and their abusers span the entire range of cultural, educational, racial, religious and socioeconomic strata. The Office for National Statistics (ONS 2018) reveal that in England and Wales, around 1.3 million women between the ages of 16 and 59 years experienced domestic violence compared with 695,000 men, which also indicates there has been little change in the prevalence in recent years. In some instances, the consequences of domestic abuse can result in homicide. In the triennium 2015–17, it was reported that 3% of all maternal deaths in the UK (equivalent to seven women per 100,000 maternities) were as a result of murder that occurred during pregnancy and up to 6 weeks following the birth of their baby; all by a partner or former partner (Knight et al. 2019). This fact reaffirms the important role midwives and other healthcare professionals working in maternity care services play in being vigilant in identifying cases of domestic abuse in order to prevent these women's deaths. It is known that women who have a physical disability are twice as susceptible in experiencing domestic abuse than physically able women; some of whom may also be pregnant (Public Health England, PHE 2015).

Pregnancy can be a trigger for domestic abuse and existing abuse may get worse during the childbirth continuum (Duxbury 2014), which can affect antenatal care attendance leading to poor outcomes, including an increase in low birth weight babies and pre-term birth (Shah and Shah 2010). There are many reasons for an increase in abuse at this time, including feelings of over-possessiveness, jealousy and denial of the woman being anything other than spouse, on the part of the perpetrator. Furthermore, the fetus may be perceived as an intruder to the perpetrator who, as a result of reduced sexual activity and possible increasing financial challenges, becomes violent to the woman.

The rate of detection has improved during pregnancy, since routine enquiry for domestic abuse, which has enabled women who have disclosed their experiences, to seek help and support early (NICE 2014). When abuse is suspected, the midwife should in the first instance ensure the environment is safe before questioning the woman directly to confirm there is abuse, in order to protect the unborn baby and support the woman (DH 2014) (Box 2.9).

All cases of current domestic abuse should be referred via local safeguarding procedures. Researchers have found that domestic abuse can have lifelong detrimental effects on children's development in addition to physical risks (National Society for the Prevention of Cruelty to Children, NSPCC 2019). Confidential information can be disclosed if it is justified in the public interest, i.e. to protect individuals from the risk of significant harm (NMC 2018a).

Physical abuse

Physical abuse occurs when an adult or child is deliberately assaulted and hurt, causing injuries such as cuts, bruises, burns and broken bones. It can involve hitting, kicking, shaking, throwing, poisoning, burning or scalding, drowning and suffocating. Situations where a parent or carer invents or deliberately induces the symptoms of illness in children is also considered

---

BOX 2.9   Domestic Abuse

Raising the Subject of Domestic Abuse and Violence with Women

Ensure it is safe to ask
- Consider the environment
  - Is it conducive to ask?
  - Is it safe to ask?
  - Never ask in the presence of another family member, friend or child over the age of 2 years
- Create the opportunity to ask the question
- Use an appropriate professional interpreter (never a family member).

Ask
Frame the topic first then ask a direct question.
Framing: 'As violence in the home is so common we now ask about it routinely'.
Direct Question: 'Are you in a relationship with someone who hurts or threatens you?'
'Has someone hurt you?'
'Did someone cause those injuries to you?'

Validate
Validate what is being said by the woman and send important messages to her:

'You are not alone'.
'You are not to blame for what is happening to you'.
'You do not deserve to be treated in this way'.

Assess the woman's safety by asking:
'Is your partner here with you?'
'Where are your children?'
'Do you have any immediate worries?'
'Do you have a place of safety?'

Action
Use your knowledge of domestic violence, support, and be responsive to the woman's needs.
Know how to contact your local domestic violence agency and local independent domestic violence advisor.
Be familiar with the supportive leaflets, referral agencies and safeguarding procedures

Document
Ensure that your documentation is in line with the principles of confidentiality, defined by your organization.

Adapted from Department of Health. (2014) Health visiting and school nursing programmes: supporting implementation of the new service model. No 5: Domestic Violence and Abuse – Professional Guidance. London: DH.

to be a form of physical abuse, such as giving them medicine they do not require that results in them becoming ill. This is known as *fabricated or induced illness (FII)*.

Emotional/psychological abuse

In situations where there is continual emotional maltreatment of an individual that involves deliberately trying to scare, humiliate, isolate or ignore them, the consequences are likely to cause serious psychological damage to the recipient. If this occurs in childhood, the impact can be extremely damaging to the long-term mental health and psychological development. This form of abuse can equally apply to an adult in an abusive relationship.

Neglect

Neglect is the persistent failure of a parent, guardian or carer, to meet a child's basic physical and/or psychological needs, that is likely to result in the serious impairment of the child's mental and physical health or development. Neglect may occur during pregnancy as a result of maternal substance abuse. Once the baby is born, if neglect continues, it may manifest in the mother/parent **failing to:**

- provide adequate food, clothing and shelter for the child (including exclusion from the home or even abandonment)
- protect the child from physical and emotional harm or danger
- ensure adequate supervision of the child (including the use of inadequate caregivers)
- ensure access to appropriate medical care or treatment
- respond to a child's basic emotional needs.

Sexual abuse

Where an adult or child is forced or enticed to take part in sexual activities is classified as sexual abuse. However, this type of abuse does not necessarily involve violence and the individual, particularly in the case of a child, may not fully understand that the situation they have found themselves in, is indeed an abusive one. Child sexual abuse can either be non-contact abuse or contact abuse and in some cases may be both. Non-contact sexual abuse is likely to occur through sharing of a child's details and sexual images through social media.

Contact sexual abuse occurs when the abuser makes physical contact with the child and may include a range of activities as listed below:

- forcing or encouraging the child to take part in sexual activity
- sexual touching of any part of the child's body either through their clothing or bare skin
- forcing the child to remove their clothes, touch someone else's genitals or masturbate
- rape or penetration by putting a body part or an object inside the child's mouth, vagina or anus.

Female genital mutilation, genital cutting or female circumcision

Female genital mutilation (FGM), genital cutting or female circumcision is defined as the partial or total removal of the female external genitalia for non-medical reasons (see Chapter 17). In practice, the term 'cutting' is now preferred rather than mutilation, to avoid alienating communities who believe the ritual is sacred to their culture. While genital cutting may be considered abhorrent in many western cultures, midwives should always be respectful of all women regardless of their deep rooted traditions, as many will have been deeply traumatized by this 'abuse' and should therefore be offered psychological support.

According to the WHO (2018) FGM is practised in approximately 30 countries in Africa, the Middle East and Asia, with over 200 million women having undergone the procedure. With increasing immigration and refugee migration, women who have experienced FGM present all over the world. It is therefore essential that healthcare professionals should be aware of the traditional practice of genital cutting and its implications in childbirth and in safeguarding the next generation of female children, as well as being proactive in totally eradicating this harmful cultural practice. In the UK, genital cutting is often seen among immigrants from: Eritrea, Ethiopia, Mali, Nigeria, Sierra Leone, Somalia and Sudan.

The age at which girls undergo genital cutting varies and is dependent on the community in which it is undertaken. It may be carried out when the girl is newborn, in childhood, adolescence, at marriage or during the first pregnancy. The most common time is between 4 and 8 years of age. In such communities, genital cutting is seen as a rite of passage into womanhood and girls are usually compliant to having the procedure done, as they believe they would otherwise be classed as an outcast. However, as anaesthetics and antiseptic techniques are not usually used and the procedure is undertaken with basic tools such as circumcision knives, scalpels, scissors, pieces of glass and razor blades, there are potentially serious physical and psychological health consequences for these young girls, both at the time of the procedure and in later life (see Chapter 17).

Legislation on Female Genital Mutilation. The Prohibition of Female Circumcision Act 1985 made it an offence to carry out FGM in the UK or to aid, abet or procure the service of another person. This Act was replaced in England, Wales and Northern Ireland by the Female Genital Mutilation Act 2003, which made it illegal for FGM to be performed anywhere in the world on UK permanent residents of any age and extended the maximum sentence from 5 years' to 14 years' imprisonment. This was to deter people from taking girls abroad for mutilation. Further legislation in the form of the Serious Crimes Act 2015 resulted in the:

- extension of extra-territorial jurisdiction to include FGM performed outside the UK, by a UK national or a person resident in the UK
- preservation of the anonymity of individuals over their lifetime to encourage more reporting of FGM
- introduction of a new offence for failing to protect a girl from FGM. This means that if an offense is committed against a girl under the age of 16 years, each person who is responsible for the girl at the time the cutting occurred, will be liable. (A responsible person is classed as: the mother, father, guardian or a family member assuming the responsibility of a parent to whom the girl may be sent to stay during the summer holidays).

Female Genital Mutilation Protection Order. At the Girl Summit in July 2014, there was overwhelming support to introduce a specific civil law measure to protect potential or actual victims of FGM, closely modelled on the forced marriage protection orders in the Family Law Act 1986. As a consequence, the Serious Crimes Act 2015 provides for Female Genital Mutilation Protection Orders (FGMPOs) to protect a girl against the commission of a genital mutilation offence or to protect a girl against whom such an offence has been committed. Breach of an FGMPO is a criminal offence with a maximum penalty of 5 years' imprisonment or as a civil breach, is punishable by up to 2 years' imprisonment. The courts may make a FGMPO on application by the girl who is to be protected by a third party.

An FGMPO may also contain prohibitions, restrictions or other requirements for the purposes of protecting the girl. This may include provisions to surrender a person's passport or other travel documents and not to enter any arrangements in the UK or abroad for FGM to be performed on the person to be protected.

The Serious Crimes Act 2015 also includes a mandatory reporting duty requiring specified regulated professionals from health, social care and education, in England and Wales to make a report to the police where they have discovered that FGM appears to have been carried out on a girl under the age of 18 years at the time of the discovery.

The duty applies where the professional either:

- is informed by the girl that an act of FGM has been carried out on her or
- observes physical signs that appear to show an act of FGM has been carried out and has no reason to believe the act was necessary for the girl's physical or mental health or for purposes connected with labour or birth.

Midwives must be vigilant in enquiry and mindful of other female children in the family who may also be at risk, as well as be aware of local safeguarding policies and procedures to act upon as necessary.

Human trafficking and modern slavery

Human trafficking refers to the trade of humans, particularly women and children for the purpose of forced labour, sexual slavery or commercial exploitation for the trafficker or others. This could involve providing a spouse in the context of a forced marriage or the extraction of organs and tissues, including for surrogacy and ova removal. It can occur within a country or transnationally and is a crime against the person due to the victim's rights of movement through coercion and their commercial exploitation. Most people are trafficked to the UK from overseas, but there is also a significant number of British nationals in slavery. As many as 1 in 4 women who are victims of trafficking are pregnant (Brotherton 2016). The most common countries of origin are Albania, Vietnam, Nigeria, Poland and Romania (Anti-Slavery International 2019).

Many individuals who become victims of trafficking wish to escape poverty, improve their lives and provide for their families. They are usually offered a well-paid job abroad or in another region and borrow money from their traffickers in advance to pay for arranging the job, travel and accommodation. The reality is that the job does not exist or the conditions are completely different; their passports are often taken away and they are forced to work until their debt is paid off.

The *Modern Slavery Act 2015* is more focused on the policing of the activity of trafficking and slavery rather than providing protection for the victims, with many being treated as immigration offenders rather than victims of serious crime. They are also less likely to act as witnesses in court to help prosecute the traffickers. Midwives have a duty to identify victims of trafficking when it concerns childbearing women and work with safeguarding specialists, social care and the police to protect both mother and baby. Some of these women may have been prevented from receiving antenatal care and first present in established labour, thus placing both mother and baby at risk. Furthermore, for some victims of trafficking, becoming a parent may be a positive change in their life, but, for others, whose pregnancy is as a result of rape or other sexual violence, the birth experience can be traumatic and psychologically hinder their recovery.

Child sex exploitation/grooming

The key factor that distinguishes cases of child sexual exploitation (CSE) from other forms of child sexual abuse is the concept of exchange, whereby the child or young person is coerced or manipulated into engaging in sexual activity in return for something they need or desire and/or for the gain of those perpetrating or facilitating the abuse. What the child or young person receives in return may include tangible rewards such as drugs and alcohol and/or less tangible things such as attention, perceived love and affection or a sense of value or belonging. By the child or young person receiving something in return is a key part of the abusive process, convincing them that they are in control of the situation. Fear of what might happen if they do not comply, can also be a significant influencing factor to the child (Barnados 2019). A series of high-profile child sexual exploitation cases in recent years involving large groups of offenders and victims worldwide has highlighted the need for better understanding of, and responses to, this phenomenon, triggering widespread recognition and changes in local safeguarding policy to protect vulnerable children.

ETHICAL ISSUES AND THE MIDWIFE

Although the area of ethics is complex and perceived as difficult and daunting, it is a major part of midwifery education and practice and should be seen as a daily tool to support a midwife's decision-making with childbearing women. Being ethically aware is a step towards being an autonomous practitioner: taking responsibility, empowering others and facilitating professional growth and development. The language and terminology, however, can be hard to comprehend and needs greater explanation (Box 2.10).

Ethics is often about exploring values and beliefs and clarifying what people understand, think and feel in a certain situation, often from what they say as much as what they do – such actions being underpinned by morality. Beliefs and values are very personal and dependent on many things, such as a person's background, the society they have been brought up in and the principles and concepts learned since early childhood, such as veracity (truth-telling). It is important to reflect on these issues and be open and honest about the dilemmas faced in practice. A potential area of conflict is that of law, as law and ethics are often seen as complementary to one another, yet they can also be placed at opposite ends of the spectrum, either creating overlap or creating conflict. Exploring ethics provides a framework to aid resolution of such dilemmas.

Ethical Frameworks and Theories

There are many ethical frameworks that could be adopted for use in clinical situations and Edwards (1996) advocates a four-level system of moral thinking, based on the work of Melia (1989) that can assist in

---

BOX 2.10 Terminology

Informed consent	Information regarding options for care/treatment
Rights	Justified claim to a demand
Duty	A requirement to act in a certain manner
Justice	Being treated fairly
Candour	Being open and honest, frank
Best interests	Deciding on the best course for an individual
Utilitarian	Greatest good for the greatest number
Deontological	Duty of care
Beneficence	Doing good
Non-maleficence	Avoiding harm

> **BOX 2.11   Edwards' Levels of Ethics (1996)**
>
> | | |
> |---|---|
> | **Level one** | Judgements |
> | **Level two** | Rules |
> | **Level three** | Principles |
> | **Level four** | Ethical theories |

formulating arguments and discussions and ultimately solving moral dilemmas (Box 2.11).

Level one: Judgements

Judgements are usually readily made, based on information on individual gains. Such judgements may have no real foundation except the belief of the individual who made it. They may therefore be biased and not necessarily well thought through or based on all the available evidence. What informs a judgement is often linked to personal values and beliefs, societal influences, as well as experiences of similar past events. It is important that midwives reflect on past judgements to consider if in retrospect, they were well-founded or based on personal bias or prejudice.

Level two: Rules

Rules govern our daily lives and are determined by the society or culture in which we live. In terms of ethics, rules are what guide the midwife's practice and control their actions. According to Beauchamp and Childress (2019), rules come in different forms:

- *Substantive rules*: cover issues such as privacy, confidentiality or truth-telling
- *Authority rules*: are determined by those in power and enforced on a country or section of society
- *Procedural rules*: define a set course of action or line that should be followed.

The midwife should recognize that rules can be enabling in that they define clear limits or boundaries of practice, allowing freedom to act, knowing the safe limits of those actions. Box 2.2 highlights a number of statutory rules that are bound by the Nursing and Midwifery Order 2001 and its subsequent amendments, but which can guide and enable practice when used appropriately and as a consequence ease any ethical dilemmas. *The Code* (NMC 2018a) is less formal or obligatory than rules and is viewed as a set of standards and guidelines to support safe practice among midwives as well as nurses and nursing associates.

Level three: Principles

There are four main principles, which are usually applied specifically within health care and midwifery practice:

- *Respect for autonomy*: respecting another's right to self-determine a course of action, e.g. placing women at the centre of maternity care where their views and wishes are seen as key to the decision-making process in care delivery.
- *Non-maleficence*: *Primum non nocere* – above all, do no harm or cause no hurt.
- *Beneficence*: compassion, taking positive action to do good or balance the benefits or harm in a given situation. This principle can cause a particular dilemma when a woman chooses a course of action that may not be in her and her fetus/baby's best interests.
- *Justice*: to treat everyone fairly and as equals. This principle also encompasses fair access for all women to the same level and options of health and maternity services, including place of birth.

Level four: Ethical theories

There are a number of theories that could be explored and applied to health care and midwifery practice, e.g. liberalism, ethical relativism, feminism and casuistry are just some of them. The two main normative ethical theories that are at either end of the spectrum are *utilitarianism* (consequentialism) and *deontology*.

Utilitarianism. This theory considers actions in terms of their probable consequences and originates from the Greek *telos* meaning *end* or *purpose*, such that this theory is sometimes referred to as *teleological theory*. Although the original theory's aim was for all actions to create the greatest happiness for the greatest number of people, the word *happiness* has been criticized, as for some individuals actions may result in a degree of *unhappiness*. It is therefore more apt to consider this theory as substituting *happiness* for the word *good* or *benefit*: that is, *the greatest good/benefit for the greatest number*.

Many aspects of midwifery practice have been implemented on utilitarian principles, e.g. antenatal and neonatal screening tests are offered to all women irrespective of need or individual assessment to benefit society as a whole. However, midwives do need to be mindful that, while the majority of women may opt for the testing to identify any potential health risks and consequential

> **BOX 2.12   Duty of Care to …**
>
> - Self
> - Colleagues
> - Women (mothers)/patients
> - Relatives
> - Fetus/baby
> - Employer
> - Profession (NMC).

treatment, *unhappiness* may be evoked for some women as fear and anxiety is associated with the choice to accept or decline such a test.

There are two types of this theory: *act utilitarianism* and *rule utilitarianism*. *Act utilitarianism* was developed by Bentham, Mill and Sidgwick in the 18th and 19th centuries and is the purer form of the two types. The theory expects every potential action to be assessed according to its predicted outcomes in terms of benefit. In comparison, *rule utilitarianism* considers moral rules that are intended to ensure the greatest benefit, such that each act is assessed on how it conforms to the rules. Practically, utilitarianism theory is attractive in that it can aid decision-making for the masses, such that an action is good if it provides benefits for the majority.

Deontology. This particular ethical theory derives from the Greek term *deon*, meaning *duty*, *rule or obligation*, and was formulated around the right thing to do *without regard to the consequences*, by the German metaphysician, Immanuel Kant. All health professionals would appreciate they have a duty towards their patients/clients, but as shown in Box 2.12, they may have duties in other areas that they need to consider and balance, in order to make appropriate decisions to take the best course of action. How duty is interpreted may vary according to the individual's personal situation, their values or beliefs with some individuals basing their duty on natural laws, religion and the Ten Commandments (*traditional deontology*).

The philosophy behind Kant's theory reflects that to act morally is concerned with truth-telling and out of respect for duty, *regardless* of the circumstances. Kant believed that the actions of an individual should always be rational and stem from goodwill, that is to say, duty for its own sake, namely the *categorical imperative*, which is expressed as follows:

- Act only according to that maxim by which you can also will that it would become a universal law.

- Act in such a way that you always treat humanity, whether in your own person or in the person of any other, never simply as a means, but always at the same time as an end.

This highlights that an action can only be moral if it can be applied to everyone universally, i.e. if everyone was to do it. Kant believed all individuals to be autonomous and rational and should be treated with respect, rather merely as a means to an end. Beauchamp and Childress (2019) consider that if an action necessitates treating someone *without* respect, then it is the *action that is wrong*. In maternity care, respecting women as individuals with their own personal experiences is fundamental to the role of the midwife.

Although the NHS and other healthcare providers are generally utilitarian, midwifery, nursing, medicine and other such disciplines adopt a more deontological approach. *The duty of care* which is the duty that health professionals are most familiar with is in essence embedded in the text of *The Code* (NMC 2018a).

Conflicting duties can cause dilemmas in deciding the best course of action. **Casuistry** is a system that can assist in prioritizing duties according to the circumstances. However, most people deal with conflicts and dilemmas in their lives without having an appreciation of these theories. Nevertheless, whether midwives opt to utilize formal or informal approaches to assist their ethical decision-making in practice, to have knowledge of each of them is important in order to understand how some decisions are made. Furthermore, having knowledge of ethical theories can help midwives to appreciate why certain approaches are taken by the employing organization/management, when changes or implementation of innovations are proposed in practice.

EMPLOYER-LED SUPERVISION OF MIDWIVES

For over 100 years, statutory supervision of midwives that included a regulatory, supportive and advocacy function for midwives and childbearing women had been integral to professional practice within the UK. Following high profile maternity cases, where supervision of midwifery was implicated in governance failures and the subsequent reports and recommendations (PHSO 2013; PSA 2014; Kirkup 2015; Baird et al. 2015), the decision was taken by the NMC to disestablish midwifery supervision from statute (House of Lords Hansard 2017; the Nursing and Midwifery (Amendment) Order 2017) as previously discussed in more detail.

Many organizations have argued that less emphasis should be placed on the use of external pressures such as regulation, to improve health services with a requirement to improve collective and collaborative responsibility, not only from individual health professionals but also from their employers as well as service-users and policy-makers (Bell and Jarvie 2015). Following the removal of the regulatory function of midwifery supervision, the need to maintain a supportive structure, that benefited midwives, maternity services and childbearing women, was a key consideration in the development of the various employer-led models of supervision based on the principles set out by the DH (2016) that have subsequently emerged in each of the four nations of the UK.

The DH (2016) recommended each UK country set up a task force to develop the new non-regulatory model of midwifery supervision. NHS England proceeded to set up a Midwifery Supervision Task Force to develop the new model of clinical supervision and oversee the transition to the new model across the UK, but due to the variations in demographics and size, it was decided that although each nation would operationalize the model differently, they would all be based on a consistent set of principles. As a result, the employer-led models of supervision support midwives in promoting reflective practice, self-efficacy, advocacy and professional leadership through clinical supervision, revalidation and peer review; elements that were exemplified in the former model of statutory supervision of midwives (Purdy and Read 2019). Table 2.2 presents a summary and comparisons of the tenets of the employer-led model of clinical supervision adopted by the four nations, which will be discussed in the following sections.

The Employer-Led Model of Supervision in England

The new model of midwifery supervision in England, A-EQUIP (Advocating for Education and Quality Improvement) was developed following extensive consultation with a range of stakeholders, namely: women, midwives, educationalists, midwifery and nurse leaders and managers, commissioners and the Royal College of Midwives. The consultation recommended that the model should:

- have a supportive function
- build professional resilience
- support the advocacy role of the midwife
- support all midwives to provide high-quality care and seek to improve it
- include strategies that value, develop and invest in midwives
- allow flexibility for local organizational application
- not create additional financial pressure on providers.

TABLE 2.2	**The Four Nations at a Glance**
England	The PMA role is either full-time, or combined with clinical practice. Ratio of PMAs to midwives is set by each employer according to local needs. Mandated minimum of 1 h/year supervision.
Wales	Full-time supervisors with 20% of their time working on labour wards. Mandated ratio of 1:125 (supervisor to midwives). Four hours of supervision a year, with 2 h of this being group supervision. Further *ad hoc* sessions available as needed.
Scotland	Supervisors combine role with clinical practice. Individual Boards set the ratio of supervisors to midwives. One mandatory group session a year with individual support as needed.
Northern Ireland	Experienced, additionally trained midwives provide supervision. Ratio of 1:15 (supervisors to midwives) maintained. Midwives entitled to at least one supervisory meeting a year, plus round-the-clock access to advice as needed.

Adapted from Purdy S, Read J. (2019) Employer-led models of midwifery supervision. In: JE Marshall (ed.) Myles professional studies for midwifery education and practice: concepts and challenges. Edinburgh: Elsevier, pp. 159–73.

The A-EQUIP model (NHS England 2017) is based on Proctor's (1986) three function model of clinical supervision adapted by Hawkins and Shohet (2012). The A-EQUIP model is made up of four distinct supportive functions: monitoring, evaluation and quality control (normative), clinical supervision (restorative), personal action for quality improvement and education and development (formative). Fig. 2.3 illustrates the four functions of the model.

Monitoring, evaluation and quality control (normative)

This function of the A-EQUIP model is focused on evaluation and quality control aspects of professional practice; referred to by Proctor (1986) as the *accountability* or *normative* function. Through reflection and discussion with others, this element benefits the midwife by promoting a sense of personal and professional accountability, increasing self-awareness, identifying enhancements in performance leading to the delivery of service improvements.

Clinical supervision (restorative)

Restorative clinical supervision (RCS) has been found to address the emotional needs and wellbeing of staff and to support the development of resilience. Stephen and Pettit (2015) affirm that RCS provides for the creation of space that allows the practitioner to physically and mentally slow down while restoring their thinking capacity and ability to understand and process thoughts, enabling them to consider different perspectives and inform their decision-making. The RCS approach has been found to have a positive impact on physical and emotional wellbeing, reduce stress, improve relationships with colleagues and increase job satisfaction; this can be undertaken in either one-to-one or group sessions.

Personal action for quality improvement

Personal action for quality improvement should follow the midwife's progress through peer review, feedback from service-users and RCS. As the midwife identifies aspects of their practice that would benefit from improvement, the next step is to identify how that action to improve will benefit women and their families. According to NHS England (2017), action to improve quality of care, such as through audit and research, should become an intrinsic part of every health professional's role.

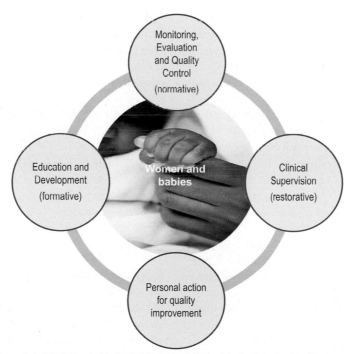

Fig. 2.3 A-EQUIP model. (NHS England. (2017) A-EQUIP a model of clinical midwifery supervision. Available at: www.england.nhs.uk/wp-content/uploads/2017/04/a-equip-midwifery-supervision-model.pdf.)

Education and development (formative)

This function of the A-EQUIP model is seen to support the NMC process of revalidation, employer-led appraisal and leadership development. The *formative* process can be guided by peer review and reflection and is seen to increase self-awareness and self-confidence.

Professional midwifery advocates

The responsibility for implementing the A-EQUIP model rests with the individual healthcare provider and NHS organization, and is undertaken by professional midwifery advocates (PMAs) (replacing the Supervisor of Midwives in England). The principles of the PMA supporting midwives to advocate for women, demonstrates the concept of accountable practice where midwives reflect on their practice, build their resilience and manage their own professional development in order to achieve the highest standard of midwifery care.

Preparing midwives to be professional midwifery advocates. Professional midwifery advocates (PMAs) are experienced midwives who have undertaken further recognized training provided by a Higher Education Institute (HEI) having been selected for the role, which can be in a full-time capacity or on a sessional basis. A PMA commands professional credibility and respect from colleagues and external stakeholders, has excellent communication skills, the ability to think strategically and effectively drive the quality improvement agenda within their workplace.

The first cohorts of PMAs were drawn from former Supervisors of Midwives (SoM) who undertook a shortened PMA 'bridging' programme designed to build on the previous learning and experience of the SoM, while providing an opportunity to develop the skills necessary to facilitate restorative clinical supervision (NHS England 2017). Midwives who do not have the SoM qualification are required to complete a longer preparation programme of at least 10 days duration, facilitated through HEIs at Framework for Higher Education Qualifications (FHEQ) academic level 7 (Master's degree level). Both the bridging and full programme ensure the new PMA meets the competency requirements detailed in the NHS England (2017) guidance. The competencies were modelled on those of the Care Quality Commission key lines of enquiry: 'safe', 'effective', 'caring', 'responsive' and 'well-led' (CQC 2017). By aligning the criteria, there is a clear acknowledgement of the PMA role in driving the NHS quality agenda.

The Employer-Led Model of Supervision in Wales

In Wales, the transition from statutory supervision to a new model of clinical supervision was different, as a full review and remodelling of services, that was part of the 'future proofing' process in 2014 had already taken place before the disestablishment of statutory supervision (Ness and Richards, 2014). This resulted in the introduction of the full-time clinical supervisor for midwives (CSfM). As a consequence, the decision was made to retain the elements of the future-proofing model, which met the requirements of the post-disestablishment supervisor remit.

The Welsh Government has mandated the provision of clinical midwifery supervision, with a ratio of one full-time supervisor to every 125 midwives, rather than devolving the role of implementation of the new model to the healthcare provider. Every supervisor is required to spend 20% of their time working clinically and support midwives to learn, reflect, review and discuss practice issues through a model of coaching and mentoring. There is a mandatory requirement for all midwives to access 4 h of clinical supervision each year, 2 h of which must be a group session. There is an All Wales CSfM Forum that provides peer support to each CSfM.

The Employer-Led Model of Supervision in Scotland

Following their review, the Scottish task force devised a very similar model of employer-led supervision to that adopted in England. The focus of the model is on restorative supervision, with an emphasis on reflection and advocacy. NHS Education for Scotland has developed an education programme for prospective supervisors similar to that already discussed for England. Part of the training involves the supervisor of midwives developing skills in group facilitation and coaching techniques to enable all midwives to get the most out of their group supervision sessions. It is an expectation that all midwives attend at least one group supervision per year.

The Employer-Led Model of Supervision in Northern Ireland

The Northern Ireland Practice and Education Council for Nursing and Midwifery were tasked with producing an overarching framework of employer-led supervision, which covers midwifery, nursing and children's safeguarding. The interim arrangements are very similar in structure to the previous, statutory supervision, with the exception of the investigatory function.

Northern Ireland has retained 24 h access to experienced clinical midwifery advice from the original supervision model, with all midwives retaining a 'named midwifery supervisor' (DH 2016), with whom they meet at least annually and which contributes to the revalidation process. Midwives are required to meet regularly with a midwifery supervisor to discuss emerging issues and promote high standards of care. Heads of Midwifery are required to maintain a list of midwifery supervisors and allocated supervisees, aiming for a ratio of 1:15.

Midwives Working in Education, Research and Management

Midwives who work in education and research historically had access to statutory supervision through the Local Supervisory Authority, whereby an SoM would be allocated to them if none were available in their workplace. Since the removal of statutory supervision, there has been no consensus on how midwives working outside institutional maternity providers should access the support of a PMA/supervisor. Although some AEIs have equipped a number of midwifery lecturers to become PMAs to be able to provide this support to midwifery staff, the DH (2016) makes a distinction between the needs of midwives working in clinical roles to those in education, research and management settings, emphasizing the need for the provision of supervision to be proportional to the risk profile of the working environment. While a form of clinical supervision is recommended for midwives who provide clinical care, a system of peer review is considered appropriate for those midwives whose roles are less exposed to the clinical practice setting.

The DH (2016) also postulates the need for HEIs to consider whether sufficient emphasis is placed within their midwifery education programmes on the advocacy role of midwives. Prior to disestablishment, SoMs could provide impartial support to women regarding their birth choices. The DH (2016) highlighted concerns that midwives may be reluctant to advocate effectively for women in their care, fearful of employer censure. It is essential that students and registered midwives fully understand the supportive role of the PMA or clinical supervisor and are effectively prepared to confidently advocate for women, especially those whose wishes deviate from recommended care pathways.

RESILIENCE IN MIDWIFERY

Resilience is a complex, dynamic, developmental process (Cicchetti 2010; Rutter 2012), which can be planned for, developed and practised. It is defined as the ability to adapt, cope positively (Hunter and Warren 2014), transform and even thrive in adversity (Wendt et al. 2011). Key factors that contribute to individual resilience include: professional identity; supportive relationships; supervision; work/life balance; spirituality; self-awareness, including emotional insight; self–compassion; hope and learning opportunities. Culture is an important consideration when attempting to understand resilience, as cultural norms influence how distress is expressed, which responses are regarded effective and which values and beliefs underpin those responses (Dutton et al. 2014). Furthermore, it is thought that resilience could be nurtured through education, and by promoting reflective learning within workplace teams (McAllister and McKinnon 2009). However, little is currently known about effective methods of developing resilience or whether attempts to develop resilience can be sustained over time.

Midwifery can be a joyous, fulfilling and rewarding profession but it can also be challenging. All those working in the maternity services need to know how to look after their emotional wellbeing. While many studies have reported on the negative implications of stress and burnout (Tetrick and Barling 1995; Turner et al. 2002), researchers are beginning to investigate the service-users/patient benefits of positive psychology at work.

Being happy at work is a two-way commitment (Austin 2017). While employers have a legal obligation to create an environment that protects the physical and emotional wellbeing of their staff, employees should develop *compassionate resilience* and find healthy ways of coping with the inevitable challenges of contemporary midwifery practice. The concept of compassionate resilience forms the basis of *The Resilience Framework* (Stephen and Pettit 2015) shown in Fig. 2.4, that was originally developed for health visiting, but its principles can have relevance to other professions, including midwifery.

The resilience framework is underpinned by compassion, resilience models, including the compassionate mind model (Gilbert 2010), self-compassion (Neff 2011), mindfulness (Berry 2014) and resilience (Hart and Heaver 2013) and the principles of the professional *Code* and the 'Six Core Values' (the 6Cs:

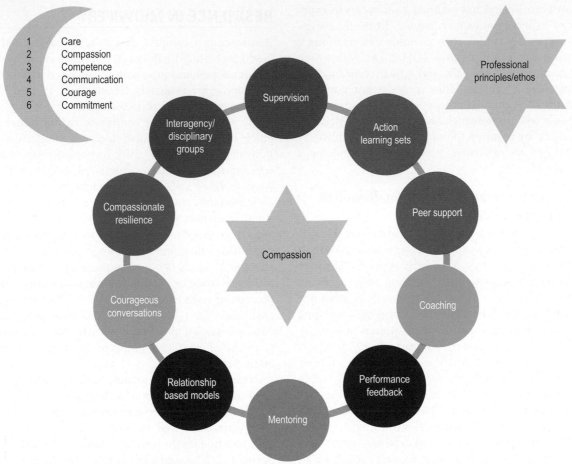

Fig. 2.4 The Resilience Framework. (Stephen R, Pettit A. (2015) Developing resilience in practice. London: Institute of Health Visiting. https://healthvisitors.files.wordpress.com/2015/03/ihv_literature-review_v9.pdf)

care, compassion, competence, communication, courage and *commitment*) (NHS Commissioning Board 2012; Francis 2013) are key components. The framework is designed to proactively support practitioners and employers to be prepared for, and cope positively with, adversity. An ecological approach to resilience incorporating individual, societal and environmental interaction and the capacities of individuals to change structures through emancipatory actions is essential. A range of 10 models and concepts of support are included and provide a menu of support to choose from: supervision, action learning, peer support, coaching, performance feedback, mentoring, relationship-based models, courageous conversations, compassionate resilience and interagency/disciplinary groups. To be effectively delivered, the framework requires compassionate and

resilient leadership, interagency education and practice and a skilled compassionate workforce (Stephen and Pettit 2015).

Six skills to support midwives in developing their ability to remain resilient and sustain compassion, even in challenging circumstances have been identified as follows:

- **Enhancing self-awareness:** Gilbert (2010) has developed a very simple model to demonstrate how brains work. Keeping this model in mind can develop awareness of personal reactions to perceived threats. It can also provide a better understanding of the reactions of others.
- **Being in the now:** Mindfulness is used as part of a wide number of psychological interventions within the NHS. It involves *paying attention without judgement*. It can reduce stress, help an

individual to regain focus and manage emotions, reduce depression, help manage pain and improve general health.

- **Developing acceptance:** Having the ability to accept that pain and suffering are an inevitable part of life and learning to accept and tolerate that they can help an individual to adjust to stress and trauma. It also helps to preserve a person's energy allowing them time to work on things that they can influence and change, as opposed to fretting about what they cannot.
- **Expressing vulnerability:** Having the ability to express feelings of vulnerability to someone who can be trusted can help an individual to manage, recognize and tolerate their emotions. Brown (2012) believes it can also facilitate growth and help develop relationships with others.
- **Building supportive relationships:** Establishing relationships that provide containment, acceptance and hope is a key factor to building resilience.
- **Fostering hope:** Having the capacity to remain hopeful by reflecting on what they are grateful for, has been identified as a contributory factor to resilience.

If individuals can be more compassionate and nurturing to themselves, they will be more able to cope with stress and deliver better and safer care. Resilience should not be viewed as a problem that needs to be *fixed* (Austin 2017). It may be that there are wider organizational issues that require attention and change. Those who have self compassion are more able to tolerate the suffering of others, stay healthier and experience successful relationships. Self-compassion skills incorporate a range of approaches such as *positive psychology* and *mindfulness*. Table 2.3 presents a summary of key recommendations to support health practitioners in developing resilience (Stephen and Pettit 2015).

CLINICAL GOVERNANCE

Clinical governance is a term used to describe the accountability processes for the *safety*, *quality* and *effectiveness* of clinical care delivered to service users and was introduced in British health policy in the late 1990s (DH 1997; Scottish Executive 1997; Welsh Office 1998; Department of Health, Social Services and Public Safety, DHSSPS 2001). It was originally defined in First Class Service (DH 1998:33) as *a framework through which NHS organizations are accountable for continuously improving the quality of their services and safeguarding high standards of care by creating an environment in which excellence in clinical care will flourish.*

The Key Components of Clinical Governance

Clinical governance has developed beyond simply being a moral principle and was made a *statutory duty* for all NHS organizations to address in the Health Act 1999, forming part of the overall drive to improve quality. It should be an integrated process in all aspects of healthcare delivery and the various processes underpinning it should in themselves be integrated with each other (Jaggs-Fowler 2011). Traditionally, clinical governance has been described according to seven key components, presented in Box 2.13, which contribute to the delivery of high-quality care. However, it may also be prudent to acknowledge that *effective leadership* and *interpersonal skills* are also vital components to the successful governance of an organization.

To assist midwives and other health and social care professionals in understanding the different tenets of clinical governance, the mnemonics identified in Box 2.14 are useful to apply in everyday practice.

Within the context of local midwifery practice, the focus of clinical governance lies in the effective partnership between women and health professionals and the establishment of midwifery networks, where the voice of service users assists in shaping local maternity services, policies, protocols, guidelines and standards. In addition, professional bodies endorse the importance of health professionals working, learning and collaborating to provide safe and effective care to childbearing women, their babies and families (RCOG/RCM/RCoA/RCPCH 2007; RCOG/RCM/RCoA 2008; RCOG 2009; RCOG/RCM 2016). Regular monitoring visits by national bodies such as the Care Quality Commission (CQC) (England), Healthcare Improvement Scotland, Healthcare Inspectorate Wales, the Regulation and Quality Improvement Authority (Northern Ireland) and assessment by the NMC through professional education programme approval and monitoring means that, from a clinical governance perspective, there can be confidence in the standard of care provided in each maternity unit.

TABLE 2.3	Summary of Key Recommendations for Developing Resilience in Midwifery Practice
Look after your physical health	Get enough sleep, eat well and find a way to fit in some exercise you enjoy.
Look after your emotional health	Build and nurture positive relationships; try to focus on the good things that have happened in your day. Build some mindfulness exercises into your busy schedule, even if it is while you are on the bus. Develop your self-awareness and emotional regulations skills. Be compassionate, kind and understanding to yourself – strengthening your inner container and silencing your inner critic. Accept your limitations and stay within your boundaries. Stay true to your values. Make time for the things you enjoy.
Recognize the importance of peer support	Help to build your team. It's the little things that are often important to building teams; offering support, expressing your own vulnerabilities makes it safe for others to do the same, remembering birthdays, having a laugh together. Look after and nurture one another. Join or start action learning sets, work discussion groups, communities of practice, etc.
Manage conflict	Remember conflict is normal in any relationship. Develop your skills in managing conflict, be brave and use conflict as an opportunity to create better understanding and strengthen your team. Don't let conflict hurt, or fester anger.
Build opportunities for job satisfaction	Build on your strengths and the work you enjoy. Develop your expertise and sense of mastery. Develop your influencing skills to ensure that those who commission and manage midwifery services recognize the importance of supporting midwives to develop relationships with women, babies and families in an unhurried way. Take responsibility for creating opportunities to develop midwifery practice. Be tenacious and bounce back quickly from set-backs. Believe in yourself.
Changing the culture you work in	Develop your knowledge on compassionate leadership and compassionate organizations. Practise with compassion – role-modelling, the approach to others. Use your knowledge to influence peers, managers, leaders, commissioners and local counsellors. Maintain hope and a belief that change is possible.
Build your formal support	Embrace opportunities to engage in formal support that is offered and seek out other opportunities, e.g. supervision, which includes a restorative function, a mentor/mentoring (remember a mentor can be useful at any point in your career), coaching, action learning and feedback. Learn to accept and welcome constructive challenges.

Adapted from Stephen R, Pettit A. (2015) Developing resilience in practice. London: Institute of Health Visiting.

Leadership in Midwifery

Within the clinical governance framework it is important to acknowledge the vital role that leadership plays. Every midwife has a key role to play in leadership, to ensure that the care provided to all childbearing women, their babies and families is safe, of high quality and their health and wellbeing optimized (NMC 2018a). The RCM have developed a *Leadership Competency Framework* (RCM 2012) based on the NHS Leadership Academy *Clinical Leadership Competency*

BOX 2.13   The Seven Key Components of Clinical Governance

Clinical Effectiveness and Research	Ensuring the best outcomes for services users and patients, i.e. the right thing to do to the right person at the right time in the right place, by:

- adopting an evidence-based approach to practice
- changing your practice, developing new protocols or guidance based on experience and evidence if current practice is shown inadequate
- implementing NICE guidelines, National Service Frameworks and other national standards to ensure optimal care (when not superseded by more recent and more effective treatments)
- conducting research to develop the body of evidence available and enhance the level of care provided to patients and service users in the future
- assessment of evidence as to whether services/treatments are cost-effective
- information systems to assess current practice and provide evidence of improvement.

Audit

The aim of the audit process is to ensure that clinical practice is continuously monitored and any deficiencies in relation to set standards of care are remedied. This is achieved through:

- quality improvement tools (such as clinical audit and evaluation) to review and improve treatments and services based on:
  - the views of patients, service users and staff
  - evidence from incidents, near-misses, clinical risks and risk analysis
  - outcomes from treatments or services
  - measurement of performance to assess whether the team/department/organization is achieving the desired goals
  - identifying areas of care that need further research.

Risk Management

This involves having robust systems in place to understand, monitor and minimize the risks to service-users, patients and staff and to learn from mistakes. When things go wrong in practice in relation to clinical care, midwives and other clinical staff should feel safe admitting it, and be able to learn, and share what they have learned. This includes:

- complying with protocols to minimize risk (e.g. hand washing, disposal of sharps, etc.)
- learning lessons from near misses
- detection and reporting of any significant adverse events via critical incident forms, examining complaints, etc.
- ensuring action is taken to prevent recurrence
- assessing the risks identified for their probability of occurrence and the impact they may have if an incident did occur
- implementing processes to reduce the risk and its impact (dependent on financial resources available and the seriousness of risk)
- promoting a blame-free culture to encourage everyone to report concerns and mistakes.

Education and Training

Appropriate support is required to enable staff to be competent in their role and to develop their knowledge and skills to keep up-to-date. Professional development should be continuous: *lifelong learning*. For midwives this relates to:

- fulfilling NMC (2019a) requirements for triennial revalidation
- peer review through employer-led supervision models (PMA or clinical supervisor)
- annual performance appraisal to identify strengths and areas for further development and improvement
- promoting individual learning and learning across the organization
  - professional development programmes
  - dissemination of good practice, ideas and innovation.

Continued

BOX 2.13   The Seven Key Components of Clinical Governance—cont'd

Patient and Public Involvement (PPI)

This aspect is about ensuring that the services provided are in accordance with the needs of the local service-user and patient population, based on their feedback that is used to develop services and improve their quality. This can be achieved through:
- local service-user/patient/carer feedback
- the involvement of the *Patient Advice and Liaison Service (PALS)* in handling concerns from the public
- national patient surveys organized by the Healthcare commission that feed into local NHS Trust rankings
- Local Involvement Networks (LINks) have been introduced to enable communities to influence healthcare services at a local level (previously known as 'Patient Forums')
- National Maternity Voices support the establishment of Maternity Voice Partnerships in reviewing and contributing to local maternity care at Local Maternity System (LMS) level
- Foundation Trust Board of Governors who are elected members of the local community and have a voice in the organization of the local Trust and the services it provides.

Using Information and Technology

This aspect is about ensuring that:
- patient data is accurate, high-quality and up-to-date
- confidentiality of patient data is always respected
- full and appropriate use of data is made to measure quality of outcomes (through audit) and to develop services according to local needs.

Staffing and Staff Management Communication

This aspect relates to:
- appropriate recruitment and management of staff
- ensuring that underperformance is identified and addressed
- encouraging staff retention by motivating and developing staff
- providing a conducive and supportive work environment.

BOX 2.14   Useful Clinical Governance Mnemonics

C	Clinical effectiveness	**P**	Patient and public involvement	**S**	Staff management
A	Audit	**I**	Information and technology	**P**	Patient and public involvement
R	Risk management	**R**	Risk management	**A**	Audit
E	Education and training	**A**	Audit	**R**	Risk management
		T	Training and education	**E**	Effectiveness (clinical)
		E	Effectiveness (clinical)	**I**	Information and technology
		S	Staff management	**T**	Training and education

Framework (NHS Leadership Academy 2011). The framework describes the following attributes that midwives should possess to deliver the governance framework:

- **Midwives show leadership by ensuring patient safety:** assess and manage the risk of patients while balancing economic considerations with the priority of patient safety
- **Midwives show leadership by critically evaluating:** think analytically to identify where service

improvements can be made, working individually or as part of a team

- **Midwives show leadership by encouraging improvement and innovation:** create a climate of continuous service improvement
- **Midwives show leadership by facilitating transformation:** contribute to the change process that leads to improvements in healthcare.

The central core of the Midwifery Leadership Competency Framework applies to all healthcare workers engaged in clinical practice and is built on the concept of shared leadership. This indicates that leadership is not restricted to individuals who hold designated leadership roles, but is where there is a shared sense of responsibility for the success of the organization and its services. As acts of leadership can come from anyone in the organization, they should be focused on the achievement of the group rather than of an individual.

Audit

Clinical audit is a process that is undertaken to review and evaluate the effectiveness of practice by measuring standards of health/midwifery care against national benchmarks. It is important to ensure that the auditing process is comprehensive, multidisciplinary and centred upon the women who receive the care and that the audit loop is closed completely. This means that, should the data collected reveal any shortfall in meeting clinical standards, strategies to rectify such a deficit should always be implemented. Furthermore, when a change in practice is implemented, there should always be an evaluation to ensure the audit cycle develops into an audit spiral, leading to improved health care.

In midwifery, local surveys should take place regularly to monitor women's satisfaction with their maternity care to ensure these achieve the expected standards as well as identify areas for improvement. Midwives have a responsibility to identify areas of clinical practice that would benefit from auditing and further inquiry/research.

To address clinical governance, each maternity unit/service is expected to publish its local statistics and monitor generic indicators of the effectiveness and efficiency of health care. Such outcomes include healthcare-acquired infection (HCAI), infant mortality, neonatal mortality and stillbirths, women's experiences of childbirth and admission of full-term babies to neonatal care.

RISK MANAGEMENT

Risk management is the systematic identification, analysis and control of any potential and actual risk and of any circumstances that put individuals at risk of harm. The concept was introduced in the mid-1990s with the principal aim of reducing litigation costs. Organizations such as the UK NHS are expected to adhere to the legislation pertaining to health and safety in the workplace and other legal principles such as *the duty of care* to both the public and employees as part of their

risk management strategy (CQC 2010; NHS Resolution 2017). Managing risk is therefore a fundamental component of clinical governance.

When a risk is evaluated, it is not only important to consider the *probability* of something adverse happening but also the consequences if it should happen. In the context of health care, risk is usually associated with health risks, injury and death. More specifically within the context of maternity care, the *risk of harm* would include injury to a woman and/or her baby during childbirth or to a health professional engaged in providing maternity care. The *risk of detriment* is associated with some form of economic/social loss, which may not only include a valuation of harm to individuals but also damage on a much wider scale, such as adverse publicity for the local maternity services. All health service managers are expected to be conversant in risk management theory in order to identify and manage risk, so that the probability of harm or detriment is lessened and the consequences of risk are reduced. Part of risk management is to keep a Risk Register that should be reviewed regularly. The organization's Board is responsible for monitoring the risks identified in the organization's Risk Register. A traffic light system is often used to indicate the level of risk pertaining to each indicator:

- GREEN: indicates the goal has been achieved.
- AMBER: the goal is not met and action is required to prevent movement into the RED zone.
- RED: the goal is not met and the upper threshold is breached. Urgent action is required from the highest level to maintain safety and restore quality care.

Risks can be identified through a range of sources such as incident reporting (internal) and complaints from service-users and patients (external). Midwives are responsible for identifying incidents and taking steps to reduce risk of harm to women and babies (NMC 2018a). An investigation and root-cause analysis of each clinical incident are essential in identifying the contributory factors, including those human factors that have resulted in harm to the woman and baby. It is also useful to identify themes/trends from clinical incidents such that similar incidents may be investigated together. Recommendations arising from investigations and any subsequent actions should always be logged and recorded when completed.

Policies, Protocols, Guidelines and Standards

All healthcare providers are required to have policies, protocols, guidelines and standards in place to govern safe, effective and quality care to the public. It is important that midwives understand the differences between these definitions in order to utilize them appropriately in their clinical practice.

Policies are general principles or directions, usually without the mandatory approach for addressing an issue. They are a means of ensuring a consistent standard of care to avoid any confusion over practice and are often set at national level, for example: *National Maternity Review: Better Births: Improving outcomes of maternity services in England – A five year forward view for maternity services* (NHS England 2016) and *The Best Start review: a five year forward plan for neonatal and maternity services in Scotland* (Scottish Government 2017). Policies should make clear the procedures that will be followed by midwives, doctors and support staff. There are differing views about the benefits of policies, ranging from ensuring safe practice and providing consistency, to restricting midwives' autonomy. Indeed, if a midwife's clinical judgement on an individual woman's care is at odds with policy, she may be in breach of her contract of employment unless she can justify her actions.

The term *protocol* is often used interchangeably with *guideline*. A 'protocol' is usually regarded as a local initiative that practitioners are expected to follow, but may also vary in meaning, e.g. a written agreement between parties, a multidisciplinary action plan for managing care or an action plan for a clinical trial. Protocols therefore determine individual aspects of practice and should be based on the latest evidence. Most protocols are binding on employees, as they usually relate to the management of individuals with urgent, life-threatening conditions, for example antepartum haemorrhage, such that if the practitioner does not work within the protocol, they would be deemed to be in breach of their contract of employment. However, it would not be expected to have protocols for the care of healthy women experiencing a physiological labour and birth.

Guidelines are usually less specific than protocols and may be described as suggestions for criteria or levels of performance that are provided to implement agreed *standards*. Both 'guidelines' and 'standards' should be based on contemporary, reliable research findings and include specific outcomes, which act as performance indicators, upon which progress can be measured as evidence of achievement within an agreed timescale. The National Institute for Health and Care Excellence (NICE) sets guidelines for clinical practice in all areas of health care,

including maternity and neonatal care, to provide good practice guidance for midwives and obstetricians. NICE guidance officially applies to England only, however, it has agreements to provide certain product and services to Wales, Scotland and Northern Ireland. The devolved administrations make the decisions on how NICE guidance applies in these countries.

The interpretation and application of a guideline remains the responsibility of individual practitioners, as each midwife should be aware of local circumstances and the needs and wishes of informed women. Guidelines are therefore tools to assist the midwife in making the most appropriate clinical decision in partnership with the woman, based on best available evidence.

It is acknowledged that there is a plethora of 'clinical guidelines' not only produced by NICE but also organizations such as the Scottish Intercollegiate Guidelines Network (SIGN), RCOG and RCM. However, as variations in outcomes persist, it is essential that commissioners build into their contracts, the requirements to deliver services to national standards and to manage performance against these. It is the responsibility of the Care Quality Commission (CQC) in England, Healthcare Improvement Scotland (HIS), the Regulation and Quality Improvement Authority in Northern Ireland (RQIA) and Healthcare Inspectorate Wales (HIW) to monitor health services against national standards in the respective UK countries.

Clinical Negligence Scheme for Trusts

The Clinical Negligence Scheme for Trusts (CNST) is a voluntary risk-pooling scheme for negligence claims arising out of incidents occurring after 1 April 1995. The scheme has been administered by NHS Resolution since April 2017 (formerly NHS Litigation Authority, NHSLA) and its purpose is to provide expertise to the NHS to resolve concerns fairly, share learning for improvement and preserve resources for patient care. All NHS Trusts including Foundation Trusts belong to the Scheme by paying an insurance premium based on their individual compliance to certain incentives general standards. There are equivalent schemes in Scotland (Clinical Negligence and Other Risks Indemnity Scheme, CNORIS), in Wales (the Welsh Risk Pool) and Northern Ireland. These schemes help to resolve disputes and claims between patients and the NHS as well as aim to keep legal actions out of court to keep the cost down.

BOX 2.15   The 10 Maternity Safety Actions (NHS Resolution 2019)

Safety action 1   Are you using the National Perinatal Mortality Review Tool to review perinatal deaths to the required standard?

Safety action 2   Are you submitting data to the Maternity Services Data Set to the required standard?

Safety action 3   Can you demonstrate that you have transitional care facilities to support the *Avoiding Term Admissions into the Neonatal Units Programme*?

Safety action 4   Can you demonstrate an effective system of medical workforce planning to the required standard?

Safety action 5   Can you demonstrate an effective system of midwifery workforce planning to the required standard?

Safety action 6   Can you demonstrate compliance with all four elements of the *Saving Babies' Lives Care Bundle*?

Safety action 7   Can you demonstrate that you have a patient feedback mechanism for maternity services and that you regularly act on feedback?

Safety action 8   Can you evidence that 90% of each maternity unit staff group have attended an in-house multiprofessional maternity emergencies training session within the last training year?

Safety action 9   Can you demonstrate that the trust safety champions (obstetricians and midwife) are meeting bi-monthly with Board level champions to escalate locally identified issues?

Safety action 10   Have you reported 100% of qualifying (year) incidents under *NHS Resolution's Early Notification Scheme*?

It has been reported by NHS Resolution (2019) that within 2018–19, of the clinical negligence claims notified, obstetric claims represented 10% (1068) of clinical claims by number but 50% of the total value of new claims: £2465.5 million of the total £4931.8 million. The Maternity Safety Strategy set out the Department of Health and Social Care's strategy to reward those who have taken action to improve maternity safety. This includes the maternity incentive scheme that rewards Trusts who meet 10 safety actions designed to improve the delivery of best practice in maternity and neonatal services as shown in Box 2.15. The 10 actions have been agreed in partnership with the Collaborative Advisory Group which was established by NHS Resolution. The Collaborative Advisory Group includes:

- The Department of Health and Social Care
- NHS Digital
- NHS England
- NHS Improvement
- Royal College of Obstetricians and Gynaecologists
- Royal College of Midwives
- Mothers and Babies: Reducing Risk through Audit and Confidential Enquiries (MBRRACE)
- Royal College of Anaesthetists
- Care Quality Commission.

Trusts that demonstrate they have achieved all of the 10 safety actions will recover the element of their contribution to the CNST maternity incentive fund and also receive a share of any unallocated funds. Trusts that do not meet the 10-out-of-10 threshold will not recover their contribution to the CNST maternity incentive fund, but may be eligible for a small discretionary payment from the scheme to help them make progress against those actions they have not achieved. This payment will be at a much lower level than the 10% contribution to the incentive fine.

REFLECTIVE ACTIVITY FOR SELF-ASSESSMENT

1. With reference to the four themes contained within *The Code* (NMC 2018a) and the *Enabling Professionalism Framework* (NMC 2017b), identify how you fulfil these standards when caring for childbearing women and their babies. Provide examples of how you demonstrate *advocacy, accountability, competence* and *leadership* in your current role and position within the organization you work.

2. How does your employing organization address the requirements of the Human Medicines Regulations (2012) in respect of midwifery practice? Select a woman from your caseload who has required medicines during the childbirth continuum, identify each category of medicines they each fall under and reflect upon your role in their supply, prescription and administration.

3. You suspect a woman in your care is in an abusive relationship. What are your professional and legal obligations in such a case to safeguard the woman and her baby? From whom may you gain support and guidance in this instance?

4. What is your professional, legal and ethical responsibility towards providing a safe and harmonious working environment? How do you support new staff and students to feel part of the midwifery team and the wider multiprofessional team in your workplace?

5. Review the social media sources that you use. Select a number of items from each source that have been posted and with reference to the NMC *Code* and *guidance on using social media responsibly,* determine to what extent they have been posted responsibly and uphold the reputation of the midwifery profession. What factors have you taken into consideration to reach your decisions? Should you be concerned about a particular post that in your opinion fails to uphold the professional standards of practice and behaviour of midwives, what would your subsequent action(s) be as a responsible registrant?

REFERENCES

Anti-Slavery International. (2019). *Slavery in the UK.* Available at: www.antislavery.org/slavery-today/slavery-uk.

Austin, J. A. (2017). What a difference a day makes. *Midwives* 20(Summer):68–69.

Baird, B., Murray, R., Seale, B., et al. (2015). *Midwifery regulation in the United Kingdom.* Available at: www.nmc.org.uk/globalassets/sitedocuments/councilpapersanddocuments/council-2015/kings-fund-review.pdf.

Barnados. (2019). *Child sexual exploitation.* Available at: www.barnardos.org.uk/what_we_do/our_work/sexual_exploitation/about-cse/cse-our-work.htm.

Beauchamp, T. L., & Childress, J. F. (2019). *Principles of biomedical ethics* (8th ed.). Oxford: Oxford University Press.

Bell, D., & Jarvie, A. (2015). Preventing 'where next'. Patients, professionals and learning from serious failings in care. *Journal of the Royal College of Physicians of Edinburgh, 45,* 4–8.

Bergman, R. (1981). Accountability: Definition and dimensions. *International Nursing Review, 28*(2), 3–9.

Berry, C. (2014). Wellbeing in four policy areas. *Report by the all-party parliamentary group on wellbeing economics.* London: New Economics Foundation.

Brotherton, V. (2016). *Time to deliver: Considering pregnancy and parenthood in the UK's response to human trafficking.* London: The Anti-Trafficking Monitoring Group.

Brown, B. (2012). *Daring greatly: How the courage to be vulnerable transforms the way we live, love, parent and lead.* London: Penguin Books Ltd.

CQC (Care Quality Commission). (2010). *Guidance about compliance: Essential standards of quality and safety.* London: CQC.

CQC (Care Quality Commission). (2017). *Key lines of enquiry, prompts and ratings characteristics for healthcare services.* Available at: www.cqc.org.uk/guidance-providers/healthcare/key-lines-enquiry-healthcare-services.

Castro Lopes, S., Nove, A., Ten Hoope-Bender, P., et al. (2016). A descriptive analysis of midwifery education, regulation and association in 73 countries: The baseline for a post-2015 pathway. *Human Resources for Health, 14*(1), 37.

Cicchetti, D. (2010). Resilience under conditions of extreme stress: A multi-level perspective. *World Psychiatry, 9,* 145–154.

DH (Department of Health). (1997). *The new NHS: Modern dependable.* London: TSO.

DH (Department of Health). (1998). *First class service.* London: HMSO.

DH (Department of Health). (2006). The regulation of the non-medical healthcare professions. *A review by the Department of Health.* Chair: Andrew Foster. Available at: www.pmguk.co.uk/data/page_files/publications%20and%20reports/2006/R.RegulationNon-medicalHealthProf.pdf.

DH (Department of Health). (2007). *Trust, assurance and safety: The regulation of health professions in the 21st century.* CM7013. London: TSO.

DH (Department of Health). (2009). *Reference guide to consent for examination or treatment* (2nd ed.). London: DH.

DH (Department of Health). (2014). *Health visiting and school nursing programmes: Supporting implementation of the new service model. No 5: Domestic violence and abuse – Professional guidance.* London: DH.

DH (Department of Health). (2016). *Proposals for changing the system of midwifery supervision in the UK.* London: DH. Available at: www.gov.uk/government/publications/changes-to-midwife-supervision-in-the-uk.

DHSSPS (Department of Health, Social Services and Public Safety). (2001). *Best practice – best care: A framework for setting standards, delivering services and improving monitoring and regulation in the HPSS.* Belfast: DHSSPS.

Donaldson, L. (2006). *Good doctors, safer patients: Proposals to strengthen the system to assure and improve the performance of doctors and to protect the safety of the public.* London: DH.

Dutton, J. E., Workman, K. M., & Hardin, A. E. (2014). Compassion at work. *Annual Review of Organisational Psychology and Organisational Behaviour, 1*, 277–304.

Duxbury, F. (2014). Domestic violence and abuse. In S. Bewley, & J. Welch (Eds.), *ABC of domestic and sexual violence* (pp. 9–16). Chichester: John Wiley and Sons.

Edwards, S. D. (1996). *Nursing ethics: A principle-based approach*. Basingstoke: Macmillan.

Equality and Human Rights Commission. (2016). *Equality Act guidance*. Available at: www.equalityhuman-rights.com/en/advice-and-guidance/equality-act-guidance#h1.

Francis, R. (2013). *Report of the mid staffordshire NHS foundation trust public inquiry. Chairman: Robert Francis QC*. London: The Stationery Office.

Gilbert, P. (2010). *The compassionate mind: A new approach to life's challenges*. London: Constable.

Gillman, L. J., & Lloyd, C. (2015). *Re-framing midwifery supervision: A discussion paper*. Available at: www.rcm.org.uk/sites/default/files/Re framing%20supervision%20-paper%20for%20discussion%-20final%2023%203%202015.pdf.

GMC/NMC (General Medical Council and Nursing and Midwifery Council). (2015). *Openness and honesty when things go wrong: The professional duty of candour*. London: GMC and NMC.

Hart, A., & Heaver, B. (2013). Evaluating resilience-based programs for schools using a systematic consultative review. *Journal of Child and Youth Development, 1*(1), 27–53.

Hawkins, P., & Shohet, R. (2012). *Supervision in the helping professions* (4th ed.). Maidenhead: Open University Press.

HM Government. (2018a). *Information sharing advice for practitioners providing safeguarding services to children, young people, parents and carers*. London: DfE. Available at: https://assets.publishing.service.gov.uk/government/uploads/system/uploads/attachment_data/file/721581/Information_sharing_advice_practitioners_safeguarding_services.pdf.

HM Government. (2018b). *Working together to safeguard children: A guide to inter-agency working to safeguard and promote the welfare of children*. London: DfE. Available at: https://assets.publishing.service.gov.uk/government/uploads/system/uploads/attachment_data/file/779401/Working_Together_to_Safeguard-Children.pdf.

Hunter, B., & Warren, L. (2014). Midwives experience of workplace resilience. *Midwifery, 30*(8), 926–934.

ICM (International Confederation of Midwives). (2011). *Global standards for midwifery regulation*. The Hague: ICM. Available at: www.internationalmidwives.org/assets/files/general-files/2018/04/global-standards-for-midwifery-regulation-eng.pdf.

ICM (International Confederation of Midwives). (2013). *Global standards for midwifery education*. Available at: www.internationalmidwives.org/assets/uploads/documents/CoreDocuments/ICM%20Standards%20Guidelines_ammended2013.pdf.

ICM (International Confederation of Midwives). (2019). *Essential competencies for midwifery practice*. The Hague: ICM. Available at: www.internationalmidwives.org/assets/files/general-files/2019/03/icm-competencies-en-screens.pdf.

Jaggs-Fowler, R. M. (2011). Clinical governance. *InnovAiT: Education and Inspiration for General Practice, 4*(10), 592–595.

J. M. Consulting (1998). *The regulation of nurses, midwives and health visitors: Report on a review of the nurses, midwives and health visitors Act 1997*. Bristol: JM Consulting Ltd.

Kennedy, I. (2001). The Report of the Public Inquiry into Children's Heart Surgery at the Bristol Royal Infirmary 1984–95: Learning from Bristol. Chair: Professor Ian Kennedy. London: The Stationery Office.

Kirkup, B. (2015). *The Report of the Morecambe Bay Investigation*. Preston, Lancashire: The Stationery Office. Available at: www.gov.uk/government/uploads/system/uploads/attachment_data/file/408480/47487_MBI_Accessible_v0.1.pdf.

Knight, M., Bunch, K., Tuffnell, D., et al. (Eds.) (2019); on behalf of MBRRACE-UK. *Saving Lives Improving Mothers' Care – Lessons learned to inform maternity care from the UK and Ireland Confidential Enquiries into Maternal Deaths and Morbidity 2015–2017*. Oxford: National Perinatal Epidemiology Unit, University of Oxford. Available at: www.npeu.ox.ac.uk/downloads/files/mbrrace-uk/reports/MBRRACE-UK%20Maternal%20Report%202018%20-%20Web%20Version.pdf.

Law, Society (2012). *Equality Act 2010 practice notes*. Available at: www.lawsociety.org.uk/support-services/advice/practice-notes/equality-act-2010.

Melia, K. (1989). *Everyday nursing ethics*. London: Macmillan.

McAllister, M., & McKinnon, J. (2009). The importance of teaching and learning resilience in the health disciplines: A critical review of the literature. *Nurse Education Today, 29*(4), 371–379.

National Advisory Group on the Safety of Patients in England. (2013). Chair: Berwick D. *A promise to learn – a commitment to act: Improving the safety of patients in England*. London: DH. Available at: www.gov.uk/government/uploads/system/uploads/attachment_data/file/226703/Berwick_Report.pdf.

NHS Commissioning Board. (2012). *Compassion in practice: Nursing, midwifery and care staff our vision and strategy*. London: DH.

NHS England. (2017). *A-EQUIP: a model of clinical midwifery supervision*. Available at: www.england.nhs.uk/wp-content/uploads/2017/04/a-equip-midwifery-supervision-model.pdf.

NHS England. (2016). *National maternity review. Better births: Improving outcomes of maternity services in England: A five year forward view for maternity care.* London: NHS England. Available at: www.england.nhs.uk/wp-content/uploads/2016/02/national-maternity-review-report.pdf.

NHS England and NHS Improvement. (2015). *Safeguarding Policy.* Available at: www.england.nhs.uk/wp-content/uploads/2019/09/safeguarding-policy.pdf.

NHS Leadership Academy. (2011). *Clinical Leadership Competency Framework.* Coventry: NHS Leadership Academy. Available at: www.leadershipacademy.nhs.uk/wp-content/uploads/2012/11/NHSLeadership-Leadership-Framework-Clinical-Leadership-Competency-Framework-CLCF.pdf.

NHS Resolution. (2017). *Delivering fair resolution and learning from harm: Our strategy to 2022.* London: NHS Resolution.

NHS Resolution. (2019). *Maternity Incentive Scheme.* Available at: https://resolution.nhs.uk/services/claims-management/clinical-schemes/clinical-negligence-scheme-for-trusts/maternity-incentive-scheme.

NICE (National Institute for Health and Care Excellence). (2014). *Domestic violence and abuse: Multi-agency working. PH50.* London: NICE. Available at: www.nice.org.uk/guidance/ph50/resources/domestic-violence-and-abuse-multiagency-working-pdf-1996411687621.

NSPCC (National Society for the Prevention of Cruelty to Children). (2019). *Domestic abuse.* Available at: www.nspcc.org.uk/what-is-child-abuse/types-of-abuse/domestic-abuse/#effects.

Neff, K. (2011). Self-compassion, self-esteem and wellbeing. *Social and Personality Psychology Compass, 5*(1), 1–12.

Ness, V., & Richards, J. (2014). Future proofing supervision in Wales: Improving the quality of statutory supervision. *British Journal of Midwifery, 22*(4), 276–280.

NMC (Nursing and Midwifery Council). (2009). *Survey of European midwifery regulation.* London: NMC.

NMC (Nursing and Midwifery Council). (2012). *Midwives rules and standards.* London: NMC.

NMC (Nursing and Midwifery Council). (2017a). *Practising as a midwife in the UK. An overview of midwifery regulation.* London: NMC.

NMC (Nursing and Midwifery Council). (2017b). *Enabling professionalism in nursing and midwifery practice.* London: NMC. Available at: www.nmc.org.uk/globalassets/sitedocuments/other-publications/enabling-professionalism.pdf.

NMC (Nursing and Midwifery Council). (2018a). *The code: Professional standards of practice and behaviour for nurses, midwives and nursing associates.* London: NMC.

NMC (Nursing and Midwifery Council). (2018b). *Realising professionalism: Standards for education and training. Part1: Standards framework for nursing and midwifery education.* London: NMC.

NMC (Nursing and Midwifery Council). (2018c). *Realising professionalism: Standards for education and training. Part 2: Standards for student supervision and assessment.* London: NMC.

NMC (Nursing and Midwifery Council). (2019a). *How to revalidate with the NMC.* London: NMC. Available at: www.nmc.org.uk/globalassets/sitedocuments/revalidation/how-to-revalidate-booklet.pdfhttp://revalidation.nmc.org.uk.

NMC (Nursing and Midwifery Council). (2019b). *The NMC register: 31 March 2019.* London: NMC. Available at: www.nmc.org.uk/globalassets/sitedocuments/other-publications/nmc-register-data-march-19.pdf.

NMC (Nursing and Midwifery Council). (2019c). *Realising professionalism: Standards for education and training. Part 3: Standards for pre-registration midwifery programmes.* London: NMC.

NMC (Nursing and Midwifery Council). (2019d). *Standards of proficiency for midwives.* London: NMC.

NMC (Nursing and Midwifery Council). (2019e). *Practising as a midwife in the UK. An overview of midwifery regulation.* London: NMC.

NMC (Nursing and Midwifery Council). (2019f). *Guidance on using social media responsibly.* London: NMC. Available at: www.nmc.org.uk/globalassets/sitedocuments/nmc-publications/social-media-guidance.pdf.

ONS (Office for National Statistics). (2018). *Domestic abuse in England and Wales: Year ending March 2018. How domestic abuse is dealt with at the local level within England and Wales, using annual data from the crime survey for England and Wales, police recorded crime and a number of different organizations.* Newport: ONS.

PHSO (Parliamentary and Health Service Ombudsman). (2013). *Midwifery supervision and regulation: Recommendations for change.* Available at: www.ombudsman.org.uk/sites/default/files/Midwifery%20supervision%20and%20regulation_%20recommendations%20for%20change.pdf.

Proctor, B. (1986). Supervision: A co-operative exercise in accountability. In M. Marken, & M. Payne (Eds.), *Enabling and ensuring – supervision in practice.* Leicester: National Youth Bureau Council for Education and Training in Youth and Community Work.

PSA (Professional Standards Authority for Health and Social Care). (2014). *Written evidence for the public administration select committee follow up session on the parliamentary and health service ombudsman's* report into severe sepsis and midwifery supervision and regulation. London: PSA. Available at: www.professionalstandards.org.uk/docs/default-source/publications/consultation-response/others-consultations/2014/-pase-evidence-severe-sepsis-and-midwifery-supervision-and-regulation.pdf?sfvrsn=55a47f20_9.

PHE (Public Health England). (2015). *Disability and domestic abuse: Risk, impacts and response*. London: PHE.

Purdy, S., & Read, J. (2019). Employer-led models of midwifery supervision. In J. E. Marshall (Ed.), *Myles professional studies for midwifery education and practice: Concepts and challenges* (pp. 159–173). Edinburgh: Elsevier.

RCM (Royal College of Midwives). (2012). *Midwifery leadership competency framework*. London: RCM.

RCM (Royal College of Midwives). (2019). *Strengthening midwifery leadership; A manifesto for better maternity care*. London: RCM.

RCOG (Royal College of Obstetricians and Gynaecologists). (2009). *Improving patient safety: Risk management for maternity and gynaecology: Clinical governance advice 2*. London: RCOG Press.

RCOG/RCM (Royal College of Obstetricians and Gynaecologists, Royal College of Midwives). (2016). *Joint RCOG/RCM statement on multi-disciplinary working and continuity of carer*. Available at: www.rcog.org.uk/en/news/joint-rcogrcm-statement-on-multi-disciplinary-working-and-continuity-of-carer.

RCOG/RCM/RCoA (Royal College of Obstetricians and Gynaecologists, Royal College of Midwives, Royal College of Anaesthetists). (2008). *Standards for maternity care: Report of a working party*. London: RCOG Press.

RCOG/RCM/RCoA/RCPCH (Royal College of Obstetricians and Gynaecologists, Royal College of Midwives, Royal College of Anaesthetists, Royal College of Paediatrics and Child Health). (2007). *Safer childbirth: Minimum standards for the organisation and delivery of care in labour*. London: RCOG Press.

Rutter, M. (2012). Resilience as a dynamic concept. *Development and Psychopathology, 24*(2), 335–344.

Scottish Executive. (1997). *Designed to care: Renewing the national health service in Scotland*. Edinburgh: Scottish Executive Health Department.

Scottish Government. (2017). *The best start review: A five year forward plan for neonatal and maternity services in Scotland*. Edinburgh: The Scottish Government. Available at: www.gov.scot/publications/best-start-five-year-forward-plan-maternity-neonatal-care-scotland.

Shah, P. S., & Shah, J. (2010). Maternal exposure to domestic violence and pregnancy and birth outcomes. A systematic review and meta-analysis. *Journal of Women's Health, 19*(11) 2017–31.

Smith, J. (2004). *The Shipman inquiry: Fifth report, safeguarding patients lessons from the past – proposals for the future. Chair: Dame Janet Smith*. London: The Stationery Office.

Stephen, R., & Pettit, A. (2015). *Developing resilience in practice*. London: Institute of Health Visiting. Available at: https://healthvisitors.files.wordpress.com/2015/03/ihv_literature-review_v9.pdf.

Strickland, P., & Allen, G. (2018). *Domestic violence in England and Wales: Briefing paper No. 6337*. London: House of Commons Library.

Tetrick, L. E., & Barling, J. (Eds.). (1995). *Changing employment relations: Behavioural and social perspective*. Washington DC: American Psychological Association.

Turner, N., Barking, J., Etpitropaki, O., Butcher, V., & Milner, C. (2002). Transformational leadership and moral reasoning. *Journal of Applied Psychology, 87*(2), 304–311.

UNICEF-UK. (2019). *Guide to the UNICEF-UK Baby Friendly Initiative University Standards* (2nd ed.). Available at: www.unicef.org.uk/babyfriendly/wp-content/uploads/sites/2/2019/07/Guide-to-the-Unicef-UK-Baby-Friendly-Initiative-University-Standards.pdf.

UNFPA/ICM/WHO (United Nations Population Fund, International Confederation of Midwives and World Health Organization). (2014). *The state of the world's midwifery 2014: A universal pathway. A woman's right to health*. New York: UNFPA.

Walshe, K. (2003). *Inquiries: Learning from failure in the NHS?* London: The Nuffield Trust.

Walshe, K. (2009). Regulating health professionals. In J. Healy, & P. Dugdale (Eds.), *Patient safety first: Responsive regulation in healthcare* (pp. 144–166). New South Wales: Allen and Unwin.

Welsh Office. (1998). *NHS Wales quality care and clinical excellence*. Cardiff: Welsh Office.

Wendt, S., Tuckey, M. R., & Prosser, B. (2011). Thriving, not just surviving, in emotionally demanding fields of practice. *Health and Social Care in the Community, 19*(3), 317–325.

WHO (World Health Organization). (2018). *Female genital mutilation: Fact sheet*. Geneva: WHO. Available at: www.who.int/news-room/fact-sheets/detail/female-genital-mutilation.

CASES

Bolam v. Friern Hospital Management Committee [HMC] 1957 1 WLR 582

Gillick v. West Norfolk and Wisbech AHA 1985 3 All ER 402

Montgomery v. Lanarkshire Health Board [2015] UKSC 11

STATUTES, ORDERS AND DIRECTIVES

Charities Act 2011, London: HMSO

Children Act 1989 (Chapter 41: England and Wales), London: HMSO

Children (Scotland) Act 1995, London: HMSO

Children (Northern Ireland) Order 1995, London: HMSO

Children Act 2004 (Chapter 31), London: HMSO

Congenital Disabilities (Civil Liability) Act 1976 Chapter 28, London: HMSO

Directive 2013 /55/EU *(the 'Modernised' Directive)* of the European Parliament and of the Council of 20 November 2013 amending Directive 2005/36/EC on the recognition of professional qualifications and Regulation EU No 1024/2012 on administrative cooperation through the Internal Market Information System (*'the IMI Regulation'*)

Equality Act 2010 (Chapter 15), London: HMSO

EU General Data Protection Regulation (GDPR) 2018

European Communities Act 1972

European Convention for the Protection of Human Rights and Fundamental Freedoms 1951, London: HMSO

Family Law Act 1986 (Chapter 55), London: HMSO

Female Genital Mutilation Act 2003 (Chapter 31), London: HMSO

Health Care and Associated Professions (Indemnity Arrangements) Order 2014 SI 2014 N0 1887 (*The Indemnity Order*)

House of Lords Hansard (2017) Nursing and Midwifery (Amendment) Order 28 February 2017: Vol. 779. Available at: https://hansard.parliament.uk/Lords/2017-02–28/debates/1B4AAA1D-1823–4038-B24D-7523943A9F37/NursingAndMidwifery(Amendment)Order2017.

Health Act 1999 (Chapter 8), London: HMSO.

Health Care and Associated Professions (Indemnity Arrangements) Order 2014 [The Indemnity Order], London: TSO.

Health and Safety at Work Act 1974, London: HMSO.

Health and Social Care Act 2012, London: TSO

Human Medicines Regulations 2012 Statutory Instrument 2012 No 1916, London: TSO

Human Medicines (Amendment) Regulations 2019 Statutory Instruments 2019 No. 62, London: TSO

Human Rights Act 1998, London: HMSO

Medical Act 1858 London: HMSO

Medicines Act 1968, London: HMSO

Mental Capacity Act 2005, London: TSO

Midwives Act 1902 (England and Wales), London: HMSO

Midwives (Scotland) Act 1915, London: HMSO

Midwives (Ireland) Act 1918, London: HMSO

Midwives Act 1926, London: HMSO

Midwives Act 1934, London: HMSO

Midwives Act 1936, London: HMSO

Midwives Act 1950, London: HMSO

Midwives Act 1951, London: HMSO

Midwives (Scotland) Act 1951, London: HMSO

Modern Slavery Act 2015 Chapter 30, London: HMSO

Nurses, Midwives and Health Visitors Act 1979, London: HMSO

Nurses, Midwives and Health Visitors Act 1992, London: HMSO

Nurses, Midwives and Health Visitors Act 1997, London: HMSO

Nurses Registration Act (England and Wales) 1919, London: HMSO

Nursing and Midwifery Council (Education, Registration and Registrations Appeals) Rules 2004 Statutory Instrument 2004 No. 1767, London: TSO

Nursing and Midwifery Council (Fitness to Practise) (Education, Registration and Registrations Appeals) Amendment Rules Order of Council 2015, Statutory Instrument 2015 No. 52, London: TSO

Nursing and Midwifery Order 2001 Statutory Instrument 2002 No. 253 [The Order], London: TSO

Nursing and Midwifery (Amendment) Order 2017 Statutory Instrument 2017 No. 321, London: TSO

Pharmacy Act 1852, London: HMSO

Prohibition of Female Circumcision Act 1985 Chapter 35, London: HMSO

Safeguarding Vulnerable Groups Act 2006 (Controlled Activity and Miscellaneous Provisions) Regulations 2010 Statutory Instrument 2010 No. 1146, London: TSO

Serious Crimes Act 2015 Chapter 9, London: HMSO

United Nations Conventions on the Rights of the Child 1989

ANNOTATED FURTHER READING

Beauchamp, T. L., & Childress, J. F. (2019). *Principles of biomedical ethics* (8th ed.). Oxford: Oxford University Press.

This popular best-selling text provides a highly original, practical and insightful guide to morality in the health professions. Drawing from contemporary research and integrating detailed case studies and vivid real-life examples and scenarios, the authors demonstrate how ethical principles can be expanded to apply to various conflicts and dilemmas in clinical practice, including delivering bad news.

Marshall, J. E. (2019). *Myles professional studies for midwifery education and practice: Concepts and challenges.* Edinburgh: Elsevier.

This text explores the non-clinical areas of midwifery education and practice, such as ethics and law, employer-led supervision, the principles of coaching and continuing professional development, in a helpful and user-friendly format. The inclusion of real-life case studies and reflective activities assist the reader in applying the theory to practice.

USEFUL WEBSITES

Against violence and abuse: https://avaproject.org.uk

Anti-Slavery International: www.antislavery.org

Barnardos: www.barnardos.org.uk

Care Quality Commission (CQC) (England): www.cqc.org.uk

Department for Education: www.gov.uk/government/organisations/department-for-education

Department of Health and Social Care: www.gov.uk/government/organisations/department-of-health-and-social-care

Healthcare Improvement (Scotland): www.healthcareimprovementscotland.org

Healthcare Inspectorate (Wales): https://hiw.org.uk

International Confederation of Midwives (ICM): www.internationalmidwives.org

Kings Fund: www.kingsfund.org.uk

MBRRACE-UK: Mothers and Babies: Reducing Risk through Audits and Confidential Enquiries across the UK: www.npeu.ox.ac.uk/mbrrace-uk

Medicines and Healthcare Products Regulatory Agency (MHPRA): www.gov.uk/government/organisations/medicines-and-healthcare-products-regulatory-agency

National Health Service Improving Quality https://improvement.nhs.uk/improvement-hub/quality-improvement

National Health Service [NHS] England: www.england.nhs.uk

National Health Service [NHS] Leadership Academy: www.leadershipacademy.nhs.uk

National Health Service [NHS] Resolution: https://resolution.nhs.uk

National Institute for Health and Care Excellence: www.nice.org.uk

Nursing and Midwifery Council (NMC): www.nmc.org.uk

Parliamentary and Health Service Ombudsman: www.ombudsman.org.uk

Professional Standards Authority (PSA): www.professionalstandards.org.uk

Public Health England: www.gov.uk/government/organisations/public-health-england

Regulation and Quality Improvement Authority (Northern Ireland): https://rqia.org.uk

Royal College of Anaesthetists: www.rcoa.ac.uk

Royal College of Midwives: www.rcm.org.uk

Royal College of Obstetricians and Gynaecologists: www.rcog.org.uk

Royal College of Paediatrics and Child Health: www.rcpch.ac.uk

Scottish Intercollegiate Guidelines Network (SIGN): www.sign.ac.uk

The Scottish Government: www.gov.scot

United Nations Population Fund (UNFPA): www.unfpa.org

World Health Organization: www.who.int

Human Anatomy and Reproduction

3

The Female Pelvis and the Reproductive Organs

Ranee Thakar, Abdul H. Sultan

CHAPTER CONTENTS

It is important that midwives are well versed in the applied anatomy of the female pelvis and understand the processes of reproduction.

THE CHAPTER AIMS TO

- cover the basic anatomy of the female and male reproductive system

- identify the main functions of the internal and external female and male genital organs.

FEMALE EXTERNAL GENITAL ORGANS

The female external genitalia (the vulva) include: the mons pubis, labia majora, labia minora, clitoris, vestibule, the greater vestibular glands (Bartholin's glands) and bulbs of the vestibule (Fig. 3.1).

- The mons pubis is a rounded pad of fat lying anterior to the symphysis pubis. It is covered with pubic hair from the time of puberty.
- The labia majora ('greater lips') are two folds of fat and areolar tissue, which are covered with skin and

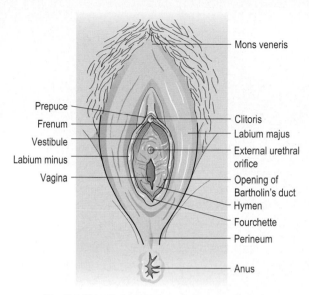

Fig. 3.1 Female external genital organs (vulva).

pubic hair on the outer surface and have a pink, smooth inner surface.

- The labia minora ('lesser lips') are two small subcutaneous folds, devoid of fat, that lie between the labia majora. Anteriorly, each labium minus divides into two parts: the upper layer passes above the clitoris to form, along with its fellow, a fold, the prepuce, which overhangs the clitoris. The prepuce is a retractable piece of skin which surrounds and protects the clitoris. The lower layer passes below the clitoris to form with its fellow, the frenulum of the clitoris.
- The clitoris is a small rudimentary sexual organ corresponding to the male penis. The visible knob-like portion is located near the anterior junction of the labia minora, above the opening of the urethra and vagina. Unlike the penis, the clitoris does not contain the distal portion of the urethra and functions solely to induce the orgasm during sexual intercourse.
- The vestibule is the area enclosed by the labia minora in which the openings of the urethra and the vagina are situated.
- The urethral orifice lies 2.5 cm posterior to the clitoris and immediately in front of the vaginal orifice. On either side lie the openings of the Skene's ducts, two small blind-ended tubules 0.5 cm long running within the urethral wall.
- The vaginal orifice, also known as the introitus of the vagina, occupies the posterior two-thirds of the vestibule.

The orifice is partially closed by the hymen, a thin membrane that tears during sexual intercourse. The remaining tags of hymen are known as the *carunculae myrtiformes* because they are thought to resemble myrtle berries.

- The greater vestibular glands (Bartholin's glands) are two small glands that open on either side of the vaginal orifice and lie in the posterior part of the labia majora. They secrete mucus, which lubricates the vaginal opening. The duct may occasionally become blocked, which can cause the secretions from the gland to accommodate within it and form a cyst.
- The bulbs of the vestibule are two elongated erectile masses flanking the vaginal orifice.

Blood Supply

The blood supply comes from the internal and the external pudendal arteries. The blood drains through corresponding veins.

Lymphatic Drainage

Lymphatic drainage is mainly via the inguinal glands.

Innervation

The nerve supply is derived from branches of the pudendal nerve.

THE PERINEUM

The perineum corresponds to the outlet of the pelvis and is somewhat lozenge-shaped. Anteriorly, it is bound by the pubic arch, posteriorly by the coccyx, and laterally by the ischiopubic rami, ischial tuberosities and sacrotuberous ligaments. The perineum can be divided into two triangular parts by drawing an arbitrary line transversely between the ischial tuberosities. The anterior triangle, which contains the external urogenital organs, is known as the *urogenital triangle* and the posterior triangle, which contains the termination of the anal canal, is known as the *anal triangle*.

The Urogenital Triangle

The urogenital triangle (Fig. 3.2A) is bound anteriorly and laterally by the pubic symphysis and the ischiopubic rami. The urogenital triangle has been divided into two compartments: the superficial and deep perineal spaces, separated by the perineal membrane, which

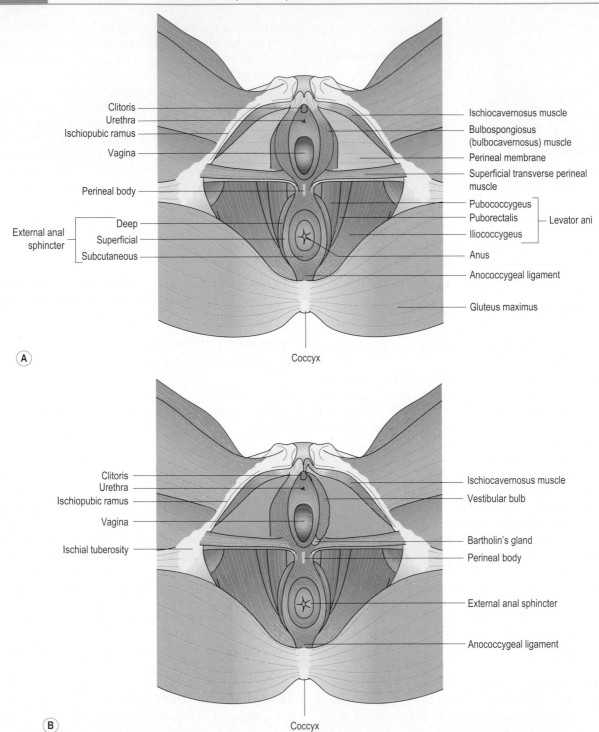

Fig. 3.2 (A) Diagram of the perineum demonstrating the superficial muscles of the perineum. The superficial transverse perineal muscle, the bulbospongiosus and the ischiocavernosus form a triangle on either side of the perineum with a floor formed by the perineal membrane. (B) The left bulbospongiosus muscle has been removed to demonstrate the vestibular bulb and the Bartholin's gland.

spans the space between the ischiopubic rami. The levator ani muscles are attached to the cranial surface of the perineal membrane. The vestibular bulb and clitoral crus lie on the caudal surface of the membrane and are fused with it. These erectile tissues are covered by the bulbospongiosus and the ischiocavernosus muscles.

Superficial Muscles of the Perineum

Superficial transverse perineal muscle. The superficial transverse muscle is a narrow slip of a muscle that arises from the inner and forepart of the ischial tuberosity and is inserted into the central tendinous part of the perineal body (Fig. 3.2A). The muscle from the opposite side, the external anal sphincter (EAS) from behind, and the bulbospongiosus in the front, all attach to the central tendon of the perineal body.

Bulbospongiosus muscle. The bulbospongiosus (previously known as 'bulbocavernosus') muscle runs on either side of the vaginal orifice, covering the lateral aspects of the vestibular bulb anteriorly and the Bartholin's gland posteriorly (Fig. 3.2B). Some fibres merge posteriorly with the superficial transverse perineal muscle and the EAS in the central fibromuscular perineal body. Anteriorly, its fibres pass forward on either side of the vagina and insert into the corpora cavernosa clitoridis, a fasciculus crossing over the body of the organ, so as to compress the deep dorsal vein. This muscle diminishes the orifice of the vagina and contributes to the erection of the clitoris.

Ischiocavernosus muscle. The ischiocavernosus muscle is elongated, broader at the middle than at either end and is situated on the side of the lateral boundary of the perineum (Fig. 3.2A). It arises by tendinous and fleshy fibres from the inner surface of the ischial tuberosity, behind the crus clitoridis, from the surface of the crus and from the adjacent portions of the ischial ramus.

Innervation

The nerve supply is derived from branches of the pudendal nerve.

The Anal Triangle

This area includes the anal canal, the anal sphincters and the ischioanal fossae.

Anal Canal

The rectum terminates in the anal canal (Fig. 3.3). The anal canal is attached posteriorly to the coccyx by the anococcygeal ligament, a midline fibromuscular structure that runs between the posterior aspect of the EAS and the coccyx. The anus is surrounded laterally and posteriorly by loose adipose tissue within the ischioanal fossae, which is a potential pathway for spread of perianal sepsis from one side to the other. The pudendal nerves pass over the ischial spines at this point and can be accessed for injection of local anaesthetic into the pudendal nerve at this site. Anteriorly, the perineal body separates the anal canal from the vagina.

The anal canal is surrounded by an inner epithelial lining, a vascular subepithelium, the internal anal sphincter (IAS), the EAS and fibromuscular supporting tissue. The lining of the anal canal varies along its length due to its embryologic derivation. The proximal anal canal is lined with rectal mucosa (columnar epithelium) and is arranged in vertical mucosal folds called the columns of Morgagni (Fig. 3.3). Each column contains a terminal radical of the superior rectal artery and vein. The vessels are largest in the left lateral, right-posterior and right-anterior quadrants of the wall of the anal canal where the subepithelial tissues expand into three *anal cushions*. These cushions seal the anal canal and help maintain continence of flatus and liquid stools. The columns are joined together at their inferior margin by crescentic folds called anal valves. About 2 cm from the anal verge, the anal valves create a demarcation called the dentate line. Anoderm covers the last 1–1.5 cm of the distal canal below the dentate line and consists of modified squamous epithelium that lack skin adnexal tissues such as hair follicles and glands, but contains numerous somatic nerve endings. Since the epithelium in the lower canal is well supplied with sensory nerve endings, acute distension or invasive treatment of haemorrhoids in this area causes profuse discomfort, whereas treatment can be carried out with relatively few symptoms in the upper canal lined by insensate columnar epithelium. As a result of tonic circumferential contraction of the sphincter, the skin is arranged in radiating folds around the anus and is called the anal margin. These folds appear to be flat or ironed out when there is underlying sphincter damage. The junction between the columnar and squamous epithelia is referred to as the anal transitional zone, which

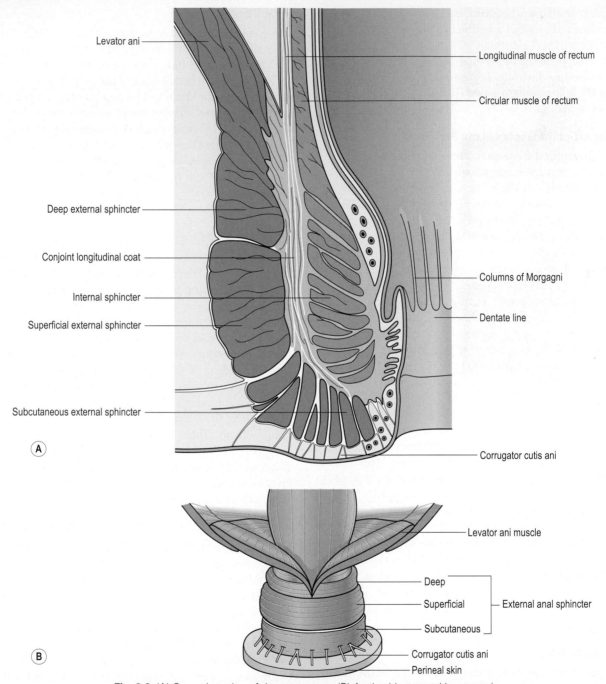

Levator ani

Deep external sphincter

Conjoint longitudinal coat

Internal sphincter

Superficial external sphincter

Subcutaneous external sphincter

Longitudinal muscle of rectum

Circular muscle of rectum

Columns of Morgagni

Dentate line

Corrugator cutis ani

(A)

Levator ani muscle

Deep

Superficial   External anal sphincter

Subcutaneous

Corrugator cutis ani

Perineal skin

(B)

Fig. 3.3 (A) Coronal section of the anorectum. (B) Anal sphincter and levator ani.

is variable in height and position and often contains islands of squamous epithelium extending into columnar epithelium. This zone probably has a role to play in continence by providing a highly specialized sampling mechanism.

Anal Sphincter Complex

The anal sphincter complex consists of the EAS and IAS separated by the conjoint longitudinal coat (Fig. 3.3). Although they form a single unit, they are distinct in structure and function.

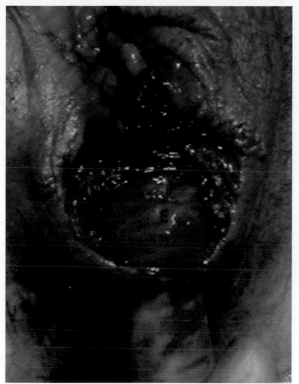

Fig. 3.4 An intact external anal sphincter (E), which is red in colour and appears like raw red meat.

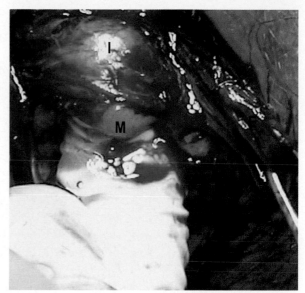

Fig. 3.5 The internal anal sphincter (I) is pale in colour and appears like raw white meat. (E) is the external anal sphincter; (M) is the mucosa.

External anal sphincter. The EAS comprises of striated muscle and appears red in colour (similar to raw red meat) (Fig. 3.4). As the EAS is normally under tonic contraction, it tends to retract when completely torn. A defect of the EAS can lead to urgency and/or urge faecal incontinence. In contrast to the male, the external sphincter in the female is shorter anteriorly. This is clinically relevant during clinical or sonographic assessment of anal sphincter injuries.

Internal anal sphincter. The IAS is a thickened continuation of the circular smooth muscle of the bowel and terminates with a well-defined rounded edge 6–8 mm above the anal margin at the level of the superficial and subcutaneous EAS junction. In contrast to the EAS, the IAS has a pale appearance to the naked eye (Fig. 3.5). A defect of the IAS can lead to passive soiling of stools and flatus incontinence.

The longitudinal layer and the conjoint longitudinal coat. The longitudinal layer is situated between the EAS and IAS and consists of a fibromuscular layer, the conjoint longitudinal coat and the intersphincteric space with its connective tissue components (Fig. 3.3).

Innervation of the Anal Sphincter Complex

The nerve supply is derived from branches of the pudendal nerve.

Vascular Supply

The anorectum receives its major blood supply from the superior haemorrhoidal (terminal branch of the inferior mesenteric artery) and inferior haemorrhoidal (branch of the pudendal artery) arteries, and to a lesser degree, from the middle haemorrhoidal artery (branch of the internal iliac), forming a wide intramural network of collaterals. The venous drainage of the upper anal canal mucosa, IAS and conjoint longitudinal coat passes via the terminal branches of the superior rectal vein into the inferior mesenteric vein. The lower anal canal and the EAS drain via the inferior rectal branch of the pudendal vein into the internal iliac vein.

Lymphatic Drainage

The anorectum has a rich network of lymphatic plexuses. The dentate line represents the interface between

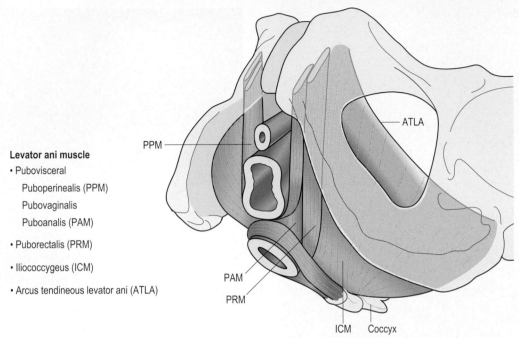

Levator ani muscle
- Pubovisceral
   Puboperinealis (PPM)
   Pubovaginalis
   Puboanalis (PAM)
- Puborectalis (PRM)
- Iliococcygeus (ICM)
- Arcus tendineous levator ani (ATLA)

Fig. 3.6 The levator muscle. Schematic view of the levator ani muscles from below after the vulvar structures and perineal membrane have been removed showing the arcus tendineus levator ani (ATLA); puboanal muscle (PAM); perineal body uniting the two ends of the puboperineal muscle (PPM); iliococcygeal muscle (ICM); puborectal muscle (PRM). Note that the urethra and vagina have been transected just above the hymenal ring. (Courtesy Professor John DeLancey.)

the two different systems of lymphatic drainage. Above the dentate line (the upper anal canal), the IAS and the conjoint longitudinal coat drain into the inferior mesenteric and internal iliac nodes. Lymphatic drainage below the dentate line, which consists of the lower anal canal epithelium and the EAS, proceeds to the external inguinal lymph nodes.

The Ischioanal Fossa

The ischioanal fossa (previously known as the 'ischiorectal fossa') extends around the anal canal and is bound anteriorly by the perineal membrane, superiorly by the fascia of the levator ani muscle and medially by the EAS complex at the level of the anal canal. The ischioanal fossa contains fat and neurovascular structures, including the pudendal nerve and the internal pudendal vessels.

The Perineal Body

The perineal body is the central point between the urogenital and the anal triangles of the perineum (Fig. 3.2A). Within the perineal body there are interlacing muscle

fibres from the bulbospongiosus, superficial transverse perineal and EAS muscles. Above this level there is a contribution from the conjoint longitudinal coat and the medial fibres of the puborectalis muscle. Therefore, the support of the pelvic structures, and to some extent the hiatus urogenitalis between the levator ani muscles, depends upon the integrity of the perineal body.

THE PELVIC FLOOR

The pelvic floor is a musculotendinous sheet that spans the pelvic outlet and consists mainly of the symmetrically paired levator ani muscle (LAM) (Fig. 3.6), which is a broad muscular sheet of variable thickness attached to the internal surface of the true pelvis. Although there is controversy regarding the subdivisions of the muscle, it is broadly accepted that it is subdivided into parts according to their attachments, namely the pubovisceral (also known as pubococcygeus), puborectal and iliococcygeus. The pubovisceral part is further subdivided according to its relationship to the viscera, i.e. puboperinealis, pubovaginalis and puboanalis. The puborectalis muscle is located lateral to the pubovisceral muscle, cephalad to the deep component of the EAS, from which it is inseparable posteriorly.

The muscles of the levator ani differ from most other skeletal muscles in that they:

- maintain constant tone, except during voiding, defaecation and the Valsalva manoeuvre
- have the ability to contract quickly at the time of acute stress (such as a cough or sneeze) to maintain continence
- distend considerably during parturition to allow the passage of the term infant, and then contract after birth to resume normal functioning.

Until recently, the concept of pelvic floor trauma was attributed largely to perineal, vaginal and anal sphincter injuries. However, in recent years, with advances in magnetic resonance imaging (MRI) and three-dimensional (3D) ultrasound, it has become evident that LAM injuries form an important component of pelvic floor trauma. LAM injuries occur in 13–36% of women who have a vaginal birth. Injury to the LAM is attributed to vaginal birth resulting in reduced pelvic floor muscle strength, enlargement of the vaginal hiatus and pelvic organ prolapse. There is inconclusive evidence to support an association between LAM injuries and stress urinary incontinence and there seems to be a trend towards the development of faecal incontinence.

Innervation of the Levator Ani

The levator ani is supplied on its superior surface by the sacral nerve roots (S2–S4) and on its inferior surface by the perineal branch of the pudendal nerve.

Vascular Supply

The levator ani is supplied by branches of the inferior gluteal artery, the inferior vesical artery and the pudendal artery.

THE PUDENDAL NERVE

The pudendal nerve is a mixed motor and sensory nerve and derives its fibres from the ventral branches of the second, third and fourth sacral nerves and leaves the pelvis through the lower part of the greater sciatic foramen. It then crosses the ischial spine and re-enters the pelvis through the lesser sciatic foramen. It accompanies the internal pudendal vessels upward and

forward along the lateral wall of the ischioanal fossa, contained in a sheath of the obturator fascia termed 'Alcock's canal' (Fig. 3.7). It is presumed that during a prolonged second stage of labour, the pudendal nerve is vulnerable to stretch injury due to its relative immobility at this site.

The inferior haemorrhoidal (rectal) nerve then branches off posteriorly from the pudendal nerve to innervate the EAS. The pudendal nerve then divides into two terminal branches: the perineal nerve and the dorsal nerve of the clitoris. The perineal nerve divides into posterior labial and muscular branches. The posterior labial branches supply the labium majora. The muscular branches are distributed to the superficial transverse perineal, bulbospongiosus, ischiocavernosus and constrictor urethrae muscles. The dorsal nerve of the clitoris, which innervates the clitoris, is the deepest division of the pudendal nerve (Fig. 3.8).

THE PELVIS

Knowledge of anatomy of a normal female pelvis is key to midwifery and obstetric practice, as one of the ways to estimate a woman's progress in labour is by assessing the relationship of the fetus to certain bony landmarks of the pelvis. Understanding the normal pelvic anatomy helps to detect deviations from normal and facilitate appropriate care.

The Pelvic Girdle

The pelvic girdle is a basin-shaped cavity and consists of two innominate bones (hip bones), the sacrum and the coccyx. It is virtually incapable of independent movement except during childbirth, as it provides the skeletal framework of the birth canal. It contains and protects the bladder, rectum and internal reproductive organs. In addition, it provides an attachment for trunk and limb muscles. Some women experience pelvic girdle pain in pregnancy and need referral to a physiotherapist (see Chapter 17).

Innominate Bones

Each innominate bone or hip bone is made up of three bones that have fused together: the ilium, the ischium and the pubis (Fig. 3.9). On its lateral aspect is a large, cup-shaped acetabulum articulating with the femoral head, which is composed of the three fused bones in the following proportions: two-fifths ilium, two-fifths

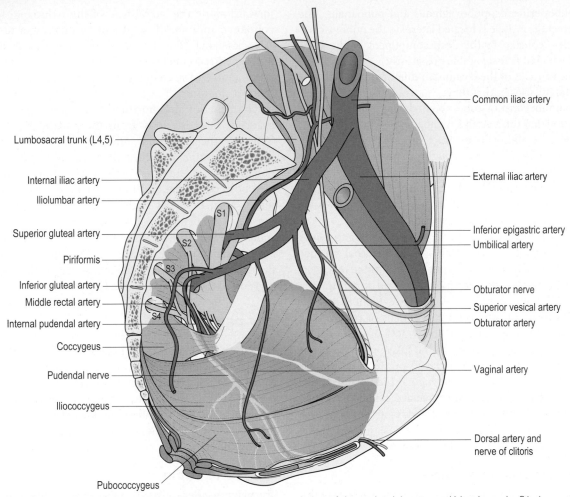

Lumbosacral trunk (L4,5)

Internal iliac artery

Iliolumbar artery

Superior gluteal artery

Piriformis

Inferior gluteal artery

Middle rectal artery

Internal pudendal artery

Coccygeus

Pudendal nerve

Iliococcygeus

Pubococcygeus

S1

S2

S3

S4

Common iliac artery

External iliac artery

Inferior epigastric artery

Umbilical artery

Obturator nerve

Superior vesical artery

Obturator artery

Vaginal artery

Dorsal artery and
nerve of clitoris

Fig. 3.7 Sagittal view of the pelvis demonstrating the pathway of the pudendal nerve and blood supply. S1–4, sacral nerve roots.

ischium and one-fifth pubis (Fig. 3.9). Anteroinferior to this is the large oval or triangular obturator foramen. The bone is articulated with its fellow to form the pelvic girdle.

The ilium has an upper and lower part. The smaller lower part forms part of the acetabulum and the upper part is the large flared-out part. When the hand is placed on the hip, it rests on the iliac crest, which is the upper border. A bony prominence felt in front of the iliac crest is known as the anterior superior iliac spine. A short distance below it is the anterior inferior iliac spine. There are two similar points at the other end of the iliac crest, namely the posterior superior and the posterior inferior iliac spines. The internal concave anterior surface of the ilium is known as the iliac fossa.

The ischium is the inferoposterior part of the innominate bone and consists of a body and a ramus. Above, it forms part of the acetabulum. Below its ramus, it ascends anteromedially at an acute angle to meet the descending pubic ramus and complete the obturator foramen. It has a large prominence known as the ischial tuberosity on which the body rests when sitting. Behind and a little above the tuberosity is an inward projection, the ischial spine. This is an important landmark in midwifery and obstetric practice, as in labour, the station of the fetal head is estimated in relation to the ischial spines allowing assessment of progress of labour.

The pubis forms the anterior part. It has a body and two oar-like projections, the superior ramus and the inferior ramus. The two pubic bones meet at the symphysis

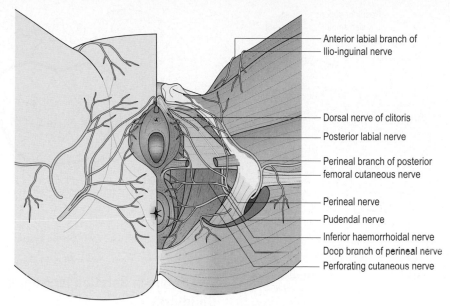

Fig. 3.8 Branches of the pudendal nerve.

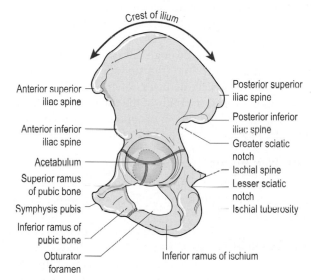

Fig. 3.9 Lateral view of the innominate bone showing important landmarks.

pubis and the two inferior rami form the pubic arch, merging into a similar ramus on the ischium. The space enclosed by the body of the pubic bone, the rami and the ischium is called the 'obturator foramen'.

The Sacrum

The sacrum is a wedge-shaped bone consisting of five fused vertebrae, and forms the posterior wall of the pelvic cavity as it is wedged between the innominate bones. The caudal apex articulates with the coccyx and the upper border of the first sacral vertebra (sacral promontory) articulates with the first lumbar vertebra. The anterior surface of the sacrum is concave and is referred to as the hollow of the sacrum. Laterally, the sacrum extends into a wing or ala. Four pairs of holes or foramina pierce the sacrum and, through these, nerves from the cauda equina emerge to innervate the pelvic organs. The posterior surface is roughened to receive attachments of muscles.

The Coccyx

The coccyx is a vestigial tail. It consists of four fused vertebrae, forming a small triangular bone, which articulates with the fifth sacral segment.

Pelvic Joints

There are four pelvic joints: one symphysis pubis, two sacroiliac joints and one sacrococcygeal joint.
- **The symphysis pubis** is the midline cartilaginous joint uniting the rami of the left and right pubic bones.
- **The sacroiliac joints** are strong, weight-bearing synovial joints with irregular elevations and depressions that produce interlocking of the bones. They join the sacrum to the ilium and as a result connect the spine to the pelvis. The joints allow a limited backward

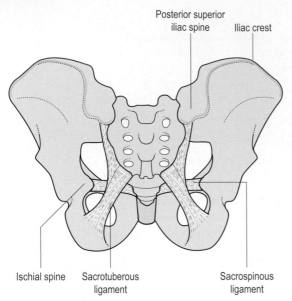

Posterior superior
iliac spine   Iliac crest

Ischial spine   Sacrotuberous   Sacrospinous
                 ligament   ligament

Fig. 3.10 Posterior view of the pelvis showing the ligaments.

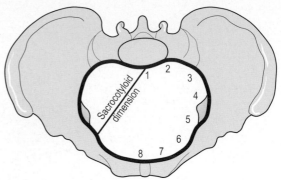

Fig. 3.11 Brim of female pelvis (see text for details of 1–8).

and forward movement of the tip and promontory of the sacrum, sometimes known as 'nodding' of the sacrum.

- **The sacrococcygeal** joint is formed where the base of the coccyx articulates with the tip of the sacrum. It permits the coccyx to be deflected backwards during the birth of the fetal head.

Pelvic Ligaments

The pelvic joints are held together by very strong ligaments that are designed not to allow movement. However, during pregnancy the hormone relaxin gradually loosens all the pelvic ligaments allowing slight pelvic movement thereby providing more room for the fetal head as it passes through the pelvis. A widening of 2–3 mm at the symphysis pubis during pregnancy above the normal gap of 4–5 mm is normal but if it widens significantly, the degree of movement permitted may give rise to pain on walking.

The ligaments connecting the bones of the pelvis with each other can be divided into four groups:

- those connecting the sacrum and ilium – the sacroiliac ligaments
- those passing between the sacrum and ischium – the sacrotuberous ligaments and the sacrospinous ligaments (Fig. 3.10)
- those uniting the sacrum and coccyx – the sacrococcygeal ligaments

- those between the two pubic bones – the inter-pubic ligaments.

The Pelvis in Relation to Pregnancy and Childbirth

The term 'pelvis' is applied to the skeletal ring formed by the innominate bones and the sacrum, the cavity within and even the entire region where the trunk and the lower limbs meet. The pelvis is divided by an oblique plane, which passes through the prominence of the sacrum, the arcuate line (the smooth rounded border on the internal surface of the ilium), the pectineal line (a ridge on the superior ramus of the pubic bone) and the upper margin of the symphysis pubis, into the true and the false pelvis.

The True Pelvis

The true pelvis is the bony canal through which the fetus must pass during birth. It is divided into a brim, a cavity and an outlet.

The Pelvic Brim

The superior circumference forms the brim of the true pelvis, the included space being called 'the inlet'. The brim is round except where the sacral promontory projects into it.

Midwives need to be familiar with the fixed points on the pelvic brim that are known as its landmarks. Commencing posteriorly, these are (Fig. 3.11):

- sacral promontory (1)
- sacral ala or wing (2)
- sacroiliac joint (3)
- iliopectineal line, which is the edge formed at the inward aspect of the ilium (4)

- iliopectineal eminence, which is a roughened area formed where the superior ramus of the pubic bone meets the ilium (5)
- superior ramus of the pubic bone (6)
- upper inner border of the body of the pubic bone (7)
- upper inner border of the symphysis pubis (8).

The Pelvic Cavity

The cavity of the true pelvis extends from the brim superiorly to the outlet inferiorly. The anterior wall is formed by the pubic bones and symphysis pubis and its depth is 4 cm. The posterior wall is formed by the curve of the sacrum, which is 12 cm in length. Because there is such a difference in these measurements, the cavity forms a curved canal. With the woman upright, the upper portion of the pelvic canal is directed downward and backward, and its lower course curves and becomes directed downward and forward. Its lateral walls are the sides of the pelvis, which are mainly covered by the obturator internus muscle.

The cavity contains the pelvic colon, rectum, bladder and some of the reproductive organs. The rectum is placed posteriorly, in the curve of the sacrum and coccyx; the bladder is anterior behind the symphysis pubis.

The Pelvic Outlet

The lower circumference of the true pelvis is very irregular; the space enclosed by it is called the outlet. Two outlets are described: the anatomical and the obstetrical. The anatomical outlet is formed by the lower borders of each of the bones together with the sacrotuberous ligament. The obstetrical outlet is of greater practical significance because it includes the narrow pelvic strait through which the fetus must pass. The narrow pelvic strait lies between the sacrococcygeal joint, the two ischial spines and the lower border of the symphysis pubis. The obstetrical outlet is the space between the narrow pelvic strait and the anatomical outlet. This outlet is diamond-shaped.

The False Pelvis

It is bounded posteriorly by the lumbar vertebrae and laterally by the iliac fossae, and in front by the lower portion of the anterior abdominal wall. The false pelvis varies considerably in size according to the flare of the iliac bones. However, the false pelvis has no significance in midwifery.

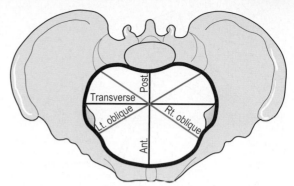

Fig. 3.12 View of pelvic brim showing diameters.

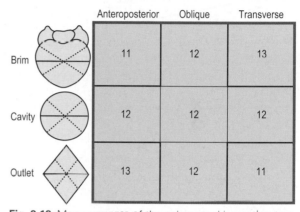

	Anteroposterior	Oblique	Transverse
Brim	11	12	13
Cavity	12	12	12
Outlet	13	12	11

Fig. 3.13 Measurements of the pelvic canal in centimetres.

Pelvic Diameters

Knowledge of the diameters of the normal female pelvis is essential in the practice of midwifery because contraction of any of them can result in malposition or malpresentation of the presenting part of the fetus.

Diameters of the Pelvic Inlet

The brim has four principal diameters: the anteroposterior diameter, the transverse diameter and the two oblique diameters (Figs 3.12, 3.13).

The anteroposterior or conjugate diameter extends from the midpoint of the sacral promontory to the upper border of the symphysis pubis. Three conjugate diameters can be measured: the anatomical (true) conjugate, the obstetrical conjugate and the internal or diagonal conjugate (Fig. 3.14).

The anatomical conjugate, which averages 12 cm, is measured from the sacral promontory to the uppermost point of the symphysis pubis. The obstetrical conjugate, which averages 11 cm, is measured from the sacral

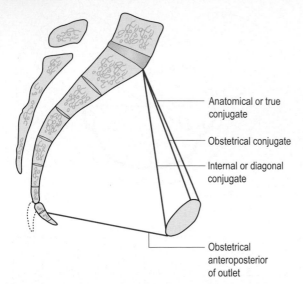

Fig. 3.14 Median section of the pelvis showing anteroposterior diameters.

- Anatomical or true conjugate
- Obstetrical conjugate
- Internal or diagonal conjugate
- Obstetrical anteroposterior of outlet

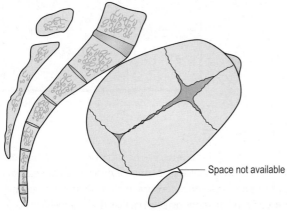

- Space not available

Fig. 3.15 Fetal head negotiating the narrow obstetrical conjugate.

promontory to the posterior border of the upper surface of the symphysis pubis. This represents the shortest anteroposterior diameter through which the fetus must pass and is hence of clinical significance to midwives (Fig. 3.15). The obstetrical conjugate cannot be measured with the examining fingers or any other technique.

The diagonal conjugate is measured anteroposteriorly from the lower border of the symphysis to the sacral promontory.

The transverse diameter is constructed at right-angles to the obstetric conjugate and extends across the greatest width of the brim; its average measurement is about 13 cm.

Each oblique diameter extends from the iliopectineal eminence of one side to the sacroiliac articulation of the opposite side; its average measurement is about 12 cm. Each takes its name from the sacroiliac joint from which it arises, so the left oblique diameter arises from the left sacroiliac joint and the right oblique from the right sacroiliac joint.

Another dimension, the sacrocotyloid (Fig. 3.11), passes from the sacral promontory to the iliopectineal eminence on each side and measures 9–9.5 cm. Its importance is concerned with posterior positions of the occiput when the parietal eminences of the fetal head may become caught (see Chapter 23).

Diameters of the Cavity

The cavity is circular in shape and although it is not possible to measure its diameters exactly, they are all considered to be 12 cm (Fig. 3.13).

Diameters of the Outlet

The outlet, which is diamond-shaped, has three diameters: the anteroposterior diameter, the oblique diameter and the transverse diameter (Fig. 3.13).

The anteroposterior diameter extends from the lower border of the symphysis pubis to the sacrococcygeal joint. It measures 13 cm; as the coccyx may be deflected backwards during labour, this diameter indicates the space available during birth.

The oblique diameter, although there are no fixed points, is said to be between the obturator foramen and the sacrospinous ligament. The measurement is taken as being 12 cm.

The transverse diameter extends between the two ischial spines and measures 10–11 cm. It is the narrowest diameter in the pelvis. The plane of least pelvic dimensions is said to be at the level of the ischial spines.

Orientation of the Pelvis

In the standing position, the pelvis is placed such that the anterior superior iliac spine and the front edge of the symphysis pubis are in the same vertical plane, perpendicular to the floor. If the line joining the sacral promontory and the top of the symphysis pubis were to be extended, it would form an angle of 60 degrees with the horizontal floor. Similarly, if a line joining the centre of the sacrum and the centre of the symphysis pubis were to be extended, the resultant angle with the floor would be 30 degrees. The angle of inclination of the outlet is

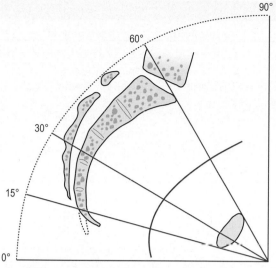

Fig. 3.16 Median section of the pelvis showing the inclination of the planes and the axis of the pelvic canal.

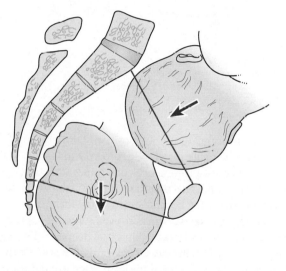

Fig. 3.17 Fetal head entering plane of pelvic brim and leaving plane of pelvic outlet.

15 degrees (Fig. 3.16). When in the recumbent position, the same angles are made as in the vertical position; this fact should be kept in mind when carrying out an abdominal examination.

Pelvic Planes

Pelvic planes are imaginary flat surfaces at the brim, cavity and outlet of the pelvic canal at the levels of the lines described above (Fig. 3.17).

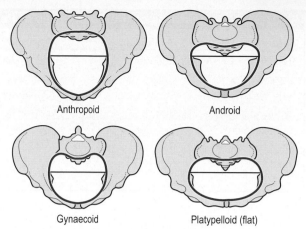

Fig. 3.18 Characteristic brim of the four types of pelvis.

Axis of the Pelvic Canal

A line drawn exactly half-way between the anterior wall and the posterior wall of the pelvic canal would trace a curve known as the curve of Carus. The midwife needs to become familiar with this concept in order to make accurate observations on vaginal examination and to facilitate the birth of the baby.

The Four Types of Pelvis

The size of the pelvis varies not only in the two sexes, but also in different members of the same sex. The height of the individual does not appear to influence the size of the pelvis in any way, as women of short stature, in general, have a broad pelvis. Nevertheless, the pelvis is occasionally equally contracted in all its dimensions, so much so that all its diameters can measure 1.25 cm less than the average. This type of pelvis, known as a 'justo minor' pelvis, can result in normal labour and birth if the fetal size is consistent with the size of the maternal pelvis. However, if the fetus is large, a degree of cephalopelvic disproportion will result. The same is true when a malpresentation or malposition of the fetus exists (see Chapter 23).

The principal divergences, however, are found at the brim (Fig. 3.18) and affect the relation of the anteroposterior to the transverse diameter. If one of the measurements is reduced by 1 cm or more from the normal, the pelvis is said to be contracted and may give rise to difficulty in labour or necessitate caesarean section.

Classically, pelves have been described as falling into four categories: the gynaecoid pelvis, the android pelvis, the anthropoid pelvis and the platypelloid pelvis (Table 3.1).

TABLE 3.1 Features of the Four Types of Pelvis

Features	Gynaecoid	Android	Anthropoid	Platypelloid
Brim	Rounded	Heart-shaped	Long oval	Kidney-shaped
Forepelvis	Generous	Narrow	Narrowed	Wide
Side walls	Straight	Convergent	Divergent	Divergent
Ischial spines	Blunt	Prominent	Blunt	Blunt
Sciatic notch	Rounded	Narrow	Wide	Wide
Subpubic angle	90°	<90°	>90°	>90°
Incidence	50%	20%	25% (50% in non-Caucasian)	5%

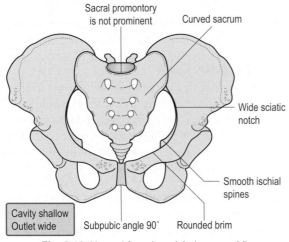

Fig. 3.19 Normal female pelvis (gynaecoid).

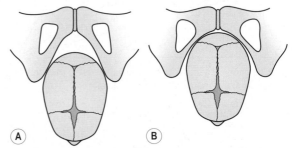

Fig. 3.20 (A) Outlet of android pelvis. The fetal head, which does not fit into the acute pubic arch, is forced backwards onto the perineum. (B) Outlet of the gynaecoid pelvis. The head fits snugly into the pubic arch.

The Gynaecoid Pelvis

This is the best type for childbearing as it has a rounded brim, generous forepelvis, straight side walls, a shallow cavity with a well-curved sacrum and a subpubic arch of 90° (Fig. 3.19).

The Android Pelvis

The android pelvis is so called because it resembles the male pelvis. Its brim is heart-shaped, it has a narrow forepelvis and its transverse diameter is situated towards the back. The side walls converge, making it funnel-shaped, and it has a deep cavity and a straight sacrum. The ischial spines are prominent and the sciatic notch is narrow. The subpubic angle is less than 90°. It is found in short and heavily built women, who have a tendency to be hirsute.

Because of the narrow forepelvis and the fact that the greater space lies in the hindpelvis, the heart-shaped brim favours an occipitoposterior position. Furthermore, funnelling in the cavity may hinder progress in labour. At the pelvic outlet, the prominent ischial spines sometimes prevent complete internal rotation of the head and the anteroposterior diameter becomes caught on them, causing a deep transverse arrest. The narrowed subpubic angle cannot easily accommodate the biparietal diameter (Fig. 3.20) and this displaces the head backwards. Because of these factors, this type of pelvis is the least suited to childbearing.

The Anthropoid Pelvis

The anthropoid pelvis has a long, oval brim in which the anteroposterior diameter is longer than the transverse diameter. The side walls diverge and the sacrum is long and deeply concave. The ischial spines are not prominent and the sciatic notch and the subpubic angle are very wide. Women with this type of pelvis tend to be tall, with narrow shoulders. Labour does not usually present any difficulties, but a direct occipitoanterior or direct occipitoposterior position is often a feature and the position adopted for engagement may persist to birth.

The Platypelloid Pelvis

The platypelloid (flat) pelvis has a kidney-shaped brim in which the anteroposterior diameter is reduced and the transverse diameter increased. The sacrum is flat and the cavity shallow. The ischial spines are blunt, and the sciatic notch and the subpubic angle are both wide. The head must engage with the sagittal suture in the transverse diameter, but usually descends through the cavity without difficulty. Engagement may necessitate lateral tilting of the head, known as 'asynclitism', in order to allow the biparietal diameter to pass the narrowest anteroposterior diameter of the brim (Box 3.1).

Other Pelvic Variations

High assimilation pelvis occurs when the 5th lumbar vertebra is fused to the sacrum and the angle of inclination of the pelvic brim is increased. Engagement of the head is difficult but, once achieved, labour progresses normally.

Malformed pelvis may result from a developmental anomaly, dietary deficiency, injury or disease (Box 3.2).

THE FEMALE REPRODUCTIVE SYSTEM

The female reproductive system consists of the external genitalia, known collectively as the vulva, and the internal reproductive organs: the vagina, the uterus, two uterine tubes and two ovaries. In the non-pregnant state, the internal reproductive organs are situated within the true pelvis.

The Vagina

The vagina is a hollow, distensible fibromuscular tube that extends from the vestibule to the cervix. It is approximately 10 cm in length and 2.5 cm in diameter (although there is wide anatomical variation). During sexual intercourse and when a woman gives birth, the vagina temporarily widens and lengthens.

The vaginal canal passes upwards and backwards into the pelvis with the anterior and posterior walls in close contact along a line approximately parallel to the plane of the pelvic brim. When the woman stands upright, the vaginal canal points in an upward–backward direction and forms an angle of slightly more than 45 degrees with the uterus.

Function

The vagina allows the escape of the menstrual fluids, receives the penis and the ejected sperm during sexual intercourse, and provides an exit for the fetus during birth.

BOX 3.1 Negotiating the Pelvic Brim in Asynclitism

Anterior Asynclitism

The anterior parietal bone moves down behind the symphysis pubis until the parietal eminence enters the brim. The movement is then reversed and the head tilts in the opposite direction until the posterior parietal bone negotiates the sacral promontory and the head is engaged.

Posterior Asynclitism

The movements of anterior asynclitism are reversed. The posterior parietal bone negotiates the sacral promontory prior to the anterior parietal bone moving down behind the symphysis pubis.

Once the pelvic brim has been negotiated, descent progresses, normally accompanied by flexion and internal rotation.

Relations

Knowledge of the relations of the vagina to other pelvic organs is essential for the accurate examination of the pregnant woman and the safe birth of the baby (Figs 3.22, 3.23).

- **Anterior** to the vagina lie the bladder and the urethra, which are closely connected to the anterior vaginal wall.
- **Posterior** to the vagina lie the pouch of Douglas, the rectum and the perineal body, which separates the vagina from the anal canal.
- **Laterally** on the upper two-thirds are the pelvic fascia and the ureters, which pass beside the cervix; on either side of the lower third are the muscles of the pelvic floor.
- **Superior** to the vagina lies the uterus.
- **Inferior** to the vagina lies the external genitalia.

Structure

The posterior wall of the vagina is 10 cm long, whereas the anterior wall is only 7.5 cm in length; this is because the cervix projects into its upper part at a right-angle.

The upper end of the vagina is known as the vault. Where the cervix projects into it, the vault forms a circular recess that is described as four arches or fornices. The posterior fornix is the largest of these because the vagina is attached to the uterus at a higher level behind than in front. The anterior fornix lies in front of the cervix and the lateral fornices lie on either side.

Layers

The vaginal wall is composed of three layers: mucosa, muscle and fascia. The mucosa is the most superficial layer and

BOX 3.2   Malformed Pelves

Developmental anomalies

The Naegele and Robert pelves are rare malformations caused by a failure in development. In the Naegele pelvis, one sacral ala is missing and the sacrum is fused to the ilium causing a grossly asymmetric brim. The Robert pelvis has similar malformations that are bilateral. In both instances, the abnormal brim prevents engagement of the fetal head.

Dietary deficiency

Deficiency of vitamins and minerals necessary for the formation of healthy bones is less frequently seen today than in the past but might still complicate pregnancy and labour to some extent.

A *rachitic pelvis* is a pelvis deformed by rickets in early childhood, as a consequence of malnutrition. The weight of the upper body presses downwards on to the softened pelvic bones, the sacral promontory is pushed downwards and forwards and the ilium and ischium are drawn outwards resulting in a flat pelvic brim similar to that of the platypelloid pelvis (Fig. 3.21). The sacrum tends to be straight, with the coccyx bending acutely forward. Because the tuberosities are wide apart, the pubic arch is wide. The clinical signs of rickets are bow legs and spinal deformity.

If severe contraction is present, caesarean section is required to deliver the baby. The fetal head will attempt to enter the pelvis by asynclitism.

Osteomalacic pelvis. The disease osteomalacia is rarely encountered in the UK. It is due to an acquired deficiency of calcium and occurs in adults. All bones of the skeleton soften because of gross calcium deficiency. The pelvic canal is squashed together until the brim becomes a Y-shaped slit. Labour is impossible. In early pregnancy, incarceration of the gravid uterus may occur because of the gross deformity.

Injury and disease

Trauma. A pelvis that has been fractured will develop callus formation or may fail to unite correctly. This may lead to reduced measurements and therefore to some degree of contraction. Conditions sustained in childhood such as fractures of the pelvis or lower limbs, congenital dislocation of the hip and poliomyelitis may lead to unequal weight-bearing, which will also cause deformity.

Spinal deformity. If kyphosis (forward angulation) or scoliosis (lateral curvature) is evident, or is suggested by a limp or deformity, the midwife must refer the woman to a doctor. Pelvic contraction is likely in these cases.

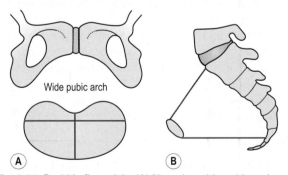

Fig. 3.21 Rachitic flat pelvis. (A) Note the wide pubic arch and kidney-shaped brim. (B) The lateral view shows the diminished anteroposterior diameter of the brim and the increased anteroposterior diameter of the outlet.

consists of stratified, squamous non-keratinized epithelium, thrown in transverse folds called 'rugae'. These allow the vaginal walls to stretch during intercourse and childbirth. Beneath the epithelium lies a layer of vascular connective tissue. The muscle layer is divided into a weak inner coat of circular fibres and a stronger outer coat of longitudinal fibres. Pelvic fascia surrounds the vagina and adjacent pelvic organs and allows for their independent expansion and contraction.

There are no glands in the vagina; however, it is moistened by mucus from the cervix and a transudate that seeps out from the blood vessels of the vaginal wall.

In spite of the alkaline mucus, the vaginal fluid is strongly acid (pH 4.5) owing to the presence of lactic acid formed by the action of Döderlein's bacilli on glycogen found in the squamous epithelium of the lining. These lactobacilli are normal inhabitants of the vagina. The acid deters the growth of pathogenic bacteria.

Blood Supply

The blood supply comes from branches of the internal iliac artery and includes the vaginal artery and a descending branch of the uterine artery. The blood drains through corresponding veins.

Lymphatic Drainage

Lymphatic drainage is via the inguinal, the internal iliac and the sacral glands.

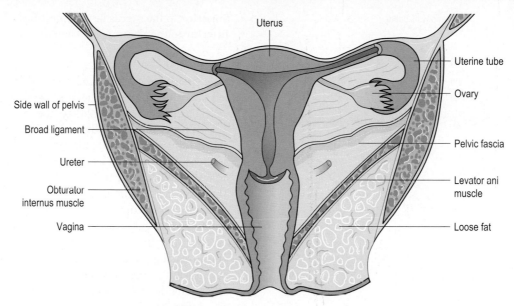

Fig. 3.22 Coronal section through the pelvis.

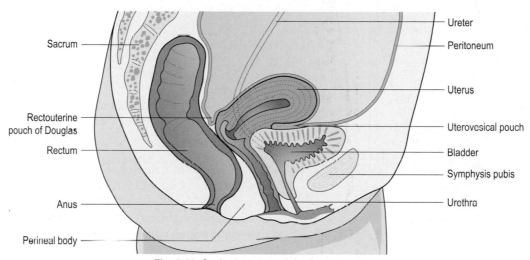

Fig. 3.23 Sagittal section of the female pelvis.

Nerve Supply

The nerve supply is derived from the pelvic plexus. The vaginal nerves follow the vaginal arteries to supply the vaginal walls and the erectile tissue of the vulva.

The Uterus

The uterus is a hollow, pear-shaped muscular organ located in the true pelvis between the bladder and the rectum. The position of the uterus within the true pelvis is one of anteversion and anteflexion. Anteversion means that the uterus leans forward and anteflexion means that it bends forwards upon itself. When the woman is standing, the uterus is in an almost horizontal position with the fundus resting on the bladder if the uterus is anteverted (Fig. 3.23).

Function

The main function of the uterus is to nourish the developing fetus prior to birth. It prepares for pregnancy each month and following pregnancy expels the products of conception.

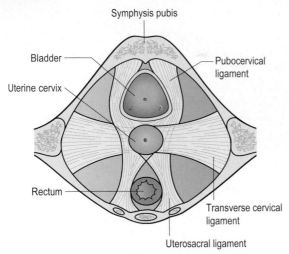

Fig. 3.24 Supports of the uterus, at the level of the cervix.

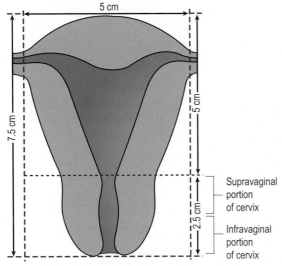

Fig. 3.25 Measurements of the uterus.

Relations

Knowledge of the relations of the uterus to other pelvic organs (Figs 3.24, 3.25) is desirable, particularly when giving women advice about bladder and bowel care during pregnancy and childbirth.

- **Anterior** to the uterus lie the uterovesical pouch and the bladder.
- **Posterior** to the uterus are the rectouterine pouch of Douglas and the rectum.
- **Lateral** to the uterus are the broad ligaments, the uterine tubes and the ovaries.
- **Superior** to the uterus lie the intestines.
- **Inferior** to the uterus is the vagina.

Supports

The uterus is supported by the pelvic floor and maintained in position by several ligaments, of which those at the level of the cervix (Fig. 3.24) are the most important.

- The transverse cervical ligaments fan out from the sides of the cervix to the side walls of the pelvis. They are sometimes known as the 'cardinal ligaments' or 'Mackenrodt's ligaments'.
- The uterosacral ligaments pass backwards from the cervix to the sacrum.
- The pubocervical ligaments pass forwards from the cervix, under the bladder, to the pubic bones.
- The broad ligaments are formed from the folds of peritoneum, which are draped over the uterine tubes. They hang down like a curtain and spread from the sides of the uterus to the side walls of the pelvis.
- The round ligaments have little value as a support but tend to maintain the anteverted position of the uterus; they arise from the cornua of the uterus, in front of and below the insertion of each uterine tube, and pass between the folds of the broad ligament, through the inguinal canal, to be inserted into each labium majus.
- The ovarian ligaments also begin at the cornua of the uterus but behind the uterine tubes and pass down between the folds of the broad ligament to the ovaries.

It is helpful to note that the round ligament, the uterine tube and the ovarian ligament are very similar in appearance and arise from the same area of the uterus. This makes careful identification important when tubal surgery is undertaken.

Structure

The non-pregnant uterus is 7.5 cm long, 5 cm wide and 2.5 cm in depth, each wall being 1.25 cm thick (Fig. 3.25). The cervix forms the lower-third of the uterus and measures 2.5 cm in each direction. The uterus consists of the following parts:

- The cornua are the upper outer angles of the uterus where the uterine tubes join.
- The fundus is the domed upper wall between the insertions of the uterine tubes.
- The body or corpus makes up the upper two-thirds of the uterus and is the greater part.

- The cavity is a potential space between the anterior and posterior walls. It is triangular in shape, the base of the triangle being uppermost.
- The isthmus is a narrow area between the cavity and the cervix, which is 7 mm long. It enlarges during pregnancy to form the lower uterine segment.
- The cervix or neck protrudes into the vagina. The upper half, being above the vagina, is known as the supravaginal portion while the lower half is the infravaginal portion.
- The internal os (mouth) is the narrow opening between the isthmus and the cervix.
- The external os is a small round opening at the lower end of the cervix. After childbirth, it becomes a transverse slit.
- The cervical canal lies between these two ostia and is a continuation of the uterine cavity. This canal is shaped like a spindle, narrow at each end and wider in the middle.

Layers

The uterus has three layers: the endometrium, the myometrium and the perimetrium, of which the myometrium, the middle muscle layer, is by far the thickest.

The endometrium forms a lining of ciliated epithelium (mucous membrane) on a base of connective tissue or stroma. In the uterine cavity, this endometrium is constantly changing in thickness throughout the menstrual cycle (see Chapter 5). The basal layer does not alter but provides the foundation from which the upper layers regenerate. The epithelial cells are cubical in shape and dip down to form glands that secrete an alkaline mucus.

The cervical endometrium does not respond to the hormonal stimuli of the menstrual cycle to the same extent. Here, the epithelial cells are tall and columnar in shape and the mucus-secreting glands are branching racemose glands. The cervical endometrium is thinner than that of the body and is folded into a pattern known as the 'arbor vitae' (tree of life). This is thought to assist the passage of the sperm. The portion of the cervix that protrudes into the vagina is covered with squamous epithelium similar to that lining the vagina. The point where the epithelium changes, at the external os, is termed the 'squamocolumnar junction'.

The myometrium is thick in the upper part of the uterus and is sparser in the isthmus and cervix. Its fibres run in all directions and interlace to surround the blood vessels and lymphatics that pass to and from the endometrium. The outer layer is formed of longitudinal fibres that are continuous with those of the uterine tube, the uterine ligaments and the vagina.

In the cervix, the muscle fibres are embedded in collagen fibres, which enable it to stretch in labour.

The perimetrium is a double serous membrane, an extension of the peritoneum, which is draped over the fundus and the anterior surface of the uterus to the level of the internal os. It is then reflected onto the bladder forming a small pouch between the uterus and the bladder called the 'uterovesical pouch'. The posterior surface is covered to where the cervix protrudes into the vagina and is then reflected onto the rectum forming the rectouterine pouch. Laterally, the perimetrium extends over the uterine tubes forming a double fold, the broad ligament, leaving the lateral borders of the body uncovered.

Blood Supply

The uterine artery arrives at the level of the cervix and is a branch of the internal iliac artery. It sends a small branch to the upper vagina, and then runs upwards in a twisted fashion to meet the ovarian artery and form an anastomosis with it near the cornu. The ovarian artery is a branch of the abdominal aorta, leaving near the renal artery. It supplies the ovary and uterine tube before joining the uterine artery. The blood drains through corresponding veins (Fig. 3.26).

Lymphatic Drainage

Lymph is drained from the uterine body to the internal iliac glands and from the cervical area to many other pelvic lymph glands. This provides an effective defence against uterine infection.

Nerve Supply

The nerve supply is mainly from the autonomic nervous system, sympathetic and parasympathetic, via the inferior hypogastric or pelvic plexus.

Uterine Malformations

The prevalence of uterine malformation is estimated to be 6.7% in the general population. The female genital tract is formed in early embryonic life when a pair of ducts develops. These paramesonephric or Müllerian ducts come together in the midline and fuse into a Y-shaped canal. The open upper ends of this structure

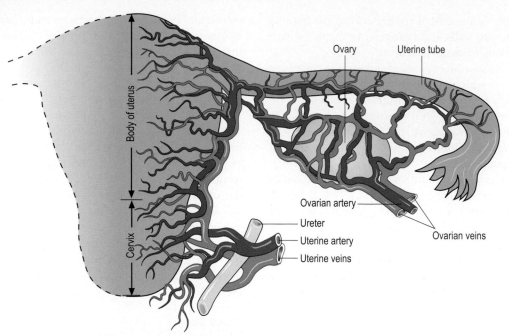

Fig. 3.26 Blood supply of the uterus, uterine tubes and ovaries.

BOX 3.3   Uterine Malformations

Types of uterine malformation

Various types of structural abnormality can result from failure of fusion of the Müllerian ducts. Three of these abnormalities can be seen in Fig. 3.27. A double uterus with an associated double vagina will develop where there has been complete failure of fusion. Partial fusion results in various degrees of duplication. A single vagina with a double uterus is the result of fusion at the lower end of the ducts only. A bicornuate uterus (one with two horns) is the result of incomplete fusion at the upper portion of the uterovaginal area. In rare cases, one Müllerian duct regresses and the result is a uterus with one horn – termed a 'unicornuate uterus'.

---

lead into the peritoneal cavity and the unfused portions become the uterine tubes. The fused lower portion forms the uterovaginal area, which further develops into the uterus and vagina. Abnormal development of the Müllerian duct(s) during embryogenesis can lead to uterine abnormalities (Box 3.3 and Fig. 3.27).

Structural abnormality of the uterus can lead to various problems during pregnancy and childbirth. The outcome depends on the ability of the uterus to accommodate the growing fetus. A problem exists only if the tissue is insufficient to allow the uterus to enlarge for a full-term fetus lying longitudinally. If there is insufficient hypertrophy, the possible difficulties are miscarriage, premature labour and abnormal lie of the fetus. In labour, poor uterine function may be experienced. Minor defects of structure cause little problem and might pass unnoticed, with the woman having a normal outcome to her pregnancy. Occasionally problems arise when a fetus is accommodated in one horn of a double uterus and the empty horn has filled the pelvic cavity. In this situation, the empty horn has grown owing to the hormonal influences of the pregnancy, and its size and position will cause obstruction during labour. Caesarean section would be the mode of birth.

The Fallopian Tubes

The uterine tubes, also known as fallopian tubes, oviducts and salpinges, are two very fine tubes leading from the ovaries into the uterus.

Function

The uterine tube propels the ovum towards the uterus, receives the spermatozoa as they travel upwards and provides a site for fertilization. It supplies the fertilized ovum with nutrition during its continued journey to the uterus.

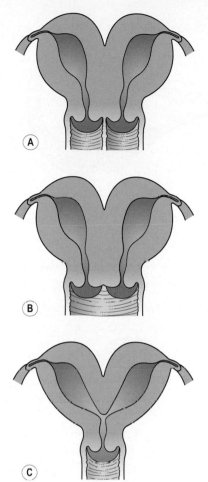

Fig. 3.27 Uterine malformations. (A) Double uterus with duplication of body of uterus, cervix and vagina. (B) Duplication of uterus and cervix with single vagina. (C) Duplication of uterus with single cervix and vagina.

Position

The uterine tubes extend laterally from the cornua of the uterus towards the side walls of the pelvis. They arch over the ovaries, the fringed ends hovering near the ovaries in order to receive the ovum.

Relations

- **Anterior**, posterior and superior to the uterine tubes are the peritoneal cavity and the intestines.
- **Lateral** to the uterine tubes are the side walls of the pelvis.
- **Inferior** to the uterine tubes lie the broad ligaments and the ovaries.
- **Medial** to the two uterine tubes lies the uterus.

Supports

The uterine tubes are held in place by their attachment to the uterus. The peritoneum folds over them, draping down below as the broad ligaments and extending at the sides to form the infundibulopelvic ligaments.

Structure

Each tube is 10 cm long. The lumen of the tube provides an open pathway from the outside to the peritoneal cavity. The uterine tube has four portions (Fig. 3.28):

- **The interstitial portion** is 1.25 cm long and lies within the wall of the uterus. Its lumen is 1 mm wide.
- **The isthmus** is another narrow part that extends for 2.5 cm from the uterus.
- **The ampulla** is the wider portion, where fertilization usually occurs. It is 5 cm long.
- **The infundibulum** is the funnel-shaped fringed end that is composed of many processes known as fimbriae. One fimbria is elongated to form the ovarian fimbria, which is attached to the ovary.

Layers

The lining of the uterine tubes is a mucous membrane of ciliated cubical epithelium that is thrown into complicated folds known as plicae. These folds slow the ovum down on its way to the uterus. In this lining are goblet cells that produce a secretion containing glycogen to nourish the oocyte.

Beneath the lining is a layer of vascular connective tissue.

The muscle coat consists of two layers: an inner circular layer and an outer longitudinal layer, both of smooth muscle. The peristaltic movement of the uterine tube is due to the action of these muscles.

The tube is covered with peritoneum but the infundibulum passes through it to open into the peritoneal cavity.

Blood Supply

The blood supply is via the uterine and ovarian arteries, returning by the corresponding veins.

Lymphatic Drainage

Lymph is drained to the lumbar glands.

Nerve Supply

The nerve supply is from the ovarian plexus.

The Ovaries

The ovaries are components of the female reproductive system and the endocrine system.

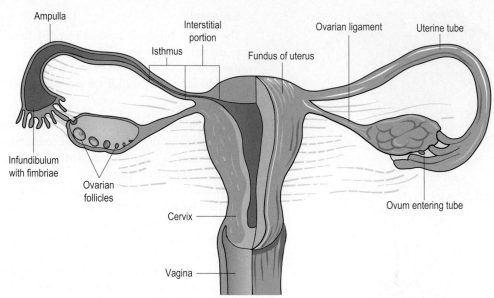

Fig. 3.28 The uterine tubes in section. Note the ovum entering the fimbriated end of one tube.

Function

The ovaries produce oocytes and the hormones, oestrogen and progesterone.

Position

The ovaries are attached to the back of the broad ligaments within the peritoneal cavity.

Relations

- **Anterior** to the ovaries are the broad ligaments.
- **Posterior** to the ovaries are the intestines.
- **Lateral** to the ovaries are the infundibulopelvic ligaments and the side walls of the pelvis.
- **Superior** to the ovaries lie the uterine tubes.
- **Medial** to the ovaries lie the ovarian ligaments and the uterus.

Supports

The ovary is attached to the broad ligament but is supported from above by the ovarian ligament medially and the infundibulopelvic ligament laterally.

Structure

The ovary is composed of a medulla and cortex, covered with germinal epithelium.

- **The medulla** is the supporting framework, which is made of fibrous tissue; the ovarian blood vessels,

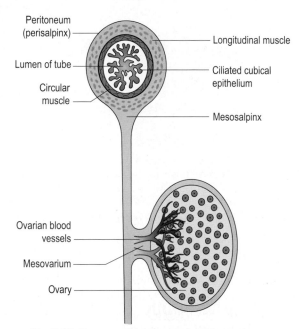

Fig. 3.29 Cross-section of a uterine tube and ovary.

lymphatics and nerves travel through it. The hilum where these vessels enter lies just where the ovary is attached to the broad ligament and this area is called the mesovarium (Fig. 3.29).

- **The cortex** is the functioning part of the ovary. It contains the ovarian follicles in different stages of development, surrounded by stroma. The outer

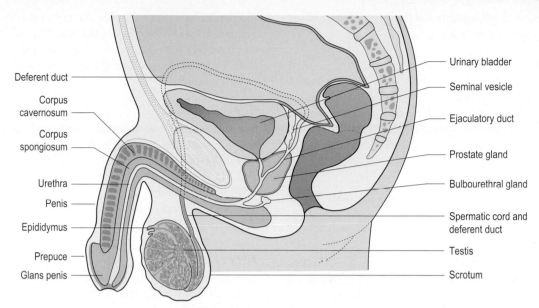

Fig. 3.30 Male reproductive system.

Labels (left side, top to bottom): Deferent duct, Corpus cavernosum, Corpus spongiosum, Urethra, Penis, Epididymus, Prepuce, Glans penis

Labels (right side, top to bottom): Urinary bladder, Seminal vesicle, Ejaculatory duct, Prostate gland, Bulbourethral gland, Spermatic cord and deferent duct, Testis, Scrotum

layer is formed of fibrous tissue known as the tunica albuginea. Over this lies the germinal epithelium, which is a modification of the peritoneum.

- The cycle of the ovary is described in Chapter 5.

Blood Supply

Blood is supplied to the ovaries from the ovarian arteries and drains via the ovarian veins. The right ovarian vein joins the inferior vena cava, but the left returns its blood to the left renal vein.

Lymphatic Drainage

Lymphatic drainage is to the lumbar glands.

Nerve Supply

The nerve supply is from the ovarian plexus.

THE MALE REPRODUCTIVE SYSTEM

The male reproductive system (Fig. 3.30) consists of a set of organs that are partly visible and partly hidden within the body. The visible parts are the scrotum and the penis. Inside the body are the prostate gland and tubes that link the system together. The male organs produce and transfer sperm to the female for fertilization. The organs are the scrotum, testis, rete and epididymis, ductus deferens, seminal vesicles, prostate gland, bulbourethral glands and penis with the urethra.

The Scrotum

The scrotum is part of the external genitalia. Also called the scrotal sac, the scrotum is a thin-walled, soft, muscular pouch located below the symphysis pubis, between the upper parts of the thighs behind the penis.

Function

The scrotum forms a pouch in which the testes are suspended outside the body, keeping them at a temperature slightly lower than that of the rest of the body. A temperature around 34.4°C enables the production of viable sperm, whereas a temperature of or above 36.7°C can be damaging to sperm count.

Structure

The scrotum is formed of pigmented skin and has two compartments, one for each testis.

The Testes

Like the ovaries, to which they are homologous, the testes (also known as testicles) are components of both the reproductive system and the endocrine system. Each testis weighs about 25 g.

Function

The testes produce and store spermatozoa, and are the body's main source of the male hormone testosterone.

Testosterone is responsible for the development of secondary sex characteristics.

Position

In the embryo, the testes develop high up in the lumbar region of the abdominal cavity. In the last few months of fetal life they descend through the abdomen, over the pelvic brim and down the inguinal canal into the scrotum outside the body. The testes are contained within the scrotum.

Structure

Each testis is an oval structure about 5 cm long and 3 cm in diameter.

Layers

There are three layers to the testis:

- **The tunica vasculosa** is an inner layer of connective tissue containing a fine network of capillaries.
- **The tunica albuginea** is a fibrous covering, ingrowths of which divide the testis into 200–300 lobules.
- **The tunica vaginalis** is the outer layer, which is made of peritoneum brought down with the descending testis when it migrated from the lumbar region in fetal life.

The duct system within the testes is highly intricate:

- **The seminiferous** ('seed-carrying') tubules are where spermatogenesis, or production of sperm, takes place. There are up to three of them in each lobule. Between the tubules are interstitial cells that secrete testosterone. The tubules join to form a system of channels that lead to the epididymis.
- **The epididymis** is a comma-shaped, coiled tube that lies on the superior surface and travels down the posterior aspect to the lower pole of the testis, where it leads into the deferent duct or vas deferens.

The Spermatic Cord

The spermatic cord is the name given to the cord-like structure consisting of the vas deferens and its accompanying arteries, veins, nerves and lymphatic vessels.

Function

The function of the deferent duct is to carry the sperm to the ejaculatory duct.

Position

The cord passes upwards through the inguinal canal, where the different structures diverge. The deferent duct then continues upwards over the symphysis pubis and arches backwards beside the bladder. Behind the bladder, it merges with the duct from the seminal vesicle and passes through the prostate gland as the ejaculatory duct to join the urethra.

Blood Supply

The testicular artery, a branch of the abdominal aorta, supplies the testes, scrotum and attachments. The testicular veins drain in the same manner as the ovarian veins.

Lymphatic Drainage

Lymphatic drainage is to the lymph nodes round the aorta.

Nerve Supply

The nerve supply to the spermatic cord is from the 10th and 11th thoracic nerves.

The Seminal Vesicles

The seminal vesicles are a pair of simple tubular glands.

Function

The function of the seminal vesicles is production of a viscous secretion to keep the sperm alive and motile. This secretion ultimately becomes semen.

Position

The seminal vesicles are situated posterior to the bladder and superior to the prostate gland.

Structure

The seminal vesicles are 5 cm long and pyramid-shaped. They are composed of columnar epithelium, muscle tissue and fibrous tissue.

The Ejaculatory Ducts

These small muscular ducts carry the spermatozoa and the seminal fluid to the urethra.

The Prostate Gland

The prostate is an exocrine gland of the male reproductive system.

Function

The prostate gland produces a thin lubricating fluid that enters the urethra through ducts.

Position

The prostate gland surrounds the urethra at the base of the bladder, lying between the rectum and the symphysis pubis.

Structure

The prostate gland measures 4 × 3 × 2 cm. It is composed of columnar epithelium, a muscle layer and an outer fibrous layer.

The Bulbourethral Glands

The bulbourethral glands are two very small glands, which produce yet another lubricating fluid that passes into the urethra just below the prostate gland.

The Penis

The penis is the male reproductive organ and additionally serves as the external male organ of urination.

Functions

The penis carries the urethra, which is a passage for both urine and semen. During sexual excitement it stiffens (an erection) in order to be able to penetrate the vagina and deposit the semen near the woman's cervix.

Position

The root of the penis lies in the perineum, from where it passes forward below the symphysis pubis. The lower two-thirds are outside the body in front of the scrotum.

Structure

The penis has three columns of erectile tissue:
- **The corpora cavernosa** are two lateral columns that lie one on either side in front of the urethra.
- **The corpus spongiosum** is the posterior column that contains the urethra. The tip is expanded to form the glans penis.

The lower two-thirds of the penis are covered in skin. At the end, the skin is folded back on itself above the glans penis to form the prepuce or foreskin, which is a movable double fold. The penis is extremely vascular and during an erection the blood spaces fill and become distended.

The Male Hormones

The control of the male gonads is similar to that in the female, but it is not cyclical. The hypothalamus produces

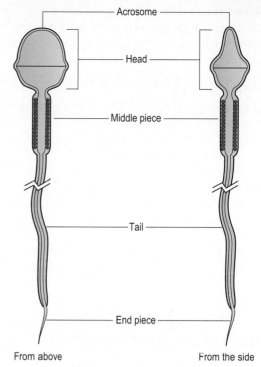

Fig. 3.31 Spermatozoon.

gonadotrophin-releasing factors. These stimulate the anterior pituitary gland to produce follicle stimulating hormone (FSH) and luteinizing hormone (LH). FSH acts on the seminiferous tubules to bring about the production of sperm, whereas LH acts on the interstitial cells that produce testosterone.

Testosterone is responsible for the secondary sex characteristics: deepening of the voice, growth of the genitalia and growth of hair on the chest, pubis, axilla and face.

Formation of the Spermatozoa

Production of sperm begins at puberty and continues throughout adult life. Spermatogenesis takes place in the seminiferous tubules under the influence of FSH and testosterone. The process of maturation is a lengthy one and takes some weeks. The mature sperm are stored in the epididymis and the deferent duct until ejaculation. If this does not happen, they degenerate and are reabsorbed. At each ejaculation, 2–4 mL of semen is deposited in the vagina. The seminal fluid contains about 100 million sperm/mL, of which 20–25% are likely to be abnormal. The remainder move at a speed of 2–3 mm/ min. The individual spermatozoon has a head, a body and a long, mobile tail that lashes to propel the sperm along (Fig. 3.31). The tip of the head is covered by an acrosome; this contains enzymes to dissolve the covering of the oocyte in order to penetrate it.

REFLECTIVE ACTIVITY FOR SELF-ASSESSMENT

1. Name the superficial muscles of the perineum and their anatomical location.
2. Name the levator ani muscles of the pelvic floor and state their anatomical location.
3. List the functions of the internal and external anal sphincters.
4. Use the unlabelled Fig. 3.11 here to label the eight landmarks of the pelvic brim.

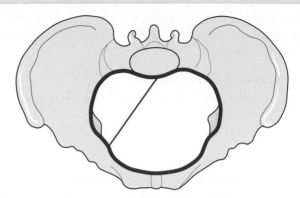

ANNOTATED FURTHER READING

Kearney, R., Sawhney, R., & DeLancey, J. O. (2004). Levator ani muscle anatomy evaluated by origin-insertion pairs. *Obstetrics and Gynecology, 104,* 168–173.
A comprehensive and up-to-date description of levator ani muscle anatomy.
Schwertner-Tiepelmann, N., Thakar, R., Sultan, A. H., et al. (2012). Obstetric levator ani muscle injuries – current status. *Ultrasound in Obstetrics and Gynecology, 39,* 372–383.
This review article critically appraises the diagnosis of obstetric LAM injuries, to establish the relationship between LAM injuries and pelvic floor dysfunction and to identify risk factors and preventive strategies to minimize such injuries.
Rankin, J. (Ed.). (2017). *Physiology in childbearing: with anatomy and related biosciences* (4th edn.) Edinburgh: Baillière Tindall.
This textbook presents a comprehensive and clear account of anatomy and physiology and related biosciences at all stages of pregnancy and childbirth.

Standring, S. (Ed.). (2016). *Gray's anatomy: The anatomical basis of clinical practice* (41st ed.) London: Elsevier Churchill Livingstone.
This large volume, with detailed information about the anatomy of every part of the human body, provides the reader with much more insight into the structure and function of the reproductive organs. This edition includes specialist revision of topics such as the anatomy of the pelvic floor.
Sultan, A. H., Thakar, R., & Fenner, D. E. (2007). *Perineal and anal sphincter trauma: diagnosis and clinical management.* London: Springer-Verlag.
This is a comprehensive text that focuses on the maternal morbidity associated with childbirth. It is essential reading for anyone involved in obstetric care such as obstetricians, midwives and family practitioners but will also be of interest to colorectal surgeons, gastroenterologists, physiotherapists, continence advisors and lawyers.

4

The Female Urinary Tract

Jean Rankin

CHAPTER CONTENTS

The midwife must have a sound knowledge of the anatomy of the structures of the urinary tract and the basics of normal renal physiology to then understand the changes taking place during pregnancy and how these changes may impact on the health and wellbeing of the childbearing woman.

THE CHAPTER AIMS TO

- provide an overview of the anatomy and functions of the various structures of the urinary system
- describe the processes of excretion, elimination and homeostatic regulation of the volume and solute concentration of blood plasma
- explain how urine is produced in the kidneys and eliminated through the process of micturition
- provide an overview of how the physiological effects of pregnancy and its hormonal influences may impact on the functioning of the urinary tract.

THE KIDNEYS

The kidneys are excretory glands with both endocrine and exocrine functions. They perform the excretory functions of the urinary system by removing metabolic waste products from the circulation to produce urine. The kidneys also have a major role in the maintenance of homeostasis

109

BOX 4.1   Functions of the Kidney

- Regulation of water balance
- Regulation of blood pressure (renin–angiotensin system)
- Regulation of pH (acid–base balance) and inorganic ion balance (potassium K^+, sodium Na^+ and calcium Ca^{++})
- Regulation of volume and chemical makeup of the blood
- Control of formation of red blood cells (via erythropoietin)
- Secretion of hormones – renin, erythropoietin, 1,25-dihydroxyvitamin D3 (1,25-dihydroxycholecalciferol, synthetic version is named calcitriol) and prostaglandins
- Conversion of vitamin D to the active form and calcium balance
- Gluconeogenesis (formation of glucose from amino acids and other precursors)
- Excretion of metabolic and nitrogenous waste products (urea from protein, uric acid from nucleic acids, creatinine from muscle creatine and haemoglobin breakdown products)
- Removal of toxins, metabolic waste and excess ions through the formation and excretion of urine.

---

within the internal environment through the regulation of volume and composition of body fluids (Box 4.1).

A typical adult kidney is a bean-shaped reddish-brown organ. Each kidney is about 10 cm long, 6.5 cm wide, 3 cm thick and weighs about 100 g (Coad and Dunstall 2011). Although similar in shape, the left kidney is a longer and slimmer organ than the right kidney. Congenital absence of one or both kidneys, known as unilateral or bilateral renal agenesis, can occur (Jones et al. 2015). Although uncommon, bilateral renal agenesis is a serious failure in the development of both kidneys in the fetus. It is one causative agent of the Potter sequence (also known as *Potter syndrome*). This absence of fetal kidneys causes *oligohydramnios*, a deficiency of amniotic fluid in a pregnant woman, which can place extra pressure on the developing fetus and can cause further malformations. Non-pregnant adults with unilateral renal agenesis have a considerably higher risk of developing hypertension, which will become even more pronounced during pregnancy.

Position and Relations

The kidneys are situated in the posterior part of the abdominal cavity, one on either side of the vertebral column between the eleventh thoracic vertebra (T11) and the third lumbar vertebra (L3) (Jones et al. 2015). The right kidney is slightly lower than the left kidney owing to its relationship to the liver (Coad and Dunstall 2011). The anterior and posterior surfaces of the kidneys are related to numerous structures, some of which come into direct contact with the kidneys whereas others are separated by a layer of peritoneum:

- *Posteriorly*, the kidneys are related to rib 12 and the diaphragm, psoas major, quadratus lumborum and transversus abdominis muscles.
- *Anteriorly*, the right kidney, is related to the liver, duodenum, ascending colon and small intestine. The left kidney is related to the spleen, stomach, pancreas, descending colon and small intestine.

The triangular-shaped adrenal (suprarenal) glands are situated in the upper pole of the kidneys (Coad and Dunstall 2011).

Supports

The kidneys are maintained in position within the abdominal cavity by the overlying peritoneum, contact with adjacent visceral organs, such as the gastrointestinal tract and by supporting connective tissue (Martini et al. 2018).

Structure

Each kidney has a smooth surface covered by a tough fibrous capsule. There is a concave side facing medially. On this medial aspect is an opening called the *hilum*. The hilum is the point of entry for the renal artery and renal nerves, and the point of exit for the renal vein and the ureter (Fig. 4.1). Internally, the hilum is continuous with the renal sinus.

Each kidney is enclosed by a thick fibrous capsule and has two distinct layers: the reddish-brown renal *cortex*, which has a rich blood supply, and the inner renal *medulla* where the structural and functional units of the kidney are located (Coad and Dunstall 2011). The renal medulla lies below the renal cortex and consists of between 8 and 18 distinct cone-shaped structures called *medullary* or *renal pyramids*. Each renal pyramid (which is striped in appearance) together with the associated overlying renal cortex forms a *renal lobe*. The base of each pyramid is broad and faces the cortex, while the pointed apex (*papilla*) projects into a minor *calyx*. Several minor calyces open into each of two or three major calyces, which then open into the *renal pelvis*. The renal

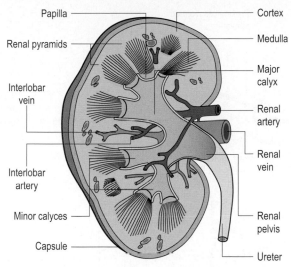

Fig. 4.1 Longitudinal section of the kidney.

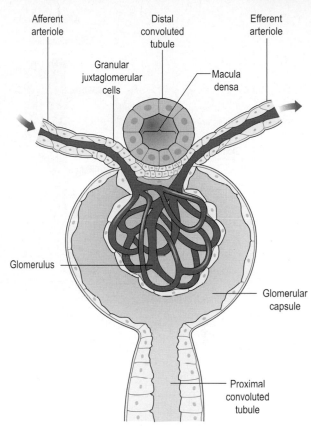

Fig. 4.2 A glomerular body.

pelvis is a flat funnel-shaped tube that is continuous with the *ureter*. Urine produced by the kidney flows continuously from the renal pelvis into the ureter and then into the bladder for storage (Rankin 2017).

The Nephron

Each kidney has over 1 million nephrons, which are the functional units of the kidney. The nephron is approximately 3 cm long and is a tubule that is closed at one end and opens into the collecting duct at the other (Coad and Dunstall 2011). The nephron has five distinct regions, each of which is adapted to a specific function:

- *Bowman's capsule* containing the glomerulus (renal corpuscle)
- the proximal convoluted tubule
- the *loop of Henle*
- the distal convoluted tubule and
- the collecting duct (Jones et al. 2015).

There are two types of nephrons: *cortical nephrons* and *juxtamedullary nephrons*. The majority are cortical nephrons (85–90%) and these have short loops of Henle. The main function of the cortical nephrons is to control plasma volume during normal conditions. The juxtamedullary nephrons have longer loops of Henle extending into the medulla. These nephrons facilitate increased water retention when there is restricted water available (Coad and Dunstall 2011).

Each nephron begins at the renal corpuscle, which comprises the Bowman's capsule (a blind-ended

cup-shaped chamber), and the glomerulus, a coiled arranged capillary network incorporated within the capsule (Fig. 4.2).

Blood enters the renal corpuscle by way of the afferent arteriole, which delivers blood to the glomerulus, with blood leaving by way of the efferent arteriole. This is the only place in the body where an artery collects blood from capillaries. The pressure within the glomerulus is increased because the afferent arteriole has a wider bore than the efferent arteriole and this factor forces the filtrate out of the capillaries into the capsule. At this stage, any substance with a small molecular size will be filtered out.

The cup of the capsule is attached to the tubule of the nephron (Fig. 4.3). The proximal convoluted tubule initially winds and twists through the cortex, then forms a straight loop of Henle that dips into the medulla (descending arm), rising up into the cortex again (ascending arm) to wind and turn as the distal convoluted tubule before joining the straight collecting tubule.

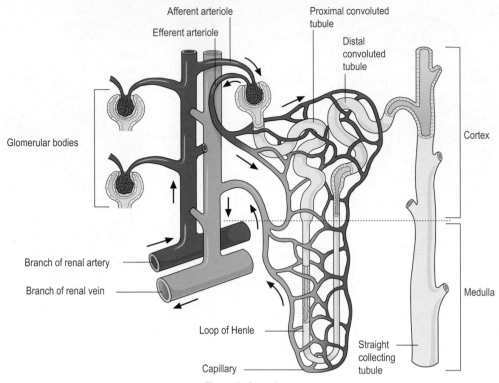

Fig. 4.3 A nephron.

The straight collecting tubule runs from the cortex to a *medullary pyramid* where it forms a *medullary ray* and receives urine from many nephrons along its length (Martini et al. 2018).

The distal convoluted tubule returns to pass alongside granular cells (also known as *juxtaglomerular cells*) of the afferent arteriole and this part of the tubule is called the *macula densa* (Fig. 4.2). The granular cells and macula densa are known as the juxtaglomerular apparatus. The granular cells secrete renin whereas the macula densa cells monitor the sodium chloride concentration of fluid passing through.

Blood Supply

The kidneys receive about 20–25% of the total cardiac output (Jones et al. 2015). In healthy individuals, about 1200 mL of blood flows through the kidneys each minute. This is a phenomenal amount of blood for organs that have a combined weight of <300 g (Martini et al. 2018).

Each kidney receives blood through the renal artery, which originates from the lateral surface of the descending abdominal aorta near the level of the superior mesenteric artery. The artery enters at the renal hilum, transmitting numerous branches into the cortex to form the glomerulus for each nephron. Blood is collected up and returned via the renal vein.

Lymphatic Drainage

A rich supply of lymph vessels lies under the cortex and around the urine-bearing tubules. Lymph drains into large lymphatic ducts that emerge from the hilum and lead to the aortic lymph glands.

Nerve Supply

The kidneys are innervated by renal nerves. A renal nerve enters each kidney at the hilum and follows tributaries of renal arteries to reach individual nephrons. The sympathetic innervation adjusts rates of urine formation by changing blood flow and blood pressure at the nephron and mobilizes the release of renin, which ultimately restricts loss of water and salt in the urine by stimulating reabsorption at the nephron (Martini et al. 2018).

TABLE 4.1	Characteristics of Urine
Characteristics	**Normal Range**
pH	4.5–8.0 (average 6.0)
Specific gravity	1.010–1.030
Osmotic concentration (osmolarity)	855–1335 mOsmol/L
Water content	93–97%
Volume	Varies depending on intake but usually 1000–1500 mL/day
Colour	Clear pale straw (dilute)
	Dark brown (very concentrated)
	Clear (in babies)
Odour	Varies with composition
Bacterial content	None (sterile)

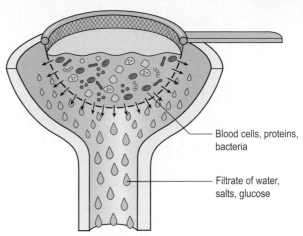

Fig. 4.4 Filtration: larger molecules stay in the sieve (glomerulus) and smaller molecules filter out (into the glomerular capsule).

Labels: Blood cells, proteins, bacteria; Filtrate of water, salts, glucose

Endocrine Activity

The kidney secretes two hormones: *renin* and *erythropoietin*. Renin is produced in the afferent arteriole and is secreted when the blood supply to the kidneys is reduced and in response to lowered sodium levels. It acts on *angiotensinogen* (present in the blood) to form angiotensin, which raises blood pressure and encourages sodium reabsorption. The kidneys produce the hormone erythropoietin, in response to low oxygen levels that stimulate an increase in the production of red blood cells from the bone marrow (Coad and Dunstall 2011).

URINE

Urine is usually acid and should not contain glucose or ketones or carry blood cells or bacteria. The amber colour is due to the bile pigment *urobilin* and the colour varies depending on the concentration (Table 4.1). In the newborn baby, it is almost clear. The volume and final concentration of urea and solutes depend on fluid intake. An adult can usually void between 1000 mL and 1500 mL of urine daily (this amount varies). Urine has a characteristic smell, which is not unpleasant when fresh. Strong odour or cloudiness generally indicates a bacterial infection.

Women are susceptible to urinary tract infection, usually due to ascending infection acquired via the urethra. A colony bacterial count >100,000/mL is considered to be pathologically significant and is often referred to as bacteraemia (Coad and Dunstall 2011).

The Production of Urine

The production of urine takes place in three stages: *filtration*, *selective reabsorption* and *secretion*.

Filtration

Filtration is a largely passive, non-selective process that occurs through the semipermeable walls of the glomerulus and glomerular capsule. Fluids and solutes are forced through the membrane by hydrostatic pressure. The passage of water and solutes across the filtration membrane of the glomerulus is similar to that in other capillary beds; moving down a pressure gradient. However, the glomerular filtration membrane is thousands of times more permeable to water and solutes, and glomerular pressure is much higher than normal capillary blood pressure (Rankin 2017). Water and small molecules such as glucose, amino acids and vitamins easily pass through the filter as the *filtrate* and enter the nephron, whereas blood cells, plasma proteins and other large molecules are prevented from passing through by the capillary pores and retained in the blood (Fig. 4.4). The content of the Bowman's capsule is referred to as the *glomerular filtrate* (GF) and the rate at which this is formed is referred to as the *glomerular filtration rate* (GFR). The kidneys form about 180 L of dilute filtrate each day (125 mL/min). Most of this is selectively reabsorbed so that the final volume of urine produced daily is about 1000–1500 mL/day (Coad and Dunstall 2011).

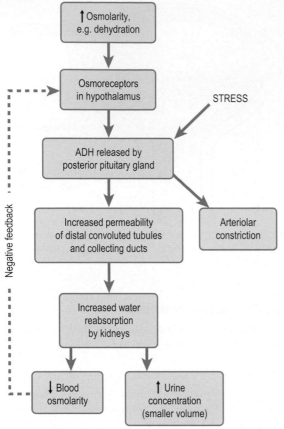

Fig. 4.5 The action of the antidiuretic hormone (ADH).

Selective Reabsorption

Substances from the glomerular filtrate are reabsorbed from the rest of the nephron into the surrounding capillaries. Some substances, such as amino acids and glucose, are completely reabsorbed and are not normally present in urine. The reabsorption of other substances is under the regulation of several hormones. Water balance is mainly regulated by the *antidiuretic hormone* (ADH) produced by the posterior lobe of the pituitary gland. This is regulated through a negative feedback loop (Fig. 4.5).

The secretion of ADH is initiated by an increase in plasma osmolality, by a decrease in circulating blood volume and by lowered blood pressure (e.g. through reduced fluid intake or sweating). The action of ADH is to increase permeability of the renal tubular cells. More water is reabsorbed, resulting in reduced volume of more concentrated urine. When the body has sufficient fluid intake and physiological

parameters are within normal range, then the production of ADH is inhibited and urine increases in volume and is more dilute. One interesting exception relates to the consumption of alcohol, which inhibits the effect of ADH on the kidneys, thereby inducing diuresis that is out of proportion to the volume of fluid ingested. Newborn babies have poor ability to concentrate and dilute their urine and this is even more so for preterm infants. For this reason, preterm infants are unable to tolerate wide variations in their fluid intake.

Minerals are selected according to the body's needs. Calcitonin increases calcium excretion and parathyroid hormone enhances reabsorption of calcium from the renal tubules (Coad and Dunstall 2011). The reabsorption of sodium is controlled by aldosterone, which is produced in the cortex of the suprarenal gland. The interaction of aldosterone and ADH maintains water and sodium balance. It is vital that the pH of the blood is controlled in the body and if it is tending towards acidity, then acids will be excreted in urine. However, if the opposite situation arises then alkaline urine will be produced. Often, this is the result of an intake of an alkaline substance. A diet high in meat and cranberry juice will keep the urine acidic while a diet rich in citrus fruit, most vegetables and legumes will keep the urine alkaline. Bacteria causing a urinary tract infection or bacterial contamination will also produce alkaline urine.

Secretion

Tubular secretion is an important mechanism in clearing the blood of unwanted substances. Secreted substances into the urine include hydrogen ions, ammonia, creatinine, drugs and toxins.

THE URETERS

The ureters are hollow muscular tubes. The upper end is funnel-shaped and merges into the renal pelvis, where urine is received from the renal tubules.

Function

The ureters transport urine from the kidneys to the bladder by waves of peristalsis. About every 30 s, a peristaltic contraction begins at the renal pelvis and sweeps along the ureter, forcing urine towards the urinary bladder (Martini et al. 2018).

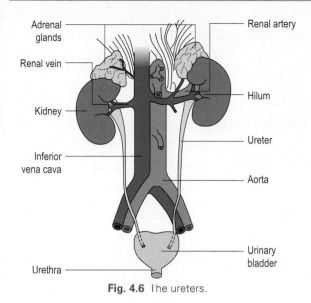

Fig. 4.6 The ureters.

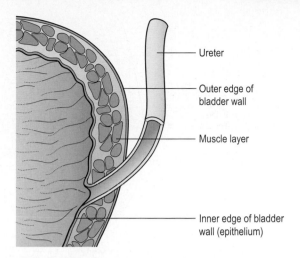

Fig. 4.7 Diagram showing the entry of the ureter into the posterior wall of the bladder.

Structure

Each ureter is about 0.3 cm in diameter and 25–30 cm long, running from the renal hilum to the posterior wall of the bladder (Fig. 4.6).

The ureters extend inferiorly and medially, passing over the anterior surfaces of the *psoas major muscle* and are firmly attached to the posterior abdominal wall. At the pelvic brim the ureters descend along the side walls of the pelvis to the level of the ischial spines and then turn forwards to pass beside the uterine cervix and enter the bladder from behind (Fig. 4.7). The ureters penetrate the posterior wall of the urinary bladder without entering the peritoneal cavity. They pass through the bladder wall at an oblique angle, and the ureteral openings are slit-like rather than rounded. This shape helps prevent the backflow of urine toward the ureter and kidneys when the urinary bladder contracts (Martini et al. 2018).

Layers

The ureters are composed of three layers: an *inner lining*, a *middle muscular layer* and an *outer coat* (Martini et al. 2018). The inner lining comprises of transitional epithelium arranged in longitudinal folds. This type of epithelium consists of several layers of pear-shaped cells and makes an elastic and waterproof inner coat. The middle muscular layer is made up of longitudinal and circular bands of smooth muscle. The outer coat comprises fibrous connective tissue that is continuous with the fibrous capsule of the kidney.

Blood Supply

The blood supply to the upper part of the ureter is similar to that of the kidney. In its pelvic portion, it derives blood from the common iliac and internal iliac arteries and from the uterine and vesical arteries, according to its proximity to the different organs. Venous return is along corresponding veins.

Lymphatic Drainage

Lymph drains into the internal, external and common iliac nodes.

Nerve Supply

The nerve supply is from the renal, aortic, superior and inferior hypogastric plexuses.

THE BLADDER

The bladder is a distensible, hollow, muscular, pelvic organ that functions as a temporary reservoir for the storage of urine until it is convenient for it to be voided. Pregnancy and childbirth can affect bladder control and thus midwives need to be familiar with the anatomy and physiology of the bladder.

Position, Shape and Size

The empty bladder lies in the pelvic cavity and is described as being *pyramidal* with its triangular base resting on the upper half of the vagina and its apex directed towards the symphysis pubis. However, as it fills with urine it rises up

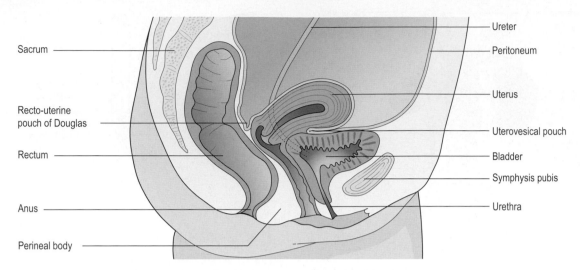

Fig. 4.8 Sagittal section of the pelvis showing the relations of the bladder.

out of the pelvic cavity becoming an abdominal organ and more globular in shape as its walls are distended. It can be palpated above the symphysis pubis when full. As the fetus descends into the pelvic cavity during labour, the bladder is displaced to become an abdominal organ.

The empty bladder is of similar size to the uterus, but when full of urine it becomes much larger. The normal capacity of the bladder is approximately 500 mL, although the capacity in individuals does vary between 300 mL and 700 mL (Rankin 2017).

Relations

Details are shown in Fig. 4.8.

- *Anterior* to the bladder is the symphysis pubis, which is separated from it by a space filled with fatty tissue called the *Cave of Retzius.*
- *Posterior* to the bladder are the cervix and ureters.
- *Laterally* are the lateral ligaments of the bladder and the side walls of the pelvis.
- *Superiorly* lie the intestines and peritoneal cavity. In the non-pregnant female, the anteverted, anteflexed uterus lies partially over the bladder.
- *Inferior* to the bladder is the urethra and the muscular diaphragm of the pelvic floor, which forms its main support, and on which its function partly depends.

Supports

There are five ligaments attached to the bladder (Rankin 2017). A fibrous band called the *urachus* extends from

the apex of the bladder to the umbilicus. Two *lateral ligaments* extend from the bladder to the side walls of the pelvis. Two *pubovesical ligaments* attach from the bladder neck anteriorly to the pubic bones. These ligaments also form part of the pubocervical ligaments of the uterus.

Structure

The base of the bladder is termed the *trigone*. It is situated at the back of the bladder, resting against the vagina. The three angles include the exit of the urethra below and the two slit-like openings of the ureters above. The apex of the trigone is thus at its lowest point, which is also termed *the neck* (Fig. 4.9).

The anterior part of the bladder lies close to the symphysis pubis and is termed the *apex of the bladder*. From the apex of the bladder, the urachus runs up the anterior abdominal wall to the umbilicus. In fetal life, the urachus is the remains of the yolk sac but in the adult it is simply a fibrous band.

Layers

The lining of the bladder, similar to the ureter, is formed of transitional epithelium, which helps to allow the distension of the bladder without losing its water-holding effect. The lining, except over the trigone, is thrown into *rugae*, which flatten out as the bladder expands and fills. The mucous membrane lining lies on a submucous layer of areolar tissue that carries blood vessels, lymph vessels and nerves.

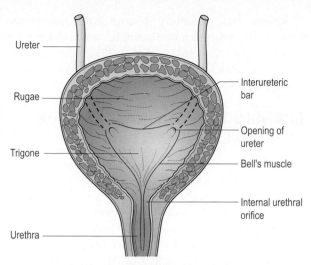

Ureter

Rugae

Trigone

Urethra

Interureteric bar

Opening of ureter

Bell's muscle

Internal urethral orifice

Fig. 4.9 Section through the bladder.

The epithelium over the trigone is smooth and firmly attached to the underlying muscle. The musculature of the bladder consists chiefly of the large *detrusor muscle* with the function to expel urine. This muscle has three coats of smooth muscle: an *inner longitudinal, a middle circular* and an *outer longitudinal* layer. Around the neck of the bladder, the circular muscle is thickened to form the internal urethral sphincter (Rankin 2017). The general elasticity of the numerous muscle fibres around the bladder neck tends to keep the urethra closed (Standring and Tunstall 2015). In the trigone, the muscles are somewhat differently arranged. A band of muscle between the ureteric openings forms the *interureteric bar*. The *urethral dilator muscle* lies in the ventral part of the bladder neck and the walls of the urethra and it is thought to be of significance in overcoming urethral resistance to micturition (Standring and Tunstall 2015).

The outer layer of the bladder is formed of visceral pelvic fascia, except on its superior surface, which is covered with peritoneum (Fig. 4.8).

Blood Supply

Blood supply is from the superior and inferior vesical arteries and drainage is by the corresponding veins.

Lymphatic Drainage

Lymph drains into the internal iliac and the obturator nodes.

Nerve Supply

The nerve supply is parasympathetic and sympathetic and comes via the *Lee–Frankenhauser pelvic plexus* in the pouch of Douglas. The stimulation of sympathetic nerves causes the internal urethral sphincter to contract and the detrusor muscle to relax, whereas the parasympathetic nerve fibres cause the sphincter to relax and the bladder to empty.

THE URETHRA

The female urethra is a narrow tube, about 4 cm long, and runs embedded in the lower half of the anterior vaginal wall. It passes from the internal meatus of the bladder to the vestibule of the vulva, where it opens externally as the urethral meatus. The internal sphincter surrounds the urethra as it leaves the bladder. As the urethra passes between the levator ani muscles (see Chapter 3), it is enclosed by bands of striated muscle known as the membranous sphincter of the urethra, which is under voluntary control (Rankin 2017).

Structure

The urethra forms the junction between the urinary tract and the external genitalia. The epithelium of its lining reflects this. The upper half is lined with transitional epithelium whereas the lower half is lined with squamous epithelium. The lumen is normally closed unless urine is passing down it or a catheter is *in situ*. When closed, it has small longitudinal folds. Small blind ducts called urethral crypts (of which the two largest are the *paraurethral glands* or *Skene's ducts*) open into the urethra near the urethral meatus (Martini et al. 2018).

The submucous coat of the urethra is composed of epithelium, which lies on a bed of vascular connective tissue. The musculature of the urethra is arranged as an inner longitudinal layer, continuous with the inner muscle fibres of the bladder, and an external circular layer. The *inner muscle fibres* help to open the internal urethral sphincter during micturition.

The *outer layer* of the urethra is continuous with the outer layer of the vagina and is formed of connective tissue.

At the lower end of the urethra, voluntary, striated muscle fibres form the so-called 'membranous sphincter' of the urethra. Although this is not a true sphincter, it gives some voluntary control to the woman when she desires to resist the urge to void urine. The powerful levator ani muscles (see Chapter 3), which pass on either side of the uterus, also assist in controlling continence of urine.

Blood Supply

The blood to the urethra is circulated by the inferior vesical and pudendal arteries and veins.

Lymphatic Drainage

Lymph drains through the internal iliac glands.

Nerve Supply

The internal urethral sphincter is supplied by sympathetic and parasympathetic nerves but the membranous sphincter is supplied by the pudendal nerve and is under voluntary control.

MICTURITION

The process of micturition (urination) is a coordinated response that is due to the contraction of the muscular wall of the bladder, reflex relaxation of the internal sphincter of the urethra and voluntary relaxation of the external sphincter (Coad and Dunstall 2011). As the bladder fills with urine, stretch receptors in the wall of the urinary bladder are stimulated which then relay parasympathetic sensory nerve impulses to the brain generating awareness of fluid pressure in the bladder. This usually occurs when the bladder contains approximately 200–300 mL of urine (with increasing discomfort as the volume increases). The urge to micturate can be voluntarily resisted and postponed until a suitable time. This is due to the conscious descending inhibition of the reflex bladder contraction and relaxation of the external sphincter. If the urge to micturate is not voluntarily resisted, then the bladder will empty of urine by the muscle wall contracting, the internal sphincter opening by the action of Bell's muscles (Fig. 4.9) and voluntary relaxation of the external sphincter. This is assisted by the increased pressure in the pelvic cavity as the diaphragm is lowered and the abdominal muscles contract. The tone of the external sphincter is also affected by psychological stimuli (such as waking or leaving home) and external stimuli (such as the sound of running water). Any factor that raises the intra-abdominal and intravesicular pressures (such as laughter or coughing) in excess of the urethral closing pressure can result in incontinence (Coad and Dunstall 2011).

Infants lack voluntary control over micturition because the necessary corticospinal connections have yet to be established (Martini et al. 2018). Cortical control of micturition occurs from learned behaviour and is usually achieved by about 2 years of age.

CHANGES TO THE URINARY TRACT IN PREGNANCY AND CHILDBIRTH

The urinary system can be markedly stressed by pregnancy, mostly because of its close proximity to the reproductive organs and the major changes in fluid balance resulting in fluid retention during pregnancy (Coad and Dunstall 2011). In pregnancy, the enlarging uterus affects all the parts of the urinary tract (see Chapter 10) at various times. In early pregnancy, bladder capacity is compromised by the growing uterus within the pelvic cavity, which is relieved when the uterus becomes an abdominal organ. Once the presenting part engages through the pelvic brim in late pregnancy, this again restricts space

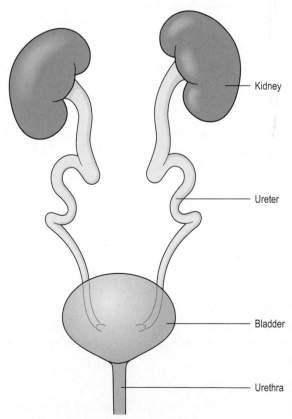

Fig. 4.10 Dilated, kinked ureters in pregnancy.

available for bladder capacity. The hormones of pregnancy also have an influence on the urinary tract. Under the influence of progesterone, bladder capacity can increase to about 1000 mL by late pregnancy and the walls of the ureters relax, which allows them to dilate, bend or 'kink' (Fig. 4.10). If this occurs in the ureters, then it tends to result in a slowing down or stasis of urinary flow, causing women to be more at risk from infection.

During pregnancy, large amounts of urine are produced due to an increase in glomerular filtration as this helps to eliminate the additional wastes created by maternal and fetal metabolism. During labour, as the bladder is drawn up into the abdomen, the urethra becomes elongated extending several centimetres.

During the postnatal period (see Chapter 28) there is a rapid and sustained loss of sodium and a major diuresis occurs, especially between the 2nd and 5th postnatal day. A normal urine output for a woman during this time may be up to 3000 mL/day with voiding of 500–1000 mL at any one micturition (Rankin 2017).

CONCLUSION

The kidneys are excretory glands with both endocrine and exocrine functions. Urine produced by the kidney flows continuously from the renal pelvis into the ureter and then into the bladder for storage. The three major functions are: excretion, elimination and homeostatic regulation of the volume and solute concentration of blood plasma. Water balance is mainly regulated by the antidiuretic hormone (ADH) through a negative feedback loop.

During pregnancy, the urinary system can be markedly stressed, mostly because of its close proximity to the reproductive organs, the major changes in fluid balance and the hormones of pregnancy. The midwife needs to recognize what effects these changes can have on childbearing women to offer them appropriate advice and support in relieving any discomfort.

▍ REFLECTIVE ACTIVITY FOR SELF-ASSESSMENT

1. Reflecting on the female urinary system what three anatomical factors does the midwife need to consider during pregnancy, childbirth or postpartum?
2. What are the key physiological changes that may occur in the urinary system during or following pregnancy?
3. What could be the significance of a range of abnormal characteristics (e.g. blood, protein, glucose) you may find present in the urine sample of a pregnant woman?

REFERENCES

Coad, J., & Dunstall, M. (2011). *Anatomy and physiology for midwives* (3rd ed.). Edinburgh: Churchill Livingstone.

Jones, T. L., Harris, K. P. G., & Horton-Szar, D. (2015). *Crash course: Renal and urinary system* (4th ed.). London: Mosby Elsevier.

Martini, F. H., Nath, J. L., & Bartholomew, E. F. (2018). *Fundamentals of anatomy and physiology* (10th ed.). (Global edition). Harlow: Pearson International.

Rankin, J. (2017). *Physiology in childbearing with anatomy and related biosciences* (4th ed.). London: Elsevier.

Standring, S., & Tunstall, R. (2015). *Gray's anatomy: The anatomical basis of clinical practice* (41st ed.). New York: Churchill Livingstone.

ANNOTATED FURTHER READING

Coad, J., & Dunstall, M. (2011). Anatomy and physiology for midwives (3rd ed.). Edinburgh: Churchill Livingstone.
Chapter 2 of this book includes several stylized diagrams related to urine production. The diagrams are detailed and well explained and may help the individual who prefers visual representation. The updated edition is due early 2020.

Rankin, J. (2017). Physiology in childbearing with anatomy and related biosciences (4th ed.). London: Elsevier.
Chapter 19 provides a fuller and more in-depth account of the physiology related to the renal and urinary system, including the physiological and physical changes in pregnancy and a short account of the postnatal period.

5

Hormonal Cycles: Fertilization and Early Development

Jenny Bailey

CHAPTER CONTENTS

Monthly physiological changes take place in the ovaries and the uterus, regulated by hormones produced by the hypothalamus, anterior pituitary gland and ovaries. These monthly cycles commence at puberty and occur simultaneously, and together are known as the female reproductive cycle.

THE CHAPTER AIMS TO

- explore in detail the events that occur during the ovarian and menstrual cycles
- describe in detail the process of fertilization followed by the subsequent development of the conceptus into the pre-embryonic period

- introduce the different methods of assisted conception.

INTRODUCTION

The functions of the female reproductive cycle are to prepare the *egg*, often referred to as the *gamete* or *oocyte*, for fertilization by the *spermatozoon* (sperm), and to prepare the uterus to receive and nourish the fertilized oocyte. If fertilization has not taken place, the inner lining of the uterus or endometrium and the oocyte are shed, bleeding occurs per vagina, and the cyclic events begin again.

Before the onset of puberty, luteinizing hormone (LH) and follicle stimulating hormone (FSH) levels are low. Pulsatile increases in gonadotrophin releasing hormone (GnRH), initially at night, cause increases in FSH and LH secretion. As puberty advances, pulsatile surges also occur during the day and increase in frequency over a 3–4-year period until an adult pattern develops. These increasing surges of FSH and LH are established prior to menarche (Tortora and Derrickson 2014). It is also thought that the interaction of leptin with GnRH may have a role in the initiation of puberty. The first-ever occurrence of cyclic events is termed *menarche*, meaning the first menstrual bleeding. The average age of menarche is 12 years, although between the ages of 8 and 16 is considered normal. The onset of menstrual bleeding ('periods' or menses) is a major stage in a girl's life, representing the maturation of the reproductive system and physical transition into womanhood. For many women, this monthly phenomenon signals and embodies the quintessence of being a 'woman'. Similarly, for other women it is regarded as an inconvenience, causing pain, shame and embarrassment (Chrisler 2011). Cultural and religious traditions affect how women and their communities feel about menstruation. The advent of hormonal contraception affords women, especially those in Western society, an element of control over their periods. Factors such as heredity, diet, anorexia, obesity and overall health can accelerate or delay menarche. Interference with the hormonal–organ relationship prior to and during the reproductive years is likely to cause menstrual cycle dysfunction, which may result in failure to ovulate. The cessation of cyclic events is referred to as the *menopause* and signifies the end of reproductive life. Each woman has an individual reproductive cycle that varies in length, although the average cycle is normally 28 days long, and recurs regularly from puberty to the menopause except when pregnancy intervenes (Fig. 5.1).

THE OVARIAN CYCLE

The ovarian cycle (Fig. 5.2) is the name given to the physiological changes that occur in the ovaries essential for the preparation and release of an oocyte. The ovarian cycle consists of three phases, all of which are under the control of hormones.

The Follicular Phase

The formation of oogonia in the germinal epithelium of the ovaries is known as *oogenesis*. Primordial germ cells differentiate into oogonia in the ovaries during fetal life. These diploid stem cells divide mitotically and proliferate into millions of germ cells. Most of the germ cells degenerate (by atresia), however some develop further into *primary oocytes*, and enter the prophase of meiosis I cell division. Meiotic arrest occurs, and the process does not continue until after puberty (further meiotic division takes place at ovulation of the secondary oocyte and the process is only completed if fertilization occurs). While in this arrested prophase stage of meiosis I the primary oocyte is surrounded by follicular cells and is hence known as the *primordial follicle*. There are up to 2 million primary oocytes in each ovary at birth and due to atresia, the number is reduced to approximately

40,000 at puberty; 400 of these will mature and ovulate during the woman's lifetime (Moore et al. 2016a). Following puberty, FSH and LH further stimulate the development of primordial follicles into *primary* and *secondary follicles* and subsequently into large *preovulatory* or *Graafian follicles* (Fig. 5.3) by a process known as 'folliculogenesis'.

Low levels of oestrogen and progesterone stimulate the hypothalamus to produce GnRH. This releasing hormone causes the production of FSH and LH by the anterior pituitary gland. FSH controls the growth and maturity of the Graafian follicles. The Graafian follicles begin to secrete oestrogens, which comprises beta oestradiol, oestrone and oestriol. Rising levels of beta oestradiol cause a surge in LH. When beta oestradiol reaches a certain peak, the secretion of FSH is inhibited. The reduced FSH secretion causes a slowing in follicle growth and eventually leads to follicle death, known as *atresia*. The largest and dominant follicle secretes *inhibin*, which further suppresses FSH. This dominant follicle prevails and forms a bulge near the surface of the ovary, and soon becomes competent to ovulate. The time from the growth and maturity of the Graafian follicles to ovulation is normally around 1 week. Occasionally, the follicular phase may take longer if the dominant follicle does not ovulate, and the phase will begin again. The differing lengths of menstrual cycle reported between individual women are as a result in the varying timespans in this preovulatory phase. It can last from day 6 to day 13 in a 28-day cycle (Tortora and Derrickson 2014).

Ovulation

High oestrogen levels cause a sudden surge in LH around day 12–13 of a 28-day cycle, and can last for approximately 48 h. This matures the oocyte and weakens the wall of the follicle and causes *ovulation* to occur on day 14.

Ovulation is the process whereby the dominant Graafian follicle ruptures and discharges the secondary oocyte into the pelvic cavity. Fimbriae guide it into the ampulla region of the uterine tube where it awaits fertilization. During the time of ovulation, meiotic cell division resumes and the diploid oocyte becomes haploid (with a first polar body). The expelled secondary oocyte is surrounded by the *zona pellucida* and the *corona radiata*. During ovulation, some women experience varying degrees of abdominal pain known as *mittelschmerz*, which can last several hours. There may be some light

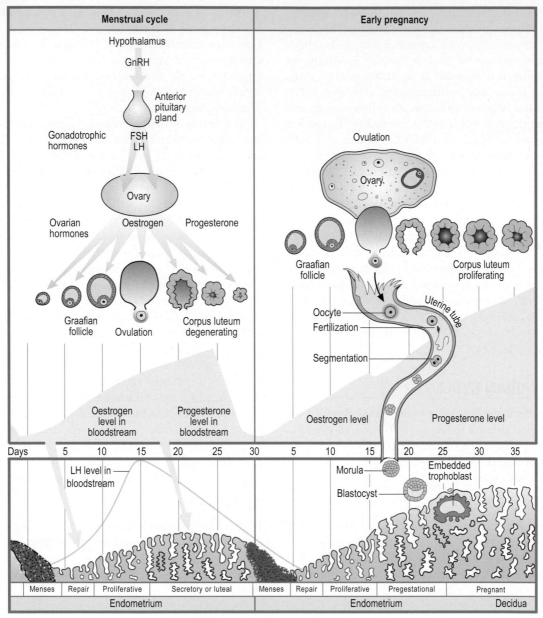

Fig. 5.1 The female reproductive cycle.

bleeding caused by the hormonal changes taking place. Stringy clear mucus appears in the cervix, ready to accept the sperm from intercourse. Following ovulation, the fertilized or unfertilized oocyte travels to the uterus.

The Luteal Phase

The *luteal phase* is the process whereby the cells of the residual ruptured follicle proliferate and form a yellow

irregular structure known as the *corpus luteum*. The corpus luteum produces predominantly progesterone but also oestrogen, relaxin and inhibin for approximately 2 weeks, to develop the endometrium of the uterus, which awaits the fertilized oocyte. Small amounts of relaxin cause uterine quiescence, which is an ideal environment for the fertilized oocyte to implant. The corpus luteum continues its role until

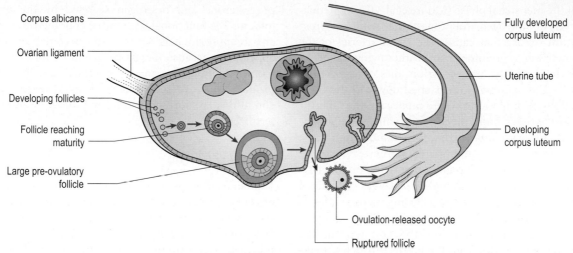

Corpus albicans

Ovarian ligament

Developing follicles

Follicle reaching maturity

Large pre-ovulatory follicle

Fully developed corpus luteum

Uterine tube

Developing corpus luteum

Ovulation-released oocyte

Ruptured follicle

Fig. 5.2 The cycle of a Graafian follicle in the ovary.

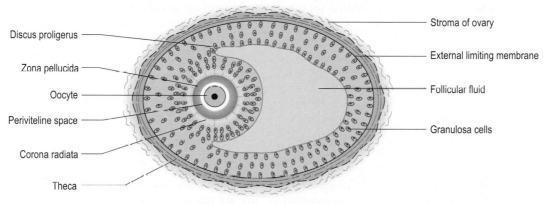

Discus proligerus

Zona pellucida

Oocyte

Periviteline space

Corona radiata

Theca

Stroma of ovary

External limiting membrane

Follicular fluid

Granulosa cells

Fig. 5.3 A ripe Graafian follicle.

the placenta is adequately developed to take over. During the luteal phase, the cervical mucus becomes sticky and thick. In the absence of fertilization, the corpus luteum degenerates and becomes the corpus albicans (white body), and progesterone, oestrogen, relaxin and inhibin levels decrease. In response to low levels of oestrogen and progesterone the hypothalamus produces GnRH. The rising levels of GnRH stimulate the anterior pituitary gland to produce FSH and the ovarian cycle commences again (Rankin and Matthews 2017). The luteal phase is the most constant part of the ovarian cycle, lasting 14 days out of a 28-day cycle, from day 15 to day 28 (Tortora and Derrickson 2014).

THE MENSTRUAL OR ENDOMETRIAL CYCLE

The *menstrual cycle* is the name given to the physiological changes that occur in the endometrial layer of the uterus, and which are essential to receive the fertilized oocyte. The menstrual cycle consists of three phases.

The Menstrual Phase

This phase is often referred to as *menstruation*, *bleeding*, *menses* or a *period*. Physiologically, this is the terminal phase of the reproductive cycle of events and is simultaneous with the beginning of the follicular phase of the ovarian cycle. The first day of menstruation is the first day of the menstrual phase (Moore et al. 2016a). Reducing levels of oestrogen and progesterone stimulate prostaglandin release that causes the spiral arteries of the endometrium to go into spasm, withdrawing the blood supply to it, and the endometrium dies, referred to as *necrosis*. The endometrium is shed down to the basal layer along with blood from the capillaries, the unfertilized oocyte tissue fluid, mucus and epithelial cells. Failure to menstruate (*amenorrhoea*) is an indication that a woman may have become pregnant. The term *eumenorrhoea* denotes normal, regular menstruation that lasts for typically 3–5 days, although 2–7 days is considered normal. The average blood loss during menstruation is 50–150 mL. The blood is inhibited from clotting due to the enzyme plasmin contained in the endometrium. The menstrual flow passes from the uterus through the cervix and the vagina to the exterior. The term *menorrhagia* denotes heavy bleeding. Some women experience uterine cramps caused by muscular contractions to expel the tissue. Severe uterine cramps are known as *dysmenorrhoea*.

The Proliferative Phase

This phase follows menstruation, is simultaneous with the follicular phase of the ovary and lasts until ovulation. There is the formation of a new layer of endometrium in the uterus, referred to as the proliferative endometrium. This phase is under the control of oestradiol and other oestrogens secreted by the Graafian follicle and consist of the regrowth and thickening of the endometrium in the uterus. During the first few days of this phase the endometrium is reforming, described as the *regenerative phase*. At the completion of this phase, the endometrium consists of three layers. The *basal layer* lies immediately above the myometrium and is approximately 1 mm thick. It contains all the necessary rudimentary structures for building new endometrium. The *functional layer*, which contains tubular glands, is approximately 2.5 mm thick and lies on top of the basal layer. It changes constantly according to the hormonal influences of the ovary. The *layer of cuboidal ciliated epithelium* covers the functional layer. It dips down to line the tubular glands of the functional layer. If fertilization occurs, the fertilized oocyte implants itself within the endometrium.

The Secretory Phase

This phase follows the proliferative phase and is simultaneous with ovulation. It is under the influence of progesterone and oestrogen secreted by the corpus luteum. The functional layer of the endometrium thickens to approximately 3.5 mm and becomes spongy in appearance because the glands are more tortuous. The blood supply to the area is increased and the glands produce nutritive secretions such as glycogen. These conditions last for approximately 7 days, awaiting the fertilized oocyte.

FERTILIZATION

Human fertilization, known as conception, is the fusion of genetic material from the haploid sperm cell and the secondary oocyte (now haploid), to form the zygote (Fig. 5.4). The process takes approximately 12–24 h and normally occurs in the ampulla of the uterine tube. Fertilization is a series of complex, coordinated molecular events that begins with the sperm and egg meeting and ends with mixing of maternal and paternal chromosomes during metaphase I division of the zygote (Moore et al. 2016a). Following ovulation, the oocyte, which is about 0.15 mm in diameter, passes into the uterine tube. The oocyte, having no power of locomotion, is wafted along by the cilia and by the peristaltic muscular contraction of the uterine tube. At the same time the cervix, which is under the influence of oestrogen, secretes a flow of alkaline mucus that attracts the spermatozoa. In the fertile male at intercourse, approximately 200 million sperm are deposited in the posterior fornix of the vagina. Approximately 2 million reach the loose cervical mucus, survive and propel themselves towards the uterine tubes, while the rest are destroyed by the acid medium of the vagina. Approximately 200 sperm will ultimately reach the oocyte (Tortora and Derrickson 2014). Sperm swim from the vagina and through the cervical canal using their whip-like tails (flagella). Prostaglandins from semen and uterine contractions as a result of intercourse facilitate the passage of the sperm into the uterus and beyond. Once inside the uterine tubes (within minutes of intercourse), the sperm undergo a process known as *capacitation*. This process takes up to 7 h. Influenced by secretions from the uterine tube, the sperm undergo changes to the plasma membrane, resulting in the removal of the glycoprotein coat and increased flagellation. The zona pellucida of the oocyte produces chemicals that attract capacitated sperm only. The acrosomal layer of the capacitated sperm becomes reactive and releases the enzyme hyaluronidase known

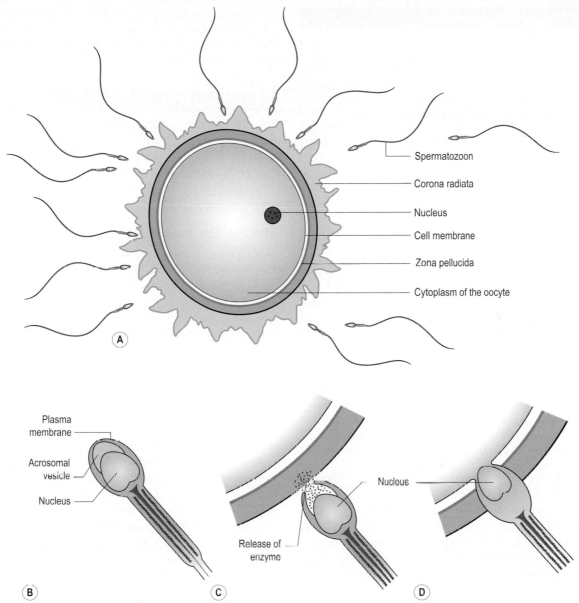

Fig. 5.4 Fertilization. Diagrammatic representation of the fusion of the oocyte and the spermatozoon. (*Note*: B, C and D are more greatly magnified than A.)

as the *acrosome reaction*, which disperses the corona radiata (the outermost layer of the oocyte) allowing access to the zona pellucida (Fig. 5.4C). Many sperm are involved in this process. The proteolytic enzyme acrosin and other enzymes such as esterases and neuraminidase produce an opening in the zona pellucida. The first spermatozoon that reaches the zona pellucida binds to it and subsequently penetrates it (Fig. 5.4D).

Upon penetration, the oocyte releases corticol granules; this is known as the *cortical reaction*. The cortical reaction and depolarization of the oocyte cell membrane makes the zona pellucida impermeable to other sperm. This is important as there are many sperm surrounding the oocyte at this time. Only the head and tail of the penetrating spermatozoon enter the cytoplasm of the oocyte, its plasma membrane and mitochondria are left

BOX 5.1 Chromosomes

Each human cell has a complement of 46 chromosomes arranged in 23 pairs, of which one pair are sex chromosomes. The remaining pairs are known as autosomes. During the process of maturation, both gametes shed half their chromosomes, one of each pair, during a reduction division called *meiosis*. Genetic material is exchanged between the chromosomes before they split up. In the male, meiosis starts at puberty and both halves re-divide to form four sperm in all. In the female, meiosis commences during fetal life, but the first division is not completed until many years later at ovulation. The division is unequal; the larger part will eventually go on to form the oocyte while the remainder forms the first polar body. At fertilization the second division takes place and results in one large cell, which is now mature, and a much smaller one, the second polar body. At the same time, division of the first polar body creates a third polar body.

When the gametes combine at fertilization to form the zygote, the full complement of chromosomes is restored. Subsequent division occurs by mitosis where the chromosomes divide to give each new cell a full set.

Sex determination

Females carry two similar sex chromosomes, XX; males carry two dissimilar sex chromosomes, XY. Each sperm will carry either an X or a Y chromosome, whereas the oocyte always carries an X chromosome. If the oocyte is fertilized by an X-carrying sperm a female is conceived, if by a Y-carrying one, a male.

behind. The spermatozoon and oocyte fuse. The oocyte at this stage completes its second meiotic division and becomes mature, with a *haploid* number of chromosomes (23) in its pronucleus. On entry to the oocyte, the tail of the sperm degenerates and there is the formation of the male pronucleus, which contains a haploid number of chromosomes (23). The male and female pronuclei fuse to form a new nucleus that is a combination of 23 pairs of chromosomes from both the sperm and oocyte, referred to as a *diploid* cell. The male and the female gametes each contribute half the complement of chromosomes to make a total of 46 (Box 5.1). This new cell is called a *zygote*.

Dizygotic twins (fraternal twins) are produced from two oocytes released independently but in the same timeframe fusing with two different sperm; they are genetically different from each other. Monozygotic twins

develop from a single zygote for a variety of reasons, where cells separate into two embryos, usually before 8 days following fertilization. These twins are genetically identical (see Chapter 16).

DEVELOPMENT OF THE ZYGOTE

The development of the zygote can be divided into three periods. The first 2 weeks after fertilization, referred to as the *pre-embryonic period*, includes the implantation of the zygote into the endometrium; weeks 2–8 are known as the *embryonic period*; and weeks 8 to birth are known as the *fetal period*.

The Pre-Embryonic Period

During the first week, the zygote travels along the uterine tube towards the uterus. At this stage a strong membrane of glycoproteins called the 'zona pellucida' surrounds the zygote. The zygote receives nourishment, mainly glycogen, from the goblet cells of the uterine tubes and later the secretory cells of the uterus. During their travel, the zygote undergoes repeated mitotic cellular replication and division referred to as *cleavage*, resulting in the formation of smaller cells known as *blastomeres*. The zygote divides into two cells at 1 day, then four at 2 days, eight by 2.5 days, 16 by 3 days, now known as the *morula*. The cells bind tightly together in a process known as *compactation*. Next, *cavitation* occurs whereby the outermost cells secrete fluid into the morula and a fluid-filled cavity or *blastocoele* appears in the morula. This results in the formation of the blastula or *blastocyst*, comprising 58 cells. The process from the development of the morula to the development of the blastocyst is referred to as *blastulation* and has occurred by around day 4 (Fig. 5.5).

The zona pellucida remains during the process of cleavage, so that despite an increase in number of cells the overall size remains that of the zygote and constant at this stage. The zona pellucida prevents the developing blastocyst from increasing in size and therefore getting stuck in the uterine tube; it also prevents embedding occurring in the tube rather than the uterus, which could result in an ectopic pregnancy. Around day 4, the blastocyst enters the uterus. Endometrial glands secrete glycogen-rich fluid into the uterus, which penetrates the zona pellucida. This and nutrients in the cytoplasm of the blastomeres provides nourishment for the developing cells. The blastocyst digests its way out of the zona pellucida once it enters the uterine cavity. The blastocyst possesses

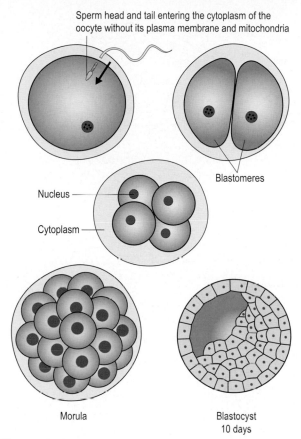

Sperm head and tail entering the cytoplasm of the oocyte without its plasma membrane and mitochondria

Blastomeres

Nucleus

Cytoplasm

Morula

Blastocyst
10 days

Fig. 5.5 Diagrammatic representation of the development of the zygote.

an *inner cell mass* or *embryoblast*, and an *outer cell mass* or *trophoblast*. The trophoblast becomes the placenta and chorion, while the embryoblast becomes the embryo, amnion and umbilical cord (Moore et al. 2016a).

During week 2, the trophoblast proliferates and differentiates into two layers: the outer *syncytiotrophoblast* or *syncytium* and the inner *cytotrophoblast* (cuboidal dividing cells) (Fig. 5.6). Implantation of the trophoblast layer into the endometrium, known as the *decidua*, begins. Implantation is usually to the upper posterior wall. At the implantation stage, the zona pellucida will have totally disappeared. The syncytiotrophoblast layer invades the decidua by forming finger-like projections called *villi* that make their way into the decidua and spaces called *lacunae* that fill up with the mother's blood. The villi begin to branch, and contain blood vessels of the developing embryo, thus allowing gaseous exchange between the mother and embryo. Implantation is assisted

by both apoptosis of localized decidual tissue and proteolytic enzymes secreted by the syncytiotrophoblast cells that erode the decidua; the degeneration of decidual stroma cells assists with the nutrition of the embryo. The syncytiotrophoblast cells also produce human chorionic gonadotrophin (hCG), a hormone, which enters maternal blood via the lacunae and that prevents menstruation and maintains pregnancy by sustaining the function of the corpus luteum. It also maintains the development of the spiral arteries in the myometrium and formation of the syncytiotrophoblast. Human chorionic gonadotrophin forms the basis of pregnancy tests.

Simultaneous to implantation, the embryo continues developing. The cells of the embryoblast differentiate into two types of cells: the *epiblast* (closest to the trophoblasts) and the *hypoblast* (closest to the blastocyst cavity). These two layers of cells form a flat disc known as the *bilaminar embryonic disc*. A process of *gastrulation* turns the bilaminar disc into a trilaminar embryonic disc (three layers). Gastrulation is the beginning of morphogenesis – the development of body form and structure of the various organs and body parts (Moore et al. 2016a). During gastrulation, cells rearrange themselves and migrate due to predetermined genetic coding. Three primary germ layers are the main embryonic tissues from which various structures and organs will develop. The first appearance of these layers, collectively known as the primitive streak, is around day 15, the beginning of the 3rd week of human development.

The primitive streak appears on the dorsal aspect of the embryonic disc due to proliferation and migration of cells from the epiblast. Once the primitive streak appears, it is possible to identify the cranial (head) and caudal (tail) ends of the embryo. Further elongation of the caudal end is accompanied by the cranial end forming the *primitive node*. Also, a primitive groove appears in the primitive streak, ending in the *primitive pit*. Soon after the primitive streak is formed cells migrate to form mesoderm, which is loose connective embryonic tissue known as *mesenchyme*. This forms the supporting tissues of the embryo. Several embryonic growth factors cause further epiblast cell migration through the primitive groove to become the *endoderm* and *mesoderm*.

The epiblast separates from the trophoblast and forms the floor of a cavity, known as the *amniotic cavity*. The amnion forms from the cells lining the cavity. The cavity is filled with fluid, and gradually enlarges and folds around the bilaminar disc to enclose it. This

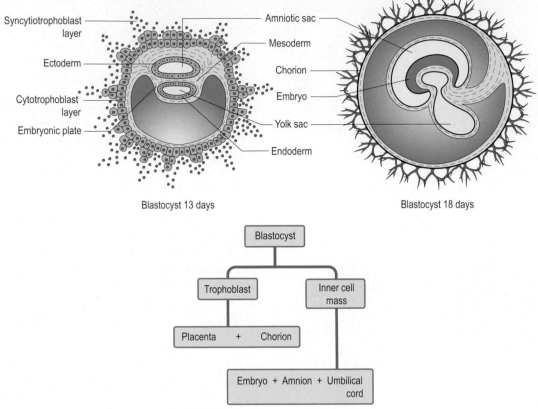

Fig. 5.6 The development of the blastocyst.

amniotic cavity fills with fluid (amniotic fluid) derived initially from maternal filtrate; later the fetus contributes by excreting urine. Fetal cells can be found in the amniotic fluid and can be used in diagnostic testing for genetic conditions via a procedure known as amniocentesis (see Chapter 13).

At about 16 days, mesenchymal cells migrate cranially and form a cellular cord in the midline called the *notochordal process*; it soon acquires a lumen, the *notochordal canal*. The notochord process grows cranially between the ectoderm and endoderm layers until it reaches the *prechordal plate*. This is responsible for organizing head and neck development in the embryo. Mesenchymal cells from the primitive streak and notochordal process migrate laterally until they meet the edges of the embryonic disc. The mesenchymal cells are continuous with the *extraembryonic mesoderm* that covers the amnion and umbilical cord. Other cells from the primitive streak migrate to form cardiogenic mesoderm

where the heart primordium begins to develop (Moore et al. 2016a).

Specialized inducing cells and responding tissues cause development of the vertebral bodies and intervertebral discs to occur. The neural tube is developed from further cell migration, differentiation and folding of embryonic tissue. This occurs in the middle of the embryo and develops towards each end. The whole process is known as *neurulation*. The notochord mostly degenerates and disappears, although some is found as part of the forming vertebral bodies. Teratogens, diabetes or folic acid deficiency may lead to neural tube defects. The notochord is the primary inductor in the early embryo; it induces the embryonic ectoderm to thicken and form the neural plate.

The hypoblast layer of the embryoblast gives rise to extraembryonic structures only, such as the yolk sac. Hypoblast cells migrate along the inner cytotrophoblast lining of the blastocoele, secreting extracellular tissue which becomes the yolk sac. The yolk sac is lined with extraembryonic endoderm, which in turn is lined with extraembryonic mesoderm. The yolk sac serves as a primary nutritive function, carrying nutrients and oxygen to the embryo until the placenta fully takes over this role. The endoderm and mesoderm cells contribute to the formation of some organs, such as the primitive gut arising out of the endoderm cells. At about day 16, an outpouching of the endodermic tissue forms the *allantois*; it runs from the caudal wall of the umbilical vessel into the connecting stalk. The allantois is responsible for early blood formation and the urinary bladder. The blood vessels of the allantois become the umbilical arteries and veins (Moore et al. 2016a). Blood islands that later go on to develop blood cells arise from the mesodermal layer; the remaining yolk sac resembles a balloon floating in front of the embryo until it atrophies by the end of the 6th week when blood-forming activity transfers to embryonic sites. After birth, all that remains of the yolk sac is a vestigial structure in the base of the umbilical cord, known as the *vitelline duct*.

In the 3rd week, the main three layers of the trilaminar disc form various areas of the embryo's body.

- The **ectoderm** is the start of tissue that covers most surfaces of the body: the epidermis layer of the skin, hair and nails. Additionally, it forms the nervous system.
- The **mesoderm** forms the muscle, skeleton, dermis of skin, connective tissue, the urogenital glands, blood vessels, and blood and lymph cells.
- The **endoderm** forms the epithelial lining of the digestive, respiratory and urinary systems, and glandular cells of organs such as the liver and pancreas.

The pre-embryonic period is crucial in terms of initiation and maintenance of the pregnancy and early embryonic development. Inability to implant properly can results in ectopic pregnancy or miscarriage. Additionally, chromosomal defects and abnormalities in structure and organs can occur during this time (Moore et al. 2016b).

During embryological development, stem cells under predetermined genetic control become specialized giving rise to further differentiation with a varying functionality according to their predefined role (Box 5.2).

BOX 5.2 Stem Cells

- Stem cells are unspecialized and give rise to specialized cells.
- The zygote can give rise to a whole organism, known as a *totipotent* stem cell.
- Stem cells such as those in the inner cell mass can give rise to many different types of cells and are consequently known as *pluripotent*.
- Further specialization of pluripotent stem cells gives rise to cells with more specific functions, known as *multipotent* stem cells.

Stem cells in adult organs (also known as adult stem cells, somatic or tissue-specific cells) have the potential to become *any* type of cell in a specific organ – multipotent. These cells facilitate repair of a damaged or diseased organ. Adult stem cells may have some 'plasticity' and may have the potential to be used in other organs of the body.

In the UK, cell cleavage up to 14 days after fertilization can be used for research. This tends to be undertaken at 5–6 days. As research occurs on the cells at this stage, the embryo does not exist as a 3D entity and its properties are changed – in essence it is no longer an 'embryo'.

Stem cell harvesting

Stem cells from an embryo, if transferred into another individual where there is no genetic match, will cause rejection issues similar to tissue transplantation.

Stem cells found in the umbilical cord, which can be collected, have originated in the fetal liver; most stem cells found in the cord are progenitor cells and have differentiated further – usually into haematopoietic stem cells.

These cells may cause transplant issues if used in other people unless there is a very close genetic match, such as a sibling. The cells could then be used to treat acute lymphoblastic leukaemia.

In the UK, the Human Tissue Authority (HTA 2018) and the Royal College of Obstetricians and Gynaecologists/ Royal College of Midwives (RCOG/RCM 2011) have produced useful guidance papers to help inform midwifery practice around the issue of stem cell harvesting and routine commercial umbilical cord blood collection.

METHODS OF ASSISTED CONCEPTION

In the UK, the Human Fertilisation and Embryology Authority (HFEA) regulates fertility treatment. The National Institute for Health and Care Excellence (NICE) provide additional clinical guidelines about applying the

BOX 5.3   Different IVF Egg and Sperm Combinations

OEPS – IVF treatment cycles using a patient's own eggs and their partner's sperm.

OEDS – IVF treatment cycles using a patient's own eggs and donor sperm.

DEPS – IVF treatment cycles using donor eggs and the patient's partner's sperm.

DEDS – IVF treatment cycles using donor eggs and donor sperm.

regulations. They produce guidance on access to fertility treatment, factors which predict success and long-term health and safety outcomes (NICE 2018).

In Vitro Fertilization and Embryo Transfer

In vitro fertilization (IVF) is a treatment where a woman's eggs are fertilized with sperm in a laboratory (HFEA 2018). IVF was pioneered by Robert Edwards and Patrick Steptoe in 1978, culminating in the world's first 'test tube baby', Louise Brown being born (Moore et al. 2016b). IVF of oocytes and transfer of cleaving zygotes enables many parents unable to have children to do so. Often several embryos are collected, those not used initially may be frozen for future use (crypto-preservation) with successful transfer after thawing now ubiquitous. Egg freezing can also be used by cancer patients and transgender people for fertility preservation (HFEA 2018).

Different combinations of individuals' own and/or donor eggs and sperm can be used for IVF treatment cycles (Box 5.3).

IVF and embryo transfer involve several processes (Box 5.4).

Preimplantation genetic diagnosis (PGD) is a treatment that allows people with a serious inheritable genetic condition in the family to avoid passing it on by testing the embryo(s) approximately 5 days prior to implantation (HFEA 2018; Moore et al. 2016a).

More recently, the Human Fertilisation and Embryology Act has been amended to include regulations regarding mitochondrial replacement therapies (HFEA 2015). The therapies aim to prevent transmission of mitochondrial disease to children from their genetically-related biological mother. Mitochondrial DNA (mtDNA) IVF is a relatively new treatment (Box 5.5).

BOX 5.4   Processes Involved in an IVF Cycle

- Controlled stimulation of ovarian follicles (avoiding hyperstimulation syndrome)
- Aspiration of mature oocytes from ovarian follicles by laparoscopy or transvaginal ultrasonography-guided needle. Conscious sedation should be offered for the latter (NICE 2018).
- Sperm collection and mixing oocytes with capacitated sperm and culture medium
- Fertilization of oocytes and cleavage monitored for 3–5 days
- Early blastocysts transferred into the uterus
- Any remaining embryos stored in liquid nitrogen (cryopreservation)
- The woman lies supine for several hours afterwards. Women should be offered luteal phase support (progesterone) for up to 8 weeks' gestation (NICE 2018).
- Increased chance of multiple pregnancy or miscarriage following this procedure.

BOX 5.5   Mitochondrial DNA IVF

Most DNA is contained within a cell's nucleus. However, 0.1% of the total amount of DNA is contained within the mitochondria (Castro 2016). This means there are multiple copies of mtDNA within a single cell. In addition to energy production, mitochondria regulate other cell functions including: apoptosis, production of haem and cholesterol. To undertake their functions, they need their own specialized DNA. Mitochondrial DNA contains 37 genes; 13 for enzymes for energy production and the remaining 24 for manufacturing transfer RNA and ribosomal RNA. These types of RNA are essential for assembling protein building blocks. Despite the small percentage of DNA in mitochondria, devastating consequences can occur because of mitochondrial mutation. Mutations can affect some or all the copies of mtDNA. Thus, individuals are affected in highly variable ways; depending on which organs are affected they can be mildly or severely affected. During fertilization, the oocyte provides all of the cytoplasm for the embryo, therefore mitochondrial diseases are only inherited from the female line. In the UK, the average number of births per year among women at risk for transmitting mtDNA disease is 152 (Gorman et al. 2015). Mitochondrial replacement therapy uses healthy mitochondria from a donor egg.

With regard to IVF in general, Moore et al. (2016b) report that several studies have shown an increased incidence in birth abnormalities such as embryonic tumours or chromosomal changes in children conceived as a result of assisted reproductive technologies. HFEA (2018) state that multiple births (twins and triplets) are the single biggest risk to the health of women and babies undergoing IVF, followed by severe reaction to the fertility drugs used.

Between 2014 and 2016, the percentage of IVF treatments that resulted in a live birth in the UK (HFEA 2018) was:

- 29% for women under 35
- 23% for women aged 35–37
- 15% for women aged 38–39
- 9% for women aged 40–42
- 3% for women aged 43–44
- 2% for women aged over 44.

Intracytoplasmic Sperm Injection (ICSI)

A single sperm is injected directly into the cytoplasm of a mature oocyte. This method can be used when sperm are few, where uterine tubules are blocked or where IVF has previously failed.

Donor Insemination (DI)

Donor sperm is placed directly into the uterus. It is used for several reasons, such as by single women or same sex couples who do not have fertility problems but need to use donated sperm in treatment, or for couples with male fertility problems.

Intrauterine Insemination (IUI)

Where partner sperm is placed directly into the uterus.

Assisted *In Vivo* Fertilization

Sometimes known as gamete intrafallopian (intratubal) transfer (GIFT) or zygote intrafallopian (intratubal) transfer (ZIFT). This employs some of the processes of IVF, however several oocytes and sperm (GIFT) or the zygote itself (ZIFT) are placed directly in the uterine tubules. Due to increased success rates in IVF treatments, GIFT is now rarely used in the UK.

Sperm Washing

This service has been developed for couples who wish to have a child where the male partner is human immunodeficiency virus (HIV)-positive, but the female is HIV-negative (referred to as HIV discordant couple status). This prevents the risk of HIV transmission to the woman via unprotected intercourse, as HIV is transmitted via the seminal fluid and not the sperm. The HIV infected seminal fluid is separated from the sperm by centrifugation and 'washing'. The 'washed' sperm is then combined with nutritional fluid, tested for HIV using a sensitive test called a 'polymerase chain reaction' (PCR) assay, and provided this is negative, inseminated into the female partner when she is ovulating and most likely to become pregnant. In couples with fertility problems, washed sperm can be used in other fertility treatments such as IVF (Chelsea and Westminster Hospital NHS Foundation Trust 2018).

Surrogacy

Surrogacy is when a woman carries a baby on behalf of another person or couple. Surrogacy may be appropriate for those women with a medical condition that makes it impossible or a high risk for them to become pregnant and give birth. It is also a popular option for male same-sex couples who want to have a family. HFEA do not regulate surrogacy in the UK, however data is collected from clinics when a woman is registered as a surrogate and undergoes IVF or DI treatment (HFEA 2018).

Legislation around surrogacy is not universal; for example surrogacy contracts are not enforced by UK law, even if a contract has been signed with a surrogate and expenses have been paid. It is illegal to pay a surrogate in the UK, except for their reasonable expenses. Further rights of the mother and father in the UK can be found at: www.gov.uk/legal-rights-when-using-surrogates-and-donors.

REFLECTIVE ACTIVITY FOR SELF-ASSESSMENT

1. When would be the optimum time for a couple to conceive if the woman has a regular 28-day cycle?
2. At the antenatal 'booking' appointment why is it important to establish the timing, duration and characteristics of the woman's last bleed?
3. The protective effect of folate against neural tube defects is well documented. When is the optimum time for a woman to take folic acid supplementation?

REFERENCES

Castro, R. (2016). Mitochondrial replacement therapy: The UK and US regulatory landscapes. *Journal of Law and the Biosciences*, 3(3), 726–735.

Chelsea and Westminster Hospital NHS Foundation Trust. (2018). Sperm-washing. Available at: www.chel-west.nhs.uk/services/womens-health-services/assisted-conception-unit-acu/treatment-options/sperm-washing.

Chrisler, J. C. (2011). Leaks, lumps, and lines: Stigma and women's bodies. *Psychology of Women Quarterly*, 35(2), 202–214.

Gorman, G., Grady, J., Ng, Y., et al. (2015). Mitochondrial donation — how many women could benefit? *New England Journal of Medicine*, 372, 885–887.

HFEA (Human Fertilisation and Embryology Authority). (2015). *The human fertilisation and embryology (mitochondrial donation) regulations 2015 No. 572*. Available at: www.legislation.gov.uk/ukdsi/2015/9780111125816/contents.

HFEA (Human Fertilisation and Embryology Authority). (2018). Fertility treatment 2014–2016 Trends and figures. Available at: www.hfea.gov.uk.

HTA (Human Tissue Authority). (2018). *Guide to quality and safety assurance for human tissues and cells for human treatment, April 2018*. Available at: www.hta.gov.uk/sites/default/files/HTA%20guide%20to%20Quality%20and%20Safety%20Assurance%20for%20Human%20Tissue%20and%20Cells%20for%20Patient%20Treatment%20v2%20April%202018.pdf.

Moore, K. L., Persaud, T. V. N., & Torchia, M. (2016a). *Before we are born: Essentials of embryology and birth defects* (9th ed.). Philadelphia: Elsevier/Saunders.

Moore, K. L., Persaud, T. V. N., & Torchia, M. (2016b). *The developing human. Clinically orientated embryology* (10th ed.). Philadelphia: Elsevier/Saunders.

NICE (National Institute of Health and Care Excellence). (2018). *NICE Pathway: In vitro fertilisation treatment for people with fertility problems*.

Rankin, J., & Matthews, L. (2017). The female reproductive system. In J. Rankin (Ed.), *Physiology in childbearing with anatomy and related biosciences* (4th ed.). Edinburgh: Elsevier.

RCOG/RCM (Royal College of Obstetricians and Gynaecologists/Royal College of Midwives). (2011). Statement on umbilical cord blood collection and banking. Available at: www.rcog.org.uk.

Tortora, G. J., & Derrickson, B. (2014). *Principles of anatomy and physiology (EMEA edition)* (14th ed.). Hoboken: Wiley.

ANNOTATED FURTHER READING

Coad, J., & Dunstall, M. (2011). *Anatomy and Physiology for Midwives* (3rd ed.). Edinburgh: Churchill Livingstone.

A very full and clear explanation of endocrine activity is given in Chapter 3. Chapter 4 addresses the reproductive cycles in similar detail with clear diagrams to assist the reader.

Johnson, M. H. (2018). *Essential Reproduction* (8th ed.). Oxford: Wiley-Blackwell Science.

This authoritative volume provides the interested reader with a much greater depth of information than is possible in the present book and is recommended for those who wish to study the hormonal patterns of reproduction in detail.

Rankin, J. (Ed.). (2017). *Physiology in Childbearing With Anatomy and Related Biosciences* (4th ed.) Edinburgh: Elsevier.

See Chapter 7 regarding infertility.

Schoenwolf, G. C., Bleyl, S. B., Brauer, P. R., & Francis-West, P. H. (2015). *Larsen's Human Embryology* (5th ed.). Philadelphia: Churchill Livingstone.

Detailed embryology for those students wanting greater depth.

USEFUL WEBSITES

British Fertility Society: https://britishfertilitysociety.org.uk/
Human Tissue and Embryology Authority: www.hfea.gov.uk/
National Institute for Health and Care Excellence: www.nice.org.uk
The Visible Embryo: www.visembryo.com

The Placenta

Jenny Bailey

CHAPTER CONTENTS

This chapter discusses the development of the placenta – a complex organ, deriving from two separate individuals, the mother and the fetus. It is formed from the merging of the chorion and the allantois (see Chapter 5) in early pregnancy. The process of forming a placenta (known as placentation) involves prevention of immune rejection, transfer of nutrients and waste products and the secretion of hormones to maintain the pregnancy. In addition, the chapter includes details of anatomical variations of the placenta and umbilical cord, highlighting their significance to midwifery practice (Tortora and Derrickson 2014; Rampersad et al. 2011).

THE CHAPTER AIMS TO

- outline the development of the placenta

- explore variations of the placenta and umbilical cord and highlight their significance to midwifery practice.

EARLY DEVELOPMENT

Within a few days of fertilization, the trophoblasts (see Chapter 5) begin to produce human chorionic gonadotrophin (hCG), ensuring that the endometrium will be receptive to the implanting embryo. The endometrium increases in vascularity and undergoes a series of structural changes in a process known as *decidualization* in preparation for implantation; hence the endometrium is referred to as the *decidua* in pregnancy. Interconnecting arteriovenous shunts form between the maternal spiral arteries and veins which persist into the immediate postpartum period. A reduction of the number of shunts leading to narrower uterine arteries is involved with complications of pregnancy such as pre-eclampsia (Burton et al. 2009).

The decidua has regions named according to its relationship to the implantation site and these are helpful in diagnosing early pregnancy during ultrasound scan.

- The *decidua basalis* lies between the developing embryo and the stratum basalis of the uterus at the implantation site and forms the maternal part of the placenta.
- The *decidua capsularis* covers the developing embryo.
- The *decidua vera* (otherwise known as the *decidua parietalis*) lines the remainder of the uterine cavity.

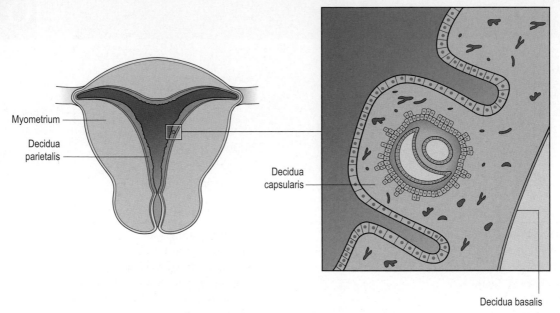

Myometrium

Decidua
parietalis

Decidua
capsularis

Decidua basalis

Fig. 6.1 Early implantation of the blastocyst.

Under the influence of increasing progesterone levels, the endometrial connective tissue cells enlarge and differentiate into *decidual cells*, filled with glycogen and lipids (Moore et al. 2016).

Uterine glands secrete nutrients such as glycogen, to maintain the developing conceptus until the intraplacental blood flow is fully developed, some 10–12 weeks later. The cellular and vascular changes that occur in the endometrium as the blastocyst implants, are known as the *decidual reaction*.

In pregnancy a sophisticated immune adaptation occurs to prevent rejection of the fetus. The decidua is invaded by macrophages, which become immunosuppressive. Adapted T-regulator cells, known as 'Tregs', become less effective as part of the specific hormonal response to antigens and the effect of natural killer (NK) cells is reduced such that their cytotoxicity becomes impaired and they are less likely to destroy any foreign cells. It is also thought that the newly formed decidual cells arise from stem cells, which migrate from fetal haemopoietic organs (liver) and bone marrow during early stages of development (Moore et al. 2016).

Microchimerism is the term for the presence of a small number of cells in one individual that originated in a different individual. Some fetal cells

actively move into the mother's circulation, tissues and organs in the first trimester of pregnancy without triggering an immune response. The role of these cells in maternal systems is unclear. They could have an immunosuppressant effect to protect the fetus and they also can facilitate growth and repair in maternal systems.

Implantation

Implantation involves two stages: prelacunar and lacunar.

Prelacunar Stage

Seven days post-conception, the blastocyst makes contact with the decidua (*apposition*) and the process of placentation begins (Fig. 6.1). The process of implantation is extremely aggressive: chemical mediators, prostaglandins and proteolytic enzymes are released by both the decidua and the trophoblasts and maternal connective tissue is invaded. Nearby maternal blood vessels ensure there is optimum blood flow to the placenta. At this stage, the cytotrophoblasts form a double layer and further differentiate into various types of syncytiotrophoblasts. The supply of syncytiotrophoblasts is as a result of continued mitotic proliferation of the cytotrophoblastic layer below.

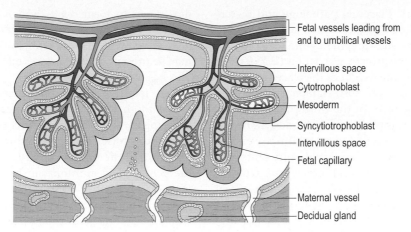

Fetal vessels leading from and to umbilical vessels

Intervillous space

Cytotrophoblast

Mesoderm

Syncytiotrophoblast

Intervillous space

Fetal capillary

Maternal vessel

Decidual gland

Fig. 6.2 Chorionic villi.

Lacunar Stage

Increasing numbers of syncytiotrophoblasts surround the blastocyst and small lakes form within these cells known as *lacunae*, which will become the *intervillous spaces* between the villi (Fig. 6.2) and will be bathed in blood as maternal spiral arteries are eroded some 10–12 weeks following conception. Prior to this, the embryo is nourished from uterine glands (see Chapter 5).

The trophoblasts have a potent invasive capacity, which if left unchecked would spread throughout the uterus. This potential is moderated by the decidua, which secretes cytokines and protease inhibitors that modulate trophoblastic invasion. The *layer of Nitabusch* is a collagenous layer between the endometrium and myometrium, which assists in preventing invasion further than the decidua. At birth, the placenta separates from this layer. Trophoblastic invasion into the myometrium can give rise to a morbidly adhered placenta, known as *placenta accreta* (see Chapter 14).

The Chorionic Villous Tree

Chorionic villi are finger-like projections of chorion surrounded by cytotrophoblastic and syncytiotrophoblastic layers. Initially, new blood vessels develop from progenitor cells within the chorionic villi of the placenta (known as 'vasculogenesis'). A relatively low level of oxygen promotes this. Further growth of these vessels (angiogenesis) produces a vascular network that ultimately connects with those blood vessels developed independently in the embryo via the umbilical arteries and vein through the connecting stalk.

Each chorionic villus is a branching structure, like a tree arising from one stem (anchoring villus). Its centre consists of mesoderm and fetal blood vessels, as well as branches of the umbilical arteries and vein. These are covered by a single layer of *cytotrophoblast* cells and the external layer of the villus is the *syncytiotrophoblast* (Fig. 6.2). This means that four layers of tissue separate the maternal blood from the fetal blood making it impossible for the two circulations to mix unless any villi are damaged.

The villi proliferate and branch out approximately 3 weeks after fertilization. Over time, the villi can differentiate and specialize, resulting in different functions. Villi become most profuse in the area where the blood supply is richest, the *decidua basalis*. This part of the trophoblastic layer, which is known as the *chorion frondosum*, eventually develops into the placenta. The villi under the decidua capsularis gradually degenerate due to lack of nutrition, forming the *chorion laeve*, which is the origin of the chorionic membrane (Fig. 6.3). As the fetus enlarges and grows, the decidua capsularis is pushed towards the decidua vera on the opposite wall of the uterus until, at about 27 weeks' gestation, the decidua capsularis subsequently disappears.

THE PLACENTA AT TERM

At term, the placenta is discoid in shape, about 20 cm in diameter and 2.5 cm thick at its centre and weighing approximately 470 g, which is directly proportional to the weight of the fetus. Rampersad et al. (2011) state that, by term, the ratio of fetal size to that of the placenta is about 7:1. Placental pathology and maternal disease can affect this ratio: such sequelae being diabetes, pre-eclampsia, pregnancy-induced hypertension or intrauterine growth restriction (IUGR) (see Chapters 15 and 34). The weight of the placenta may be affected by early or delayed cord clamping, physiological or active management of the third stage of labour owing to the varying amounts of fetal blood retained in the vessels. The placenta is no longer routinely weighed in clinical practice; however, some maternity units may do so as part of clinical trials and research activities.

The maternal surface of the placenta (i.e. the *basal plate*) is dark red in colour due to maternal blood and partial separation of the basal decidua (Fig. 6.4A). The surface is arranged in up to 40 cotyledons (lobes), which are separated by *sulci* (furrows), into which the decidua

dips down to form *septa* (walls). The cotyledons are made up of lobules, each of which contains a single villus with its branches. Sometimes, deposits of lime salts may be present on the surface, making it slightly gritty. This has no clinical significance.

The fetal surface of the placenta (i.e. the *chorionic plate*) has a shiny appearance due to the amnion covering it (Fig. 6.4B). Branches of the umbilical vein and arteries are visible, spreading out from the insertion of the umbilical cord, which is normally in the centre. The amnion can be peeled off the surface of the chorion as far back as the umbilical cord, whereas the chorion, being derived from the same trophoblastic layer as the placenta, cannot be separated from it.

Functions

The placenta performs a variety of functions for the developing fetus, which can be determined by the pneumonic SERPENT (Fig. 6.5).

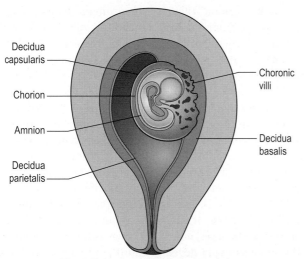

Fig. 6.3 Implantation site at 3 weeks.

Decidua capsularis
Chorion
Amnion
Decidua parietalis
Choronic villi
Decidua basalis

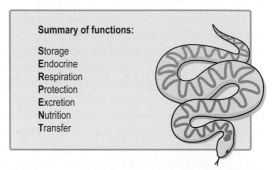

Summary of functions:

Storage
Endocrine
Respiration
Protection
Excretion
Nutrition
Transfer

Fig. 6.5 Summary of the functions of the placenta (SERPENT).

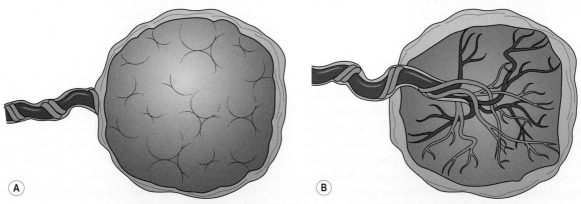

Ⓐ   Ⓑ

Fig. 6.4 The placenta at term. (A) Maternal surface. (B) Fetal surface.

Storage

The placenta metabolizes glucose, stores it in the form of glycogen and reconverts it to glucose as required. It can also store iron and the fat-soluble vitamins.

Endocrine

The many and varied endocrine functions of the placenta are complex, requiring maternal and fetal input. Both types of trophoblasts produce steroidal hormones (oestrogens and progesterone) in addition to many placental protein hormones necessary for pregnancy (Kay et al. 2011).

Steroid hormones. There are three important oestrogens: *oestrone*, *beta oestradiol* and *oestriol*. Both maternal and fetal adrenal production provide precursors for oestrogen production by the placenta. *Pregnalone sulphate* is converted to oestriol by the fetoplacental unit from 6 to 12 weeks onwards, rising steadily until term. Oestrogens influence uterine blood flow, enhance ribonucleic acid (RNA) and protein synthesis and aid growth of uterine muscle. They also increase the size and mobility of the maternal nipple and cause alveolar and duct development of the breast tissue. Serial serum (mmol/L) oestriol measurements can indicate the level of fetoplacental wellbeing.

Progesterone production is maintained by the corpus luteum for approximately 8 weeks until the placenta takes over this function and is dependent on maternal cholesterol stores. Progesterone is thought to play an important part in immunosuppression to maintain the pregnancy (Kay et al. 2011). Progesterone is produced in the syncytial layer of the placenta in increasing quantities until immediately before the onset of labour when its level falls. It maintains the myometrium in a quiescent state, during pregnancy. It is involved in preparing breast tissue during pregnancy and when levels reduce after birth of the placenta, prolactin stimulates lactation.

Protein hormones. *Human chorionic gonadotrophin* (hCG) is produced under the influence of placental gonadotrophic releasing hormone (GnRH) by the trophoblasts. Initially, it is present in very large quantities, with peak levels being achieved by the 8th week, but these gradually reduce as the pregnancy advances. The function of hCG is to stimulate the corpus luteum to produce mainly progesterone. It also increases *fetal Leydig cells* to affect male sexual development prior to fetal luteinizing hormone (LH) production (Kay et al. 2011). Human chorionic gonadotrophin forms the basis of the many pregnancy tests available, as it is excreted in the mother's urine.

Human placental lactogen (hPL) is sometimes known as *human chorionic somatomammotropin hormone* (hCS) as it not only stimulates somatic growth but also stimulates proliferation of breast tissue in preparation for lactation. In early pregnancy, hPL stimulates food intake and weight gain, mobilizing free fatty acids, and functions with prolactin to increase circulating insulin levels (Barbour et al. 2007; Kay et al. 2011). Human placental lactogen is no longer considered the primary agent of insulin resistance as other growth hormones, such as human placental growth hormone (hPGH), appear to be the main determinants for this. Levels of hPL have been used as a screening tool in pregnancy to assess placental function.

Human placental growth hormone (hPGH) levels rise throughout pregnancy. This hormone is involved with hPL as a determinant of insulin resistance in late pregnancy. It mobilizes maternal glucose for transfer to the fetus and contributes to lipolysis, lactogenesis and fetal growth.

Human chorionic thyrotropin and human choroid corticotropin are also synthesized by the placenta. There are also many other factors, such as *insulin growth factor* (IGF) and *vascular endothelial growth factor* (VEGF), playing a variety of roles in metabolism, growth, vasculogenesis and regulation of uteroplacental blood flow.

Respiration

Gaseous exchange to and from the fetus occurs as a result of diffusion. Transfer of gases is assisted by a slight maternal respiratory alkalosis in pregnancy. The fetal haemoglobin level is high *in utero* to facilitate transport of gases. The fetal haemoglobin also has a high affinity for oxygen.

Protection

The placenta provides a limited barrier to infection. Few bacteria can penetrate with the exception of the Treponema of syphilis and the tubercle bacillus. However, many types of virus can penetrate the placental barrier, such as human immunodeficiency virus (HIV), hepatitis strains, Parvovirus B19, human cytomegalovirus (CMV) and rubella. In addition to this, some parasitic and protozoal diseases, such as malaria and toxoplasmosis, will cross the placenta.

The placenta filters substances of a high molecular weight, therefore some drugs and medicines may transfer to the fetus. Although such drugs will cross the placental barrier to the fetus, many will be harmless, and others, such as antibiotics administered to a pregnant woman with syphilis, are positively beneficial (see Chapter 13). Substances including alcohol and some chemicals associated with smoking cigarettes and recreational drug use are not filtered out. These substances can cross the placental barrier freely and may cause congenital malformations and subsequent problems for the baby.

Immunoglobulins will be passed from mother to fetus transplacentally in late pregnancy, providing about 6–12 weeks of naturally acquired passive immunity to the baby.

In the case of Rhesus disease, if sensitization occurs and fetal blood cells enter the maternal circulation, responding antibodies produced by the mother may cross the placenta and destroy fetal surface antigens and consequently fetal cells, causing haemolysis, hydrops fetalis and potential fetal demise.

Excretion

The main substance excreted from the fetus is carbon dioxide. Bilirubin will also be excreted as red blood cells are replaced relatively frequently. There is very little tissue breakdown apart from this and the amounts of urea and uric acid excreted are very small.

Nutrition

The fetus requires nutrients for its ongoing development, such as amino acids and glucose, which are required for growth and energy, calcium and phosphorus for bones and teeth and iron and other minerals for blood formation. These nutrients are actively transferred from the maternal to the fetal blood through the walls of the villi. The placenta is able to select those substances required by the fetus, even depleting the mother's own supply in some instances. Water, vitamins and minerals also pass to the fetus. Fats and fat-soluble vitamins (A, D and E) cross the placenta only with difficulty and mainly in the later stages of pregnancy. Some substances, including amino acids, are found at higher levels in the fetal blood than in the maternal blood.

Transfer of Substances

Substances transfer to and from the fetus by a variety of transport mechanisms, as stated below:
- simple diffusion of gases and lipid soluble substances
- water pores transfer water-soluble substances as a result of osmotic and potentially hydrostatic forces

- facilitated diffusion of glucose using carrier proteins
- active transport against concentration gradients of ions, calcium (Ca) and phosphorus (P)
- endocytosis (pinocytosis) of macromolecules.

Placental Circulation
Maternal Placental Circulation

The syncytiotrophoblasts surrounding the villi erode the walls of maternal vessels opening them up and forming a lake of maternal blood in which the villi float. Maternal blood from 80–100 eroded spiral endometrial arteries pulses between the intervillous spaces and is temporarily outside of maternal circulation. The blood entering is at a higher pressure than that already in the intervillous spaces, so blood spurts towards the chorionic plate; as pressure dissipates, the blood flows slowly over the branch villi. Approximately 150 mL of blood flows into the intervillous spaces, being 3–4 times/min (Moore et al. 2016). The maternal blood circulates, enabling some of the villi to absorb nutrients and oxygen and to excrete waste. These are known as the *nutritive villi*; the blood returns to maternal circulation via endometrial veins. A few villi are more deeply attached to the decidua and are called *anchoring villi*. Reductions in uteroplacental blood flow can result in fetal hypoxia and intrauterine growth restriction (IUGR); severe reduction can result in death.

Fetal Placental Circulation

Umbilical arteries transport poorly oxygenated blood to the placenta. Where the umbilical cord attaches to the placenta, the umbilical arteries subdivide into chorionic arteries that branch outwards and downwards to the chorionic plate and ultimately into the chorionic villi. Here there is a large surface area for gaseous and metabolic exchange of substances through an extensive arteriocapillary-venous system. The well oxygenated fetal blood in the fetal capillaries passes into thin walled veins. At the site of attachment of the umbilical cord to the placenta the veins converge into one umbilical vein transporting highly oxygenated blood (Fig. 6.6).

The Membranes

The basal and chorionic plates come together and meet at the edges to form the *chorioamnion membrane* where the amniotic fluid is contained. The chorioamnion membrane is composed of two membranes: the *amnion* and the *chorion*.

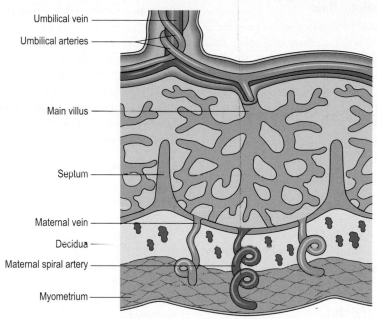

Umbilical vein

Umbilical arteries

Main villus

Septum

Maternal vein

Decidua

Maternal spiral artery

Myometrium

Fig. 6.6 Blood flow around chorionic villi.

The *amnion* is the inner membrane derived from the inner cell mass and consists of a single layer of epithelium with a connective tissue base. It is a tough, smooth and translucent membrane, continuous with the outer surface of the umbilical cord which moves over the chorion aided by mucous. The amnion contains amniotic fluid, which it produces in small quantities as well as prostaglandin E2 (PGE2), which plays a role in the initiation of labour. In rare instances, the amnion can rupture, causing amniotic bands that can affect the growth of fetal limbs.

The *chorion*, which is the outer membrane that is continuous with the edge of the placenta, is composed of mesenchyme, cytotrophoblasts and vessels from the extended spiral arteries of the decidua basalis. It is a rough, thick, fibrous, opaque membrane, which lines the decidua vera during pregnancy, although loosely attached. It produces enzymes that can reduce progesterone levels and also produces prostaglandins, oxytocin and platelet-activating factor, which stimulate uterine activity. This membrane is friable and can rupture easily, so it can be retained in the uterus following birth.

Amniotic Fluid

Amniotic fluid is a clear alkaline and slightly yellowish liquid contained within the amniotic sac. It is derived initially from the cells of the amnion and subsequently from the maternal circulation across the placental membranes and exuded from the fetal surface. Fluid and solutes are passed to and from the fetus and amniotic fluid via the skin prior to keratinization; as a result amniotic fluid is very similar to fetal tissue fluid. The fetus also contributes to the amniotic fluid through metabolism via small quantities of urine, fluid from the GI tract and fluid from its lungs. This fluid is returned to the fetus by intramembranous flow across the amnion into the fetal vessels and through the mechanism of the fetus swallowing.

Functions of the Amniotic Fluid

Amniotic fluid distends the amniotic sac allowing for the growth and free movement of the fetus and permitting symmetrical musculoskeletal development, also helping to prevent adherence to the amnion. It also allows for normal lung development. It equalizes pressure and protects the fetus from jarring and injury. The fluid maintains a constant intrauterine temperature, protecting the fetus from heat loss and providing it with small quantities of nutrients. In labour, so long as the membranes remain intact the amniotic fluid protects the placenta and umbilical cord from the pressure of uterine contractions. It also aids effacement of the cervix and dilatation of the uterine os, particularly where the presenting part is poorly applied.

Constituents of the amniotic fluid

Amniotic fluid consists of 99% water with the remaining 1% being dissolved solid matter, including food substances and waste products. In addition, the fetus sheds skin cells, *vernix caseosa* and *lanugo* into the fluid. Abnormal constituents of the liquor, such as *meconium* in the case of fetal compromise, may give valuable diagnostic information about the condition of the fetus. Aspiration of amniotic fluid for diagnostic examination is termed *amniocentesis*. Research has found that amniotic fluid is a plentiful source of non-embryonic stem cells (Moraghebi et al. 2017).

Volume of amniotic fluid

During pregnancy, amniotic fluid increases in volume as the fetus grows from 30 mL at 10 weeks, 350 mL at 20 weeks, to approximately 700–1000 mL at term. The water content changes every 3 h.

The Umbilical Cord (Funis)

The umbilical cord, which extends from the fetal surface of the placenta to the umbilical area of the fetus, is formed by the 5th week of pregnancy. It originates from the duct that forms between the amniotic sac and the yolk sac, which transmits the umbilical blood vessels (see Chapter 5).

Functions

The umbilical cord transports oxygen and nutrients to the developing fetus and removes waste products.

Structure

The umbilical cord contains two arteries and one vein (Fig. 6.7), which are continuous with the blood vessels in the chorionic villi of the placenta. The blood vessels are enclosed and protected by *Wharton's jelly*, a gelatinous substance formed from primary mesoderm. The whole cord is covered in a layer of amnion that is continuous with that covering the placenta. There are no nerves in the umbilical cord, so cutting it following the birth of the baby is not painful.

The presence of only two vessels in the cord may indicate renal or cardiac malformations in the fetus; however, in some instances this has little significance to the subsequent health of the baby.

Measurements

The cord is approximately 1–2 cm in diameter and 50 cm in length. This length is sufficient to allow for the birth of the baby without applying any traction to the placenta.

A cord is considered *short* when it measures <40 cm. There is no specific agreed length for describing a cord as *too long*, but the disadvantages of a very long cord are that it may become wrapped round the neck or body of the fetus or become knotted. Either event could result in occlusion of the blood vessels, especially during labour. Long cords are also more prone to prolapsing.

Compromise of the fetal blood flow through the umbilical cord vessels can have serious detrimental effects on the health of the fetus and baby. *True knots* should always be noted on examination of the cord, but they must be distinguished from *false knots*, which are lumps of Wharton's jelly on the side of the cord and do not have any physiological significance.

Anatomical Variations of the Placenta and Cord

A *succenturiate lobe* of placenta is the most significant of the variations in conformation of the placenta. A small extra lobe is present that is separate from the main placenta and joined to it by blood vessels that run through the membranes to connect it (Fig. 6.8). The danger is that this small lobe may be retained *in utero* after the

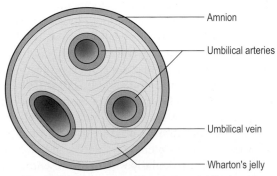

Fig. 6.7 Cross-section through the umbilical cord.

Amnion
Umbilical arteries
Umbilical vein
Wharton's jelly

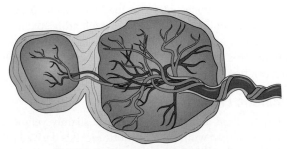

Fig. 6.8 Succenturiate lobe of placenta.

placenta is expelled, and if it is not removed, it may lead to haemorrhage and infection. Every placenta must be examined for evidence of a retained succenturiate lobe, which can be identified by a hole in the membranes with blood vessels running to it.

In a *circumvallate* placenta, an opaque ring is seen on the fetal surface of the placenta. It is formed by a doubling back of the fetal membrane onto the fetal surface of the placenta and may result in the membranes leaving the placenta nearer the centre instead of at the edge as usual (Fig. 6.9). This placental variation is associated with *placental abruptio* and intrauterine growth restriction (IUGR).

In a *bipartite placenta*, there are two complete and separate lobes where the main cord bifurcates to supply both parts (Fig. 6.10). A *tripartite placenta* is similar to a bipartite placenta, but it has three distinct parts.

In a *battledore* insertion of the cord, the cord is attached at the very edge of the placenta, and where the attachment is fragile, it may cause significant problems with active management of the third stage of labour (Fig. 6.11).

A *velamentous* insertion of the cord, occurs when the cord is inserted into the membranes some distance from the edge of the placenta. The umbilical vessels run through the membranes from the cord to the placenta (Fig. 6.12). If the placenta is normally situated, no harm

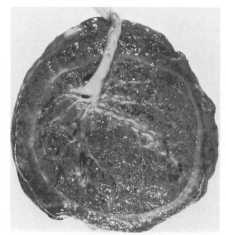

Fig. 6.9 Circumvallate placenta.

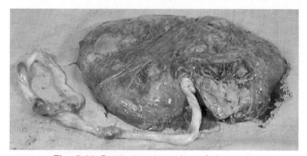

Fig. 6.11 Battledore insertion of the cord.

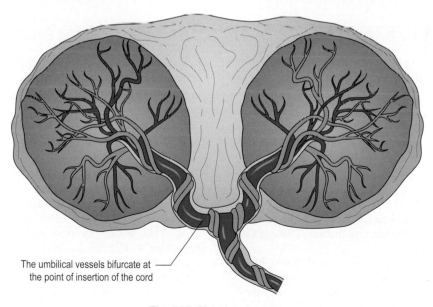

The umbilical vessels bifurcate at the point of insertion of the cord

Fig. 6.10 Bipartite placenta.

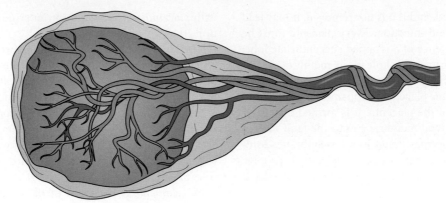

Fig. 6.12 Velamentous insertion of the cord.

will result to the fetus, but the cord is likely to become detached upon applying traction during active management of the third stage of labour. However, if the placenta is low-lying, the vessels may pass across the uterine os (*vasa praevia*). In this case, there is great danger to the fetus when the membranes rupture and even more so during artificial rupture of the membranes, as the vessels may be torn, leading to rapid exsanguination of the fetus. If the onset of haemorrhage coincides with rupture of the membranes, fetal haemorrhage should be assumed and the birth expedited. It is possible to distinguish fetal blood from maternal blood by Singer's alkali-denaturation test, although, in practice, time is so short that it may not be possible to save the life of the baby. If the baby survives, haemoglobin levels should be estimated after birth and blood transfusion considered.

CONCLUSION

Development of the placenta requires complex processes involving enzymes, hormones and growth factors, which remodel maternal tissue in addition to constructing new tissue specifically for the sustenance of the fetus. The placenta acts as a life support system for the developing embryo and fetus until birth.

▋ REFLECTIVE ACTIVITY FOR SELF-ASSESSMENT

1. Without the immunological adaptions during pregnancy, why would the mother reject the developing fetus?
2. What effect do you think smoking will have on implantation of the blastocyst and on the placenta?
3. How does the timing of cord clamping affect the neonate?

REFERENCES

Barbour, L. A., McCurdy, C. E., Hernandez, T. L., et al. (2007). Cellular mechanisms for insulin resistance in normal pregnancy and gestational diabetes. *Diabetes Care, 30*(Suppl. 2), 112–119.

Burton, G. J., Woods, A. W., Jauniaux, E., et al. (2009). Rheological and physiological consequences of conversion of maternal spiral arteries for uteroplacental blood flow during human pregnancy. *Placenta, 30*(6), 473–482.

Kay, H. H., Nelson, D. M., & Wang, Y. (2011). *The placenta: From development to disease*. Oxford: Blackwell.

Moore, K. L., Persaud, T. V. N., & Torchia, M. (2016). *Before we are born: Essentials of embryology and birth defects* (9th ed.). Philadelphia: Elsevier/Saunders.

Moraghebi, R., Kirkeby, A., Chaves, P., et al. (2017). Term amniotic fluid: An unexploited reserve of mesenchymal stromal cells for reprogramming and potential cell therapy applications. *Stem Cell Research & Therapy, 8*(1), 190.

Rampersad, R., Cerva-Zivkovic, M., & Nelson, D. M. (2011). Development and anatomy of the human placenta. In H. H. Kay, D. M. Nelson, & Y. Wang (Eds.), *The placenta: From development to disease*. Oxford: Blackwell.

Tortora, G. J., & Derrickson, B. (2014). *Principles of anatomy and physiology (EMEA edition)* (14th ed.). Hoboken NJ, USA: John Wiley & Sons Inc.

ANNOTATED FURTHER READING

Coad, J., & Dunstall, M. (2011). *Anatomy and physiology for midwives* (3rd ed.). London: Churchill Livingstone/Elsevier. *Chapter 8 of this comprehensive text provides a detailed account of the placenta.*

Kay, H. H., Nelson, D. M., & Wang, Y. (2011). *The placenta: From development to disease*. Oxford: Blackwell. *Chapters 3 and 4 provide details regarding placental development for students who wish a more in-depth knowledge.*

Oats, J. K., & Abraham, S. (2016). *Llewellyn-Jones fundamentals of obstetrics and gynaecology* (10th ed.). London: Elsevier. *This book has a section on the placenta (Chapter 3) that the reader may find useful.*

Rankin, J. (Ed.). (2017). *Physiology in childbearing with anatomy and related biosciences* (4th ed.). Edinburgh: Elsevier. *See section 2A, in Chapter 12, that considers the placenta, membranes and amniotic fluid.*

USEFUL WEBSITES

NICE: Antenatal care for uncomplicated pregnancies. Clinical guideline [CG62] Published March 2008. Last updated: January 2017: www.nice.org.uk/guidance/cg62/chapter/1-guidance

Placenta – the Official Journal of the International Federation of Placenta Associations: www.journals.elsevier.com/placenta

Placenta development: https://embryology.med.unsw.edu.au/embryology/index.php/Placenta_Development#Introduction

7

The Fetus

Jenny Bailey

CHAPTER CONTENTS

This chapter provides a system-by-system approach for the reader to appreciate the complexities surrounding embryonic and fetal development and the subsequent changes that occur in the baby at the time of birth. In addition, discussion of the fetal skull and the significance of its diameters in late pregnancy and during labour in influencing an optimum birth outcome is provided. An understanding of the detail is of value to the midwife when providing parents with information about the effects of maternal lifestyle, such as diet, smoking, alcohol intake, drug use and exercise, on fetal growth and development (see Chapter 9) and when a baby is born before term (see Chapter 34).

THE CHAPTER AIMS TO

- outline the early development of the embryo and subsequent development of the fetus
- discuss the fetal circulation and the changes that occur at birth
- discuss the significance of the fetal skull and the significance of its diameters in determining a successful birth outcome.

TIME SCALE OF DEVELOPMENT

Embryological development is complex and occurs from the 2nd to the 8th week of pregnancy and includes the development of the *zygote* in the first 2–3 weeks following fertilization. *Fetal* development occurs from the 8th week until birth. The interval from the beginning of the last menstrual period (LMP) until fertilization is not part of pregnancy, however this period is important for the calculation of the expected date of birth. Fig. 7.1 illustrates the comparative lengths of these prenatal events.

A summary of embryological and fetal development categorized into 4-week periods is provided in Box 7.1. This should be used to complement the text below.

FETAL GROWTH AND MATURATION

From the 9th week of pregnancy, fetal growth is rapid. Tissues grow by cell proliferation, cell enlargement and accretion of extracellular material. An adequate supply of nutrients and oxygen from the placenta to the fetus is crucial for growth. In developed countries, the average

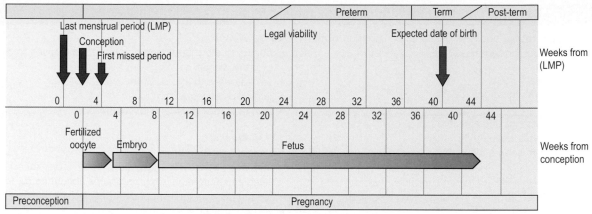

Fig. 7.1 Timescales of prenatal events.

BOX 7.1 Summary of Embryological and Fetal Development

Embryo

0–4 Weeks:

- blastocyst implants
- primitive streak appears
- conversion of bilaminar disc into trilaminar disc
- primitive axial skeleton and vertebral column develops
- some body systems laid down in primitive form
- primitive central nervous system forms (*neurulation*)
- blood vessels appear in the wall of umbilical vessel, allantois, chorion and embryo
- fetal erythrocytes develop from haematopoietic precursors
- primitive heart develops and begins to beat on day 22
- covered with a layer of skin
- limb buds form
  - optic vessels develop
  - gender determined.

4–8 Weeks:

- very rapid cell division, folding of tissues from a flat disc into a cylindrical embryo
- more body systems laid down in primitive form and continue to develop
- spinal nerves begin to develop
- blood is pumped around the vessels
- lower respiratory system begins to develop
- kidneys begin to develop
- skeletal ossification begins developing
- developing brain incorporated into the cranial end of embryo; head and facial features develop
- early movements
- embryo is visible on ultrasound from 6 weeks
- main organ systems are established by 8th week.

Fetus

8–12 Weeks:

- rapid weight gain
- eyelids meet and fuse
- urine formation occurs and is passed, contributing to the amniotic fluid
- swallowing begins
- distinguishing features of external genitalia appear nearer to 12 weeks
- some primitive reflexes present
- erythropoiesis occurs initially in the fetal liver then in the spleen by the 12th week.

12–16 Weeks:

- development of primary ossification centres; rapid skeletal development – visible on ultrasound; limb movements become coordinated
- rapid growth occurs
- meconium present in gut
- nasal septum and palate fuse
- external genitalia fully differentiate into male or female by week 12
- fetus capable of sucking thumb
- in females, ovaries are differentiated and contain primordial ovarian follicles and their oogonia.

16–20 Weeks:

- constant weight gain
- 'quickening' – mother feels fetal movements
- fetal heart heard on auscultation
- vernix caseosa and lanugo both appear
- skin cells begin to be renewed
- brown adipose tissue (BAT) forms

BOX 7.1   Summary of Embryological and Fetal Development—cont'd

- in males, testes begin to descend; canalization of the vagina occurs in females.

20–24 Weeks:
- most organs functioning well
- eyes complete
- periods of sleep and activity
- ear apparatus developing
- responds to sound, blink/startle reflexes approx. 22–23 weeks
- skin red and wrinkled, blood capillaries visible
- surfactant secreted in the lungs from week 20
- fingernails develop.

24–28 Weeks:
- legally viable and survival may be expected if born
- eyelids open
- respiratory movements
- increase in white fat to 3.5% body weight
- bone marrow takes over from spleen as site of erythropoiesis.

28–32 Weeks:
- begins to store fat and iron; white fat increases to 8% of body weight
- testes descend into scrotum
- lanugo disappears from face
- skin becomes paler and less wrinkled.

32–36 Weeks:
- weight gain 25 g/day
- increased white fat makes the body more rounded; head and abdominal circumferences almost equal
- lanugo disappears from body
- hair on fetal head lengthens
- nails reach tips of fingers and toes
- ear cartilage soft
- plantar creases visible.

36 Weeks to birth:
- birth is expected
- body round and plump; abdominal circumference can be greater than head
- skull formed but soft and pliable.

---

birth weight is around 3400 g, of which 50% is acquired by 30 weeks' gestation. The fetus gains approximately 25 g/day between weeks 32 and 40. A visual representation of growth in terms of height is provided in Fig. 7.2.

As fetal growth is an indicator of fetal health and wellbeing, monitoring of growth is crucial. This is done by visual observation of the uterus for size, symphysis fundal height measurements and ultrasonography.

The Cardiovascular System

The early development of the cardiovascular system in the 3rd week of pregnancy coincides with the lack of the yolk sac, and the urgent need to supply the growing embryo with oxygen and nutrients from the maternal blood through the placenta.

The cardiovascular system is the first system to function in the embryo. The heart and vascular system commences development in the 3rd week, and by the 4th week (approx. 6 weeks after the last menstrual period), a primitive heart is visible by ultrasound scan and is beginning to function, beating at day 21 or 22 days (Moore et al. 2016a). Initially a vascular plexus is formed in the embryo, which is continually remodelled into a system of arteries and veins to accommodate the growing and developing embryo. The first signs of the heart are the appearance of paired endothelial strands in the cardiogenic mesoderm, which canalize to become heart tubes and then fuse to become a tubular-shaped heart. The tubular heart joins with blood vessels within the embryo, connecting stalk, chorion and umbilical vessel; this forms the basis of the primordial cardiovascular system. Major architectural and dynamic cell elongation in the heart is coordinated with extension of the foregut (Kidokoro et al. 2018).

The development of the heart continues to include remodelling and septation, while the heart continues to beat. The embryonic heart rate (EHR) is determined by growth of the cardiovascular system and the embryo's size. A 2 mm embryo EHR should be 75 bpm; 5 mm 100 bpm; 10 mm 120 bpm; and 15 mm 130 bpm (Coulam et al. 1996).

Ultrasound assessment of the structural development of the fetal heart occurs in the UK at 20 weeks' gestation (Box 7.2), as part of the fetal anomaly screening programme [FASP] (Public Health England 2019).

Blood is pumped around the vessels from the 4th week, by which time three major vascular systems have developed (see below). Vascular endothelial growth

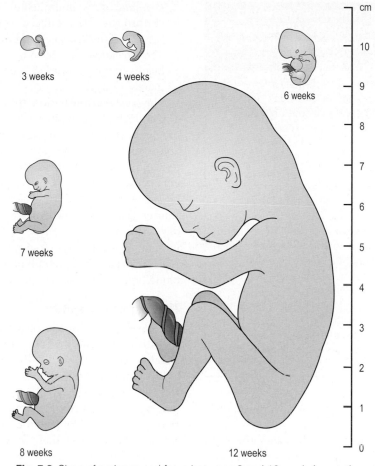

Fig. 7.2 Sizes of embryos and fetus between 3 and 12 weeks' gestation.

factor is a protein that causes vasculogenesis and subsequent angiogenesis to occur. Vasculogenesis commences in the extraembryonic mesoderm of the umbilical vessel, connecting stalk and chorion. By the end of the 3rd week a primordial uteroplacental circulation has also developed.

Mesenchymal cells differentiate into *angioblasts which form into clusters known as 'blood islands'*. Cavities arise in these blood islands; the angioblasts then flatten, providing an endothelium and line the cavities, becoming the forerunners of vessels. The vessels bud and branch into surrounding non-vascularized tissues and ultimately fuse to form a network. Mesenchymal cells surrounding the primitive endothelial blood vessels also differentiates into the muscular and connective tissue components of the blood vessels.

Arteries

Vitelline arteries link the aorta with the yolk sac, which subsequently supplies the gut and other arteries in the neck and thorax. Mid-gestation, they are remodelled to form three main arteries, which supply the gastrointestinal tract.

Two *umbilical* arteries deliver deoxygenated blood to the placenta.

Veins

The embryo has three major venous systems draining into the tubular-shaped heart: vitelline, umbilical and cardinal (Schoenwolf et al. 2014).

The *vitelline* veins return poorly oxygenated blood from the gut and yolk sac. The hepatic veins and the portal vein develop from the vitelline veins and their networks. A temporary shunt, the *ductus venosus*, also develops from these veins.

Umbilical veins form in the body stalk. The right umbilical vein anastomoses with the ductus venosus shunting oxygenated placental blood into the inferior vena cava leaving the left umbilical vein to continue carrying oxygenated blood from the placenta to the embryo. Between 5–7 weeks of pregnancy, the foramen ovale is formed. From here on, there is shunting of highly oxygenated blood from the right to left atrium, bypassing the right ventricle and pulmonary system, allowing the higher oxygenated blood to be pumped immediately to the brain and upper body.

The *cardinal* veins drain the head, neck and body wall into the heart.

Development over time ensures that the three systems develop into the adult pattern, while maintaining some temporary structures in the fetus which resolve at, or soon after, birth.

There are three phases of red blood cell formation (*haematogenesis*) (Moore et al. 2016b):
• The *yolk sac* period where blood develops from haematopoietic stem cells arising from specialized haemangiogenic endothelium of the yolk sac. Some erythrocytes are produced from the blood vessels at the end of the 3rd week and the dorsal aorta.
• The *hepatic/liver* period, where haematogenesis begins in the primordial liver and spleen at approximately 12 weeks.
• The *bone marrow* period, from the 24–28th week.

The *erythrocytes* contain fetal haemoglobin. Fetal haemoglobin (HbF) has a much greater affinity for oxygen and is found in greater concentrations (18–20 g/dL at term) in the blood than adult haemoglobin (HbA), thus enhancing the transfer of oxygen across the placental site. Fetal erythrocytes have a life span of 90 days, shorter than adult erythrocytes, which is around 120 days. The short life span of fetal erythrocytes contributes to neonatal physiological jaundice (see Chapter 37). Genes passed from both parents determine the fetal blood type and Rhesus factor.

The Respiratory System

The development of the respiratory system begins in the 4th week. The lower respiratory tract and lungs develop simultaneously. The lungs originate from a 'lung bud' growing out of the caudal aspect of the foregut, which repeatedly subdivides to form the branching structure of the bronchial tree. Cartilaginous plates form from surrounding *splanchnic mesenchyme*, as does bronchial smooth muscle, connective tissue, pulmonary connective tissue and capillaries. As the lungs continue to develop, the visceral pleura is formed. The parietal pleura is formed from the thoracic body lining; the space between the two pleura is the *pleural cavity*.

Maturation of the lungs goes through histological stages:
• The pseudoglandular period (5–17 weeks): all major components of the lungs are formed, except those that deal with gaseous exchange. Respiration is not possible.
• The canalicular period (16–25 weeks): lung tissue is well vascularized; increase in size of lumen of bronchi and terminal bronchioles, which subdivide to form two or more respiratory bronchioles with primordial alveolar ducts and thin walled terminal sacs. Respiration is now possible as gaseous exchange can occur, though respiratory system is very immature.
• The terminal saccular period (24 weeks–term): further development of alveoli occurs. Close contact

between terminal sac squamous epithelial cells (type I pneumocytes) and endothelial cells creates a blood–air barrier, where gaseous exchange can occur.

- The development of type II pneumocyte cells commences around 20 weeks of fetal life. These cells are necessary to produce *surfactant*, a lipoprotein that reduces the surface tension in the alveoli and assists gaseous exchange. The amount of surfactant increases until the alveoli mature between 36 weeks and birth.
- The alveolar period (term–8 years of age): approximately 95% mature alveoli develop in the postnatal period and their development is completed by approximately the age of 3 years. New alveoli may be added up until 8 years of age.
- There is some movement of the thorax from the 12th week of fetal life and more definite, rhythmic diaphragmatic movements from the 24th week coordinated by the developing central nervous system. This does not constitute breathing as gaseous exchange is via the placenta.
- At term, the lungs contain about 100 mL of lung fluid. About one-third of this is expelled during birth and the rest is absorbed and transported by the lymphatics and blood vessels as air takes its place.
- Babies born before 24 weeks of pregnancy have a reduced chance of survival owing to the immaturity of the capillary system in the lungs and the lack of surfactant (see Chapter 37).

The Urogenital System

The urogenital system is divided functionally into the *urinary/renal* system and the *genital/reproductive* system. Both systems develop from the *intermediate mesoderm*. There are three successive sets of kidneys which develop in the fetus in the first trimester. *Pronephroi* develop from the 4th week of fetal life; these are non-functional, degenerate and are used by the second set of kidneys – the *mesonephroi*. These appear at the end of the 4th week, below the pronephros location. Forty glomeruli and mesonephric tubules and ducts are present opening into the *cloaca*. *Mesonephroi* produce small amounts of urine between the 6th and 10th week, when the permanent kidneys take over. *Metanephroi* start to develop in the 5th week and become more functional around the 9th week when more urine is produced. The urine does not constitute a route for excretion, as elimination of waste products is via the placenta. The urine forms

much of the amniotic fluid and production increases with fetal maturity. As the fetus develops, the kidneys change location, reaching their adult destination by the 9th week. Continued development of nephrons collecting tubules occurs; glomeruli grow into the tubule area and vessels surround the nephrons. By week 36, each kidney contains approximately 2 million nephrons.

The superior vesical arteries arise from the first few centimetres of the hypogastric arteries, which lead to the umbilical arteries. A single umbilical artery at birth is suggestive of malformations of the renal tract (see Chapter 36).

The sex of the embryo is determined at fertilization: either two X chromosomes (in the female) or one X and one Y chromosome (in the male) are inherited. Prior to the 7th week, the gonads are identical in both sexes and are known as 'indifferent gonads'. The gonads develop from the 5th week from the mesodermal epithelium. In the two sexes, genital development is similar and is referred to as the *indifferent state of sexual development*. Testis determining factor (TDF)) on the sex determining region on the Y gene (SRY) controls the subsequent male development pattern (Moore et al. 2016b). Differentiation occurs from the 7th week in the male, but female gonad development occurs slowly and under the influence of *pro-ovarian* genes and the ovaries may not be identifiable until the 10th week. Active mitosis produces millions of oogonia during fetal life. Many oogonia degenerate, however 2 million enlarge and become primary oocytes before birth. The external genitalia in both sexes develop in the 9th week, but males and females are not fully distinguishable until about the 12th week. By 18 weeks, the female uterus is formed, and the vagina starts to canalize.

The Endocrine System

The adrenal glands develop from mesoderm and neural crest cells from the 6th week of fetal life and grow to 10–20 times larger than the adult adrenals. Their size regresses during the first year of life. They produce the precursors for placental formation of oestriols and influence maturation of the lungs, liver and epithelium of the digestive tract. It is also thought that the fetal adrenal glands play a part in the initiation of labour. Corticotropin releasing hormone (CRH) is secreted by the fetal hypothalamus, stimulating adrenocorticotropic hormone from the fetal pituitary gland. This in turn causes cortisol and oestrogens to be secreted from the fetal suprarenal cortex. Oestrogens increase myometrial contractility.

The posterior area of the forebrain (see below) develops swellings in the walls of the 3rd ventricle, which become the thalamus, hypothalamus and epithalamus. The pineal and pituitary gland also develop in this area. The pituitary gland arises from two embryonic areas, hence it has an anterior and posterior lobe. The fetal pituitary produces gonadotrophins, i.e. luteinizing hormone (LH) and follicle stimulating hormone (FSH) from weeks 13–14, and human growth hormone (hGH) is present by weeks 19–20.

The Digestive System

The primitive gut develops from the endodermal layer of the yolk sac in the 4th week of fetal life. It begins as a straight tube, and proceeds on several levels: foregut, midgut and hindgut.

By the 5th week, the *foregut* (oesophagus, stomach and duodenum) is visible. Foregut extension is coordinated with heart elongation (Kidokoro et al. 2018). The liver, gallbladder and pancreas bud form the gut tube around the 4th to 5th week of fetal life. The liver grows rapidly from the 5th week and by the 10th week occupies much of the abdominal cavity, constituting about 10% of the fetal weight by the 9th week. During the 6th week, haematopoiesis occurs and various types of blood cells are developed. Towards the end of pregnancy, iron stores are laid down in the liver and the liver cells produce bile from the 12th week. Insulin is secreted from 10 weeks of fetal life and glucagon from 15 weeks, both of which rise steadily with increasing fetal age.

The *midgut* (small intestine, caecum and vermiform appendix, ascending colon and transverse colon) undertakes much of its development in the 6th week. Defects near the median plane of the abdominal wall will allow the viscera to protrude into the amniotic cavity (*gastroschisis*) and can be seen on ultrasound scan (see Chapter 36).

The *hindgut* (rectum and anal canal) completes its development in the 7th week of fetal life. Muscular, connective tissue and all other layers for all of the alimentary tract arise from splanchnic mesenchyme surrounding the primordial gut.

Around 12 weeks, the digestive tract is well formed, and the lumen is patent. Most digestive juices are present before birth and act on the swallowed substances to form *meconium*. Bile enters the duodenum from the bile duct during the 13th week, giving the intestinal contents a dark green colour. Meconium is *normally* retained in the gut until after birth when it is passed as the first stool of the baby.

The Nervous System

The brain begins to develop from the 3rd week and appears as the neural plate and neural groove (see Chapter 5). The neural tube is derived from the *ectoderm*, which folds inwards by a complicated process to form the neural tube, which is then covered over by skin. Closure of the neural tube is essential and takes place by 26 days. This process is occasionally incomplete, leading to open neural tube defects (see Chapter 36). In the UK, a nuchal scan (nuchal translucency, NT scan) is offered between 11 weeks and 2 days, and 14 weeks and 1 day of pregnancy, as part of the FASP. The thickness of fluid in the tissue space within the nape of the fetal neck is where the nuchal translucency is measured. An increased amount of fluid may indicate that the fetus has Down syndrome or a structural or genetic anomaly. By combining the mother's age and the gestation of the pregnancy with information from the scan, an individual statistical chance of an anomaly can be given for that pregnancy. Guidance from Public Health England (2018) recommends that if the chance is 1 in 150 or higher a diagnostic test, such as chorionic villus sampling CVS, will be offered in accordance with FASP (see Chapter 13).

The meninges develop during days 20–35 covering the brain and spinal cord (Moore et al. 2016b); the pia mater and choroid plexuses secrete fluid into the ventricles; this becomes cerebrospinal fluid (CSF). Signalling from the choroid plexuses and signalling morphogens in the CSF are necessary for brain development.

Brain development occurs simultaneously with neural tube development, some of the neural tube developing into the brain. Various bending and folding occurs within the brain giving rise to three main structures: *forebrain*, *midbrain* and *hindbrain*. Various areas of the hindbrain become the medulla oblongata, pons and cerebellum. Myelination of nerve fibres does not occur until late pregnancy and continues up to 1 year of age.

The development of the sense organs, including the transmission of sensory input to the brain and output from the brain, occurs under complex processes. The eyes and ears are associated with the development of the head and neck, which begin early and continue until the cessation of growth in the late teens. Although the eyes develop from around 22 days, for normal vision to occur, many complex structures within the eye must properly relate to neighbouring structures. The eye is completely formed by 20 weeks, rapid eye movements occur at 21 weeks; blink/startle responses have been noted at 22–23 weeks (Moore et al. 2016b) but the eyelids are fused until around 24 weeks. The developing eyes are sensitive to light from about 30 weeks.

The development of the inner ear, which contains the structures for hearing and balance, commences early in embryological life but is not complete until around 25 weeks.

Motor output controlled by the basal ganglia in the form of movement, begins around 8 weeks, however these movements are not usually felt by the mother until around 16 weeks, and are referred to as *quickening*. As the nervous system matures, fetal behaviour becomes more complex and more defined. The fetus develops behavioural patterns: sleep with no eye or body movements; sleep with periodic eye and body movements, known as *REM sleep*; wakefulness with subtle eye and limb movements; active phase with vigorous eye and limb movements.

Integumentary, Skeletal and Muscular Systems

Integumentary. The epidermis develops from a single layer of ectoderm to which other layers are added. By the end of 4 weeks, a thin outer layer of flattened cells covers the embryo. Further development continues until 24 weeks. Brown adipose tissue (BAT) develops from 17–20 weeks' gestation; this plays an important part in thermoregulation after birth. From 18 weeks, the fetus is covered with a white, creamy substance called *vernix caseosa*, which protects the skin from the amniotic fluid and from any friction against itself. Hair begins to develop between the 9th and 12th week. By 20 weeks, the fetus is covered with a fine downy hair called *lanugo*; at the same time, the hair on the head and eyebrows begin to form. Lanugo is shed from 36 weeks and by term, there is little left. Fingernails develop from about 10 weeks, but the toenails do not form until about 18 weeks. By term, the nails usually extend beyond the fingertips therefore it is not unusual to see scratches on the baby's face.

Skeletal. Most skeletal tissue arises from the mesodermal and neural crest cells but skeletal tissue in different parts of the body are diverse in morphology and tissue architecture. Skeletal development is stimulated by mechanical forces generated by fetal kicks. This stimulation is critical for musculoskeletal development. Absence or abnormal movement has been associated with multiple congenital disorders (Verbruggen et al. 2018).

The skull develops during the 4th week from the mesenchyme surrounding the developing brain. It consists of two major parts: the *neurocranium*, which forms the bones of the skull, and the *viscerocranium*, which forms the bones of the face (Tortora and Derrickson 2014; Moore et al. 2016b). The neurocranium forms flat bones at the roof and sides of the skull. Ossification here is intramembranous and the membranous separations between the flat bones are known as *sutures* and *fontanelles*. The functions of these will be discussed later in the chapter.

THE FETAL CIRCULATION

The placenta is the source of oxygenation, nutrition and elimination of waste for the fetus. There are several temporary structures in addition to the placenta and the umbilical cord that enable the fetal circulation to occur (Fig. 7.3). These include:

- the *ductus venosus*, which connects the umbilical vein to the inferior vena cava
- the *foramen ovale*, which is an opening between the right and left atria
- the *ductus arteriosus*, which leads from the bifurcation of the pulmonary artery to the descending aorta
- the *hypogastric arteries*, which branch off from the internal iliac arteries and become the umbilical arteries when they enter the umbilical cord.

The fetal circulation takes the following course: *oxygenated blood* from the placenta travels to the fetus in the umbilical vein. The umbilical vein divides into two branches – one that supplies the portal vein in the liver, the other anastomosing with the ductus venosus and joining the inferior vena cava. Most of the oxygenated blood that enters the right atrium passes across the foramen ovale to the left atrium, which mixes with a very small amount of blood returning from the lungs from where it passes into the left ventricle via the bicuspid valve, and then the aorta. The head and upper extremities receive approximately 50% of this blood via the coronary and carotid arteries, and the subclavian arteries,

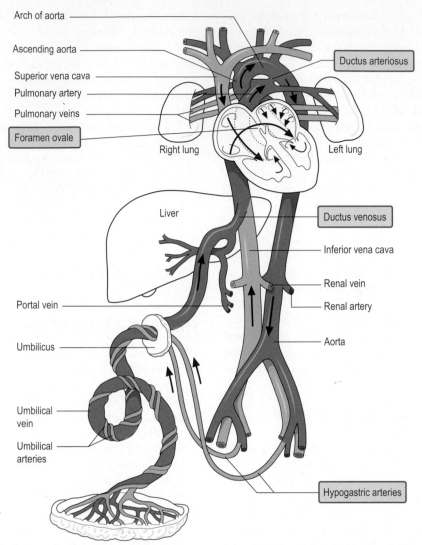

Arch of aorta

Ascending aorta

Superior vena cava

Pulmonary artery

Pulmonary veins

Foramen ovale

Right lung

Ductus arteriosus

Left lung

Liver

Ductus venosus

Inferior vena cava

Renal vein

Renal artery

Portal vein

Aorta

Umbilicus

Umbilical vein

Umbilical arteries

Hypogastric arteries

Fig. 7.3 A diagram of the fetal circulation. The arrows show the course taken by the blood. The temporary structures are labelled in colour.

respectively. The rest of the blood travels down the descending aorta, mixing with deoxygenated blood from the right ventricle via the ductus arteriosus. *Deoxygenated blood* collected from the head and upper parts of the body returns to the right atrium via the superior vena cava. Blood that has entered the right atrium from the superior vena cava enters at a different angle to the blood that enters from the inferior vena cava and heads towards the foramen ovale.

Hence there are two distinct blood flows entering the right atrium. Most of the lesser oxygenated blood entering the right atrium from the superior vena cava

passes behind the flow of highly oxygenated blood going to the left atrium and enters the right ventricle via the tricuspid valve. There is a small amount of blood mixing where the two blood flows meet in the atrium. From the right ventricle a little blood travels to the lungs in the pulmonary artery, for their development. Most blood, however, passes from the pulmonary artery through the ductus arteriosus into the descending aorta. This blood, although low in oxygen and nutrients, is sufficient to supply the lower body of the fetus. It is also by this means that deoxygenated blood travels back to the placenta via the internal iliac arteries, which lead into the hypogastric arteries, and ultimately into the umbilical arteries. This circulation means that the fetus has a well-oxygenated and perfused head, brain and upper body compared with its lower extremities.

ADAPTATION TO EXTRAUTERINE LIFE

At birth, there is a dramatic alteration to the fetal circulation and an almost immediate change occurs. The cessation of umbilical blood flow causes a cessation of flow in the ductus venosus and a fall in pressure in the right atrium. As the baby takes its first breath, blood is drawn along the pulmonary system via the pulmonary artery and therefore, pressure increases in the left atrium due to the increased blood supply returning to it via the pulmonary veins. The alteration of pressures between the two atria causes a mechanical closure of the foramen ovale. In addition, the neonate's first breath results in the inflation of the lungs, and there is a rapid fall in pulmonary vascular resistance of approximately 80%, a slight reverse flow of oxygenated aortic blood along the ductus arteriosus and a rise in the oxygen tension. This causes the smooth muscle in the walls of the ductus arteriosus to contract and constrict, usually within 24 h following birth at term, though it can remain patent for a few days.

As these structural changes become permanent, the following fetal structures arise:
- The umbilical vein becomes the *ligamentum teres*.
- The ductus venosus becomes the *ligamentum venosum*.
- The ductus arteriosus becomes the *ligamentum arteriosum*.
- The foramen ovale becomes the *fossa ovalis*.
- The hypogastric arteries become the *obliterated hypogastric arteries* except for the first few centimetres, which remain open and are known as the *superior vesical arteries*.

Adaptation to extrauterine life also involves (Rankin 2017):
- maintenance of a nutritional state through the establishment of breastfeeding
- elimination of waste via the kidneys and gastrointestinal system
- establishment of the portal and liver circulation
- temperature control

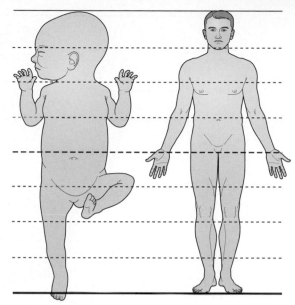

Fig. 7.4 Comparison of a baby's proportions to those of an adult. The baby's head is wider than the shoulders and one-quarter of the total length.

- communication developed through parent–baby interactions.

THE FETAL SKULL

The fetal head is large in relation to the fetal body compared with the adult (Fig. 7.4). Additionally, it is large in comparison with the maternal pelvis and is the largest part of the fetal body to be born.

Adaptation between the skull and the pelvis is necessary to allow the head to pass through the pelvis during labour without complications. The bones of the vault are thin and pliable, and if subjected to great pressure damage to the underlying delicate brain may occur. Important intracranial membranes, venous sinuses and structures can be seen in Figs 7.5, 7.6.

Divisions of the Fetal Skull

The skull is divided into the *vault*, the *base* and the *face* (Fig. 7.7).
- The *vault* is the large, dome-shaped part above an imaginary line drawn between the orbital ridges and the nape of the neck.
- The *base* comprises bones that are firmly united to protect the vital centres in the medulla oblongata.

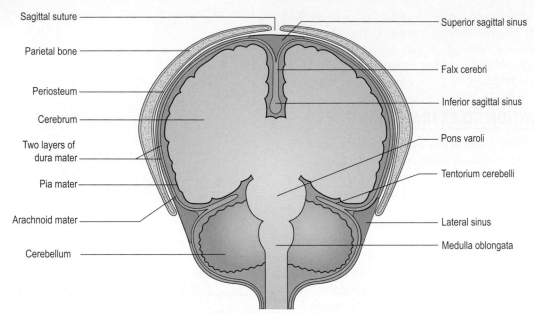

Fig. 7.5 Coronal section through the fetal head to show intracranial membranes and venous sinuses.

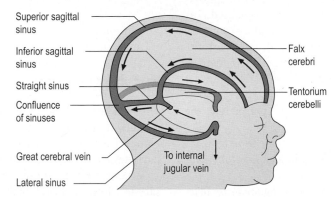

Fig. 7.6 Diagram showing intracranial membranes and venous sinuses. Arrows show direction of blood flow.

- *The face* is composed of 14 small bones that are also firmly united and non-compressible.

The Bones of the Vault

The bones of the vault (Fig. 7.8) are laid down in membrane. They harden from the centre outwards in a process known as *ossification*. Ossification is incomplete at birth, leaving small gaps between the bones, known as the *sutures* and *fontanelles*. The ossification centre on each bone appears as a *protuberance*. Ossification of the skull is not complete until early adulthood.

The bones of the vault consist of:

- The *occipital bone*, which lies at the back of the head. Part of it contributes to the base of the skull as it contains the *foramen magnum*, which protects the spinal cord as it leaves the skull. The ossification centre is the *occipital protuberance*.
- The two *parietal bones*, which lie on either side of the skull. The ossification centre of each of these bones is called the *parietal eminence*.
- The two *frontal bones*, which form the forehead or *sinciput*. The ossification centre of each bone is the

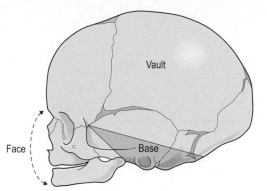

Fig. 7.7 Divisions of the skull showing the large, compressible vault and the non-compressible face and base.

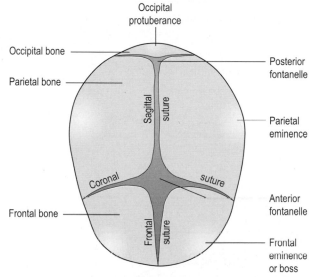

Fig. 7.8 View of fetal head from above (head partly flexed), showing bones, sutures and fontanelles.

frontal eminence. The frontal bones fuse into a single bone by 8 years of age.

- The upper part of the *temporal bone* on both sides of the head forms part of the vault.

Sutures and fontanelles

The *sutures* are the cranial joints formed where two bones meet. Where two or more sutures meet, a *fontanelle* is formed (Fig. 7.8). The sutures and fontanelles described below permit a degree of overlapping of the skull bones during labour, which is known as *moulding.*

- The *lambdoidal suture* separates the occipital bone from the two parietal bones.
- The *sagittal suture* lies between the two parietal bones.
- The *coronal suture* separates the frontal bones from the parietal bones, passing from one temple to the other.
- The *frontal suture* runs between the two halves of the frontal bone. Whereas the frontal suture becomes obliterated in time, the other sutures eventually become fixed joints.
- The *posterior fontanelle* or *lambda* (shaped like the Greek letter lambda λ) is situated at the junction of the lambdoidal and sagittal sutures. It is small, triangular in shape and can be recognized vaginally because a suture leaves from each of the three angles. It normally closes by 6 weeks of age.
- The *anterior fontanelle* or *bregma* is found at the junction of the sagittal, coronal and frontal sutures. It is broad, kite-shaped and recognizable vaginally because a suture leaves from each of the four corners. It measures 3–4 cm long and 1.5–2 cm wide and normally closes by 18 months of age. Pulsations of cerebral vessels can be felt through this fontanelle.

Regions and Landmarks of the Fetal Skull

The skull is further separated into regions, and within these, there are important landmarks as shown in Fig. 7.9. These landmarks are useful to the midwife when undertaking a vaginal examination, as they help ascertain the position of the fetal head.

- The *occiput region* lies between the foramen magnum and the posterior fontanelle. The part below the *occipital protuberance* (landmark) is known as the *suboccipital region.*
- The *vertex region* is bounded by the posterior fontanelle, the two parietal eminences and the anterior fontanelle.
- The *forehead/sinciput region* extends from the anterior fontanelle and the coronal suture to the orbital ridges.
- The face extends from the orbital ridges and the root of the nose to the junction of the *chin* or *mentum* (landmark) and the neck. The point between the eyebrows is known as the *glabella.*

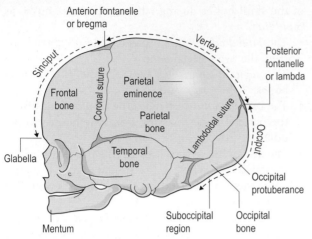

Fig. 7.9 Fetal skull showing regions and landmarks of clinical importance.

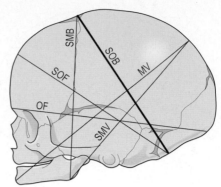

Fig. 7.10 Diagram showing the longitudinal diameters of the fetal skull (see text).

Diameter	Length (cm)
SOB, suboccipitobregmatic	9.5
SOF, suboccipitofrontal	10.0
OF, occipitofrontal	11.5
MV, mentovertical	13.5
SMV, submentovertical	11.5
SMB, submentobregmatic	9.5

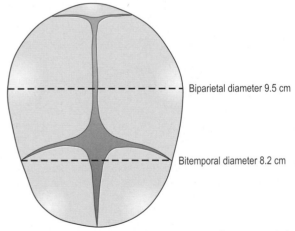

Fig. 7.11 Diagram showing the transverse diameters of the fetal skull.

Diameters of the Fetal Skull

Knowledge of the diameters of the skull alongside the diameters of the pelvis allows the midwife to determine the relationship between the fetal head and the mother's pelvis.

There are six longitudinal diameters (Fig. 7.10). These are:

- The *suboccipitobregmatic* (SOB) diameter (9.5 cm) measured from below the occipital protuberance to the centre of the anterior fontanelle or bregma.
- The *suboccipitofrontal* (SOF) diameter (10 cm) measured from below the occipital protuberance to the centre of the frontal suture.
- The *occipitofrontal* (OF) diameter (11.5 cm) measured from the occipital protuberance to the glabella.
- The *mentovertical* (MV) diameter (13.5 cm) measured from the point of the chin to the highest point on the vertex.
- The *submentovertical* (SMV) diameter (11.5 cm) measured from the point where the chin joins the neck to the highest point on the vertex
- The *submentobregmatic* (SMB) diameter (9.5 cm) measured from the point where the chin joins the neck to the centre of the bregma (anterior fontanelle).

There are also two transverse diameters, as shown in Fig. 7.11.

- The *biparietal diameter* (9.5 cm) – the diameter between the two parietal eminences.
- The *bitemporal diameter* (8.2 cm) – the diameter between the two furthest points of the coronal suture at the temples.

Knowledge of the diameters of the trunk is also important for the birth of the shoulders and breech (as detailed in Box 7.3).

Presenting Diameters

Some presenting diameters are more favourable than others for easy passage through the maternal pelvis and this will depend on the attitude of the fetal head. This term *attitude* is used to describe the degree of flexion or extension of the fetal head on the neck. The attitude of the head determines which diameters will present in labour and therefore influences the outcome.

The presenting diameters of the head are those that are at right-angles to the *curve of Carus* of the maternal pelvis. There are always two: a *longitudinal* diameter and a *transverse* diameter. The presenting diameters determine the *presentation* of the fetal head, of which there are three:

BOX 7.3 Diameters of the Fetal Trunk

Bisacromial Diameter 12 cm
This is the distance between the acromion processes on the two shoulder blades and is the dimension that needs to pass through the maternal pelvis for the shoulders to be born. The articulation of the clavicles on the sternum allows forward movement of the shoulders, which may reduce the diameter slightly.

Bitrochanteric Diameter 10 cm
This is measured between the greater trochanters of the femurs and is the presenting diameter in breech presentation.

---

1. *Vertex presentation.* When the head is well flexed the suboccipitobregmatic diameter (9.5 cm) and the biparietal diameter (9.5 cm) present (Fig. 7.12). As these two diameters are the same length the presenting area is circular, which is the most favourable shape for dilating the cervix and birth of the head. The diameter that distends the vaginal orifice is the suboccipitofrontal diameter (10 cm). When the head is deflexed, the presenting diameters are the occipitofrontal (11.5 cm) and the biparietal (9.5 cm). This situation often arises when the occiput is in a posterior position. If it remains so, the diameter distending the vaginal orifice will be the occipitofrontal (11.5 cm).

2. *Face presentation.* When the head is completely extended (i.e. hyperextended resulting in the occiput coming into contact with the fetal back as the lie of the fetus is longitudinal) the presenting diameters are the submentobregmatic (9.5 cm) and the bitemporal (8.2 cm). The submentovertical diameter (11.5 cm) will distend the vaginal orifice. At term and when the woman is in labour, the most common position is mentoanterior, which favours a vaginal birth. Mentoposterior or mentotransverse positions are least common and more likely to result in a caesarean section (Pilliod and Caughey 2017) (see Chapter 23).

3. *Brow presentation.* When the head is partially extended, the mentovertical diameter (13.5 cm) and the bitemporal diameter (8.2 cm) present. If this presentation persists, vaginal birth is unlikely.

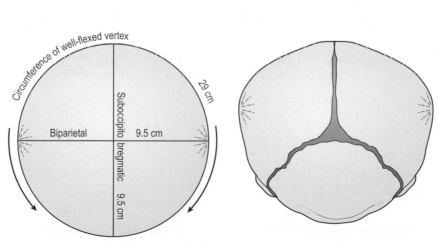

Fig. 7.12 Diagram showing the dimensions presenting when the fetal head is well flexed in a vertex presentation.

Moulding

The term *moulding* is used to describe the change in shape of the fetal head that takes place during its passage through the birth canal. Alteration in shape is possible because the bones of the vault allow a slight degree of bending and the skull bones are able to override at the sutures. This overriding allows a considerable reduction in the size of the presenting diameters, while the diameter at right-angles to them is able to lengthen owing to the give of the skull bones (Fig. 7.13). The shortening of the fetal head diameters may be by as much as 1.25 cm. The dotted lines in Figs 7.14–7.19 illustrate moulding in the various presentations.

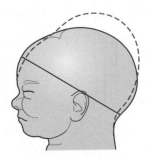

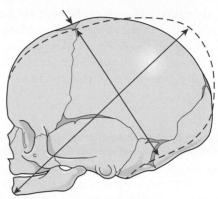

Fig. 7.13 Demonstration of the principle of moulding. The diameter compressed is diminished; the diameter at right-angles to it is elongated.

Fig. 7.14 Moulding in a normal vertex presentation with the head well flexed. The suboccipitobregmatic diameter is reduced and the mentovertical elongated.

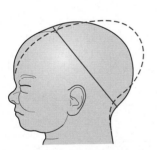

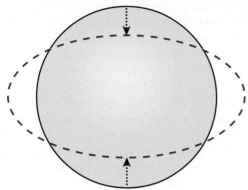

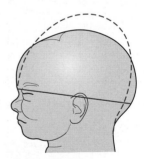

Fig. 7.15 Vertex presentation, head well-flexed.

Fig. 7.16 Vertex presentation, head partially flexed.

Fig. 7.17 Vertex presentation, head deflexed.

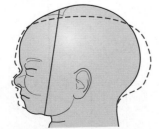

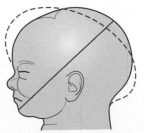

Fig. 7.18 Face presentation.

Fig. 7.19 Brow presentation.

Figs. 7.15–7.19 Series of diagrams showing moulding when the head presents. Moulding is shown by the dotted line.

Additionally, moulding is a protective mechanism and prevents the fetal brain from being compressed providing it is not excessive, too rapid or in an unfavourable direction. The skull of the preterm infant is softer and has wider sutures than that of the term baby, and hence may mould excessively should labour occur prior to term.

Venous sinuses are closely associated with the intracranial membranes, as shown in Fig. 7.6, and if membranes are torn due to excessive moulding or precipitate labour there is danger of bleeding. A tear of the tentorium cerebelli may result in bleeding from the great cerebral vein.

CONCLUSION

Embryonic and fetal development occurs alongside placental development. The process is dynamic and there is constant growth and remodelling of cells, tissues, organs and systems prior to birth. Several temporary structures in the fetus support systems *in utero*; these consequently become redundant at birth and they either disappear or become ligaments. At birth, all organs are functioning, but some may be immature and continue to develop as part of extra-uterine life.

REFLECTIVE ACTIVITY FOR SELF-ASSESSMENT

1. How are cardiac anomalies screened for in pregnancy?
2. How does a knowledge of presenting diameters of the fetal skull help the midwife to provide optimal care for a woman during labour?
3. What does the 20-week anomaly scan performed between 18 weeks + 0 days and 20 weeks + 6 days of pregnancy assess for?

REFERENCES

Coulam, C. B., Britten, S., & Soenksen, D. M. (1996). Early (34–56 days from last menstrual period) ultrasonographic measurements in normal pregnancies. *Human Reproduction*, *11*(8), 1771–1774.

Fetal Anomaly Screening Programme. (2015) Available at: www.gov.uk/government/publications/fetal-anomaly-screening-programme-handbook.

Kidokoro, H., Yonei-Tamura, S., Tamura, K., et al. (2018). *The heart tube forms and elongates through dynamic cell rearrangement coordinated with foregut extension.* Available at: http://dev.biologists.org/content/early/2018/02/21/dev.152488.

Moore, K. L., Persaud, T. V. N., & Torchia, M. (2016a). The developing human. *Clinically orientated embryology* (10th ed.). Philadelphia: Elsevier/Saunders.

Moore, K. L., Persaud, T. V. N., & Torchia, M. (2016b). *Before we are born: Essentials of embryology and birth defects* (9th ed.). Philadelphia: Elsevier/Saunders.

Pilliod, R. A., & Caughey, A. B. (2017). Fetal malpresentation and malposition: Diagnosis and management. *Obstetrics & Gynecology Clinics of North America*, *44*(4), 631–643.

Public Health England (PHE). (2018). *Fetal anomaly screening programme handbook.* Available at: www.gov.uk/government/publications/fetal-anomaly-screening-programme handbook.

Public Health England (PHE). (2019). *Fetal anomaly screening programme: Standards (FASP).* Available at: https://www.gov.uk/government/publications/fetal-anomaly-screening-programme-standards.

Rankin, J. (2017). *Physiology in childbearing with anatomy and related biosciences* (4th ed.). Edinburgh: Elsevier.

Schoenwolf, G., Bleyl, S., Brauer, P., et al. (2014). *Larsen's human embryology* (5th ed.). Philadelphia: Churchill Livingstone.

Skelton, E. (2017). A clearer picture. *Midwives*, *20*, 44–46.

Tortora, G. J., & Derrickson, B. (2014). *Principles of anatomy and physiology* (EMEA edition). Hoboken NJ, USA: John Wiley & Sons Inc.

Verbruggen, S., Kainz, B., Shelmerdine, S., et al. (2018). Stresses and strains on the human fetal skeleton during development. *Journal of the Royal Society Interface*, *15*(138), 20170593.

ANNOTATED FURTHER READING

Coad, J., & Dunstall, M. (2011). *Anatomy and physiology for midwives* (3rd ed.). London: Churchill Livingstone/Elsevier.

A detailed discussion of embryonic and fetal development appears in Chapter 9. The fetal circulation and transition to neonatal life are addressed in Chapter 15.

England, M. A. (1996). *Life before birth* (2nd ed.). London: Mosby–Wolfe.

Although this is now a historical text it still has currency serving to illustrate embryological and fetal development in photographic form. For the student who requires a detailed understanding of prenatal events and in particular the hormonal influences, this book is unsurpassed..

Public Health England PHE. (2018). *Fetal anomaly screening programme handbook.* Available at: www.gov.uk/government/publications/fetal-anomaly-screening-programme-handbook.

The purpose of this handbook is to bring together in one publication, the Fetal Anomaly Screening Programme's (FASP) guidelines and recommendations that relate to the screening pathway and are not covered in detail in the other handbooks.

Schoenwolf, G. C., Bleyl, S. B., Brauer, P. R., et al. (Eds.). (2014). *Larsen's human embryology* (5th ed.) Philadelphia: Churchill Livingstone.

Originating in a series of Christmas lectures at the Royal Institution, this text explores the unifying principles that may account for the way embryos develop. Written for the non-specialist, it invites the reader to think broadly and aims to inspire as well as instruct.

USEFUL WEBSITES

National Institute for Health and care Excellence (NICE) Antenatal care for uncomplicated pregnancies: www.nice.org.uk/guidance/CG62

Newborn and Infant Physical Examination (NIPE) clinical guidance: www.gov.uk/government/collections/newborn-and-infant-physical-examination-clinical-guidance

The Visible Embryo: www.visembryo.com

Pregnancy

Designing and Implementing High Quality Midwifery Care: Evidence, Policy and Models of Care

Mary J. Renfrew, Mary Ross-Davie

CHAPTER CONTENTS

Policy shapes the care and services that women, newborn infants and families receive. It is a powerful mechanism to drive large-scale change. Policy can influence decisions and practice at local and national levels, and it has a direct influence on what practitioners and managers do every day. Good policy that is well informed and well implemented can transform the quality of care and the experiences of women, newborn infants and families. The absence of policy, or ill-informed policy, can make it very difficult, if not impossible, to improve the quality of care and can hold back practice and service development and improvement. This chapter explores how policy that aims to strengthen the quality of care can be effectively developed and implemented. The quality care needed by women and newborn infants worldwide is examined, and the key elements required for the successful translation of policy into practice is discussed. Two examples of recent evidence-informed national policy developments that situate midwifery as central to the provision of safe, effective, care, and that are creating positive, system-wide change are presented. Resources are provided to support the development and effective implementation of evidence-informed midwifery and maternity policy.

THE CHAPTER AIMS TO

- examine the evidence that supports quality midwifery care as being essential to improving the health and wellbeing of all childbearing women, their infants and their families worldwide
- describe how policy that aims to strengthen the quality of care can be effectively developed and implemented

- give examples of recent national policy developments that are aiming to transform the way maternity services are being designed and provided
- discuss the key elements required for the successful translation of policy into practice
- provide information regarding important resources on quality maternal and newborn care within the national and international context.

INTRODUCTION AND BACKGROUND

Quality Matters

All women and all infants require good quality care, regardless of where they live, or their circumstances. Quality care is far from universally available, however. Despite important improvements in the provision of care globally over the past 25 years, the number of women and children dying as a result of mainly preventable complications of pregnancy and birth remains unacceptably high (Box 8.1). The great majority of these deaths occur in low- and middle-income countries. There is also a marked inequality in provision of quality care, with women and children from deprived backgrounds being more likely to die and to have complications in all countries. This is the case even in the United Kingdom (UK), where currently black, Asian and minority ethnic (BAME) women are five times more likely to die as a result of complications than white women (Knight et al. 2019).

Evidence Matters

Evidence shows that good quality midwifery care can improve survival, reduce complications and enhance women's experiences (Renfrew et al. 2014; Homer et al. 2014; van Lerberghe et al. 2014; Sandall et al. 2016; ten Hoope-Bender et al. 2014; Bohren et al. 2017). With skilled midwifery care, more women and infants will not only survive childbirth, but they are more likely to be healthy, to have better psychosocial outcomes, to breastfeed and to establish close family relationships. They are also less likely to experience routine, unnecessary and potentially harmful interventions (Boerma et al. 2018). Good quality midwifery care is not widely available globally, however. A recent review found that only 15% of 'skilled birth attendants' in low- and middle-income countries identified themselves as 'midwives' (Hobbs et al. 2019), and it is not known if these respondents met international standards for midwives (International Confederation of Midwives, ICM 2018). Significant barriers to midwifery care have been identified in international reports, including professional, sociocultural and economic barriers, all underpinned by gender inequality (Filby et al. 2016; World Health Organization, WHO 2016).

As a result of the evidence that has shown the positive impact of midwifery, significant work is now being conducted internationally to strengthen midwifery, and

> **BOX 8.1 Mortality Statistics**
>
> - The maternal mortality rate fell by over 40% between 1990 and 2015, but over 300,000 women still die as a result of pregnancy and birth each year, mainly of preventable causes (www.who.int/news-room/fact-sheets/detail/maternal-mortality).
> - The number of newborn infants dying in the first month of life is around 2.6 million, 1 million of these in the first day of life (www.who.int/gho/child_health/mortality/neonatal_text/en/).
> - Around 2.6 million stillbirths occur each year (www.who.int/maternal_child_adolescent/epidemiology/stillbirth/en/).
> - In the UK, 9.2 women per 100,000 die in pregnancy or around childbirth, with heart disease, the leading cause of women dying during or up to 6 weeks after the end of pregnancy. Most women who died had multiple health problems or other vulnerabilities, such as addiction, abuse or domestic violence (see: https://www.npeu.ox.ac.uk/downloads/files/mbrrace-uk/reports/MBRRACE-UK%20Maternal%20Report%202019%20-%20WEB%20VERSION.pdf).

in particular, midwifery education (WHO 2019). Countries including India, Bangladesh, Nepal and Somalia are all working to introduce or to strengthen international-standard midwifery, within the context of interdisciplinary working and the whole health system.

Policy Matters

Health systems, including maternity systems, have developed over many years. The process by which models of care and service provision evolves is not necessarily linear, planned or coherent. Local variations in practice, norms and models of care develop over time, shaped by a variety of factors. One factor is the nature and extent of health policy. Health policy may be guided by short-term political considerations rather than by long-term evidence-based goals. This results in maternity systems and practice that are extremely variable within and between countries. Furthermore, national health systems do not consistently have processes that enable the national translation of evidence into practice. The process that most countries have is through the development of policy.

Global and national policy is key to improving the quality of care for women and infants. The development and implementation of policy is a way of seeking to develop a greater level of consistency of quality across a whole system. Policy shapes the care and services that women, newborn infants and families receive. It can be a powerful mechanism to drive large-scale change, especially if grounded in evidence (Ridde and Yaméogo 2018). Policy can influence decisions and practice at local and national levels, and it has a direct influence on what practitioners and managers do every day. Good policy, that is well informed and well implemented, can transform the quality of care and the experience of women and families (Renfrew 2016). The absence of policy, or ill-informed policy, can make it very difficult, if not impossible, to improve the quality of care, and can hold back development and improvement. Policy is not enough on its own; it needs a proactive implementation plan, to be well-resourced and supported.

This chapter will commence by examining the quality care that all women, infants and families need. A description is then be provided as to how policy that aims to strengthen the quality of care can be effectively developed and implemented. Included are examples of recent national policy developments that are transforming the way maternity services are being designed and implemented. Their evidence-informed recommendations situate midwifery as central to the provision of safe, effective care that focuses on the needs, views and preferences of women, newborn infants, partners and families.

WHAT IS QUALITY MATERNAL AND NEWBORN CARE?

The WHO defines quality care as *'the extent to which health care services provided to individuals and patient populations improve desired health outcomes. In order to achieve this, health care must be safe, effective, timely, efficient, equitable and people-centred'* (www.who.int/maternal_child_adolescent/topics/quality-of-care/definition/en/).

Furthermore, in 2014, *The Lancet Series on Midwifery* examined the quality care that childbearing women, newborn infants and families need (Renfrew et al. 2014). It defined quality midwifery care as shown in Box 8.2.

A framework for quality maternal and newborn care was developed, drawing on evidence from hundreds of studies, both qualitative and quantitative. This framework focused on the needs of women and infants across the whole continuum of care, from pre-pregnancy, pregnancy, labour

> **BOX 8.2 Definition of Midwifery from** *The Lancet Series on Midwifery*
>
> *Skilled, knowledgeable and compassionate care for childbearing women, newborn infants and families across the continuum from pre-pregnancy, pregnancy, birth, postpartum and the early weeks of life. Core characteristics include optimising normal biological, psychological, social and cultural processes of reproduction and early life, timely prevention and management of complications, consultation with and referral to other services, respecting women's individual circumstances and views, and working in partnership with women to strengthen women's own capabilities to care for themselves and their families.*
>
> (Renfrew et al. 2014, p. 1130. Reprinted with permission from Elsevier (*The Lancet*, 2014, *384*, 1129–1145).)

and birth and beyond. It was based on a human rights approach, considering the quality care that all women and infants need, without exception (United Nations, UN 2000). The framework is shown in Fig. 8.1.

This framework distinguishes between the key components of quality care. First, it shows the **practices** that all women and newborn infants need, whatever their circumstances. These are:

- education, information and health promotion – to enable and support women to care for themselves and to seek information and support
- assessment, screening and care planning – to ensure that the needs, views and preferences of women and newborn infants are identified and met
- promotion of normal processes, prevention of complications – to promote and support women's own abilities and avoid interfering with physiological processes unnecessarily.

Then, it identifies the additional practices that women and infants with complications would need. These are:

- first-line management of complications – ensuring a timely and effective response to complications when they occur
- medical, obstetric and neonatal services – inter-professional working to provide the interventions that women and infants need to treat complications.

The framework then includes the important aspect of **organization of care**. Services must be available,

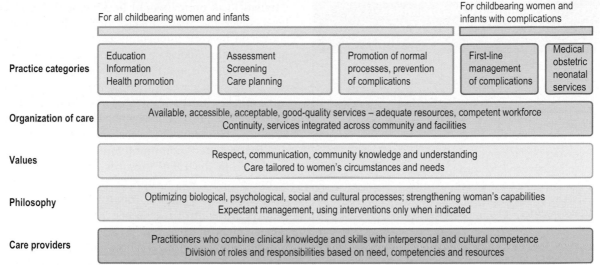

	For all childbearing women and infants			For childbearing women and infants with complications	
Practice categories	Education Information Health promotion	Assessment Screening Care planning	Promotion of normal processes, prevention of complications	First-line management of complications	Medical obstetric neonatal services
Organization of care	Available, accessible, acceptable, good-quality services – adequate resources, competent workforce Continuity, services integrated across community and facilities				
Values	Respect, communication, community knowledge and understanding Care tailored to women's circumstances and needs				
Philosophy	Optimizing biological, psychological, social and cultural processes; strengthening woman's capabilities Expectant management, using interventions only when indicated				
Care providers	Practitioners who combine clinical knowledge and skills with interpersonal and cultural competence Division of roles and responsibilities based on need, competencies and resources				

Fig. 8.1 The framework for Quality Maternal and Newborn Care (QMNC). (From Renfrew et al. (2014) Midwifery and quality care: Findings from a new evidence-informed framework for maternal and newborn care. Reprinted with permission from Elsevier (*The Lancet*, 2014, *384*, 1129–1145).

accessible, acceptable and of good quality for all. They must be adequately resourced and provided by a competent workforce. Continuity is important, to ensure that services are seamless across the continuum of care and between community and facilities.

Next, the framework illustrates that *values* are essential. These include the provision of:

- respectful care
- good communication with women and families
- community knowledge and understanding to help women identify the resources they need
- tailoring care to individual women's circumstances and needs.

The *philosophy* of care is also of importance and includes:

- optimizing normal processes and strengthening women's own capabilities
- using interventions when, and only when, indicated, avoiding unnecessary interventions.

Finally, the *care providers* who work with women, infants and families need to combine clinical knowledge and skills with interpersonal and cultural competence. Different disciplines need to work together to provide seamless care, with a division of responsibilities based on need, on competencies and available resources. To meet the needs and preferences of

women, infants and families, strong and effective interdisciplinary working is essential. These factors combined, result in quality care. The great majority of this care can be provided by midwives who are educated and trained to international standards, as long as they are supported and enabled to provide the full scope of this care. The evidence shows that if all women and newborn infants worldwide received this quality of care, over 80% of maternal and newborn mortality, and of stillbirths, could be prevented. Over 50 outcomes could be improved (Box 8.3).

The current challenge is how to implement this standard of care, consistently for all women, infants and families. Key to achieving this is the development and implementation of policy.

THE IMPORTANCE OF POLICY AND ITS IMPLEMENTATION

In maternity and midwifery, policy documents set out the way in which care and services should be provided for women, newborn infants and families. These can be local documents that outline the way care should be provided in one particular organization, or they can be national or international documents that set the direction of travel, the goals and plans that all health services

---

BOX 8.3 Summary of Outcomes Improved by the Full Scope of Midwifery Care

Summarized from *The Lancet Series on Midwifery* (Renfrew et al. 2014. Reprinted with permission from Elsevier (*The Lancet*, 2014, *384*, 1129–1145).):

- Maternal mortality
- Stillbirth
- Low birth weight
- Interventions in labour
- Birth spacing and contraceptive use
- Hospital stays and referrals
- Newborn mortality
- Preterm birth
- Maternal morbidity
- Psychosocial outcomes
- Breastfeeding initiation and duration
- Attendance by known midwife.

BOX 8.4 Definitions of General Policy and of Health Policy

In **general terms**, policy includes principles, rules, recommendations and guidelines formulated or adopted by a government or organization to reach its long-term goals. Policy is designed to influence and determine all major decisions and actions in regard to a particular topic. It should be published and made widely accessible (see: www.businessdictionary.com/definition/policies-and-procedures.html).

In the **field of health**, policy plays an essential role in defining a country's vision and strategies for ensuring the health of its population (see: www.who.int/national-policies/nationalpolicies/en/).

---

must adhere to (Box 8.4). Issues covered can be very specific, such as preventing and treating infection, or very broad, such as how to organize maternity services. Policy should then inform the development of specific guidance and guidelines, and produce a plan to implement it effectively in all settings.

Examples of topics covered by local and national policy in maternity care and midwifery include infection control, informed consent, child protection and non-medical prescribing.

The focus on the development and implementation of national policy for maternity and midwifery care and service is known as the *macro* level, whereas detailed local policy would be known as the **micro** level. Over the years, macro-level policy has been shown to be very important, as it has a substantial impact on the quality of care provided for everyone. In the 1960s, 70s and 80s, for example, UK national maternity policy was aimed at women giving birth in hospital, with the result that very limited services were available for women who wished to give birth at home. Consequently, services were fragmented, divided between community and hospital (Davis 2013). From the 1990s onwards, evidence-informed women's choice was recognized as a key principle in national maternity policy, along with increased continuity and control by women over their own care (Department of Health, DH 1993). This innovative policy resulted in some positive changes, but the lack of resources and support for implementation limited these to local developments, many of which were not sustained or up-scaled to create the national, system-wide change needed. In order to effect successful policy implementation, the following are considered to be essential elements:

- evidence-informed policy development
- consensus of multiprofessional leadership
- strategic national leadership
- proactive stakeholder engagement and participation, including a core focus on the needs, views, preferences and decisions of women, infants and families and the needs, views and preferences of the midwives and other professionals providing the care
- focused work-streams to lead implementation of particular recommendations
- outreach face-to-face sessions by policy leaders
- local leadership and project management
- educational resources and publications to support knowledge and implementation
- ring-fenced funding for training and workforce development
- appropriate equipment and environments to support new ways of working
- ongoing monitoring and evaluation of the change and the impact on outcomes for women, infants, partners, families and for the health service in general.

Even when all of these elements are in place, it is unlikely that large-scale system change will be able to flourish unless the maternity services in which the changes are taking place are adequately funded and appropriately staffed.

How to Develop Positive, System-Wide Change Through Effective National Policy

Well-informed and well-implemented policy can create a positive environment for effective system change. It is possible, however, to develop policy that inadvertently causes harm through recommending inappropriate actions or not fully exploring the possible consequences. It is also possible to develop good policy, but for it not to be implemented through lack of resources, lack of government support, or lack of leadership. To avoid harm, and to maximize the potential for the best possible outcomes, health policy development needs to be informed by important key principles (Gavine et al. 2018), which are outlined as follows:

- Assessing the opportunity for change and its timeliness, the leadership needed to drive the change, and how it fits with the current government agenda:
  - Policy does not work in a vacuum. It relates to other existing policy, to the appetite of key decision-makers to create change, and to the resources available. It may be necessary to work to develop these preconditions before more detailed work on the specific policy can begin.
- Being clear about the values and principles that underpin the policy, and clarifying the aims and objectives:
  - *Values*: Using a human rights perspective to ensure equity and to promote accessible, available, appropriate, good quality care for all is important in any health policy (UN 2000). This will require consideration of those who may be most vulnerable as a result, for example, of poverty, geography, disability, or culture. If equity is not considered as a core value, policy can result in some people being excluded or receiving inferior care, while more affluent and able people have better access to improved services. This can increase inequalities. Tackling this will require that services are tailored to need, and plans made to proactively reach out to all.
  - *Aims and objectives*: Identifying and agreeing these at the start is essential to make sure that the ambition of the policy is clear and focused, aligned with the evidence, and with sufficient political will to support the recommendations through the inevitable range of barriers.
- Using up-to-date, good quality evidence on effective care and on the experiences of those providing and receiving care, and developing knowledge and understanding of the current context and need for change:
  - This should include searching for all the relevant quantitative and qualitative evidence, and data on the current situation and the potential for change. Together, this information helps to identify problems with the current system, and what is needed to tackle these.
- Ensuring the participation of those with experience of receiving care, and of those who provide it, in informing and shaping the policy recommendations:
  - This could include, for example, organizing a survey, conducting focus groups and interviews and ensuring that a wide range of those likely to be affected are included.
  - Committees that work on policy development should include people from all perspectives, and collaboration and positive participation should be expected and enabled.
  - Both national and local implementation groups should include representatives from all involved professions and women and families with recent experience of receiving maternity care in the area.
- Setting clear, deliverable goals and timescales, and with recommendations that are realistic and affordable:
  - Any national policy that is over-aspirational, or that develops recommendations that will not be supported by decision-makers, the public or practitioners and managers, is likely to fail.
- Realistic policy implementation should be considered as the recommendations are developed:
  - It is important to assess the current context and the readiness for change. This could include variations across the country, such as urban and rural locations, or areas of deprivation, or current staffing levels.
  - An implementation plan will assist everyone to see the steps needed, any preparation required and the timescales, and will help to scope out the level of resource needed.
- Monitoring and evaluation should be planned from the start:
  - This is needed to ensure that the new policy is doing what was intended, and that no unexpected harmful consequences are occurring.
  - The findings can then be included in further implementation planning, in a cycle of continuous improvement.

DEVELOPING AND IMPLEMENTING EVIDENCE-INFORMED MATERNITY POLICY

In this section, examples of recent policy developments in Scotland and in England are used to show how policy can be effectively developed and implemented to improve the design and delivery of care and services, and to introduce an evidence-informed model of care. A definition of a model of care has been provided by Davidson et al. (2006) (highlighted in Box 8.5). In both of these examples, midwifery continuity of carer (MCoC) and family-centred care are the key models of care that the policies recommend. The first of these examples drew on the method of policy development described in the previous section (Gavine et al. 2018).

How Evidence-Informed National Maternity Policy can be Developed

Healthcare provision and health policy have been devolved from the UK Government to the Scottish Government since the Scotland Act of 1998. In 2015, the Scottish Government instigated a national review of maternity and neonatal services, which lasted 18 months and culminated in the publication of the 'Best Start five year forward plan for maternity and neonatal care in Scotland', with 76 recommendations (Scottish Government, 2017).The vision for a maternity and neonatal service built around the needs, views and preferences of women and families is radical and transformational.

The policy sets out a plan for a maternity service in which all women have the opportunity to build a relationship with a primary midwife who provides the majority of their care; where women can access high quality antenatal, intrapartum and postnatal care as close to home as possible; where women have access to a range of birthplace options including homebirth, birth in a midwife-led care setting or obstetric unit birth; and where women with increased medical, obstetric, psychological or social need are able to access the care and support they need through well-developed multidisciplinary teams and multiagency networks.

The *Best Start* vision for neonatal care also places the needs of the family at the centre, with an emphasis on the central importance of keeping mothers and babies together, providing the majority of care locally, with intensive care provided in a smaller number of centres of excellence. One of the eight key principles upon which the review recommendations were based is that of the pressing need to reduce the impact of inequalities on health and improve the health of future generations.

The vision described in the policy grew from the existence of several of the key preconditions set out earlier in the chapter; political will, timeliness and evidence. The *Best Start* recommendations sit well in the context of the Scottish Government's wider agenda in relation to health care: that is, an integrated health and social care service, where most care is provided in the community rather than in large hospitals; where specialist care is centred in a smaller number of specialist centres, with the reduction of inequalities being a focus; and where the needs of those being cared for are at the centre of service strategy and design (National Health Service, NHS Scotland 2010) and delivery (Scottish Government 2016).

It is too soon to determine whether all of the key principles set out above are being fully operationalized to support successful implementation within the Scottish context. However, it is vital that all professions who work together to provide maternity care also work collaboratively on implementation, alongside women and families with recent experience of the care. It is also imperative that goals and aims are regularly reviewed to ensure that they remain realistic and achievable and that appropriate investment is secured. It is essential that the principle of co-production and consultation with those who will be delivering the care is embedded.

The development of the *Scottish Best Start* policy (Scottish Government, 2017) is an example of how a national maternity policy is shaped by the country specific context alongside the international evidence base.

The review process included a number of interconnected elements:

BOX 8.5   Definition of a Model of Care

*… an overarching design for the provision of a particular type of health care service that is shaped by a **theoretical basis**, **evidence based practice**, and **defined standards***

(Adapted from Davidson et al. Beyond the rhetoric: what do we mean by a 'model of care'? *Australian Journal of Advanced Nursing* 2006:23.).

1. *Establishment of core values and principles*

The establishment of an overarching *Review Board* made up of all key stakeholders including government civil servants, senior health service managers, experienced health professionals, leaders of the professional associations and service user representatives and advocates. This Review Board identified an overarching set of principles and values for the review process, which were rooted in the framework for Quality Maternal and Newborn Care (Renfrew et al. 2014), as shown in Fig. 8.1.

2. *Identification of key work areas*

The establishment of working subgroups of the Board made up to lead the review of evidence and the development of recommendations in four key areas:

- Maternal models of care
- Neonatal models of care
- Evidence and data
- Workforce planning and development.

3. *Engagement with all key stakeholders*

A series of stakeholder engagement events were conducted by the review team throughout Scotland. This included consulting with maternity care professionals including midwives, obstetricians, neonatologists and anaesthetists in each of the 14 Health Board areas to hear their views about what was working well in the current system and what the challenges were. Engagement with women and their families to hear their views about the care they received from maternity and neonatal services was undertaken through a written service user survey (Cheyne et al. 2015) and through focus groups (Scottish Health Council 2017).

4. *The review of evidence*

An independent team of researchers with experience of undertaking systematic evidence reviews and of maternity and neonatal care was asked to undertake a series of rapid evidence reviews on a range of issues to inform the work of the subgroups in developing their recommendations. Each of the subgroups set out a number of key questions that required further exploration of the evidence to effectively answer. The rapid evidence reviews reflected the eight-stage process adapted from the work of Gavine et al. (2018), shown in Box 8.6.

The key areas chosen by the working groups for the rapid evidence reviews were:

- Models of care for women requiring maternity critical care
- Models of care for infants requiring neonatal services and their families
- Improving care, services, and outcomes for women and babies from vulnerable population groups
- Continuity models of care

- Place of maternity care, including place of birth
- Organization of services for childbearing women across the continuum (including methods for assessment/triage in early labour)
- Improving multidisciplinary working.

Table 8.1 identifies the ways in which recommendations in two key areas: **place of birth** and **continuity of care**, were shaped by the evidence.

How Evidence-Informed National Maternity Policy can be Implemented

The Maternity Review for England was undertaken using a broadly similar approach to that described above for the Scottish review, and resulted in the publication of *Better Births: Improving outcomes of maternity services in England – a five year forward view for maternity care* (NHS England 2016). Many of the central recommendations are very similar to those set out in *Best Start* (Scottish Government 2017), including an emphasis on the centrality of family-centred care, continuity of carer, community-based care and choice.

A key difference between the English and Scottish reviews is in the nature of the implementation process. Scotland remains a centrally commissioned national

---

BOX 8.6 Eight Stages of an Efficient Evidence Review for Policy-Making

1. Establishing a review team with expertise both in the issues and in systematic reviewing
2. Clarifying the review questions with policy-makers and subject experts who acted as review sponsors
3. Development of review protocol to systematically identify quantitative and qualitative evidence
4. Agreeing a framework to structure the analysis of the reviews around a consistent set of key concepts and outcomes
5. Developing an iterative process between policy-makers, reviewers and review sponsors
6. Rapid searches and retrieval of literature
7. Analysis of identified literature, which was mapped to the framework and included review sponsor input
8. Production of recommendations mapped to the agreed framework and presented as *'summary top-sheets'*.

Adapted from Gavine, A., MacGillivray, S., Ross-Davie, M., Campbell, K., White, L., & Renfrew, M. J. (2018). Maximising the availability and use of high-quality evidence for policymaking: collaborative, targeted and efficient evidence reviews. Palgrave Communications, 4(5) Available at: https://www.nature.com/articles/s41599-017-0054-8.)

TABLE 8.1   Shaping Policy: Recommendations from the Evidence

Rapid Evidence Reviews	Key Findings from Reviews	Recommendation in *Best Start* (Scottish Government 2017)
Place of Birth:	Giving birth is generally very safe.	Midwifery care settings offer a safe alternative to consultant hospital settings for many women.
England Birthplace study reports (NPEU) 2010–2015, 13 papers:	Low-risk women who plan birth in a midwife-led care setting have no more adverse outcomes for them or their babies than women planning to give birth in an obstetric-led care setting.	Women should have the full range of choices of place of birth, including home birth, midwifery-led care setting and obstetric-led unit, wherever they live in Scotland.
Brocklehurst et al. (2011)		
Li et al. (2014, 2015)		
Hollowell et al. (2014, 2015a, 2015b)	Low-risk women planning birth in a midwife-led care setting experience fewer medical interventions during labour.	
Kurinczuk et al, (2015)		
Lukasse et al. (2014)		
McCourt et al. (2012)	For women having their first baby, planning birth at home brings some increased risk of poor outcomes for the baby compared with planning birth in a midwife-led or obstetric-led care setting.	
Rowe et al. (2012, 2013, 2014)		
Schroeder et al. (2012)		
Cochrane reviews:		
Hodnett et al. (2012)		
Olsen and Clausen (2012)	For women having their second or subsequent baby, planning birth at home has no greater adverse outcomes than planning birth in other settings.	
NICE guidelines:		
Antenatal care for uncomplicated pregnancies (NICE 2019)		
Intrapartum care of healthy women and babies (NICE 2017)	For women having a first baby, there is a fairly high probability of transferring to an obstetric unit during labour or immediately after the birth.	
13 × quantitative studies of birthplace outside of the UK:		
Blix et al. (2016)		
Cheyney et al. (2014)		
Davis et al. (2011, 2012)		
Halfdansdottir et al. (2015)		
Hendrix et al. (2009)		
Janssen et al. (2009, 2015)		
Lindgren et al. (2008)		
Overgaard et al. (2012)		
Schroeder et al. (2012)		
Van der Kooy et al. (2011)		
Wax et al. (2010)		
3 × RCOG Guidelines:		
RCOG (2013)		
RCOG/RCM/RCoA/RCPCH (2007, 2008)		
4 × large scale surveys with service users:		
NPEU (2014)		
NFWI/NCT (2013)		
Cheyne et al. (2013, 2015)		

TABLE 8.1 Shaping Policy: Recommendations from the Evidence—cont'd

Rapid Evidence Reviews	Key Findings from Reviews	Recommendation in *Best Start* (Scottish Government 2017)
Continuity of care: ***3 × high quality systematic reviews/reviews of reviews:*** Sutcliffe et al. (2012) Sandall et al. (2016) Turienzo et al. (2016) ***NICE guidelines:*** *Antenatal care for uncomplicated pregnancies* (NICE 2019) *Postnatal care up to 8 weeks after birth* (NICE 2015) ***5 × RCM and RCOG guidelines:*** RCM 2016 RCOG 2013 RCOG/RCM 2016 RCOG/RCM/RCoA/RCPCH 2007, 2008 ***4 × large scale reviews of women's views:*** NPEU (2014) NFWI/NCT (2013) Cheyne et al. (2013, 2015)	No adverse outcomes from mid-wife-led continuity models vs standard care. Lower rates of premature labour, fetal loss and a range of medical interventions. Higher rates of normal birth and satisfaction. Women find fragmented care difficult and value continuity of carer.	Maternity care in Scotland should be relationship-based care. Maternity systems across Scotland should be redesigned to offer continuity of care and carer across the maternity journey.

health service made up of 14 Health Boards, where policy, service organization and systems are largely centrally directed. The English National Health Service in comparison, has undergone a significant programme of decentralization over recent years, with the creation of local commissioning through Clinical Commissioning groups (CCGs) of which there are 211 across England. The Maternity Transformation Programme (MTP), which is the delivery programme resulting from the *Better Births* review, led to the establishment of Local Maternity Systems (LMS), in which NHS Trusts providing maternity care have grouped together into 42 systems to plan the design and delivery of services. The work of the MTP has been divided into nine concurrent work-streams, which are depicted in Fig. 8.2. While it is expected transformation will take place locally, it is supported by national enabling action. As a consequence, this has led to the creation of an overarching Maternity Transformation Programme Board that is supported by a stakeholder group, established to scrutinize the work of the Board.

In late 2018, the Maternity Transformation Programme was embedded into the NHS England's overarching long-term plan (NHS England 2019). In comparison to *Better Births* (NHS England 2016), the long-term plan set out more explicitly the need to focus on continuity of carer, especially on those women living with particular vulnerabilities and risks who require it the most (NHS England 2019). Box 8.7 provides a definition and elements of a Midwifery Continuity of Carer system.

The national MTP team has sought to support implementation through a programme of face-to-face activities, publications, social media engagement and funding of education and training. This has included outreach engagement sessions across England, including all local maternity systems in order to develop understanding of the aims of the programme among health professionals.

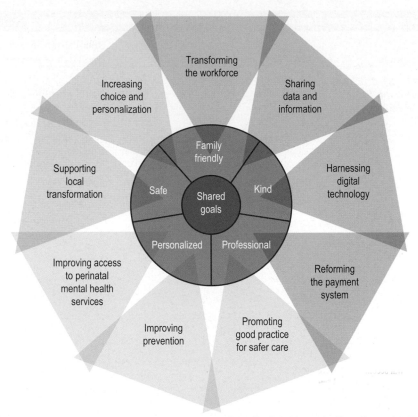

Fig. 8.2 The key shared goals and the nine work-streams of the English Maternity Transformation Programme.

During 2017 and 2018, the MTP team developed and commissioned a number of guidance documents to support implementation (NHS England 2017; Sandall 2018), the development of an online learning module on *Continuity of Carer* as well as running a series of webinars with experts. Significant funding for local maternity systems to buy local training on the implementation of Continuity of Carer from a range of approved trainers has been made available through the NHS England MTP team.

Such strategic national support for the implementation of a maternity policy from both Government and the professional association and trade union for midwives in the UK, the Royal College of Midwives (RCM), represents a significant shift from earlier maternity policies, such as *Changing Childbirth* (DH 1993). Earlier policies have tended to be published and then local maternity services were left to lead implementation with little strategic support or direction, leading to a patchy and variable spread of recommendations.

BOX 8.7 A Maternity System Built Around Continuity of Carer

Definition: *Midwifery Continuity of Carer* (MCoC) is a model of maternity care that:

- enables a pregnant woman to build a relationship with a midwife (and a small team of midwives) through her maternity journey
- provides a pregnant woman with a primary or named midwife who will give the majority of her antenatal, intrapartum and postnatal care
- enables midwives to build relationships with the women in their care.

Royal College of Midwives (RCM 2018a). Position statement on continuity of midwife-led care. London: RCM. Available at: https://www.rcm.org.uk/media/2946/midwifery-continuity-of-carer-mcoc.pdf

Local Implementation of National Policy

The implementation of the MTP at a local level has been led by seven early adopter sites through Sustainability and Transformation Partnerships (STP) and Integrated

Care Systems (ICS): Birmingham and Solihull United Maternity and Newborn Pathway (BUMP), Cheshire and Merseyside, Dorset, North Central London, North West London, Somerset and Surrey Heartlands. The early adopter sites chose which of the nine work-streams they would focus on, rather than trying to implement all nine areas simultaneously. Pace and depth of change has varied significantly between early adopter sites. Meanwhile, all local maternity services are charged with identifying the current proportion of women in their service who receive continuity of carer from a lead named midwife. Targets for increasing the proportion of women booked to receive a continuity pathway were set at 20% from March 2019, increasing annually to ensure that by 2021, the majority of women are receiving continuity of carer.

Risks to Maternity Policy Implementation

The *Best Start* (Scottish Government 2017) and *Better Births* (NHS England 2016) policies are in the early stages of their implementation and so it is not yet known whether the implementation of all key recommendations will be achieved. Furthermore, whether *Continuity of Carer* (Box 8.8) will become the central model of maternity care for women in England and Scotland in a sustained way, is not yet clear. A range of local and national frameworks and approaches will be used to evaluate the success or otherwise of the implementation process. These will include national maternity service user surveys to identify trends and changes in women's perceptions of care; local service user surveys; local audit of processes to identify what care is provided, where, when and by whom; local surveys with health professionals about their experiences of providing care, and collection of data for national databases on key clinical outcomes (McInnes et al. 2018; Sandall 2018).

As the implementation of the recommendations of the policies gather pace across both England and Scotland, a number of key risks to successful implementation are emerging. If large scale, sustainable and safe implementation is to be achieved, it will be vital that the Governments and all key stakeholders with a role in implementation acknowledge the risks and develop strategies and responses to mitigate these risks. Key factors include:

1. **Adequate workforce.** In 2019, significant pressures exist in the midwifery workforce across the UK. England continues to have a shortfall of at least 3000 midwives (RCM 2018b) and Scotland has seen a significant rise in the number of unfilled vacancies and retirements (RCM 2018c). The significant service

---

BOX 8.8 Midwifery Continuity of Carer Recommendations in *Best Start* (Scottish Government 2017) and *Better Births* (NHS England 2016)

- The caseload proposed in both policies is around 35 women a year per midwife.
- Smaller caseloads for women with more complex needs. Out of hours and intrapartum care should be covered by a small team of midwives working with the primary midwife. These teams will be made up of between four and eight midwives.
- Each continuity team should work to develop a shared philosophy, build team trust and support, and should have the opportunity to largely self-manage the way in which on-calls and rotas are worked.
- Women should have the opportunity to meet all members of the small team of midwives during pregnancy – through drop-in sessions and preparation for parenthood classes.
- Most continuity teams will be based in the community. Each team should be linked with an obstetrician and general practitioner (GP) where medical or obstetric needs arise. Some continuity teams may be based in hospitals if they are providing care to women with complex needs. These teams will be multidisciplinary including obstetricians as well as midwives.
- Any continuity model of care will require a strong core midwifery staffing of hospital maternity units to ensure that there is 24 hours/7 days/week staffing in place to respond to unexpected admissions, emergencies and to support continuity teams during particularly busy periods.
- Any model of care should be set up in such a way as to be accessible, appropriate and able to provide quality services for all: proactively reaching out, leaving no-one behind, regardless of socioeconomic or clinical circumstances.

National Health Service (NHS) England. (2016). National Maternity Review. Better Births: Improving outcomes of maternity services in England: A Five Year Forward View for maternity care. London: NHS England. Available at: https://www.england.nhs.uk/wp-content/uploads/2016/02/national-maternity-review-report.pdf.

---

redesign heralded in the English and Scottish maternity policies requires a focus on addressing these workforce issues. Midwives require training and time to adapt to working in very different settings.

2. **Adequate funding.** Transformational change requires appropriate ring-fenced resources. The changes recommended in the UK maternity policies require investment in staffing, training, equipment

and environments to be implemented safely. It is not yet clear whether appropriate, targeted and sustained funding will be made available across *all* areas of England and Scotland in all of these key areas of need.

3. **Safeguarding the needs of the workforce.** The needs of all staff to have adequate rest and work–life balance as well as having a choice regarding their preferred ways of working, must be respected through any change process. Successful implementation requires co-production with the staff who provide the direct care. Any new model of care needs to reflect the need and desire of many midwives to work flexibly or part-time. Not all midwives are willing or able to work in a continuity model of care and alternative ways of working should be possible within the wider system. The traditional approaches to system change and management that have evolved over many years in the NHS will clearly need to adapt to enable models that encourage self-management, high levels of flexibility and choice for the workforce to develop.

4. **Evaluation.** Real-time evaluation of the processes and outcomes of any new model of care must be built in to any new policy implementation process, to ensure that change is taking place, and that no adverse consequences are developing. This evaluation must inform the ongoing implementation process through an assessment of the impact of the changes on the women and families receiving the new model, the impact on those women and families who are not receiving the new model, and the impact on the staff providing the care. Evaluation and measurement frameworks have been devised to inform local processes, but the extent to which the lessons from evaluations will be learned and fed forward to inform future implementation are still to be determined.

A New Look Maternity System Based on the Review Recommendations

In addition to the Midwifery Continuity of Carer recommendations (Scottish Government 2017; NHS England 2016), Box 8.9 provides details as to how a maternity system built around the needs of women and their families, enables the woman to choose where she wishes to birth her baby. This involves the midwife being conversant with the evidence-based information (highlighted in this chapter) that all women should be provided with

in order to make that decision, as well as knowledge of change management theories and tools (Polenz et al. 2019). Recognizing the challenges this may pose for some maternity services, ideas are presented that can support moving to a *new look* maternity system where all women can choose the place of birth, and enable it to work in practice.

BOX 8.9   A Maternity System that Enables Women to have a Choice about Place of Birth

What choice?
Home, midwife-led care setting (freestanding or alongside), obstetric unit.

What Information do Women Need to Make an Informed Decision About Place of Birth?
Evidence-based advice and guidance from health professionals:
- Results of the Birthplace England study and an explanation of how those results relate to their own personal situation.
- Written information about the potential benefits and risks of different places of birth.
- Information about transfer times and arrangements in their own area.
- Ability to see all the different environments. It is helpful to have the opportunity to meet women who have experienced different places of birth.

What is Required to Make this Work?
Resources and capital spending to create different birth place settings:
- Each obstetric unit should have an alongside midwife-led unit; creation of 'community hubs' may include a birth room.
- Freestanding midwife-led units need to be up-to-date, comfortable, with equipment to manage arising emergencies.
- Midwives need to have confidence in their ability to provide safe care in all settings; for some, this will mean time spent shadowing colleagues, further training and time to embed new practices.
- Support from the multidisciplinary team (MDT); collaborative working to develop guidelines, transfer arrangements and mutual respect between professions.
- Support from senior management and the core midwifery team in the obstetric receiving unit.

If the key central elements of continuity of carer and choice of birthplace were universally implemented, imagine what this would look like and the benefits this would have for women, their babies and families, as well individual midwives and the midwifery profession as a whole.

CONCLUSION

Quality maternal and newborn care saves lives and improves health and wellbeing, with **midwifery** being the key to delivering best quality care that focuses on the needs, views and preferences of women, infants, partners and families. Ensuring the provision of best quality care needs a combination of evidence, policy and change management (Polenz et al. 2019) to ensure effective implementation. Everyone has a part to play in this: policy-makers; managers; professional associations and trade unions; midwives and other health professionals; advocacy groups; women and families; and the public. Evidence-informed national and local policy is essential to enable and support the development of maternity and newborn care that meets the needs of women, infants, partners and families. Without strong and evidence-informed policy, it is very hard for practitioners to make the changes needed to deliver best care.

It is not enough just to develop the policy, however well informed it is. A clear plan is needed, involving all stakeholders – women and families, advocates, health professionals, managers, professional associations, trade unions and policy-makers. Ring-fenced resources should be identified to support the development and change. Realistic, measurable and achievable goals should be set, with clear project management timelines. Practical considerations for those providing the care must be addressed before ways of providing care are changed – staff and services must have the appropriate equipment, transport arrangements, physical environments (including office and clinical space). Ongoing monitoring and evaluation is needed to ensure that the change is taking place, and there are no adverse or unforeseen consequences in terms of the impact on outcomes for women, infants, partners, families and for the health service. Policy design and implementation are complex tasks – they require a huge investment of time, finances and commitment at every level. The rewards for such focused, long-term and frankly difficult work could be great – with the development of services that have not just evolved piecemeal over time, but that have been designed to provide the highest quality care for the best outcomes, evidenced by high quality research.

▌REFLECTIVE ACTIVITY FOR SELF-ASSESSMENT

1. How would you define quality midwifery care?
2. Suggest ways in which women and their families could effectively engage in developing high quality midwifery services that reflect the needs of all women, including those who are living with deprivation and are vulnerable.
3. What is health or maternity policy and why is policy important?

4. What is required in order to develop high quality health or maternity policy?
5. Consider an aspect of recent health or maternity policy that has been implemented in your workplace to improve the experiences of women, babies and families as well as the health professionals providing the care. What was needed to implement it and how will its success be measured?

REFERENCES

Blix, E., Kumle, M. H., Ingversen, K., et al. (2016). Transfer to hospital in planned home birth in four Nordic countries – a prospective cohort study. *Acta Obstetricia et Gynecologica Scandinavica*, 95(4), 420–428.

Boerma, T., Ronsmans, C., Melesse, D. Y., et al. (2018). Global epidemiology of use of and disparities in caesarean sections. *Lancet*, 392(10155), 1341–1348.

Bohren, M. A., Hofmeyr, G. J., Sakala, C., et al. (2017). Continuous support for women during childbirth. *Cochrane Database of Systematic Reviews* (7), CD003766.

Brocklehurst, P., Hardy, P., Hollowell, J., et al. (2011). Perinatal and maternal outcomes by planned place of birth for healthy women with low risk pregnancies: The Birthplace in England national prospective cohort study. *British Medical Journal*, 343, d7400.

Cheyne, H., Critchley, A., Elders, A., et al. (2015). *Having a baby in Scotland 2015: Listening to mothers report: An official statistics publication for Scotland.* Edinburgh: The Scottish Government. Available at: www.gov.scot/publications/having-baby-scotland-2015-maternity-care-survey.

Cheyne, H., Skar, S., Paterson, A., et al. (2013). *Having a baby in Scotland 2013: Women's experiences of maternity care.* Edinburgh: The Scottish Government. Available at: www.gov.scot/publications/having-baby-scotland-2013-womens-experiences-maternity-care/.

Cheyney, M., Bovbjerg, M., Everson, C., et al. (2014). Outcomes of care for 16,924 planned home births in the United States: The midwives Alliance of North America Statistics project, 2004 to 2009. *Journal of Midwifery & Women's Health, 59*(1), 17–27.

Davidson, P., Halcomb, E., Hickman, L., et al. (2006). Beyond the rhetoric: What do we mean by a 'model of care'? *Australian Journal of Advanced Nursing, 23*(3), 47–55.

Davis, A. (2013). Choice, policy and practice in maternity care since 1948, policy Papers: History and policy. Available at: www.historyandpolicy.org/policy-papers/papers/choice-policy-and-practice-in-maternity-care-since-1948.

Davis, D., Baddock, S., Pairman, S., et al. (2011). Planned place of birth in New Zealand: Does it affect mode of birth and intervention rates among low-risk women? *Birth, 38*(2), 111–119.

Davis, D., Baddock, S., Pairman, S., et al. (2012). Risk of severe postpartum hemorrhage in low-risk childbearing women in New Zealand: Exploring the effect of place of birth and comparing third stage management of labor. *Birth, 39*(2), 98–105.

Department of Health (1993). *Changing childbirth: Report of the expert maternity group: Part 1.* London: The Stationery Office.

Filby, A., McConville, F., & Portela, A. (2016). What prevents quality midwifery care? A systematic mapping of barriers in low and middle income countries from the provider perspective. *PLoS One, 11*(5), e0153391.

Gavine, A., MacGillivray, S., Ross-Davie, M., et al. (2018). Maximising the availability and use of high-quality evidence for policymaking: Collaborative, targeted and efficient evidence reviews. *Palgrave Communications, 4*(5). Available at: https://doi.org/10.1057/s41599-017-0054-8.

Halfdansdottir, B., Smarason, A., Olafsdottir, O., et al. (2015). Outcome of planned home and hospital births among low-risk women in Iceland in 2005–9: A retrospective cohort study. *Birth, 42*(1), 16–26.

Hendrix, M., Evers, S. M., Basten, M. C., et al. (2009). Cost analysis of the Dutch obstetric system: Low-risk nulliparous women preferring home or short-stay hospital birth: A prospective non-randomised controlled study. *BMC Health Services Research, 9*(211), 211.

Hobbs, A. J., Moller, A. B., Kachikis, A., et al. (2019). Scoping review to identify and map the health personnel considered skilled birth attendants in low-and-middle income countries from 2000–15. *PLoS One, 14*(2), e0211576.

Hodnett, E. D., Downe, S., & Walsh, D. (2012). Alternative versus conventional institutional settings for birth. *Cochrane Database of Systematic Reviews,* (8), CD000012.

Hollowell, J., Li, Y., Bunch, K., & Brocklehurst, P. (2015a). *Review of Maternity Services, NHS England.* Report 2: Perinatal and maternal outcomes by parity in midwifery-led settings. *Secondary analysis of the Birthplace in England cohort comparing outcomes in planned freestanding and alongside midwifery unit births.* Oxford: NPEU, University of Oxford. Available at: www.england.nhs.uk/wp-content/uploads/2015/07/npeu-report2-birthplace-analysis-report.pdf.

Hollowell, J., Chisholm, A., Li, Y., & Malouf, K. (2015b). *Review of maternity services England. Report 4: A systematic review and narrative synthesis of the quantitative and qualitative literature on women's birth place preferences and experiences of choosing their intended place of birth in the UK.* Oxford: National Perinatal Epidemiology Unit, University of Oxford. Available at: www.england.nhs.uk/wp-content/uploads/2015/07/npeu-report4-choices-evidence-review-synthesis.pdf.

Hollowell, J., Pillas, D., Rowe, R., et al. (2014). The impact of maternal obesity on intrapartum outcomes in otherwise low risk women: Secondary analysis of the birthplace national prospective cohort study. *BJOG, 121*(3), 343–355.

Homer, C. S., Friberg, I. K., Dias, M. A., et al. (2014). The projected effect of scaling up midwifery. *Lancet, 384*(9948), 1146–1157.

ten Hoope-Bender, P., de Bernis, L., Campbell, J., et al. (2014). Improvement of maternal and newborn health through midwifery. *Lancet, 384*(9949), 1226–1235.

ICM (International Confederation of Midwives). (2018). Essential competencies for midwifery practice. The Hague: ICM. Available at: www.internationalmidwives.org/assets/files/general-files/2019/03/icm-competencies-en-screens.pdf.

Janssen, P., Milton, C., & Aghajanian, J. (2015). Costs of planned home vs. hospital birth in British Columbia attended by registered midwives and physicians. *PLoS One, 10*(7), e0133524.

Janssen, P., Saxell, L., Page, L., et al. (2009). Outcomes of planned homebirth with registered midwife versus planned hospital birth with midwife or physician. *CMAJ Canadian Medical Association Journal, 181*(6–7), 377–383.

Knight, M., Bunch, K., Tuffnell, D., et al. (Eds.). (2019). *Saving lives, improving mothers' care – lessons learned to inform maternity care from the UK and Ireland Confidential Enquiries into maternal deaths and morbidity 2015–2017.* Oxford: National Perinatal Epidemiology Unit, University of Oxford.

Kurinczuk, J., Knight, M., Rowe, R., & Hollowell, J. (2015). *Review of maternity services England. Report 1: Summary of the evidence on safety of place of birth; and implications for policy and practice from the overall evidence review.* Oxford: National Perinatal Epidemiology Unit, University of Oxford. Available at: www.england.nhs.uk/wp-content/uploads/2015/07/npeu-report1-safety-of-birth-place-and-implications.pdf.

van Lerberghe, W., Matthews, Z., Achadi, E., et al. (2014). Country experience with strengthening of health systems and deployment of midwives in countries with high maternal mortality. *Lancet, 384*(9949), 1215–1225.

Li, Y., Townend, J., Rowe, R., et al. (2014). The effect of maternal age and planned place of birth on intrapartum outcomes in healthy women with straightforward pregnancies: Secondary analysis of the Birthplace national prospective cohort study. *BMJ Open, 4*(1), e004026.

Li, Y., Townend, J., Rowe, R., et al. (2015). Perinatal and maternal outcomes in planned home and obstetric unit births in women at 'higher risk' of complications: Secondary analysis of the birthplace national prospective cohort study. *BJOG, 122*(5), 741–753.

Lindgren, H. E., Radestad, I. J., Christensson, K., & Hildingsson, I. M. (2008). Outcome of planned home births compared to hospital births in Sweden between 1992 and 2004. A population-based register study. *Acta Obstetricia et Gynecologica Scandinavica, 87*(7), 751–759.

Lukasse, M., Rowe, R., Townend, J., et al. (2014). Immersion in water for pain relief and the risk of intrapartum transfer among low risk nulliparous women: Secondary analysis of the birthplace national prospective cohort study. *BMC Pregnancy and Childbirth, 14*(1), 60.

McCourt, C., Rayment, J., Rance, S., & Sandall, J. (2012). Organisational strategies and midwives' readiness to provide care for out of hospital births: An analysis from the Birthplace organisational case studies. *Midwifery, 28*(5), 636–645.

McInnes, R., Hollins Martin, C. J., & MacArthur, J. (2018). Midwifery continuity of carer: Developing a realist evaluation framework to evaluate the implementation of strategic change in Scotland. *Midwifery, 66*, 103–110.

NFWI/NCT (National Federation of Women's Institutes and National Childbirth Trust). (2013). *Support overdue: Women's experiences of maternity services.* London: The Women's institute. Available at: www.thewi.org.uk/__data/assets/pdf_file/0006/49857/support-overdue-final-15-may-2013.pdf.

NHS England. (2016). *National maternity review. Better births: Improving outcomes of maternity services in England: A five year forward view for maternity care.* London: NHS England. Available at: www.england.nhs.uk/wp-content/uploads/2016/02/national-maternity-review-report.pdf.

NHS England. (2017). *Implementing better births: Continuity of carer.* London: NHS England. Available at: www.england.nhs.uk/publication/implementing-better-births-continuity-of-carer/.

NHS England. (2019). *The NHS long term plan.* London: NHS England. Available at: www.longtermplan.nhs.uk/wp-content/uploads/2019/01/nhs-long-term-plan.pdf.

NHS Scotland. (2010). *The healthcare quality strategy for NHS Scotland.* Edinburgh: The Scottish Government. Available at: www2.gov.scot/resource/doc/311667/0098354.pdf.

NICE (National Institute for Health and Care Excellence). (2015). *Postnatal care up to 8 weeks after birth: Clinical guidance 37.* London: NICE.

NICE (National Institute for Health and Care Excellence). (2017). *Intrapartum care of healthy women and babies: Clinical guideline 190.* London: NICE.

NICE (National Institute for Health and Care Excellence). (2019). *Antenatal care for uncomplicated pregnancies: Clinical guideline 62.* London: NICE.

NPEU (National Perinatal Epidemiology Unit). (2014). *Safely delivered: A national survey of women's experience of maternity care.* Oxford: National Perinatal Epidemiology Unit, University of Oxford. Available at: www.npeu.ox.ac.uk/downloads/files/reports/Safely%20delivered%20NMS%202014.pdf.

Olsen, O., & Clausen, J. A. (2012). Planned hospital birth versus planned home birth. *Cochrane Database of Systematic* (9), CD000352.

Overgaard, C., Fenger-Gron, M., & Sandall, J. (2012). Freestanding midwifery units versus obstetric units: Does the effect of place of birth differ with level of social disadvantage. *BMC Public Health, 12*, 478.

Polenz, L. Y., Forman, J., & Marshall, J. E. (2019). Change and innovation in midwifery education and practice. In J. E. Marshall (Ed.), *Myles professional studies for midwifery education and practice: Concepts and challenges* (pp. 229–249). Edinburgh: Elsevier.

RCM (Royal College of Midwives). (2016). *Position statement on continuity of midwife-led care.* London: RCM.

RCM (Royal College of Midwives). (2018a). *Position statement on continuity of midwife-led care.* London: RCM. Available at: www.rcm.org.uk/media/2946/midwifery-continuity-of-carer-mcoc.pdf.

RCM (Royal College of Midwives). (2018b). *State of maternity services report 2018*. England. London: RCM. Available at: www.rcm.org.uk/media/2373/state-of-maternity-services-report-2018-england.pdf.

RCM Royal College of Midwives. (2018c). State of maternity services report 2018, Scotland. London: RCM. Available at: www.rcm.org.uk/media/2448/state-of-maternity-services-report-2018-scotland.pdf.

RCOG (Royal College of Obstetricians and Gynaecologists). (2013). *Reconfiguration of women's services. Good practice No 15*. London: RCOG. Available at: www.rcog.org.uk/globalassets/documents/guidelines/reconfiguration_good_practice_no.15_corrected_february_2014.pdf.

RCOG/RCM (Royal College of Obstetricians and Gynaecologists and Royal College of Midwives). (2016). *Joint statement on multidisciplinary working and continuity of carer*. London: RCOG. Available at: www.rcog.org.uk/en/news/joint-rcogrcm-statement-on-multi-disciplinary-working-and-continuity-of-carer/.

RCOG/RCM/RCoA/RCPCH (Royal College of Obstetricians and Gynaecologists, Royal College of Midwives, Royal College of Anaesthetists, Royal College of Paediatrics and Child Health). (2007). *Safer childbirth: minimum standards for the organisation and delivery of care in labour*. London: RCOG. Available at: www.rcog.org.uk/globalassets/documents/guidelines/wprsaferchildbirthreport2007.pdf.

RCOG/RCM/RCoA/RCPCH (Royal College of Obstetricians and Gynaecologists, Royal College of Midwives, Royal College of Anaesthetists, Royal College of Paediatrics and Child Health). (2008). *Standards for maternity care: Report of a Working Party*. London: RCOG. Available at: www.rcog.org.uk/globalassets/documents/guidelines/wprmaternitystandards2008.pdf.

Renfrew, M. J. (2016). Optimising the contribution of midwifery to preventing stillbirths and improving the overall quality of care: Co-ordinated global action needed. *Midwifery*, 35, 99–101.

Renfrew, M. J., McFadden, A., Bastos, M. H., et al. (2014). Midwifery and quality care: Findings from a new evidence-informed framework for maternal and newborn care. *Lancet*, 384(9948), 1129–1145.

Ridde, V., & Yaméogo, P. (2018). How Burkina Faso used evidence in deciding to launch its policy of free healthcare for children under five and women in 2016. *Palgrave Communications*, 4, 119.

Rowe, R. E., Fitzpatrick, R., Hollowell, J., & Kurinczuk, J. J. (2012). Transfers of women planning birth in midwifery units: Data from the birthplace prospective cohort study. *British Journal of Obstetrics and Gynaecology*, 119(9), 1081–1090.

Rowe, R. E., Townend, J., Brocklehurst, P., et al. (2013). Duration and urgency of transfer in births planned at home and in freestanding midwifery units in England: Secondary analysis of the birthplace national prospective cohort study. *BMC Pregnancy and Childbirth*, 13, 224.

Rowe, R. E., Townend, J., Brocklehurst, P., et al. (2014). Service configuration, unit characteristics and variation in intervention rates in a national sample of obstetric units in England: An exploratory analysis. *BMJ Open*, 4(5), e005551.

Sandall, J. (2018). *Measuring continuity of carer: A monitoring and evaluation framework*. London: RCM/NHS England. Available at: www.rcm.org.uk/media/2465/measuring-continuity-of-carer-a-monitoring-and-evaluation-framework.pdf.

Sandall, J., Soltani, H., Gates, S., et al. (2016). Midwife–led continuity models versus other models of care for childbearing women. *Cochrane Database of Systematic Reviews* (4), CD004667.

Schroeder, E., Petrou, S., Patel, N., et al. (2012). Cost effectiveness of alternative planned places of birth in woman at low risk of complications: Evidence from the birthplace in England national prospective cohort study. *British Medical Journal*, 344, e2292.

Scotland Act. (1998). Chapter 46. London: The Stationery Office. Available at: www.legislation.gov.uk/ukpga/1998/46/pdfs/ukpga_19980046_en.pdf.

Scottish Government. (2016). *Health and social care delivery plan*. Edinburgh: The Scottish Government. Available at: www.gov.scot/publications/health-social-care-delivery-plan/.

Scottish Government. (2017). *The best start review: A five year forward plan for neonatal and maternity services in Scotland*. Edinburgh: The Scottish Government. Available at: www.gov.scot/publications/best-start-five-year-forward-plan-maternity-neonatal-care-scotland/.

Scottish Health Council. (2017). *National review of maternity and neonatal services: Gathering views and experience of maternity and neonatal services*. Glasgow: Scottish Health Council. Available at: http://scottishhealthcouncil.org/publications/gathering_public_views/maternity_and_neonatal_review.aspx#.XOAvT8E1vD4.

Sutcliffe, K., Caird, J., Kavanagh, J., et al. (2012). Comparing midwife-led and doctor-led maternity care: A systematic review of reviews. *Journal of Advanced Nursing*, 68(11), 2376–2386.

Turienzo, C., Sandall, J., & Peacock, J. (2016). Models of antenatal care to reduce and prevent preterm birth: A systematic review and meta-analysis. *BMJ Open*, 6, e009044.

UN (United Nations). Committee on economic, social and cultural rights. (2000). *General Comment No. 14: The Right to the Highest attainable Standard of Health (Art. 12 of the Covenant)*. E/C.12/2000/4. Available at: www.refworld.org/docid/4538838d0.html.

Van der Kooy, J., Poeran, J., de Graaf, J., et al. (2011). Planned home compared with planned hospital births in The Netherlands: Intrapartum and early neonatal death in low-risk pregnancies. *Obstetrics & Gynecology*, 118(5), 1037–1046.

Wax, J. R., Lucas, F. L., Lamont, M., et al. (2010). Maternal and newborn outcomes in planned homebirth vs planned hospital births: A metaanalysis. *American Journal of Obstetrics and Gynecology*, 203(3), e1–e8 243.

WHO (World Health Organization). (2016). *Midwives' voices, midwives' realities: Findings from a global consultation on providing quality midwifery care*. Geneva: WHO. Available at: https://apps.who.int/iris/bitstream/handle/10665/250376/9789241510547-eng.pdf?sequence=1.

WHO (World Health Organization). (2019). *Strengthening quality midwifery education for Universal Health Coverage 2030: framework for action*. Geneva: WHO. Available at: https://www.who.int/maternal_child_adolescent/topics/quality-of-care/midwifery/strengthening-midwifery-education/en/.

ANNOTATED FURTHER READING

Kuhlmann, E., Blank, R., Bourgeault, I., & Wendt, C. (Eds.). (2015). *The Palgrave international handbook of healthcare policy and governance*. London: Palgrave Macmillan.

This handbook provides the reader with international examples alongside an analysis of differing approaches to healthcare policy and governance, illustrated with a variety of case studies. It is an invaluable source not only for healthcare students but also health policy researchers and policy-makers around the globe.

Marmot, M., Allen, J., Goldblatt, P., et al. (2010). *Fair society, healthy lives: Strategic review of health inequalities in England post-2010*. London: The Marmot review. Available at: www.instituteofhealthequity.org/resources-reports/fair-society-healthy-lives-the-marmot-review.

The Marmot Review (led by Professor Sir Michael Marmot) into health inequalities in England proposed an evidence-based strategy to address the social determinants of health, the conditions in which people are born, grow, live, work and age and which can lead to health inequalities. The review set out a framework for action under two policy goals: to create an enabling society that maximizes individual and community potential; and to ensure social justice, health and sustainability are at the heart of all policies. Central to the Review was the recognition that disadvantage starts before birth and accumulates throughout life, which was reflected in six policy objectives.

Midwifery Action: YouTube. www.youtube.com/user/midwiferyaction.

A useful website that provides a series of short films on The Lancet Series on Midwifery, including the development and implementation of the Framework of Quality Maternal and Newborn Care (QMNC), the principles of which can be applied worldwide to all childbearing women, their babies and families, including the most vulnerable and those with complex healthcare needs.

USEFUL WEBSITES

Cochrane Reviews: www.cochranelibrary.com/cdsr/reviews

Department of Health (and social care) England: www.gov.uk/government/organisations/department-of-health-and-social-care

International Confederation of Midwives: www.internationalmidwives.org/

Midwifery Action: YouTube: www.youtube.com/user/midwiferyaction

National Institute for Health and Care Excellence: www.nice.org.uk/

National Perinatal Epidemiology Unit (NPEU) Birthplace in England Research Programme: www.npeu.ox.ac.uk/birthplace

NHS England: www.england.nhs.uk/

NHS Scotland: www.scot.nhs.uk/

Royal College of Midwives: www.rcm.org.uk/

Royal College of Obstetricians and Gynaecologists: www.rcog.org.uk/

The Lancet Series on Midwifery: www.thelancet.com/series/midwifery

The Scottish Government: www.gov.scot/

World Health Organization: www.who.int/

9

Antenatal Education for Birth and Parenting

Mary L. Nolan

CHAPTER CONTENTS

This chapter discusses the special opportunities that antenatal education sessions provide for midwives to help mothers, fathers, partners and families make a happy and successful transition to parenthood. It explores the aims and themes of antenatal education, and describes skills and activities, which midwives can use to enable group members to acquire information, develop problem-solving skills and build a social support network to enhance their self-efficacy for birth and parenting.

THE CHAPTER AIMS TO

- support midwives to provide expectant parents with a relevant, participatory antenatal programme that enables them to build a social support network
- show midwives how they can build women's self-efficacy for labour and birth, and their partners' confidence to support them, through antenatal education sessions
- develop midwives' group-work skills so as to help mothers, fathers and partners understand the importance of sensitive, responsive parenting

- enable midwives to employ antenatal education sessions to enhance couples' understanding of each other's needs and strengthen mothers', fathers' and partners' mental health
- build midwives' confidence and skills to facilitate antenatal sessions that effectively meet the needs of women and men making the transition to parenthood.

PARENT EDUCATION FOR THE CRITICAL 1000 DAYS

The 1000 days from conception to 2 years of age is 'critical' for both children and their parents/key carers. This is the time of maximum neuroplasticity of the baby's brain and the time when the baby's attachment style is developing. Attachment has evolved to ensure that helpless human infants remain in close contact with an adult human who can protect him or her from danger. Who the baby becomes, the kind of citizen, lover, worker, parent she grows up to be, is determined by the way in which her genetic inheritance interacts with the environment into which she is born. For the new baby, and the very young child, the most influential aspects of their 'environment' are the relationships they have with the key people in their life, generally their mother and father. 'For the growing brain of a young child, the social world supplies the most important experiences influencing the expression and regulation of genes' (Siegal 2012: 32). If social experiences shape the baby's view of the world as a place of comfort and security, the baby will develop a secure attachment style, which is likely to have a strongly positive impact on her entire life trajectory. The midwife has a wonderful opportunity throughout pregnancy, during which she has regular contact with the mother and her family to support the development of a sensitive, responsive relationship between the key players in the new baby's life and the baby. Antenatal education in particular is a means of nurturing these relationships.

For parents, too, the first 1000 days of their baby's life is a period of unprecedented biological, personal, social and spiritual change. Research has shown that pregnant women undergo neurobiological changes that support developing mother–infant relationships (Kim et al. 2016). Men also undergo detectable physiological changes during pregnancy (Bartlett 2004). Levels of testosterone fall, while levels of oestradiol (the primary female sex hormone) rise (Berg and Wynne-Edwards 2001). Expectant and new parents are therefore primed to take action to provide the best possible start in life for their baby (Sher 2016; Feinberg and Kan 2008). Midwives and others working in the very early years who provide education and support for families have therefore both an exceptional opportunity and an exceptional responsibility. Gutman et al. (2009:x) are insistent that, 'The best time to target mothers is most likely during pregnancy, considering the importance of parenting for children's development. Investing in parents in the early years can have dividends that extend to the school years and beyond'.

Preparing women and fathers/partners for labour and birth has traditionally been seen by midwives as the main focus of antenatal education. Today, it remains an important focus, but the act of giving birth is located *within the continuum* of the woman's (and her partner's) evolving experience of becoming a mother, father or parent.

Research into the impact of antenatal education remains inconclusive. The 2007 Cochrane review, 'Individual or group antenatal education for childbirth or parenthood, or both' (Gagnon and Sandall 2007: Abstract), however, acknowledges that the quality of studies is generally poor:

> There are many varied ways of providing antenatal education and some may be more effective than others. The review found 9 trials involving 2284 women. Interventions varied greatly and no consistent outcomes were measured. The review of trials found a lack of high quality evidence from trials and so the effects of antenatal education remain largely unknown.

Gilmer et al. (2016: 118), in their examination of parent education interventions designed to support the transition to parenthood, also found 'no compelling evidence to suggest that a single educational programme or delivery format was effective at a universal level'. However, like Gagnon and Sandall (2007), they also highlighted serious deficiencies in the research and argued that careful consideration should be accorded to current programming and future initiatives given 'the importance of the transition to parenthood and its impact on parent and child wellbeing' (p. 119).

The Social Research Unit (2016: 2) acknowledges that there is, 'a lack of evidence about the impact of universal services, primarily because of difficulties in evaluating whether such population level approaches are effective. … This means that "what works" is "what is most likely to work".'

The fact that parents themselves seek antenatal education eagerly is clearly of considerable importance when considering whether it should be funded and universally available. The Scottish Government (2012a: ix) comments on: 'a huge appetite for clear, concise and consistent information on feeding, behaviour management, relationships, emotional wellbeing and mental health'. Kane et al. (2007) report that parents are seeking skills, understanding, acceptance and support from other parents through attending preparation for parenting sessions, and a sense of control and of being able to cope. Yet a survey of 3682 women (Nolan 2008) from all parts of the UK revealed that a large number of women had been offered no or very few antenatal education sessions during their most recent pregnancy. Many of those who had attended sessions were dissatisfied with their quality, criticizing in particular the unrealistic portrayal of labour, birth and early parenting, lack of practical skills work to help them use their own resources for coping with the pain of labour and being given no opportunity to discuss their new role as a mother. Fathers, too, have said they were side-lined during antenatal sessions and describe not being seen as important recipients of parenting information or helped to play an equal part with the mother in promoting their child's wellbeing (Scottish Government 2012a).

The UK government has been committed to supporting parents, and especially first-time parents, since the publication of the Child Health Programme in 2008 (Department of Health, DH 2008). In a more recent document, Public Health England (PHE 2014a) has stressed that nurturing emotional resilience in children starts from the first days of life, and speaks of the need for good quality parenting programmes to promote positive warm parenting (PHE 2014b). The Scottish Government (2012b), in its National Parenting Strategy, is very clear that parents are their children's first educators and that they remain the single most important influence on their child's educational aspirations and attainment throughout life.

What, therefore, should be the content of an antenatal education programme? A review by McMillan et al. (2009) of the effectiveness of antenatal education found some evidence that antenatal programmes aimed at promoting the transition to parenthood, focusing on issues such as the emotional changes that parents experience at this time, the couple's relationship, parenting skills, bonding and attachment and problem-solving skills, have a positive effect on mothers' psychological wellbeing, parents' confidence, satisfaction with the couple's relationship and the parent–infant relationship in the postnatal period. This review became the basis of a resource pack put together by an Expert Reference Group convened by the Department of Health. Entitled *Preparation for Birth and Beyond: A resource pack for leaders of community groups and activities*, it provided a raft of activities to address themes that the McMillan et al. (2009) review had suggested were important in the transition to parenthood. The rest of this chapter considers what antenatal education is aiming to achieve; what its principal themes should be; and the facilitation skills that are required to lead groups for people who are preparing for a major life transition that will impact not only their own lives, but the lives of their babies and, in time, those babies' own parenting.

AIMS OF ANTENATAL EDUCATION

No educational intervention is likely to be successful if those delivering it are not clear about what they are trying to achieve. Commissioners commissioning parent education, services delivering it and midwives leading parent education groups need to be clear about their aims, as these will determine both the content of the programme and the way in which it is provided to parents.

TO INCREASE WOMEN'S SELF-EFFICACY FOR LABOUR AND BIRTH

It is a subject for debate among midwives and other childbirth educators whether antenatal education sessions should focus exclusively on straightforward vaginal birth with no information being provided about pharmacological forms of pain relief, assisted birth or caesarean section, or whether antenatal education should devote time to all of these interventions, given the frequency with which they are used. The fear is that by including interventions in sessions about preparation for labour, the impression may be conveyed that these are a 'normal' part of having a baby in the 21st century. However, if antenatal sessions cover only the events of an uninterfered with vaginal birth, might this risk leaving women and their birth companions unprepared for alternatives to this scenario, and potentially traumatized as a result?

Globally, the caesarean section rate is of concern; for example the rate in the UK has been climbing over the last 30 years from 12% in 1990 (Parliamentary Office of Science and Technology, POST 2002) to 28% in May, 2017 (NHS Digital 2017). Yet, birth without interventions has many benefits for women's physical and mental health, and for maternity services in terms of reduced expenditure (Smith et al. 2016; Kassebaum et al. 2014; O'Mahoney et al. 2010). There is also evidence that women themselves would like to labour without drugs or medical interventions (Wharton et al. 2017; Care Quality Commission, CQC 2015).

Anecdotal evidence would suggest that women and their partners are keen to receive information about pain-relief in labour. However, if straightforward vaginal birth is to be promoted and the self-efficacy of women and their partners for normal birth is to be strengthened, antenatal education must include a strong emphasis on helping them maximize their understanding of the normal progress of labour, and of their own capacity for managing its emotions and the physical intensity of contractions. The result of increasing women's self-efficacy beliefs through antenatal education should be that there is a need for fewer obstetric interventions, as anxious women are likely to use more medications and experience more caesareans.

Best Practice
Birth Stories

Antenatal education should aim to present birth in all its diversity and richness. One means of doing this is by sharing birth stories. Stories about labours which progressed uneventfully can be told alongside stories where intervention was necessary and helpful. Women regularly tell each other 'horror stories', and there are plenty available via social media, television and the press. Hearing *positive* birth stories is less common and midwives may, with integrity, choose deliberately to invite women who have had a satisfying normal birth to visit an antenatal education session in order to rebalance women's and their partners' skewed understanding of labour. Positive birth stories can also be told through birth images displayed on the walls, of women labouring in active birth positions, without medical apparatus visible, surrounded by family members and their midwife.

Active Birth Practice

Helping women and their partners learn how to maximize the woman's own capacity to manage the intensity of labour is a major part of antenatal preparation. Non-recumbent positions for labour, massage strokes, breathing techniques and relaxation strategies such as visualization and positive affirmations, need to be practised at *every* antenatal session. It is this repeated practice that builds

the woman's confidence in her body, and her partner's understanding of how he can support her. Campbell and Nolan (2019: 79) report how highly women value regular practice of labour-management strategies:

> *It was the teaching it every week…. The calm … repeating … definitely increased my confidence. (Kirsten)*

> *What was really helpful was … she always encouraged us to try different kinds of positions … to see which position is the most comfortable for me …. It was easier to try different things [in labour] because I had tried them already during the course. (Adali)*

Birth Companions

Fathers/partners are the people most likely to make a positive or negative difference to the woman's experience of labour. Their presence at antenatal education sessions is essential so that they can understand the physical and psychological skills that are being practised in readiness for labour, and how they can support their partner to persist with coping strategies. The loving attention the partner can give during and in-between contractions, kissing and cuddling, and boosting the woman's morale, will increase her oxytocin levels and reduce her fear in facing labour (Carter 2011).

Birth Hormones and Environment

Antenatal education for labour and birth can usefully include discussion of how the hormones of labour – oxytocin, adrenalin and prolactin – work with or against each other in the different stages of labour, either to facilitate or impede its course. Understanding how birth hormones work helps women and their partners comprehend how important the environment of labour is. Oxytocin flows best when women feel safe, when their privacy is guaranteed and when they are unobserved except by those whom they choose to have near them. Discussion of the impact of the environment may persuade some couples to stay at home longer, where the conditions necessary for straightforward labour are generally more conducive than in a birth institution. Such discussion can also cover items that parents might take to hospital or the birth centre from home to personalize the environment and thereby increase their confidence that the act of giving birth is a normal human activity rather than one requiring 'the medical gaze'.

TO PROMOTE SENSITIVITY TO INFANTS

Antenatal education aims to help mothers and fathers/partners establish an enduring emotional relationship with their child, based on frequent, reciprocal, sensitive and enjoyable interactions. Many children do not have a secure attachment to one or more significant adults in their lives (Molinuevo 2013) and the legacy of poor early attachment is felt down the generations as it impacts the kind of relationships children form with other children, with adults when they grow up, and finally, with their own children.

Around 95% of women have developed a sense of their baby as 'a real person' by the third trimester of pregnancy (Brandon et al. 2009). Half of women have normal, healthy representations of their unborn baby; about one-third feel disengaged from their baby; and the rest have 'distorted' representations of their baby (Huth-Bocks et al. 2011). The way the woman thinks about her baby during pregnancy tends to persist into the postnatal period (Vreeswijk et al. 2012), with women who have unbalanced views of their unborn babies tending to be controlling as mothers, and more hostile towards their babies. Research has also found that *fathers'* imaginings of their baby during pregnancy are as vivid as mothers' although men tend to visualize their baby after he or she has been born, whereas mothers visualize the baby inside the womb (Seimyr et al. 2009).

Antenatal education aims to promote secure attachment by building the relationship between the mother and father/partner with their unborn and newborn baby, and supporting parents to be 'mind-minded', that is to see their child as a unique individual with her own mind, rather than as a (mere) dependent entity with (primarily) physical needs.

Best Practice

There are many ways in which midwives leading antenatal education sessions can help nurture a relationship between the mother, father, partner and the baby. For example, asking parents to talk about their babies' behaviour in the womb makes the point that the parents possess the primary knowledge of their baby, and also affirms the baby as a unique individual. While most expectant parents talk to their baby, some will find this a novel idea, but may be encouraged to do so if peers talk about their 'conversations' with the baby. The midwife might ask the group:

- Do you talk to your babies? What do you tell them?
- What kind of music do your babies like? Do you sing to them?
- Do you ask your babies if they're having a good day?

The midwife can also help the parents to *wonder* about their babies:

- What kind of personality do you think your baby has?
- Do you think your baby is like someone in your family?
- Do you think your babies get upset when you're upset – how do you comfort them?
- How do you think your babies are feeling at this moment?

Parents are fascinated to find out about how their baby is developing in the womb. This hunger for information is testified to by the large number of apps that offer a week-by-week description of the growing baby. Discussing what stage of development each baby has reached is an excellent topic for an antenatal session because it arouses in parents a sense of wonder at their baby's rapid growth and the increasing capacity for connecting with the outside world through, for example, hearing the parents' voices, and swallowing amniotic fluid flavoured by whatever the mother has been eating!

Antenatal education sessions provide multiple opportunities to help mothers, fathers and partners explore their thoughts and feelings about their babies and for the midwife to identify and support parents who seem to be struggling to form a relationship with their baby (Barlow 2016). Topics to help parents develop their relationship both before and after the baby is born might include:

- what the baby can see, hear, taste, touch and smell at different stages of pregnancy
- what part the baby plays in the onset of labour
- how to comfort newborn babies by recreating their experience in the womb (e.g. holding them close, skin to skin, so that they are warmed by the parent's body and can hear their heartbeat and voice clearly)
- the importance of babies' emotions being reflected in their parents' facial expressions, tone of voice and in the way they are held
- the value of reading to babies, singing and reciting nursery rhymes, as these are forms of communication that both build the baby's relationship with his parents and help to develop language
- why crying babies should be responded to – exploding the myth that picking up a distressed baby is creating 'a rod for your own back'.

TO ENHANCE PRACTICAL PARENTING SKILLS

Caring for a baby and young children is no longer part of the social stock of knowledge (Mechlin 2001). Many expectant parents in wealthy, post-industrial countries know little about how to care for a baby, and are increasingly anxious about how to manage everyday baby-care (Scottish Government 2012a). Education provided across the transition to parenthood therefore aims to build competence in the essential parenting skills of feeding, soothing, dressing and bathing babies, and to enable parents to experience self-efficacy in the knowledge that they have the information, understanding and skills to meet their baby's basic physical needs.

Best Practice

Nobody ever learned to ride a bicycle by looking at one or by watching someone else ride one! In order to acquire a practical skill, and to feel confident in using it, there has to be practise. By including hands-on learning about bathing a baby, dressing, soothing and putting the baby safely down to sleep, antenatal education sessions have an important part to play in boosting mothers', fathers' and partners' enjoyment of parenting. In addition, handling – even a doll – in order to practise how to bath a baby, makes their unborn baby 'real' for the parents and contributes to building the relationship between them.

The midwife can lead the group in demonstrating how to bath a baby – but ideally, the parents should be doing more than just watching her; they should be copying what she is doing using a doll, baby bath, towels and baby clothes provided for the session. It is important for men to be very involved in practising baby-care skills. Research (Fatherhood Institute 2010) has shown that men and partners may find 'a way in' to having a relationship with their new baby difficult, especially if the baby is being breastfed. They may also feel that women are inherently better at baby-care than men. The midwife can assure them that this is not the case – being good at baby-care is simply a reflection of how often it has been carried out. Boosting fathers' and partners' confidence by arming them with knowledge and skills of how to look after their baby may contribute to a smoother transition to parenthood for both mothers – who have help to hand – plus fathers and partners, who feel that they have a part to play in their babies' lives.

TO REDUCE PARENTAL STRESS AND SUPPORT MENTAL HEALTH

Research suggests that while in the womb, the baby is affected by and lays down memories of his mother's vital signs. By monitoring her heart rate, blood pressure and body temperature, the baby prepares body and brain to enter a world characterized by the level of threat deduced from the mother's 'emotional temperature' (diPietro et al. 2008). The pregnant woman also influences the development of her baby's brain through the stress hormones which she bathes the baby in when they cross the placenta. Raised levels of maternal dopamine and serotonin lower the baby's tolerance of stress across the life trajectory and adversely affect the immature immune system (Howerton and Bale 2012). A mother who is experiencing chronic stress as a result of poverty, domestic violence, unfamiliarity with the country in which she is living, or substance abuse, is more likely to have her baby prematurely and more likely to have a small-for-dates baby (Wadhwa et al. 1993). Prematurity and low birth weight are predictive of ill health extending into adulthood (Barker et al. 2001).

In 2014, the London School of Economics and Centre for Mental Health reported that the total economic and social long-term cost of perinatal mental health problems, is around £8.1 billion for each 1-year cohort of births in the UK (Maternal Mental Health Alliance, MMHA 2014). In the short-term, mental ill health impacts the quality of life of the mother, and therefore, of her baby and other family members, and in the long-term, continues to impact her child, with the likelihood of problems developing that persist into adulthood. The baby's physical safety, as well as his or her emotional well-being, may be endangered if stress, depression or anxiety manifest as aggression (Lieberman and Van Horn 2013). In addition, research is increasingly demonstrating that fathers' poor mental health also adversely impacts their children's emotional and behavioural development, and their peer relationships. Domoney et al. (2013) argue that increased information about the possible difficulties of becoming a father can help to normalize men's experiences and encourage disclosure of problems early on.

Relaxation

Teaching relaxation to pregnant women and their partners provides them with a skill for life, as well as more immediately, for pregnancy and labour. Indeed, many targeted antenatal education programmes, such as Baby Steps (www.nspcc.org.uk) and Mindfulness Based Birth and Parenting (Duncan and Bardacke 2010) have relaxation at their core.

Women will often ask for relaxation to be included in their antenatal education programme. They are eager to learn skills and to practise. Some midwives may find the idea of leading relaxation sessions daunting. It is important to reflect on why it seems so challenging and to discuss concerns with experienced, skilled childbirth educators.

There are many relaxation scripts available on the internet, to which midwives can turn for help if they prefer not to make up their own. Practising leading a relaxation session for colleagues, or with the family at home, boosts confidence; ideas for engaging parents in relaxation can be gained by observing colleagues who are confident in doing this.

Discussing Mental Health

Some mothers and fathers/partners who are anxious or depressed antenatally will be helped by support mediated by friendships made at antenatal education sessions. This means that midwives have to nurture an atmosphere in which group members get to know each other and become interested in and concerned about each other. Antenatal sessions can transmit positive mental health messages. For example, the midwife might pass round the Mental Health Foundation's list of 'essentials' for maintaining good mental health (MHF 2018). She can invite parents to identify how these might be impacted by the arrival of their baby and discuss how they can adapt their lifestyles to ensure positive mental health during the postnatal period. Parents can be asked what they know about depression and share information about where help is available. Even if antenatal education impacts the mental wellbeing of only a small number of mothers and fathers/partners, reduced demands on health and social care services means savings of millions of pounds.

TO STRENGTHEN THE COUPLE RELATIONSHIP

There is much research to indicate that the transition to first-time parenthood is challenging for many couples (e.g. Doss et al. 2009; Lawrence et al. 2008). New mothers and fathers may struggle with exhaustion (Petch and Halford 2008) and role overload (Perry-Jenkins et al. 2007) and regret that they have no time for previously enjoyed leisure activities and for intimacy (Feeney et al. 2001). Couples in Western societies may find themselves largely unsupported. They may live far away from grandparents, or grandparents may be working full-time and not able to help with the new baby. Friends and neighbours may not offer support in communities where 'community' is no longer a reality. Tiredness exacerbated by anxiety over their new parental roles may lead to failures of communication between the couple (Howard and Brooks-Gunn 2009; Huston and Holmes 2004) and decreasing support for each other.

Couple conflict in the postnatal period has implications beyond the immediate wellbeing of the couple. It increases the likelihood of both parents experiencing depression during the first 2 years of their child's life (Figueiredo et al. 2017) which, in turn, negatively impacts outcomes for their babies and children (El-Sheikh et al. 2009). A mother, father or partner with a depressed spouse may experience a decrease in relationship satisfaction owing to the depressed partner's making demands, or failing to help with the unfamiliar and relentless activities associated with the care of a new baby (Benazon and Coyne 2000). Conflict may impact the way in which the couple parent their baby, and the extent to which they are consistent in responding to their baby's signals.

Best Practice

The review of antenatal education by McMillan et al. (2009) found evidence that programmes focusing on strengthening the couple's relationship in preparation for parenting improved parental confidence and satisfaction with the couple relationship in the postnatal period. Each partner in the parenting couple, whether this is same-sex or heterosexual, needs to understand the other's response to conflict and to be able to manage and resolve it. In recent years, Don and Mickelson (2014) have argued that helping couples develop positive coping strategies to meet the challenges of new parenthood may help prevent or lessen decline in relationship satisfaction. Houlston et al. (2013) suggest that parent education programmes should target the couple's relationship with key areas for discussion, those being:

- expectations of each partner of the other's role as mother/father
- how each individual's current role in relation to division of household chores might change/should change after the baby is born

- how the couple currently manages conflict in their relationship
- triggers for conflict that the couple anticipate might occur following the birth of the baby
- strategies for managing conflict openly and with negotiation.

The key messages for parents-to-be to take away from a discussion on managing conflict are (OnePlusOne 2018):

- Conflict is a normal part of relationships.
- Making-up helps a couple recover from any negative impact of conflict and keeps the relationship strong.
- Children benefit from seeing conflict managed well; when conflict is not managed well, children can be harmed both in the short and long term.
- The key skills in conflict management are recognizing when it is time to stop, talking it through and working things out together.

A common trigger for conflict postnatally is the division of household and baby-care tasks between the partners. Activities and discussions that help couples to understand each other's expectations of who will do what, when, and how often after the baby arrives, may be helpful. Prioritizing is also a key skill to minimize conflict in early parenting. Couples can be invited to put lists of household tasks and baby-care activities in order according to how important they think each is. Some couples may consider having a tidy house important; for others, this is not important. Some couples may want to bath their baby daily, and others once a week. In addition, couples need to discuss with each other the importance they attach to their leisure activities, to seeing family and friends and going out together.

TO BUILD SOCIAL SUPPORT

Increasing the extent and supportiveness of individuals' social environments is an important strategy for preventing mental ill health and enhancing wellbeing (Mitchell et al. 1982). However, the decline of family and community networks in many countries over the last 50 years means that new parents may find themselves isolated following the birth of their child, as networks of support connected with work and with friends who are childless are no longer available. This shrinking of the social network occurs at exactly the time when it is most needed. Lack of social support has been found to correlate with poor parenting quality, child physical and emotional abuse, and maternal depression, while mothers with strong social networks have been found to have more positive interactions with their babies as a result of improved mental health linked to the support they are able to access (Scott et al. 2001; see also Chapter 30).

Best Practice

Parent-to-parent support appears to play a key role in promoting social and emotional wellbeing for families (Molinuevo 2013) and belonging to peer support groups is rated highly by parents (Scottish Government 2012a). Therefore, transforming the antenatal group into a social support network ready for parents' period of greatest need following the arrival of their babies is a primary prevention strategy that can be realized through sessions which focus on helping parents get to know and become interested in and concerned about each other. Providing multiple opportunities for parents to exchange feelings and ideas during small group work, making breaks as enjoyable and friendly as possible, and suggesting to parents that they form Facebook or WhatsApp groups, or meet for coffee or antenatal exercise sessions and postnatal baby groups, are all obvious means of helping the antenatal group become a postnatal support group. If nothing else is achieved as a result of parents' attendance at antenatal sessions beyond their making new friends, this, in and of itself, is an important achievement for the midwife.

Including Fathers and Partners

Cowan et al. (1985) argued over 30 years ago that there are three different experiences of the transition to parenthood: the mother's, the father's/partner's and the couple's. (The baby's experience should also be added!) It is therefore appropriate to offer parent education in pregnancy and the early postnatal period to *both* parents, and provide couples with opportunities to think *together* about their life with a new baby, rather than addressing the mother only, leaving her feeling that the major and perhaps sole responsibility for the baby lies with her. If the father/partner is led to believe that care of the baby lies principally with the mother, this may lead to disengagement from the child and a decline in relationship satisfaction. Clapton (2014) has suggested that the marginalization of fathers presents three problems:

- It implies that fathers are optional in their children's lives.

- It is detrimental to mothers as it over-burdens them when they cannot share responsibility.
- It dissuades take-up of and participation in health and care services by fathers and pushes them towards a diminished role in the life of their families.

There are various key strategies for attracting fathers and partners to antenatal education groups and for retaining their attendance. First, it is important to ensure that the invitation to attend is addressed both to the mothers and the fathers/partners. The Fatherhood Institute (2007) recommends avoiding the term *parent* as this is commonly interpreted by both men and women as meaning mothers. The Institute also recommends not using the words *classes*, *groups* or *education* in the name of the programme, but instead to use a title that indicates a practical focus, such as *How to Have a Baby and Look After It*. It is essential to provide sessions at times that make it possible for fathers and partners to attend.

Fathers and partners want to be involved from pregnancy onwards; they want gender-specific information and to be treated as active agents in terms of supporting their child's health (Scottish Government 2012a). During sessions, their perspectives need to be sought on every topic. For example, a topic such as 'onset of labour' needs to consider both how the mother may feel *and* her partner. 'Promoting mental health' needs to be about more than what the fathers and partners can do to support the mothers, but also about what they can do to look after *themselves*. It is important to make sure that visual aids depict fathers and partners, and that there are handouts and literature available that are aimed specifically at them.

LEADING ANTENATAL EDUCATION SESSIONS

Defining Learning Outcomes

There is never enough time for antenatal sessions. This being the case, it is very important that midwives are clear about what it is they want to achieve (their aims) and what they want participants to learn. Aims have already been discussed in this chapter. Learning outcomes are vital for ensuring that the group leader and the group remain on task and that parents leave the session feeling they have learned something useful. Learning outcomes for any session will include learning in various 'domains': cognitive, emotional and physical. In order to ensure that learning outcomes define the *learning* that will have taken place, rather than the learning *activities* engaged in, every learning outcome needs to begin with the stem: '*by the end of this session, participants will be able to …*' (rather than, '*by the end of this session, participants will have done such and such an activity…*').

Learning outcomes for a session covering the relationship between unborn babies and their parents; the start of labour; comfort positions for labour; healthy eating for busy parents; and avoiding couple conflict in the postnatal period, might be expressed as follows:

By the end of this session, participants will be able to …

- *describe the importance of relaxation during pregnancy*
- *utilize relaxation strategies in their everyday lives*
- *state five signs that labour is about to start or has started*
- *demonstrate three positions that might make contractions easier to manage*
- *suggest two easy-to-make, inexpensive and nutritious meals for the first months after the baby is born*
- *agree with their partners how to divide household chores and baby care.*

Sharing Information

Any antenatal group session is likely to involve information-sharing, discussion and practical skills work. Of these, the first is probably the area in which many group leaders who are health professionals feel most competent, and the one in which they are often, in fact, least. There are two pitfalls: first, to believe that the more information given, the better; and the second, that giving information will change people's behaviour.

The fact that many midwives know from personal experience that most information is forgotten as soon as students leave a lecture, does not deter them from overloading mothers and fathers with information. In order for people to retain information:

- it must be the information that they want at this moment in their lives
- it must be linked either to first-hand experiences or to experiences other people have shared with them
- it must be presented in as many different forms as possible – verbally, in illustrated format, and/or by practical demonstration.

Many topics that might be covered in antenatal sessions are potentially information-heavy, for example, 'Labour and Birth'. Yet mothers and fathers do not need to know the anatomy and physiology or the clinical management of labour and birth in the depth that a midwife needs to know these things. What group participants need to know is, 'What will it be like for me?'

A fascinating experiment was conducted in an old-fashioned 'Nightingale Ward' in the 1950s (Janis 1958), with patients undergoing prostate surgery. The patients on one side of the ward were given detailed, technical information about the surgical procedures they would undergo. The patients on the other side of the ward were given descriptions of the sensations involved in having an anaesthetic, waking up after surgery and recovering from an abdominal wound. The patients who had received this kind of information made far speedier recoveries than those given 'textbook' information.

Mothers and fathers attending antenatal sessions already know a great deal – they will be the repositories of both correct and incorrect information. The task of the midwife is to elicit what they know, so that she can reinforce what is correct and reshape what is not. Asking participants to share their own experiences of a particular aspect of labour, for example having an induction, or what they have heard about it from friends and other informants, enables her to judge the level of knowledge in the group and to find out what parents want to know. A rich learning experience is provided by exploring the details of the experience as described by members of the group, acknowledging accurate information, asking group members themselves to correct misinformation (which they are often able to do), and answering questions raised by people on a need to know basis (Box 9.1). Embedding new information in a web made up of what people already know and their shared ideas of what an experience might be like, provides the most effective means of transmitting information, so that mothers and fathers/partners can use it to make decisions.

A study by Stapleton et al. (2002) of the effectiveness of the Midwives' Information Resource Service (MIDIRS) information leaflets came to the conclusion that women did not value or use information that was presented to them 'cold'. They *did* value having the opportunity to discuss the information presented in the

---

BOX 9.1 Sharing Group Knowledge and Experience

It is often the case that group members know far more about a topic than might be expected. Finding out what the group knows, and building on that knowledge is an important skill for the group leader. The example below is taken from an actual antenatal session.

When asked to talk about friends' experiences of having a caesarean section, group members shared a lot of information and useful insights:

- There are planned caesareans and emergency ones.
- Emergency caesareans can be traumatic for both mother and father/partner (and probably for the baby, too).
- The surgery proceeds quickly until the birth of the baby; once the baby is born, the mother remains in theatre for quite a long time afterwards.
- Some fathers/partners find being present during surgery daunting.
- Often the father holds the baby first because the mother has drips in her arms.
- There is an unexpected amount of pain afterwards and it can be difficult for the mother to hold the baby for feeding.
- Some mothers recover quickly and are back to normal in a few weeks; some take months.
- Some mothers feel fine about their caesarean and some feel as if they have 'failed'.

In this session, the group leader needed to contribute little beyond answering a few questions raised by the group members and stressing the importance of asking for help with the baby on the postnatal ward, keeping the wound clean, recognizing signs of infection and not expecting to do too much once home.

---

leaflets with a midwife who could answer their questions. This research constitutes a warning to midwives who believe that information-giving is satisfactory without interaction with the recipients and discussion as to its relevance to their circumstances.

The more varied the means by which information is transmitted, the more locations in the brain are used to store it, thus increasing the likelihood that it will be retained. Giving information verbally can be supplemented by pictures that present facts visually, thereby aiding memory and enhancing enjoyment of learning, which in itself makes learning more effective. Today, there is a huge range of video material available, which can be used to present facts in a visually exciting way,

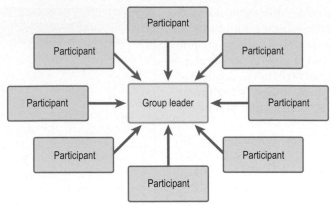

Fig. 9.1 Leader–participant interaction without group discussion.

and provide information to trigger discussion. A quick foray into YouTube will produce a multitude of video clips ideal for antenatal sessions.

Three-dimensional (3D) models that parents can handle to enable learning to take place through the hands and eyes – such as plastic pelves, dolls, different kinds of nappies and pieces of clinical equipment – help in the journey from simply knowing facts to understanding them and ultimately to applying them. Role-play is also a form of 3D modelling that is enormously effective in enriching mothers' and fathers' concept of 'what it will be like'.

Promoting Discussion

It is often mistakenly assumed that participants in an antenatal session in which the midwife gives information and the group members ask questions are having a discussion. However, a group whose interactions can be charted as in Fig. 9.1 is not having a discussion but rather, a question and answer session. A group whose interactions can be charted as in Fig. 9.2 is genuinely enjoying a discussion.

In order to have a discussion, group members need to know a little about each other and therefore to feel at ease. Ice-breakers are important to help people start to learn each other's names and something of each other's history, as well as because they make a statement that the session is going to be as much about participants talking as about the midwife talking.

A group consisting of more than six people will deter many from contributing. The midwife can break a big group into smaller ones to facilitate discussions in which everyone feels at ease to contribute.

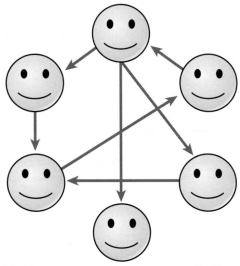

Fig. 9.2 Interactions among a group engaged in discussion.

The first 10 min of an antenatal session are an excellent learning opportunity. People are usually excited about joining the group, perhaps slightly anxious. As long as they are not paralysed with nerves, a little adrenalin primes them for learning. Ice-breakers can incorporate both a 'getting to know you' element and an exchange of ideas on topics integral to the antenatal course. Having invited group members to form small groups of three or four people, the midwife might invite them to talk about:

- what they already know about their unborn babies
- where they are planning on giving birth and why they have chosen this location
- what they think will be the most enjoyable aspects of parenting, and what the most challenging.

Sharing ideas and feelings, even if cautiously in the beginning, enables group members to appreciate that they share the same worries and concerns as other 'parents-to-be'. Establishing the commonalities that mark everyone's journey into parenthood provides a secure basis from which group members can develop friendships and engage in more profound discussions at future sessions.

Research by Nolan et al. (2012) has shown that making friends may proceed at a faster pace during pregnancy, and bypass much of the 'social chit-chat' that generally characterizes the early stages of friendship formation. An emerging appreciation of the responsibilities that parenting entails, and of the extent to which current lifestyles will change following the birth of their baby, motivates people to reach out to others for support and companionship. Perhaps the overriding duty of antenatal education sessions is to develop a social support network for parents and this is dependent on providing multiple opportunities for them to get to know each other.

Using open-ended questions such as, 'How do you feel about that?'; 'Could you say a little more?' and reflecting questions raised by individuals back to the group, e.g. 'Would anyone like to comment on that suggestion from their point of view?' are key tools in promoting discussion. Discussion may also be facilitated by prompts such as pictures and video clips, by inviting new parents to visit the group to talk about their experiences, and by engaging the group in activities that require them to do more than simply write down facts. Finding the right trigger for discussion can transform a group that appears disinterested in the session into one where everyone is contributing and learning (Box 9.2).

BOX 9.2   Promoting Valuable Discussion

A fairly reserved group of young mothers quickly began to function as a group in which quality learning was taking place when asked to discuss how to manage with a new baby on an income of only £70 a week. During the vigorous exchanges that took place, the teenagers learned from each other which shops offered the best prices for nappies and an array of household items; how to prepare a variety of easy-to-make, inexpensive (and often nutritious) meals; how to avoid bank charges; where to go to find out about benefit entitlements; and what each thought about the amount of help boyfriends and partners should give with the new baby.

Practical Skills Work

A survey by Nolan (2008) of antenatal education noted that many women wanted more time in sessions to be devoted to practising self-help skills for labour, such as breathing and other relaxation techniques, active birth positions and massage. For fathers and partners, learning baby-care skills is important and group leaders should make it a priority to help men learn how to change nappies, bathe, soothe and settle babies. High levels of father/partner involvement with their babies are strongly linked with couples' satisfaction with their relationship and with family life (Craig and Sawrikar 2006).

Many midwives are daunted at the prospect of leading practical sessions. This discomfort may be due to lack of ease with their own bodies; lack of belief that teaching such skills will make a difference in labour; a perception that group members might be reluctant to participate; and poor venues where there is insufficient space for people to move around freely. Midwives whose only preparation for antenatal education in groups has been a couple of lectures during their pre-registration training, and whose apprenticeship has been spent observing other midwives equally diffident about leading practical work, are understandably nervous. Yet labour, birth and caring for babies are intensely physical activities (as is midwifery) and people need practise to be well prepared for their role either as parent (or as midwife).

The best way to gain confidence in teaching physical skills is to observe and speak to as many confident and competent practitioners as possible. Active Birth teachers, Hypnobirthing therapists, Birth Dance teachers, antenatal teachers trained by the National Childbirth Trust (NCT) are able to demonstrate and analyse how they facilitate practical skills work.

These are some of the ways of making practical work easier for both group leaders and group members:

- Ensure that, as the group leader, you know why you are teaching certain skills, and that you have given group participants a strong rationale for why they should practise them.
- Ask everyone to try out the same active birth positions, or massage strokes, or baby-care task *at the same time*, copying you while you demonstrate.
- Support people constantly while they are practising, giving positive feedback and making suggestions to each woman or couple individually.
- Have a laugh with the group.

- If practising baby-care skills, separate the fathers/ partners from the mothers. When men are in a single sex group, they interrupt each other with supportive comments but supportive comments decrease as the number of female members in the group increases.

Group members may seem reluctant to participate in practical work, but provided that the group leader is sufficiently confident, she will be able to help people overcome their anxiety. The learning that is achieved through practical work can be dramatic (Box 9.3).

How Many in the Group?

In a study by Ho and Holroyd (2002), antenatal education sessions were attended by between 48 and 95 women. The women identified that it was impossible to engage in questioning and discussion, impossible to have their individual problems addressed, impossible to make friends and impossible for the educators to seek useful feedback from them.

Groups function best when they are composed of about 8–16 people (Sher 2016). This ensures that shy members can contribute if they want to, and gives everyone an opportunity to be heard and have his or her particular concerns addressed. It may be acceptable to offer information in a lecture style to larger groups, but it has to be questioned whether what people learn could not equally well have been learnt from a leaflet handed to them at the antenatal clinic.

How Many Sessions and How Long?

The survey of antenatal education by Nolan (2008), found that women wanted to attend more than one session. They felt that sessions held over a number of weeks gave them the opportunity to get to know the other people in the group and form friendships that would continue into the postnatal period. In addition, a single session was considered simply inadequate to cover the many topics on which they wanted to gain information and share ideas.

Information is retained according to its perceived relevance to learners. Antenatally, mothers and fathers are focused on issues relating to pregnancy, labour, birth and the first weeks of their baby's life. Following the birth, the need for more information about looking after their baby, and for support from other parents and health professionals, becomes apparent. For this reason, antenatal groups that continue into the postnatal period offer midwives a wonderful opportunity to help mothers and fathers/partners cope with problems that could only be dimly anticipated antenatally. Nolan et al. (2012) have noted that women manage anxiety about their baby's development better if they can compare notes with other women and gain a broad concept of what is 'normal'. The aim therefore should be to move away from *antenatal* education to one of *transition to parenthood* education, with sessions starting from mid-pregnancy and continuing into the first 3–6 postnatal months. It is possible that this level of support might well reduce demands on community midwives, health visitors and general practitioners (GPs), and lead to a reduction in the incidence of mental ill health and relationship breakdown following childbirth.

The length of individual sessions may well be determined by the availability of the venue and staff capacity, but whatever the length, it is important to recognize certain key features of adult learning when considering how to pace sessions. The average attention span of an adult is about 10 min. This means that activities, discussions and information-giving that continue for longer than this may result in a diminishing return as far as learning is concerned. In order to retain people's interest, every session needs a variety of learning opportunities interspersed with opportunities for reflection, to appeal to both activists and reflectors (Honey and Mumford 1982). The brain needs water, glucose and protein in order to be able to function. A break halfway through the session allows time for parents to socialize and to have a drink and something to eat – thus enhancing attention and learning capacity when the session recommences.

BOX 9.3   Practical Skills: A Significant Impact

A group that included a very young father who was clearly attending antenatal sessions under a certain amount of duress was taught some simple baby massage skills. While everyone was practising, the group leader played a compilation of nursery rhymes and talked about how massaging a baby and singing or reciting nursery rhymes would make the baby feel secure, help him or her develop language, and be a source of enjoyment for both parent and child. At the end of the session, the young father asked the group leader if she could send him the nursery rhymes she had played and tell him where he could attend baby massage sessions with his baby.

Training and Education of Practitioners

There is a popular myth, much detested by teachers that, 'those who can, do, and those who can't, teach'. Leading a group of adults may not primarily be about teaching, although there is likely to be an element of instruction. Nonetheless, ensuring that parents find the experience of attending antenatal sessions as relevant and useful as possible, demands sophisticated skills on the part of the midwife.

The quality of health and social care services has regularly been linked to the level of training of those who deliver them. For example, there is a clear link in nursery provision between how well carers have been trained to understand the needs of very small children, and children's optimal development (Department for Children, Schools and Families, DCSF 2012). The effects of parenting education for expectant and new parents have been demonstrated to vary according to the qualifications of the educators (Pinquart and Teubert 2010). In a detailed analysis of parenting support and education across Europe, Molinuevo (2013) concluded that the effective delivery of parent education services requires a workforce with adequate skills and that professionals need to devote themselves to ongoing continuing education to maintain the highest standards of best practice. Some European countries take this requirement very seriously with parent support practitioners in Austria, for example, being required to undergo a 500 hour training programme focused on parent education (Molinuevo 2013).

EVALUATION

The midwife needs to strive to achieve *balance* in each session:

- between her talking and the group members talking
- between people sitting in their seats and moving around
- between work done in the whole group and work done in small groups
- between focusing on pregnancy and birth and focusing on life with a new baby
- between group participants determining the agenda and how long to give to each topic, and the midwife managing the session.

Effective evaluation of any session could be carried out using the above list. If the programme being delivered is either a manualized programme or one that has been dictated by the institution, the midwife could ask herself the following (Social Research Unit 2016: 23):

- *Was each component of the session delivered? (Adherence)*
- *How well was each component delivered? (Quality)*
- *Was the right amount of time allocated to each component? (Dose)*
- *Did group members engage with the session? (Engagement).*

CONCLUSION

Transition to parenthood education is a primary means of building a culture of health and creating stability in communities, as these things are dependent in large part on the wellbeing of families (Verbiest et al. 2016). It is the aspiration of such education to 'level the playing field' by helping children born into under-privileged families to enjoy the same degree of physical, emotional and cognitive wellbeing, and therefore, to have as good a chance of leading a healthy, enjoyable, financially and socially secure life, as children born into easier circumstances. Scotland's National Parenting Strategy (Scottish Government 2012b) states that the most significant influence on a child's life-time opportunities is the way in which she or he is parented. Donkin et al. (2014: 89) describe the aim of early parenting education as 'to flatten the social gradient' by:

> *Improving parenting skills ... by communicating 'what works' to all parents.*

Gutman and Feinstein (2010: 555) argue that disadvantaged children are more likely to do well if they enjoy 'involved, engaged parenting' and therefore, programmes which help parents to interact sensitively with their babies and toddlers foster the positive development of less privileged children, thereby reducing inequalities dependent on social circumstances. However, parenting programmes are *not* a magic wand (Public Health England, PHE 2014b) and cannot be expected to remedy all social ills. They are one means by which outcomes for children across the life trajectory might be improved; a raft of other strategies to support new families is also required. Nonetheless, early parenting education, including antenatal education, and support should be seen as a social investment (Molinuevo 2013) and as a means of achieving social justice by improving all parents' experience and enjoyment of the transition to parenthood.

■ REFLECTIVE ACTIVITY FOR SELF-ASSESSMENT

1. To what extent do you feel that your clinical practice and your practice as an educator are focused on building the relationship between the mother and her unborn/newborn baby?
2. Have the antenatal education sessions that you have observed, or led, focused on the transition to parenthood rather than solely on labour and birth?
3. Is the midwife's educational role in preparing mothers, fathers and partners for early parenting sufficiently recognized by your profession as well as by the Trusts in which you have worked?

REFERENCES

Baby Steps (undated) Available at: www.nspcc.org.uk/services-and-resources/childrens-services/baby-steps.

Barker, D. J. P., Forsen, T., Uutela, A., et al. (2001). Size at birth and resilience to effects of poor living conditions in adult life: Longitudinal study. *British Medical Journal, 323*(1273), 1.

Barlow, J. (2016). The relationship with the unborn baby: Why it matters. *International Journal of Birth and Parent Education, 4*(1), 5–10.

Bartlett, E. E. (2004). The effects of fatherhood on the health of men: A review of the literature. *Journal of Men's Health & Gender, 1*(2–3), 159–169.

Benazon, N. R., & Coyne, J. C. (2000). Living with a depressed spouse. *Journal of Family Psychology, 14,* 71–79.

Berg, S. J., & Wynne-Edwards, K. E. (2001). Changes in testosterone, cortisol, and estradiol levels in men becoming fathers. *Mayo Clinic Proceedings, 76*(6), 582–592.

Brandon, A. R., Pitts, S., Denton, W. H., et al. (2009). A history of the theory of prenatal attachment. *Journal of Prenatal & Perinatal Psychology & Health, 23*(4), 201–222.

Campbell, V., & Nolan, M. L. (2019). 'It definitely made a difference': A grounded theory study of yoga for pregnancy and women's self-efficacy for labour. *Midwifery, 68,* 74–83.

Carter, S. (2011). The healing power of love: An oxytocin hypothesis. *Neuroscience Research, 71,* e14.

Clapton, G. (2014). The birth certificate, 'father unknown' and adoption. *Adoption and Fostering, 38*(3), 209–222.

Cowan, C. P., Cowan, P. A., Heming, G., et al. (1985). Transition to parenthood: His, hers and theirs. *Journal of Family Issues, 6,* 451–481.

CQC (Care Quality Commission). (2015). *Survey of women's experiences of maternity care.* London: Care Quality Commission.

Craig, L., & Sawrikar, P. (2006). Work and family balance: Transitions to high school. *Unpublished Draft final report.* University of New South Wales: Social Policy Research Centre.

DCSF (Department for Children, Schools and Families). (2012). *The early years: Foundations for life, health and learning.* London: DCSF.

DH (Department of Health). (2008). *The child health promotion programme: Pregnancy and the first five years of life.* London: DH/DCSF.

diPietro, J. A., Costigan, K. A., Nelson, P., et al. (2008). Fetal responses to induced maternal relaxation during pregnancy. *Biochemical Psychiatry, 77*(1), 11–19.

Domoney, J., Iles, J., & Ramchandani, P. (2013). Paternal depression in the postnatal period: Reflections on current knowledge and practice. *International Journal of Birth and Parent Education, 1*(3), 17–20.

Donkin, A., Roberts, J., Tedstone, A., et al. (2014). Family socio-economic status and young children's outcomes. *Journal of Children's Services, 9*(2), 83–95.

Don, B. P., & Mickelson, K. D. (2014). Relationship satisfaction trajectories across the transition to parenthood among low-risk parents. *Journal of Marriage and Family, 76*(3), 677–692.

Doss, B. D., Rhoades, G. K., Stanley, S. M., et al. (2009). The effect of the transition to parenthood on relationship quality: An 8-year prospective study. *Journal of Personality and Social Psychology, 96,* 601–609.

Duncan, L., & Bardacke, N. (2010). Mindfulness-based childbirth and parenting education: Promoting family mindfulness during the perinatal period. *Journal of Child and Family Studies, 19*(2), 190–202.

El-Sheikh, M., Kouros, C. D., Erath, S., et al. (2009). Marital conflict and children's externalizing behavior: Interactions between parasympathetic and sympathetic nervous system activity. *Monographs of the Society for Research in Child Development 74*(1), vii, 1–79.

Fatherhood Institute. (2007). *Including new fathers: A guide for maternity professionals.* Available at: www.fatherhoodinstitute.org/uploads/publications/246.pdf.

Fatherhood Institute. (2010). Fathers and family health in the perinatal period: A briefing on the benefits of paternal engagement. *The Fatherhood Institute (formerly Fathers Direct) 2007. Including new fathers: A guide for maternity professionals.* London: Fathers Direct.

Feeney, J. A., Hohaus, L., Noller, P., et al. (2001). *Becoming parents: Exploring the bonds between mothers, fathers and their infants*. New York: Cambridge University Press.

Feinberg, M. E., & Kan, M. L. (2008). Establishing Family Foundations: Intervention effects on coparenting, parent/infant well-being, and parent-child relations. *Journal of Family Psychology, 22*(2), 253–263.

Figueiredo, B., Canario, C., Tendais, I., et al. (2017). Couple relationship moderates anxiety and depression trajectories over the transition to parenthood. *European Journal of Public Health, 27*(Suppl. 3).

Gagnon, A. J., & Sandall, J. (2007). Individual or group antenatal education for childbirth or parenthood, or both. *Cochrane Database of Systematic Reviews* (3), CD002869.

Gilmer, C., Buchan, J. L., Letourneau, N., et al. (2016). Parent education interventions designed to support the transition to parenthood: A realist review. *International Journal of Nursing Studies, 59*, 118–133.

Gutman, L., Brown, J., & Akerman, R. (2009). *Nurturing parenting capability: The early years*. London: Centre for Research on the Wider Benefits of Learning Research: Report No. 30.

Gutman, L., & Feinstein, L. (2010). Parenting behaviours and children's development from infancy to early childhood: Changes, continuities and contributions. *Early Child Development and Care, 180*(4), 535–556.

Ho, I., & Holroyd, E. (2002). Chinese women's perceptions of the effectiveness of antenatal education in the preparation for motherhood. *Journal of Advanced Nursing, 38*(1), 74–85.

Honey, P., & Mumford, A. (1982). *Manual of learning styles*. London: Honey Publications.

Houlston, C., Coleman, L., & Mitcheson, J. (2013). Changes for the couple relationship during the transition to parenthood: Risk and protective factors. *International Journal of Birth and Parent Education, 1*(1), 18–22.

Howard, K. S., & Brooks-Gunn, J. (2009). Relationship supportiveness during the transition to parenting among married and unmarried parents. *Parenting Science and Practice, 9*, 123–142.

Howerton, C. L., & Bale, T. L. (2012). Prenatal programing: At the intersection of maternal stress and immune activation. *Hormones and Behavior, 62*(3), 237–242.

Huston, T., & Holmes, E. K. (2004). Becoming parents. In A. Vangelisti (Ed.), *Handbook of family communication* (pp. 105–133). Mahwah NJ: Erlbaum.

Huth-Bocks, A. C., Theran, S. A., Levendosky, A. A., et al. (2011). A social-contextual understanding of concordance and discordance between maternal prenatal representations of the infant and infant-mother attachment. *Infant Mental Health Journal, 34*(4), 405–426.

Janis, I. L. (1958). *Psychological stress: Psychoanalytic and behavioral studies of surgical patients*. New York: Academic Press.

Kane, G. A., Wood, V. A., & Barlow, J. (2007). Parenting programmes: A systematic review and synthesis of qualitative research. *Child: Care, Health and Development, 33*(6), 784–793.

Kassebaum, N. J., Bertozzi-Villa, A., Coggeshall, M. S., et al. (2014). Global, regional, and national levels and causes of maternal mortality during 1990–2013: A systematic analysis for the Global burden of Disease study 2013. *Lancet, 384*(9947), 980–1004.

Kim, P., Strathearn, L., & Swain, J. E. (2016). The maternal brain and its plasticity in humans. *Hormones and Behavior, 77*, 113–123.

Lawrence, E., Rothman, A. D., Cobb, R., et al. (2008). Marital satisfaction across the transition to parenthood. *Journal of Family Psychology, 22*, 41–50.

Lieberman, A. F., & Van Horn, P. (2013). Infants and young children in military families: A conceptual model for intervention. *Clinical Child and Family Psychological Review, 16*, 282–293.

McMillan, A. S., Barlow, J., & Redshaw, M. (2009). *Birth and beyond: A review of the evidence about antenatal education*. Warwick: University of Warwick.

Mechlin, J. (2001). Advice to historians on advice to mothers. *Journal of Social History, 9*(1), 44–62.

MHF (Mental Health Foundation). (2018). *How to look after your mental health – 10 top tips*. Available at: www.mental-health.org.uk/publications/how-to-mental-health.

Mitchell, R. E., Billings, A. G., & Moos, R. H. (1982). Social support and well-being: Implications for prevention programs. *Journal of Primary Prevention, 3*(2), 77–98.

MMHA (Maternal Mental Health Alliance). (2014). *Costing perinatal mental health and understanding cost-effectiveness*. London: Maternal Mental Health Alliance.

Molinuevo, D. (2013). *Parenting support in Europe*. Dublin: European Foundation for the Improvement of Living and Working Conditions.

NHS Digital. 2017 Maternity services monthly statistics – May 2017. Available at: https://digital.nhs.uk/data-and-information/publications/statistical/maternity-services-monthly-statistics/may-2017.

Nolan, M. (2008). Antenatal survey (1). What do women want? *The Practising Midwife, 11*(1), 26–28.

Nolan, M., Mason, V., Snow, S., et al. (2012). Making friends at antenatal classes: A qualitative exploration of friendship across the transition to motherhood. *The Journal of Perinatal Education, 21*(3), 178–185.

OnePlusOne. (2018). *How to argue better*. Available at: www.oneplusone.space/how-to-argue-better/.

O'Mahoney, F., Hofmeyr, G. J., & Menon, V. (2010). Choice of instruments for assisted vaginal delivery. *Cochrane Database of Systematic Reviews, 2010,* (11). Available at: www.cochranelibrary.com/cdsr/doi/10.1002/14651858.CD005455.pub2/abstract.

Perry-Jenkins, M., Goldberg, A. E., Pierce, C. P., et al. (2007). Shift work, role overload and the transition to parenthood. *Journal of Marriage and Family, 68*, 123–138.

Petch, J., & Halford, W. K. (2008). Psycho-education to enhance couples' transition to parenthood. *Clinical Psychology Review, 28*, 1125–1137.

PHE (Public Health England). (2014a). *Improving the home to school transition*. London: PHE Publications.

PHE (Public Health England). (2014b). *Good quality parenting programmes*. London: PHE Publications.

Pinquart, M., & Teubert, D. (2010). Effects of parenting education with expectant and new parents: A meta-analysis. *Journal of Family Psychology, 24*(3), 316–327.

POST (Parliamentary Office of Science and Technology). (2002). *Caesarean sections*. London: POST.

Scott, D., Brady, S., & Glynn, P. (2001). New mother groups as a social network intervention: Consumer and maternal and child health nurse perspectives. *Australian Journal of Advanced Nursing, 18*(4), 23–29.

Scottish Government. (2012a). *Bringing up children: Your views*. Edinburgh: The Scottish Government.

Scottish Government. (2012b). *National parenting strategy: Making a positive difference to children and young people through parenting*. Edinburgh: The Scottish Government.

Seimyr, L., Sjögren, B., Welles-Nyström, B., et al. (2009). Antenatal maternal depressive mood and parental-fetal attachment at the end of pregnancy. *Archives of Women's Mental Health, 12*, 269–279.

Sher, J. (2016). Missed periods: A primer on preconception health, education and care. *An independent report commissioned by NHS Greater Glasgow and Clyde*. Glasgow: Public Health.

Siegal, D. J. (2012). *The Developing Mind* (2nd ed.). New York: Guildford Press.

Smith, H., Peterson, N., Lagrew, D., et al. (2016). *Toolkit to support vaginal birth and reduce primary cesareans: A quality improvement toolkit*. Stanford: CMQCC.

Social Research Unit. (2016). *Better evidence for a better start*. Dartington: SRU.

Stapleton, H., Kirkham, M., & Thomas, G. (2002). Qualitative study of evidence based leaflets in maternity care. *British Medical Journal, 324*, 639.

Verbiest, S., Malin, C. K., Drummonds, M., et al. (2016). Catalyzing a reproductive health and social justice movement. *Maternal and Child Health Journal, 20*, 741–748.

Vreeswijk, C. M. J. M., Maas, A. J. B. M., & van Bakel, H. J. A. (2012). Parental representations: A systematic review of the working model of the child Interview. *Infant Mental Health Journal, 33*(3), 314–328.

Wadhwa, P. D., Sandman, A., Porto, M., et al. (1993). The association between prenatal stress and infant birth weight and gestational age at birth: A prospective investigation. *American Journal of Obstetrics and Gynecology, 169*(4), 858–865.

Wharton, K. R., Ecker, J. L., & Wax, J. R. (2017). Approaches to limit intervention during labor and birth. Committee on Obstetric Practice. *Obstetrics & Gynecology, 129*(2), e20–e28.

ANNOTATED FURTHER READING

Department of Health. (2011). *Preparation for birth and beyond: A resource pack for leaders of community groups and activities*. London: DH. Available at: www.dh.gov.uk/en/Publicationsandstatistics/Publications/PublicationsPolicyAndGuidance/DH_130565.

Lots of practical activities for use with diverse groups of parents are described in this manual and copyright-free worksheets can be downloaded.

Dempsey, R. (2013). *Birth with confidence: Savvy choices for normal birth*. Australia: Boat House Press.

This innovative book describes a series of pivotal moments in labour when women may lose confidence in their ability to birth their babies. It demonstrates how sensitive support can make the difference to the outcome of labour.

Leech, P. (2017). *Transforming infant wellbeing: Research, policy and practice for the first 1001 critical days*. London: Routledge.

This book brings together contemporary research involving pregnancy, birth and infancy and shows the gap between what is known and what is being done. It argues that acting on the research would make a positive difference to individuals, families and society as a whole from one generation to the next.

Daws, D., & de Rementeria, A. (2015). *Finding your way with your baby*. London: Routledge.

This is a book for parents but it is invaluable reading for midwives, describing the complex experience of motherhood and fatherhood and the emotional life of the baby in the first year.

USEFUL WEBSITES

NCT (National Childbirth Trust): www.nct.org.uk

National Society for the Prevention of Cruelty to Children: www.nspcc.org.uk – provides useful resources such as video clips about the social baby available at: https://learning.nspcc.org.uk/research-resources/pre-2013/social-baby/

The Fatherhood Institute (UK): www.fatherhoodinstitute.org

10

Change and Adaptation in Pregnancy

Irene Murray, Jenny Hendley

CHAPTER CONTENTS

Anatomical and physiological adaptations occurring throughout pregnancy affect virtually every body system. The timing and intensity of the changes vary between systems but all are designed to support fetal growth and development, and prepare the woman for birth and motherhood. Many of the changes originate in the luteal phase of the menstrual cycle. These are accentuated following conception, orchestrated by a complex interplay of progressive neurohormonal adaptive responses. The midwife's appreciation of pregnancy adaptations is essential to avoid misinterpretation and to ensure the recognition of abnormal findings, enabling her to provide appropriate midwifery care to each woman, including those affected by pre-existing illness. A common feature of these changes is the dynamic and symbiotic partnership between the uteroplacental unit and the woman influenced by physical, mechanical, genetic and hormonal factors. Studies on pregnancy have been relatively few but as maternal health and the appropriate adaptation to pregnancy will determine the health of the next generation, there is a driving need for intense research in every area of physiological adaptation to pregnancy (Thornburg et al. 2015). (Changes in the breast are detailed in Chapter 27 and changes in the woman's emotional state due to hormonal factors are discussed in Chapter 30.)

- provide an overview of the adaptation of each body system during pregnancy and the underlying hormonal changes
- identify the physiological changes that mimic or mask disease in pregnancy
- provide the rationale for common disorders in pregnancy in order for the midwife to facilitate appropriate advice
- review the diagnosis of pregnancy.

PHYSIOLOGICAL CHANGES IN THE REPRODUCTIVE SYSTEM

During pregnancy, the uterus undergoes immense changes to provide the optimal environment for the protection and nurturing of the embryo and growing fetus, and to provide the mechanisms for safe parturition (Myers and Elad 2017). These structural and functional changes take place mainly in the *endometrium* for embryo implantation and fetal growth, and the *myometrium* for structural support and contractions during labour (Wu et al. 2018). The *perimetrium*, which partially covers the myometrium becomes greatly stretched and distorted as the uterus grows (Ahluwalia et al. 2018).

Perimetrium

The perimetrium is the outermost layer of the uterus. Mostly made of loose connective tissue, it protects the uterus from friction with other organs in the body (Baah-Dwomoh et al. 2016). Stretching from the pelvic walls to the uterus, the perimetrium drapes over both uterus and uterine tubes, where it forms deep supportive parallel folds known as *broad ligaments* (van Baal et al. 2016) (see Chapter 3). The broad ligament opens out to accommodate the massive increase in the sizes of the uterine and ovarian vessels, lymphatics and nerves (Standring 2016). The uterine veins, in particular, can reach about 1 cm in diameter and they appear to act as a significant reservoir for blood during uterine contractions (Standring 2016).

Myometrium

The myometrium is the muscular wall of the uterus that undergoes dramatic remodelling during pregnancy in order to: provide support for the growing fetus; expel the fetus and placenta during labour; contract after birth to prevent maternal haemorrhage; and finally to remodel by involution to the non-pregnant status within

4 weeks of birth (Myers and Elad 2017). The myometrium is composed of millions of smooth muscle cells known as *myocytes* (Myers and Elad 2017). The myocytes are elongated, spindle-shaped cells which, when relaxed in the non-pregnant state, are around 5 μm in width and 50 μm in length, increasing 10-fold in volume throughout pregnancy (Myers and Elad 2017). Individual myocytes are grouped together into *bundles* giving the uterus its contractile functionality. Connective tissue sheaths containing elastic fibres, blood vessels, lymphatics and nerves surround and connect the neighbouring bundles. Several dozens of myocyte bundles embedded within an extracellular matrix (ECM) of collagen, elastin, proteoglycans and other adhesion molecules forms the *fasciculus*, the predominant macroscopic structural element of the myometrium (Myers and Elad 2017). Each fasciculus is 1–2 mm in diameter and several centimetres long and directs the contractile force of its myocytes. Fasciculi run in circumferential, longitudinal and oblique directions within the myometrium (Myers and Elad 2017).

Myometrial layers

The classic description of the three layers of myometrium (*stratum supravasculare*, *stratum vasculare* and *stratum subvasculare*) found in most major texts was observed during research in other species such as the rat and mouse. In spite of extensive investigation since the end of the 19th century, researchers continue to have difficulty in describing and agreeing on the directional planes of human myometrial muscle fibres, finding some layers to be 'almost indescribable' (Escalante and Pino 2017).

The three layers described here follow the classic description:

1. The outermost layer (*stratum supravasculare*) lying beneath the perimetrium and containing longitudinal fibres, which arch over the fundus and extend into the various ligaments (Sheldon et al. 2015) (Fig. 10.1).

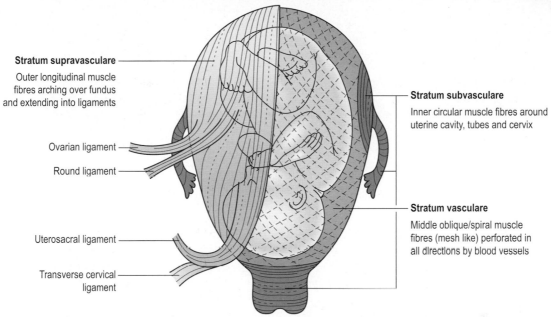

Stratum supravasculare
Outer longitudinal muscle fibres arching over fundus and extending into ligaments

Ovarian ligament

Round ligament

Uterosacral ligament

Transverse cervical ligament

Stratum subvasculare
Inner circular muscle fibres around uterine cavity, tubes and cervix

Stratum vasculare
Middle oblique/spiral muscle fibres (mesh like) perforated in all directions by blood vessels

Fig. 10.1 Myometrium showing inner, middle and outer layers of the pregnant uterus with the outer layer extending into ligaments.

2. The middle layer (*stratum vasculata*) forms the largest part of the myometrium and is comprised of a dense network of muscle fibres perforated in all directions by blood vessels. Each myocyte has a double curve forming a figure of 8 – an arrangement crucial to the contraction of the myocytes following birth in order to constrict blood vessels and halt bleeding (Cunningham et al. 2018).

3. The inner myometrium (*stratum subvasculare*) lies immediately under the endometrium and consists of bundles of smooth muscle cells arranged as a circular layer, which wraps around the uterine cavity and cervix (Kashgari et al. 2015). Sphincter-like fibres surround the orifices of the uterine tube and cervical os (Cunningham et al. 2018).

Phases of myometrial development. Myometrial growth in pregnancy is due mainly to *hyperplasia* (the rapid 10-fold increase in myocytes) and *hypertrophy* (increase in the size of myocytes). Hyperplasia occurs during the first half of pregnancy (*proliferative phase*), while hypertrophy and remodelling of the extracellular matrix (ECM) occurs during the latter half of pregnancy (*synthetic phase*) (Mesiano et al. 2015). It occurs mainly in the body of the uterus, being minimal within the cervical myometrium (Cunningham et al. 2018).

The lower uterine segment is formed from the *isthmus*, which does not undergo hypertrophy and becomes increasingly thin and distensible (Norwitz et al. 2014). Between 12 and 16 weeks' gestation a gradual unfolding of the internal os occurs and by 20 weeks, the entire isthmic part forms the inferior part of the body of the uterus. The uterus becomes more spherical, allowing for expansion of the amniotic sac with minimal uterine stretching (Myers and Elad 2017). At term, the upper part of the lower segment has stretched to about 10 cm above the internal os. It is thinner and less vascular than the upper segment and the muscle fibres are arranged mainly transversely (Rawal 2016).

The uterus grows dramatically during pregnancy mostly due to increased vascularity and fluid retention in the myometrium. Growth is driven by a combination of mechanical stretching and the combined actions of progesterone and oestrogens produced by the maternal ovary or placenta (Standring 2016). In the first 12 weeks of pregnancy, growth is due mainly to hypertrophy of myometrial cells (Menon et al. 2016) induced by the mechanical load that pregnancy imposes on the uterine wall. Some hyperplasia occurs due to the growth of myometrial arteries and veins promoted by growth factors such as insulin-like growth factor-1 (IGF-1) interacting

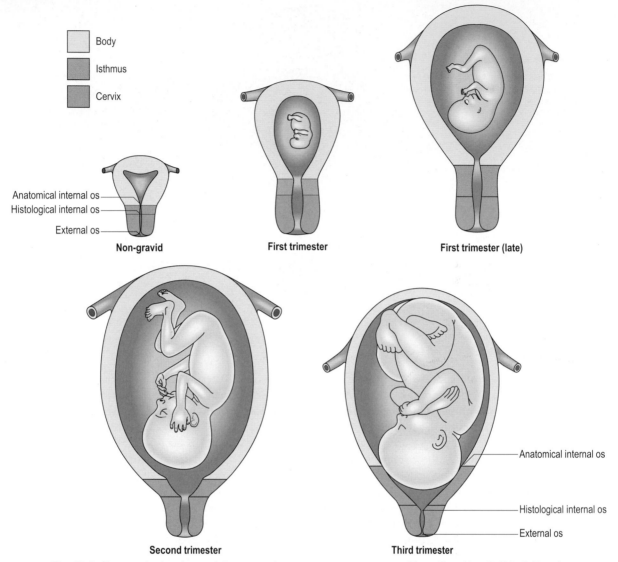

Body
Isthmus
Cervix

Anatomical internal os
Histological internal os
External os

Non-gravid

First trimester

First trimester (late)

Anatomical internal os
Histological internal os
External os

Second trimester

Third trimester

Fig. 10.2 Changes in the shape of the uterus from non-pregnant to term. (From Standring S. (2016) Female reproductive system. In: Gray's anatomy (41st ed.). London: Elsevier.)

with oestrogen (Standring 2016). Up to the 4th month the uterus increases its muscular mass by 30 times (Marani and Koch 2014). After 20 weeks, fetal growth rate accelerates and mechanical distension causes the uterus to rapidly elongate and the walls begin to thin (Myers and Elad 2017). Its height grows more quickly than its width, particularly between 20 and 32 weeks. From 28 weeks until term when fetal growth rate is at its maximum, the uterus slows its tissue growth while continuing to stretch and thin (Myers and Elad 2017).

During the third trimester the myometrium transitions from hyperplasia to hypertrophy, rapidly stretching and thinning as fetal growth exceeds growth of the uterus (Menon et al. 2016) (Fig. 10.2).

During most of pregnancy the myometrium is relatively unresponsive to additional endocrine stimulation and is in a passive, non-contractile state of relaxation or quiescence (Standring 2016) while it grows, unfolds and stretches to accommodate the enlarging fetus and placenta (Myers and Elad 2017). The balance between quiescent and contractile states are controlled by the relaxing influences of progesterone and the repression of inflammation within the myometrium (Brubaker et al. 2016). Minor factors involved in maintaining uterine quiescence are prostacyclin, relaxin, parathyroid hormone, calcitonin, vasoactive intestinal peptide and nitric oxide, all of which inhibit the release of intracellular calcium for myometrial contractility (Vannuccini et al. 2016).

Progesterone, as its name implies, is a 'pro-gestation' hormone that is essential for the establishment and maintenance of pregnancy. It is secreted by the placenta into the maternal circulation, in large amounts. It promotes myometrial relaxation, cervical closure and decidual quiescence (Menon et al. 2016). It stimulates uterine nitric oxide (NO) (a major factor in uterine quiescence), inhibits the production of prostaglandin and the development of calcium channels and oxytocin receptors, and is in dynamic balance with oestrogen in the control of uterine activity (Vannuccini et al. 2016). Progesterone and relaxin decrease the density and permeability of *gap junctions*, which are specialized channels that facilitate electrical and metabolic communication between adjacent myometrial cells. During Phase 0, gap junctions are scant and poorly electrically connected, resulting in the myometrium producing only weak and uncoordinated contractile activity (Mesiano et al. 2015). Spontaneous, poorly-coordinated uterine contractions were first described by Braxton Hicks in 1872. These contractions appear unpredictably and sporadically and are usually non-rhythmic, only becoming more frequent as term approaches (Cunningham et al. 2018). They are not effective in dilating the cervix and are likely the myometrial response to distention (Mesiano et al. 2015). Late in pregnancy they may cause discomfort and be confused with so-called 'false labour' (Cunningham et al. 2018).

In contrast to most species, human parturition is triggered by a functional rather than a systemic withdrawal of progesterone causing target cells in the uterus to be desensitized to its pro-gestational actions (Menon et al. 2016). Progesterone levels remain high throughout labour, decreasing only after expulsion of the placenta (Sivarajasingam et al. 2016). The switch from the contractures of the quiescent phase to the contractions associated with activation of uterine function (Phase 1) may start weeks prior to the onset of active labour. It involves an increase in myometrial contractility and cervical softening with inflammation of the tissues (Mesiano et al. 2015). A rise in oestrogen and

TABLE 10.1 Increases in Weight and Size of the Uterus during Pregnancy

	Nulliparous	Parous	At Term
Weight of uterus (g)	70	110	1100
Size of uterus (cm)	7 × 5 × 2.5	8 × 6 × 3.5	30 × 23 × 20
Volume of uterus (mL)	10		5L

From Cunningham G, Leveno K, Bloom S, et al. (Eds) (2018) Williams obstetrics. London: McGraw-Hill Education; Menon R, Bonney E, Condon J, et al. (2016).

corticotrophic releasing hormone (CRH) along with mechanical stretch is thought to trigger the activation of connexin 43, prostaglandin and oxytocin receptors, all of which are required for contractions (Vannuccini et al. 2016).

During Phase 2, oestrogen, oxytocin and prostaglandins increase the density and permeability of the gap junctions between the myometrial cells (Sheldon et al. 2015). The increase in the number of gap junctions coincides with the onset of the coordinated, rhythmic, forceful contractions of active labour with progressive cervical softening and dilatation, and birth of the fetus and placenta. Following the birth of the fetus and placenta (Phase 3) the myometrium sustains forceful contractions to constrict the spiral arterioles and control bleeding under the influence of oxytocin (Mesiano et al. 2015).

The shape of the gravid uterus is strikingly different between women. It contains irregular and asymmetric features and undergoes large changes with the growth of the fetus (Menon et al. 2016).

For the first few weeks, the uterus maintains its original pear-shape but by 12 weeks' gestation the corpus and fundus become globular and almost spherical (Table 10.1). Subsequently, it grows more rapidly in length than width and becomes ovoid (Cunningham et al. 2018). During the first trimester the isthmus hypertrophies like the uterine body, and triples in length to become about 3 cm long (Standring 2016) (Fig. 10.2).

Wall thickness. During pregnancy, the uterus is transformed into a thin-walled muscular organ capable of accommodating the fetus, placenta and amniotic fluid. During the first few months of pregnancy the walls of the corpus thicken up to 3 cm and lengthen considerably but after 20 weeks, with acceleration of fetal growth, they gradually thin to 1–2 cm thick by term and the fetus can usually be palpated through the soft, readily indentable uterine walls (Cunningham et al. 2018). The wall of the isthmus and the body are the same thickness from the second trimester but by the middle of the third trimester, the walls of the lower uterine segment are <1 cm thick, and are significantly thinner at term in women who have had a previous caesarean section (Ginsberg et al. 2013). The thicker myometrium in the body of the uterus is the main contractile portion that will generate the contractions of labour. The lower uterine segment is more compliant and allows for the descent of the fetus in late pregnancy and during labour. As it is thinner and less vascular than the upper uterus, it is the preferred site of incision during a caesarean section. In addition, because it is less contractile, there is a lower risk of uterine rupture in subsequent pregnancies, compared with an incision made in the body of the uterus during a 'classical' caesarean section (Standring 2016).

Endometrium (decidua). The transformation of the endometrium during Phase 0 is one of the most critical and remarkable events that occurs in pregnancy. Impairment of this process can lead to infertility, recurrent miscarriage and uteroplacental disorders (Okada et al. 2017). During the secretory phase of each menstrual cycle, the endometrium transforms into a receptive tissue that is suitable for implantation and for supporting a pregnancy (Okada et al. 2017). This process of *decidualization* occurs in response to elevated levels of oestrogen and progesterone and is independent of an implanting blastocyst. Progesterone receptor is highly expressed in the stromal cells in pregnancy and is a prerequisite for successful implantation (Okada et al. 2017). Following implantation of the blastocyst, stromal tissue further differentiates in the *decidual reaction* of pregnancy, whereupon the endometrium is known as the 'decidua' (Degner et al. 2016). Decidualization is essential in the coordinated regulation of trophoblast invasion and placental formation (Okada et al. 2017). It begins approximately 6 days after ovulation at the onset of the assumed 'window of implantation' and occurs when the elongated fibroblast-like mesenchymal cells in the uterine stroma differentiate into rounded epithelioid-like cells. Decidualized stroma cells include fibronectin, laminin and collagen and form the ECM, which enables them to prepare the endometrium for implantation, protect it

from aggressive invasion by the trophoblast and provide nutrition for the implanting blastocyst prior to placental formation. They protect the embryo, encapsulate, enclose and protect it from stressors and from maternal immunological rejection (Okada et al. 2017). The decidua is regionalized as the *deciduas basalis* (between the blastocyst and myometrium), the *decidua capsularis* (which covers the part penetrated by the blastocyst) and the *decidua vera* (the remaining endometrial lining) (Mesiano et al. 2015). Distension of the amniotic sac gradually brings the decidua capsularis to fuse with the deciduas pareitalis (Patil and Patil 2014).

During pregnancy, the cells of the trophoblast penetrate deeply into the myometrium and change the structure of the spiral and arcuate arteries causing them to dilate greatly and to lose the muscle and elastic layer around them (Marani and Koch 2014). They start to dilate due to reduced organization of vascular smooth muscle cells long before the trophoblast reaches the vessel. This remodelling of the spiral arterioles allows for low-resistance flow into the intervillous space (Standring 2016). The spiral artery only gives the impression of spiralling – it does not spiral around its own axis but instead follows a tortuous course. By the end of 5 weeks' gestation, this spiralling of the uterine vessels is more pronounced as a result of axial longitudinal growth of the vessel in excess to the increase in endometrial thickness. The increase in vessel wall diameter and thinning of the vessel wall is a prerequisite to trophoblastic invasion. By the end of week 10, when the decidua has become greatly thinned due to the growth of the conceptus, the spiral arteries follow an oblique or diagonal course rather than radial. The tortuosity of the uterine vessels increases due to further lengthwise growth and their accommodation with a relatively narrower, thinner uterine wall (Degner et al. 2016).

During the second trimester, spiralling is further intensified and by 18–24 weeks the increased thickness of the uterine wall causes the apparent coils of the uterine arteries to straighten out and assume an undulating course. This growth and expansion of the vessel continues as gestation advances (Degner et al. 2016). By mid-pregnancy, the diameter of the arcuate arteries exceeds that of the uterine vessels. Thus, the pressure in the arcuate arteries is lower than that of the uterine arteries, which facilitates vasodilation in the uterine wall and a reduction in the systemic vascular resistance and pressure (Marani and Koch 2014). Following vascular remodelling, the spiral arteries are known as the utero-placental vessels. These vessels provide blood to the intervillous space where the maternal blood is free to interact with the fetal villous tree. The diameter of the uteroplacental arteries have a mean diameter of 500 microns – a significant increase compared with the 200 micron-diameter in non-pregnant uterine spiral arteries (Degner et al. 2016).

Until the beginning of the second trimester, trophoblast plugs block the spiral arteries, which occludes the flow of oxygenated maternal red blood cells to the intervillous space of the placenta. Trophoblasts also invade uterine glands and open them towards the intervillous space ensuring nutrition for the embryo prior to the onset of a functioning placenta (Weiss et al. 2016). From 6 to 11 weeks' gestation, the plugs gradually disintegrate allowing maternal blood to perfuse the intervillous space and oxygen concentration to rise. This process is not completed until around week 18 when the spiral arteries are converted into wide bore openings, which slows the velocity of blood flow entering the intervillous space to a rate that is conducive to maximal exchange. The maternal blood does not seep passively from these vessels but rather it leaves the artery mouth in a jet-like stream, which ensures penetration of maternal blood deep into the placental tissue (James et al. 2017).

Blood supply to the uterus increases nearly 10 times from 50–100 mL/min to 500–800 mL/min but diminishes after the 6th month (Marani and Koch 2014). The uterine and ovarian arteries hypertrophy greatly in pregnancy (Cunningham et al. 2018). There is a 10-fold increase in uterine blood flow – from 2% of cardiac output in the non-pregnant state to 17% at term. The blood is redistributed within the uterus and as pregnancy progresses, 80–90% goes to the placenta and the remainder is equally distributed between the myometrium and endometrium (Norwitz et al. 2014). The passage of blood through the dilated uterine vessels produces a soft, blowing sound known as the *uterine souffle*. It is heard most distinctly near the lower portion of the uterus and is synchronous with the maternal pulse. In contrast the *funic souffle*, a sharp, whistling sound synchronous with the fetal pulse, is caused by the rush of blood through the umbilical arteries and may not be heard consistently (Cunningham et al. 2018).

The site of placental attachment and implantation of the blastocyst in the uterus is determined by many different factors. In early pregnancy, it often appears to be situated near the internal os but in the majority of cases as the uterus grows and stretches, it draws the placenta upwards and away from the cervix (Standring 2016). An endometrial thickness of 8 mm or more is necessary for successful implantation. By 6 weeks, the endometrial thickness beneath the implanted embryo is around 5 mm and by 14 weeks' gestation, the endometrium regresses to 1 mm thick (Burton et al. 2017).

Changes in uterine shape and size

Although fruit sizes are variable, comparing the uterus with fruit on bimanual examination in early pregnancy is an established method of estimating gestational age. At 5 weeks' gestation, the uterus is approximately the size of a small unripe *pear*. The 6-week pregnant uterus feels like a *small orange*. By 8 weeks, it feels like a *large orange*. By 12 weeks, the pregnant uterus feels like a *grapefruit* (Morgan and Cooper 2018). Traditionally, gestational age was assessed by comparing uterine height with abdominal landmarks such as the umbilicus and the xiphisternum on abdominal palpation (Robert Peter et al. 2015). This method is very subjective with wide inter-observer differences. International standards for serial symphysis–fundal height measurement are now recommended as a first level screening tool for monitoring fetal growth (Papageorghiou et al. 2016) (see Chapter 13).

12th week of pregnancy. The fundus becomes palpable just above the pubic symphysis at the end of the 12th week (Bouyou et al. 2015). For the first few weeks of pregnancy, the uterus maintains its original pear-shape but as pregnancy advances, the corpus and fundus become globular and by 12 weeks, it is almost spherical. Thereafter it increases more rapidly in length than in width and becomes ovoid in shape and tension is exerted on the broad and round ligaments (Cunningham et al. 2018). From the 3rd month onwards it continues to grow by 4 cm each month (Marani and Koch 2014). The uterine tubes are displaced upwards and laterally and the ovaries are lifted high in the pelvis (Standring 2016).

16th week of pregnancy. Between 12 and 16 weeks' gestation, the fundus – a previously flattened convexity between tubal insertions – becomes dome-shaped (Cunningham et al. 2018). As it extends out of the pelvis it contacts the anterior abdominal wall and displaces the intestines laterally and superiorly (Cunningham et al. 2018). The uterine isthmus unfolds and is taken up into the corpus to create the *lower uterine segment* (Fig. 10.2).

BOX 10.1 **Supine Hypotensive Syndrome**

In later pregnancy (from 24 weeks) the gravid uterus occludes the inferior vena cava and laterally displaces the subrenal aorta, this is particularly so when the mother lies supine. This *aortocaval* compression has a profound effect on venous return to the heart (Humphries et al. 2017).

Turning from a lateral to a supine position can reduce maternal cardiac output by 10–30% (Lee and Landau 2017). The event is often concealed, because only 10% of pregnant women will exhibit supine hypotension syndrome (Humphries et al. 2017). The majority of women are able to compensate by raising systemic vascular resistance and heart rate. Blood from the lower limbs may also return through the development of paravertebral collateral circulation, however if these are not well developed or adequately perfused, the pregnant woman may experience *supine hypotensive syndrome*. This occurs in around 10% of the childbearing population and consists of *hypotension, bradycardia, dizziness, light-headedness* and *nausea*, if the woman remains in the supine position too long. The fall in blood pressure may be severe enough for the woman to lose consciousness due to reduced cerebral blood flow. Compression of the aorta may lead to reduced uteroplacental and renal blood flow and fetal compromise but can be relieved by placing a wedge under the woman's hip or by tilting the operating table to displace the uterus (Lee and Landau 2017).

The uterus then becomes more spherical, allowing expansion of the amniotic sac (Myers and Elad 2017). As the uterus rises it is normal for it to rotate to the right (*dextrorotation*) due to the recto-sigmoid colon on the left side of the pelvis. Rotation of >45 degrees, however, would represent torsion of the uterus (Hoffmann and Jayaratnam 2018). The ovaries more than double their size in pregnancy and by 14 weeks' gestation, they become partly abdominal structures (Standring 2016).

20th week of pregnancy. By the 20th week of pregnancy, the uterine fundus is at the level of the umbilicus and by 24 weeks, the distance between the pubic symphysis and the uterine fundus generally corresponds to the number of gestational weeks and is often used in clinical care as a screening method to detect a pregnancy that is measuring suspiciously larger or smaller than expected. If there is more than a 2 cm discrepancy, a more accurate, sonographic assessment of fetal size and amniotic fluid volume is indicated (Standring 2016). As the uterus expands there is increasing stress and tension on the round ligaments, which hypertrophy and increase considerably in length and diameter (Standring 2016). This can cause severe pelvic and low back pain, which may occur suddenly, and often at night on changing positions in bed (Shasteen and Pontius 2017). This pain is considered to be physiological in normal pregnancy and usually resolves spontaneously with rest (Chaudhry and Chaudhry 2018).

30th week of pregnancy. In the supine position, the enlarging uterus can cause aortocaval compression, leading to reduced venous return to the heart and decreased cardiac output. In some women, this can lead to symptomatic hypotension and symptoms of nausea and faintness (Standring 2016) (Box 10.1). By 32 weeks, the appendix lies above the iliac crest and the right tube and ovary is displaced posteriorly behind the uterus. The left tube and ovary are displaced behind the small bowel and sigmoid colon (Bouyou et al. 2015). Upward and lateral displacement of the appendix in later pregnancy can cause difficulties in the diagnosis of appendicitis.

The uterine tubes and ovaries are totally abdominal structures and lie vertically behind and lateral to the parous uterus (Standring 2016).

36th week of pregnancy. At 36 weeks, the uterus reaches the level of the xiphisternum and about half of the cervical canal is incorporated into the lower uterine segment. Bladder and rectum space is reduced and the uterus lies against the ureters (Marani and Koch 2014). Intraperitoneal organs are displaced making the localization of pain and peritoneal signs more challenging to diagnose (Ahluwalia et al. 2018).

38th week of pregnancy. By term, the fundus almost reaches the liver and only the lower-third of the cervical canal and external os remain to be dilated in the first stage of labour. The rising height of the uterus causes further tension on broad and round ligaments. The abdominal wall supports the uterus and maintains a longitudinal axis corresponding to the pelvic inlet axis unless the wall is lax (Cunningham et al. 2018). Towards the end of pregnancy the jejunum, ileum and transverse colon tend to be displaced upwards by the enlarging uterus, and the sigmoid colon is displaced posteriorly and to the left (Standring 2016). The uterus lies alongside the greater omentum and it displaces the stomach posteriorly. On the right, it lies in contact with the inferior border of the liver and gallbladder (Bouyou et al. 2015). The increase in intra-abdominal pressure produced by the gravid uterus may produce eversion of the umbilicus. In multiparous women, diastasis (divarication) of right and left rectus abdominis may occur to further accommodate the enlarging uterus (Standring 2016).

UTERINE DIVISIONS

The lower segment myometrium is unique from that in the upper uterine segment, resulting in distinct roles for each near term and during labour (Cunningham et al. 2018). The upper segment contracts, retracts during contractions, whereas the lower segment is softer, distended and more passive to develop into a greatly expanded, thinned-out tube through which the fetus can pass (Cunningham et al. 2018). By term, the upper boundary of the lower uterine segment is about 10 cm above the internal os (Zara and Depuis 2017). The area of loose attachment of the peritoneum on the front of the uterus and upper limit is marked by the firm attachment of the peritoneum and corresponds to the site of the *physiological retraction ring*, which marks the boundary between upper and lower uterine segments and lies about two fingers above the pubic hair but is not palpable in normal labour (Rawal 2016).

As the lower uterine segment becomes fully developed, the fetal head descends into the pelvic brim; this is known as *lightening*. The abdomen commonly undergoes a shape change, sometimes described by women as 'the baby dropped' (Cunningham et al. 2018). There is usually a decrease in fundal height and the woman may report a decrease in pregnancy symptoms related to intra-abdominal pressure, however there is likely an increase in gastrointestinal symptoms related to fetal pressure within the pelvis (Edmonds and Zabbo 2017). Descent of the fetal head into the pelvic brim (*engagement*) at 38 weeks' gestation in the primigravida has traditionally been considered a reassuring sign that labour will proceed normally. The unengaged or 'floating' head at term or onset of labour has been considered an important risk factor for cephalopelvic disproportion (Pahwa et al. 2018). In many multigravidae, however,

and some primigravidae, the fetal head is freely movable, or 'floating' above the pelvic brim at the onset of labour. However, this does not appear to affect vaginal birth rates (Cunningham et al. 2018).

The Cervix

The cervix is normally 3 cm long and 2.5 cm in diameter, although these dimensions vary considerably between women depending on ethnicity, race, maternal age and parity. The cervix is considered 'short' with an increased risk of preterm labour if it is <2.5 cm long (Norwitz et al. 2014). Its function is to resist the downward push of the amniotic sac and the upward pull of the uterine wall. The transition between the muscular uterus to the collagenous cervix is seamless with smooth muscle cell content declining towards the external os (Norwitz et al. 2014). The cervix can be divided into three compartments: the *ectocervix*, that projects into the vagina and is lined by epithelial cells; the *endocervix* that forms the lining of the cervical canal; *stromal fibroblasts* that form the body of the cervix that connects to the myometrium. The main role of the stromal fibroblasts is to produce collagen-rich ECM that confers rigidity to regulate the size of the cervical canal. During pregnancy, the ectocervical epithelial cells proliferate and form endocervical glands that extend and branch deeply into the fibrous connective tissue of the cervical wall. By late in the third trimester, endocervical glands occupy up to 50% of the entire cervical mass (Myers et al. 2015).

The primary function of the cervix during pregnancy is to remain rigid and unyielding in order to maintain the fetus within the uterus. This requires withstanding multiple forces from the uterus including the weight of the growing fetus and amniotic sac and passive pressure from the uterine wall (Myers et al. 2015). Unlike the body of the uterus, cervical tissue contains little smooth muscle and is composed mainly of endocervical fibroblasts and a small number (10–15%) of myometrial cells (Nott et al. 2016). The fibroblasts produce a dense and rigid ECM composed of collagen, elastin and fibronectin, which acts as a scaffold providing stability and strength (Vink and Myers 2018). This helps to keep the cervix closed during normal pregnancy as it resists tensile forces generated by myometrial contractions (Mesiano et al. 2015).

The rigidity of the cervix appears to be related to the orientation and length of its collagen fibres within the

ECM (Standring 2016). Closely parallel collagen bundles with fibre lengths of at least 20 μm augment tissue rigidity while short collagen fibres in a disarrayed configuration decrease tissue rigidity (Mesiano et al. 2015). The rigidity of the cervix in the first few months of pregnancy progressively decreases after mid-gestation without losing tensile strength. This process involves restructuring of the collagen, increased vascularity and oedema, hypertrophy and hyperplasia of the cervical glands and generalized growth (Mesiano et al. 2015). There are however discrepancies on the reported data for collagen content of the cervix in term pregnant tissue (Marani and Koch 2014).

During pregnancy, cervical tissue is responsive to hormones and to stretch, and it remodels itself to facilitate drastic tissue softening necessary for the safe birth of the baby (Myers and Elad 2017). Cervical remodelling includes property changes that result in anatomical changes. The wall thickness of the cervix decreases until it reaches 0.4 cm thickness at term (Marani and Koch 2014). Under hormonal control, the cervix is transformed from a closed, rigid, non-distensible, collagen-dense structure responsible for maintaining a pregnancy, to a soft, distensible and nearly indistinguishable ring of tissue capable of stretching and dilating to permit the passage of a fetus at term (Antony et al. 2017). As the cervix remodels, the tissue softens and causes the collagen scaffold to become disorganized and unstable. This remodelling process takes place in four phases: softening, ripening, dilation and repair (Baah-Dwomoh et al. 2016).

Softening of the collagen-rich cervical stroma begins soon after conception by disruption of the collagen fibre network (Baah-Dwomoh et al. 2016). As early as one month after conception, the increased vascularity within the cervical stroma creates an ectocervical violet-blue tint that is characteristic of *Chadwick's sign*. Cervical oedema leads to softening known as *Goodell's sign*, whereas softening of the isthmus between the cervix and the uterus is known as *Hegar's sign*, which was once used to diagnose pregnancy (Cunningham et al. 2018). Cervical glands also secrete substances that affect the integrity of the ECM. After mid-gestation, the cervical gland area begins a gradual decline that correlates with progressive cervical softening and shortening of the cervical canal (Mesiano et al. 2015). Cervical remodelling is progressive throughout pregnancy and gradual softening and shortening continue in the weeks preceding labour (Standring 2016).

CERVICAL RIPENING

Cervical ripening is an inflammatory process controlled by nitric oxide and brought about by the combination of cervical stretch and pressure exerted by the fetus, and hormones such as progesterone, oestrogen, oxytocin and relaxin (Norwitz et al. 2014). *Ripening* precedes the onset of active labour by several weeks and is accompanied by tissue vascularization. The connective tissue becomes more elastic and there is increased water content and dispersion of collagen fibres (Norwitz et al. 2014). This leads to a loss of structural integrity and tensile strength, making the cervix soft, thin, pliable and easily distensible and decreasing its load-bearing capacity (Mesiano et al. 2015).

CERVICAL SHORTENING AND EFFACEMENT

Further alterations in collagen organization in the cervix takes place as labour approaches, resulting in the structural and mechanical changes of effacement and dilatation (Myers et al. 2015).

Taking-up or *effacement* of the cervix is the shortening of the cervical canal from about 3 cm in length to a circular orifice with paper-thin edges. Muscle fibres at the level of the internal os are pulled upwards to become part of the lower uterine segment (Cunningham et al. 2018).

Cervical shortening usually takes place from above downwards in a wedge-shaped fashion. It begins at the internal os where the cervix starts to dilate leading to a *funnelled* cervical canal. It is thought that the internal os dilates first because tissue stresses are higher there compared with the external os (Myers et al. 2015). Muscle fibres at the internal cervical os are 'taken-up' to become an anatomical and physiological part of the lower uterine segment (Nott et al. 2016). Only the lower-third of the cervical canal and external os remain to be dilated in the first stage of labour. Effacement often takes place in the multigravida at the same time as dilatation of the cervical os before active labour begins, whereas in the primigravida, full effacement takes place before dilatation of the external os (Cunningham et al. 2018) (see Chapter 19).

Situated at the internal os between the muscular corpus and the predominantly fibrous cervix is the *fibromuscular junction*, the point at which the endometrium changes to become endocervical columnar epithelium. During pregnancy, the junction migrates up the wall of the lower uterine segment, which explains why many low-lying placentas are no longer praevia by the end of pregnancy (Rawal 2016).

Vink et al. (2016) have recently suggested that the internal os may be compared with a specialized sphincter that may be involved in propagating uterine contractions and cervical remodelling. They found that the internal os contained approximately 50–60% smooth muscle and the bundles were arranged circumferentially around the endocervical canal. Also the smooth muscle content gradually decreased at the mid-point of the cervix and the external os was composed mostly of collagen and 10% muscle cells. This is a novel and exciting possibility in the quest to understand premature cervical failure leading to preterm birth, and calls into question the long-held belief that the cervix is a mainly collagenous structure and a *passive bystander* in the process of parturition (Vink and Myers 2018).

The cervix protects the interior of the uterus from ascending infection and is the final barrier to protecting the fetus during pregnancy (Dubey et al. 2016). When cervical mucus is spread and dried on a glass slide, the test may produce a crystallization pattern that resembles a fern. This *ferning* or arborization pattern (a branching, tree-like arrangement) may also be observed in spontaneous rupture of membranes when there is crystallization of sodium chloride derived from amniotic fluid (Patil and Patil 2014). Columnar epithelial cells of the cervix undergo marked proliferation and secrete mucus that acts as plug called the *operculum,* which provides a protective seal against the entry of pathogens and also has antibacterial properties. Late in the softening phase and before or during early labour the cervical canal may dilate by up to 3 cm and the operculum is released as a blood-tinged mucous discharge known as the *show* (Dubey et al. 2016).

The appearance of the cervix on colposcopy changes dramatically during pregnancy due to high levels of circulating progesterone. Cyanosis of the stroma causes a dusky appearance (Mehta and Singla 2014). There is cuffing of gland openings and a progressive process called *eversion* of endocervical epithelium onto the ectocervix. Eversion of the endocervical glands is known as *cervical ectropion.* This tissue tends to bruise easily, and gentle touch as on coitus or *Papanicolaou smear* (Pap test) tends to cause bleeding (Reichman et al. 2014).

Cervical ectropion is normal in pregnancy and makes it easier to visualize the squamocolumnar junction and the transformational zone. These changes can make the interpretation of cytological smears in pregnancy challenging, however the accuracy of the Pap test is the same in pregnancy as in the non-pregnant state (Nigam et al. 2017). The remaining elements involved in cervical remodelling (dilatation and repair) are discussed in Chapters 19 and 28.

THE VAGINA

As early as the 4th week of pregnancy there is increased vascularity and softening of the vaginal portion of the cervical mucosa (Goodell's sign) (Ramos-e-Silva et al. 2016). By the 8th week of pregnancy, there is increased vascularity and hyperaemia in the skin and muscles of the perineum and vulva, and the underlying connective tissue softens. This augmented vascularity mostly affects the vagina and cervical stroma and creates an ectocervical blue or violet tint that is characteristic of *Chadwick's sign.* In preparation for the distension that occurs in labour, the vaginal walls undergo striking changes: the epithelial mucosa thickens, connective tissue loosens and smooth muscle cells hypertrophy (Cunningham et al. 2018).

Vaginal discharge in pregnancy is common but distinguishing abnormal vaginal discharge from the normal leucorrhoea of pregnancy is challenging (Ibrahim et al. 2016). Cervical secretions, which are greatly increased during pregnancy, form a thick, white discharge, which at times may be confused with leakage of amniotic fluid (Cunningham et al. 2018). Metabolism of glycogen to lactic acid by *Lactobacilli* in the vagina contributes to the maintenance of a low vaginal pH (<4.5), which inhibits the growth of pathological vulvo-vaginal organisms, particularly during the second and third trimesters (Romero et al. 2014). This ensures greater resilience to ascending infection during pregnancy, which is a risk factor for preterm birth and other conditions that compromise the fetus (Romero et al. 2014).

CHANGES IN THE CARDIOVASCULAR SYSTEM

During pregnancy, profound but predominantly reversible changes occur in maternal haemodynamics and cardiac function. These complex adaptations are necessary to:

TABLE 10.2   A Summary of the Key Components of the Cardiovascular System and Adaptations in Pregnancy

Component	Key Change in Pregnancy
The heart	Increases in size Shifted upwards and to the left
Arteries	Dramatic systemic and pulmonary vasodilatation to increase blood flow
Capillaries	Increased permeability
Veins	Vasodilatation and impeded venous return in lower extremities
Blood	Haemodilution Increased capacity for clot formation

Adapted from Torgersen KL, Curran CA. (2006) A systematic approach to the physiologic adaptations of pregnancy. Critical Care Nursing Quarterly 29:2–19.

- meet evolving maternal changes in physiological function
- promote the growth and development of the utero-placental–fetal unit
- compensate for blood loss at the end of labour.

These physiological adaptations are extensive, with all components undergoing a degree of modification in pregnancy, as highlighted in Table 10.2. In most women, achieving this critical balance between fetal requirements and maternal tolerance is effectively accommodated by physiological adaptations without compromising the mother. However, the challenges these evoke on the cardiovascular system may unmask predispositions for future maternal disease and impact fetal-programming of cardiac function in their offspring (Ventura et al. 2018).

Anatomical Changes in the Heart and Blood Vessels

The heart is enlarged by chamber dilatation and a degree of physiological hypertrophy in early pregnancy (Fu 2018) leading to a 10–15% increase in ventricular wall muscle. The progressive rise in blood volume throughout pregnancy results in increased end diastolic volume (particularly in the left ventricle) and progressive distension of the heart chambers (Martin et al. 2017). Despite cardiac enlargement, efficiency is maintained by lengthening of myocardial fibres and reduction in afterload facilitated by peripheral vasodilatation. These structural changes in the heart mimic *exercise-induced cardiac remodelling* (Chung and Leinwand 2014), which occurs in response to physical training, and similarly, they are reversible after pregnancy. This remodelling, as seen in healthy athletes and normal pregnancy, is determined primarily by physiological volume overload driven by the need to ensure adequate blood, oxygen and nutrient supplies (Ghossein-Doha et al. 2017).

The enlarging uterus raises the diaphragm, and the heart is correspondingly displaced upward and to the left to produce a slight anterior rotation of the heart on its long axis. This partially accounts for pregnancy variations in key parameters used for cardiac assessment, including electrocardiography (ECG) and radiographic assessments and can give an exaggerated impression of cardiac enlargement (Fu 2018). Atrial or ventricular extra systoles are relatively common in pregnancy along with increased susceptibility to supraventricular tachycardia, and arrhythmias (Boriani et al. 2017) however, it is imperative that signs of severe disease such as angina or resting dyspnoea are not overlooked (Adamson et al. 2011).

Within 5 weeks of conception, changes in maternal blood vessels are evident, including an increase in aortic size and venous blood volume. Compliance of the entire vasculature is increased, partially due to the softening of the collagen and smooth muscle hypertrophy (Blackburn 2018). While influenced by progesterone, relaxin and endothelial-derived relaxant factors such as nitric oxide and prostacyclin, the exact mechanism underlying these changes is not yet fully understood (Fu 2018).

Alongside these anatomical changes, widespread haemodynamic adaptations occur, these are realized through a multifactorial rebalancing of homeostatic mechanisms (Table 10.3). One explanation offered for these haemodynamic changes is that pregnancy 'resets' both volume and osmoreceptors (Tkachenko et al. 2014). The precise mechanism through which this is achieved is not fully understood, but the first step is widely accepted to be peripheral vasodilatation facilitated by a systemic and renal vasodilator unique to pregnancy. The interplay between some of these proposed mechanisms is summarized in Fig. 10.3.

The cumulative result of these adaptations is *widespread peripheral vasodilatation resulting in the high flow, low resistance haemodynamic state with marked haemodilution characteristic of a healthy pregnancy.*

TABLE 10.3   Key Physiological Changes in the Cardiovascular System in Pregnancy

Parameter	Adaptation	Magnitude	Non-Pregnant (Average Value)	Timing of Peak/ Average Peak Value
Oxygen consumption	Increase	20–30%	180 mL/min	Term
Total body water	Increase	6–8 L		Term
Plasma volume	Increase	45–50%	2600 mL	32–34 weeks; 3850 mL
Red cell mass	Increase	20–30%	1400 mL	Term 1650 mL
Total blood volume	Increase	30–50%	4000 mL	32 weeks; 5500 mL
Cardiac output	Increase	30–50%	4.9 L/min	28 weeks; / L/min
Stroke volume	Increase			20 weeks
Heart rate	Increase	10–20 bpm	75 bpm	Trimester 1; 90 bpm
Systemic vascular resistance	Decrease	21%	–	Trimester 2
Pulmonary vascular resistance	Decrease	35%	–	34 weeks
Diastolic blood pressure	Decrease, returning to normal by term	10–15 mmHg	–	24 weeks
Systolic blood pressure	Minimal, no decrease	5–10 mmHg	–	24 weeks
Serum colloid osmotic pressure	Decrease	10–15%	–	14 weeks

Nelson-Piercy C. (2015) Handbook of obstetric medicine (5th ed.). London: Taylor and Francis; Blackburn S. (2018) Maternal, fetal and neonatal physiology (5th od.). Philadelphia: Saunders

Blood Volume

The increase in total blood volume (TBV) is essential to:
- meet the demands of the enlarged uterus with a significantly hypertrophied vascular system and to provide extra blood flow for placental perfusion
- supply extra metabolic needs of the fetus
- protect the woman (and fetus) against the potential harmful effects of impaired venous return
- provide extra perfusion of maternal organs
- counterbalance the effects of increased arterial and venous capacity
- safeguard against adverse effects of excessive maternal blood loss at birth.

Plasma volume expansion begins prior to the development of an intact placenta and is initiated by a modification of the renin-angiotensin-aldosterone system (RAAS, the hormone signalling cascade that regulates blood pressure and systemic electrolyte and fluid balance). The dramatically vasodilated, uteroplacental vasculature contributes to this change supported by evidence that fetal weight correlates directly with the rise in blood volume (Blackburn 2018). This only partially explains the reduced systemic vascular resistance, since a significant proportion of the decrease occurs outside the uteroplacental circulation and prior to complete placentation. Relaxin, the peptide hormone produced by the corpus luteum and placenta, causes systemic and renal vasodilation and plays a key important role in the regulation of the haemodynamics and water metabolism in pregnancy (Leo et al. 2017). Vasodilatation is also partly mediated the upregulation of nitric oxide production by oestradiol and possibly vasodilatory prostaglandins (PGI2) (Tkachenko et al. 2014).

Vasodilatation causes an *underfilling* of the maternal circulation which subsequently initiates fluid and electrolyte retention, expansion of the plasma and extracellular fluid volumes. This initiates a concurrent increase in cardiac output and parallel increase in renal blood flow and glomerular filtration rate. The impact of this profound vasodilation on fluid balance and osmoregulation

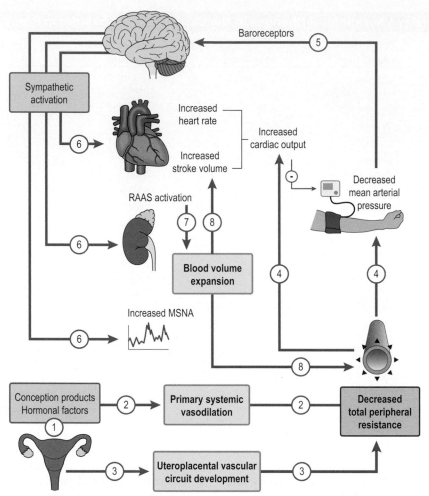

Fig. 10.3 An overview of the possible mechanisms underlying maternal haemodynamic adaptations in a health pregnancy. (From Fu Q. (2018) Hemodynamic and electrocardiographic aspects of uncomplicated singleton pregnancy. In: P Kerkhof, V Miller (Eds) Sex-specific analysis of cardiovascular function. Advances in experimental medicine and biology, Vol. 1065. Amsterdam: Springer, with permission of Springer ebooks.)

is mediated through RASS and the autonomic nervous system (Fu 2018). It has been postulated that raised oestrogen levels increase sympathetic activity through a central mechanism to compensate for systemic vasodilation and subsequently, raise blood pressure towards term (Fu 2018). Despite this marked sympathetic activation, vasoconstrictor responsiveness is blunted during uncomplicated pregnancy predominantly due to increased nitric oxide bioavailability and vasodepressor effect of prostacyclin on angiotensin II (Fu 2018). Thus, pregnancy results in a modification of the RAAS, which is intensified by the increase in Angiotensin (1–7), a vasodilator that appears to counterbalance the rise in

angiotensin II (Yamaleyeva et al. 2014). Recent studies suggest that over-activation of the sympathetic nervous system and failure to modify RAAS may mediate the increased vasoconstriction associated with pre-eclampsia (Lumbers and Pringle 2013; Spradley 2018).

Oestrogen reduces the transcapillary escape rate of albumin, which promotes intravascular protein retention and shifts extracellular fluid volume distribution while lowering the osmotic threshold for antidiuretic hormone (ADH) release. Levels of ADH appear to remain relatively stable despite heightened production, owing to a three- to four-fold increase in metabolic clearance as a consequence of the placental enzyme

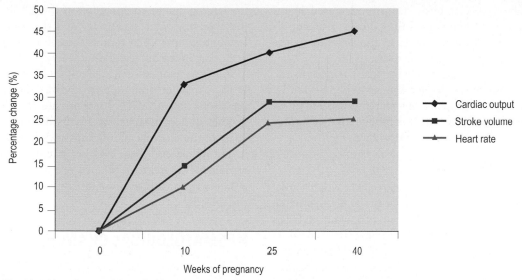

Fig. 10.4 Key changes in cardiac function in pregnancy. (Data from Cunningham G, Leveno K, Bloom S, et al. (Eds). (2018) Williams obstetrics. London: McGraw-Hill Education.)

vasopressinase, which inactivates ADH and oxytocin. Sodium homeostasis is maintained through additional homeostatic modifications with notable increases in atrial natriuretic factor and relaxin, which both mediate sodium levels in pregnancy.

Cardiac Output

The profound increase in cardiac output (30–50%) ensures blood flow to the brain and coronary arteries is maintained, while distribution to other organs is modified as pregnancy advances. While the literature reports a marked variation in the timing, linearity and extent of this increase (Meah et al. 2016), there is agreement that this is ultimately caused by increases in stroke volume and heart rate. The relative contributions of these vary with gestational age and parity (Iizuka et al. 2016) (Fig. 10.4). Stroke volume increases during the first half of pregnancy, partially due to increased ventricular wall muscle mass (Nelson-Piercy 2015), reaching a peak at 20 weeks, this declines slightly by term. The accompanying increase in heart rate contributes to early changes in cardiac output, further augmented by the plasma volume expansion. Cardiac output changes are detectable at 6–8 weeks and have been shown to positively correlate with birth weight (Mahendru et al. 2017).

Cardiac output in pregnancy is extremely sensitive to changes in body position; this increases with advancing pregnancy, as the gravid uterus impinges on the inferior

vena cava, thereby decreasing blood return to the heart (Box 10.1). Inconsistencies in study findings may be due to postural effects of aortocaval compression by the enlarged uterus on maternal haemodynamics (Meah et al. 2016).

Blood Pressure and Vascular Resistance

While cardiac output is raised, arterial blood pressure is reduced by 10% in early pregnancy. The decrease in systemic vascular resistance by 30–40% accounts for this, particularly in the peripheral vessels (Fu 2018). The decrease begins at 5 weeks' gestation, reaches a nadir in the second trimester (a 21% reduction) and then gradually rises as term approaches (Blackburn 2018). Numerous modifications occur in the mechanisms controlling vascular activity. Agents responsible for peripheral vasodilatation include prostacyclin, nitric oxide and progesterone and vasoactive prostaglandins. The changes are not limited to the uteroplacental circulation but are apparent throughout the body in a healthy pregnancy. Increased heat production further contributes to the reduced resistance, stimulating vasodilatation in peripheral vessels.

Early pregnancy is associated with a marked decrease in diastolic blood pressure of 10–15 mmHg by 24 weeks' gestation but minimal reduction in systolic pressure, dropping just 5–10 mmHg below baseline levels. Thereafter, blood pressure gradually rises, returning to the pre-pregnant levels at term. Despite increased blood volume systemic venous pressures do not rise significantly. The exception to this is in the legs due to the gravid uterus impeding venous return.

It is important to acknowledge that haemodynamic changes in pregnancy do not appear to be affected by parity but they are influenced by maternal age and physical characteristics (Fu 2018), subsequently the figures quoted in this chapter are approximations.

Regional Blood Flow

As blood volume increases with gestation, a substantial proportion (10–20%) is distributed to the uteroplacental unit. Renal vasodilatation early in pregnancy initiated prior to implantation in the luteal phase (Conrad 2011) results in a significant increase in renal blood flow and glomerular filtration rate which facilitates efficient excretion.

As a percentage of total cardiac output blood flow to the brain, coronary arteries and liver is reduced, the overall increase in cardiac output compensates for this and the blood flow to these regions is not significantly changed. Pulmonary blood flow increases secondary to the increase in cardiac output, further facilitated by reduced pulmonary vascular resistance. Blood flow in the lower limbs decelerates in late pregnancy by compression of the iliac veins and inferior vena cava by the enlarging uterus and the hydrodynamic effects of increased venous return from the uterus. Reduced venous return and increased venous pressure in the legs contributes to the increased distensibility and pressure in the veins of the legs, vulva, rectum and pelvis, leading to dependent oedema, varicose veins of the legs, vulva and anus (Box 10.2). These changes are more pronounced in

the left leg due to compression of the left iliac vein by the overlying right iliac artery and the ovarian artery, accounting for 85% of venous thrombosis in pregnancy occurring in the left leg (Nelson-Piercy 2015).

A rise in temperature by 0.2–0.4°C occurs as a result of the effects of progesterone and the increased basal metabolic rate (BMR). To eliminate the excess heat produced there is an increased blood flow to the capillaries of the mucous membranes and skin, particularly in the hands and feet. This peripheral vasodilatation explains why pregnant women are often heat-intolerant, more prone to perspire, to nasal congestion and to nosebleeds.

HAEMATOLOGICAL CHANGES

In parallel with the increase in maternal blood volume, plasma volume increases by approximately 45% over the course of the pregnancy (Fu 2018), followed by a relatively smaller increase in red blood cell volume (Table 10.4). These changes are responsible for the *haemodilution of pregnancy* leading to numerous modifications of the blood cellular components and plasma constituents commonly assessed in blood tests (Table 10.5). Most notable is the net decrease in red blood cell volume and total circulating plasma proteins. Plasma

---

BOX 10.2 Varicosities

Varicosities develop in approximately 40% of women and are usually seen in the veins of the legs, but may also occur in the vulva and as haemorrhoids in the anal area.

The effects of progesterone and relaxin on the smooth muscles of the vein walls and the increased weight of the growing uterus all contribute to the increased risk of valvular incompetence. A family tendency is also a factor (Blackburn 2018).

Some suggestions for alleviating them include: spraying the legs with hot and cold water, resting with the legs elevated and wearing supportive stockings.

TABLE 10.4 Key Haematological Changes in Pregnancy

	Non-Pregnant	WEEKS OF PREGNANCY		
		20	30	40
Plasma volume (mL)	2600	3150	3750	3850
Red cell mass (mL)	1400	1450	1550	1650
Total blood volume (mL)	4000	4600	5300	5500
Haematocrit (PCV) (%)	35–47	32.0	29.0	30.0
Haemoglobin (g/L)	115–165	110	105	110

From Oats J, Abraham S. (2017) Llewellyn-Jones fundamentals of obstetrics and gynaecology (10th ed.). Edinburgh: Elsevier.

TABLE 10.5 Normal Values in Pregnant/Non-Pregnant Women

Test	Non-Pregnant (Typical Range)	Pregnant (Typical Range)	Comments
Biochemistry			
Alanine transaminase (ALT) (U/L)	7–41	Slight drop 2–33	Raised levels indicate liver damage
Alkaline phosphatase (IU/L)	40–120 33–96	Doubled by late pregnancy 38–229	Usually elevated in the third trimester due to placental production of enzyme
Bile acids (total) (µmol/L)	<10	Unchanged	Values of total bile acids ≥14 µmol/L are viewed as abnormal, indicating severe cholestasis when >40
Bilirubin (µmol/L)	5–22.2	Minimal drop	Little change in non-pregnant range
Creatinine (µmol/L)	44–80	Slight drop	Lower in early pregnancy but rises towards term
Potassium (mmol/L)	3.5–5.0	Slight drop	
Albumin (g/L)	35–46	28–37 lowest towards term	Total protein and albumin are both lower in pregnancy
Urea (mmol/L)	2.5–7.5	Usually ≤4.5	Lower in pregnancy
Uric acid (µmol/L)	150–350	10 × gestational age in weeks is approximately the upper limit of normal	Lower in early pregnancy but rises towards term
24-h protein mg/24 h	>1.5	>0.3	
Haematology			
Clotting time (min)	12	8	Observe for clotting or oozing from venepuncture sites in women of higher risk
Fibrin degradation products (µg/mL)	Mean 1.04	High values in the third trimester and especially around the time of birth	
Fibrinogen (g/L)	1.7–4.1	By term 2.9–6.2	Marked increase in pregnancy especially in third trimester and around the time of birth
Haemotocrit (%)	35–47	31–35	Lower in pregnancy
Haemoglobin (g/L)	115–165	100–120 should be >100 in the third trimester	Good iron stores needed to maintain pregnancy levels. Fall in the first trimester whether or not iron and folate taken
Platelets (×10⁹/L)	150–400	Slight decrease in pregnancy; lower limit of normal = 120	No functional significance
White cell count (×10⁹/L)	4.0–11.0	9.0–15.0; higher values up to 25.0 around the time of birth	Normal increase in pregnancy Rise in infections

Data from Perinatology.com (2019) Available at: http://perinatology.com/Reference/Reference%20Ranges/Reference%-20for%20Serum.htm.

volume begins to increase prior to blastocyst implantation. The steepest increase is seen mid-pregnancy, with a peak around 30–32 weeks (Fu 2018). Excessive increases in plasma volume have been associated with multiple pregnancy, prolonged pregnancy, maternal obesity and large for gestational age babies, while inadequate increases have been associated with pre-eclampsia (Blackburn 2018).

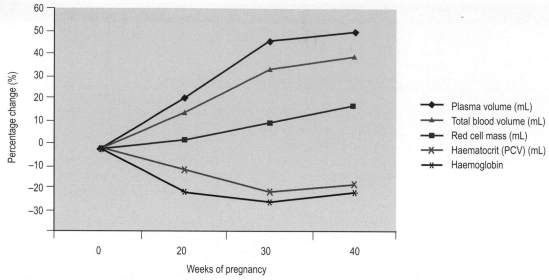

Fig. 10.5 Key haematological changes in pregnancy. (Data from Cunningham G, Leveno K, Bloom S, et al. (Eds). (2018) Williams obstetrics. London: McGraw-Hill Education.)

Total red blood cell volume increases during pregnancy by approximately 20% in response to increased levels of erythropoietin stimulated by maternal hormones (prolactin, progesterone, human placental lactogen and oestrogen) and increased oxygen requirements of maternal and placental tissue (Cunningham et al. 2018). This homeostatic mechanism is discrete from that which controls fluid balance and increased plasma volume. Therefore, in spite of the increased production of red blood cells, the marked increase in plasma volume causes dilution of many circulating factors. As a result, the red cell count, haematocrit and haemoglobin concentration all decrease, resulting in *apparent anaemia*, characteristic of a healthy pregnancy (Fig. 10.5). This trend reverses towards term as red cell mass continues to increase after 30 weeks when the plasma volume expansion has plateaued. The disproportionate increase in plasma volume is advantageous; i.e. by reducing blood viscosity, resistance to blood flow is reduced leading to improved placental perfusion and reduced maternal cardiac effort (Cunningham et al. 2018).

Red blood cells become more spherical with increased diameter due to the fall in plasma colloid pressure encouraging more water to cross the erythrocyte cell membrane. Mean cell volume (MCV) also increases due to the higher proportion of young larger

BOX 10.3   Pregnancy Laboratory Values

One consequence of the physiological changes occurring in a normal pregnancy are the significant alterations in certain laboratory values which in a non-pregnant woman would be considered distinctly abnormal. Laboratories do not usually report normal values for 'females', much less for pregnant women. A common example is expected lower haemoglobin concentrations from physiological haemodilution. Subsequently, most reports of these pregnancy-induced variations are drawn from studies of a limited number of analyses, making it challenging to determine accurate reference ranges.

red blood cells (reticulocytes). The exact increase in red cell mass remains inconclusive, partly because assessments have been influenced by routine iron medication.

While total haemoglobin increases from 85 g to 150 g the mean haemoglobin decreases. In healthy women with adequate iron stores this reduces by about 20 g/L from an average of 133 g/L in the non-pregnant state to 110 g/L in early pregnancy (Box 10.3). It is at its lowest at around 32 weeks' gestation when plasma volume expansion is maximal, and after this time rises by approximately 5 g/L, returning to 110 g/L around the 36th week of pregnancy. A haemoglobin level below

105 g/L at 28 weeks should be investigated (National Institute for Health and Care Excellence; NICE 2018a) (see Chapter 15).

Iron Metabolism

Iron requirements increase significantly in pregnancy, with the average net pregnancy related iron loss, estimated to be 740 mg (Fisher and Nemeth 2017). While there is an initial net saving from amenorrhoea, in late pregnancy, iron requirements increase dramatically to 3–8 mg iron/day. About 450 mg are required to increase the maternal red blood cell mass, 360 mg are transported to the fetus and placenta, and the remaining 230 mg are utilized in compensating for insensible loss in skin, stool and urine. In spite of the moderate increase in iron absorption from the gut, to accommodate the requirements of pregnancy, women require an iron-rich diet to supplement the approximate 500 mg of stored iron prior to conception. Since this amount is not available from body stores in most women, the red cell volume and haemoglobin level decrease with the rising plasma volume.

Many women conceive with insufficient iron reserves, but research to date has not fully established the benefits and drawbacks of iron supplementation or the optimal biomarkers for interpreting circulating iron status. In spite of this apparent imbalance, even with severe maternal iron deficiency anaemia, the placenta is able to provide sufficient iron from maternal serum for fetal production of haemoglobin. Hepcidin has been identified as a key hormone in the homeostasis of maternal, placental and fetal iron levels; the reduced concentrations during pregnancy ensure greater bioavailability of iron to the mother and fetus (Vricella 2017).

Plasma Protein

Haemodilution leads to a decrease in total serum protein content within the first trimester, which remains low throughout pregnancy. Despite oestrogen reducing the transcapillary escape rate of albumin, concentration declines abruptly in early pregnancy and then more gradually towards term (Table 10.5). Albumin is important as a carrier protein for hormones, drugs, free fatty acids and unconjugated bilirubin, and its influence in decreasing colloid osmotic pressure. A 10–15% fall in colloid osmotic pressure allows water to move from the plasma into the cells or out of vessels and plays a part in the increased fragility of red blood cells and oedema of the lower limbs (Nelson-Piercy 2015). It is now accepted that peripheral oedema in the lower limbs in late pregnancy is a feature of physiological, uncomplicated pregnancy.

Clotting Factors

In pregnancy, adaptations occur in the coagulation system to protect the woman from peripartum haemorrhage, while also maintaining the uteroplacental interface. The cumulative effect of these is commonly described as the *characteristic hypercoagulable state of pregnancy*. The increased tendency to clot is caused by increases in clotting factors and fibrinogen accompanied by reduced plasma fibrinolytic activity and an increase in circulating fibrin degradation products in the plasma. Due to these changes, pregnant women have a five- to six-fold increased risk for thromboembolic disease (Nelson-Piercy 2015); see Chapter 15.

From 12 weeks' gestation, there is a 50% increase in synthesis of plasma fibrinogen concentration (Factor I) rising to 200% pre-pregnancy levels at term. This is critical for the prevention of haemorrhage at the time of placental separation. The development of a fibrin mesh to cover the placental site to control the bleeding requires 5–10% of all the circulating fibrinogen. When this process is impaired, for example by inadequate uterine action or incomplete placental separation, compounded by placental blood flow of up to 700 mL/min at term, there is rapid depletion of fibrinogen reserves, putting the woman at risk of haemorrhage (see Chapters 21 and 25).

Coagulation factors VII, VIII and X increase in pregnancy, while factors II (prothrombin) and V remain constant or show a slight fall. Both the prothrombin time (normal 10–14 s) and the partial thromboplastin time (normal 35–45 s) are slightly shortened as pregnancy advances. The clotting times of whole blood, however, are not significantly different in pregnancy to non-pregnant values. The platelet count declines slightly as pregnancy advances, which is explained by haemodilution and increased consumption in the uteroplacental circulation. The increased production of platelets results in a slight increase in mean platelet volume (MPV), which is due to immature platelets being larger than old ones, resulting in an overall increase in average size. Substantial increases in MCV could indicate excessive platelet consumption and has been used as a marker for hypertensive disease.

A decrease in some endogenous anticoagulants (anti-thrombin, protein S and activated protein C resistance) occur in pregnancy along with the physiological vasodilatation of pregnancy, this contributes to the increased risk of thromboembolism in pregnancy.

White blood cells (leucocytes) and immune function

Pregnancy presents a paradox for the woman's immune system as the mechanisms that are essential to protect her from infection have the potential to destroy the genetically disparate conceptus. It is clear that the immunological relationship between the mother and the fetus involves a two-way communication involving fetal antigen presentation and maternal recognition of and reaction to these antigens by the immune system (PrabhuDas et al. 2015). There is evidence that progesterone plays a major role in the immunological tolerance seen in pregnancy.

The total white cell count rises from 8 weeks' gestation and reaches a peak at 30 weeks. This is mainly because of the increase in numbers of neutrophil polymorphonuclear leucocytes, monocytes and granulocytes; the latter two producing a far more active and efficient phagocytosis function. This enhances the blood's phagocytic and bactericidal properties. Numbers of eosinophils, basophils, monocytes, lymphocytes and circulating T cells and B cells remain relatively constant. Lymphocyte function is depressed, and natural killer cytokine activity is downregulated by progesterone, particularly in the latter stages of pregnancy. Chemotaxis is suppressed resulting in a delayed response to some infections. There is decreased resistance to viral infections such as herpes, influenza, rubella, hepatitis, poliomyelitis and malaria. The metabolic activity of granulocytes increases during pregnancy, probably initiated by rising oestrogen and cortisol levels. Immature granulocytes counts have been shown to increase significantly during healthy pregnancy, especially in the second and third trimesters (Yu et al. 2016). These are useful markers for infection. It is therefore critical that reference intervals according to pregnancy trimester are used to guide clinical decisions.

The maternal immune response is biased toward an enhancement of innate (humoral) immunity and away from cell-mediated response that could be harmful to the fetus. The stimulus for these changes is predominantly hormonal, involving progesterone, human placental lactogen (hPL), prostaglandins, corticosteroids, human chorionic gonadotrophin (hCG), prolactin and serum proteins.

CHANGES IN THE RESPIRATORY SYSTEM

To accommodate increased oxygen requirements and the physical impact of the enlarging uterus, intricate changes occur in respiratory physiology. These are mediated by an interaction of hormonal, biochemical and mechanical factors and are summarized in Table 10.6. Progressive increases in maternal and fetal metabolic demands are reflected in a marked increase in resting oxygen consumption reaching a 20–30% peak from non-pregnant values at term.

The driving force for change is the respiratory stimulatory effect of progesterone initiating hyperventilation by increasing sensitivity to carbon dioxide through lowering the threshold at which the respiratory centre is stimulated. This causes arterial oxygen tension to increase and arterial carbon dioxide tension to decrease, accompanied by a compensatory decline in serum bicarbonate; mild respiratory alkalosis is consequently physiologically normal in pregnancy (Mehta et al. 2015) (Box 10.4).

To counteract the effect of the enlarging pregnant uterus and elevated diaphragm, the diameter of the chest increases and subcostal angle widens, thus altering but not compromising pulmonary function (Blackburn 2018). This commences in early pregnancy; the overall shape of the chest alters as the anteroposterior and transverse diameters increase by about 2 cm resulting in a 5–7 cm expansion of the chest circumference. The lower ribs flare outwards prior to any mechanical pressure from the growing uterus. This progressively increases the subcostal angle, from 68° in early pregnancy to 103° at term (Fig. 10.6). Although the expanding uterus causes the diaphragm to rise by up to 4 cm above its usual resting position, diaphragmatic movement during respiration is not impaired as chest wall mobility increases and lower ribs flare, increasing the thoracic space. Changes are mediated by progesterone and relaxin, which increase ribcage elasticity by relaxing ligaments in a similar mechanism to that occurring in the pelvis. Forced vital capacity (FVC) increases significantly after 14–16 weeks' gestation, FVC% is significantly higher in parous than primigravid women, which suggests these changes in FVC persist postpartum (Grindheim et al. 2012).

Progesterone also facilitates bronchial and tracheal smooth muscle relaxation, thereby reducing airway resistance. This improves air flow and explains why the health of women with existing respiratory problems rarely deteriorates in pregnancy.

TABLE 10.6 Summary of Changes in Respiratory Function

Parameter	Adaptation	Magnitude (%)	Non-Pregnant (Average Value)	Timing of Peak/Average Peak Value
Oxygen consumption	Increase	18–20	250 mL/min	300 mL/min
Metabolic rate	Increase	15		Peaks at term with increases up to eight-fold reported
Resting minute volume: amount of air/min moved into and out of the lungs	Increase	40–50	7.5 L/min	Peaks at term; 10.5 L/min
Tidal volume: amount of air inspired and expired with normal breath	Increase	40	500 mL	700 mL
Vital capacity: maximum amount of air that can be forcibly expired after maximum inspiration	No change	–	3200 mL	3200 mL
Functional residual capacity: amount of air in lungs at resting expiratory level	Decrease	20	1700 mL	3rd trimester 1350 mL
Blood gas analysis:				
Arterial oxygen tension (PaO_2)	Increase		95–100 mmHg	Peak end trimester 1; 106–8 mmHg
Arterial carbon dioxide tension ($PaCO_2$)	Decrease		35–40 mmHg	27–32 mmHg
Serum bicarbonate	Decrease			18–22 mmol/L
Arterial Ph	Small increase			7.44 (a mild respiratory alkalosis)

Nelson Piercy C. (2015) Handbook of obstetric medicine (5th ed.). London: Taylor and Francis; Blackburn S. (2018) Maternal, fetal and neonatal physiology (5th ed.). Philadelphia: Saunders.

BOX 10.4 Breathlessness

The respiratory changes can be extremely uncomfortable and may lead to dyspnoea, dizziness and altered exercise tolerance. Up to 75% of pregnant women with no underlying pre-existing respiratory disease experience some degree of subjective feeling of breathlessness, possibly due to an increased awareness of the physiological hyperventilation (Nelson-Piercy 2015). This physiological dyspnoea often occurs early in pregnancy and does not interfere with daily activities and usually diminishes as term approaches. Although mechanical impediment by the uterus is often blamed, hyperventilation is due to altered sensitivity to CO_2. Although it is not usually associated with pathological processes, care must be taken not to dismiss this lightly and miss a warning sign of cardiac or pulmonary disease (Soma-Pillay et al. 2016).

Breathlessness can be alleviated by maintaining an upright posture and holding hands above the head while taking deep breaths. Women may need to modify their physical activity levels to accommodate these symptoms, however studies have shown that exercising in pregnancy can help to alleviate them (Barakat et al. 2015).

Expansion of the rib cage causes the tidal volume to increase by 30–50% gradually rising from approximately 8 weeks' gestation to term (Mehta et al. 2015). Studies report that the normal respiratory rate of 14–15 breaths/min may demonstrate minimal increase in pregnancy, though pregnant women do breathe more deeply, even at rest. The minute volume, which facilitates gas exchange is increased by 30–40%, from 7.5–10.5 L/min baseline, and minute oxygen uptake increases appreciably as pregnancy advances (Cunningham et al. 2018).

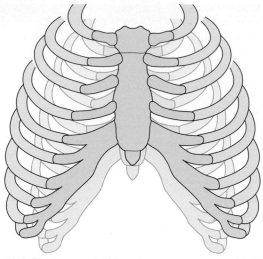

Fig. 10.6 Displacement of the ribcage in pregnancy (dark) and the non-pregnancy state (light) showing elevated diaphragm, the increased transverse diameter and circumference, flaring out of ribs and the increased subcostal angle. (From de Swiet M. (1998) The respiratory system. In: G Chamberlain, F Broughton Pipkin (Eds) Clinical physiology in obstetrics (3rd ed.). Oxford: Blackwell Science, with permission from Wiley Publishing Ltd.)

The enhanced tidal volume contributes to an increase in inspiratory capacity while vital capacity is unchanged. As a result, the functional residual capacity is decreased by 20%. This reduces the amount of used gas mixing with each new inspiration, thereby enhancing alveolar gas exchange by 50–70%. Reductions in these parameters may be explained by the upward tilt of the diaphragm caused by the enlarging uterus, resulting in a decreased negative intrapleural pressure and reduction in the alveolar partial pressure of carbon gas caused by hyperventilation during pregnancy (Pastro et al. 2017). While making ventilation more efficient, this may result in rapid falls in arterial oxygen tension even with short periods of apnoea, which is further compounded by the reduced buffering capacity. Whether from obstruction of the airway or inhalation of a hypoxic mixture of gas the consequence of these adaptations is that pregnant women have less reserve if they become hypoxic.

Blood volume expansion and vasodilatation of pregnancy result in hyperaemia and oedema of the upper respiratory mucosa, which predispose the pregnant woman to nasal congestion, epistaxis and even changes in voice. The changes to the upper respiratory tract may lead to upper airway obstruction and bleeding, making both mask anaesthesia and tracheal intubation more difficult. These can be further exacerbated by fluid overload or oedema associated with pregnancy-induced hypertension or pre-eclampsia (see Chapter 15).

Blood Gases

Changes in respiratory function result in a state of compensated respiratory alkalosis. Arterial oxygen partial pressure (PaO_2) is slightly increased from non-pregnant values (98–100 mmHg) to pregnant values (101–104 mmHg). In addition, the *hyperventilation of pregnancy* causes a 15–20% decrease in maternal arterial carbon dioxide partial pressure ($PaCO_2$) from an average of 35–40 mmHg in the non-pregnant woman to ≤30 mmHg in late pregnancy. Because fetal $PaCO_2$ is 44 mmHg, these changes not only safeguard adequate oxygenation but also maintain an exaggerated carbon dioxide gradient from fetus to mother. This facilitates the transfer of CO_2 from the fetus to the mother and the subsequent expiration of CO_2 from the maternal lungs. It is important that clinicians consider these changes when undertaking assessment of maternal blood gases. A $PaCO_2$ of 35–40 mmHg, which might ordinarily be considered borderline low, is markedly abnormal in a pregnant woman and can even represent impending respiratory failure (Mehta et al. 2015).

The body has a considerable capacity for storing carbon dioxide in blood, largely as bicarbonate. To compensate for the reduction in CO_2, renal excretion of bicarbonate is significantly increased, which may limit the buffering capacity in pregnancy. The fall in $PaCO_2$ is matched by an equivalent fall in plasma bicarbonate concentration. Although maternal arterial pH changes very little, the resulting *mild alkalaemia* (arterial pH 7.40–7.45) further facilitates oxygen release to the fetus.

Changes in the Central Nervous System

Adaptations of the central nervous system (CNS) are probably the least well understood compared with other body systems. The adaptive changes encompass diverse scientific disciplines, including neuroendocrinology, neuroscience, physiology and psychology, such that failure of adaptation can lead to disorders that have profound and long-lasting consequences for the woman. Progression of pregnancy is signalled to the brain by the pattern of secretion of these hormones culminating in a complex interplay of communications between the mother and fetoplacental unit.

Hoekzema et al. (2017) affirm that human pregnancy is associated with substantial alterations in maternal brain structure, notably reductions in grey matter volume primarily in the cerebral cortex. They propose these serve a social adaptive purpose for pending motherhood. Anecdotal evidence that the majority of pregnant women report symptoms of 'baby brain' were confirmed in a recent meta-analysis (Davies et al. 2018). This concluded that, consistent with the findings of long-term reductions in brain grey matter volume during pregnancy, overall cognitive functioning was significantly poorer in pregnant than in control women, particularly in the third trimester. Studies suggest these changes are reversible and women demonstrate a restoration/rejuvenation effect postpartum (Luders et al. 2018).

Adaptations in neural circuitry in the maternal brain are initiated by pregnancy hormones, which remodel the female brain, increasing the size of neurones in some regions and producing structural changes in others. Oestrogen and progesterone readily enter the brain to act on nerve cells changing the balance between inhibition and stimulation. The pregnancy hormones, such as relaxin, prolactin and lactogen, also have an impact on hormonal fluctuations occurring throughout pregnancy.

The raised levels of human chorionic gonadotropin and progesterone are soporific, stimulating daytime sleepiness and early sleep onset (Won 2015). However, pregnant women commonly experience poor sleep quality, insufficient night-time sleep, significantly disrupted sleep, and significant daytime sleepiness. A large (N=2427) internet-based survey found that 76% of pregnant women were poor sleepers, a much higher rate than for women in the general population (Mindell and Jacobson 2014). A pregnant woman's sleep pattern can be affected by mechanical and hormonal influences including nocturia, dyspnoea, nasal congestion, stress and anxiety, as well as muscular aches and pains, leg cramps and fetal activity (Box 10.5).

Studies of microchimerism (presence of fetal cells in the maternal body) suggest that pregnancy can leave a long-lasting footprint by altering the neuroplastic potential of the hippocampus and the brain's response to sex hormones. In middle age, verbal memory and global cognition may be enhanced while circulating hormones are reduced; male microchimerism increases the risk of autoimmune diseases but decreases the risk of some cancers and Alzheimer's disease (Boddy et al. 2015).

BOX 10.5 **Sleep Disturbances**

Various hormonal and mechanical influences promote insomnia leading to disturbed sleep during pregnancy, i.e. sleep fragmentation with greater amounts of light sleep and fewer periods of deep sleep. These disturbances tend to worsen as pregnancy advances, with up to 90% of women reporting frequent night awakenings (Won 2015) that for some continue postpartum. As a consequence, sleep disturbance has been associated with increased labour length and caesarean section rates and may also contribute to the tendency for some women becoming depressed postpartum compared with other periods in their life.

Interventions include establishing sleep–wake habits, avoiding caffeine, relaxation techniques, massage, heat and support for lower back pain, modifying sleep environment, limiting fluids in the evening and avoiding passive smoking. Sleep medications should be avoided, although psycho-educational interventions are being explored as a potentially effective alternative (Mindell and Jacobson 2014).

CHANGES IN THE URINARY SYSTEM

Major changes occur in the urinary system, which are critical for an optimal pregnancy outcome. Renal plasma flow rises early in pregnancy due to increased cardiac output and lowered renal afferent and efferent arteriolar resistance (Colombo 2017). The 40% reduction in systemic vascular resistance by week 6 of gestation creates a state of under-filling because 85% of the volume remains in the venous circulation. This is a situation unique to pregnancy (Soma-Pillay et al. 2016). By the second trimester, renal plasma flow increases by 60–80% (Nelson-Piercy 2015). The increase may be facilitated by relaxin, which boosts renal nitric oxide production (Cunningham et al. 2018). Nitric oxide plays a critical role in the decrease in renal resistance and subsequent renal hyperaemia. Relaxin appears to be important in activating some of the effects of nitric oxide on the kidney. Failure of this crucial adaptation is associated with adverse outcomes such as pre-eclampsia and fetal growth restriction. The increase in renal plasma flow is maintained until 34 weeks' gestation when a 25% decline occurs (Antony et al. 2017). Despite this, it is still 50% greater than pre-pregnancy values at term (Nelson-Piercy 2015).

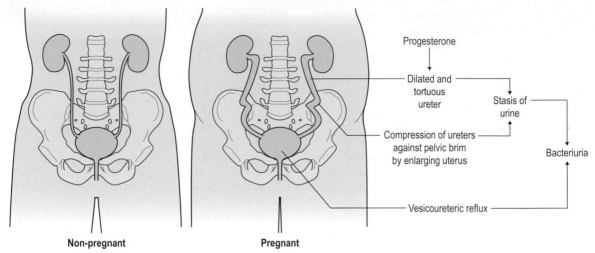

Non-pregnant   **Pregnant**

Fig. 10.7 Changes in the urinary tract in pregnancy and the factors predisposing women to urinary tract infection in pregnancy.

The increased renal blood flow causes the kidneys to enlarge by up to 30% and increase in length by 1 cm by mid-pregnancy. This results in *physiological hydronephrosis* in over 80% of women. This is often more prominent on the right side due to the right ureter crossing the iliac and ovarian vessels at an angle before entering the pelvis (Soma-Pillay et al. 2016). The kidneys, pelvis and calyceal systems all dilate due to mechanical compression on the ureters and reduced ureteral tone. Some dilatation develops before 14 weeks but this becomes more marked by mid-pregnancy. There is also some vesicoureteral reflux during pregnancy. Because of these physiological changes (Fig. 10.7), the risk of upper urinary tract infection rises (Cunningham et al. 2018).

Mild dilation of the ureters is normal in pregnancy, and is caused by progesterone-induced relaxation of smooth muscle in the walls of the ureters (Standring 2016). Dilation begins in the 2nd month of pregnancy and is maximal by the middle of the second trimester when ureteric diameter may be as much as 2 cm (Antony et al. 2017). There is also hypertrophy of smooth muscle and hyperplasia of connective tissue. These structural changes may persist for up to 4 months postpartum (Thornburg et al. 2015). Dilatation is right-sided in 86% of women with an average dilation of 15 mm on the right side and 5 mm on the left side by term (Antony et al. 2017). This may be because the left ureter is cushioned by the sigmoid colon, while the right ureter is compressed by the dextrorotated uterus. The dilated right ovarian vein complex lying obliquely over

the right ureter may also compound right ureteral dilatation (Cunningham et al. 2018). Ureteric dilatation is usually only found above the pelvic brim, which tends to suggest that dilation is mainly due to the mechanical compression of the ureters by the enlarging uterus as it rises out of the pelvis, laterally displacing and compressing them at the pelvic brim. However, the early onset of dilation suggests that progesterone is equally responsible (Antony et al. 2017).

Due to these anatomical and hormonal changes, pregnant women are more susceptible to develop urinary tract infections. Compression of the bladder as the uterus grows and increases in weight blocks the drainage of urine from the bladder (Sunil et al. 2018). Obstruction to the flow of urine leads to stasis and increases the likelihood of infection developing (Smaill and Vazquez 2015). Smooth muscle relaxation and dilation of the ureters facilitate the ascent of bacteria from the bladder to the kidney (Colombo 2017). Vesicoureteral reflux, and mechanical compression on the ureters by the growing uterus impedes flow and causes stasis of urine in the dilated collecting system (Soma-Pillay et al. 2016) and in conjunction with progesterone causes hydroureter and hydronephrosis. Differences in urine pH and osmolality and pregnancy-induced glycosuria and aminoaciduria may also facilitate bacterial growth, which may lead to asymptomatic bacteriuria, which occurs in 2–10% of pregnant women (Smaill and Vazquez 2015) (Box 10.6).

There are few anatomical changes in the bladder before 12 weeks' gestation. Thereafter, as the

BOX 10.6 Asymptomatic Bacteriuria

Asymptomatic bacteriuria is defined as the isolation of bacteria in at least 1×10^5 colony-forming units/mL on a cultured mid-stream specimen of urine in the absence of signs or symptoms of a urinary tract infection (Kazemier et al. 2015). Colonization of the urinary tract results from ascending infection from the perineum and may be related to sexual intercourse (Nelson-Piercy 2015). It is usually caused by *Escherichia coli* (*E. coli*) probably derived from the large bowel. If not treated, up to 40% of women will develop symptoms of a lower urinary tract infection (UTI), and approximately 25% of infected women will develop symptomatic infection during pregnancy (Cunningham et al. 2018). Treating asymptomatic bacteriuria reduces the risk of preterm birth, and low birth-weight babies (Nelson-Piercy 2015). A recent study controversially shows, however, that low-risk women with untreated asymptomatic bacteriuria, although at increased risk of symptomatic urinary tract infection during pregnancy, have only a 2.4% risk of pyelonephritis and that these women are not at increased risk of giving birth to a preterm or small for gestational age baby (Kazemier et al. 2015). This highlights the need for revised guidance on the management of pregnant women with asymptomatic bacteriuria. The initial antenatal appointment in the form of urine analysis and culture is now questioned on the grounds of efficacy and cost, as is the length of antibiotic treatment as both 4- and 7-day courses are considered effective (Johnstone et al. 2017).

BOX 10.7 Urinary Incontinence

Urinary incontinence affects nearly 20% of women during the first trimester and by the third trimester, at least half of all pregnant women experience some degree of urinary incontinence (Cunningham et al. 2018). The increasing pressure of the growing uterus and fetal weight on pelvic-floor muscles throughout pregnancy, together with pregnancy-related hormonal changes lead to reduced strength of pelvic floor supportive and sphincteric functions. Mobility of the bladder neck and urethra lead to urethral sphincter incompetence (Sangsawang and Sangsawang 2013). Risk factors for stress urinary incontinence (SUI) development are first pregnancy, maternal age >30 years, obesity, smoking, constipation, gestational diabetes mellitus and previous vaginal birth (Cunningham et al. 2018). Pelvic floor muscle exercises are a safe and effective treatment for SUI during pregnancy, without significant adverse effects (Sangsawang and Sangsawang 2013).

Encouraging uptake of a structured antenatal pelvic floor muscle training programme may decrease the risk and prevent the onset of urinary incontinence in late pregnancy and postpartum (Woodley et al. 2017). The possibility of urinary incontinence should be considered in the differential diagnosis of ruptured membranes (Cunningham et al. 2018).

uterus grows, the bladder trigone is elevated and the intraureteric margin thickens due to the hyperplasia of bladder muscle and connective tissues and generalized hyperaemia of all pelvic organs. Marked deepening and widening of the trigone continues until term (Cunningham et al. 2018). There is an increase in vascular size and tortuosity throughout the bladder, which can cause haematuria in a small proportion of women (Antony et al. 2017). Bladder capacity reduces and there is an increase in urinary frequency, urgency and incontinence due to the increasing size of the uterus (Antony et al. 2017). To compensate for reduced bladder capacity the urethral length increases. At the same time, maximal intraurethral pressure rises, thus continence is maintained. In spite of this, at least half of pregnant women experience some degree of urinary incontinence by the third trimester (Cunningham et al. 2018) (Box 10.7). Bladder pressure in primigravidae increases from 8 cm H_2O early in pregnancy to 20 cm H_2O at term. When the presenting part engages, the entire base of the bladder is pushed anteriorly and superiorly, which impairs blood and lymph drainage from the bladder base, often rendering the area oedematous, easily traumatized, and possibly more susceptible to infection. The normally convex surface of the bladder is converted into a concavity (Cunningham et al. 2018).

Due to the increase in renal plasma flow and renal vasodilation glomerular filtration rate is 50% higher than in the non-pregnant state by the end of the first trimester and this is maintained until the end of pregnancy (Cunningham et al. 2018). By the third trimester, renal plasma falls to non-pregnant levels whereas glomerular filtration rate continues to be elevated resulting in an increased filtration fraction. Progesterone, relaxin, renin, angiotensin and aldosterone are all implicated in these changes (Nelson-Piercy 2015). Glomerular filtration rate is best estimated in pregnancy by a 24-hour urine collection for creatinine clearance. Creatinine clearance rises in pregnancy by about 50% to values of 150 to 200 mL/min (normal is 120 mL/min). This increase occurs by 5–7 weeks' gestation and is normally maintained until the third trimester. Consequently, serum urea nitrogen and creatinine levels decrease during pregnancy to values of around 9 and 0.5 mg/dL, respectively from non-pregnant values of 13 and 0.8. A serum creatinine value of >0.8 mg/dL may therefore indicate abnormal renal function in pregnancy (Thornburg et al. 2015). Because of the rise in glomerular filtration rate (or due to decreased tubular reabsorption) uric acid excretion increases (Soma-Pillay et al. 2016). Levels of serum uric acid decline early in pregnancy until 24 weeks, reaching a nadir of 2 to 3 mg/dL. Thereafter the levels begin to rise and by the end of pregnancy, uric acid levels are at pre-pregnancy levels. The rise is caused by increased renal tubular absorption of urate and increased fetal uric acid production (Antony et al. 2017).

During pregnancy, glucose excretion increases. About 90% of pregnant women with normal blood glucose levels excrete 1 to 10 g of glucose/day (normal in the non-pregnant woman is <100 mg/day) resulting in glycosuria (Soma-Pillay et al. 2016). Glucose is freely filtered by the glomerulus and with the 50% increase in glomerular filtration rate coupled with decreased tubular glucose reabsorption in the proximal and collecting tubule, a greater load of glucose is presented to the proximal tubules (Antony et al. 2017). With this reduction in the average renal threshold for glucose (i.e. the plasma glucose level above which significant glucosuria begins to occur), glucosuria can be a feature of normal pregnancy (Cunningham et al. 2018). Glycosuria is not a reliable diagnostic tool for impaired glucose tolerance or diabetes in pregnancy (Nelson-Piercy 2015). If repetitive, women should be screened for diabetes mellitus (Antony et al. 2017).

Proteinuria and albuminuria increase as pregnancy advances. There is also an increase in excretion of amino acids in the urine and an increase in calcium excretion (Antony et al. 2017). Due to the increase in glomerular filtration rate and glomerular capillary permeability to albumen the excretion of protein may increase. In normal pregnancies, the total protein concentration in urine does not increase above the upper normal limit (Soma-Pillay et al. 2016), which is 300 mg in 24 h or a protein creatinine ratio of 30 mg/mmol (Nelson-Piercy 2015). Urinary albumin excretion often increases but remains within the normal pregnant range (Thornburg et al. 2015).

The filtered load of sodium increases but due to the increased tubular reabsorption, there is retention of about 1 g of sodium per day (Thornburg et al. 2015). Consequently, there is a physiological sodium and water retention, with 80% of pregnant women developing some oedema, which becomes more marked towards term (Nelson-Piercy 2015). Additional factors are believed to modulate sodium and water retention during pregnancy. Aldosterone secreted from the adrenal cortex is essential for normal renal sodium and potassium balance and thus indirectly regulates blood volume. The rate of aldosterone secretion and its consequent plasma levels are increased in normal gestation. The increased levels of aldosterone appear necessary to achieve this critically important adaptation of sodium and water retention (Thornburg et al. 2015). During pregnancy, urine volume is increased and nocturia is more common. In the upright position, sodium and water are retained but at night when in the recumbent position, the added water is excreted leading to nocturia. Later in pregnancy, renal function is affected by position and renal haemodynamics are decreased according to change from lateral recumbent, supine or standing positions (Antony et al. 2017).

Renal secretion of vitamin D, renin and erythropoietin are all increased in pregnancy (Nelson-Piercy 2015). Renal excretion of calcium increases during pregnancy with maximum excretion levels reached during the third trimester. Urinary excretion of calcium levels in pregnancy range between 350 and 620 mg/day (non-pregnant range 100–250 mg/day) (Swapna et al. 2015). In spite of the many physiological changes that promote increased filtration of potassium in pregnancy (volume expansion, increased renal blood flow, increased glomerular filtration rate (GFR) and activation of the renin-angiotensin-aldosterone axis), serum potassium levels remain at normal levels due to the increased levels of progesterone, which resist calcium excretion in the urine (Acelajado et al. 2016).

CHANGES IN THE GASTROINTESTINAL SYSTEM

Anatomical and physiological changes take place in each organ of the gastrointestinal system. The oral mucosa is sensitive to physiological, metabolic, hormonal and chemical changes within the body (Jain and Kaur 2015). Gingival hyperaemia and oedema of the gums occur in

Ptyalism is thought to be due to the inability of the pregnant woman to swallow saliva due to nausea rather than due to an increase in the production of saliva as previously believed. Although usually unexplained, ptyalism sometimes appears to follow salivary gland stimulation by the ingestion of starch (Antony et al. 2017). Many experts believe that ptyalism actually represents an inability of the nauseated woman to swallow normal amounts of saliva as opposed to a true increase in the saliva production (Greenspan 2018). Although ptyalism represents an unpleasant mental and physical condition, it is not thought to pose any specific risk to the health of the mother or increase adverse perinatal outcomes for the fetus (Bronshtein et al. 2018). Eating less starchy food may help decrease the amount of saliva (Antony et al. 2017). The increasing acidity of salivary pH as pregnancy advances, however, particularly in the third trimester, has been associated with increased prevalence of oral mucosal lesions, dental caries and gingivitis (Jain and Kaur 2015).

up to 75% of pregnant women. It causes the gingiva to change from dark red to blue. It may be due to hormonal changes and local irritation or nutritional deficiencies (Panicker et al. 2017). Ptyalism gravidarum is a condition of hypersalivation that affects pregnant women early in gestation. Symptoms include massive saliva volumes (up to 2 L/day), swollen salivary glands, sleep deprivation, significant emotional distress and social difficulties (Bronshtein et al. 2018) (Box 10.8).

Pregnancy gingivitis is more common in women with pre-existing gingivitis as it is aggravated by elevated progesterone and oestrogen levels resulting in increased vascular permeability and decreased immune resistance. Pregnancy gingivitis can vary from mild inflammation to severe hyperplasia, pain and bleeding. The inflammatory changes usually begin in the 2nd month and severity increases through the 8th month, after which they decline with declining hormone levels. The second trimester is considered the safest period for providing routine dental care. Importantly, pregnancy is not a contraindication to dental treatment, including dental radiographs. The importance of good oral hygiene in pregnancy should be emphasized (Ramos-e-Silva et al. 2016).

Bleeding gums can develop into a localized hyperplasia known as *pyogenic granuloma* or *pregnancy epulis*, which are lesions made of granulation tissue and inflammation (Antony et al. 2017). There is benign hyperplasia of capillaries and fibroblasts. It develops between the 2nd and 5th months of pregnancy in up to 10% of women, due to an increased inflammatory response to local irritations, then enlarges rapidly and bleeds easily, becoming hyperplastic and nodular. The lesions are usually painless and regress spontaneously postpartum, however reoccurrence is common (Ramos-e-Silva et al. 2016).

Periodontal disease occurs in up to 40% of pregnant women but there is no evidence to suggest that it increases more rapidly during pregnancy, in spite of the increased incidence of gingivitis (Antony et al. 2017). Periodontal disease has been linked previously with preterm birth, however evidence is insufficient to show an association between periodontal infection and preterm birth, nor is there evidence of improved outcomes following dental treatment during pregnancy. Nonetheless, good oral hygiene in pregnancy is recommended to improve dental health (Antony et al. 2017).

Between 50% and 90% of women have some degree of nausea with or without vomiting. Although often termed *morning sickness* – both symptoms frequently continue throughout the day (Cunningham et al. 2018). Nausea and vomiting have varying levels of severity and have far reaching effects for some women in terms of the ability to carry out day-to-day tasks, care for children and take part in full-time employment. It commonly occurs between weeks 5–18 and usually improves after 16 weeks. The causes of nausea and vomiting are unclear but may be related to increased levels of human chorionic gonadotrophin (hCG) which doubles every 48 h in early pregnancy and peaks at about 12 weeks (West et al. 2017). Women are therefore more likely to suffer from this condition if they have a multiple pregnancy, a previous history of the condition, a history of motion sickness, a relative who has also suffered from the condition, or who have a history of migraine headaches (West et al. 2017) (Box 10.9).

Biological regulation of appetite is very complex, engaging a number of tissues, organs, hormones and neural circuits throughout the body in a feedback loop between the brain and peripheral tissues. Leptin and insulin are just two of a number of hormones important in appetite regulation (MacLean et al. 2017). Leptin is secreted by adipose tissue in general and by the placenta during pregnancy. It plays an important role in fat metabolism by inhibiting hunger. During

BOX 10.9   **Nausea and Vomiting**

Treatment seldom provides complete relief, but symptoms can be minimized. Eating smaller meals at frequent intervals may help. The herbal remedy ginger is thought to be effective. Mild symptoms usually respond to vitamin B6 given along with doxylamine, but some women require phenothiazine or antiemetics (Cunningham et al. 2018). Supplemental vitamin B has been shown to be effective in relieving nausea and vomiting in pregnancy (West et al. 2017). Strategies to manage nausea, vomiting, heartburn and indigestion include: eating small, low-fat meals; eating slowly and regularly; avoiding strong food odours and foods that may cause stomach irritation such as spicy foods, citrus fruits, tomato products or peppermint; drinking fluids between meals rather than with meals; waiting 1–2 h after a meal before lying down; taking a walk after meals; brushing teeth after eating (West et al. 2017). Research has shown that supplemental vitamin B6 is effective at relieving nausea and vomiting during pregnancy. The upper level of vitamin B6 intake is 100 mg/day. Excessive amounts however, can cause numbness and nerve damage (West et al. 2017).

BOX 10.10   **Pica**

Pica items are diverse, and vary according to race/ethnicity, culture and geographic location. Most often the substances are harmless, but also may include toxic substances such as paint, pencil lead, sharp objects, sand, soap, starch and chalk, to name but a few. A mother that consumes clay is more at risk for adverse effects than a mother that consumes ice chips. Pica has been linked to both physiological and psychological impairments. Due to the related shame and stigma, it is difficult to diagnose and requires a trusting and reliable relationship between the woman and her midwife who needs to display sensitivity and empathy. Any underlying mental health concerns that may be contributing factors need to be considered. Treatment may include iron or other nutritional supplements, education, dietary advice and psychological assessment/treatment (Johnson and Gretton 2017).

pregnancy, its serum concentration rises significantly, especially in second and third trimesters. In spite of this rise in leptin levels, the appetite and food intake are still increased during pregnancy due to pregnancy-induced leptin resistance (Pusukuru et al. 2016). Some women who perceive their increased appetite is not satisfied feel they have low energy levels and feel 'wobbly' or 'faint'.

Women's gastrointestinal symptoms of pregnancy appear to be exacerbated by perceptual changes in smell, taste and texture (Swift et al. 2017). There may be an increase or a decrease in threshold in perceived tastes of sweet and sour, salty and bitter (Choo and Dando 2017). A blunted sense of taste in some women can lead to an increased desire for highly-seasoned food. Pica refers to the compulsive craving and consumption of non-food items that are non-nutritive (Box 10.10). Food cravings and aversions are commonly reported in pregnancy. Evidence suggests that the preference for savoury foods is strongest during the first trimester, while preference for sweet foods peaks in intensity during the second trimester. Both cravings and aversions can serve as motivators for increasing and/or decreasing the intake of certain foods. Food cravings have been associated with weight and eating-related pathology and are usually for foods that provide energy, whereas aversions are more often associated with the avoidance of foods that cause nausea and vomiting.

The most common cravings are for sweet foods, particularly chocolate and other high energy sugary and fatty foods, fruit dairy foods, meats and starchy foods. Many cravings are general (e.g. something sweet) while others are specific (e.g. chocolate ice cream or green apples). Others may be for unusual food combinations for example pickled onions and marmalade sandwiches (Hill et al. 2016).

Heartburn and indigestion affect two-thirds of pregnant women (Antony et al. 2017). In the third trimester, heartburn and reflux may be due to limited gastric capacity as the abdominal organs shift to accommodate the growing fetus. Other contributing factors are the combination of the upward displacement and compression of the stomach by the uterus, lower oesophageal pressure and decreased motility with relaxation of the lower oesophageal sphincter due to the effects of progesterone (West et al. 2017) (Box 10.11).

Pregnant women frequently complain of abdominal bloating and constipation. It is likely caused in pregnancy by hormonal changes that affect small bowel and colonic motility. Small bowel transit time appears to be significantly longer during pregnancy and more so

BOX 10.11 Heartburn

In most pregnant women, symptoms of heartburn are mild and relieved by eating smaller meals more frequently. Avoiding bending over or lying flat, not lying down after eating, abstaining from smoking and alcohol, elevating the head of the bed and acupuncture may all help to prevent it. So-called 'trigger' foods such as fatty foods, tomato-based foods and coffee should also be avoided. Oral antacids are first-line therapy and antacids such as aluminium hydroxide, magnesium trisilicate, or magnesium hydroxide may provide relief (Cunningham et al. 2018). Evidence on the effectiveness of the various treatments, however is limited and further research is needed to fully evaluate the effectiveness of these interventions in pregnancy. Future research should address other medications such as histamine 2-receptor antagonists, promotility drugs, proton pump inhibitors and a raft-forming alginate reflux suppressant. More research is needed on acupuncture and other complementary therapies as treatments for heartburn in pregnancy. Future research should also evaluate any adverse outcomes, maternal satisfaction with treatment and measure pregnant women's quality of life in relation to the intervention (Phupong and Hanprasertpong 2015).

BOX 10.12 Abdominal Distension

Abdominal distension may be relieved by avoiding carbonated beverages and drinking plenty of water. Regular exercise will help to reduce constipation and the accompanying build-up of gas by improving motility and transit through the intestines (Sigust 2018). The best approach is the increased use of dietary fibre by regular use of bread, fruits, vegetables and fruit juice. Non-starch polysaccharide bulking agents such as psyllium, methylcellulose, or sterculia are quite safe in pregnancy because no systemic absorption occurs. Some women may find it helpful to avoid dairy products or reduce fibre intake. Medication as advised by a doctor may be necessary to ease distension (Sigust 2018).

in both the second and third trimesters of pregnancy compared with the first trimester. Increased progesterone concentration has been shown to decrease the activity of colonic smooth muscle activity and possibly is also responsible for reduced concentration of plasma motilin, which is a stimulatory gastrointestinal hormone. Also, the pregnant uterus can impede the transit time in the small bowel particularly in late pregnancy (Bianco 2017) (Box 10.12).

STOMACH AND INTESTINES

The stomach and intestines are displaced as the uterus grows and the tone and motility of the stomach and gastro-oesophageal sphincter are decreased due to the effects of progesterone and oestrogen. Newer studies suggest that oestrogen-induced nitric oxide released from nerves that supply the gastrointestinal tract may also be implicated in the relaxation of the muscles (Antony et al. 2017). Scientific evidence regarding delayed gastric emptying, however, remains inconclusive. A study by Barboni et al. (2016) has shown that in pregnant women at term, the stomach does not seem to be able to expand immediately after a meal and the transit of food is completed later than in non-pregnant women. Other evidence suggests that it appears to be unchanged in the three trimesters of pregnancy compared with non-pregnant women and the only delay is seen in labour, possibly due to the pain and stress of labour (Antony et al. 2017) when the administration of opioids delays gastric emptying time considerably. Consequently, debate continues regarding the length of fasting required to avoid the dangers of general anaesthesia for birth, which could lead to regurgitation and aspiration of either food-laden or highly acidic gastric contents (Cunningham et al. 2018). Alterations in the motility of the small intestines and colon can result in either constipation or diarrhoea. The motility of the small intestines is reduced in pregnancy with increased oral-caecal transit times. Increased transit time allows for more efficient water and sodium absorption in the colon (Antony et al. 2017).

Constipation affects up to 50% of women during pregnancy. It is associated with straining, hard stools and incomplete evacuation (West et al. 2017). It can be very debilitating and decrease productivity and quality of life as well as inducing permanent pelvic muscle dysfunction. It can also delay recovery time of digestion postpartum and increase the prevalence of haemorrhoids (Hestiantoro and Baida 2018). Progesterone does not appear to alter colonic transit time and the cause of constipation is probably mainly due to the enlarged uterus mechanically limiting colonic emptying. In addition, the increased water absorption from the large intestine further slows gut motility (West et al. 2017) (Box 10.13).

BOX 10.13 Constipation and Haemorrhoids

Constipation has a range of consequences from reduced quality of life and perception of physical health. It is often accompanied by gastrointestinal discomfort, a bloated feeling, an increase in haemorrhoids and heartburn and decreased appetite. It can also be aggravated by iron supplements. Strategies for managing constipation in pregnancy include: increasing fluid intake and drinking more water, herbal teas and decaffeinated drinks, increasing the fibre intake including fruit and vegetables, increasing physical activity, and if necessary, taking stool softeners (West et al. 2017). The Cochrane review by Rungsiprakarn et al. (2015) reviewed interventions for treating constipation in pregnancy. From the little evidence that was found they suggest that dietary fibre supplementation may increase the frequency of stools, and that stimulant laxatives may relieve constipation better than bulk-forming laxatives although the former may cause more abdominal discomfort and diarrhoea. They conclude that more research in this area is needed (Rungsiprakarn et al. 2015).

Haemorrhoids develop during pregnancy due to high levels of progesterone, which decreases the strength of the muscle walls of the veins and reduces venous tone. A combination of increased intra-abdominal pressure, increased venous congestion from the weight of the fetus, and obstruction of venous return contributes to their incidence (Åhlund et al. 2018). While it is clear that the prevention of constipation and straining is paramount, further research is needed to determine the best treatment for haemorrhoids since the study by Beksac et al. (2018), found that haemorrhoid complaints increased despite dietary recommendations and physiotherapy interventions. Women with haemorrhoids may have on-going problems for more than a year after the birth of the baby and have described it as a neglected area by the healthcare system (Åhlund et al. 2018; Rungsiprakarn et al. 2015).

APPENDIX

The appendix is usually progressively displaced upward and outwards from the right lower quadrant by the growing uterus. At times, it may reach the right flank (Cunningham et al. 2018). These anatomical changes may obscure classic signs of appendicitis thereby confounding the diagnosis (Greenspan 2018).

GALLBLADDER

During normal pregnancy, progesterone inhibits the contraction of the smooth muscle of the gallbladder leading to reduced contractility. The rate at which the gallbladder empties is much slower in pregnancy and after the first trimester the fasting and residual volumes are twice as great (Antony et al. 2017). Impaired emptying, subsequent stasis and the increased cholesterol saturation of bile in pregnancy contribute to the increased prevalence of cholesterol gallstones in multiparas (Cunningham et al. 2018).

There is a progressive rise in serum bile acids with advancing pregnancy probably due to a combination of gestational signals that act on bile acid metabolism and transport in the liver and gut (McIlvride et al. 2017). Most women stay below the upper limit of the normal reference range (10–14 μmol/L). If serum levels rise above this range accompanied by hepatic impairment and pruritus that is not explained by any other disorder, a diagnosis is made of intrahepatic cholestasis of pregnancy (ICP), a specific disease associated with adverse fetal outcomes including stillbirth (McIlvride et al. 2017). It is vital therefore that pruritus gravidarum is differentiated from generalized itch of greater severity commonly affecting hands and feet with deterioration during the night – which is frequently connected with ICP (Szczęch et al. 2017).

LIVER

Liver size is unchanged in pregnancy, however many clinical signs associated with liver disease are evident (Antony et al. 2017). Estimates of hepatic blood flow in normal pregnancy have demonstrated a significant rise in portal blood flow compared with pre-pregnancy values. This occurs via an increase in the diameter of the intra- and extra-hepatic branches of the portal vein, despite a reduction in mean blood velocity (Bissonnette et al. 2015). Some laboratory test results of hepatic function are altered in normal pregnancy. Biochemical and haematological indices taken during pregnancy need to be interpreted in light of these altered normal ranges (Table 10.5). Maternal alkaline phosphatase (ALP) increases in the third trimester (Westbrook et al. 2016) and serum aspartate transaminase (AST), alanine transaminase (ALT), γ-glutamyl transpeptidase (GGT) and bilirubin levels are slightly lower compared with non-pregnant values (Cunningham et al. 2018). Understanding these physiological changes in liver function tests during normal pregnancy is essential for identifying pathological conditions of the liver.

Changes in Metabolism

Numerous and intense metabolic changes in carbohydrate, protein and fat metabolism occur during pregnancy. These changes provide for the needs of the rapidly growing fetus and placenta and prepare the woman for subsequent lactation and care of the baby (Longo 2018). By the third trimester, maternal basal metabolic (BMR) rate rises by 20% compared with the non-pregnant state (Cunningham et al. 2018). The total maternal energy requirements for a full term pregnancy to support the maternal cardiovascular, renal and respiratory systems are estimated at 80,000 kcal, or 300 kcal/day. This accounts for the increased metabolic activity of maternal and fetal tissues as well as for the growth of fetus and placenta (West et al. 2017).

Guidelines for energy requirements in pregnancy in many countries agree that additional requirements are relatively modest after allowance for the physical and metabolic adaptations for pregnancy. Furthermore, increases in caloric intake in well-nourished women are not distributed equally throughout the antenatal period (Swift et al. 2017). The Institute of Medicine (2009) and World Health Organization (WHO 2016) recommend that pregnant women of normal weight with a singleton pregnancy in the general obstetric population in developed countries do not need to increase energy intake in the first trimester when energy expenditure does not change greatly. However, in the second and third trimesters, daily caloric intake should be increased by 340 and 450 additional kcal/day, respectively, above the non-pregnant energy requirements for appropriate weight gain (West et al. 2017). As energy requirements may also vary by physical activity as well as age, weight and height, recommendations regarding energy intake may require to be individualized (Garner 2019). However, the Royal College of Obstetricians and Gynaecologists (RCOG 2015) recommends that since one in five pregnant women in the UK are obese, energy needs do not change until the last 12 weeks of pregnancy when women need only a modest increase of 200 kcal/day – an approximate 10% increase from the 1940 kcal/day recommendation in the non-pregnant adult woman (Ho et al. 2016).

Most women in pregnancy require a significant increase in food intake, particularly in early to mid-gestation to promote uteroplacental development (Thornburg et al. 2015). Women require advice to ensure they achieve the most balanced diet possible, as what a woman eats during pregnancy can have a profound and lasting effect on her health and that of her child (Koenig 2017). There is clear evidence that reduced fetal growth prior to birth can lead to chronic disease as adults (Thornburg et al. 2015).

In order to give appropriate and culturally sensitive advice on diet and nutrition, clinicians should be aware of the impact of dietary practices, which vary from society to society and are passed from one generation to the next, often deeply rooted in religious, cultural and traditional beliefs. For example, despite healthcare professional advice, Muslim women may prefer to observe daylight fasting during Ramadan, even though according to the Quran it is not considered mandatory for pregnant women (D'Souza et al. 2016). Prenatal exposure to maternal fasting during Ramadan has been shown to lead to increased risks for the fetus of chronic diseases in adulthood. It is important therefore that midwives are educated to proactively address this sensitive religious topic with women to ensure they make an informed decision about fasting (Leimer et al. 2018).

The accumulation of white fat (lipogenesis) in response to the rise in insulin secretion provides essential energy sources for both mother and fetus and serves as an energy reservoir for breastmilk synthesis during lactation. Fat storage occurs mostly in the second trimester and is mainly central rather than in peripheral sites. With the accumulation of water and electrolytes, the growth of some organs and fat deposition, the average weight gain during pregnancy is 12.5 kg (Longo 2018). Adiponectin is a protein produced by the maternal and fetal adipose tissue and plays a role in the modulation of glucose and lipid metabolism in insulin-sensitive tissues and the developing of gestational diabetes. Maternal adiponectin levels are generally decreased during pregnancy, especially in the third trimester of pregnancy when compared with the non-gravid state. This results in increased production of glucose by the liver (Pusukuru et al. 2016).

Pregnancy is described as a *diabetogenic state* and the adaptation in glucose metabolism allows shunting of glucose to the fetus to promote development while maintaining adequate maternal nutrition. Hyperplasia of pancreatic beta cells results in increased insulin secretion and increased insulin sensitivity in early pregnancy followed by progressive insulin resistance. While insulin production doubles from the end of the first trimester to the third trimester, pregnancy is a state of physiological insulin resistance and relative glucose intolerance. Resistance to the action of insulin on glucose uptake and utilization means there is decreased ability of target tissues such as liver, adipose tissue and muscle to respond to normal circulating concentrations of insulin. Maternal insulin resistance serves as a physiological adaptation of the mother to ensure adequate carbohydrate supply for the rapidly growing fetus. It leads to more use of fats than carbohydrates for energy by the mother and spares carbohydrates for the fetus (Sonagra et al. 2014).

In the first trimester, insulin sensitivity increases but in the second and third trimesters, there is progressive insulin resistance as a result of increasing secretion of human placental lactogen (hPL), growth hormone, progesterone, cortisol and prolactin. These hormones cause a decrease in insulin sensitivity in the peripheral tissues such as adipocytes and skeletal muscle by interfering with insulin receptor signalling (Nelson-Piercy 2015). In late normal pregnancy, insulin action is 50% lower than in the non-pregnant state. Oestrogen and progesterone may partly be responsible for this insulin resistance and placental lactogen may also play a part (Longo 2018). Hypoglycaemia results in lipolysis allowing the pregnant woman to use fat for fuel, preserving the available glucose and amino acids for the fetus and minimizing protein catabolism (Soma-Pillay et al. 2016). Screening of all pregnant women for insulin resistance is recommended as early interventions may help to reduce the associated complications. Insulin sensitivity can be improved by modifying diet, lifestyle, amount and type of physical activity, avoidance of sedentary lifestyle and increasing amount of activity before, during and after pregnancy (Sonagra et al. 2014).

Normal pregnancy is characterized by a state of mild fasting hypoglycaemia, postprandial hyperglycaemia, and hyperinsulinaemia (Longo 2018). After an oral glucose meal, the pregnant woman demonstrates prolonged hyperglycaemia and hyperinsulinaemia and a greater suppression of glucagon. This reflects the pregnancy-induced state of peripheral insulin resistance, which ensures a sustained postprandial supply of glucose to the fetus. Insulin sensitivity in late normal pregnancy is 30–70% lower than that of non-pregnant women (Cunningham et al. 2018).

Overnight, the pregnant woman changes from a postprandial state characterized by elevated and sustained glucose levels to a fasting state characterized by decreased plasma glucose and some amino acids. Plasma concentrations of free fatty acids, triglycerides and cholesterol are also higher in the fasting state. This pregnancy-induced switch in fuels from glucose to lipids has been called *accelerated starvation*, and when fasting is prolonged in the pregnant woman, these alterations are exaggerated and ketonaemia rapidly appears (Cunningham et al. 2018). Pregnant women skipping meals quickly reach states similar to those of 'accelerated starvation' (Leimer et al. 2018).

Fasting glucose levels are decreased due to increased storage of tissue glycogen, increased peripheral glucose use, decrease in glucose production by the liver and uptake of glucose by the fetus. The placenta allows transfer of glucose, amino acids and ketones to the fetus but is impermeable to large lipids. Gestational diabetes develops when the woman is unable to overcome the insulin resistance associated with pregnancy (Soma-Pillay et al. 2016). Normal glucose ranges for the majority of healthy individuals are 4.0–5.4 mmol/L when fasting but may rise to 7.8 mmol/L 2 h after eating. Gestational diabetes is diagnosed if the woman has either a fasting blood glucose level of 5.6 mmol/L or above, or a 2-h post-prandial blood glucose level of 7.8 mmol/L or above (NICE 2018b).

The concentrations of lipids, lipoproteins and apolipoproteins in plasma rise appreciably during pregnancy. Increased insulin resistance and oestrogen stimulation during pregnancy are responsible for the appreciable rise maternal hyperlipidaemia causing maternal fat accumulation during the first two trimesters. In the third trimester, however, fat storage declines or ceases due to enhanced lipolytic activity, which reduces circulating triglyceride uptake into adipose tissue. Cholesterol levels are also increased in the third trimester. This allows maternal use of lipids as an energy source and spares glucose and amino acids for the fetus. Maternal hyperlipidaemia is one of the most consistent and striking changes of lipid metabolism during late pregnancy (Cunningham et al. 2018).

The growing fetus and placenta places great demands on requirements for protein (Longo 2018). Amino acids are actively transported across the placenta to fulfil the needs of the developing fetus and protein catabolism is decreased as fat stores are used to provide for energy metabolism (Soma-Pillay et al. 2016). However, increased intake of protein is required during pregnancy for fetal, placental and maternal tissue development. Protein recommendations are increased from 46 g/day for an adult non-pregnant woman to 71 g/day throughout pregnancy (West et al. 2017). Pregnant women are advised by the Food and Drug Administration (FDA) to consume 200–300 mg/day of protein. This is important for fetal brain development, which is best sourced by consuming 1–2 servings of fish per week (West et al. 2017).

Maternal intestinal calcium absorption is doubled during pregnancy from 12 weeks' gestation to meet the significant need of the fetus for calcium. The fetus requires about 30 g calcium to maintain its physiological processes, 80% of which is deposited during the third trimester. To help compensate, sufficient calcium is required in the diet to prevent excess depletion from the mother. This is especially important for pregnant adolescents, in whom bones are still developing (Cunningham et al. 2018). The early increase in calcium absorption may allow the maternal skeleton to store calcium in advance. Increased calcium absorption is associated with an increase in calcium excretion in the urine and these changes begin from 12 weeks. During periods of fasting urinary calcium values are low or normal confirming that hypercalcaemia is the consequence of increased absorption. Pregnancy is therefore a risk factor for kidney stones (Soma-Pillay et al. 2016).

Vitamin D supplementation is essential for proper absorption of calcium, normal bone health and skeletal homeostasis during pregnancy and it is critical for fetal growth and development. Low maternal vitamin D status has been associated with reduced intrauterine long-bone growth, shorter gestation, congenital rickets and fractures in the newborn. It may also be helpful in preventing pre-eclampsia and promoting neonatal wellbeing. The recommended intake of vitamin D during pregnancy and lactation is 600 IU/day. Supplementation with 1000 to 4000 IU/day of vitamin D is advised for women who are strict vegetarians, black women, those with limited access to sunlight and those who avoid dairy foods (West et al. 2017).

Vitamin C (ascorbic acid) is needed for iron uptake. Women who smoke have an increased need for vitamin C. Pregnant women are recommended to consume 85 mg/day of vitamin C to ensure that adequate amounts are transported to the fetal circulation (West et al. 2017).

MATERNAL WEIGHT

A variety of components contribute to weight gain during pregnancy (Table 10.7). Normal weight gain during pregnancy is more likely to be associated with optimal reproductive outcome, fetal and infant growth and development. It varies considerably between individuals, with very low or very high weight gains being associated with poorer outcomes compared with moderate weight gain. Less weight gain is recommended with each step increase in pre-pregnancy BMI (Thornburg et al. 2015). Pre-conception health is strongly linked to the outcome of pregnancy and research identifies the preconception period as crucial for health across generations (Stephenson et al. 2018). Starting pregnancy at an appropriate pre-gravid weight is therefore very important. Although variable between women, it is generally considered that gestational weight gain is comprised of the accumulation of the following: the fetus 27%, the placenta 5%, amniotic fluid 6%, uterus 10%, breasts 3%, blood volume and extravascular fluid 22%, and maternal fat stores 27% (Triunfo and Lanzone 2015). The degree to which pregnant women deposit additional adipose tissue in visceral (central) and subcutaneous (peripheral) adipose tissue depots varies considerably

TABLE 10.7 Distribution of Average Increase in Weight

	WEIGHT GAIN	
	(kg)	**(lb)**
Maternal		
Uterine hypertrophy	0.9	2
Breast enlargement	0.5–1.4	1–3
Fat stores	2.7–3.6	6–8
Increased blood volume	1.4–1.8	3–4
Increased extravascular fluid volume	0.9–1.4	2–3
Fetal		
Fetus	3.2–3.6	7–8
Placenta	0.7	1.5
Amniotic fluid	0.9	2
Total	11.00–14.00	24.5–31.5

From Poston L. (2018) Gestational weight gain. UpToDate. Waltham, MA. Available at: www.uptodate.com/contents/gestational-weight-gain.

but is important because of the potential contribution to future chronic disease (Gilmore et al. 2015). The majority of the maternal fat deposited during pregnancy is subcutaneous and is deposited mainly in the hips, back and upper thighs, a pattern unique to pregnancy. Fat deposition occurs mainly during the first 30 weeks of gestation under progesterone stimulation. This early fat deposit acts as an energy store for late pregnancy and during lactation (Donangelo and Bezerra 2016).

The total amount of weight gained during pregnancy, regardless of preconception BMI classification, has dramatically increased over the last 4 decades from 10 kg to 15 kg. In the USA for example, more than 48% of all women exceed the American Institute of Medicine (IOM 2009) guidelines for appropriate weight gain during pregnancy. The number of women entering pregnancy as either overweight or obese has increased significantly. This presents a major public health concern and evidenced-based prevention programmes are needed on a wide scale (Gilmore et al. 2015).

The IOM (2009) guidelines recommend that women of normal weight (BMI 18.5–24.9) should gain 11.5–16 kg; obese women (BMI ≥30) should gain only 5–9 kg; overweight women (BMI 25–29.9) should gain 11–7 kg; and underweight women (BMI <18.5) (should gain <12.5–18 kg (Rasmussen and Yaktine 2009). Gestational weight gain below or above the IOM guidelines is associated with higher risk of adverse maternal and infant outcomes (Goldstein et al. 2017). However, these recommendations were issued without firm scientific evidence to support them, and their value remains unproven (Cunningham et al. 2018). In the UK, NICE guidelines do not recommend specific gestational weight gain targets, which makes it difficult to advise women on appropriate weight gain in pregnancy (Olander 2015), and instead tips for healthy eating and activity are recommended. Interestingly, a large UK trial (Poston et al. 2015) recently found that limiting weight gain in pregnant women with obesity during pregnancy is not adequate to prevent gestational diabetes, or to reduce the incidence of large-for-gestational-age infants, further suggesting strong evidence is still lacking for what constitutes appropriate healthy or safe weight gain in pregnancy (Olander 2015).

One of the most significant adaptations of pregnancy is the increase in total body water of 6.5–8.5 L by the end of pregnancy. Extravascular fluid collects in the uterus, breasts and adipose tissue and contributes to overall maternal weight gain along with increased blood volume. A decline in interstitial colloid osmotic pressure induced by normal pregnancy causes oedema late in pregnancy. Pitting oedema of ankles and legs is evident in most pregnant women, especially at the end of the day during the second and third trimesters. This may amount to ≥1 L and results from greater venous pressure below the level of the uterus due to partial occlusion of the vena cava (Cunningham et al. 2018). It is accompanied by feelings of heaviness and pressure of limbs and pain. Compression stockings and regular physical exercise including aquatic exercise and foot massage may be helpful in reducing swelling, however further research is required in this area to provide evidence-based care (Ochalek et al. 2017).

Pregnancy is therefore a condition of chronic volume overload with active sodium and water retention secondary to changes in osmoregulation and the renin-angiotensin system (Antony et al. 2017). Accumulation of total body water is normal in pregnancy and mediated partly by a drop in plasma osmolality of 10 mOsm/kg, which develops early in pregnancy (Cunningham et al. 2018). This should exert an inhibitory influence on thirst mechanisms however, a reset of osmotic thresholds for thirst and vasopressin secretion occurs. Consequently, thirst perception is significantly higher in pregnant women despite plasma hypotonicity. It reaches a peak in the second trimester, remaining at that peak until term (Agoreyo and Obika 2017).

Elements of Weight Gain in Pregnancy

In the first trimester, placental growth is more rapid than that of the fetus. By 17 weeks' gestation, placental and fetal weights are approximately equal. From 20 weeks onwards there is substantial increase in fetal weight as growth is influenced by insulin and other growth factors. Fat is laid down in late pregnancy and the fetus reaches an average of 3.5 kg at term while placental weight is approximately one-sixth of fetal weight (Cunningham et al. 2018). Amniotic fluid volume increases throughout pregnancy reaching 800 mL by the mid-third trimester (Cunningham et al. 2018) and accounting for 6% of gestational weight (Donangelo and Bezerra 2016). The volume of amniotic fluid increases rapidly with gestation and averages about 50 mL at 12 weeks; 400 mL at 20 weeks; reaches a peak of nearly 1 L at 35 weeks; after which the volume decreases to a range of about 100 mL at 43 weeks (Patil and Patil

TABLE 10.8	Breast Changes in Chronological Order
Time of Occurrence	**Changes**
4–12 weeks	Breasts feel nodular and lumpy, tender and tingly due to the development in the ductal system (under the influence of oestrogen) and due to lobular formation (under the influence of progesterone). The breasts begin to increase in size
12 weeks	The nipples are more prominent and the areola develops an increased fullness and brown pigmentation (primary areola) The sebaceous and lactiferous glands, known as Montgomery's tubercles, begin to provide secretions to lubricate and protect the areola and nipple during pregnancy and lactation, become more visible and appear as raised projections. They also provide a scent to attract the newborn to the nipple
16 weeks	Colostrum is synthesized (under the influence of prolactin) but high circulating levels of progesterone prevent milk excretion
16 weeks	Blood supply increases and a network of subcutaneous veins becomes visible beneath the skin. This network increases in size and complexity throughout pregnancy
24 weeks	Further pigmentation appears around the primary areola (secondary areola) and is particularly noticeable in dark-haired women
By term	Breasts usually enlarge by 5 cm overall and increase up to 1.4 kg in weight

From Pollard M. (2017) The breasts and lactation In: J Rankin (Ed.) Physiology in childbearing. Edinburgh: Elsevier.

2014). The weight of the breasts increases during pregnancy by about 400 g, with considerable variability between women (Cunningham et al. 2018). Changes in the breasts are summarized in Table 10.8.

MUSCULOSKELETAL CHANGES

Pregnancy weight gain progressively increases the mechanical stress on the joints of the axial skeleton and pelvis. This is compounded by the position of the gravid uterus which shifts the centre of gravity, causing the spine to shift to a more posterior position accompanied by a slight lumbar lordosis. Towards term, many women accommodate these changes by adopting a typical 'pregnancy' posture and both stand and walk with their backs arched and the shoulders held backwards. The abdominal muscles are stretched to their elastic limit by the end of pregnancy and are less efficient at maintaining core stability and achieving balance recovery (Wu and Yeoh 2014). The distance between the two rectus abdominis muscles widen, and the linea alba can split under the strain resulting in diastasis recti (Thabah and Ravindran 2015).

The hormones progesterone, oestrogen, prolactin and relaxin play an important part in some of these musculoskeletal manifestations; however, their precise role and timing remain unclear. Production of relaxin from the corpus luteum increases 10-fold, its primary function is to target pelvic ligaments, enabling pelvic cavity expansion to create a better 'cradle' to support the gravid uterus. However, by increasing pelvic laxity and relaxing pelvic ligaments, it increases instability placing additional mechanical strain on the back, symphysis pubis and sacroiliac joints. Progesterone and oestrogen soften ligaments by altering ground substance and digesting collagen fibres, increasing mobility of joint capsules and pelvic joint structure in preparation for birth.

Throughout pregnancy there is a gradual accumulation of additional musculoskeletal modifications, which result in a decreased neuromuscular control and coordination, decreased abdominal strength, increased spinal lordosis and changes in mechanical loading and joint kinetics. Toward the third trimester, water retention leads to soft tissue oedema in the lower limbs and may also lead to joint effusion and cause nerve entrapment. The pelvic floor may drop as much as 2.5 cm (1 inch) leading to pudendal nerve compression from the gravid uterus. There is a permanent loss of medial arch height of foot, with concomitant increases in foot length and arch drop (Segal et al. 2013). Hormonal and biomechanical imbalances in addition to an increased functional demand on the ankle plantar flexors during pregnancy exacerbate leg cramp syndrome. This is caused by the sudden involuntary spasm of the gastrocnemius muscle. Treatment for leg cramps is not usually required.

> **BOX 10.14 Back Pain**
>
> As a result of the many changes in load and body mechanics, many women experience low back pain. The stretched abdominal muscles lose their ability to maintain posture so that the lower back has to support the majority of the weight.
>
> Women who exercise prior to and during pregnancy can strengthen abdominal, back and pelvic muscles to improve posture and increased weight-bearing ability. Exercise in the second half of pregnancy focusing on abdominal strength, pelvic tilts and water aerobics are particularly effective in reducing low back pain. Pelvic girdle support belts and corsets are also useful in supporting the back. Simple home remedies such as heat pads and over-the-counter medication may ease the pain before muscle relaxants or opioids are considered. Self-care methods such as light exercise, yoga, massage and acupressure are known to be effective interventions (Gibson 2017).

> **BOX 10.15 Hair Growth**
>
> Hair growth has been shown to follow a common pattern in pregnancy. Women commonly report a thickening and increased volume of scalp hair. Stimulated by oestrogen, the growing period (anagen) for hairs is increased in pregnancy so the woman reaches the end of pregnancy with many over-aged hairs. This ratio is reversed after birth, so that sometimes alarming amounts of hair are shed (telogen phase) during brushing or washing (Gizlenti and Ekmekci 2014). Spontaneous hair recovery takes 3–12 months (Kar et al. 2012). Actions that may help include reducing damage to the hair by not combing when it is wet, and avoiding hairstyles that pull and stress hair, using shampoos and conditioners that contain biotin and silica. Diet that is high in fruit and vegetables containing flavonoids and antioxidants may provide protection for the hair follicles and encourage growth. Mild hirsutism is common during pregnancy, particularly on the face but usually resolves after delivery (Vora et al. 2014).

Various treatments have been explored for preventing and alleviating cramps, including Vitamin B1, B6, D, E, C and magnesium, calcium supplements; to-date, no consensus has been reached (Mansouri et al. 2017)

All of these changes influence postural control and may be related to the significant increased risk of falling in pregnancy comparable with that of over 65-year-olds (Wu and Yeoh 2014). The malalignments caused by the changes in load and body mechanics result in approximately 75% of women experiencing low back pain in pregnancy (Gharaibeh et al. 2018) (Box 10.14).

SKIN CHANGES

Pregnancy causes a variety of common changes in skin, hair and nails, which in the majority of cases is a normal physiological response modulated by hormonal, immunological and metabolic factors (Box 10.15). Those attributed to hormonal changes are often also seen in women on the combined oral contraceptive pill (Handel et al. 2014), while other changes have been shown to be familial, particularly *striae gravidarum* (stretch marks) and hyperpigmentation.

Increased melanin synthesis is due to raised melanocyte stimulating hormone, progesterone and oestrogen serum levels, which lead to an increased melanin synthesis intensified by upregulation of tyrosinase by human placental lipids (Bieber et al. 2017). Almost all women note some degree of skin darkening during pregnancy. While the exact physiology remains unclear (Natale et al. 2016), it is generally attributed to a combination of hormonal factors, genetic predisposition and ultraviolet exposure (Motosko et al. 2017). Hyperpigmentation is more marked in dark-skinned women, being pronounced in areas that are normally pigmented, e.g. areola, genitalia and umbilicus but can also occur in areas prone to friction, such as the axillae and inner thighs, and in recent scars. The *linea alba* is a line that lies over the midline of the rectus muscles from the umbilicus to the symphysis pubis, hyperpigmentation causes it to darken resulting in the distinct *linea nigra*.

Pigmentation of the face affects up to 50–70% of pregnant women and is known as *chloasma* or *melasma*. It is more common in women with darker complexions (Ikino et al. 2015). Numerous factors have been implicated in its aetiology: pregnancy hormones, cosmetics, photosensitizing medications, endocrinopathies (e.g. hypothyroidism), emotional stress and anticonvulsants, along with a genetic predisposition and exposure to sunlight. Ultimately it is caused by melanin deposition into epidermal or dermal macrophages, further exacerbated by sun exposure (Tamega et al. 2013). The chloasma usually regresses postpartum but may persist in approximately 10% of women and may be aggravated by oral contraceptives, which should be avoided in susceptible women (Handel et al. 2014).

As maternal size increases in pregnancy, stretching occurs in the collagen layer of the skin, particularly over the breasts, abdomen and thighs. In some women, this results in *striae gravidarum* caused by thin tears occurring in the dermal collagen. These appear as red or purple stripes changing to glistening, silvery white lines, approximately 6 months postpartum. The aetiology of striae has yet to be defined but may be compounded by adrenocorticoids, oestrogens and relaxin, which modify collagen and possibly elastic tissue. Other predisposing factors include raised BMI, familial history and birth weight (Kasielska-Trojan et al. 2015). Longstanding attempts to identify an effective treatment remain inconclusive (Korgavkar and Wang 2015).

Pruritus in pregnancy is characterized by intense itching either with or without a rash. It occurs in up to 20% of pregnancies (Nelson-Piercy 2015) with numerous potential differential diagnoses, including infection, eczema or is related to drug therapy.

Angiomas or *vascular spiders* (minute red elevations on the skin of the face, neck, arms and chest) and palmar erythema (reddening of the palms) frequently occur, possibly as a result of high oestrogen levels. They are rarely of clinical significance and usually resolve spontaneously within a few months postpartum. Nevertheless, changes may mask more serious conditions such as malignant neoplasms or herpes gestationis. It is therefore imperative to assess for specific dermatoses of pregnancy that may be associated with maternal disease and fetal mortality and morbidity if severe and left untreated (Motosko et al. 2017).

CHANGES IN THE ENDOCRINE SYSTEM

The changes in all compartments of the endocrine system and their timing are critical for the initiation and maintenance of pregnancy, for fetal growth and development and for parturition (see Chapter 5). Hormone levels are influenced by and vary according to parity, BMI, age, gestation, ethnicity and smoking.

Placental Hormones

Human chorionic gonadotrophin (hCG) is the earliest hormone produced by the new conceptus and is produced as early as 7 days after implantation. Its primary importance is immediately after conception and during the first few weeks of pregnancy when it prevents regression of the corpus luteum and thus maintains the

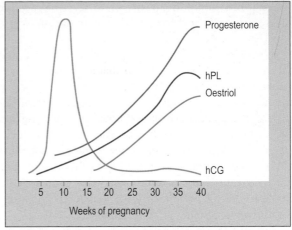

Fig. 10.8 Variations in plasma hormone concentrations during a normal pregnancy. (From Oats J, Abraham S. (2017) Llewellyn-Jones fundamentals of obstetrics and gynaecology. (10th edn.). Edinburgh: Elsevier.)

continued secretion of progesterone, oestrogen and relaxin (Kuo et al. 2018). This continues throughout pregnancy, however its endocrine function is largely replaced by the placenta after 8 weeks' gestation (Standring 2016). Before 5 weeks, hCG is expressed both in the syncytiotrophoblast and in cytotrophoblasts. Later, in the first trimester when maternal serum levels peak, hCG is produced almost solely in the syncytiotrophoblast. hCG likely enters maternal blood at the time of blastocyst implantation. Plasma levels rise rapidly after implantation, doubling every 2 days in the first trimester. Secretion of hCG peaks at concentrations of 100,000 mIU/mL at 10 weeks, after which plasma levels begin to decline, and a nadir of 30,000 mIU/mL is reached by approximately 14 weeks (Fig. 10.8) and this lower level is maintained for the remainder of gestation (Cunningham et al. 2018).

Measurement of hCG has many useful functions, not least it is the basis of the pregnancy test (Kuo et al. 2018). Maternal urine also contains hCG and concentrations follow the same general pattern in the urine as that in maternal plasma, peaking at approximately 10 weeks' gestation (Cunningham et al. 2018). Serial hCG measurements can assist in establishing the viability of an uncertain gestation as well as a possible ectopic pregnancy. Pregnancies with trisomies 13, 18 and 21 secrete either too high or too low levels of hCG and molar pregnancy secretes very high hCG levels (Kuo et al. 2018). Total hCG levels may differ according to maternal BMI, smoking, parity, ethnicity, child gender, placental weight and hyperemesis gravidarum symptoms (Korevaar et al. 2015).

Relaxin is secreted by the corpus luteum, decidua and placenta in a pattern similar to that of hCG. Its secretion supports many physiological adaptations, such as enhanced renal haemodynamics, lowered serum osmolality and increased arterial compliance (Cunningham et al. 2018). It is also involved in endometrial vascularization, remodelling of connective tissue and softening of the cervix in preparation for birth (Vannuccini et al. 2016). Despite its name, serum relaxin levels do not contribute to greater peripheral joint laxity or pelvic girdle pain during pregnancy (Cunningham et al. 2018).

Human placental lactogen (hPL) is secreted by the syncytiotrophoblast and can be detected in the maternal circulation as early as the 3rd week of gestation. Concentrations rise steadily until reaching a plateau around 36 weeks. HPL influences maternal metabolism by promoting lipolysis, which increases circulating free fatty acid levels. This provides an energy source for maternal metabolism and fetal nutrition. It also acts as an appetite stimulant and promotes growth of mammary glandular tissue in preparation for lactation. Its action as an insulin antagonist thereby raising maternal blood glucose is now in question, since placental growth hormone is believed to have a more important role in this respect (Burton et al. 2017).

The principal role of oestrogens in pregnancy is to stimulate uterine growth and increase blood flow. Oestrogens also affect breast development in preparation for lactation. The major oestrogen formed during pregnancy is oestriol, which constitutes >90% of the oestrogen in pregnancy urine (Mesiano 2018). In addition, significant levels of oestriol and oestradiol are found in the maternal circulation, and levels also rise, particularly late in gestation. During the first 2–4 weeks of pregnancy, oestradiol is produced in the corpus luteum under the influence of rising hCG levels. After the 7th week of pregnancy, there is a significant drop in the production of both progesterone and oestrogens in the maternal ovaries. By the 7th week, more than half of the oestrogen entering the maternal circulation is produced in the placenta. It continues to produce vast amounts so that at term, pregnancy is a hyper-oestrogenic state. This terminates abruptly after delivery of the placenta (Cunningham et al. 2018). Oestrogen promotes uterine quiescence by advancing progesterone responsiveness and at the end of pregnancy it

aids processes leading to parturition. Oestrogen, along with progesterone, placental lactogen, prolactin, cortisol and insulin, all appear to act together to stimulate the growth and development of the milk-secreting cells. After the birth of the placenta, oestrogen levels decline abruptly and profoundly. This drop removes the inhibitory influence of progesterone and stimulates the production of milk (Cunningham et al. 2018).

As the name implies, progesterone is a pro-gestational hormone and has been aptly called the 'hormone of pregnancy' because it is essential for the establishment and maintenance of pregnancy (Mesiano 2018). Progesterone is mainly derived from the corpus luteum in the first few weeks of pregnancy but as the placental mass increases it takes over the production, contributing about 250 mg/day (Burton et al. 2017). Progesterone maintains pregnancy by promoting myometrial relaxation, cervical closure and decidual quiescence. Large amounts of progesterone are produced throughout pregnancy. It is not systemic progesterone withdrawal that initiates parturition but rather a functional progesterone withdrawal whereby progesterone target cells (myometrial, cervical, decidual) desensitize to the pro-pregnancy actions of progesterone and this signals myometrial contractility and cervical softening and dilatation (Kuo et al. 2018). Throughout this chapter, the numerous effects of progesterone-induced relaxation of smooth muscle during pregnancy have been identified in almost every system of the body.

THE PITUITARY GLAND AND ITS HORMONES

The anterior pituitary undergoes a two- to three-fold enlargement during pregnancy, primarily because of hyperplasia and hypertrophy of lactotroph cells (Tal et al. 2015). The upper surface of the gland becomes more convex superiorly. Its height increases steadily throughout pregnancy and by term, it can be 10 mm high and approach the optic chasm (Bonneville 2016). This increase may compress the optic chiasma to reduce visual field although this is rare (Cunningham et al. 2018). Simultaneously with enlargement of the gland, lactotrophs increase dramatically within the gland from 20% in the non-pregnant gland to 60% at term. Serum prolactin levels begin to rise at 5–8 weeks, reach 40 ng/mL at the end of the first trimester and are 10 times higher at 200–400 ng/mL by term (Bonneville 2016; Antony et al.

2017). Prolactin along with progesterone, oestrogen, cortisol and insulin all appear to act together to stimulate the growth and development of the milk-secreting apparatus. The principal function of maternal prolactin is to prepare the breasts for lactation (see Chapter 27). Pulsatile bursts of prolactin secretion are a response to suckling during early lactation (Cunningham et al. 2018).

In the first trimester, growth hormone is secreted predominantly from the maternal pituitary gland. However, as the placenta becomes the principal source of growth hormone secretion around 20 weeks, maternal pituitary growth hormone production is suppressed. Maternal serum growth hormone levels rise slowly from approximately 3.5 ng/mL at 10 weeks to plateau at about 14 ng/mL after 28 weeks (Cunningham et al. 2018). Increasing secretion of growth hormone contributes to maternal insulin resistance along with hPL progesterone, cortisol and prolactin (Soma-Pillay et al. 2016). With this increase in overall growth hormone activity, insulin-like growth factor 1 levels increase in the second half of pregnancy contributing to the acromegaloid features of some pregnant women. Through negative feedback, pituitary growth hormone levels consequently decline in the second half of gestation (Molitch 2015).

ADRENAL GLAND

In normal pregnancy, the adrenal glands undergo little change. Levels of circulating adrenocorticotropic hormone (ACTH), also known as corticotropin, are dramatically reduced in early pregnancy but as it progresses, ACTH levels rise and there is a two- to three-fold increase in free cortisol levels (Cunningham et al. 2018). Despite this, pregnant women do not exhibit any overt signs of hypercortisolism, likely due to the anti-glucocorticoid activities of the elevated levels of progesterone (Tal et al. 2015). Plasma renin substrate levels are increased as a result of the effects of oestrogen on the liver. The higher levels of renin and angiotensin during pregnancy lead to elevated angiotensin II levels and markedly elevated levels of aldosterone (Tal et al. 2015). Increased levels of the renin-angiotensin-aldosterone axis, which is intimately involved in blood pressure control via sodium and water balance, are important in first-trimester blood pressure maintenance (Cunningham et al. 2018). Water retention exceeds sodium excretion and although an additional 900 mEq of sodium is retained during pregnancy due to enhanced tubular reabsorption, serum levels of sodium decrease by 3–4 mmol/L. Over half of the additional sodium is contained within the fetoplacental unit, including amniotic fluid (Antony et al. 2017). Plasma osmolality is decreased. The threshold for thirst and vasopressin release changes early in pregnancy and by 5–8 weeks, there is an increased intake of water leading to increased urine volume but with a net increase in total body water. After 8 weeks' gestation, the new state for osmolality is established with little subsequent change resulting in reduced polyuria. Pregnant women respond to dehydration normally with changes in thirst but this occurs at a new, lower 'osmostat' (Antony et al. 2017).

During pregnancy, apart from a slight rise in LH levels in the first trimester (to maintain the corpus luteum), the levels secreted of both LH and FSH are low until birth. The inhibited production of those two hormones probably results from the persistently elevated levels of oestrogen and progesterone (Chang et al. 2014).

Two hormones *vasopressin* and *oxytocin* are secreted from the posterior pituitary gland. Levels of vasopressin (the antidiuretic hormone) do not change during pregnancy. Oxytocin is synthesized centrally in the hypothalamus and released into the bloodstream via the posterior pituitary gland during labour and lactation (Prevost et al. 2014). It acts directly on the myometrium to cause uterine contractions and on the myoepithelial cells of the alveoli in the breast to cause them to contract and eject the milk (Newton 2017). The study by Prevost et al. (2014) found that oxytocin levels varied considerably between individuals, ranging from 50 pg/mL to over 2000 pg/mL. For most women, oxytocin levels rose from the first to the third trimester and fell during the postpartum period. The specific roles of oxytocin in parturition and lactation are discussed in Chapter 27.

Thyroid Function

The fetus relies on maternal thyroxine, which crosses the placenta in small quantities to maintain normal fetal thyroid function. Early exposure to thyroid hormone is essential for the development of the fetal nervous system (Cunningham et al. 2018). To meet maternal and fetal needs, the thyroid gland boosts production of thyroid hormones by 40–100% (Moleti et al. 2014) (Fig. 10.9). The glandular hyperplasia and greater vascularity required to achieve this causes the thyroid gland to enlarge moderately during pregnancy. Mean thyroid volume increases from 12 mL in the first trimester to 15 mL at term (Cunningham et al. 2018).

As a result of this enlargement, production of thyroid hormones increases, mostly in the first half of gestation, plateauing around 20 weeks until term. There is a massive increase in upregulation of thyroid binding globulin driven by high levels of oestrogen and reduced hepatic clearance. This results in an increase in total thyroxine (T4) and triiodothyronine (T3), while the free forms of the hormones (fT4 and fT3) remain relatively stable and within normal limits (Costantine 2014). Free T_3 and T_4 are the physiologically important hormones and are the main determinants of whether a woman is euthyroid. Maternal free T4 (fT4) and free T3 (fT3) rather than total hormone concentrations must be measured in pregnancy. It is only the fT3 and fT4 fraction (not the bound fraction) that can enter cells and modify metabolism (Soma-Pillay et al. 2016). Negative feedback from peripheral T3 and T4 causes a decrease in thyroid stimulating hormone (TSH) in the first trimester in most women however, they still remain in the normal range for non-pregnant women (Cunningham et al. 2018). A normal value of TSH during the first half of pregnancy is between 0.5 and 2.5 mIU/L compared with an upper limit of normal value for TSH of 5 mIU/L in the non-pregnant state (Costantine 2014). This is in response to the thyrotropic effects of increased levels of human chorionic gonadotropin. Levels of TSH increase again at the end of the first trimester, and the upper limit

in pregnancy is raised to 5.5 µmol/L (Soma-Pillay et al. 2016). Secretion of T4 and T3 is not the same for all pregnant women. Approximately one-third of women experience relative hypothyroxinaemia and higher, albeit normal, serum TSH levels. Thus, thyroidal adjustments during normal pregnancy may vary considerably (Cunningham et al. 2018).

Other factors that affect thyroid hormones metabolism and levels in pregnancy include: the higher maternal metabolic demands and rate during pregnancy; the increase in transfer of thyroid hormones to the fetus early in pregnancy; and the increase in maternal renal iodine excretion (secondary to increase in GFR) (Costantine 2014). Pregnancy is therefore associated with a relative iodine deficiency, and iodine requirements increase predominantly due to an increase in renal iodide clearance and the use of iodine for thyroid hormone production. The causes for this are active transport of iodine from the mother to the fetoplacental unit and increased iodine excretion in the urine. If iodine intake is maintained in pregnancy, the size of the thyroid gland remains unchanged, however in women who are iodine deficient, the thyroid gland is 25% larger and goitres occur in 10% of women. The WHO (2016) recommends that iodine intake be increased from 100 mg/day to 200 mg/day. The development of an apparent goitre in pregnancy must be investigated (Antony et al. 2017), as iodine deficiency in pregnancy may be associated with neuro-developmental deficits that can result in hypothyroidism in the offspring (Cunningham et al. 2018). Evidence-based recommendations for optimal screening, prompt diagnosis and adequate treatment of congenital hypothyroidism via the routine neonatal 'blood spot' screening test are available (Léger et al. 2014).

Standard thyroid function test reference intervals should not be used for pregnant women due to the risk of misclassification of women with subclinical hypothyroidism as 'normal' in the first trimester. Trimester-specific reference ranges for thyroid hormones and TSH are still needed, particularly as ethnicity may also have a significant effect on TSH and fT4 reference limits in pregnancy (McNeil and Stanford 2015).

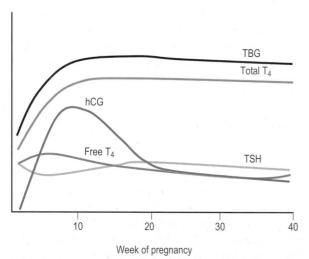

Fig. 10.9 Changes in maternal thyroid function during pregnancy. (From Antony K, Racusin D, Aagaard K, Dildy G. (2017) Maternal physiology. In: SG Gabbe, JR Neibyl, JL Simpson, et al. Obstetrics. Normal and problem pregnancies (7th ed.). Edinburgh: Elsevier.)

Diagnosis of pregnancy

Pregnancy is usually diagnosed when a woman presents with a positive home urine pregnancy test and possibly some presumptive signs. Typically, these women receive confirmation of pregnancy via a blood test for levels of human chorionic gonadotropin (hCG). Amenorrhoea is not a reliable pregnancy indicator until 10 days or more after the expected menstrual period have passed. Occasionally, implantation bleeding that mimics menstruation is noted after conception and may be described as an atypical last menstrual period. Other symptoms such as nausea and vomiting, breast tenderness and fullness, urinary frequency and fatigue, which develop early in pregnancy (Cunningham et al. 2018) could all have other causes, hence their categorization as 'possible signs' (Table 10.9). Other issues that may confuse the diagnosis of early pregnancy are the use of contraception and a history of irregular periods. Similarly, 'presumptive signs' cannot be relied upon in the diagnosis of pregnancy. Although they may still be of value in some parts of the world, they have generally been rendered obsolete in the developed world by more modern and sophisticated methods. They are described here purely for historical interest.

Chadwick's sign or Jacquemier's sign. This is the ectocervical violet-blue tint that develops as early as one month after conception due to the increased vascularity within the cervical stroma (Cunningham et al. 2018).

Hegar's sign. This is the softening of the isthmus between the cervix and uterus. Hegar (1895) first described palpable softening of the lower uterine segment at 4–6 weeks' gestation, and this sign was once used to diagnose pregnancy (Cunningham et al. 2018).

Goodell's sign. This is cervical oedema that leads to softening of the tissues (Cunningham et al. 2018).

TABLE 10.9 Signs of Pregnancy

Sign	Time of Occurrence	Differential Diagnosis
Possible (presumptive) signs		
Early breast changes (*unreliable in multigravida*)	3–4 weeks +	Contraceptive pill
Amenorrhoea	4 weeks +	Hormonal imbalance Emotional stress Illness
Nausea and vomiting	5–18 weeks	Gastrointestinal disorders Pyrexial illness Cerebral irritation, etc.
Bladder irritability	6–12 weeks	Urinary tract infection Pelvic tumour
Quickening	16–20 weeks +	Intestinal movement, wind
Probable signs		
Presence of human chorionic gonadotrophin (hCG) in:		
Blood	9–10 days	Hydatidiform mole
Urine	14 days	Choriocarcinoma
Softened isthmus (Hegar's sign)	6–12 weeks	
Blueing of vagina (Chadwick's sign)	8 weeks +	
Pulsation of fornices (Osiander's sign)	8 weeks +	Pelvic congestion Tumours
Changes in skin pigmentation	8 weeks +	
Uterine souffle	12–16 weeks	Increased blood flow to uterus as in large uterine myomas or ovarian tumours
Braxton Hicks contractions	16 weeks	
Ballottement of fetus	16–28 weeks	

Continued

TABLE 10.9	Signs of Pregnancy—cont'd	
Sign	Time of Occurrence	Differential Diagnosis
Positive signs		
Visualization of gestational sac by:		
Transvaginal ultrasound	4.5 weeks	
Transabdominal ultrasound	5.5 weeks	
Visualization of heart pulsation by:		
Transvaginal ultrasound	5 weeks	
Transabdominal ultrasound	6 weeks	
Fetal heart sounds by:		
Doppler	11–12 weeks	
Fetal stethoscope	20 weeks +	No alternative diagnosis
Fetal movements		
Palpable	22 weeks +	
Visible	Late pregnancy	
Fetal parts palpated	24 weeks +	
Visualization of fetus by X-ray (superseded by ultrasound)	16 weeks +	

Osiander's sign. This is the increased pulsation of the uterine artery felt in the lateral vaginal fornices from the 6th week of pregnancy (Alinsky and Goldstein 2017). This may also occur in the non-pregnant woman due to pelvic inflammation (Khadilkar and Patil 2014).

Quickening. This is the term used for the first fetal movements felt by the mother. They alert the pregnant woman to her growing fetus *in utero*. It usually occurs between 16 and 22 weeks. It is called a presumptive sign of pregnancy because it can be confused with peristalsis, flatus and abdominal muscle contractions. A multiparous woman will usually notice the gentle fluttering movements as early as 16 weeks, while a primigravid woman may not feel anything until 20–22 weeks. Around 20 weeks' gestation, fetal movements can be palpated externally through the abdomen, and this is considered a positive sign of pregnancy (Bryant and Thistle 2018) (Table 10.9).

Early pregnancy detection is critical as it allows antenatal care to begin during the most vulnerable stages of fetal development. The latest WHO (2016) guidelines continually emphasize the importance of accessing antenatal care early in pregnancy in order to identify and reduce risk and improve outcomes for mother and baby. Over-the-counter pregnancy test kits have been available since the early 1970s, but not all are as accurate as advertised. A detection limit of 12.5 mIU/mL would be required to diagnose 95% of pregnancies at the time of missed menses, but it is reported that only one brand has this degree of sensitivity and another two brands give false-positive or invalid results. The ultrasound scan is now generally accepted as the definitive method of diagnosing pregnancy and determining an accurate gestational age (Cunningham et al. 2018).

Common disorders arising from adaptations to pregnancy

Throughout this chapter, reference has been made to the multitude of symptoms produced by the physiological changes occurring in pregnancy. While deemed physiological, women may experience these as unpleasant, and even distressing or debilitating, leading to decreased quality of life (Kazemi et al. 2017). Having differentiated clearly between physiological and potentially pathological symptoms, midwives must be able to provide information about physiology, prevention and self-care for pregnancy discomforts with kindness and compassion in order to relieve anxiety and fear and promote a more emotionally satisfying outcome for mother, infant, and family (Gamel et al. 2017; Renfrew et al. 2014).

REFLECTIVE ACTIVITY FOR SELF-ASSESSMENT

The chapter started by describing how the female reproductive tract changes in pregnancy.

1. How might a midwife use this knowledge in practice?
2. What are the main differences you would expect to see if you compared a pregnant woman's blood results taken at 30 weeks with a set of results taken prior to pregnancy?
3. Identify all the clinical details identified throughout the chapter as being normal for pregnancy, but which could be confused with a medical condition?

REFERENCES

Acelajado, M., Culpepper, M., & Bolton, W. (2016). Hyperemesis gravidarum in undiagnosed Gitelman's syndrome. *Case Reports in Medicine, 8*, 1–4.

Adamson, D., Dhanjal, M., & Nelson-Piercy, C. (2011). *Heart disease in pregnancy*. Oxford: Oxford University Press.

Agoreyo, F., & Obika, L. (2017). Thirst perception and fluid intake in pregnant female humans in the three trimesters of pregnancy. *European Journal of Biology and Medical Science Research, 5*(4), 33–48.

Åhlund, S., Rådestad, I., Zwedberg, S., et al. (2018). Haemorrhoids – a neglected problem faced by women after birth. *Sexual & Reproductive Healthcare, 18*, 30–36.

Ahluwalia, A., Moshiri, M., Bahett, A., et al. (2018). MRI of acute and abdominal and pelvic non-obstetric conditions in pregnancy. *Current Radiology Reports, 6*(8), 25.

Alinsky, R., & Goldstein, M. (2017). Adolescent pregnancy. In M. Goldstein (Ed.), *The mass general Hospital for children adolescent medicine handbook* (2nd ed.) (p. 181). Boston: Springer.

Antony, K., Racusin, D., Aagaard, K., & Dildy, G. (2017). Maternal physiology. In S. G. Gabbe, J. R. Neibyl, J. L. Simpson, et al. (Eds.), *Obstetrics. Normal and problem pregnancies* (7th ed.) (Vol. 56) (pp. 49–54, 59). Edinburgh: Elsevier.

Baah-Dwomoh, A., McGuire, J., Tan, T., & De Vita, R. (2016). Mechanical properties of female reproductive organs and supporting connective tissues: A review of the current state of knowledge. *Applied Mechanics Reviews, 68*(6), 060801–060812.

van Baal, J., van de Vijver, K., Nieuwland, R., et al. (2016). The histophysiology and pathophysiology of the peritoneum. *Tissue and Cell, 49*, 95–105.

Barakat, R., Perales, M., Garatachea, N., et al. (2015). Exercise during pregnancy. A narrative review asking: What do we know? *British Journal of Sports Medicine, 49*, 1377–1381.

Barboni, E., Mancinelli, P., Bitossi, U., et al. (2016). Ultrasound evaluation of the stomach and gastric emptying in pregnant women at term: A case-control study. *Minerva Anestesiologica, 82*(5), 543–549.

Beksac, B., Aydin, E., Uzelpasaci, E., et al. (2018). Hemorrhoids and related complications in primigravid pregnancy. *Journal of Coloproctology, 38*(3), 179–182.

Bianco, A. (2017). Maternal adaptations to pregnancy: Gastrointestinal tract. *UpToDate*. Available at: www.uptodate.com/contents/maternal-adaptations-to-pregnancy-gastrointestinal-tract.

Bieber, A. K., Martires, K. J., Stein, J. A., et al. (2017). Pigmentation and pregnancy: Knowing what is normal. *Obstetrics & Gynecology, 129*(1), 168–173.

Bissonnette, J., Durand, F., de Raucourt, E., et al. (2015). Pregnancy and vascular liver disease. *Journal of Clinical and Experimental Hepatology, 5*(1), 41–50.

Blackburn, S. (2018) *Maternal, fetal and neonatal physiology* (5th ed.). Philadelphia: Saunders.

Boddy, A. M., Fortunato, A., Wilson Sayres, M., et al. (2015). Fetal microchimerism and maternal health: A review and evolutionary analysis of cooperation and conflict beyond the womb. *BioEssays, 37*(10), 1106–1118.

Bonneville, J. (2016). Normal pituitary gland and pregnancy. In *MRI of the pituitary gland* (Ch.7). Cham: Springer International Publishing.

Boriani, G., Lorenzetti, S., Cerbai, E., et al. (2017). The effects of gender on electrical therapies for the heart: Physiology, epidemiology, and access to therapies. *EP Europace, 19*(9), 1418–1426.

Bouyou, J., Gaujoux, S., Marcellin, L., et al. (2015). Abdominal emergencies during pregnancy. *Journal of Visceral Surgery, 152*, S105–S115.

Bronshtein, M., Gover, A., Beloosesky, R., et al. (2018). Characteristics and outcomes of ptyalism gravidarum. *Israeli Medical Association Journal, 20*(9), 573–575.

Brubaker, D., Barbaro, A., Chance, M., & Mesiano, S. (2016). A dynamical systems model of progesterone receptor interactions with inflammation in human parturition. *BMC Systems Biology, 10,* 79.

Bryant, J., & Thistle, J. (2018). Fetal movement. In *StatPearls.* Treasure Island: StatPearls Publishing. Available at: www.ncbi.nlm.nih.gov/books/NBK470566.

Burton, G., Sibley, C., & Jauniaux, E. (2017). Placental anatomy and physiology. In S. G. Gabbe, J. R. Neibyl, J. L. Simpson, et al. (Eds.), Obstetrics. *Normal and problem pregnancies* (7th ed.) (pp. 20–21). London: Elsevier.

Chang, C., Tsai, M., Lin, C., et al. (2014). The association between nonylphenols and sexual hormones levels among pregnant women: A cohort study in Taiwan. *PLoS One, 9*(8), e104245.

Chaudhry, S., & Chaudhry, K. (2018). Anatomy, abdomen and pelvis, uterus round ligament. In *StatPearls.* Treasure Island: StatPearls Publishing. Available at: www.ncbi.nlm.nih.gov/books/NBK499970.

Choo, E., & Dando, R. (2017). The impact of pregnancy on taste function. *Chemical Senses, 42,* 279–286.

Chung, E., & Leinwand, L. A. (2014). Pregnancy as a cardiac stress model. *Cardiovascular Research, 101*(4), 561–570.

Colombo, F. (2017). Renal disease in pregnancy. In S. G. Gabbe, J. R. Neibyl, J. L. Simpson, et al. (Eds.), Obstetrics. *Normal and problem pregnancies* (7th ed.) (pp. 850–851). London: Elsevier.

Conrad, K. P. (2011). Emerging role of relaxin in the maternal adaptations to normal pregnancy: Implications for pre-eclampsia. *Seminars in Nephrology, 31*(1), 15–32.

Costantine, M. (2014). Physiologic and pharmacokinetic changes in pregnancy. *Frontiers in Pharmacology, 5*(65).

Cunningham, G., Leveno, K., Bloom, S., et al. (Eds.). (2018). *Williams obstetrics.* London: McGraw-Hill Education.

Davies, S. J., Lum, J. A., Skouteris, H., et al. (2018). Cognitive impairment during pregnancy: A meta-analysis. *Medical Journal of Australia, 208*(1), 35–40.

Degner, K., Magness, R., & Shah, S. (2016). Establishment of the human uteroplacental circulation: A historical perspective. *Reproductive Sciences, 24*(5), 753–761.

Donangelo, C., & Bezerra, F. (2016). Pregnancy: Metabolic adaptations and nutritional requirements. In B. Caballero, P. Finglas, & F. Toldrá (Eds.), *The encyclopedia of food and health 4* (pp. 484–490). Oxford: Academic Press.

Dubey, V., Mythirayee, S., Gaharwar, U., et al. (2016). Cervical mucus helps in the fertilisation in women. *World Journal of Pharmacy and Pharmaceutical Science, 5*(10), 242–250.

D'Souza, L., Jayaweera, H., & Pickett, K. (2016). Pregnancy diets, migration, and birth outcomes. *Health Care for Women International, 37*(9), 964–978.

Edmonds, J., & Zabbo, G. (2017). Women's descriptions of labour onset and progression before hospital admission. *Nursing for Women's Health, 21*(4), 251–258.

Escalante, N., & Pino, J. (2017). Arrangement of muscle fibers in the myometrium of the human uterus: A mesoscopic study. *MOJ Anatomy and Physiology, 4*(2), 280–283.

Fisher, A. L., & Nemeth, E. (2017). Iron homeostasis during pregnancy. *American Journal of Clinical Nutrition, 106*(Suppl. 6) 1567S–74S.

Fu, Q. (2018). Hemodynamic and electrocardiographic aspects of uncomplicated singleton pregnancy. In P. Kerkhof, & V. Miller (Eds.), Sex-specific analysis of cardiovascular function. *Advances in experimental medicine and biology.* Amsterdam: Springer.

Gamel, W., Fathy, T., El-Nemer, A., & Shabana, K. (2017). Utilization of self-care brochure for relieving mother's minor discomforts during pregnancy. *Journal of Nursing and Women's Healthcare, 108.*

Garner, D. (2019). *Nutrition in pregnancy.* Waltham, MA: UpToDate. Available: www.uptodate.com/contents/nutrition-in-pregnancy.

Gharaibeh, A. A., Wadiya, E., Qdhah, et al. (2018). Prevalence of low back pain in pregnant women and the associated risk factors. *Journal of Orthopedics & Bone Disorders, 2*(1), 1–7.

Ghossein-Doha, C., Khalil, A., & Lees, C. C. (2017). Maternal hemodynamics: A 2017 update. *Ultrasound in Obstetrics and Gynecology, 49,* 10–14.

Gibson, L. (2017). Pregnancy related low back pain. *International Journal of Childbirth Education, 32*(1), 27–29.

Gilmore, L., Klempel-Donchenko, M., & Redman, L. (2015). Pregnancy as a window to future health: Excessive gestational weight gain. *Seminars in Perinatology, 39*(4), 296–303.

Ginsberg, Y., Goldstein, I., Lowenstein, L., & Weiner, Z. (2013). Measurements of the lower uterine segment during gestation. *Journal of Clinical Ultrasound, 41*(4), 214–217.

Gizlenti, S., & Ekmekci, T. R. (2014). The changes in the hair cycle during gestation and the post–partum period. *Journal of the European Academy of Dermatology and Venereology, 28*(7), 878–881.

Goldstein, R., Abell, S., Ranasinha, S., et al. (2017). Association of gestational weight gain with maternal and infant outcomes a systematic review and meta-analysis. *Journal of the American Medical Association, 317*(21), 2207–2225.

Greenspan, P. (2018). Maternal anatomical and physiological adaptation to pregnancy. In P. Greenspan (Ed.), *The diagnosis and management of the acute abdomen in pregnancy.* Cham: Springer International Publishing. Ch. 1.

Grindheim, G., Toska, K., Estensen, M. E., et al. (2012). Changes in pulmonary function during pregnancy: A longitudinal cohort study. *BJOG: An International Journal of Obstetrics and Gynaecology, 119,* 94–101.

Handel, A. C., Lima, P. B., Tonolli, V. M., et al. (2014). Risk factors for facial melasma in women: A case–control study. *British Journal of Dermatology, 171*(3), 588–594.

Hestiantoro, A., & Baida, P. (2018). The prevalence and risk factors of constipation in pregnancy. *Indonesian Journal of Obstetrics and Gynecology, 6*(2), 84–88.

Hill, A., Cairnduff, V., & McCance, D. (2016). Nutritional and clinical associations of foodcravings in pregnancy. *Journal of Human Nutrition and Dietetics, 29*, 281–289.

Hoekzema, E., Barba-Müller, E., Pozzobon, C., et al. (2017). Pregnancy leads to long-lasting changes in human brain structure. *Nature Neuroscience, 20*(2), 287–296.

Hoffmann, S., & Jayaratnam, S. (2018). Uterine torsion – a case report and literature review. *Global Journal of Reproductive Medicine, 5*(2), 555–664.

Ho, A., Flynn, A., & Pasupathy, D. (2016). Nutrition in pregnancy. *Obstetrics, Gynecology and Reproductive Medicine, 26*(9), 259–264.

Humphries, A., Stone, P., & Mirjalili, S. A. (2017). The collateral venous system in late pregnancy: A systematic review of the literature. *Clinical Anatomy, 30*, 1087–1095.

Ibrahim, S., Buka, M., & Audu, B. (2016). Management of abnormal discharge in pregnancy. In A. Darwish (Ed.), Genital infections and infertility. *IntechOpen* (p. 48) Ch. 4.

Iizuka, M., Miyasaka, N., Hirose, Y., et al. (2016). Is there a differential impact of parity on factors regulating maternal peripheral resistance? *Hypertension Research, 39*(10), 737–743.

Ikino, J. K., Nunes, D. H., Silva, V., et al. (2015). Melasma and assessment of the quality of life in Brazilian women. *Anais Brasileiros de Dermatologia, 90*(2), 196–200.

Institute of Medicine. (2009). *Weight gain during pregnancy: Re-examining the guidelines*. Washington, DC: National Academics Press.

Jain, K., & Kaur, H. (2015). Prevalence of oral lesions and measurement of salivary pH in the different trimesters of pregnancy. *Singapore Medical Journal, 58*(1), 53–57.

James, J., Chamley, L., & Clark, A. (2017). Feeding your baby in utero: How the uteroplacental circulation impacts pregnancy. *Physiology, 32*, 234–249.

Johnson, D., & Gretton, K. (2017). Pica during pregnancy. *International Journal of Childbirth Education, 32*(1), 45–47.

Johnstone, C., Johnston, M., Corke, A., & Davies, M. (2017). A likely urinary tract infection in a pregnant woman. *British Medical Journal, 357*, j1777.

Kar, S., Krishnan, A., & Shivkumar, P. V. (2012). Pregnancy and skin. *Journal of Obstetrics and Gynecology of India, 62*(3), 268–275.

Kashgari, F., Oraif, A., & Bajouh, O. (2015). The uterine junctional zone. *Life Science Journal, 12*(2), 101–105.

Kasielska-Trojan, A., Sobczak, M., & Antoszewski, B. (2015). Risk factors of striae gravidarum. *International Journal of Cosmetic Science, 37*, 236–240.

Kazemier, B., Koningstein, F., Schneeberger, C., et al. (2015). Maternal and neonatal consequences of treated and untreated asymptomatic bacteriuria in pregnancy: A prospective cohort study with an embedded randomised controlled trial. *The Lancet Infectious Diseases, 15*(11), 1324–1333.

Kazemi, F., Nahidi, F., & Kariman, N. (2017). Disorders affecting quality of life during pregnancy: A qualitative study. *Journal of Clinical and Diagnostic Research, 11*(4), QC06–10.

Khadilkar, S., & Patil, D. (2014). Physiological changes. In M. Arora, & A. Sharma (Eds.), *A practical guide to first trimester of pregnancy*. London: Jaypee. Ch.1.

Koenig, M. (2017). Nutrient intake during pregnancy. *Journal of Obstetric, Gynecologic, and Neonatal Nursing, 46*(1), 120–122.

Korevaar, T., Steegers, E., de Rijke, Y., et al. (2015). Reference ranges and determinants of total hCG levels during pregnancy: The generation R study. *European Journal of Epidemiology, 30*(9), 1057–1066.

Korgavkar, K., & Wang, F. (2015). Stretch marks during pregnancy: A review of topical prevention. *British Journal of Dermatology, 172*(3), 606–615.

Kuo, K., Hackney, D., & Mesiano, S. (2018). The endocrine control of human pregnancy. In A. Belfiore, & D. LeRoith (Eds.), *Principles of endocrinology and hormone action*. Cham: Springer International. Ch. 25.

Lee, A., & Landau, R. (2017). Aortocaval compression syndrome: Time to revisit certain dogmas. *Anesthesia & Analgesia, 125*, 1975–1985.

Léger J, Olivieri A, Donaldson M, et al.; On behalf of the congenital hypothyroidism consensus conference Group. (2014) European society for Paediatric Endocrinology consensus guidelines on screening, diagnosis and management of congenital hypothyroidism. *Hormone Research in Paediatrics 81*, 80–103.

Leimer, B., Pradella, F., Fruth, A., et al. (2018). Ramadan observance during pregnancy in Germany: A challenge for prenatal care. *Geburtshilfe und Frauenheilkunde, 78*(7), 684–689.

Leo, C. H., Jelinic, M., Ng, H., et al. (2017). Vascular actions of relaxin: Nitric oxide and beyond. *British Journal of Pharmacology, 174*, 1002–1014.

Longo, L. (2018). *The rise of fetal and neonatal physiology, perspectives in physiology* (2nd ed.). New York: Springer. Ch. 10.

Luders, E., Gingnell, M., Poromaa, I. S., et al. (2018). Potential brain age reversal after pregnancy: Younger brains at 4–6 weeks postpartum. *Neuroscience, 386*, 309–314.

Lumbers, E. R., & Pringle, K. G. (2013). Roles of the circulating renin-angiotensin-aldosterone system in human pregnancy. *American Journal of Physiology - Regulatory, Integrative and Comparative Physiology, 306*(2), R91–R101.

MacLean, P., Blundell, J., Mennella, J., & Batterham, R. (2017). Biological control of appetite: A daunting complexity. *Obesity*, *25*(Suppl. 1), S8–S16.

Mahendru, A. A., Foo, F. L., & McEniery, C. M. (2017). Change in maternal cardiac output from preconception to mid–pregnancy is associated with birth weight in healthy pregnancies. *Ultrasound in Obstetrics and Gynecology*, *49*(1), 78–84.

Mansouri, A., Mirghafourvand, M., Charandabi, S., et al. (2017). The effect of vitamin D and calcium plus vitamin D on leg cramps in pregnant women: A randomized controlled trial. *Journal of Research in Medical Sciences*, *22*, 24.

Marani, E., & Koch, W. (2014). The birth canal. In E. Marani, & W. Koch (Eds.), *The pelvis – structure, gender and society*. London: Springer. Ch. 3.

Martin, R., Nelson, D., Stewart, R., et al. (2017). Left and right atrial changes during pregnancy measured using cardiac MRI. *American Journal of Obstetrics and Gynecology*, *216*(1), S299–S300.

McIlvride, S., Dixon, P., & Williamson, C. (2017). Bile acids and gestation. *Molecular Aspects of Medicine*, *56*, 90–100.

McNeil, A., & Stanford, P. (2015). Reporting thyroid function tests in pregnancy. *Clinical Biochemist Reviews*, *36*(4), 109–126.

Meah, V. L., Cockcroft, J. R., Backx, K., et al. (2016). Cardiac output and related haemodynamics during pregnancy: A series of meta-analyses. *Heart*, *102*, 518–526.

Mehta, N., Chen, K., Hardy, E., et al. (2015). Respiratory disease in pregnancy. Best practice & research. *Clinical Obstetrics & Gynaecology*, *29*(5), 598–611.

Mehta, S., & Singla, A. (2014). Colposcopic examination in pregnancy. In S. Mehta, & P. Sachdeva (Eds.), *Colposcopy of the female genital tract*. Singapore: Springer. Ch. 13.

Menon, R., Bonney, E., Condon, J., et al. (2016). Novel concepts on pregnancy clocks and alarms: Redundancy and synergy in human parturition. *Human Reproduction Update*, *22*(5), 535–560.

Mesiano, S. (2018). Endocrinology of human pregnancy and fetal-placental neuroendocrine development. In J. Strauss, R. Barbieri, & A. Gargiulo (Eds.), *Yen & Jaffe's reproductive endocrinology: Physiology, pathophysiology, and clinical management* (8th ed.) (p. 269). Philadelphia: Elsevier.

Mesiano, S., DeFranco, E., & Muglia, L. (2015). Parturition. In T. Plant, & A. Zeleznik (Eds.), *Knobil and Neill's physiology of reproduction* (4th ed.) (pp. 1879–1888). London: Elsevier Inc.

Mindell, J. A., & Jacobson, B. J. (2014). Sleep disturbances during pregnancy. *Journal of Obstetric, Gynecologic, and Neonatal Nursing*, *29*(6), 590–597.

Moleti, M., Trimarchi, F., & Vermiglio, F. (2014). Thyroid physiology in pregnancy. *Endocrine Practice*, *20*, 589–596.

Molitch, M. (2015). Pituitary and adrenal disorders of pregnancy. In K. Feingold, B. Anawalt, A. Boyce, et al. (Eds.), *Endotext. South Dartmouth*. MDText.com, Inc. 2000.

Morgan, J., & Cooper, D. (2018). Pregnancy dating. In *StatPearls*. Treasure Island: StatPearls Publishing Available at: www.ncbi.nlm.nih.gov/books/NBK442018.

Motosko, C. C., Bieber, A. K., Pomeranz, M. K., et al. (2017). Physiologic changes of pregnancy: A review of the literature. *International Journal of Women's Dermatology*, *3*(4), 219–224.

Myers, K., & Elad, D. (2017). Biomechanics of the human uterus. *WIREs Systems Biology and Medicines*, *9*(5), e1388.

Myers, K., Feltovich, H., Mazza, E., et al. (2015). The mechanical role of the cervix in pregnancy. *Journal of Biomechanics*, *48*, 1511–1523.

Natale, C. A., Duperret, E. K., Zhang, J., et al. (2016). Sex steroids regulate skin pigmentation through nonclassical membrane-bound receptors. *ELIFE*, *5*, e15104.

Nelson-Piercy, C. (2015). *Handbook of obstetric medicine* (5th ed.). London: Taylor and Francis.

Newton, E. (2017). Lactation and breastfeeding. In S. G. Gabbe, J. R. Neibyl, J. L. Simpson, et al. (Eds.), *Obstetrics. Normal and problem pregnancies* (7th ed.) (p. 519). London: Elsevier.

NICE (National Institute for Health and Care Excellence). (2018a). *Antenatal care: Routine care for the healthy pregnant woman: CG 62*. London: NICE.

NICE (National Institute for Health and Care Excellence). (2018b). *2018 surveillance of diabetes in pregnancy: Management from pregnancy: Management from preconception to the postnatal period preconception to the postnatal period (NICE guideline NG3)*. London: NICE.

Nigam, A., Sharma, S., & Saxena, P. (2017). Preinvasive lesions in pregnancy and menopause. In S. Mehta, & P. Sachdeva (Eds.), *Colposcopy of the female genital tract* (p. 144). Singapore: Springer.

Norwitz, E., Mahendroo, M., & Lye, S. (2014). Biology of parturition. In R. Creasey, R. Resnik, J. Iams, et al. (Eds.), *Creasey and Resnik's maternal-fetal medicine* (7th ed.) (pp. 66–79). Philadelphia: Elsevier.

Nott, J., Bonney, E., Pickering, J., & Simpson, N. (2016). The structure and function of the cervix during pregnancy. *Translational Research in Anatomy*, *2*, 1–7.

Ochalek, K., Pacyga, K., Curyło, M., et al. (2017). Risk factors related to lower limb edema, compression, and physical activity during pregnancy: A retrospective study. *Lymphatic Research and Biology*, *15*(2), 166–171.

Okada, H., Tsuzuki, T., & Murata, H. (2017). Decidualization of the human endometrium. *Reproductive Medicine and Biology*, *17*(3), 220–227.

Olander, E. (2015). Weight management in pregnancy. *Nursing in practice. City Research Online.* Available at: http://openaccess.city.ac.uk/.

Pahwa, S., Kaur, A., & Nagpal, M. (2018). Obstetric outcome of floating head in primigravida at term. *International Journal of Reproduction, Contraception, Obstetrics and Gynecology, 7*(1), 242–247.

Panicker, V., Riyaz, N., & Balachandran, P. (2017). A clinical study of cutaneous changes in pregnancy. *Journal of Epidemiology and Global Health, 7,* 63–70.

Papageorghiou, A., Ohuma, E., Gravett, M., et al. (2016). International standards for symphysis-fundal height based on serial measurements from the fetal growth longitudinal study of the INTERGROWTH – 21st project: Prospective cohort study in eight countries. *British Medical Journal, 355,* i5662.

Pastro, L., Lemos, M. M., Fernandes, F., et al. (2017). Longitudinal study of lung function in pregnant women: Influence of parity and smoking. *Clinics, 72*(10), 595–599.

Patil, S., & Patil, V. (2014). Maternal and foetal outcomes in premature rupture of membranes. *IOSR Journal of Dental and Medical Sciences, 13*(12), 56–83.

Phupong, V., & Hanprasertpong, T. (2015). Interventions for heartburn in pregnancy. *Cochrane Database of Systematic Reviews, 9,* CD011379.

Poston L, Bell R, Croker H, et al.; UPBEAT trial Consortium. (2015) Effect of a behavioural intervention in obese pregnant women (the UPBEAT study): A multicentre, randomised controlled trial. *Lancet* 3(10):767–777.

PrabhuDas, M., Bonney, E., Caron, K., et al. (2015). Immune mechanisms at the maternal-fetal interface: Perspectives and challenges. *Nature Immunology, 16*(4), 328.

Prevost, M., Zelkowitz, P., Tulandi, T., et al. (2014). Oxytocin in pregnancy and the postpartum: Relations to labor and its management. *Frontiers in Public Health, 2*(1).

Pusukuru, R., Shenoi, A., Kyada, P., et al. (2016). Evaluation of lipid profile in second and third trimester of pregnancy. *Journal of Clinical and Diagnostic Research, 10*(3), QC12–QC16.

Ramos-e-Silva, M., Martins, N., & Kroumpouzos, G. (2016). Oral and vulvovaginal changes in pregnancy. *Clinics in Dermatology, 34,* 353–358.

Institute of medicine; National research Council. In K. Rasmussen, & A. Yaktine (Eds.), (2009). *Weight gain during pregnancy: Re-examining the guidelines.* Washington, DC: National Academies Press.

Rawal, A. (2016). The lower segment of the uterus – a critical area in childbirth and resulting trauma. In A. Gandhi, N. Malhotra, J. Malhotra, et al. (Eds.), *Principles of critical care in obstetrics* (Vol. 1). New Delhi: Springer. Ch.18.

RCOG (Royal College of Obstetricians and Gynaecologists). (2015). *RCOG statement: Advice on nutrition in pregnancy.* London: RCOG.

Reichman, O., Gal, M., Leibovici, V., & Samueloff, A. (2014). Evaluation of vaginal complaints during pregnancy: The approach to diagnosis. *Current Dermatology Reports, 3*(3), 159–164.

Renfrew, M., McFadden, A., Bastos, M., et al. (2014). Midwifery and quality care; Findings from a new evidence-informed framework for maternal and newborn care. *Lancet, 384*(9948), 1129–1145.

Robert Peter, J., Ho, J., Valliapan, J., & Sivasangari, S. (2015). Symphysial fundal height (SFH) measurement in pregnancy for detecting abnormal fetal growth. *Cochrane Database of Systematic Reviews* (9), CD008136.

Romero, R., Hassan, S., Gajer, P., et al. (2014). The composition and stability of the vaginal microbiota of normal pregnant women is different from that of non-pregnant women. *Microbiome, 2*(4).

Rungsiprakarn, P., Laopaiboon, M., Sangkomkamhang, U., et al. (2015). Interventions for treating constipation in pregnancy. *Cochrane Database of Systematic Reviews* (9), CD011448.

Sangsawang, B., & Sangsawang, N. (2013). Stress urinary incontinence in pregnant women: A review of prevalence, pathophysiology, and treatment. *International Urogynecology Journal, 24*(6), 901–912.

Segal, N. A., Boyer, E. R., Teran-Yengle, P., et al. (2013). Pregnancy leads to lasting changes in foot structure. *American Journal of Physical Medicine & Rehabilitation, 92*(3), 232–240.

Shasteen, M., & Pontius, E. (2017). Non-obstetric abdominal pain in pregnancy. In J. Borhart (Ed.), *Emergency department management of obstetric complications. E.book* (p. 151). Springer International Publishing.

Sheldon, R., Shmygol, A., van den Berg, H., & Blanks, A. (2015). Functional and morphological development of the womb throughout life. *Science Progress, 98*(2), 103–127.

Sigust, A. (2018). How to reduce bloating and discomfort in the belly when pregnant. Livestrong.com. Available at: www.livestrong.com/article/548532-how-to-reduce-bloating-discomfort-in-the-belly-when-pregnant/.

Sivarajasingam, S., Imami, N., & Johnson, M. (2016). Myometrial cytokines and their role in the onset of labour. *Journal of Endocrinology, 231,* R101–R119.

Smaill, F., & Vazquez, C. (2015). Antibiotics for asymptomatic bacteriuria in pregnancy. *Cochrane Database of Systematic Reviews, 8,* CD000490.

Soma-Pillay, P., Nelson-Piercy, C., Tolppanen, H., et al. (2016). Physiological changes in pregnancy. *Cardiovascular Journal of Africa, 27*(2), 89–94.

Sonagra, A., Biradar, S. M., Dattatreya, K., & Murthy, D. S. J. (2014). Normal pregnancy – a state of Insulin resistance. *Journal of Clinical and Diagnostic Research, 8*(11), CC01–CC03.

Spradley, F. T. (2018). Sympathetic nervous system control of vascular function and blood pressure during pregnancy and preeclampsia. *Journal of Hypertension, 37*(1) 10.10.

Female reproductive system. In S. Standring (Ed.), (2016). *Gray's anatomy – the anatomical basis of clinical practice* (41st ed.) (pp. 1288–1313). London: Elsevier.

Stephenson, J., Heslehurst, N., Hall, J., et al. (2018). Before the beginning: Nutrition and lifestyle in the preconception period and its importance for future health. *Lancet, 391*(10132), 1830–1841.

Sunil, S., Nair, A., Sharifi, S., & Thomas, T. (2018). A review on urinary tract infection in pregnancy. *International Journal of Pharma Research & Review, 7*(5), 1–6. Available at: https://ijpr.in/Data/Archives/2018/may/0805201801.pdf.

Swapna, V., Triveni, J., & Jayaprakash Murthy, D. (2015). Study of urinary calcium and urinary creatinine levels and urinary calcium/creatinine ratio in gestational hypertensive patients. *Journal of Evolution of Medical and Dental Sciences, 4*(53), 9145–9150.

Swift, J., Langley-Evans, S., Pearce, J., et al. (2017). Antenatal weight management: Diet, physical activity, and gestational weight gain in early pregnancy. *Midwifery, 49*, 40–46.

Szczęch, J., Wiatrowski, A., Hirnle, L., & Reich, A. (2017). Prevalence and relevance of pruritus in pregnancy. *BioMed Research International.* https://doi.org/10.1155/2017/4238139.

Tal, R., Taylor, H., Burney, R., et al. (2015). Endocrinology of pregnancy. In L. De Groot, G. Chrousos, K. Dungan, et al. (Eds.), *Endotext. South Dartmouth (MA)* Available at: www.ncbi.nlm.nih.gov/books/NBK278962.

Tamega, A., Miot, L., Bonfietti, C., et al. (2013). Clinical patterns and epidemiological characteristics of facial melasma in Brazilian women. *Journal of the European Academy of Dermatology and Venereology, 27*, 151–156.

Thabah, M., & Ravindran, V. (2015). Musculoskeletal problems in pregnancy. *Rheumatology International, 35*(4), 581–587.

Thornburg, K., Bagby, S., & Giraud, G. (2015). Maternal adaptations to pregnancy. In T. Plant, & A. Zeleznik (Eds.), *Knobil and Neill's physiology of reproduction* (4th ed.). London: Elsevier Inc. Ch. 43.

Tkachenko, O., Shchekochikhin, D., & Schrier, R. W. (2014). Hormones and hemodynamics in pregnancy. *International Journal of Endocrinology and Metabolism, 12*(2), e14098.

Triunfo, S., & Lanzone, A. (2015). Impact of maternal nutrition on obstetric outcomes. *Journal of Endocrinological Investigation, 38*(1), 31–38.

Vannuccini, S., Bocci, C., Sveeri, F., et al. (2016). Endocrinology of human parturition. *Annals of Endocrinology, 77*, 105–113.

Ventura, N. M., Li, T. Y., Tse, M. Y., et al. (2018). Developmental origins of pregnancy-induced cardiac changes: Establishment of a novel model using the atrial natriuretic peptide gene-disrupted mice. *Molecular and Cellular Biochemistry, 449*(1–2), 227–236.

Vink, J., & Myers, K. (2018). Cervical alterations in pregnancy. *Best Practice & Research Clinical Obstetrics & Gynaecology, 52*, 88–102.

Vink, J., Qin, S., Clifton, B., et al. (2016). A new paradigm for the role of smooth muscle cells in the human cervix. *American Journal of Obstetrics and Gynecology, 215*(478), e1–11.

Vora, R. V., Gupta, R., Mehta, M., et al. (2014). Pregnancy and skin. *Journal of Family Medicine and Primary Care, 3*(4), 318–324.

Vricella, L. K. (2017). Emerging understanding and measurement of plasma volume expansion in pregnancy. *American Journal of Clinical Nutrition, 106*(Suppl. 6), 1620S–1625S.

Weiss, G., Sundi, M., Glasner, A., & Huppertz, B. (2016). The trophoblast plug during early pregnancy: A deeper insight. *Histochemistry and Cell Biology, 146*, 749–756.

Westbrook, R., Dusheiko, G., & Williamson, C. (2016). Pregnancy and liver disease. *Journal of Hepatology, 64*(4), 933–945.

West, E., Hark, L., & Catalano, P. (2017). Nutrition during pregnancy. In S. G. Gabbe, J. R. Neibyl, J. L. Simpson, et al. (Eds.), *Obstetrics. Normal and problem pregnancies* (7th ed.). Philadelphia: Elsevier. Ch.7.

WHO (World Health Organization). (2016). *WHO recommendations on antenatal care for a positive pregnancy experience.* Geneva: WHO.

Won, C. H. (2015). Sleeping for two: The great paradox of sleep in pregnancy. *Journal of Clinical Sleep Medicine, 11*(6), 593–594.

Woodley, S., Boyle, R., Cody, J., et al. (2017). Pelvic floor muscle training for prevention and treatment of urinary and faecal incontinence in antenatal and postnatal women. *Cochrane Database of Systematic Reviews, 12*, CD007471.

Wu, S., Li, R., & DeMayo, F. (2018). Progesterone receptor regulation of uterine adaptation for pregnancy. *Trends in endocrinology and metabolism, 29*(7), 481–491.

Wu, X., & Yeoh, H. T. (2014). Intrinsic factors associated with pregnancy falls. *Workplace Health & Safety, 62*(10), 403–408.

Yamaleyeva, L. M., Merrill, D. C., Ebert, T. J., et al. (2014). Hemodynamic responses to angiotensin-(1–7) in women in their third trimester of pregnancy. *Hypertension in Pregnancy, 33*(4), 375–388.

Yu, L. L., Jin, Y. M., Li, M. M., et al. (2016). Changes and reference intervals of immature granulocytes in the peripheral blood of women according to pregnancy trimester. *International Journal of Clinical and Experimental Medicine*, 9(5), 8169–8175.

Zara, F., & Depuis, O. (2017). Uterus – biomechanical modelling of uterus. Application to a childbirth simulation. In Y. P. J. Ohayon (Ed.), *Biomechanics of living organs: Hyperelastic constitutive laws for finite element modeling*. London: Elsevier. Ch. 15.

ANNOTATED FURTHER READING

Blackburn, S. (2018). *Maternal, fetal & neonatal physiology. E-book*. Maryland Heights: Elsevier/Saunders.

This textbook provides an extremely thorough account of physiological changes across the whole childbearing period including neonatal physiology. It includes expert insight and clinically relevant examples providing sound foundation for assessment and therapeutic interventions. It also provides detailed synthesis of the latest research to support evidence-based practice including key pharmacology with clinical examples of drug effects.

Rankin, J. (Ed.). (2017). *Physiology in childbearing*. Edinburgh: Elsevier.

This edited book provides many excellent chapters relevant to the physiological adaptations in pregnancy and is presented in an easily readable format. It includes the application of theory to practice to demonstrate how a knowledge of physiology can enhance the evidence-based care given to mothers and babies It is very well illustrated with figures and tables

and helpfully provides a list of 'main points' at the end of each chapter.

Nelson-Piercy, C. (2015). *Handbook of obstetric medicine* (5th ed.). London: Taylor and Francis.

This handbook is described as 'an essential on-the-spot guide for all professionals involved in the care of the childbearing woman', be they already in practice or in training. It is designed to address the most common and serious medical conditions encountered in pregnancy. In addition to a description of each condition, there are also sections on the differential diagnoses of common pregnancy symptoms. An appendix lists normal laboratory values in pregnancy according to trimester. Each chapter is in an easy-to-use design and includes 'points to remember' boxes for ease of reference.

USEFUL WEBSITES

Several videos in the following series by Professor Ajit Virkud published in June 2018 give detailed, illustrated and animated overviews of the maternal adaptations to pregnancy, e.g.:

Maternal Adaptations to Pregnancy Part 1: www.youtube.com/watch?v=HUB85S2AtF8

Maternal Adaptations to Pregnancy Part 2: www.youtube.com/watch?v=BWzP1cQULSo&list=PLtY-ix5Q-7z_bTyT_Pzn_HS0D8BNV1yGtU&index=2&t=0s

Maternal Adaptations to Pregnancy CVS: www.youtube.com/watch?v=DIguS6KsyJE&t=51s

Maternal Adaptations Respiratory System: www.youtube.com/watch?v=NJcl-X4QBz4

Maternal Adaptations Renal System: www.youtube.com/watch?v=W52bOLJo17U

11

Antenatal Care

Helen Baston

CHAPTER CONTENTS

Antenatal care is the care given to a pregnant woman from the time conception is confirmed until the beginning of labour. The midwife facilitates woman-centred care by providing her with accessible and relevant information to help inform her decisions throughout pregnancy. The foundation of this process is the development of a trusting relationship in which the midwife engages with the woman and listens to her story.

THE CHAPTER AIMS TO

- describe current models of antenatal care
- explore the role of the midwife in providing woman-centred care, identifying the woman's physical, psychological and sociological needs

- discuss the initial assessment visit, define its objectives and consider the significance of the woman's health and social history
- describe the physical examination and psychological support of the woman provided throughout pregnancy.

THE AIM OF ANTENATAL CARE

The aim of antenatal care is to monitor the progress of pregnancy to optimize maternal and fetal health. To achieve this, the midwife critically evaluates the physical, psychological and sociological effects of pregnancy on the woman and her family. This process requires engagement by the midwife, as outlined in Box 11.1.

BOX 11.1 Key Principles of Antenatal Care by the Midwife

- Developing a trusting relationship with the woman
- Providing a holistic approach to the woman's care that meets her individual need
- Making a comprehensive assessment of the woman's health and social status, accessing all relevant sources of information
- Promoting an awareness of the public health issues for the woman and her family
- Exchanging information with the woman and her family, enabling them to make informed choices about pregnancy and birth
- Being an advocate for the woman and her family during her pregnancy, supporting her right to choose care appropriate for her own needs and those of her family
- Identifying potential risk factors and taking the appropriate measures to minimize them
- Timely sharing of information with relevant agencies and professionals
- Accurate, contemporaneous documentation of assessments, plans, care and evaluation
- Recognizing complications of pregnancy and appropriately referring women to the obstetric team or relevant health professionals or other organizations (see Chapters 12–16)
- Preparing the woman and her family to meet the challenges of labour and birth, and facilitating the development of a birth plan
- Facilitating the woman to make an informed choice about methods of infant feeding and giving appropriate and sensitive advice to support her decision (see Chapter 27)
- Offering parenthood education within a planned programme or on an individual basis (see Chapter 9).

Historical Background

Antenatal care has been provided in the UK for almost a century and was first offered in the late 1920s (Ministry of Health 1929). The model of antenatal care followed a regime of monthly visits until 28 weeks' gestation; then fortnightly visits until 36 weeks; then weekly visits until the birth of the baby. This model continued for decades but was eventually challenged in the 1980s by Hall et al. (1980), whose retrospective analysis demonstrated that conditions requiring hospitalization, including pre-eclampsia, were neither prevented nor detected by antenatal care; and intrauterine growth restriction was over-diagnosed. It was felt that reducing visits for those who did not need them would mean that more support could be given to vulnerable women to improve their outcomes.

To evaluate the impact of reduced antenatal visiting, Sikorski et al. (1996) conducted a randomized controlled trial, with low-risk pregnant women, to compare the acceptability and effectiveness of a reduced antenatal visit schedule of six to seven routine visits, with the traditional 13 routine visits. No differences in clinical outcome between the two groups were found, but twice as many women in the reduced-visit group were dissatisfied with the frequency of attendance, compared with women who received the full range of visits. The World Health Organization trialled a system of four routine antenatal visits for women assessed as being low risk (Villar et al. 2001). They found no statistically significant differences between the outcomes of pre-eclampsia, severe anaemia, urinary tract infection and low birth-weight infants between the intervention group and standard care, in the 24,678 women enrolled in the study.

Patterns of visiting continue to be investigated and Dowswell et al. (2010) compared standard care with reduced visiting schedules investigated in seven randomized controlled trials. They concluded that for high income countries there was no difference between the groups but for low to medium income countries, perinatal mortality was increased in those receiving reduced visits and the authors conclude that visits should not be reduced without close monitoring of the impact on neonatal outcome. While previous research had demonstrated (Clement et al. 1996; Villar et al. 2001) that women prefer more scheduled visits, other models where virtual care is combined with traditional care, have proved preferable for women who already have children (Pflugeisen and Mou 2017). Creative and alternative antenatal care models will need to continue to evolve and be evaluated as the use of technology becomes increasingly acceptable.

In England, the National Institute for Health and Care Excellence (NICE 2008a/2019) has endorsed a schedule of seven visits for parous women and 10 for primigravid women and this pattern is often reflected in the service specification commissioned (see Box 11.2 for the NICE 2008a/2019 recommended visiting pattern). The midwife must continue to use her knowledge and judgement when providing care, as there will be situations where deviation from the pathway will be necessary to ensure safety for either the woman or her unborn baby. In such situations, the midwife should clearly document her rationale and ensure that she continues to evaluate the care she provides or has requested from other members of the team. If the deviation falls outside the midwife's current remit, she is obliged to 'ask for help from a suitably qualified and experienced professional to carry out any action or procedure that is beyond the limits of your competence' (Nursing and Midwifery Council, NMC 2018: 13).

Current Practice

National evidence-based guidelines, in relation to antenatal care have been developed and circulated in the UK since 2003. They were updated in 2008 and again in 2019. In addition to full national care guidance, NICE also produce 'Quality Standards' that are 'a concise set of statements designed to drive and measure priority quality improvements within a particular area of care' (NICE 2012, 2018). The Antenatal Quality Standard comprises 12 statements and these are detailed in Box 11.3. They are a useful framework for examining maternity services and provide benchmarks for audit and commissioning purposes, although most of them relate to women with risk factors.

Better births

Following extensive consultation with women, healthcare professionals and commissioners in England, a 5-year strategy for maternity care was delivered in 2016

TABLE 11.1 Key Principles of *Better Births*

	Principle	Description in brief
1.	Personalized care	All women should have: A personalized care plan, access to their own digital notes, choose a provider and the place of birth
2.	Continuity of carer	A midwife who is part of a small team of 4–6 midwives based in the community, with an identified obstetrician
3.	Safer care	Rapid referral and access to the right care in the right place from the right person. Quality outcomes data should be collected
4.	Better postnatal and perinatal mental health care	Smooth transition between midwife, obstetric and neonatal care to the ongoing care of the GP and health visitor
5.	Multiprofessional working	Multiprofessional learning should be core to pre-registration training and continuous professional development for midwives and obstetricians
6.	Working across boundaries	Community hubs should be established where antenatal and postnatal services are provided alongside other health and social services
7.	Payment system	Reformation to ensure maternity services are incentivized for efficiency and paid appropriately for the services they provide

Adapted from *Better Births,* National Maternity Review. (2016) Better Births. Improving outcomes for maternity services in England. Available at: www.england.nhs.uk/wp-content/uploads/2016/02/national-maternity-review-report.pdf.

(*Better Births*, National Maternity Review 2016). It comprised seven key aspirations as outlined in Table 11.1. Of particular relevance to antenatal care is that continuity of care should be coordinated by a named midwife working as part of a small team throughout the childbirth continuum. To this end, a range of pilot schemes are currently running and being evaluated in order to meet local needs. For example, in some areas, continuity of care is being provided to women who smoke, whereas in other areas it is being provided to women who are having an elective caesarean (NHS England 2017). These aspirations are not without challenge to maternity services, and various tools and support documents are available to aid implementation (Royal College of Midwives, RCM 2018). The ultimate aim is that most women in the UK will receive care in a continuity model by 2020/21 (NHS England 2017), see Chapter 8 for further details of this approach to care.

Public health role of the midwife

Midwives have always held a privileged position in relation to their ability to influence the health and wellbeing of women and their families. With access to women at a time in their life when they may be open to change their behaviour to achieve a healthy baby, midwives can offer support, information and referral. The public health remit of midwives was strengthened when their unique position to address inequality was formally recognized in the government White Paper *Saving Lives: Our Healthier Nation* (Department of Health, DH 1999). It has since been recognized as a significant part of the midwife's role and deeply embedded in the Midwifery 2020 strategy (McNeill et al. 2010) and government policy (DH/NHS 2014).

There are a range of health behaviours that impact on life chances and these follow a social gradient. By addressing these public health issues and working together with other agencies, midwives can influence the future health of the population. Extending the boundaries of midwifery care to offer social support can result in positive outcomes in terms of lifestyle, employment and the growth and development of children (Leamon and Viccars 2007). The Marmot Review (2010) examined strategies that could be implemented in order to reduce inequalities in health. It focused on the challenges people face throughout the life course and highlighted the importance of children getting 'the best start in life' (2010: 173). A detailed analysis of systematic reviews of maternal and infant wellbeing globally, concluded that 'survival and health can be improved by practices that lie within the scope of midwifery' (Renfrew et al. 2014: 1132). Addressing reproductive health issues is now a strong theme of the Royal College of Midwives (RCM 2017) and Public Health England's activity and resource development (PHE 2018).

Access to Care

Early contact with the maternity services, ideally by 10 weeks' gestation, is important so that appropriate and valuable advice relating to screening, nutrition and optimum care of the developing fetus can be given. Medical conditions, infections and lifestyle behaviours may all have a profound and detrimental effect on the fetus during this time. Late booking can be a symptom of vulnerability and is often a feature of reported maternal deaths in the UK (Knight et al. 2018).

Women are encouraged to access their midwife through their local health or family centre on confirmation or suspicion of a positive pregnancy test and should be facilitated to do this. They do not require a formal referral from a GP. It has been a longstanding conundrum that the people who are most likely to need or benefit from health services are least likely to access them. Often referred to as 'hard to reach' groups, it might be more accurate to describe some *services* as 'hard to reach' and particularly useful to do this when considering how access to services can be increased.

For some women, late booking cannot be avoided if they have arrived only recently into the country. However, these women are particularly vulnerable, as they may be naive about how maternity services work, not knowing where they are located, be unable to negotiate public transport and not speak English. Services can be made more accessible if community-based outreach workers and bilingual link/advocacy workers recruited from the target population are employed to provide care (Hollowell et al. 2012).

Maternity services can also be difficult to access for indigenous women. They may not recognize the importance of attending early for care to enable valuable health and social care screening to be undertaken. They may be juggling childcare demands with work and financial pressures. Centralization of services may mean that the consultant maternity unit is located in towns or cities, many miles from home. While low-risk women receive the majority of their care in the community, closer to home, for those where there is a complication or a medical condition that requires close monitoring, regular attendance at the consultant unit can be a real challenge.

A flexible approach to the timing of visits and the place of consultation has been incorporated into many maternity services and in the UK, it is a requirement of current maternity strategy that care should be available in local community hubs where a range of services can be provided (National Maternity Review 2016). However, it is equally important that women perceive antenatal care as a valuable resource and an opportunity to receive effective, relevant care from staff who treat them with respect and kindness.

Models of Midwifery Care

Women can choose from a variety of midwifery care options depending on local availability and their level of risk. The majority of low-risk women receive antenatal care in the community, either at a family Centre, Community hub, GP surgery or in their own home. Hospital- or community-based clinics are available for women who receive care from an obstetrician or physician in addition to their midwife. Midwifery teams, case-loading and independent midwifery (IM) are all examples of how antenatal care can be provided flexibly to meet the needs of individual women.

Options for place of birth include the home, a birth centre (standalone or alongside) or a consultant-led unit. National maternity policy promotes birth at home as an option for all women with low-risk pregnancies (DH 2016), but fundamental to this is women's choice and local configuration of services. Women who have identified risk factors or develop complications during pregnancy will usually plan for a hospital birth. However, some women with potentially complex needs may request midwifery-led care, for a range of reasons. They should have the opportunity to discuss their hopes and expectations so that a mutually acceptable plan can be agreed and supported by appropriately skilled midwives.

THE INITIAL ASSESSMENT (BOOKING VISIT)

The purpose of this visit is to initiate the development of a trusting relationship that facilitates the positive engagement of the woman with the maternity service; this is the most important element of antenatal care. While it is crucial that risk assessment and identification of clinically relevant information is obtained, none of these can be undertaken if the woman does not feel able to communicate with the midwife.

BOX 11.4 Objectives for the Initial Assessment (Booking Visit)

- to build the foundation for a trusting relationship in which the woman and midwife are partners in care
- to assess health by taking a detailed history and offering appropriate screening tests
- to ascertain baseline recordings of blood pressure, urinalysis, blood values, uterine growth and fetal development to be used as a standard for comparison as the pregnancy progresses
- to identify risk factors by taking accurate details of past and present midwifery, obstetric, medical, family and personal history
- to provide an opportunity for the woman and her family to express and discuss any concerns they might have about the current pregnancy and previous pregnancy loss, labour, birth or puerperium
- to give public health advice pertaining to pregnancy in order to maintain the health of the mother and fetus
- to make appropriate referral where additional health care or support needs have been identified.

BOX 11.5 Factors that may Require Additional Antenatal Support or Referral to an Obstetrician/Physician/Other Health Professional (NICE 2008b/2019)

Initial assessment
- Age less than 18 years or 40 years and over
- Grande multiparity
- Vaginal bleeding at any time during pregnancy
- Unknown or uncertain expected date of birth
- Late booking.

Past obstetric history
- Stillbirth or neonatal death
- Baby small (<5th centile or <2.5 kg) or large baby (>95 centile or >4.5 kg)
- Congenital abnormality
- Rhesus isoimmunization
- Pregnancy-induced hypertension
- Two or more terminations of pregnancy
- Three or more spontaneous miscarriages
- Previous pre-term labour
- Cervical cerclage in past or present pregnancy
- Previous caesarean section or uterine surgery
- Ante- or postpartum haemorrhage
- Precipitate labour
- Multiple pregnancy.

Maternal health
- Previous history of deep vein thrombosis or pulmonary embolism
- Chronic illness, e.g. epilepsy, severe asthma, hepatic or renal disease, cystic fibrosis
- HIV or HBV infection
- Malignancy
- Hypertension, cardiac disease
- History of infertility
- Uterine anomalies
- Family history of diabetes or genetic disorders
- Type I or Type II diabetes
- Substance abuse (drugs, alcohol or smoking)
- Psychological or psychiatric disorders requiring medication.

Examination at the initial assessment
- Blood pressure ≥140/90 mmHg
- Maternal obesity (BMI >30 kg/m^2) or underweight (BMI <18 kg/m^2)
- Blood disorders.

MEETING THE MIDWIFE

The woman's first introduction to midwifery care is crucial in forming her initial impressions of the maternity service. A friendly, professional approach will enable the development of a positive partnership between the woman and the midwife. The initial visit focuses on the exchange of information (Box 11.4) and identification of factors that may require referral to another member of the multiprofessional team (Box 11.5). It is a key opportunity for the midwife and the woman to get to know each other. The midwife may meet other members of the family and in this way, gain a more informed view of the woman's circumstances. However, the midwife will also recognize that there are occasions when the woman may need to spend time alone with her to facilitate discussion, which she may not feel able to have in the presence of family members.

Communication

The midwife requires many skills to provide optimal antenatal care: the ability to communicate effectively and sensitively is a key element of all of them (Baston and Hall 2018). Listening skills involve focusing on what the woman is saying and how she is saying it, considering the content and tone. In addition, non-verbal responses, including facial expression, body position and eye contact, will influence the quality of the interaction and have the potential to enhance or detract from the development of a positive relationship between woman and midwife (Allison 2012).

The midwife can promote communication with the woman during discussion by gentle questioning, open-ended statements and reflecting back keywords from what is said, to encourage and facilitate exploration of what is meant (Rungapadiachy 1999). Midwives also need to be aware of the language they use, avoiding unnecessary jargon and technical language, so that the woman understands the options available and their implications (Mobbs et al. 2018). Communication encompasses writing accurate, comprehensive and contemporaneous records of information given and received, and the plan of care that has been agreed; using terms that can be understood (NMC 2018). The midwife must also communicate relevant information with the multiprofessional team, other services and agencies where relevant (Knight et al. 2018) adhering to data protection principles also referred to as 'GDPR' or 'General Data Protection Regulation' (Data Protection Act 2018).

Taking an antenatal booking history involves a lot of questioning and data collection. However, while completing the documentation, the midwife must be mindful that she needs to have eye contact with the woman in order to facilitate discussion and observe her responses to particular questions. General conversation about the woman's experiences can be a more useful way of sharing information between woman and midwife rather than asking a list of questions or filling in computer data in a mechanistic manner (McCourt 2006).

Personal Information

As part of getting to know each other, the midwife will introduce herself as the woman's named midwife. She will then clarify the woman's name and the relationship to her of anyone accompanying her. Important details such as date of birth, address and current occupation are written down and provide a useful means of breaking the ice. The woman's age should be considered in relation to local guidelines. For example, it may be a recommendation that women who are 40 years of age or more are offered induction of labour at term, as such an intervention has been shown to reduce the stillbirth risk by 75% compared with expectant management (Knight et al. 2017). Every woman needs to know what her care pathway will be so that she can be fully involved in all decisions. The midwife should explain that she will be asking lots of questions, and encourage the woman to ask if anything is unclear.

Social Circumstances

It is useful to explore the woman's response to the pregnancy. Some women may be overwhelmed by having to care for a new baby along with other children, or they may be isolated or living in poverty. The woman may be a teenager, and experiencing conflict with her parents, social stigma and accommodation concerns. The midwife needs to have a contemporary knowledge of local services and initiatives, social services and voluntary agencies and to make appropriate referrals, in partnership with the woman.

Many women live in complex circumstances and the midwife sometimes needs to ask a range of questions to untangle the details. For example, what are their living arrangements, are there any children from previous relationships and who has custody, to identify if there are any safe-guarding concerns that may need further follow-up.

If the woman appears to have difficulty understanding the information that is being given, she may have a learning disability or difficulty. It is important to liaise closely with her GP to establish if any diagnosis has been made. Further referral and engagement with social care services may be necessary to ensure that appropriate advocacy and assessment is put in place. There are also many useful visual aids that can support communication where the written word is inappropriate.

Domestic abuse is also a possible concern, with severe consequences including miscarriage, fetal and maternal death, as well as the emotional, financial and relationship costs. It is important for the midwife to explore this issue sensitively and be aware of the signs or symptoms of domestic abuse. The woman may only disclose information if she is alone, hence the midwife should endeavour to provide such opportunities and do so in a secure environment (NICE 2008a/2019). Women may not disclose vital information at the first time of being asked, but exploring the issue may help her to understand that she can disclose it at a later date if she feels the need (Salmon et al. 2015). Support can then be offered in collaboration with a multiagency team and information sharing systems should be in place (Knight et al. 2018).

It may become clear that the woman and her unborn baby are potentially vulnerable, for a range of reasons. It is important that the midwife does not display a negative attitude to vulnerable women and she should be non-judgemental in her approach (NICE 2018). There are a range of agencies that can be engaged to provide additional support, including link workers, social workers, health visitors and doulas, depending on local provision. The midwife may need to consider use of an Early Help Assessment tool (EHA) to gather holistic information about a family and coordinate multiagency support (DFE 2018). This should be undertaken after the booking appointment in-line with local policy and with the mother's consent. Any immediate cause for concern should also be escalated in-line with national guidelines and local policy.

Menstrual History and Expected Date of Birth

The next topic of conversation should be the reason that has brought the woman to this appointment. An accurate menstrual history helps estimate the expected date of birth (EDB), enables the midwife to predict a birth date and subsequently estimate gestational age for ultrasound referral purposes. This is particularly important for the timing of fetal anomaly screening and measuring fetal growth and will be confirmed or amended following the initial dating scan.

The EDB is calculated by adding 9 calendar months and 7 days to the date of the first day of the woman's last menstrual period (known as Naegele's rule) (see Chapter 5). This method assumes that:

- the woman takes regular note of regularity and length of time between periods
- conception occurred 14 days after the first day of the last period; this is true only if the woman has a regular 28-day cycle
- the last period of bleeding was true menstruation; implantation of the ovum may cause slight bleeding
- breakthrough bleeding and anovulation can be affected by the contraceptive pill thus impacting on the accuracy of a last menstrual period (LMP).

The duration of pregnancy based on Naegele's rule is 280 days. However, if the woman has a 35-day cycle, then 7 days should be added; if her cycle is <28 days, then the appropriate number of days is subtracted. A definitive EDB will be given when the woman attends for her 'dating' ultrasound scan at around 12 weeks of pregnancy.

Obstetric History

Previous childbearing history is important in considering the possible outcome of the current pregnancy and also in relation to how the woman feels about the future. In order to give a summary of a woman's childbearing history, the descriptive terms *gravida* and *para* are used. 'Gravid' means 'pregnant'; 'gravida' means 'a pregnant woman', and a subsequent number indicates the number of times she has been pregnant regardless of outcome. 'Para' means 'having given birth'; a woman's parity refers to the number of times that she has given birth to a child, live or stillborn, excluding termination of pregnancy. A 'grande multigravida' is a woman who has been pregnant five times or more, irrespective of outcome. A 'grande multipara' is a woman who has given birth five times or more.

Previous childbearing experiences

A sympathetic non-judgemental approach is required to elicit information and encourage the woman to talk freely about her experiences of previous births, miscarriages or terminations. Confidential information may be recorded in a clinic-held summary of the pregnancy but not in the woman's handheld record, if she requests this. Where a woman has had a previous traumatic birth experience, subsequent pregnancy may evoke panic and fear (Ayers et al. 2016). This impending birth has the potential to heal or harm and the woman may benefit from being able to talk through what happened and/or engage with a psychological intervention to enable her to achieve closure (Furuta et al. 2018). Where a woman or her partner has lost a child due to Sudden Infant Death Syndrome (SIDS) or has a close relative who has had this experience, she is likely to be very anxious about the prospect of this happening again. Care of the Next Infant (CONI) is a programme of support facilitated by the Lullaby Trust and provided by health visitors (Lullaby Trust 2018). Eligible parents are offered training in resuscitation, monitoring equipment and extra visits and it is paramount that they are referred to the scheme in the antenatal period to ensure that this care can be facilitated in a timely way, to allay anxiety.

Repeated spontaneous fetal loss may indicate such conditions as genetic malformations, hormonal imbalance or incompetent cervix (see Chapter 14). The woman and her partner are likely to be worried about the pregnancy, and continuity of carer in these circumstances will be particularly valuable. If there is a history of unexplained stillbirth, the woman should be referred for consultant antenatal care, for possible additional surveillance and early intervention, although any obstetric action should be carefully weighed up with any potential risks (Royal College of Obstetricians and Gynaecologists, RCOG 2010/2017). There is a need for care that takes account of the parents' particular psychosocial needs (Wojcieszek et al. 2018). Some maternity units have special clinics for women who have experienced late fetal loss, and most have some means of alerting staff that a woman has previously lost a baby, often with tear-drop sticker in the hospital case notes (the Stillbirth and Neonatal Death Society, SANDS 2018). Staff do need to be mindful of painful anniversaries and be prepared for parents to express a range of emotions, depending on their own particular circumstances (see Chapter 31).

Medical and Surgical History

During pregnancy, both the mother and the fetus may be affected by a medical condition, or a medical condition may be altered by the pregnancy; if untreated there may be serious consequences for the woman's health (Knight et al. 2018). For example:

- Women with a history of thrombosis are at greater risk of recurrence during pregnancy, more so when there is presence of risk factors, including: aged over 35 years; a body mass index (BMI) >30; prolonged bed rest; a family history of venous thromboembolism (VTE); heart disease; diabetes; have had an emergency caesarean birth; infection or pre-eclampsia (Testa et al. 2014). Thromboembolism is the leading cause of direct maternal death up to 6 weeks after the pregnancy, in the UK (Knight et al. 2019). All women should have a documented risk assessment for VTE at booking, using a structured tool, and repeated if hospitalized (RCOG 2015). Appropriate thromboprophylaxis and expert referral can be initiated depending on the level of risk identified (see Chapter 15).
- Hypertensive disorders encompass: chronic hypertension (prior to 20 weeks); gestational hypertension (after 20 weeks, no significant proteinuria); pre-eclampsia (after 20 weeks with significant proteinuria) and eclampsia (convulsions associated with pre-eclampsia). NICE (2017) have produced evidence-based guidelines to support monitoring, referral and care (see Chapter 15).

- Other conditions, including asthma, epilepsy, infections and psychiatric disorders may require medication, which may adversely affect fetal development and require medical review. Major medical complications such as diabetes and cardiac conditions require the involvement and support of a medical specialist (see Chapter 15).
- In the UK, suicide is a leading cause of direct maternal mortality occurring within a year after the end of pregnancy (Knight et al. 2018), therefore any psychiatric illness prior to the pregnancy must be fully explored so that the most appropriate multidisciplinary care can be offered (NICE 2014/2018) (see Chapter 30). Screening for current mental ill health should include assessment for depression using the Whooley questions and assessment for anxiety using the two-item Generalized Anxiety Disorder scale (GAD-2) (NICE 2014/2018) and a woman's emotional wellbeing should continue to be monitored throughout pregnancy.
- Previous surgery should be documented, as it may highlight previous problems with anaesthesia or other conditions or complications of relevance. Any surgery of the spine should be noted, as this may have an impact on the woman's ability to have an epidural or spinal block in labour. Breast surgery may impact on her ability to breastfeed depending on the technique involved. Previous pelvic or abdominal surgery may have consequences requiring specialist advice.
- The woman should be asked if she is taking any medication, either prescribed or over the counter. She should be advised not to take supplements that contain vitamin A and seek advice from the pharmacist before taking any medication throughout pregnancy and when breastfeeding.

Family History

Birth outcomes are multifactorial and may relate to familial or ethnic predisposition as well as economic and social deprivation. In the UK, the stillbirth rate (per 1000 births) for Asian and black mothers is 6.1 and 8.3, respectively, compared with 3.7 to white mothers (Draper et al. 2018). The Confidential Enquiry into Maternal Deaths (Knight et al. 2018) reported that, overall, 36% of direct deaths were from minority ethnic or black groups; Asian women were twice as likely, and black women five times more likely, to die than white women (Knight et al. 2018, 2019).

Genetic disease in the baby is more likely to occur if the biological parents are close relatives such as first cousins (Shawky et al. 2013). While there is an increased risk of recessive genetic disorders in babies born to married cousins, most babies are healthy. However, there is a lack of information for parents at risk and professionals often have fixed views about the social and religious values of couples (Teeuw et al. 2012). Where it has been identified that a couple are first cousins, genetic counselling should be offered.

Diabetes, although not inherited, leads to a predisposition in other family members, particularly if they become pregnant or obese. Screening for gestational diabetes is now recommended for women with a BMI of ≥30; a previous baby weighing ≥4.5 kg; previous gestational diabetes, a first-degree relative with diabetes and when belonging to a family origin with a high prevalence of diabetes (NICE 2015). Hypertension also has a familial component and multiple pregnancy has a higher incidence in certain families. Some conditions such as sickle cell anaemia and thalassaemia, are more common in those of black Caribbean, African-Caribbean, African, Pakistani, Cypriot, Bangladeshi and Chinese ethnicity (NICE 2008a/2019); and the Family Origin Questionnaire (FOQ) is used at the booking visit to screen couples at risk (see Chapter 13).

Lifestyle
Healthy eating
General health should be discussed and good habits reinforced, giving further advice when required. All women should be provided with information about healthy eating, and vitamin D supplementation of 10 μg/day (10 micrograms per day) is suggested for all women during pregnancy and breastfeeding to maintain bone and teeth health (NICE 2008a/2019). Particular recommendation should be given to women at risk of deficiency, including women who cover their skin, have a darker skin or who remain indoors for long periods of time (NICE 2008a/2019).

All women should take 400 μg of folic acid each day prior to pregnancy and until 12 weeks' gestation, to reduce the risk of a neural tube defects. Some women such as those on anticonvulsant medication, especially sodium valproate, women with diabetes or at >30 BMI, are at increased risk of having a fetus affected by a neural tube defect. In such cases, it is recommended that the woman consults her GP and takes a higher dose of 5 milligrams (5 mg) of folic acid.

The midwife should advise the woman about eating a balanced diet during pregnancy and not 'eating for two' (NICE 2010a/2019). It is currently not recommended that women attempt to lose weight during pregnancy (NICE 2008a/2019). Women should also be informed about which foods they should avoid, e.g. pate, liver products and soft cheeses; food to limit, e.g. tuna, caffeine; and foods where precaution is needed, e.g. sushi and raw eggs (if non-Lion coded in the UK). Full details can be found on the NHS Choices website: www.nhs.uk.

Exercise
NICE (2008a/2019) require health professionals to discuss how physically active a woman is at her first antenatal visit, providing her with tailored information and advice and informing her that moderate exercise is not associated with adverse outcomes. Usual aerobic or strength conditioning exercise should be continued, and where a woman is not currently active, she should be encouraged to start gradually and listen to her body. Not only will this enhance general wellbeing, but also reduce stress and anxiety and prepare her body for the challenge of labour. Any activity that could cause trauma or physical injury to the woman or fetus, such as contact sports and scuba diving should be avoided (NICE 2008a/2019). Public Health England (PHE 2017) recommends at least 150 min of moderate intensity activity every week, and muscle strengthening activities twice a week. Sexual intercourse during an uncomplicated pregnancy can continue to be enjoyed.

Sleeping position
Women should be advised to try and avoid going to sleep on their back after 28 weeks of pregnancy. Research has shown that supine going to sleep position is linked with a 2.3 times increased risk of stillbirth (Heazell et al. 2017a). Women should be reassured that they may wake up on their back, but it is the going to sleep position that is the longest held, and that they should resume a side-lying position to return to sleep.

Smoking
Approximately 10.8% of women are smokers at the time they give birth (NHS Digital 2018), however the rate varies between cities and between wards within cities. Although approximately 50% of pregnant smokers will try to quit during pregnancy (Cooper et al. 2014), the social norms in communities can make it very

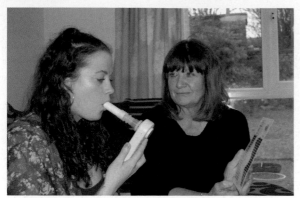

Fig. 11.1 Carbon monoxide (CO) monitoring of a woman by the midwife.

challenging for women to quit smoking. Pregnancy provides the opportunity to engage in a supported journey to a smoke-free life (Smoking in Pregnancy Challenge group 2018) and the midwife can be influential in motivating the woman to quit smoking by complying with NICE (2010b) guidelines. She should offer carbon monoxide (CO) screening to all women at each antenatal contact and refer women to a stop smoking service; a reading >5 ppm (parts per million) is associated with reduced fetal growth (Gomez et al. 2005). CO screening provides an opportunity to provide non-judgemental advice and support (Grice and Baston 2011). The recommendation for all smokers is to stop rather than cut down (Royal College of Physicians, RCP 2018). Cutting down leads to compensatory smoking, where the smoker takes a more sustained draw on the cigarette and inhales more deeply (Hughes 2000) (Fig. 11.1).

Smoking in pregnancy is associated with 35 adverse outcomes including: birth defects; low birth weight; intellectual impairment; respiratory dysfunction; stillbirth; premature birth; antepartum haemorrhage; and pre-eclampsia (RCP 2018). *The Saving Babies' Lives Care Bundle* (NHS England 2016) recommends that women at high risk of fetal growth restriction, including smokers, should have serial ultrasound scans for assessment of fetal weight and umbilical Doppler from 26–28 weeks until the birth.

Nicotine replacement therapy should be discussed with women having difficulty quitting smoking (NICE 2010) but only used if they are abstaining from smoking. While licensed products are preferable, if a woman chooses to use an E-cigarette to help her stay smoke-free, 'she should not be discouraged from doing so'

(Smoking in Pregnancy Challenge group 2017: 3) The woman, her partner and other family members should be informed about the direct and passive effects of smoking on the baby and aim to have a smoke-free home. Family members should be directed to Stop Smoking Services, as having a partner who smokes makes it very difficult for pregnant women to quit (Román-Gálvez et al. 2018).

Alcohol and drug misuse

The effects of excessive maternal alcohol on the fetus are marked, particularly in the first trimester, when fetal alcohol spectrum disorder can develop. This condition consists of restricted growth, facial malformations, central nervous system problems and behavioural and learning difficulties, and is entirely preventable (Bower et al. 2017). It is recommended that pregnant women abstain from alcohol throughout pregnancy as a precautionary measure (DH 2016). The midwife also needs to ask prospective parents if they take illicit drugs, regardless of their social status. Many maternity units have a substance misuse team that can support the care of women who abuse alcohol/drugs. Such care should be provided by a named midwife or doctor who has specialized knowledge and experience in this field (NICE 2010c/2018).

Risk Assessment

The booking assessment shapes the direction of a woman's antenatal pathway. The information gathered regarding the woman's obstetric, medical, psychosocial history and current pregnancy enables the midwife to assess her risk status. The midwife must also seek additional information from the GP and access previous case notes to elicit all the relevant information. If a risk factor is identified (Box 11.4), the woman should be referred to a consultant obstetrician, who will discuss a plan of care for her based on the need to access additional expertise and resources. Place of birth may also be influenced by the risk assessment but in all cases the ultimate decision is taken by the woman. Where a woman chooses a path of care that could cause significant harm to her or her baby, the midwife should discuss the evidence with her, document these discussions and inform someone senior of her concerns. The midwife should listen to a woman's rationale for requesting a particular path of care and respect her right to decline treatment (NMC 2018).

PHYSICAL EXAMINATION

Prior to conducting the physical examination of a pregnant woman, her consent and comfort are primary considerations. Observation of physical characteristics is important. Poor posture and gait can indicate back problems or previous trauma to the pelvis. The woman may be lethargic, which could be an indication of extreme tiredness, anaemia, malnutrition or depression. It is therefore important to look holistically at the woman and her family and assess fetal growth and development in conjunction with this knowledge.

Weight

Obesity is literally a growing problem, with 58% of women of childbearing age in England in 2014 being overweight or obese (PHE 2015). There are no evidence-based UK guidelines regarding what constitutes normal weight gain in pregnancy (NICE 2010a). However, in the USA it is recommended that women of normal BMI should gain between 11.5 and 16 kg, based on the Institute of Medicine (IOM) guidance (Rasmussen and Yaktine 2009). Referral to an obstetrician should be made if the woman's BMI is <18 kg/m^2 or ≥30 kg/m^2 (NICE 2008, 2018). Women with a BMI in the obese range are more at risk of complications of pregnancy. These may include gestational diabetes, pregnancy-induced hypertension (PIH) and shoulder dystocia. There may also be difficulty in palpating the fetal parts and defining presentation, position or engagement of the fetus. Overweight or underweight women should be carefully monitored, have additional care from an obstetrician, and be offered appropriate support, including nutritional counselling within the multiprofessional team (see Chapter 15). Women with a BMI of ≥30 should be offered a 75 g, 2 h oral glucose tolerance test (OGTT) at 24–28 weeks (NICE 2015). There is evidence that maternal and neonatal outcomes can be improved by lifestyle and dietary interventions that reduce gestational weight gain (GWG) (Rogozińska et al. 2017), however is not current practice in the UK to advise women to lose weight during pregnancy.

Blood Pressure

Blood pressure is taken in order to ascertain normality and provide a baseline reading for comparison throughout pregnancy. Systolic blood pressure does not alter significantly in pregnancy, but diastolic blood pressure falls in mid-pregnancy and rises to near non-pregnant levels at term. The systolic recording may be falsely elevated if a woman is nervous or anxious, if a small cuff is used on a large arm, the arm is unsupported or if the bladder is full. The woman should be comfortably seated or resting in a lateral position on the couch for the measurement. Brachial artery pressure is highest when the subject is sitting and lower when in the recumbent position. Current opinion is that Korotkoff V should be used (NICE 2008a/2019). See Chapter 15 for further information.

Urinalysis

At the first visit, the woman should be offered screening to exclude asymptomatic bacteriuria because the condition is asymptomatic and treatment could reduce the risk of pyelonephritis labour (NICE 2008, 2018/2019). Urinalysis is performed at every visit to exclude proteinuria, which may be a symptom of pre-eclampsia (NICE 2008a/2019) (see Chapter 15). When routine urine testing for glycosuria detects 2+ or above on one occasion or of 1+ or above on two or more occasions, further testing for gestational diabetes should be considered NICE (2008, 2015).

Blood Tests

The midwife should explain why blood tests are carried out at the booking visit to facilitate informed decision-making about the tests that are available. There are many views as to the ethical issues involved in screening. It is important to gain informed consent for any blood tests undertaken (NMC 2018) and offer appropriate counselling before and after the screening is carried out.

The midwife should be fully aware of the difference between screening and diagnostic tests, and their accuracy, and discuss these options with women. Blood tests offered at the initial assessment are covered in further detail in Chapter 13, and include the following.

ABO blood group and Rhesus (Rh) factor

It is important to identify the blood group, RhD status and red cell antibodies in pregnant women, so haemolytic disease of the newborn (HDN) can be prevented and preparations made for blood transfusion if it becomes necessary. Blood will be taken at booking and again at 28 weeks to determine if antibodies are present (NICE 2008a/2019). Since 2002 in the UK, all Rh-negative women have been offered routine antenatal anti-D prophylactic (RAADP) however, this has meant that some women who have Rh-negative babies (and therefore not at risk of HDN) have been offered a blood product unnecessarily. It is now recommended that non-invasive prenatal testing (NIPT) is used to identify the blood group of the fetus to inform if Anti-D is needed (NICE 2016). When the fetus is known to be Rh-positive, threatened miscarriage, amniocentesis, chorionic villus sampling, external cephalic version or any other uterine trauma are indications for the administration of anti-D gamma globulin within 72 hours of the event in pregnancy, in addition to any RAADP that might have already been given. A Kleihauer test should be undertaken to assess how much anti-D is required. If the titration demonstrates a rising antibody response then more frequent assessment will be made in order to plan management by a specialist in Rhesus disease.

Full blood count

This is taken to observe the woman's general blood condition and includes haemoglobin (Hb) estimations for anaemia at booking and again at 28 weeks of pregnancy and should be >110 g/L and 105 g/L, respectively. If the mean cell volume (MCV) is found to be low on the full blood count result, serum ferritin levels are also taken in order to assess the adequacy of iron stores. Iron supplementation is not considered necessary in women who are taking adequate dietary iron and who have a normal Hb and MCV at the initial assessment.

There is evidence that supplementing non-anaemic women with iron can increase the risk of hypertension and the small for gestational age birth rate (Ziaei et al. 2007). The decision to use supplements should be made on an individual woman's circumstances and include clear information about dietary iron sources. Maximum absorption of iron in meat or green leafy vegetables will be achieved by consuming vitamin C at the same time and avoiding caffeine. The intestinal mucosa has a limited ability to absorb iron and when this is exceeded, extra iron is excreted in the stools.

Other Screening Tests
Venereal disease research laboratory test

The venereal disease research laboratory (VDRL) test is performed for syphilis. Not all positive results indicate active syphilis; early testing will enable a woman to be treated in order to prevent infection of the fetus.

HIV antibodies

Routine screening to detect HIV infection should be offered in pregnancy (PHE 2016), as treatment in

pregnancy is beneficial in reducing vertical transmission to the fetus. Specialist teams should be involved in the subsequent care and management of women with a positive diagnosis.

Haemoglobinopathies

All women should be offered screening for sickle cell disease or thalassaemia by 10 weeks of pregnancy. Some ethnic groups have a higher incidence than others and the type of screening will depend on the prevalence (NICE 2008a/2019). If a woman either has or is a carrier of one of these diseases, her partner's blood should also be tested. The couple will be offered genetic counselling, and management during pregnancy will be explained.

Hepatitis B

Screening is offered in pregnancy so that infected women can be offered postnatal intervention to reduce the risk of mother-to-baby transmission (NICE 2008a/2019).

Screening for fetal anomaly

The midwife will also explain to the woman the current options regarding fetal anomaly screening and provide her with written information to enable her to make an informed choice. She will inform her about the routine dating and anomaly scans, which are part of the screening programme.

Infections *not* routinely screened for in pregnancy

Rubella. The screening programme for rubella ceased in 2016, as it no longer meets the criteria set by the UKNSC. Women who have not been vaccinated should be advised to avoid contact with anyone with the disease, because of the risk of congenital rubella syndrome in babies exposed to the virus in the first 8 weeks of pregnancy. The live vaccination should then be offered postnatally, and subsequent pregnancy must be avoided for at least 3 months.

Hepatitis C. This is currently not recommended as a routine screening test in pregnancy because there is insufficient evidence regarding the prevalence and effectiveness of treatments to reduce transmission to the baby (UKNSC 2018a).

Chlamydia. It is not recommended that all women are routinely screened for chlamydia (UKNSC 2018b), however women under 25 years of age are offered this as part of the National Chlamydia Screening Programme (PHE 2014).

Cytomegalovirus and toxoplasmosis. These are not routinely tested in pregnancy (UKNSC 2017) because tests do not currently determine which pregnancies may result in an infected fetus (NICE 2008a/2019). Toxoplasmosis screening is not recommended because the risks of screening may outweigh the benefits; however, women need to be informed of how to avoid contracting the infection.

Group B streptococcus. The UKNSC (2017) reviewed this guidance and concluded that screening should not be offered currently. However, the Royal College of Obstetricians and Gynaecologists recommended that all women should receive an information leaflet (Hughes et al. 2017).

THE MIDWIFE'S EXAMINATION

The midwife's general examination of the woman should be holistic and encompass the woman's physical, social and psychological wellbeing. This antenatal contact gives the midwife an opportunity to look at the woman's face and assess her health and general wellbeing, including demeanour and signs of fatigue. If at any time the midwife notices any sign of ill health, she should discuss this with the woman, and advocate referral to the most appropriate health professional (NMC 2018).

The midwife should facilitate discussion about infant feeding, recognizing a baby's needs and forming a positive relationship with her baby, throughout pregnancy (United Nations International Children's Emergency Fund, UNICEF 2018). Where breastfeeding peer support is available, introductions should be made so that antenatal and postnatal support can be more easily accessed. Breastfeeding should be promoted in a sensitive manner, and information given about the benefits to both mother and baby (see Chapter 27). Most women will not require an examination of their breasts. Current evidence does not support the benefits of nipple preparation (see Chapter 27). The midwife may also discuss the woman's experiences of breast changes so far in her pregnancy, and expected changes as pregnancy progresses.

Some women will appreciate information about the body changes taking place during pregnancy. Increasing abdominal size may be an acceptable body change but breast changes may not have been anticipated. For most women, breast size and appearance are an important part of their body image. Partners may also be affected by the changes and the midwife can encourage open and honest discussion between the woman and her partner to help to resolve anxieties.

Bladder and bowel function may be discussed; dietary advice may be necessary at this visit or later in the pregnancy, with reference to how hormonal changes may alter normal bowel and kidney function. Early referral within the multidisciplinary team will be necessary if treatment is required or problems identified. Vaginal discharge (leucorrhoea) increases in pregnancy; the woman may discuss any increase or changes with the midwife. If the discharge is itchy, causes soreness, is any colour other than creamy-white or has an offensive odour, then infection is likely, and should be investigated further. Later in pregnancy the woman may report a change from leucorrhoea to a heavier mucous discharge.

Early bleeding is not uncommon, however if this is reported, the woman can be referred to an Early Pregnancy Assessment Unit for confirmation of pregnancy and advice and appropriate care and follow-up. Ultrasound will usually confirm a diagnosis. The woman may require anti-D immunoglobulin if she is Rhesus-negative within 72 h (see Chapter 25 for management of antepartum haemorrhage).

In the past in developed and resource rich countries such as the UK, midwives have palpated the uterus once it has entered the abdomen, from about 12 weeks' gestation; however, current guidelines suggest that because of sophisticated scanning techniques there is no benefit in palpating the uterus prior to 24 weeks' gestation, at which time uterine growth can be measured (NICE 2008a/2019).

Oedema

This should not be evident during the initial assessment but may occur as the pregnancy progresses. Physiological oedema occurs after rising in the morning and worsens during the day; it is often associated with daily activities or hot weather. At visits later in pregnancy, the midwife should observe for oedema and ask the woman about symptoms. Often the woman may notice that her rings feel tighter and her ankles are swollen. Pitting oedema in the lower limbs can be identified by applying gentle fingertip pressure over the tibial bone: a depression will remain when the finger is removed. If oedema reaches the knees, affects the face or is increasing in the fingers, it may be indicative of hypertension of pregnancy if other markers are also present (see Chapter 15).

Varicosities

These are more likely to occur during pregnancy and are a predisposing cause of deep vein thrombosis. The woman should be asked if she has any pain in her legs. Reddened areas on the calf may be due to varicosities, phlebitis or deep vein thrombosis. Areas that appear white as if deprived of blood could be caused by deep vein thrombosis. The woman should be asked to report any tenderness that she feels either during the examination or at any time during the pregnancy. Referral should be made to medical colleagues as appropriate (NMC 2018). Support stockings will help alleviate symptoms, although not prevent varicose veins occurring (NICE 2008a/2019). Any vulval varicosities reported by the woman should be inspected and recorded.

Abdominal Examination

Abdominal examination is carried out from 24 weeks' gestation to establish and affirm that fetal growth is consistent with gestational age during the pregnancy. The specific aims are to:

- observe the signs of pregnancy
- assess fetal size and growth
- auscultate the fetal heart when indicated
- locate fetal parts
- detect any deviation from normal
- determine the presenting part (from 36 weeks).

Preparation

The woman should be asked to empty her bladder before making herself comfortable. A full bladder will make the examination uncomfortable; this can also make the measurement of fundal height less accurate. The midwife washes her hands and exposes only that area of the abdomen she needs to palpate and covers the remainder of the woman to promote privacy and protect her dignity. The woman should be lying comfortably with her arms by her sides to relax the abdominal muscles. The midwife should discuss her findings throughout the abdominal examination with the woman.

Inspection

The uterus is first assessed by observation. A full bladder, distended colon or obesity may give a false impression of fetal size. The shape of the uterus is longer than it is broad when the lie of the fetus is longitudinal, as occurs in the majority of cases. If the lie of the fetus is transverse, the uterus is low and broad.

The multiparous uterus may lack the snug ovoid shape of the primigravid uterus. Often it is possible to see the shape of the fetal back or limbs. If the fetus is in an occipitoposterior position, a saucer-like depression may be seen at or below the umbilicus. The midwife may observe fetal movements, or the mother may feel them; this can help the midwife determine the position of the fetus. The woman's umbilicus becomes less dimpled as pregnancy advances and may protrude slightly in later weeks.

Lax abdominal muscles in the parous woman may cause the uterus to sag forwards; this is known as pendulous abdomen or anterior obliquity of the uterus. In the primigravida it is a significant sign as it may be due to pelvic contraction.

Skin changes. Stretch marks from previous pregnancies appear silvery and recent ones appear pink. A linea nigra may be seen; this is a normal dark line of pigmentation running longitudinally in the centre of the abdomen below and sometimes above the umbilicus. Scars may indicate previous obstetric or abdominal surgery or self-harm.

Palpation

The midwife's hands should be clean and warm; cold hands do not have the necessary acute sense of touch, they tend to induce contraction of the abdominal and uterine muscles and the woman may find palpation uncomfortable. Arms and hands should be relaxed and the pads, not the tips, of the fingers used with delicate precision. The hands are moved smoothly over the abdomen to avoid causing contractions.

Measuring fundal height. In order to determine the height of the fundus the midwife places her hand just below the xiphisternum. Pressing gently, she moves her hand down the abdomen until she feels the curved upper border of the fundus (Fig. 11.2).

Clinically assessing the uterine size to compare it with gestation does not always produce an accurate result, although there are landmarks that can be used as an approximate guide (Fig. 11.3). From 24 weeks of pregnancy, the midwife should commence serial symphysis fundal height (SFH) measurements (Fig. 11.4). She uses a tape measure (with the centimetres facing the mother's abdomen) held at the fundus and extended down to the symphysis pubis, to take a single measurement. This should be recorded in the pregnancy record and plotted on a growth chart (NICE 2008a/2019). The

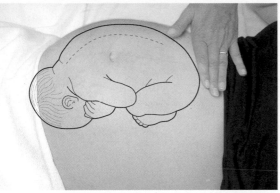

Fig. 11.2 Assessing the fundal height in finger-breadths below the xiphisternum.

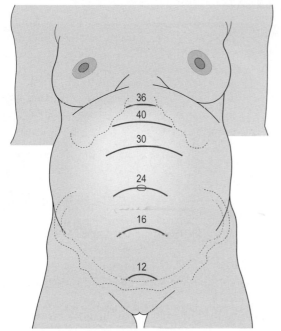

Fig. 11.3 Growth of the uterus, showing the fundal heights at various weeks of pregnancy.

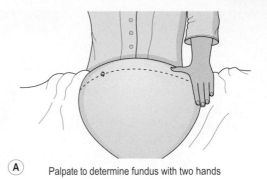

(A) Palpate to determine fundus with two hands

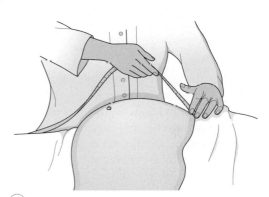

(B) Secure tape with hand at top of fundus

Fig. 11.4 Measuring fundal height. (Reproduced with permission from Morse K, Williams A, Gardosi J. (2009) Fetal growth screening by fundal height measurement. Best Practice & Research Clinical Obstetrics and Gynaecology 23:809–818.)

'Saving Babies' Lives Care Bundle' (NHS England 2016), which aims to reduce the incidence of stillbirth, states that this can be on a customized (generated for the individual mother taking into account her ethnicity, height, weight and parity) or other growth chart, rather than a population-based chart. Customized antenatal growth charts, as part of a package of education and training, have been heralded as reducing the incidence of avoidable stillbirths (Gardosi et al. 2018) and are recommended by the RCOG (2013/2014).

Further investigation is warranted and an ultrasound scan will usually be required alongside appropriate medical referral, if:

• a single measurement plots below the 10th centile; *or*
• serial measurements show slow growth by crossing centiles; *or*
• there appears to be static growth; *or*
• excessive growth/polyhydramnios is suspected.

If the uterus is unduly big, the fetus may be large or it may indicate multiple pregnancy or polyhydramnios. When the uterus is smaller than expected, the LMP date may be incorrect, or the fetus may be small for gestational age (SGA). Fetal growth restriction (FGR) is associated with stillbirth and is often linked to placental insufficiency (Silver 2018).

Fundal palpation. This determines the presence of the breech or the head in the fundus. This information will help to diagnose the lie and presentation of the

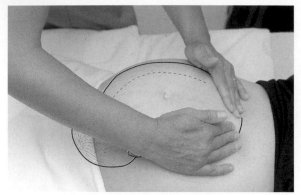

Fig. 11.5 Fundal palpation. Palms of hands on either side of the fundus and fingers held close together palpate the upper pole of the uterus.

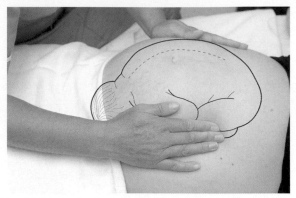

Fig. 11.6 Lateral palpation. Hands placed at umbilical level on either side of the uterus. Pressure is applied alternately with each hand.

fetus. Talking through the palpation with the woman and making eye contact with her during the procedure, the midwife lays both hands on the sides of the fundus, fingers held close together and curving round the upper border of the uterus. Gentle, yet deliberate pressure is applied using the palmar surfaces of the fingers to determine the soft consistency and indefinite outline that denotes the breech. Sometimes the buttocks feel rather firm but they are not as hard, smooth or well-defined as the head. With a gliding movement, the fingertips are separated slightly in order to grasp the fetal mass, which may be in the centre or deflected to one side, to assess its size and mobility. The breech cannot be moved independently of the body but the head can (Fig. 11.5). The head is much more distinctive in outline than the breech, being hard and round; it can be balloted with care (moved from one hand to the other) between the fingertips of the two hands because of the free movement of the neck.

Lateral palpation. This is used to locate the fetal back in order to determine position. The hands are placed on either side of the uterus at the level of the umbilicus (Fig. 11.6). Gentle pressure is applied with alternate hands in order to detect which side of the uterus offers the greater resistance. More detailed information is obtained by feeling along the length of each side with the fingers. This can be done by sliding the hands down the abdomen, while feeling the sides of the uterus alternately. Some midwives prefer to steady the uterus with one hand, and using a rotary movement of the opposite hand, to map out the back as a continuous smooth resistant mass from the breech down to the neck; on

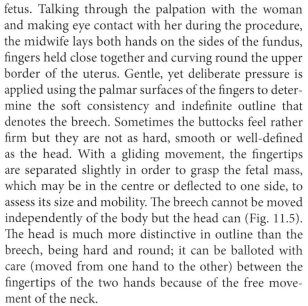

Fig. 11.7 'Walking' the fingertips across the abdomen to locate the position of the fetal back.

the other side, the same movement reveals the limbs as small parts that slip about under the carefully examining fingers.

'Walking' the fingertips of both hands over the abdomen from one side to the other is another method of locating the fetal back (Fig. 11.7).

Pelvic palpation. Pelvic palpation will identify the pole of the fetus in the pelvis; it should not cause discomfort to the woman. NICE (2008a/2019) recommend this is done only from 36 weeks onwards.

The midwife should ask the woman to bend her knees slightly in order to relax the abdominal muscles and also suggest that she breathe steadily; relaxation may be helped if she sighs out slowly. The sides of the uterus just below umbilical level are grasped snugly between the palms of the hands with the fingers held close together, pointing downwards and inwards (Fig. 11.8).

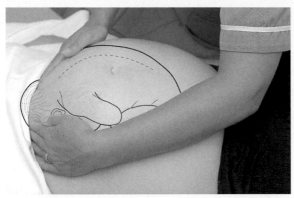

Fig. 11.8 Pelvic palpation. The fingers are directed inwards and downwards.

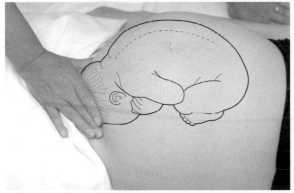

Fig. 11.9 Pawlik's manoeuvre. The lower pole of the uterus is grasped with the right hand, the midwife facing the woman's head.

If the head is presenting (towards the lower part of the uterus), a hard mass with a distinctive round smooth surface will be felt. The midwife should also estimate how much of the fetal head is palpable above the pelvic brim to determine engagement. This two-handed technique appears to be the most comfortable for the woman and gives the most information.

Pawlik's manoeuvre, where the practitioner grasps the lower pole of the uterus between her fingers and thumb, which should be spread wide enough apart to accommodate the fetal head (Fig. 11.9), is sometimes used to judge the size, flexion and mobility of the head, but undue pressure must not be applied. It should be used only if absolutely necessary as it can be very uncomfortable for the woman. There is no research evidence to support one method over the other.

Engagement

Engagement is said to have occurred when the widest presenting transverse diameter of the fetal head has passed through the brim of the pelvis. In cephalic presentations, this is the 'biparietal' diameter and in breech presentations, the 'bitrochanteric' diameter (see Chapter 20). In a primigravid woman, the head normally engages at any time from about 36 weeks of pregnancy, but in a multipara, this may not occur until after the onset of labour. Engagement of the fetal head is usually measured in fifths palpable above the pelvic brim. When the vertex presents and the head is engaged the following will be evident on clinical examination:

- only two- to three-fifths of the fetal head is palpable above the pelvic brim (Fig. 11.10)
- the head will not be mobile.

On rare occasions, the head is not palpable abdominally because it has descended deeply into the pelvis. If the head is not engaged, the findings are as follows:

- more than half of the head is palpable above the brim
- the head may be high and freely movable (ballotable) or partly settled in the pelvic brim and consequently immobile.

In a primigravid woman, it is usual for the head to engage by 37 weeks' gestation; however this is not always the case. When labour starts, the force of labour contractions encourages flexion and moulding of the fetal head and the relaxed ligaments of the pelvis allow the joints to give. This is usually sufficient to allow engagement and descent. Causes of a non-engaged head at term include:

- occipitoposterior position
- full bladder
- wrongly calculated gestational age
- polyhydramnios
- placenta praevia or other space-occupying lesion
- multiple pregnancy
- pelvic malformations
- fetal malformations.

Presentation

Presentation refers to the part of the fetus that lies at the pelvic brim or in the lower pole of the uterus. Presentations can be vertex, breech, shoulder, face or brow (Fig. 11.11). Vertex, face and brow are all head or cephalic presentations.

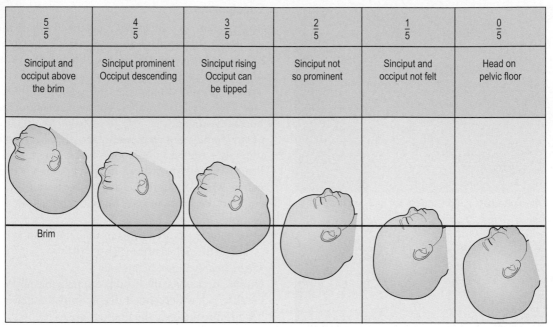

$\frac{5}{5}$	$\frac{4}{5}$	$\frac{3}{5}$	$\frac{2}{5}$	$\frac{1}{5}$	$\frac{0}{5}$
Sinciput and occiput above the brim	Sinciput prominent Occiput descending	Sinciput rising Occiput can be tipped	Sinciput not so prominent	Sinciput and occiput not felt	Head on pelvic floor

Fig. 11.10 Descent of the fetal head estimated in fifths palpable above the pelvic brim.

When the head is flexed, the vertex presents; when it is fully extended, the face presents; and when it is partially extended, the brow presents (Fig. 11.12). It is more common for the head to present because the bulky breech finds more space in the fundus, which is the widest diameter of the uterus, and the head lies in the narrower lower pole. The muscle tone of the fetus also plays a part in maintaining its flexion and consequently its vertex presentation.

Auscultation

Listening to the fetal heart has historically been an important part of the process. However, in the UK, NICE (2008a/2019) does not recommend routine listening other than at maternal request because there is no clinical benefit. A Pinard fetal stethoscope will enable the midwife to hear the fetal heart directly and determine that it is fetal and not maternal. The stethoscope is placed on the mother's abdomen, at right-angles to it, over the fetal back (Fig. 11.13). The ear must be in close, firm contact with the stethoscope but the hand should not touch it while listening because then extraneous sounds are produced. The stethoscope should be moved about until the point of maximum intensity is located where the fetal heart is heard most clearly. The midwife

should count the beats per minute (beats/min), which should be in the range of 110–160. The midwife should take the woman's pulse at the same time as listening to the fetal heart to enable her to distinguish between the two. In addition, ultrasound equipment (e.g. a Sonicaid or Doppler) can be used for this purpose so that the woman and her partner/children may also hear the fetal heartbeat.

Lie

The lie of the fetus is the relationship between the long axis of the fetus and the long axis of the uterus (Figs 11.14–11.16). In the majority of cases, the lie is longitudinal due to the ovoid shape of the uterus; the remainder are 'oblique' or 'transverse'. Oblique lie, when the fetus lies diagonally across the long axis of the uterus, must be distinguished from obliquity of the uterus, when the whole uterus is tilted to one side (usually the right) and the fetus lies longitudinally within it. When the lie is transverse, the fetus lies at right angles across the long axis of the uterus. This is often visible on inspection of the abdomen.

Attitude

Attitude is the relationship of the fetal head and limbs to its trunk. The attitude should be one of flexion. The fetus

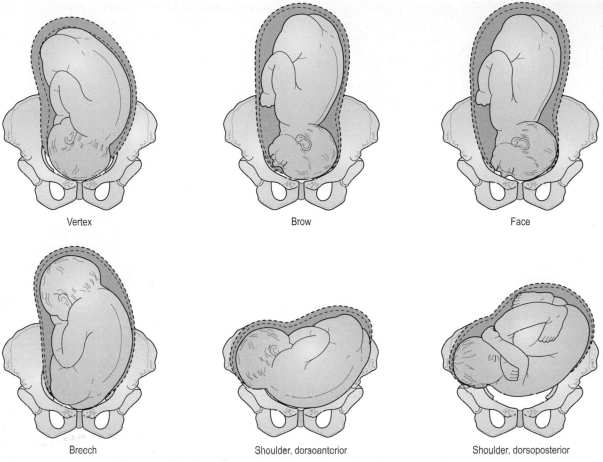

Fig. 11.11 The five presentations. Vertex, Brow, Face, Breech and Shoulder.

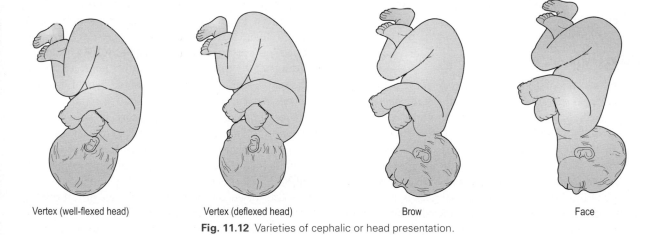

Fig. 11.12 Varieties of cephalic or head presentation.

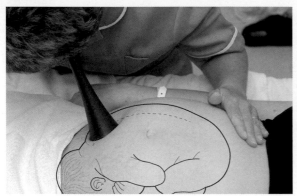

Fig. 11.13 Auscultation of the fetal heart. Vertex right occipitoanterior.

is curled up with chin on chest, arms and legs flexed, forming a snug, compact mass, which utilizes the space in the uterine cavity most effectively. If the fetal head is flexed, the smallest diameters will present and, with efficient uterine action, labour will be most effective.

Denominator

'Denominate' means 'to give a name to'; the denominator is the name of the part of the presentation, which is used when referring to fetal position. Each presentation has a different denominator and these are as follows:

- in the vertex presentation, it is the *occiput*
- in the breech presentation, it is the *sacrum*
- in the face presentation, it is the *mentum*.

Although the shoulder presentation is said to have the 'acromion' process as its denominator, in practice the 'dorsum' is used to describe the position. In the brow presentation, no denominator is used.

POSITION

The position is the relationship between the denominator of the presentation and six points on the pelvic brim (Fig. 11.17). In addition, the denominator may be found in the midline either anteriorly or posteriorly, especially late in labour. This position is often transient and is described as direct anterior or direct posterior.

Anterior positions are more favourable than posterior positions because when the fetal back is at the front of the uterus, it conforms to the concavity of the mother's abdominal wall and the fetus can flex more easily. When the back is flexed, the head also tends to flex and a smaller diameter presents to the pelvic brim. There is

also more room in the anterior part of the pelvic brim for the broad biparietal diameter of the head. The positions in a vertex presentation are summarized in Box 11.6 and shown in Fig. 11.18.

In breech and face presentations, the positions are described in a similar way using the appropriate denominator.

Findings

The findings from the abdominal palpation should be considered part of the holistic assessment of the pregnant woman's health and fetal wellbeing. The midwife collates all the information she has gathered from inspection, palpation and auscultation and relays this to the woman. Deviation from the expected growth and development should be discussed with the woman and referral to an obstetrician or appropriate professional arranged and documented as appropriate (NMC 2018).

ONGOING ANTENATAL CARE

The information gathered during the antenatal visits will enable the midwife and pregnant woman to determine the appropriate pattern of antenatal care (NICE 2008a/2019). The timing and number of visits will vary according to individual need and changes should be made as circumstances dictate (e.g. as demonstrated in Box 11.7).

Indicators of Maternal Wellbeing

Surveillance for symptoms of pre-eclampsia is ongoing throughout pregnancy. It has been recommended by NICE (2008a/2019: 1.9.2.5) that if there is a 'single diastolic blood pressure of 110 mmHg or two consecutive readings of 90 mmHg at least 4 hours apart and/or significant proteinuria (1+)', there should be an increase in surveillance (see Chapter 15).

The woman's general health and wellbeing is observed throughout, and the midwife must remain vigilant for signs of domestic abuse, emotional fragility and social instability. Endeavouring to maintain continuity of carer will be a key process for identifying impending problems and for encouraging free exchange of information between the woman and her midwife. There should be clear referral pathways for the midwife to follow when she has cause for concern regarding a woman's obstetric, social or emotional wellbeing.

Longitudinal lie

Breech   Vertex   Vertex

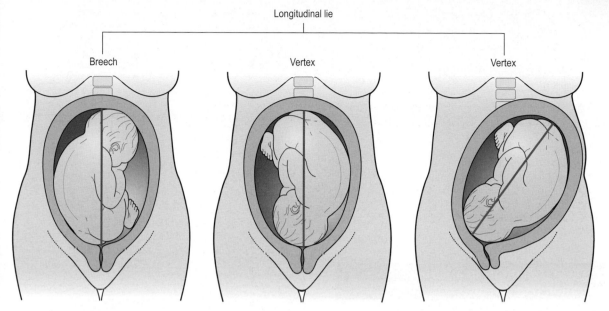

Fig. 10.14 The lie of the fetus. The longitudinal lie. Confusion sometimes exists regarding the lie seen (right-most diagram), which gives the impression of an oblique lie, but the fetus is longitudinal in relation to the uterus and merely moving the uterus abdominally rectifies the presumed obliquity.

Oblique lie   Transverse lie

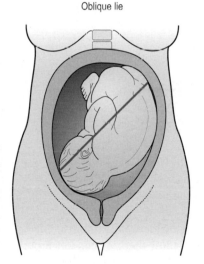 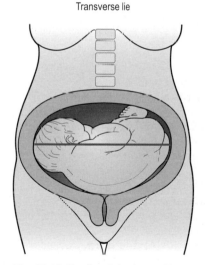

Fig. 10.15 The lie of the fetus. Shows an oblique lie because the long axis of the fetus is oblique in relation to the uterus.

Fig. 10.16 The lie of the fetus. Shows a transverse lie with shoulder presentation.

Indicators of Fetal Wellbeing

These include:

- increasing uterine size compatible with the gestational age of the fetus
- fetal heart rate that is regular and variable with a rate between 110 and 160 beats/min
- fetal movements that follow a regular pattern from the time when they are first felt.

Recurrent reduction in fetal movements (RFM) is associated with a poor fetal outcome; women who experience stillbirth are more likely than other women to have experienced abnormalities in their baby's movements in

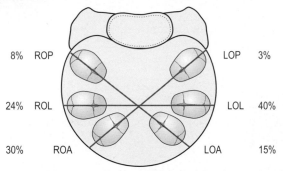

Fig. 11.17 Diagrammatic representation of the six vertex positions and their relative frequency. LOA, left occipitoanterior; LOL, left occipitolateral; LOP, left occipitoposterior; ROA, right occipitoanterior; ROL, right occipitolateral; ROP, right occipitoposterior.

BOX 11.6   Positions in a Vertex Presentation (Fig. 11.18)

- **Left occipitoanterior (LOA)** The occiput points to the left iliopectineal eminence; the sagittal suture is in the right oblique diameter of the pelvis.
- **Right occipitoanterior (ROA)** The occiput points to the right iliopectineal eminence; the sagittal suture is in the left oblique diameter of the pelvis.
- **Left occipitolateral (LOL)** The occiput points to the left iliopectineal line midway between the iliopectineal eminence and the sacroiliac joint; the sagittal suture is in the transverse diameter of the pelvis.
- **Right occipitolateral (ROL)** The occiput points to the right iliopectineal line midway between the iliopectineal eminence and the sacroiliac joint; the sagittal suture is in the transverse diameter of the pelvis.
- **Left occipitoposterior (LOP)** The occiput points to the left sacroiliac joint; the sagittal suture is in the left oblique diameter of the pelvis.
- **Right occipitoposterior (ROP)** The occiput points to the right sacroiliac joint; the sagittal suture is in the right oblique diameter of the pelvis. And:
- **Direct occipitoanterior (DOA)** The occiput points to the symphysis pubis; the sagittal suture is in the anteroposterior diameter of the pelvis.
- **Direct occipitoposterior (DOP)** The occiput points to the sacrum; the sagittal suture is in the anteroposterior diameter of the pelvis.

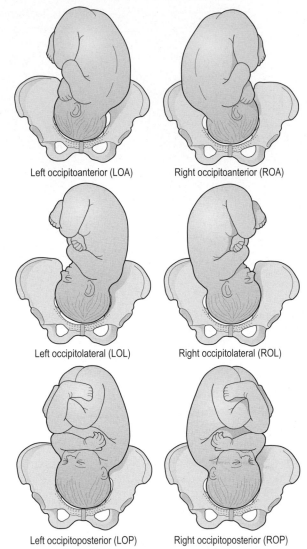

Fig. 11.18 Six positions in vertex presentation.

the previous 2 weeks (Heazell et al. 2017b). However, subsequent research has shed doubt on this practice; the AFFIRM study (Norman et al. 2018) concluded that a package of intervention designed to enhance women's reporting of RFM combined with a management plan, did not reduce the incidence of stillbirth. Further research is needed and until then, discussion around what to expect with regard to a pregnant woman noticing her baby move should continue to be an integral part of antenatal care. Eliciting information about recent fetal movements reminds the woman of the importance of noticing this feedback from her baby. Women should be reminded that there should be no reduction in fetal movements in the last trimester and to contact their midwife if they notice a change in their baby's usual pattern. Indeed, unusual 'crazy' movements should also be reported and investigated (Heazell et al. 2017b). NICE (2008, 2018), does not recommend routine fetal

BOX 11.7 Risk Factors that May Arise During Pregnancy

- any chronic or acute illness or disease in the woman
- Hb <105 g/L
- proteinuria
- blood pressure: single diastolic of 110 mmHg or two of 90 mmHg at least 4 h apart; two systolic of >160 mmHg at least 4 h apart
- uterus large or small for gestational age
- excess or decreased liquor
- malpresentation
- fetal movement pattern significantly reduced or changed
- any vaginal, cervical or uterine bleeding
- premature labour
- infection
- sociological or psychological concerns.

movement counting as there is insufficient evidence that it improves fetal wellbeing.

Preparation for Labour

Perineal massage

Women should be informed that there is evidence that perineal massage from 35 weeks of pregnancy is effective in reducing the likelihood of perineal damage during the birth (Beckmann and Stock 2013) (see Chapter 17). This can be undertaken by the woman or her partner just once or twice a week with a significant positive impact on her perineal integrity and postnatal pain (see Chapter 28).

Stretch and sweep

NICE guidelines (NICE 2008a/2019) recommend that the midwife offers a membrane sweep to women who have not given birth by 41 weeks. The Antenatal Quality Standard (NICE 2012/2016) recommends it at 40 and 41 weeks for a primigravida (Box 11.2). This procedure has been shown to reduce the number of women who require induction of labour, and although this can be uncomfortable it is a safe and simple technique (Boulvain et al. 2005) (see Chapter 22).

Birth plans

During the latter weeks of pregnancy, expectations and plans for labour and birth will be a focus of discussion. Women should know when they should contact a midwife and how to do so. If the woman has planned a home birth, she will be visited by her midwife to make final preparations. Most maternity units provide a list of items that women will need to bring with them if they are planning to birth away from home. In all situations, it is important to ensure that women know how to get advice if they have any concerns.

A birth plan can be instrumental in assisting the woman towards having the birth experience of her choice and to consider what she might like to do during labour and what is important to her. NICE (2008a/2019) recommend a birth plan should be discussed before or at 36 weeks of pregnancy. Birth plans are part of ensuring personalized care and likely to be most effective if they are written with the midwife sharing information to enable the woman to make plans that are informed by what is available locally and what is considered current best practice and care.

Flexibility and adaptability should be built into the labour and birth plans to ensure an individual approach is adopted and the woman's wishes are carefully considered (National Maternity Review 2016). Parents' wishes should be revisited when labour commences and discussions recorded in the labour notes. Each woman should be aware that it may be necessary to adapt her plans depending on the circumstances at the time but be reassured that she will be fully involved in all decisions made.

Home Visit and Safe Sleeping Advice

It is practice in many units to undertake one of the antenatal visits at the woman's home, in order to discuss arrangements for caring for the baby when it is born. This may include seeing where the baby will sleep and advising on safe sleeping principles. It provides another opportunity to discuss keeping a smoke-free home and ensuring that the woman knows how and when to make contact when labour starts.

REFLECTIVE ACTIVITY FOR SELF-ASSESSMENT

1. Consider the women who access your local maternity services. What information is available for them to find out about antenatal care and the importance of receiving early screening and health advice. How does this information address the diverse cultural and social needs of the community?

2. Think about your own personal views about women who continue to smoke during pregnancy. How can

you ensure that you provide non-judgemental care when caring for women addicted to nicotine? What specialist services are available to support women and their partners to stop smoking in pregnancy?

3. Abdominal palpation is a fundamental midwifery skill. Reflect on learning and practice while observing

how a midwife palpates the uterus of women at different gestations. How does she amend her conversation to personalize this activity? What additional information might she be gleaning in addition to fetal wellbeing?

REFERENCES

Allison, R. (2012). Language matters. *Practising Midwife*, *15*(1), 14–16.

Ayers, S., Bond, R., Bertullies, S., & Wijma, K. (2016). The aetiology of post-traumatic stress following childbirth: A meta-analysis and theoretical framework. *Psychological Medicine*, *46*(6), 1121–1134.

Baston, H., Hall, J., & Midwifery essentials (2018). (2nd ed.). *Antenatal* (Vol. 2). Edinburgh: Elsevier.

Beckmann, M., & Stock, O. (2013). Antenatal perineal massage for reducing perineal trauma. *Cochrane Database of Systematic Reviews* (4), CD005123.

Boulvain, M., Stan, C., & Irion, O. (2005). Membrane sweeping for induction of labour. *Cochrane Database of Systematic Reviews*, *1*, CD000451.

Bower, C., Elliott, E., Zimmet, M., et al. (2017). Australian guide to the diagnosis of foetal alcohol spectrum disorder: A summary. *Journal of Paediatrics and Child Health*, *53*(10), 1021–1023.

Clement, S., Candy, B., Sikorski, J., et al. (1996). Does reducing the frequency of routine antenatal visits have long term effects? Follow up of participants in a randomized controlled trial. *British Journal of Obstetrics and Gynaecology*, *106*(4), 367–370.

Cooper, S., Taggar, J., Lewis, S., et al. (2014). Effect of nicotine patches in pregnancy on infant and maternal outcomes at 2 years: Follow-up from the randomised, double-blind, placebo controlled snap trial. *Lancet: Respiratory Medicine*, *2*, 728–737.

Data Protection Act. (2018). Available at: www.gov.uk/data-protection.

DFE. (2018). *Working together to safeguard children*. Available at: https://assets.publishing.service.gov.uk/government/uploads/system/uploads/attachment_data/file/729914/Working_Together_to_Safeguard_Children-2018.pdf.

(Department of Health), D. H. (1999). *Our healthier nation: Reducing health inequalities: An action report*. London: DH.

(Department of Health), D. H. (2016). *UK Chief Medical Officers' Alcohol Guidelines Review*. Summary of the proposed guidelines. Available at: https://assets.publishing.service.gov.uk/government/uploads/system/uploads/attachment_data/file/489795/summary.pdf.

DH/NHS. (2014). *Midwifery Public health contribution in Practice through maximizing wellbeing and improving health in women, babies and families*. Available at: https://assets.publishing.service.gov.uk/government/uploads/system/uploads/attachment_data/file/208824/Midwifery_strategy_visual_B.pdf.

Dowswell, T., Carroli, G., Duley, L., et al. (2010). Alternative versus standard packages of antenatal care for low-risk pregnancy. *Cochrane Database of Systematic Reviews*, *10*, CD000934.

Draper E, Gallimore I, Kurinczuk J, et al.; on behalf of the MBRRACE-UK Collaboration. (2018) MBRRACE-UK Perinatal Mortality Surveillance Report, UK Perinatal Deaths for Births from January to December 2016. Leicester: The Infant Mortality and Morbidity Studies, Department of Health Sciences, University of Leicester.

Furuta, M., Horsch, A., Ng, E., et al. (2018). Effectiveness of trauma-focused psychological therapies for treating post-traumatic stress disorder symptoms in women following childbirth: A systematic review and meta-analysis. *Frontiers in Psychiatry*, *9*(2018):591.

Gardosi, J., Francis, A., Turner, S., & Williams, M. (2018). Customized growth charts: rationale, validation and clinical benefits. *American Journal of Obstetrics and Gynecology*, *218*(2S), S609–S618.

Gomez, C., Berlin, I., Marquis, P., & Delcroix, M. (2005). Expired air carbon monoxide concentration in mothers and their spouses above 5 ppm is associated with decreased fetal growth. *Preventive Medicine*, *40*(1), 10–15.

Grice, J., & Baston, H. (2011). Carbon monoxide screening in pregnancy. *Practising Midwife*, *14*(10), 36–41.

Hall, M. H., Cheng, P. K., & MacGillivray, I. (1980). Is routine antenatal care worthwhile? *Lancet*, *2*, 78–80.

Heazell, A., Li, J., Thompson, B., et al. (2017a). Association between maternal sleep practices and late stillbirth – findings from a stillbirth case–control study. *BJOG: An International Journal of Obstetrics & Gynaecology*, *125*(2), 254–262.

Heazell, A., Warland, J., Stacey, T., et al. (2017b). Stillbirth is associated with perceived alterations in fetal activity – findings from an international case control study. *BMC Pregnancy and Childbirth*, *17*, 11.

Hollowell, J., Oakley, L., Vigurs, C., et al. (2012). Increasing the early initiation of antenatal care by Black and Minority Ethnic women in the United Kingdom: A systematic review and mixed methods synthesis of women's views and the literature on intervention effectiveness. *Final Report*. Oxford: Perinatal Epidemiology Unit, University of Oxford. Available at: www.npeu.ox.ac.uk/downloads/files/infant-mortality/Infant-Mortality-DIVA-final-report-Oct-2012.pdf.

Hughes, J. (2000). Reduced smoking: An introduction and review of the evidence. *Addiction, 95*(Suppl. 1), S3–S7.

Hughes, R. G., Brocklehurst, P., Steer, P. J., et al.; On behalf of the Royal College of Obstetricians and Gynaecologists. (2017). Prevention of early-onset neonatal group B streptococcal disease. Green-top Guideline No 36. BJOG 124:e280–e305.

Knight, H., Cromwell, D., Gurol-Urganci, I., et al. (2017). Perinatal mortality associated with induction of labour versus expectant management in nulliparous women aged 35 years or over: An English national cohort study. *PLoS Medicine, 14*(11), E1002425.

Knight, M., Bunch, K., Tuffnell, D., et al. (Eds); on behalf of MBRRACE-UK. (2018). *Saving Lives, Improving Mothers' Care – Lessons learned to inform maternity care from the UK and Ireland Confidential Enquiries into Maternal Deaths and Morbidity, 2014–2016*. Oxford: National Perinatal Epidemiology Unit, University of Oxford.

Knight, M., Bunch, K., Tuffnell, D., et al. (Eds); on behalf of MBRRACE-UK. (2018). *Saving Lives, Improving Mothers' Care – Lessons learned to inform maternity care from the UK and Ireland Confidential Enquiries into Maternal Deaths and Morbidity, 2015–2017*. Oxford: National Perinatal Epidemiology Unit, University of Oxford.

Leamon, J., & Viccars, A. (2007). *West Howe midwifery evaluation: The with me study*. Bournemouth: Bournemouth University.

Lullaby Trust (2018). *Care of next infant (CONI)*. Available at: www.lullabytrust.org.uk/bereavement-support/how-we-can-support-you/our-care-of-next-infant-scheme.

Marmot Review. (2010). *Fair society, healthy lives. A strategic review of health inequalities in England post-2010*. Available at: www.instituteofhealthequity.org/resources-reports/fair-society-healthy-lives-the-marmot-review/fair-society-healthy-lives-full-report-pdf.pdf.

McCourt, C. (2006). Supporting choice and control? Communication and interaction between midwives and women at the antenatal booking visit. *Social Science and Medicine, 62*(6), 1307–1318.

McNeill J, Lynn F, Alderdice F. (2010) *Systematic review of reviews: The public health role of the midwife*. School of Nursing & Midwifery, Queen's University Belfast.

Ministry of Health. (1929). Maternal mortality in childbirth. *Antenatal clinics: Their conduct and scope*. London: HMSO.

Mobbs, N., Williams, C., & Weeks, A. D. (2018). *A humanising birth: Does the language we use matter?* Available at: https://blogs.bmj.com/bmj/2018/02/08/humanising-birth-does-the-language-we-use-matter.

NICE (National Institute for Health and Care Excellence). (2008a /2019) Updated 2019. Antenatal care for uncomplicated pregnancies. Clinical Guideline 62. Available at: www.nice.org.uk/guidance/cg62/resources/antenatal-care-for-uncomplicated-pregnancies-pdf-975564597445.

NICE (National Institute for Health and Care Excellence). (2008b/2019). Updated 2019. Maternal and child health. Public Health Guideline: PH 11. Available at: www.nice.org.uk/guidance/PH11.

NICE (National Institute for Health and Care Excellence). (2010a/2019). Weight management before, during and after pregnancy. *Public Health Guidance, 27*. Available at: www.nice.org.uk/guidance/ph27.

NICE (National Institute for Health and Care Excellence). (2010b). Quitting smoking in pregnancy and following childbirth. *Public Health Guidance, 26*. Available at: www.nice.org.uk/guidance/ph26.

NICE (National Institute for Health and Care Excellence). (2010c). Updated 2018. Pregnancy and complex social factors: A model for service provision for pregnant women with complex social factors. *Clinical Guideline CG 110*. Available at: www.nice.org.uk/guidance/cg110/chapter/Key priorities-for-implementation.

NICE (National Institute for Health and Care Excellence). (2012). *Updated 2016. Antenatal quality standard: Quality statements*. Available at: www.nice.org.uk/guidance/qs22

NICE (National Institute for Health and Care Excellence). (2013). *Hypertension in pregnancy. Quality Standard: QS35*. Available at: www.nice.org.uk/guidance/qs35.

NICE (National Institute for Health and Care Excellence). (2014). Updated 2018. *Antenatal and postnatal mental health. Clinical Management and Service Guidance: CG 192*. Available at: www.nice.org.uk/guidance/cg192.

NICE (National Institute for Health and Care Excellence). (2015). *Diabetes in pregnancy: Management from preconception to the postnatal periodDiabetes in pregnancy: Management from preconception to the postnatal period. NICE Guideline. NG3*. Available at: www.nice.org.uk/guidance/NG3/chapter/1-Recommendations#gestational-diabetes-2.

NICE (National Institute for Health and Care Excellence). (2016). *High-throughput non-invasive prenatal testing for fetal rhd genotype. diagnostics guidance: DG25*. Available at: www.nice.org.uk/guidance/dg25/chapter/1-Recommendations.

NICE (National Institute for Health and Care Excellence). (2017). *Surveillance report 2017 –Hypertension in pregnancy: Diagnosis and management in pregnancy (2010).* NICE Guideline: CG 107. (2010). Available at: www.nice.org.uk/guidance/cg107/resources/surveillance-report-2017-hypertension-in-pregnancy-diagnosis-and-management-2010-nice-guideline-cg107-pdf-3546403325413.

National Maternity Review. (2016). *Better Births: Improving outcomes for maternity services in England.* Available at: www.england.nhs.uk/wp-content/uploads/2016/02/national-maternity-review-report.pdf.

NHS England. (2016). *Saving Babies' Lives: A care bundle for reducing stillbirth.* Available at: www.england.nhs.uk/wp-content/uploads/2016/03/saving-babies-lives-car-bundl.pdf.

NHS England. (2017) Implementing Better Births: Continuity of carer. Available at: www.england.nhs.uk/publication/local-maternity-systems-resource-pack/ (March 2017).

NHS Choices. Your pregnancy and baby guide. Foods to avoid in pregnancy. Available at: www.nhs.uk/conditions/pregnancy-and-baby/foods-to-avoid-pregnant.

NHS Digital. (2018). *Statistics on women's smoking status at time of delivery.* England – quarter 4, 2017–18. Available at: https://digital.nhs.uk/data-and-information/publications/statistical/statistics-on-women-s-smoking-status-at-time-of-delivery-england/statistics-on-womens-smoking-status-at-time-of-delivery-england--quarter-4-october-2017-to-december-2017.

Norman, J., Heazell, A., Rodriguez, A., et al. (2018). Awareness of fetal movements and care package to reduce fetal mortality (AFFIRM): A stepped wedge, cluster-randomised trial. *Lancet,* 392(10158), 1629–1638.

NMC (Nursing and Midwifery Council). (2018). *The Code: Professional standards of practice and behaviour for nurses, midwives and nursing associates.* Available at: www.nmc.org.uk/globalassets/sitedocuments/nmc-publications/nmc-code.pdf.

Pflugeisen, B., & Mou, J. (2017). Patient satisfaction with virtual obstetric care. *Maternal and Child Health Journal,* 21(7), 1544–1551.

PHE (Public Health England). (2014). *Opportunistic chlamydia screening in young adults in England. An evidence summary.* Available at: https://assets.publishing.service.gov.uk/government/uploads/system/uploads/attachment_data/file/740182/Opportunistic_Chlamydia_Screening_Evidence_Summary_April_2014.pdf.

PHE (Public health England). (2015). *Childhood obesity: Applying all our health.* Available at: www.gov.uk/government/publications/childhood-obesity-applying-all-our-health/childhood-obesity-applying-all-our-health#fn:1.

PHE (Public Health England). (2016). *NHS infectious diseases in pregnancy screening programme handbook, 2016 to 2017.* Available at: https://assets.publishing.service.gov.uk/government/uploads/system/uploads/attachment_data/file/542492/NHS_IDPS_Programme_Handbook_2016_to_2017.pdf.

PHE (Public Health England). (2017). *Physical activity for pregnant women.* Available at: https://assets.publishing.service.gov.uk/government/uploads/system/uploads/attachment_data/file/622335/CMO_physical_activity_pregnant_women_infographic.pdf.

PHE (Public Health England). (2018). *Health matters: Reproductive health and pregnancy planning.* Available at: https://publichealthmatters.blog.gov.uk/2018/06/26/health-matters-reproductive-health-and-pregnancy-planning.

Rasmussen, K., & Yaktine, A. (Eds.). (2009). *Committee to re-examine the Institute of Medicine Pregnancy Weight Guidelines. (Weight gain during pregnancy: Re-examining the guidelines).* Available at: www.nap.edu/read/12584/chapter.

Renfrew, M., McFadden, A., Bastos, H., et al. (2014). Midwifery and quality care: Findings from a new evidence-informed framework for maternal and newborn care. *Lancet,* 384, 1129–1145.

Rogozińska, E., Marlin, N., Jackson, L., et al. (2017). Effects of antenatal diet and physical activity on maternal and fetal outcomes: Individual patient data meta-analysis and health economic evaluation. *Health Technology Assessment,* 21(41), 1–158.

Román-Gálvez, R., Amezcua-Prieto, C., Olmedo-Requena, R., et al. (2018). Partner smoking influences whether mothers quit smoking during pregnancy: A prospective cohort study. *BJOG: An International Journal of Obstetrics & Gynaecology,* 125(7), 820–827.

RCM (Royal College of Midwives). (2017). *Stepping up to public health.* Available at: www.rcm.org.uk/new-resources-available-for-stepping-up-to-public-health.

RCM (Royal College of Midwives). (2018). *RCM launches i-learn resource to support members in developing their understanding of continuity of carer.* Available at: www.rcm.org.uk/news-views-and-analysis/news/rcm-releases-continuity-of-carer-statement-and-learning-game.

RCOG (Royal of Obstetricians and Gynaecologists). (2010) Updated 2017. Green top guideline No. 55. Late intrauterine fetal death and stillbirth. Available at: www.rcog.org.uk/en/guidelines-research-services/guidelines/gtg55.

RCOG (Royal College of Obstetricians and Gynaecologists). (2013) Updated 2014. Green-top Guideline No 31. The investigation and management of the small for gestational age fetus. Available at: www.rcog.org.uk/en/guidelines-research-services/guidelines/gtg31.

RCOG (Royal College of Obstetricians and Gynaecologists), 2015 RCOG (Royal College of Obstetricians and Gynaecologists). (2015) Reducing the risk of venous thromboembolism during pregnancy and the puerperium. Green-top Guideline No 37a. Available at: www.rcog.org.uk/globalassets/documents/guidelines/gtg-37a.pdf.

RCP (Royal College of Physicians). (2018). *Hiding in plain sight: Treating tobacco dependency in the NHS.* London: RCP.

Rungapadiachy, D. (1999). *Interpersonal communication and psychology.* Oxford: Butterworth Heinemann.

Salmon, D., Baird, K., & White, P. (2015). Women's views and experiences of antenatal enquiry for domestic abuse during pregnancy. *Health Expectations, 18*(5), 867–878.

SANDS (Stillbirth and Neonatal Death Society). (2018). Available at: www.sands.org.uk/professionals/professional-resources/teardrop-stickers.

Shawky, R., Elsayed, S., Zaki, M., et al. (2013). Consanguinity and its relevance to clinical genetics. *Egyptian Journal of Medical Human Genetics, 14*(2), 157–164.

Sikorski, J., Wilson, J., Clement, S., et al. (1996). A randomized controlled trial comparing two schedules of antenatal visits: the antenatal care project. *British Medical Journal, 312*(7030), 546–553.

Silver, R. (2018). Examining the link between placental pathology, growth restriction, and stillbirth. Best Practice & Research. *Clinical Obstetrics & Gynaecology, 49,* 89–102.

Smoking in Pregnancy Challenge Group. (2017). *Use of electronic cigarettes in pregnancy. A guide for midwives and other healthcare professionals.* Available at: http://smokefreeaction.org.uk/wp-content/uploads/2017/06/eCig-SIP.pdf.

Smoking in Pregnancy Challenge group. (2018). *Review of the challenge.* Available at: http://ash.org.uk/information-and-resources/reports-submissions/reports/smoking-in-pregnancy-challenge-group-review-of-the-challenge-2018.

Teeuw, M., Hagelaar, A., & Ten, K. (2012). Challenges in the care for consanguineous couples: an exploratory interview study among general practitioners and midwives. *BMC Family Practice, 13*(1), 105.

Testa, S., Passamonti, S., Paoletti, M., et al. (2014). The 'Pregnancy Health-care Program' for the prevention of venous thromboembolism in pregnancy. *Internal and Emergency Medicine, 10*(2), 129–134.

UKNSC. (2017) (hosted by Public Health England). The UK NSC recommendation on cytomegalovirus screening in newborns. Available at: https://legacyscreening.phe.org.uk/cytomegalovirus.

UKNSC. (2018a) (hosted by Public Health England). The UK NSC recommendation on Hepatitis C screening in pregnancy. Available at: https://legacyscreening.phe.org.uk/hepatitisc-pregnancy.

UKNSC. (2018b) (hosted by Public Health England) The UK NSC recommendation on chlamydia screening in pregnancy. Available at: https://legacyscreening.phe.org.uk/chlamydia-pregnancy.

UNICEF. (2018). *UNICEF UK Baby Friendly Initiative. Guide to the standards* (2nd ed.). Available at: www.unicef.org.uk/babyfriendly/wp-content/uploads/sites/2/2014/02/Guide-to-the-Unicef-UK-Baby-Friendly-Initiative-Standards.pdf.

Villar, J., Hassan, B., Piaggio, G., et al. (2001). Who antenatal care randomized trial for the evaluation of a new model of routine antenatal care. *Lancet, 357*(9268), 1551–1564.

Wojcieszek, A., Boyle, F., Belizán, J., et al. (2018). Care in subsequent pregnancies following stillbirth. An international survey of parents. *BJOG: An International Journal of Obstetrics & Gynaecology, 125*(2), 193–201.

Ziaei, S., Norozzi, M., Faghihzadeh, S., et al. (2007). A randomized placebo-controlled trial to determine the effect of iron supplementation on pregnancy outcome in pregnant women with haemogloblin ≥13.2 g/dL. *BJOG: An International Journal of Obstetrics and Gynaecology, 114*(6), 684–688.

ANNOTATED FURTHER READING

Divall, B., Spiby, H., Nolan, M., & Slade, P. (2017). Plans, preferences or going with the flow: An online exploration of women's views and experiences of birth plans. *Midwifery, 54,* 29–34.

An interesting paper highlighting the importance of a personalized approach when supporting women in the writing and use of birth plans.

Lori, J., Munro, M., & Chuey, M. (2016). Use of a facilitated discussion model for antenatal care to improve communication. *International Journal of Nursing Studies, 54,* 84–94.

This article examines how antenatal care can be facilitated using picture cards and enhanced information sharing for pregnant women with low literacy.

Marshall, J., Baston, H., & Hall, J. (2019). Public health in midwifery. *Midwifery Essentials* (Vol. 7). Edinburgh: Elsevier.

A useful handbook that explains the midwifery context for public health and provides a jigsaw model for holistic care.

Wiggins, M., Sawtell, M., Wiseman, O., et al. (2018). Testing the effectiveness of reach pregnancy circles group antenatal care: Protocol for a randomized controlled pilot trial. *Pilot Feasibility Studies, 10*(4), 169.

A paper discussing the background to a study exploring the value of providing antenatal care to groups within the NHS.

Wilkinson, R., & Pickett, K. (2018). The inner level. *How more equal societies reduce stress, restore sanity and improve everyone's well-being.* Milton Keynes: Allen Lane.

An evidence-based exploration of the impact of inequality on health and wellbeing.

USEFUL WEBSITES

Child and Maternal Health Intelligence Network: www.chimat.org.uk

Cochrane Library – database of systematic reviews: www.thecochranelibrary.com

Kicks count: empowering mums-to-be with knowledge & confidence: www.kickscount.org.uk/your-babys-movements

Lullaby Trust – safer sleep for babies, support for families: www.lullabytrust.org.uk/

Maternity Transformation Programme: www.england.nhs.uk/mat-transformation/

National Centre for Smoking Cessation Training: www.ncsct.co.uk/publication_pregnancy_and_the_post_partum_period.php

National Institute for Health and Care Excellence: www.nice.org.uk

NHS Choices – Your Pregnancy Guide: www.nhs.uk/conditions/pregnancy-and-baby/

NHS Digital Maternity Services dashboard: https://digital.nhs.uk/data-and-information/data-collections-and-data-sets/data-sets/maternity-services-data-set/maternity-services-dashboard

NHS Fetal anomaly screening programme: www.gov.uk/topic/population-screening-programmes/fetal-anomaly

Royal College of Obstetricians and Gynaecologists – Guidance: www.rcog.org.uk/womens-health

Start for Life – Public Health: www.nhs.uk/start4life/pregnancy

Tommy's – Having a safe and healthy pregnancy: www.tommys.org/pregnancy

12

Concealed Pregnancy

Sylvia Murphy Tighe, Joan G. Lalor

CHAPTER CONTENTS

This chapter aims to promote an understanding of concealed pregnancy, for midwives and student midwives. The chapter explores the various definitions used to describe a concealed pregnancy, e.g. denial of pregnancy, and addresses recent evidence in the context of contemporary midwifery practice. The chapter highlights the association that exists in relation to concealed pregnancy and the field of traumatology, e.g. adverse childhood experiences such as child sexual abuse, sexual assault and domestic abuse/violence. The need for midwives to provide trauma-informed care in such sensitive circumstances is essential, as disclosing sexual or abusive trauma is a difficult experience for women. As traumatic and abusive events can remain undisclosed for many years, it is imperative that midwives are armed with the knowledge and skills to provide compassionate, respectful, trauma-sensitive care.

THE CHAPTER AIMS TO

- promote understanding for midwives and students in relation to meeting the needs of women who experience a concealed pregnancy antenatally, intrapartum and postnatally
- explore the various definitions used to describe a concealed pregnancy
- foster new thinking in relation to concealed pregnancy in the context of midwifery practice, research and policy
- build midwives confidence and skills to care for women who experience a concealed pregnancy
- identify the association that exists in relation to concealed pregnancy and the field of traumatology, e.g. adverse childhood experiences such as child sexual abuse, sexual assault and domestic abuse/violence.

BACKGROUND

Concealed pregnancies have occurred throughout the ages and in many jurisdictions. Women who conceal a pregnancy are sometimes assumed to have a mental illness (Murphy Tighe and Lalor 2016a). However, the literature has not substantiated this association with psychopathology, as it rarely causes concealed pregnancy (Murphy Tighe and Lalor 2019). Knowledge and understanding of concealed pregnancy has been limited by the fact that women's experiences were rarely heard. Concealed pregnancy represents a challenge for professionals in protecting the health and wellbeing of the woman and her infant. Concealed pregnancy by its nature limits the scope of professionals assistance during pregnancy and childbirth, while evidence shows that a lack of antenatal care is a concern (Wessel et al. 2003, 2007; Chen et al. 2007; Friedman et al. 2009; Schultz and Bushati 2015). The literature has identified that complications of pregnancy and unassisted childbirth can result (Conlon 2006; Wessel et al. 2007. The aim of antenatal care is to monitor the progress of pregnancy to optimize maternal and fetal health (Baston and Hall 2018) (see Chapter 11). Generally, concealed pregnancy has been viewed in terms of outcomes such as adoption, abandonment or infanticide. The outcomes of a concealed pregnancy can be serious and maternal or perinatal death is a real concern for practitioners (Murphy Tighe and Lalor 2016a). It is little wonder that the public and healthcare professionals have negative perceptions of concealed pregnancy considering the association with tragic outcomes. However, it has been argued that adaptive aspects of concealed pregnancy are rarely acknowledged (Thynne 2006). Women taking time to come to terms with a crisis pregnancy and revealing it to others is made in the context of social, relational, familial and community factors (Murphy Tighe and Lalor 2019).

DEFINITIONS OF CONCEALED PREGNANCY

Concealed pregnancy is also referred to as denied pregnancy, yet these terms vary in their meanings. Confusion and ambiguity around definitions is problematic, as it fails to offer a sound underpinning for healthcare policy or evidence for care (Murphy Tighe and Lalor 2016a). Much of the published research in the area has been informed by healthcare professionals or case notes rather than by women directly impacted by the experience. Current classifications and definitions of 'concealed' pregnancy (Conlon 2006; Spinelli 2002; Maldonado-Duran et al. 2000) and 'denied' pregnancy (Vellut et al. 2012; Beier et al. 2006; Miller 2003; Maldonado-Duran et al. 2000; Amon 2000; Kaplan and Grotowski 1996; Neifert and Bourgeois 2000; Vellut et al. 2013; Milstein and Milstein 1983; Werner et al. 1980) are inadequate for practitioners dealing with complex cases. Other terms used include negated pregnancy (Beier et al. 2006), cryptic pregnancy (Del Giudice 2007), secret pregnancy (Saunders 1989; Villeneuve-Gokalp and Jacob 2011) and conscious and unconscious denial of pregnancy (Brezinka et al. 1994; Conlon 2006). A concept analysis of concealed pregnancy (Murphy Tighe and Lalor 2016a) provides a new definition and identified attributes, antecedents and consequences (Table 12.1). Denied or denial of pregnancy has been researched and awareness of pregnancy can be suppressed or delayed in some cases (Miller 2003). Miller (2016) contends that denial of pregnancy is not normative but can occur in the absence of psychopathology with tragic outcomes sometimes being a consequence (Navarro and Urban 2004; Neifert and Bourgeois 2000; Kaplan and Grotowski 1996).

RECONCEPTUALIZING CONCEALED PREGNANCY

Historical accounts of concealed pregnancy are reminders of a sad legacy involving women and childbirth (Farrell 2013; Rattigan 2012; Ferriter 2009). In the past, women who became pregnant outside of marriage were often hidden away by families, left seeking occupational opportunities elsewhere and forced adoptions were not uncommon (Kelly 2005; Bos 2007). Keeping a pregnancy secret or private is often viewed with suspicion and as a 'risk' by health and social care professionals rather than an adaptive and personal choice due to the woman's own life experience. Pathologizing women does little to assist women faced with a crisis pregnancy they are concealing and grappling to come to terms with.

Concealed pregnancy is a complex, multidimensional and temporal process where a woman is aware of her pregnancy and copes by keeping it secret and hidden. Behaviours such as avoidance, hiding, using a cover story, staying away and secrecy are key characteristics. Fear (of others or for others) is central to the process and

TABLE 12.1 Antecedents, Attributes and Consequences of Concealed Pregnancy

Antecedents	Attributes	Consequences
• Aware of pregnancy • Fear (of others or for others) • Compares own situation to societal norms and expectations • Context – relationship/finances/culture/religiosity • Perceives a lack of support or mechanism to mother or infant	(*Internally or externally mediated*) • Secrecy • Hiding • Daytime story (cover story) • Staying away • Avoidance	**Woman** • Maternal death • Self-harm/suicide • Mothering/termination of pregnancy: forced or voluntary • Recurrence **Infant** • Neonatal death • Abandonment/neonaticide • Fostering/adoption • Parented **Society** • Increased child surveillance • Anonymous birthing • Baby hatches

From Murphy Tighe S, Lalor JG. (2016) Concealed pregnancy: a concept analysis. Journal of Advanced Nursing 72(1):50–61.

TABLE 12.2 Maternal and Neonatal Outcomes Associated with Concealed Pregnancy

Outcomes of Concealed Pregnancy for the Woman	Outcomes of Concealed Pregnancy for the Infant
• Inadequate or absence of antenatal care • Hard to detect expected date of birth (EDB); unprepared for birth • Previous concealed pregnancy • Precipitous or unassisted birth • Maternal death • Immense psychological distress, isolation, feeling judged, sense of stigma, shame • Poor obstetric outcomes: increased risk of breech presentations; pregnancy and childbirth complications • Poor adaptation postpartum	• No opportunity to detect fetal anomalies amenable to treatment • Risk of prematurity, low birth weight, small for gestational age • Birth injuries • Admission to NICU • Infant may be mothered, adoption, abandoned or neonaticide may result • Higher perinatal mortality than comparison groups • Infants often raised by grandmothers or given up for adoption • Effect on maternal–infant attachment unknown

Chen et al. 2007; Conlon 2006; Murphy Tighe and Lalor 2016a,b; Thynne 2006; Wessel et al. 2007.

an interaction with another antecedent, e.g. context/culture or a perceived lack of support to mother her infant, leads to concealing a pregnancy. It is a difficult and traumatic experience for the woman. Variations in the duration of concealed pregnancy exist and recurrence may feature in this process (Murphy Tighe and Lalor 2016a).

WHY IS CONCEALED PREGNANCY OF CONCERN?

Concealed pregnancy has previously featured in one of the UK's triennial reports: the Confidential Enquiry into Maternal Deaths (CEMD) (Lewis 2007), and more recently, in numerous Serious Case Reviews of infant deaths in the UK (Bury Local Safeguarding Children's Board 2011; Ibbetson 2014; Northumberland Safeguarding Children's Board 2012; Lewisham Local Safeguarding Children's Board 2009; North East Lincolnshire LSCB 2016) have identified concealed pregnancy as an area of concern. Risks to maternal and neonatal wellbeing include maternal and/or perinatal death (Table 12.2). Women who conceal their pregnancies experience complex psychological distress, embarrassment, stigma and isolation (Conlon 2006; Thynne 2006; Wessel et al.

2007). Delayed or absence of antenatal care may lead to serious pregnancy-related and childbirth complications (Sandoz 2011; Ali and Paddick 2009; Sadler 2002; Wessel et al. 2007; Nirmal et al. 2006). Implications of concealed pregnancy for the infant are significant including no opportunity to detect fetal anomalies amenable to treatment, risk of malpresentations, prematurity, low birth weight (LBW), small for gestational age (SGA) and birth injuries (Nirmal et al. 2006; Wessel et al. 2007). The impact of concealed pregnancy on maternal–infant attachment is unknown (Murphy Tighe and Lalor 2015).

Concealed pregnancy is closely associated with adoption (Howe et al. 1992; Bos 2007; Kelly 2005), newborn abandonment (Conlon 2006; Drescher-Burke et al. 2004; Browne 2012; Murphy Tighe and Lalor 2016a,b) and neonaticide (D'Orban 1979; Vallone and Hoffman 2003; Riley 2005; Putkonen et al. 2007; Spinelli 2010; Amon et al. 2012). Therefore, a focus on accessible and supportive services for women and infants are necessary (Murphy Tighe and Lalor 2016b). Scant attention has been paid to concealed pregnancy, its impact on the developmental trajectory of infants and mothers and on maternal-infant attachment (Murphy Tighe and Lalor 2015, 2016b,c). Recent research indicates women require supportive measures rather than surveillance (Murphy Tighe and Lalor 2019) and a dearth of care pathways was observed for women experiencing a concealed pregnancy.

REASONS WHY PREGNANCIES ARE CONCEALED

The reasons why a pregnancy is concealed are complex and multifactorial (Ali and Paddick 2009). Social isolation is a feature for women who conceal their pregnancy (Green and Manohan 1990; Conlon 2006; Thynne 2006). Reasons for concealment include social factors such as stigma (Conlon 2006) of lone motherhood, religious beliefs regarding abortion or a coping strategy (Green and Manohan 1990). Keeping a pregnancy secret enables women to maintain control over their decision-making (Mahon et al. 1998; Murphy Tighe and Lalor 2016a). Two Irish studies found fear of parental reaction was an important reason (Thynne et al. 2012), while Conlon (2006) found social stigma as a key reason for concealing a pregnancy, particularly for women pregnant outside of marriage. The literature reports that affected women come from all social classes, irrespective

of educational status or age (Wessel et al. 2002). Other reasons cited in the literature as causative factors in concealed pregnancy include: lying (Brezinka et al. 1994); hormonal causes (Wessel and Endrikat 2005); a denial of fertility (Struye et al. 2013); and psychosomatic disorders (Kenner and Nicolson 2015). An association has been identified between cyclical bleeding and corpus luteum insufficiency but causation has not been established (Wessel and Endrikat 2005).

Adolescent girls were traditionally thought to be most likely to conceal a pregnancy (Loughran and Richardson 2005). The literature reports affected women come from all social classes, irrespective of age or educational status (Wessel et al. 2002), with no clear typology (Chen et al. 2007). Nirmal et al. (2006) found in Wales that 58% of women were multiparous and 12% were married. In two studies, only 30–36% of women were primiparous (Wessel et al. 2007; Friedman et al. 2009). While Kenner and Nicolson (2015) argued that trauma has been overlooked as a factor, Navarro et al. (2011) reported in a French study of adolescents who concealed a pregnancy that trauma was a feature. Anecdotal reports of older and married women and women from various professions and in relationships concealing exist.

CONSEQUENCES OF CONCEALED PREGNANCY

There are various consequences of a concealed pregnancy (Table 12.2). A small number of studies have retrospectively examined the phenomenon (Brezinka et al. 1994; Nirmal et al. 2006; Friedman et al. 2009; Friedman and Resnick 2009) and one prospectively (Wessel et al. 2007). A concealed pregnancy may, in extreme circumstances, lead to a tragic outcome such as an unassisted birth and maternal and/or perinatal death (Murphy Tighe and Lalor 2016a). In the UK's 7th CEMD report for the triennium 2003–2005 (Lewis 2007), 17% of maternal deaths reported were related to women who had not booked for antenatal care until they were at least 5 months pregnant. A retrospective hospital record review in an Australian hospital indicates that low reports of maternal physical morbidity are possibly due to low rates of diagnosis and under-reporting (Schultz and Bushati 2015). This study examined cases from 2007 to 2013 and found a significantly increased rate of maternal morbidity with pregnancy complications such as severe pre-eclampsia necessitating admissions to intensive care unit (ICU), hence the need for responsive maternity care.

The postnatal period can be characterized by complex emotional and psychological distress, and women commonly experience feelings of embarrassment and guilt and may become isolated from family and friends (Conlon 2006; Thynne 2006; Mahon et al. 1998). If these negative feelings are sufficiently prevalent, some women may have suicidal ideation and intention (Murphy Tighe and Lalor 2016a), self-harm (Murphy Tighe and Lalor 2019) and newborn abandonment or neonaticide may ensue (Riley 2005; Murphy Tighe and Lalor 2019). Concealing a pregnancy may have profound implications for maternal and fetal health and wellbeing, however such extreme cases of abandonment or neonaticide are very rare.

In the UK, the National Institute for Health and Care Excellence (NICE 2008) recommend that women should be booked for antenatal care by the 12th week of pregnancy. Lack of antenatal care or unassisted birth may result in serious illness and trauma, not to mention severe emotional and mental distress (see Chapter 30). Women who conceal their pregnancies may be unable to access antenatal care and support (Ali and Paddick 2009; Conlon 2006). Delayed or absence of antenatal care can lead to serious pregnancy-related complications such as pre-eclampsia. Childbirth complications such as unassisted birth, postpartum haemorrhage and death may occur (Wessel et al. 2002). Recurrence of concealed pregnancy is also identified in the literature (Conlon 2006; Murphy Tighe and Lalor 2019).

A study of 16 cases of infanticide found that the effects of pregnancy or birth did not kill the infants but that the mothers were motivated by personal, social or economic reasons (Putkonen et al. 2007). Condon (1986) found in a study of 112 pregnant women that 8% acknowledged an urge to harm the fetus, and that 8% worried about harming the child when born. It is assumed that during pregnancy, women feel a connectedness to nurture and protect the fetus. However, this is not always the case and women who are ambivalent about the pregnancy have difficulties acknowledging the pregnancy, or may have experienced trauma, find pregnancy particularly challenging.

Inglis (2003) characterizes concealed pregnancy followed by giving birth in secret and then abandoning, killing or leaving the baby to die, as a final response to a crisis pregnancy. Links between concealment and infanticide are often made (Porter and Gavin 2010). A French study of the relationship between neonaticide and denial of pregnancy found psychopathology was rare. Vellut et al. (2012) explain that pathologizing women while absolving those around them has little operational value in preventing neonaticides. The pregnancy and postnatal period can be characterized by complex emotional and psychological distress and women concealing a pregnancy may experience feelings of embarrassment and guilt, and become isolated from family and friends (Conlon 2006; Thynne 2006). If these negative feelings are sufficiently prevalent, some women may have suicidal ideation/intention or thoughts of neonaticide (see Chapter 30). Meyer and Oberman's (2001) published book into mothers who kill their children shatter the illusion that such mothers are mad or monsters. Social factors that contribute to neonaticide are examined and patterns are presented, which include concealed pregnancy, recurrence and histories of neglect or trauma (Riley 2005).

Prevalence Rates

Prevalence rates of concealed pregnancy are difficult to establish with accuracy because of the nature of the phenomenon. Prevalence rates of concealed pregnancy are reported (Table 12.3) with few involving large sample sizes. Determining the incidence of concealed pregnancy is difficult because currently, data on this subject are recorded in an ad hoc manner (Conlon 2006), and due to the hidden nature of the phenomenon. Different studies report the prevalence of concealed pregnancies and only a few have involved large numbers of women (Conlon 2006; Wessel et al. 2002; Nirmal et al. 2006; Friedman et al. 2009). This data showed an epidemiologically relevant frequency of concealed pregnancies and that similar rates across many jurisdictions confirm that concealed pregnancy is not a rare event. Countries where research has identified concealed pregnancy rates are from the USA (Friedman and Resnick 2009); Ireland (Conlon 2006; Thynne 2006; Murphy Tighe and Lalor 2019); Wales (Nirmal et al. 2006); and Berlin, Germany (Wessel et al. 2002). Researchers also use varied definitions. The variation in definitions and inclusion criteria used to categorize concealed pregnancy makes comparisons difficult.

Antenatal care is considered to be an important factor, which contributes to a successful pregnancy outcome (Baston and Hall 2018). It is of concern that women who conceal a pregnancy have delayed or no

TABLE 12.3	Prevalence Rates of Concealed Pregnancy	
Place of Study	**Prevalence Rate**	**Methodology**
Ireland (rural)	1 in 146 (20 weeks' gestation)	IPA and quantitative retrospective case–control study (Thynne 2006; Thynne et al. 2012)
Ireland (rural)	1 in 403 (20 weeks' gestation)	Case study (Conlon 2006)
Ireland (urban)	1 in 625 (20 weeks' gestation) 1 in 2500 (until birth)	Case study (Conlon 2006)
Germany	1 in 475 (until birth)	Case study (Wessel et al. 2002)
USA	1 in 516 (20 weeks' gestation) 1 in 2500 (until birth)	Exploratory retrospective medical record review (Friedman et al. 2007)
Wales	1 in 2500	Retrospective population-based study over 11 years (Nirmal et al. 2006)

antenatal care. While NICE (2010) guidelines exist in the UK in relation to pregnancy and women with complex social factors, no protocol or care pathway was found to support women who experience a concealed pregnancy. Numerous guidelines identified came from a child protection perspective, where the focus is on safeguarding the infant rather than supporting the woman.

Who Conceals a Pregnancy?

The notion that only teenagers conceal their pregnancies is incorrect. In reality, concealed pregnancy crosses many boundaries and women who conceal their pregnancy are not a homogenous group (Wessel et al. 2002; Conlon 2006). Concealed pregnancy is sometimes viewed as an abnormal response to pregnancy, however the complexities involved have not been fully understood as women's perspectives are rarely heard. Some of the published literature on concealed pregnancy has a highly medicalized approach and the use of pathologizing language is noted (Jenkins et al. 2011; Sandoz 2011; Kenner and Nicolson 2015). The potential exists for women who conceal a pregnancy to become pathologized, stereotyped and demonized, as references to lying, deviancy and mental illness are made. Rather than women being supported with a crisis pregnancy they wish to keep private, it is often assumed that they have a mental health problem. Recent evidence identifies the causes of concealed pregnancy in a grounded typology (Murphy Tighe and Lalor 2019). The factors associated with concealed pregnancy may be internally or externally mediated. Internally mediated cases of concealed pregnancy relate to a controlling relationship, sexual assault, child sexual abuse or complicated attachment.

Externally mediated cases of concealed pregnancy are due to poverty, domestic abuse/violence, child protection surveillance or fear of employer.

Contemporary Cases of Concealed Pregnancy and Sequelae

Contemporary cases of concealed pregnancy are not uncommon. Women who experienced forced adoptions in many countries have experienced disenfranchised and complicated grief (Bos 2007; Dorow and Han 1999; Doka 1989; Kelly 2005). Concealed pregnancy and newborn abandonment occurs in contemporary liberal societies (e.g. *Sydney Morning Herald* 2008; BBC 2014, 2015; *Irish Times* 2015, 2018). Limited research relates to newborn abandonment (Drescher-Burke et al. 2004; Aloi 2009; Mueller and Sherr 2009; Murphy Tighe and Lalor 2016a,b) and neonaticide (Resnick 1970; D'Orban 1979; Saunders 1989; Vallone and Hoffman 2003; Riley 2005; Putkonen et al. 2007; Beyer et al. 2008; Porter and Gavin 2010; Amon et al. 2012; Vellut et al. 2012; De Bortoli et al. 2013). It must be recognized that women who abandon a newborn infant have had no health care or support during their pregnancy and some have had traumatic or adverse childhood experiences (Murphy Tighe and Lalor 2019). Unintended pregnancies can provoke ambivalent or conflicted feelings towards the infant (Kumar and Robson 1984). Some women who conceal a pregnancy have genuine fears for their safety and require protection themselves (Murphy Tighe and Lalor 2019). Women who conceal a pregnancy include those who experience rape, domestic abuse/violence and child sexual abuse (Spielvogel and Hoehener 1995; Friedman et al. 2007; Porter and Gavin 2010; Murphy

Tighe and Lalor 2019). Some women may live in vulnerable or precarious circumstances and require midwifery care that is trauma-informed. Women may continue to conceal until or after birth and this has psychological sequelae for the woman and her infant.

Women's Experiences of Concealed Pregnancy

Women have described concealed pregnancy as a bleak, desolate and lonely time in their lives. Women have described being fearful of revealing the pregnancy, which may result in avoidance of professionals (Murphy Tighe and Lalor 2016a, 2019). In a study involving 30 women who experienced a concealed pregnancy, they all confirmed they were aware of their pregnancy but reported feeling disconnected, shut down, numb and paralysed by fear. A participant in this Irish study (Murphy Tighe and Lalor 2019) who hid her pregnancy following a sexual assault said, 'my plan was to show up, have the baby, hand it over and walk away'. She went on to say 'the hospital is not set up for vulnerable women; I was clearly vulnerable. I have never experienced such a lack of empathy in my life'. As some women may have experienced adverse childhood or traumatic life experiences, it is imperative that midwives have knowledge, understanding and skills in order to respond appropriately. The necessity for trauma-informed and trauma-sensitive care is central to caring for women in a respectful and compassionate manner. Women who present late for antenatal care must have a sensitive enquiry made as to the reasons for delayed presentation. The complexity of the factors involved in concealed pregnancy mean that care pathways are urgently required, so that women are signposted to the appropriate services and not left to cope alone in secrecy and silence.

Framework for Midwives and Practitioners to Understand Concealed Pregnancy

Concealed pregnancy is a psychosocial process that is influenced by many factors. The context of concealed pregnancy is underscored by a paralysing fear and immense psychological distress and anguish most notably among women who conceal up to or very close to birth. The paralysing fear women experience influences their coping responses of avoidance (Murphy Tighe and Lalor 2019). Women sometimes hid and stayed away from family and friends and used a cover story to explain the reasons for weight gain or absences (Murphy

Tighe and Lalor 2016a). Women also outlined how they explained their avoidance to themselves. Women, rather than dealing with the pregnancy, described thoughts of cysts, tumours and abdominal or gastrointestinal conditions. Such situations can occur in the general population when individuals are faced with symptoms or circumstances that induce fear, e.g. individuals may ignore lumps, growths, infidelity in relationships, etc.

The framework developed in order to understand the process of concealed pregnancy is called *Regaining Agency and Autonomy* (Murphy Tighe and Lalor 2019). This typology (Fig. 12.1) describes the nine factors that impact concealment. Agency refers to an individual's capacity to act, while autonomy refers to one's freedom to act. Concealed pregnancy occurs in a context of social structures and patterns of expectation for women of all ages. Concealed pregnancy may be internally or externally mediated (Murphy Tighe and Lalor 2016a, 2019). Time is a critical factor in the process of concealed pregnancy and women may conceal or reveal, depending on many factors. The internally mediating factors are: controlling relationship, child sexual abuse, sexual assault, social conformity and complicated attachment. The external mediating factors are: poverty, child protection surveillance, domestic violence and employers.

The typology of concealed pregnancy recognizes *fear* as central to the process as seen in the vertical axis (Fig. 12.1). In the horizontal axis, *agency* and *autonomy* are critical factors as women's main concern was *regaining agency and autonomy* and being in charge of their own destiny. Two approaches to concealing a pregnancy were identified: *making myself invisible* (Quadrant 1) and *being made invisible* (Quadrant 4).

The typology (Fig. 12.1) identifies that concealed pregnancy may be internally or externally mediated with a trajectory of concealing and revealing over time. Women described fear as disabling, rendering them unable to seek support. For some, fear related to a violent partner, parent or fear of a social reprisal impacted coping responses of secrecy, silence and avoidance. For the purpose of clarity, it is best to consider the typology in two halves. The left-hand side considers women for whom concealed pregnancy is externally mediated. The right-hand side highlights internal mediating factors, which lead to concealed pregnancy.

Women who conceal a pregnancy (*internally mediated*) up to or close to childbirth may have a history of pre-pregnancy trauma (Quadrant 1), e.g. child sexual abuse, sexual

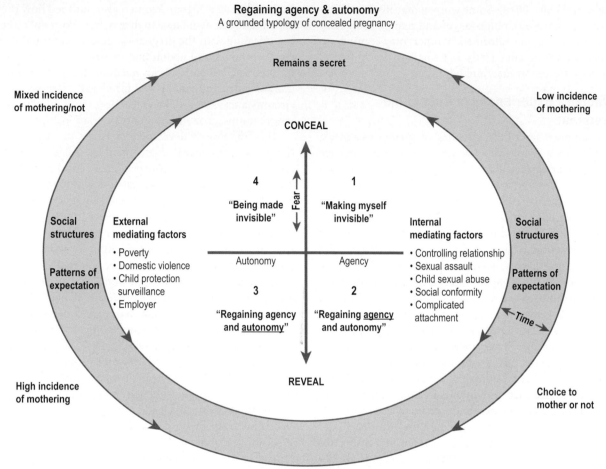

Fig. 12.1 Regaining agency and autonomy. A grounded typology of concealed pregnancy. (Reproduced with permission from Murphy Tighe S, Lalor JG. (2019) Regaining agency and autonomy: A grounded typology of concealed pregnancy. Journal of Advanced Nursing 75(3):603–15.)

assault, controlling relationships or complicated attachments. If women conceal close to or up to birth they may not mother their infants and abandonment or neonaticide may feature (Quadrant 1). Women who concealed the pregnancy themselves (Quadrant 1) described self-isolation, which was conceptualized as *making myself invisible*. The greater the fear, the more likely the woman is to stay away, hide and risk birthing alone. Among individuals who have experienced trauma, hiding may be a way of surviving (Browne 2013; Courtois and Riley 1992).

Concealed pregnancy does not end with the birth of the baby, as women negotiate their situation within the context of relationships and life events as the first circle indicates (Fig. 12.1) which may become *part of her life story*. Women with a history of abuse or complicated attachment may conceal the pregnancy and outcome for years *remains a secret*. Women with supportive relationships may be enabled to reveal earlier *regain agency and autonomy* and have the ability to choose if they wish to mother their infant or not. However, some women with complicated attachment may not be able to voice their wishes and may feel forced to mother their infants. Women experienced varying degrees of secrecy, including hidden adoptions, unassisted births, neonaticide and perinatal deaths (Murphy Tighe and Lalor 2019).

Midwifery Care for Women Experiencing a Concealed Pregnancy

Psychological distress during and after a concealed pregnancy is common and may be so extreme that a woman may self-harm or experience suicidal ideation or intent (Murphy Tighe and Lalor 2019). It may be assumed that women who proceed to mother their infant following a concealed pregnancy results in a happy outcome. Contemporary society imposes expectations on pregnant women, which discourages the expression of ambivalent or conflicted feelings. The silence and lack of discourse around conflicted feelings about an unintended or crisis pregnancy is problematic. Women require support, non-judgemental care and being enabled to feel safe in order to disclose traumatic life experiences. To assist women make a successful transition to motherhood, midwives must understand that women may experience guilt and self-blame after the infant is born because they had not presented for maternity care earlier in the pregnancy. Midwives must have a sound understanding of perinatal mental health and infant mental health issues (see Chapter 30) in order to support women who have experienced a concealed pregnancy, and signposting women to non-directive counselling is essential.

Numerous challenges posed for midwives by concealed pregnancy are: late presentation and lack of knowledge of medical history; insufficient time to prepare for labour; no antenatal care or antenatal education, birth and postnatal care; managing contact between mother and her infant and between the woman and her partner/family. Interdisciplinary guidelines are required to provide evidence-based care for women who have experienced a concealed pregnancy. It is essential that trauma-sensitive care is provided to women or re-traumatization may occur during the maternity care experience, as some may have experienced adverse life events. The distress in some women is significant and cases of self-harm, suicidal ideation and intent (Murphy Tighe and Lalor 2019) will require support from an experienced therapist or psychiatrist.

Challenging the Discourse of Denial

Researchers have questioned the discourse in relation to denial of pregnancy (Del Giudice 2007). Murphy Tighe and Lalor (2019) proposed that denial is actually avoidance (*emotional focused coping strategy*). Denial and avoidance are seen in other healthcare cases, e.g. denial following a diagnosis of terminal illness, despite being informed or avoiding/ignoring serious symptoms. However, when women are pregnant, a public surveillance or ownership of the pregnancy and fetus can mean women are marginalized and the rights of the fetus takes precedence. To substantiate this point, we draw on a case of public interest (UK), which involved a young woman who arrived to hospital with her dead newborn after an unassisted birth, denying knowledge of pregnancy. Diary extracts read in Court:

> *Please, please help me. I'm scared but trying to block it out … why can't it go away? Why can't it just go to sleep and leave me alone?*

The psychiatrists' report found the woman had no mental illness. This woman had presented late at 26 weeks for an abortion (Brooke 2007), which was a missed opportunity to assist and support her.

In a case reported in the UK, a couple in Essex were arrested and charged with concealment of birth (McLelland 2015; Gordon 2016). It transpired this woman had a spontaneous miscarriage (or stillbirth depending on the report read). The woman and her partner were charged with concealment of birth. The couple had attempted to clean up the blood on the bathroom floor, as they did not want their two young children to witness such a sight. The mother later told of a 'living nightmare' after she suffered a miscarriage and was arrested by police on suspicion of murder and her partner was accused of killing the baby. The couple spent some 34 hours behind bars at Chelmsford police station, and a further 7 months awaiting the outcome of the investigation that they had concealed a birth. The case was only dropped when a post-mortem confirmed a stillbirth. The mother said she was 'treated like a killer' and shown 'no humanity' towards her (McLelland 2015; Gordon 2016). It is vital that factual evidence and guidelines are developed so that conspiracy theories are not used and that best practice is ensured. This case of charging a couple who lost a baby illustrates how critical it is to understand the complex process of concealed pregnancy and birth. However, this has not been an isolated case of a woman charged for concealment of birth. In 2014, an Irish woman backpacking around Australia faced charges for concealment of birth in Western Australia (Lee 2014; Gardiner 2014) and the infant was also stillborn in this case. The conduct of police investigations must be respectful and sensitive. However, it does shine a light on how influential laws are, in shaping societal and official responses. It appears in some cases, there may be a rush to judgement and it is necessary to balance the rights of the woman and fetus/infant. Interdisciplinary guidelines around the management and investigation of such complex cases involving concealed pregnancy and birth are urgently required in order to ensure professional and sound interagency working and to minimize the distress and re-traumatization of the woman concerned.

Conclusion

Concealed pregnancy is a public health issue of significance and potentially a precursor to tragic outcomes such as maternal or perinatal mortality. Midwives must be aware of the importance of concealed pregnancy, and respond and support women appropriately in order to build trust and ensure they feel safe to disclose difficult experiences in their lives. Concealed pregnancy needs to urgently be reappraised from a traumatology perspective, rather than viewed through a biomedical lens. A paradigm shift is required to focus on the women, what has happened in their lives and how society can best support them at a difficult time. Institutions, state agencies, healthcare services and child protection mechanisms must not add to women's distress, as some have experienced early life trauma or may be living in controlling, violent or abusive relationships. Adverse clinical outcomes may occur, which may threaten the lives of women and their babies and that is why an urgent contemporary response is required, which is respectful and women focused. In order to ensure perinatal wellbeing, responsive maternal care must be available for women. This care must encompass midwives and other health professionals being able to sensitively enquire about and deal with emotional and traumatic issues in women's lives, *in order to provide effective support to women who have experienced a concealed pregnancy*. Integrated care pathways for women are urgently required as increasing child surveillance and child protection measures may serve to increase the fear experienced and decrease

opportunities for engagement. If it is not recognized that concealed pregnancies continue to occur, then healthcare systems will continue to fail women and their babies, as they have done in the past.

Key Points for Practice

It is recommended from a maternity care perspective that:

- care, sensitivity, dignity and privacy be afforded to women who are concealing a pregnancy
- women who present late in pregnancy for antenatal care should have a sensitive enquiry made as to who is aware of their pregnancy, if the pregnancy is concealed from close family members or intimate partners and if they have support
- screening for domestic abuse/violence and coercive control should be carried out in pregnancy and careful assessment made in relation to any aspect of concealment in order to provide appropriate supports to the woman
- where concealed pregnancy is suspected or confirmed, midwives must understand that some women may do just that due to traumatic life experiences, e.g. child sexual abuse, sexual assault or living with domestic violence or controlling relationships
- should a woman disclose she is concealing a pregnancy, it is a sensitive and private matter and the woman's wishes should be respected. Non-directive counselling will enable women to work through the crisis
- should a woman be concealing a pregnancy and discloses she is suicidal or self-harming, referral to psychiatric and psychological services must be made promptly
- education is required for midwives on the process of concealed pregnancy and on the need for trauma-sensitive care.

REFLECTIVE ACTIVITY FOR SELF-ASSESSMENT

1. Why do you think a woman might present late in pregnancy or in labour?
2. How might you as a midwife work to establish trust between yourself and a woman who is/has experienced a concealed pregnancy?
3. If you have cared for a woman who experienced a concealed pregnancy did you feel comfortable to explore the hidden nature of her pregnancy and her reasons for doing so?
4. How can you build your confidence as a midwife to explore sensitive issues involving concealed pregnancy?

REFERENCES

Ali, E., & Paddick, S. M. (2009). An exploration of the undetected pregnancy. *British Journal of Midwifery*, *17*(10), 647–651.

Aloi, J. A. (2009). Nursing the disenfranchised: Women who have relinquished an infant for adoption. *Journal of Psychiatric and Mental Health Nursing*, *16*, 27–31.

Amon, R. D. (2000). Denial of pregnancy. *Military Medicine*, *165*(12), iii–iv.

Amon, S., Putkonen, H., Weizmann-Heizmann, G., et al. (2012). Potential predictors in neonaticide: The impact of the circumstances of pregnancy. *Archives of Women's Mental Health*, *15*(3), 167–174.

Baston, H., & Hall, J. (2018). Antenatal (2nd ed.). *Midwifery essentials* (Vol. 2). Edinburgh: Elsevier.

BBC. (2014). Mother charged for abandoning baby in drain in Sydney. Available at: www.bbc.co.uk/news/world-australia-30172577.

BBC. (2015). Police probe after baby's body found in river Taff, Cardiff. London: BBC. Available at: http://tinyurl.com/hejt4np.

Beier, K. M., Wille, R. J., & Wessel, J. (2006). Denial of pregnancy as a reproductive dysfunction: A proposal for international classifications systems. *Journal of Psychosomatic Research*, *61*(5), 723–730.

Beyer, K., McAuliffe-Mack, S., & Shelton, J. (2008). Investigative analysis of neonaticide. *Criminal Justice and Behaviour*, *35*, 525–535.

Bos, P. (2007). Once a mother. Relinquishment and Adoption from the perspective of unmarried mothers in Southern India. PhD Thesis. Nijmegen.

Brezinka, C., Biebl, W., & Kinzl, J. (1994). Denial of pregnancy: Obstetrical aspects. *Journal of Psychosomatic Obstetrics and Gynaecology*, *15*(1), 1–8.

Brooke, C. (2007). Bizarre case of the mother, her secret pregnancy and a dead baby in a carrier bag. *Daily Mail*. 3rd October. Available at: www.dailymail.co.uk/news/article-485418/Bizarre-case-mother-secret-pregnancy-dead-baby-carrier-bag.html.

Browne, K. (2012). *Child abandonment and its prevention in Europe*. Nottingham: University of Nottingham.

Browne, I. (2013). *The writings of Ivor Browne steps along the road of a slow learner*. Cork: Atrium Press.

Bury Local Safeguarding Children's Board. (2011). Serious case review: Baby a (case G10): Serious case review overview report. Available at: www.Scie-Socialcareonline.Org.Uk/Serious-Case-Review-Baby-a-Case-G10-Serious-Case-Review-Report/R/A11g0000001815wiaa.

Chen, X. K., Wen, S. W., Yang, Q., & Walker, M. C. (2007). Adequacy of prenatal care and neonatal mortality in infants born to mothers with and without high-risk conditions. *The Australian and New Zealand Journal of Obstetrics and Gynaecology*, *47*(2), 122–127.

Conlon, C. (2006). *Concealed pregnancy: A case study approach from an Irish setting*. Dublin: CPA.

Condon, J. T. (1986). Psychological disability in women who relinquished a baby for adoption. *Medical Journal of Australia*, *144*(3), 117–119.

Courtois, C. A., & Riley, C. C. (1992). Pregnancy and childbirth as triggers for abuse memories: Implications for care. *Birth*, *19*(4), 222–223.

De Bortoli, L., Coles, J., & Dolan, M. (2013). A review of maternal neonaticide: A need for further research supporting evidence-based prevention. *Child Abuse Review*, *22*(5), 327–339.

Del Giudice, M. (2007). The evolutionary biology of cryptic pregnancy: A re-appraisal of the 'denied pregnancy' phenomenon. *Medical Hypotheses*, *68*(2), 250–258.

Doka, K. J. (1989). *Disenfranchised grief: Recognising hidden sorrow*. New York: Lexington Books.

Dorow, S. K., & Han, S. S. (1999). *I wish for you a beautiful life, letters from Korean mothers of Ae Ran Won to their children*. Minnesota: Yeong & Yeong.

Drescher-Burke, K., Krall, J., & Penick, A. (2004). *Discarded infants and neonaticide: A review of the literature*. California: NIARC/University of California Berkeley.

D'Orban, P. T. (1979). Women who kill their children. *British Journal of Psychiatry*, *134*, 560–571.

Farrell, E. (2013). *A most diabolical deed infanticide and Irish society*. Manchester: Manchester University Press.

Ferriter, D. (2009). *Occasions of sin: Sex and society in modern Ireland*. London: Profile Books.

Friedman, S. H., Heneghan, A., & Rosenthal, M. (2007). Characteristics of women who deny or conceal pregnancy. *Psychosomatics*, *48*(2), 117–122.

Friedman, S. H., Heneghan, A., & Rosenthal, M. (2009). Disposition and health outcomes among infants born to mothers with no prenatal care. *Child Abuse & Neglect*, *33*, 116–122.

Friedman, S. H., & Resnick, P. J. (2009). Neonaticide: Phenomenology and considerations for prevention. *International Journal of Law and Psychiatry*, *32*, 43–47.

Gardiner, A. (2014). It is almost as if there were a written script: Child murder, concealment of birth and the unmarried mother in Western Australia. *Journal of Media Culture*, *17*(5).

Gordon, A. (2016). Mother tells of her 'living nightmare' after she suffered a miscarriage and was arrested on suspicion of murder. *Daily Mail*, July.

Green, C. M., & Manohan, S. V. (1990). Neonaticide and hysterical denial of pregnancy. *British Journal of Psychiatry*, *156*, 121–123.

Howe, D., Sawbridge, P., & Hinings, D. (1992). *Half a million women mothers who lose their children by adoption*. London: Penguin.

Ibbetson, K. (2014). Serious case review. Windsor and Maidenhead local safeguarding children's board. Available at: http://library.nspcc.org.uk/HeritageScripts/Hapi.dll/search2?searchTerm0=C5052.

Inglis, T. (2003). *Truth, power and lies. Irish society and the case of the Kerry babies*. Dublin: UCD Press.

Irish Times. (2015). Gardai to issue fresh appeal for mother of baby Maria. *Irish Times*, 15 May.

Irish Times. (2018). Gardai appeal to mother of Balbriggan baby to come forward and get help. *Irish Times*, 15 December.

Jenkins, A., Millar, S., & Robins, J. (2011). Denial of pregnancy-a literature review and discussion of ethical and legal issues. *Journal of the Royal Society of Medicine, 104*, 286–291.

Kaplan, R., & Grotowski, T. (1996). Denied pregnancy (case study report). *Australian and New Zealand Journal of Psychiatry, 30*, 861–863.

Kelly, R. (2005). *Motherhood silenced the experiences of natural mothers on adoption reunion*. Dublin: Liffey Press.

Kenner, W. D., & Nicolson, S. E. (2015). Psychosomatic disorders of gravida status: False and denied pregnancies. *The Academy of Psychosomatic Medicine, 56*(2), 119–128.

Kumar, R., & Robson, K. M. (1984). A prospective study of emotional disorders in childbearing women. *British Journal of Psychiatry, 144*, 35–47.

Lee, S. (2014). Irish backpacker charged over the death of a baby she gave birth to while travelling in the Australian outback. *Daily Mail*, 8 August.

Lewis, G. (Ed.). (2007). *The confidential enquiry into maternal and child health (CEMACH) saving mothers' lives; reviewing maternal deaths to make motherhood safer 2003–2005 the seventh report on confidential enquiries into maternal deaths in the United Kingdom*. London: CEMACH.

Lewisham Local Safeguarding Children's Board. (2009). Child C: A serious case review executive summary. Available at: www.whatdotheyknow.com/Request/144101/Response/372244/Attach/6/Screxecutivesummaryc.pdf.

Loughran, H., & Richardson, V. (2005). *Mixed method adoption research. Crisis pregnancy agency report*. Dublin: CPA.

Mahon, E., Conlon, C., & Dillon, L. (1998). *Women and crisis pregnancy*. Dublin: Stationery Office.

Maldonado-Duran, M., Lartigue, T., & Feintuch, M. (2000). Perinatal psychiatry: Infant mental health interventions during pregnancy. *Bulletin of the Menninger Clinic, 64*(3), 317–327.

McLelland, E. (2015). Mother who suffered a miscarriage at her home when she was 18 weeks pregnant was arrested on suspicion of murder and thrown in the cells for a night. *Daily Mail*, November.

Meyer, C. L., & Oberman, M. (2001). *Mothers who kill their children understanding the acts of moms from Susan Smith to the 'Prom Mom'*. New York: NYU Press.

Miller, L. J. (2003). Denial of pregnancy. In M. G. Spinelli (Ed.), *Infanticide: Psychosocial and legal perspectives on mother who kill* (pp. 81–104). Washington, DC: American Psychiatric Association.

Miller, L. J. (2016). Psychological, behavioral, and cognitive changes during pregnancy and the postpartum period. In A. Wenzel (Ed.), *The Oxford handbook of perinatal psychology* (pp. 7–25). Oxford: Oxford University Press.

Milstein, K. K., & Milstein, P. S. (1983). Psychophysiologic aspects of denial in pregnancy: Case report. *Journal of Clinical Psychiatry, 44*(5), 189–190.

Mueller, J., & Sherr, L. (2009). Abandoned babies and absent policies. *Health Policy, 93*, 157–164.

Murphy Tighe, S., & Lalor, J. G. (2015). *Concealed pregnancy and newborn abandonment: A contemporary problem. Blog post published 17 May*. Available at: www.perceptionsofpregnancy.com/2015/05/17/concealed-pregnancy-newborn-abandonment-a-contemporary-Problem/.

Murphy Tighe, S., & Lalor, J. G. (2016a). Concealed pregnancy: A concept analysis. *Journal of Advanced Nursing, 72*(1), 50–61.

Murphy Tighe, S., & Lalor, J. G. (2016b). Concealed pregnancy and newborn abandonment part 1. *The Practising Midwife, 19*(6), 12–15.

Murphy Tighe, S., & Lalor, J. G. (2016c). Concealed pregnancy and newborn abandonment part 2. *The Practising Midwife, 19*(7), 14–16.

Murphy Tighe, S., & Lalor, J. G. (2019). Regaining agency and autonomy: A grounded typology of concealed pregnancy. *Journal of Advanced Nursing, 75*(3), 603–615.

Navarro, F., Delcroix, M., & Godeau, E. (2011). Le Deni de grossesse al'adolescence. *Revista de Psicologia da Criança e do Adolescente, 3*, 147–164.

Navarro, B., & Urban, R. (2004). Overkill in a case of neonaticide. *Archiv für Kriminologie, 213*(5–6), 129–137.

Neifert, P. L., & Bourgeois, J. A. (2000). Denial of pregnancy: A case study and literature review. *Military Medicine, 165*(7), 566–568.

NICE (National Institute for Health and Care Excellence). (2008). *Antenatal care for uncomplicated pregnancies. Clinical Guideline: CG 62* (updated 2019). Available at: www.nice.org.uk/guidance/cg62/resources/antenatal-care-for-uncomplicated-pregnancies-pdf-975564597445.

NICE (National Institute for Health and Care Excellence). (2010). *Pregnancy and complex social factors: A model for service provision for pregnant women with complex social factors. Clinical Guideline: CG 110.* Available at: www.nice.org.uk/guidance/cg110/resources/pregnancy-and-complex-social-factors-a-model-for-service-provision-for-pregnant-women-with-complex-social-factors-pdf-3510938271814.

Nirmal, D., Thijs, I., Bethel, J., & Bhal, P. S. (2006). The incidence and outcome of concealed pregnancy among hospital deliveries: An 11 year population-based study in Glamorgan. *Journal of Obstetrics and Gynaecology, 26*(2), 118–121.

North East Lincolnshire, L. S. C. B. (2016). Concealed pregnancy. LSCB, Sutton. *Child a serious case review overview report.* Sutton: LSCB.

Northumberland Safeguarding Children's Board. (2012). Highlighting lessons from management review. Available at: www.northumberland.go.uk/Northumberlandcountycouncil/Media/Child-Families/Management-Review-Nathanb59.pdf.

Porter, T., & Gavin, H. (2010). Infanticide and neonaticide: A review of 40 years of research literature on incidence and causes. *Trauma, Violence, & Abuse, 11*(3), 99–112.

Putkonen, H., Collander, J., & Weizzmann-Heng, G. (2007). Legal outcomes of all suspected neonaticides in Finland 1980–2000. *International Journal of Law and Psychiatry, 30*(3), 248–254.

Rattigan, C. (2012). *What else could I do: Single mothers and infanticide 1850–900.* Dublin: Irish Academic Press.

Resnick, P. J. (1970). Murder of the newborn: A psychiatric review of neonaticide. *American Journal of Psychiatry, 126*(10), 1414–1420.

Riley, L. (2005). Neonaticide: A grounded theory study. *Journal of Human Behavior in the Social Environment, 12*(4), 1–42.

Sadler, C. (2002). Mum's the word: Research into what is believed to be the largest ever study of concealed pregnancy has been carried out in Lincolnshire. *Nursing Standard, 16/37*, 14–15.

Sandoz, P. (2011). Reactive-homeostasis as a cybernetic model of the silhouette effect of denial of pregnancy. *Medical Hypotheses, 77*(5), 782–785.

Saunders, E. (1989). Neonaticides following 'secret' pregnancies: Seven case reports. *Public Health Reports, 104*(4), 368–372.

Schultz, M. J., & Bushati, T. (2015). Maternal physical morbidity associated with denial of pregnancy. *The Australian and New Zealand Journal of Obstetrics and Gynaecology, 55*(6), 559–564.

Spielvogel, A., & Hoehener, H. (1995). Denial of pregnancy: A review and case reports. *Birth, 22*(4), 220–226.

Spinelli, M. (2002). *Infanticide, psychosocial and legal perspectives on mothers who kill.* Washington: American Psychiatric Publishing Inc.

Spinelli, M. G. (2010). Denial of pregnancy: A psychodynamic paradigm. *Journal of the American Academy of Psychoanalysis and Dynamic Psychiatry, 38*(1), 117–131.

Struye, A., Zdanowicz, N., Ibrahim, C., & Reynaert, C. (2013). Can denial of pregnancy be a denial of fertility? A case discussion. *Psychiatria Danubina, 25*(Suppl. 2), S113–S117.

Sydney Morning Herald. (2008). Newborn baby found dead in public toilet. Available at: http://smh.com.au/news/baby-found-dead-in-public-toilet.

Thynne, C. (2006). Exploring the experience of women who undergo a late disclosure of pregnancy. *Doctoral thesis.* Available at: www.lenus.ie/hse/handle/10147/210730.

Thynne, C., Gaffney, G., ONeill, M., et al. (2012). Concealed pregnancy: Prevalence, perinatal measures and socio-demographics. *Irish Medical Journal, 105*(8), 263–265.

Vallone, D. C., & Hoffman, L. M. (2003). Preventing the tragedy of neonaticide. *Holistic Nursing Practice, 17*(5), 223–228.

Vellut, N., Cook, J. M., & Tursz, A. (2012). Analysis of the relationship between neonaticide and denial of pregnancy using data from judicial files. *Child Abuse & Neglect, 36*(7–8), 553–563.

Vellut, N., Simmat-Durand, L. A., & Tursz, A. (2013). The profile of neonaticide mothers in legal expertise. *Encephale, 39*(5), 352–359.

Villeneuve-Gokalp, C., & Jacob, A. (2011). Women who give birth 'Secretly' in France, 2007–2009. *Population, 66*(1), 131–168.

Werner, A., Campbell, R. J., & Frazier, S. H. (1980). *A psychiatric glossary* (5th ed.). Washington: APA.

Wessel, J., & Endrikat, J. (2005). Cyclic menstruation-like bleeding during denied pregnancy. Is there a particular hormonal cause? *Gynecological Endocrinology, 21*(6), 353–359.

Wessel, J., Endrikat, J., & Buscher, U. (2002). Frequency of denial of pregnancy: Results and epidemiological significance of a 1-year prospective study in Berlin. *Acta Obstetricia et Gynecologica Scandinavica, 81*(11), 1021–1027.

Wessel, J., Endrikat, J., & Büscher, U. (2003). Elevated risk for neonatal outcome following denial of pregnancy: Results of a one-year prospective study compared with control groups. *Journal of Perinatal Medicine, 31*(1), 29–35.

Wessel, J., Gauruder-Burmester, A., & Gerlinger, C. (2007). Denial of pregnancy – characteristics of women at risk. *Acta Obstetricia et Gynecologica Scandinavica, 86*(5), 542–546.

ANNOTATED FURTHER READING

Conlon, C. (2006). Concealed pregnancy: A case study report from an Irish setting. Crisis pregnancy agency report No 15. Available at: www.sexualwellbeing.ie/for-professionals/research/research-reports/concealed-pregnancy-a-case-study-approach-form-an-irish-setting.pdf.

This case study report looks at women's experiences of concealed pregnancy in Ireland. The research aimed to create an understanding of the psychosocial, emotional, psychological and practical factors contributing to a woman's decision to conceal her pregnancy. It documents the services that are in place for a woman trying to cope with a concealed pregnancy.

Thynne, C. (2006). Exploring the experience of women who undergo a late disclosure of pregnancy. *Thesis.* Available at: www.lenus.ie/handle/10147/210730.

This doctoral thesis explored late disclosure of pregnancy by employing in depth interviews with n=8 Irish women. The women were asked about their experiences of pregnancy and why they felt it necessary to delay disclosure. Part two of the study investigated the socioeconomic profile of women in a target group who had delayed disclosure of pregnancy (n=43), a larger normative sample (n=100) and a smaller matched group (n=30). Delayed disclosure of pregnancy emerged as a dynamic and multidimensional concept and recommendations were made for hospital and community setting.

13

Antenatal Screening of the Mother and Fetus

Kirsten Allen, Lucy Kean

CHAPTER CONTENTS

Screening has now become such a routine part of antenatal care that many women accept this, often with little thought. There is no aspect of the screening programme that does not, however, have the potential to raise huge social, emotional and health issues for pregnant women. The role of the midwife is to guide women through the wealth of tests available, with the best advice possible. This can only be achieved by excellent training and regular updates for all midwives and doctors. Screening develops and moves forward every few months and so vigilance on behalf of us all is needed to ensure we provide the best care.

THE CHAPTER AIMS TO

- discuss the principles of screening, good counselling techniques and the potential impact of positive results on women
- describe the currently available screening tests, their aims and the efficiency of each test
- define what consent is and how the consent process should be undertaken
- provide information regarding how to deal with positive tests and what negative results mean.

SCREENING PRINCIPLES

Screening of a mother and baby is now a major part of care for all pregnancies. The underlying principles of screening are that the condition being screened for must be an important health problem that is well understood. Treatment should be available and at a stage where the outcome can be changed (i.e. something that makes a difference to health and wellbeing without increasing risk). There should be an appropriate and acceptable test that is available to a defined group, and the screening should be cost-effective in reducing poorer health outcomes. Finally, there should be evidence that the screening programme is effective, with rigorous quality assurance.

The National Screening Committee of the United Kingdom (NSC 2013) defines screening as:

a process of identifying apparently healthy people who may be at an increased risk of a disease or condition, they can then be offered information, further tests and appropriate treatment to reduce their risk and/or any complications arising from the disease or condition.

Broadly speaking, the conditions that form the national programme for screening in the UK meet these criteria. When screening for currently unscreened conditions is considered (e.g. Group B streptococcus), it is weighed against these important criteria.

Screening in pregnancy can be divided into looking for conditions in the mother that, if untreated or undetected, could affect her health or the health of the baby or both, and screening for conditions in the fetus that could impact significantly on the health of the baby.

Limitations of Screening

Screening has important ethical differences from clinical practice, as the health service is targeting apparently healthy people, offering to help individuals to make better informed choices about their health. There are risks involved, however, and it is important that people have realistic expectations of what a screening programme can deliver.

While screening has the potential to save lives or improve life through early diagnosis of serious conditions, it is not a foolproof process. Equally, some screening does not influence the health of the mother at all but is directed at detecting conditions in the fetus that may lead to significant disability, in order to provide prospective parents with choices regarding continuation or otherwise of the pregnancy.

Screening can reduce the risk of developing a condition or its complications but it cannot offer a guarantee of protection. In any screening programme there will be a small number of false-positive results (wrongly reported as having the condition) and false-negative results (wrongly reported as not having the condition). The UK NSC is increasingly presenting screening as *risk reduction* to emphasize this point.

Screening can be an emotive issue. While screening for fetal problems is often considered the most emotionally charged area, it is important to realize that maternal screening can also raise issues and challenges that all health professionals involved in the service need to be equipped to help with. Imagine the emotional journey a mother embarks on when faced with a new diagnosis of human immunodeficiency virus (HIV) in early pregnancy.

Social and Psychological Impact of Screening Investigations

Pregnancy is a profound and life-changing event. During this time, the mother has to adapt physically, socially and psychologically to the forthcoming birth of her child. Many women feel more emotional than usual (Raphael-Leff 2005) and may have heightened levels of anxiety (Kleinveld et al. 2006; Raynor and England 2010). As Green et al. (2004) state, the increasing availability of fetal investigations has been shown to cause women even greater anxiety and stress. Any feelings of excitement and anticipation can quickly change when the mother is introduced to the idea that she is 'at risk' of having a baby with a particular problem (Fisher 2006).

There is evidence that mothers nearing the end of their reproductive years (with a higher risk of chromosomal malformations) experience pregnancy in a way that is different to younger women. Older mothers are often more anxious and have fewer feelings of attachment to the fetus at 20 weeks of pregnancy (Berryman and Windridge 1999). Psychologists, sociologists and health professionals now generally accept the finding that high-risk women delay attachment to the fetus until they receive reassuring test results. Rothman (1986) classically termed this the *tentative pregnancy*, in a study of women undergoing amniocentesis.

Anxiety caused by consideration of possible fetal malformation may be accompanied by moral or religious dilemmas. Tests that can diagnose chromosomal or genetic malformations also carry a risk of procedure-induced miscarriage. Many parents agonize about whether to subject a potentially normal fetus to this risk in order to obtain this information. Parents may then need to consider whether they wish to terminate or continue with an affected pregnancy. Some religious authorities only support prenatal testing so long as the integrity of the mother and fetus are maintained. There are also opposing views about the legitimacy of terminating a pregnancy, even when a serious disorder has been diagnosed. Such dilemmas are an unfortunate but inevitable cost of the choices associated with some fetal investigations.

Despite this, there are important advantages to the acquisition of knowledge about the fetus before birth. First, society greatly values the freedom of individuals to choose. People are encouraged to accept some responsibility when making decisions about treatment options, in partnership with healthcare professionals. A second advantage is that reproductive autonomy may be increased. Women can choose for themselves whether they wish to embark upon the lifelong care of a child with special needs. This may be viewed as empowering and as a means of preventing later suffering and hardship for child and family alike.

In summary, prenatal testing is a two-edged sword. It enables midwives and doctors to give people choices that were unheard of in previous generations and that may prevent much suffering. However, in some circumstances they actually increase the amount of anxiety and psychological trauma experienced in pregnancy. The long-term effects of such trauma on family dynamics are not currently understood.

HOW SCREENING IS SET UP AND THE MIDWIFE'S ROLE AND RESPONSIBILITIES

All midwives need to have a broad understanding of screening investigations because they are responsible for offering, interpreting and communicating the results. In the UK, the NMC 'Standards for Competence for Midwives' (NMC 2018a) states that midwives should communicate effectively, enabling women to make informed choices about their health and health care and encouraging them to think about how their health and

the health of their babies can be improved. The NMC (2018b) Code of Professional Practice also emphasizes the importance of prioritizing people, practicing effectively, preserving safety and promoting professionalism and trust. Some midwives specialize in discussing complex testing issues with parents and become antenatal screening coordinators.

In England, Public Health England (PHE) now oversees the Antenatal and Newborn Screening Programmes, and ensures standards are adhered to via four Regional Quality Assurance teams. The commissioning and oversight of the programmes is carried out by local screening and immunization teams. At an individual National Health Service (NHS) Trust level, dedicated screening coordinators will oversee the running of screening programmes in that Trust, as well as provide specialist advice and ensure that there is a line of referral for women whose needs are not met by routine services. Screening for pregnant women and newborn babies is now such a complex process that the role of antenatal and newborn screening coordinator has become a full-time role in most services. Standardized processes allow systems to serve women uniformly and allow good quality of care to be offered to all.

Public Health England publishes an extremely helpful timeline for antenatal and newborn screening that will help individuals to see what is required and by when (www.gov.uk/guidance/nhs-population-screening-education-and-training). To help achieve this, PHE have published service specifications for the UK Fetal Anomaly Screening Programme (PHE 2018a, service specifications 16 and 17). These aim to ensure equal access to screening, and that eligible women are provided with high quality information in order to make informed choices. PHE also publishes a leaflet entitled *Screening tests for you and your baby*, which is available in several languages on their website: www.gov.uk/government/publications/screening-tests-for-you-and-your-baby-description-in-brief. The offer of screening tests, and whether they were accepted or declined, should be recorded, and the screening tests performed in a timely fashion.

In addition to the service specifications, there are specific Fetal Anomaly Screening Programme Standards (PHE 2018b), which sets out target performance thresholds for some aspects of the screening programme. These include targets for acceptable levels of screen positive results, and time frames for the feedback of results to patients.

Each of the individual screening programmes has a number of key performance indicators (KPI) on which the performance of individual NHS Trusts is measured (PHE 2018d). Overseeing the delivery of the KPIs is the remit of the screening coordinator in each Trust, but it is the hard work of the professionals on the ground that ensures targets are met. As an example, the KPI for screening for hepatitis B states that at least 70% of pregnant women who are hepatitis B-positive should be referred and seen by an appropriate specialist within an effective timeframe (6 weeks from identification).

The KPI for screening for Down syndrome at between 10 weeks + 0 days and 20 weeks + 0 days states that the laboratory request form should be completed accurately in 97% of women who are screened. This means the form must include sufficient information for the woman to be uniquely identified, the woman's correct date of birth, maternal weight, family origin and smoking status, plus the ultrasound dating assessment in millimetres (mm), with associated gestational date and sonographer ID.

Failsafe procedures are a necessary part of the screening process. In the UK, these have been implemented to ensure all screening processes are complete. There are back-up mechanisms in addition to usual care, which ensures if something goes wrong in the screening pathway, processes are in place first to identify what is going wrong and second to determine what action should follow to ensure a safe outcome.

All professionals undertaking screening must be appropriately trained and confident in discussing the risks and benefits of all screening programmes, and in the UK, they must adhere to the NSC recommendations and standards.

Documentation

In whatever system is practised, good documentation is vital. The midwife should discuss and offer screening tests, record that the discussion has taken place, that the offer has been made and that the offer has been either accepted or declined. It is very helpful for the whole team engaged in antenatal care to understand from the documentation why screening is declined, if this is the case. Women find being persistently re-offered a screening test that they have declined frustrating and annoying, and simply documenting the discussion properly, rather than ticking a box to indicate that screening was

---

> **BOX 13.1 Principles for Obtaining Informed Consent**
>
> The midwife should provide information including:
> - the purpose of the procedure/test
> - all risks and benefits to be reasonably expected
> - details of all possible future treatments that could arise as a consequence of testing
> - disclosure of all available options (this may include tests that are offered by private providers where relevant)
> - the option of refusing any tests
> - the offer to answer any queries.

---

declined, is helpful. This can sometimes also lead on to discussion that can reveal that a woman has not understood the test, the purpose or the benefits, which can help to improve understanding.

In the event of decline for infectious diseases screening at the antenatal 'booking' appointment, a routine re-offer should be made at about 28 weeks. From a litigation perspective, it is not uncommon for women who have declined screening but experienced a poor outcome to suggest that they were not offered screening or did not understand the purpose of the test on offer. Good documentation and being able to show that written information was given can help in the comprehension of such cases.

Discussion of Options

When offering tests, it is necessary for the midwife to present and discuss the options, so that women can make an informed choice that best suits their circumstances and preferences. Midwives are required to discuss options for testing in a manner that enables shared decision-making (Nieuwenhuijze et al. 2014). This means providing the opportunity to discuss choices with a trained professional who is impartial and supportive as the women make decisions along the screening and diagnostic pathway.

There may be mixed feelings about the final decision. Sometimes it is helpful to consider what the mother's worst-case scenario would be, as that can help to decide the best way forward. The principles for consent for shared decision-making are shown in Box 13.1.

Midwives commonly recommend antenatal tests such as infectious disease screening, full blood count, or cardiotocograph for reduced fetal movements. However, tests for fetal anomaly require a non-directive approach that enables the mother to make an informed choice (Ahmed et al. 2013). Consent must be obtained prior to all tests and this must be documented.

Assumptions must never be made regarding knowledge about the conditions being screened for. Common misunderstandings are that Down syndrome cannot occur if it has not previously occurred in a family or that a woman is too young to have an affected baby. Many women (and their partners) do not understand that syphilis is a sexually transmitted infection, but that the initial result can show positive if there have been similar non-sexually transmitted infections (such as Yaws).

Women who decline first trimester screening should know that they can take up second trimester screening for Down syndrome if they change their mind. Although the second trimester screening scan for fetal anomaly at $18+^0$ to $20+^6$ weeks would still routinely be offered, this should not be regarded as a substitute for the combined or quadruple tests, as its objectives are very different (PHE 2018c).

Women who decline initial screening for infections can and should be offered screening later in the pregnancy.

Importantly, only the woman has the right to consent to or decline the screening tests. A partner or family member has no right to consent or decline on her behalf. Women can withdraw consent for testing at any time. This decision should be recorded.

The Process of Consent

Consent is a complex process not a single entity, and requires adequate time. It is important to ensure that the woman has had the time she needs to consider the information and come to a decision. There should be enough time to ask questions, so that she feels comfortable and has involved those she would wish to in reaching a decision. The extent to which women want to involve others is very variable.

The amount of information needed will vary between women. Women who do not understand English will require interpreting services and other services might be needed for some women. Not all women will have the capacity to consent. Where capacity is in doubt, there are usually local guidelines as to how this should progress forward that are beyond the scope of this chapter.

Issues to Consider when Presenting Information

When discussing tests, it is important to understand the motivations and thought processes of pregnant women. The motivation for testing is often different for mother and practitioner. For the fetal anomaly screening programme, the UK NSC rationale for testing is to identify fetal anomalies; however mothers commonly accept these tests in order to gain reassurance that their fetus is normal (Hunt et al. 2005). Mothers often think that fetal anomaly tests such as ultrasound scans are an integral or mandatory part of their antenatal care. They may also be unaware of the reasons for performing the test and this can compound the shock of finding problems or abnormalities (Åhman et al. 2016).

When women are anxious or under stress, they are less able to remember the information provided (Glover 2014). Parents may feel vulnerable and less able to ask questions. This may lead to dissatisfaction with the quality of communications with health carers. Since an unborn fetus is something of an enigma to parents, this may increase anxiety and sensitivity to real or imaginary cues. For example, professionals practising non-directive counselling may be perceived as evasive and as concealing bad news. One particular aspect of counselling that has been criticized by parents is the portrayal of risk estimates (Seror and Ville 2009).

There is much evidence that people do not make consistent decisions about undertaking tests in pregnancy on the basis of the risk information received. For instance, a mother with a risk of Down syndrome of 1:150 may perceive herself to be at a very high risk and may request amniocentesis. However, others may view that same risk as very low. The phenomenon of how parents interpret risk information is not fully understood, although it is clear that personal circumstances, preferences and beliefs are an integral part of this process. For this reason, it is vital that, with any screening, the midwife begins a consultation by investigating how much the mother knows about the condition being tested for, and what she already knows about the test risks, benefits and the consequences of results (see Box 13.2).

There are also common biases in the way people interpret risk information. The midwife should be aware of these in order to help parents choose the most appropriate course of action. For example, people tend to view an event as more likely if they can easily imagine or recall instances of it. This means that a mother whose

---

BOX 13.2   Key Aspects of the UK NSC (PHE 2016) Guidance on Antenatal Screening

- The pregnant woman must understand the condition being screened for.
- The midwife should explain about the nature, purpose, risks, benefits, timing, limitations and potential consequences of screening.
- The woman should understand that screening is optional, and understand the risks and benefits of not undergoing screening.
- In the UK, there is the choice of continuing or terminating a pregnancy for serious fetal malformations.
  Local knowledge should be shared: how, where and when the test is done and:
- what the test results mean and potential significant clinical and emotional consequences
- the decisions that might need to be made at each point along the pathway and their consequences
- how and when the results will be given
- how women progress through the pathway, including those who opt out of screening
- the possibility that screening can provide information about other conditions
- the fact that screening may not provide a definitive diagnosis
- what further tests might be needed, e.g. chorionic villus sampling (CVS) and amniocentesis
- that confirmatory/repeat testing may occasionally be required
- balanced and accurate information about the various conditions being screened should be provided.

BOX 13.3   General Principles when Providing Information

1. Be clear: explain everything in terms that are not medical jargon or complex terminology.
2. Be aware that people can remember only a limited amount of information at one time – be simple, concise and to the point.
3. Give important information first. This will then be remembered best.
4. Group pieces of information into logical categories, such as treatment, prognosis and ways to cope.
5. Information may be recalled more easily if it has been presented in several forms. For example, leaflets can be helpful.
6. Offer to answer any queries. Give contact numbers, in case people think of questions at a later date.
7. Do not make assumptions about information requirements on the basis of social class, profession, age or ethnic group.
8. Summarize, check understanding and repeat the information. Ask whether there is anything that remains unclear.

From Hunter M. (1994) *Counselling in obstetrics and gynaecology*. Leicester: British Psychological Society Books.

---

friend or neighbour has a baby with Down syndrome may be sensitized to this possibility and overestimate the chances of it happening to her. Women who experienced severe disease in childhood, or who work with those with a disability, are more likely to seek prenatal diagnosis (Sjögren 1996). Perhaps these mothers are easily able to imagine the lifelong commitment of caring for a child with special needs. This common bias in risk perception is important because it means that some mothers may not easily be reassured by reiteration of the fact that the risk of a problem may be comparatively rare.

Explaining Risk

The way in which the midwife tells a mother about risk will also greatly influence how that risk is perceived. For example, a mother who is told that her risk of a particular condition is 1 in 10 may be more alarmed than if she had been informed that there was a 90% chance of normality or 9 out of 10 babies will not be affected by the condition. This is known as the *framing* effect (Kessler and Levine 1987).

People vary considerably in the ways that they consider and understand risk, so it is important that this information is presented in a variety of ways using appropriate language. PHE (2018b) recommend the use of the word 'chance' rather than 'risk' and that the chance of the outcome (which for antenatal screening now mainly relates to screening for Down syndrome, Edwards syndrome or Patau syndrome) be given as a percentage as well as a ratio 1 in *x*. As such, a midwife discussing a 1 in 100 chance of a disorder should also point out the fact that 99% or 99 out of 100 similar people will not experience that disorder. This may help people cope when considering tests or when anxiously awaiting results.

There are other general considerations to take into account when providing information (Hunter 1994), as delineated in Box 13.3.

If a test is undertaken in pregnancy, it is good practice to ensure that the woman is clear about how, when and from whom she will be able to obtain the result. If possible, there should be some options available.

Public Health England (PHE 2018a) is clear that the person ordering the test has the responsibility to ensure that the test is properly completed and that the woman is informed of the result. It therefore requires each midwifery team to have a process for the management of tracking tests performed and the results, along with a means to inform women. It is unfortunately inevitable that, at some point the process will fail, and a test will not be performed or a sample not processed. There must then be a process of failsafe so that this is recognized in a timely enough fashion for the test to be repeated, and that the results are recorded in the woman's handheld notes.

On a logistical front, this is no mean task. Failings in the screening system are identified as serious incidents and there is a formal process in the UK that must be undertaken when failings are identified. In practice, the majority of women in whom things are missed, are those whose pregnancies do not follow the routine process, for instance those who move or whose pregnancy does not continue. These women, as much as anyone else, still should be informed of results that are important to them, such as the results of infection screening.

INDIVIDUAL SCREENING TEST CONSIDERATIONS

Antenatal screening tests are broadly divided into those that are looking directly for a problem in the fetus, or those looking for a problem in the mother that could affect her health and/or the fetus, such as an infection, the presence of a red cell antibody, or a particular haemoglobin variant.

FETAL SCREENING TESTS

Population screening of the fetus (i.e. that offered to everyone) is now directed at two areas: defining the risk of a baby having Down syndrome, Edwards syndrome or Patau syndrome (Trisomy 21, 18 or 13), and the detection of specific abnormalities.

Screening for Down Syndrome, Edwards Syndrome and Patau Syndrome

All women have a chance of having a baby affected by Down syndrome (Trisomy 21), Edwards syndrome (Trisomy 18) or Patau syndrome (Trisomy 13), and this chance increases with increasing maternal age.

Down syndrome is the most common cause of severe learning difficulty in children. In the absence of antenatal screening, around 1 in 700 births would be affected (Kennard et al. 1995). While some children with Down syndrome learn literacy skills and lead semi-independent lives, others remain completely dependent. Around one in three of these babies are born with a serious heart defect. The average life expectancy is about 60 years, although there is an increased risk of developing pathological changes in the brain (associated with Alzheimer's disease) after the age of 40 (Kingston 2002).

Edwards syndrome and Patau syndrome are not as common as Down syndrome, with <1 in 5000 live births affected by each. Sadly these syndromes are associated with significant physical health problems and learning disability, and fewer than 10% of children survive beyond their first birthday.

Screening for Down syndrome, Edwards syndrome and Patau syndrome has been driven by both health economics and maternal choice. That is not to say, however, that all mothers wish to be screened, or would act to end a pregnancy if they knew they were carrying an affected fetus. Uptake rates for screening vary depending on the population being screened. Some mothers will chose screening, despite knowing that they would not act on a result that gave them a high chance. Interestingly, the single largest factor in deciding whether to take further tests after a high chance result is the degree of magnitude of the change in risk. In other words, a mother who has a pre-test chance of trisomy 21 (based on age alone) of 1 in 100 (1%), who has a screening result of 1 in 120 (0.83%) will be less likely to wish to proceed to further testing than a woman who has a pre-test chance of 1 in 1000, who then receives a result of 1 in 120 chance, even though both are at equal risk of giving birth to a baby with Down syndrome.

The National Screening Programme in the UK offers one of two tests for chromosomal abnormalities. The first trimester combined test assesses the chance that the pregnancy is affected by Down syndrome, Edwards syndrome and Patau syndrome, whereas the second

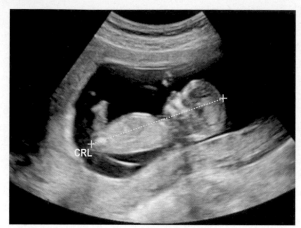

Fig. 13.1 Crown–rump length (CRL). (With permission from Landon MB, Galan HL, Jauniaux ERM, et al. (2019) Gabbe's obstetrics essentials: normal and problem pregnancies. London: Elsevier.)

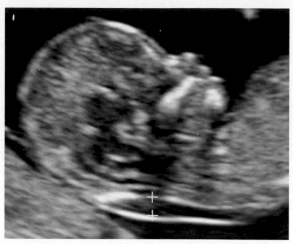

Fig. 13.2 Translucency measurement. (With permission from Coady and Bower (2014) Twining's textbook of fetal abnormalities. Expert Consult: Online and Print, 3e, Fig 2.1. London: Elsevier.)

trimester quadruple test can only be used to assess the chance of Down syndrome. Women opting for first trimester combined screening can choose to be screened for Down syndrome only, Edwards syndrome and Patau syndrome only, or all three conditions.

The gestational age window for a combined test is from $10+0$ weeks to $14+1$ weeks in pregnancy. The combined test comprises measurement of the crown–rump length (CRL) (Fig. 13.1) to estimate fetal gestational age (dating scan), measurement of the nuchal translucency (NT) space at the back of the fetal neck (Fig. 13.2) and maternal blood to measure the serum markers of pregnancy-associated plasma protein A (PAPP-A) and free beta human chorionic gonadotrophin hormone (hCG).

Using this test, 90% of fetuses affected with Down syndrome, Edwards syndrome and Patau syndrome would be expected to fall into the high-chance category (a chance of 1 in 150 or more) (the detection rate) with 2% of women carrying unaffected babies having a chance of 1 in 150 or higher (a screen positive rate of 2%).

The quadruple test window starts from $14+2$ weeks to $20+0$ weeks. A maternal blood sample is required for the analysis of hCG, alpha-fetoprotein (αFP), unconjugated oestriol (uE3) and inhibin-A. This test has a lesser detection rate for Down syndrome of 75% and a screen positive rate of <3%, but has been retained because there will always be women who book too late in pregnancy for combined testing (about 15% of the pregnant

population) and wish to have screening. Women presenting after 20 weeks are offered ultrasound for abnormality screening, which will occasionally detect an abnormality that increases the chance that the baby has Down syndrome, Edwards syndrome and Patau syndrome, but there is no population screening available at this gestation.

Women need to decide as early in their pregnancy as possible if they wish to undertake screening for Down syndrome, Edwards syndrome and Patau syndrome, as earlier testing is superior, and ease of access is important in facilitating testing.

In counselling, women need to be clear that neither screening test gives a guarantee of normality. With combined screening, 10% of affected babies will be missed and with quadruple testing, 25% of babies with Down syndrome will be missed. This is termed the *false-negative rate*.

Diagnostic Testing for Down Syndrome, Edwards Syndrome and Patau Syndrome

In the UK, women who receive a result of 1 in 150 or higher from either first or second trimester screening will be offered diagnostic testing, i.e. chorionic villus sampling (CVS) or amniocentesis. The same tests can also be offered in other circumstances such as for women with a previous pregnancy affected by a chromosomal abnormality or who carry a genetic disorder. The NHS no longer provides diagnostic testing for maternal age alone or

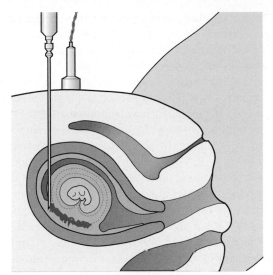

Fig. 13.3 Transabdominal chorionic villus sampling (CVS).

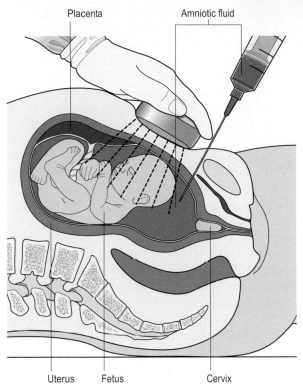

Fig. 13.4 Amniocentesis.

following a low chance screening test result, although privately available services are usually easy to access.

Chorionic villus sampling can be performed from 11 weeks of pregnancy. Usually the procedure is carried out transabdominally (Fig. 13.3), though occasionally a transcervical (TC) route is needed. The miscarriage rate is often quoted as 2–3% but in most fetal medicine units, the procedure-related loss rate is closer to 1% (although TC sampling risks are higher). A provisional result is usually issued on a direct preparation at 1–2 days. If this result shows no evidence of an extra chromosome 21, 18 or 13, it can be taken as 99.9% certain that the fetus does not have trisomy 21, 18 or 13. However, as confined placental mosaicism can rarely occur, which gives a false-negative result, definite confirmation cannot be made until the culture result of the full karyotype is available at 14–21 days.

Amniocentesis can be performed after 15 weeks (Fig. 13.4). The procedure-related loss rate is usually no higher than 1% and in many units is closer to 0.5%. Rapid testing using polymerase chain reaction or fluorescent *in situ* hybridization can usually mean that a result for trisomy 21 (and usually 13 and 18) is available in 2–3 working days.

A diagnosis of Down syndrome, Edwards syndrome and Patau syndrome can be accurately made using CVS or amniocentesis, but it cannot give certainty as to the severity of the disorder or the quality of life of a particular individual. Responses to a diagnosis will vary, according to cultural, social, moral and religious beliefs.

Non-invasive prenatal testing (NIPT) is in the process of being introduced across the UK following recommendations by the National Screening Committee. During pregnancy, cell-free DNA from the placenta crosses into the maternal circulation. As placental DNA is usually the same as fetal DNA, a maternal blood test can be carried out and the total cell-free DNA sequenced and counted. If there are increased amounts of chromosomes 21, 18 or 13 present in the sample, there is an increased likelihood that the fetus is affected by the corresponding trisomy. NIPT is already being offered by many companies privately, but will soon be offered on the NHS to women with a high-chance screening result (>1 in 150) on first or second trimester screening. NIPT has a detection rate of over 99% for Down syndrome in a high risk population. It has lower detection rates for T18 and 13 and invasive testing usually by amniocentesis will always be recommended.

Screening for Haemoglobinopathies

Haemoglobinopathies are inherited disorders of haemoglobin and are more prevalent in certain racial groups. The NHS NSC antenatal and newborn screening programmes include antenatal screening for fetal hae-moglobinopathies. Antenatal screening identifies about 22,000 carriers of sickle cell disease and thalassaemia in the UK every year (PHE 2013). This should be linked with the newborn bloodspot screening programme, which tests for sickle cell disease. Linking results of parents and babies increases health professionals' access to families with genetic disorders, allowing the results to be available throughout the individual's life, reducing repeat screening.

Currently, in the UK, antenatal screening for hae-moglobinopathy is based on population prevalence. All areas collect information on the Family Origin Questionnaire (FOQ) in their maternity population. This information is needed by laboratories to help interpret screening results. High prevalence areas, where ≥2% of booking bloods received by the laboratory are screen positive, have universal screening (offer all pregnant women electrophoresis screening for haemoglobin variants and thalassaemia trait). Low prevalence areas use the FOQ to determine genetic ancestry for the last two generations (or more if possible). Women with genetic ancestry that includes high-risk racial groups are offered electrophoresis testing. If the mother is found to be a haemoglobinopathy carrier, partner testing is then recommended and should be offered soon after the result is available. Genetic ancestry is also important when interpreting screening results. It is important to establish maternal iron levels when carrier status for thalassaemia is suspected, since iron deficiency can give rise to similar red-cell appearances (e.g. alpha thalassaemia). Most haemoglobinopathies are recessively inherited, so if both parents are carriers, the fetus would have a 1 in 4 chance of inheriting the disorder and a 1 in 2 chance of being a carrier.

Pre-Test Information for Antenatal Haemoglobinopathy Screening

- In early pregnancy, information should be supplied. In the UK, this means that all women should receive the PHE information booklet *Screening tests for you and your baby*, as early in pregnancy as possible. It is available at: https://assets.publishing.service.gov.uk/government/uploads/system/uploads/attachment_data/file/696849/Screening_tests_for_you_and_your_baby.pdf
- The information should be provided in an appropriate language or format.

- Testing should be performed as early in pregnancy as possible, ideally at 8–10 weeks' gestation, as screening decisions are often gestation-dependent.
- Women who book late in pregnancy should be offered haemoglobinopathy screening in the same way at the first point of contact. Options for ending an affected pregnancy may be limited.

Where both parents are identified as carriers, they need urgent counselling. In the UK, parents are referred urgently to a PEGASUS (Professional Education for Genetic Assessment and Screening) trained midwife for specialist counselling or to the combined obstetric/haematology clinic at the booking hospital. Diagnostic testing by CVS or amniocentesis should be offered.

Where paternity is unknown or the father of the baby is unavailable or declines testing, the woman should be offered a counselling appointment to calculate the possibility of the baby having an inherited haemoglobin disorder and an offer of diagnostic testing made if the risks warrant this. All women will be offered neonatal blood spot screening at 5 days, which will detect sickle cell disease (but not other haemoglobinopathies).

Ultrasonography for Fetal Screening

In the UK, the NSC (PHE 2018b) standards are that all pregnant women should be offered two routine ultrasound scans. These include an early pregnancy scan (usually timed to be able to perform the NT measurement if requested) and an $18+^0$ to $20+^6$ week fetal anomaly screening scan. Ultrasound works by transmitting sound at a very high frequency, via a probe, in a narrow beam. When the sound waves enter the body and encounter a structure, some of that sound is reflected back. The amount of sound reflected varies according to the type of tissue encountered; for example, fluid does not reflect sound and appears as a black image. Conversely, bone reflects a considerable amount of sound and appears as white or echogenic. Many structures appear as different shades of grey. Generally, pictures are transmitted in 'real time', which enables fetal movements to be seen.

Safety Aspects of Ultrasound

Ultrasound has been used as a diagnostic imaging tool since the 1950s, so we are now into the third generation of scanned babies. It seems reasonable to assume that any major adverse effects of this technology would have become apparent before now. However, modern machines have higher resolutions and indications for ultrasound scanning have greatly increased. This means that levels of exposure to ultrasound have increased in pregnancy. Although the technology is considered safe, it should be used with respect and only when there is good indication, and care should be taken to limit exposure time and the thermal indices should be controlled (European Committee for Medical Ultrasound Safety, ECMUS 2017). Ultrasound is a diagnostic tool, but diagnosis can only be as reliable as the expertise of the operator and the quality of the machine. As Abramowicz (2013) states, malformations may be missed or incorrectly diagnosed if the operator is inexperienced or inadequately trained.

Women's Experiences of Ultrasound

In general, women experience ultrasound as a pleasurable opportunity to have visual access to their unborn baby (Stephenson et al. 2016). Indeed, ultrasound scans have been shown to increase psychological attachment to the fetus (Sedgman et al. 2006). Parents have a profound curiosity about their baby and a scan can turn something nebulous into something that seems much more real as a living individual (Roberts 2011). This can be particularly important for a woman's partner and family, who do not have the immediate physical experience of the pregnancy. Women tend to regard their scan as providing a general view of fetal wellbeing: the fact that the fetus is alive, growing and developing. However, this reassurance is temporary and begins to wear off after a few weeks (Roberts 2011). Mothers may then seek other forms of reassurance (e.g. monitoring fetal movements, auscultation of the fetal heartbeat). This initial reassurance may also create an enthusiasm for scans when there is no clinical indication.

Scans may also cause considerable anxiety however, particularly if there is a suspected or actual problem with the fetus. There is evidence to suggest that women who miscarry after visualization of the fetus on scan may feel a heightened sense of anguish because the fetus seemed more real. This may also be the case for parents considering termination of pregnancy on the grounds of fetal malformation. However, others may view their scan as a treasured memory of the baby they lost (Asplin et al. 2013).

The identification of fetal malformation in the antenatal period has differing psychological effects for parents when the pregnancy is to continue. Some parents have reported feeling grateful that they were able to prepare for the birth of a child with a disability (Côté-Arsenault et al. 2015). However, others have reported feelings of wishing they had not known about their child's problems before birth, as they found the worry and anticipation to be far worse than the reality of caring for the baby after birth (Turner 2013). It is necessary for midwives to be mindful of the powerful psychological effects ultrasound scans have on pregnant women and their families, if sensitive and appropriate care is to be given at this potentially distressing time.

The Midwife's Role Concerning Ultrasound Scans

As for all procedures, mothers should be fully informed about the purpose of the scan. Information should be given about which conditions are being checked for and which problems the scan would be unable to detect. Because of the pleasurable aspect of seeing the fetus, ultrasound scans have traditionally been tests that mothers undertake willingly, without prior discussion and consideration of potential consequences. Ultrasound screening for fetal malformation is a screening test and as such, women should be counselled as to the purpose, choices and pitfalls of screening, so that they can decide whether or not they wish to undergo a procedure that may bring unwelcome news. Women should be aware that ultrasound scans are optional and not an inevitable part of their care.

Women should also understand that a normal 'scan' does not guarantee normality in the baby. Box 13.4 shows the detection rates for the commonly assessed malformations, which should be shared with women.

There is evidence that, although some mothers may find this information disturbing, most feel that this is outweighed by the positive aspects of seeing the baby and gaining reassurance (Oliver et al. 1996). Indeed, extra information about the purpose of the scan has been shown to increase women's understanding and satisfaction with the amount of information received, while the proportion of women accepting a scan (99%) appears to remain unchanged (Thornton et al. 1995).

Wherever scans are performed, a midwife or counsellor with a particular interest or expertise in the area should be available to discuss difficult news. All women with a suspected or confirmed fetal anomaly should be seen by an obstetric ultrasound specialist within 3 working days of the referral being made or seen by a fetal medicine unit within 5 working days

BOX 13.4 Detection Rates for Commonly Assessed Fetal Malformations

Anencephaly	98%
Open spina bifida	90%
Cleft lip	75%
Diaphragmatic hernia	60%
Gastroschisis	98%
Exomphalos	80%
Serious cardiac abnormalities	50%
Bilateral renal agenesis	84%
Lethal skeletal dysplasia	60%
Edwards syndrome (trisomy 18)	95%
Patau syndrome (trisomy 13)	95%

From UK NSC (PHE, Public Health England). (2018c) NHS fetal anomaly screening programme handbook. Valid from August 2018. Available at: www.gov.uk/government/publications/fetal-anomaly-screening-programme-handbook)

of the referral being made (PHE 2018b, Standard 4). Effective multidisciplinary team working and communication are therefore essential. It is also good practice for the midwife to liaise with the primary healthcare team, who would normally carry out the majority of antenatal care. With the increasing use of client-held records, mothers may have more opportunity to scrutinize the written results of their scan. Midwives may increasingly be called upon to explain and discuss these findings, both in hospital and in the community setting.

First Trimester Pregnancy Scans

All women should be offered a first trimester scan. The purpose of this is to establish:

- that the pregnancy is viable and intrauterine (not ectopic)
- to determine fetal number (and chorionicity or amnionicity in multiple pregnancies)
- to accurately define the gestational age
- to measure the nuchal translucency (NT) if the gestation is appropriate and screening for Down syndrome, Edwards syndrome and Patau syndrome is accepted
- to detect major fetal malformations, such as anencephaly (absence of the cranial vault).

Early ultrasound scanning is beneficial in reducing the need to induce labour for post-maturity (Whitworth et al. 2010). A gestation sac can usually be visualized from 5 weeks' gestation and a small embryo from 6 weeks. Until 13 weeks, gestational age can be accurately assessed by CRL measurement (the length of the fetus from the top of the head to the end of the sacrum). Strict criteria for the images is published for practitioners undertaking ultrasound to ensure accurate measurements. Mothers are asked to attend with a full bladder, since this aids visualization of the uterus at an early gestation.

Management of increased nuchal translucency. A nuchal translucency of >3.5 mm occurs in about 1% of pregnancies (Fig. 13.2). This is considered to be the threshold definition of an increased NT, above which the risk of other (non-chromosomal) abnormalities increases. Increased NT is associated with a risk of chromosomal abnormalities and also with other structural (mainly cardiac) abnormalities (>10% risk), genetic syndromes and an increased fetal loss rate. Where an increased NT is seen regardless of whether screening for Down syndrome, Edwards syndrome and Patau syndrome was declined, the potential for problems to be present must be discussed. Referral to specialist scanning and counselling should ideally be offered, and the option of genetic testing discussed. In the presence of a normal karyotype and if no structural malformations are found, the UK NSC (PHE 2018c) states that the incidence of adverse outcome is not increased, but also acknowledges that the chance of developmental delay is 2–4%.

Where diagnostic testing and 18–20 weeks' ultrasound is normal, it is reasonable to be optimistic regarding outcome, but it is worth recognizing that parents will carry the anxiety of uncertainty with them through and even beyond the end of the pregnancy and will often require a lot of support.

Second Trimester Ultrasound Scans

When the first pregnancy scan occurs after approximately $14+^0$ weeks of pregnancy (CRL measurement >84.0 mm), gestational age is calculated using the head circumference (HC).

The detailed fetal anomaly screening scan. This scan is usually performed at $18+^0$ to $20+^6$ weeks of pregnancy. The purpose of this scan is to reassure the mother that the fetus has no obvious structural anomalies that fall into the following categories:

- anomalies that are incompatible with life
- anomalies that are associated with significant morbidity and long-term disability
- anomalies that may benefit from intrauterine therapy

BOX 13.5 18+⁰ to 20+⁶ Weeks Fetal Anomaly Ultrasound Scan Base Menu

- spine, vertebrae and skin covering in transverse and longitudinal sections including sacrum
- head and neck: head shape and head circumference measurement, internal structures (cavum septum pellucidum, cerebellum, ventricular size at atrium), nuchal fold, face and lips
- thorax: laterality of heart, four-chamber view of heart, cardiac outflow tracts (aorta, three-vessel view, three-vessel and trachea), lungs
- abdominal shape and content: abdominal circumference measurement at level of the stomach with small portion of intrahepatic vein, abdominal wall, cord insertion, diaphragm, kidneys and bladder
- limbs: arms – three bones and hand (metacarpals); legs – three bones and foot (metatarsals)
- placental location and amniotic fluid.

From UK NSC (PHE, Public Health England). (2018c) NHS fetal anomaly screening programme handbook. Valid from August 2018. Available at: www.gov.uk/government/publications/fetal-anomaly-screening-programme-handbook)

- anomalies that may require postnatal treatment or investigation.

Detection rates should be in line with those outlined earlier. Technical difficulties, such as fetal position, multiple pregnancy, fibroids or maternal obesity may mean that a second scan before 23 weeks is offered. Some structural problems do not have sonographic signs that would be visible at this gestation or even at all. Anal atresia does not have a clear appearance on ultrasound; hydrocephalus and other bowel obstructions may not appear until later in pregnancy. Diagnosis may therefore not be possible. The UK NSC has defined which structures should be examined (Box 13.5) and which images should be stored as part of the woman's record.

Some features on ultrasound may be seen that increase the risk of another problem such as Down syndrome. An increased skin fold measurement of ≥6 mm at the level of the nuchal fold (a different entity to the nuchal translucency) should be noted as there is an associated increase in the risk for Down syndrome of at least 10-fold. Mild cerebral ventriculomegaly (≥10 mm) should be noted, as there is again an increased risk of chromosomal abnormalities of about 10%. Echogenic bowel can be associated with cystic fibrosis, fetal cytomegalovirus (CMV) infection and trisomy 21. Other structural variations will need follow-up scans as the pregnancy progresses, such as renal pelvis dilatation, which affects approximately 1% of fetuses (Hothi et al. 2009). Mild (5–9 mm) to moderate (10–15 mm) renal pelvis dilatation is more common than the severe (>15 mm) form. However, for those affected by the mild to moderate renal pelvis dilatation, there remains uncertainty about the risk of malformations and ongoing follow-up required once the baby is born.

What used to be termed 'soft markers' are no longer considered to have any significant impact on the risk of chromosomal malformation in isolation or combination. These are now termed 'normal variants' and are therefore not usually reported (choroid plexus cysts, two-vessel cord, dilated cisterna magna, echogenic cardiac focus).

Advantages and disadvantages of fetal anomaly scans. Provided the sonographer has sufficient expertise, many lethal or severely disabling conditions can be detected during the 18 to 20+⁶ week scan. Although this means that parents may be faced with difficult and unexpected decisions, it allows parents the choices that would be denied without this knowledge. Furthermore, many parents are offered reassurance that no obvious abnormalities were seen. For neonates requiring early surgical or paediatric interventions, prior knowledge of the abnormality allows a plan of care to be evolved in advance of the birth. The mother can then give birth in a unit with appropriate facilities. This has been shown to reduce morbidity in cases of gastroschisis (an abdominal wall defect, adjacent to the umbilicus, allowing the intestines and other abdominal organs to protrude outside the body), cardiac malformations and intestinal obstruction (Chen et al. 2014). For parents who choose to continue the pregnancy knowing that the baby has a life-limiting condition, careful planning regarding place of birth, care of the baby after birth and multidisciplinary support can be provided.

In summary, the 18–20 week scan appears to confer psychological and health improvement benefits in some cases, but also has the capacity to cause great anxiety and distress. Care must be taken to ensure that parents are fully informed of the purpose, benefits and limitations of ultrasound scans before they consent to this procedure.

New and Emerging Technologies

Fetal Imaging Techniques

Ultrasound scans in pregnancy have been discussed at length in this chapter, since they are important fetal investigations. Women generally see two-dimensional (2D) images of their unborn baby. However, there is a growing market for three-dimensional (3D) ultrasound imaging. As such, multiple images are stored digitally and then shaded to produce life-like pictures. This technique can assist the diagnosis of surface structural anomalies, such as cleft lip and spina bifida, and improvements are being seen in cardiac and neurological scanning (Sedgman et al. 2006; Seed 2016).

Magnetic resonance imaging (MRI) has also been applied in the examination of the fetus over the last two decades, and is now being used increasingly in clinical settings. Fetal MRI is most widely used to examine the fetal brain. There is evidence that this may provide additional information and change the counselling and management for a significant number of pregnancies where brain malformations are suspected (Glenn and Barkovich 2006). MRI is now also used to assess the cardiovascular system of the fetus where congenital heart disease is suspected (Seed 2016). A further application is that MRI offers an alternative to postmortem following termination or perinatal death. This can offer information to parents who decline postmortem because of its invasive nature (Sebire et al. 2012). MRI imaging has been used to refine the diagnosis of many other conditions including diaphragmatic hernias and sacrococcygeal teratomas (Kumar and O'Brien 2004).

SCREENING FOR MATERNAL CONDITIONS

The rationale for screening a mother is to detect conditions that are amenable to treatment and will have potential health benefits for her and her baby. In the main, in pregnancy, screening is focused on those that carry improved outcomes for the baby.

Infectious Diseases

In the UK, the NSC programme for screening of infectious diseases in pregnancy (PHE 2016) recommends that all pregnant women are screened for:
- human immune deficiency (HIV)
- syphilis
- hepatitis B (HBV)

The infectious diseases screened for meet the screening criteria, in that they are important and intervention can reduce harm. As well as allowing treatment of the mother and therefore reduction of risk to the fetus, awareness of the diagnosis can prevent unwitting infection of sexual partners.

Human Immune Deficiency Virus

Knowledge of current HIV infection allows for appropriate management in the antenatal period. This improves maternal health and reduces mother to child transfer to <1%. Screening should be offered at booking to all women, and again later in pregnancy in women at high risk (e.g. women who are paid for sex; women who have an untested partner from an area of high prevalence; intravenous drug users). Women who decline screening at booking should also be re-offered testing later in pregnancy.

Hepatitis B

Adequate immunization programmes for infants at risk of vertical transmission of hepatitis B virus (HBV) can reduce infant infection rates by 90% and improvements in maternal health can be made.

Referral to a specialist hepatologist or gastroenterologist is required for women who are found to be hepatitis B-positive. Establishing the neonatal and maternal risk will be determined by testing of antibody and antigen status and viral DNA levels. Occasionally, hepatitis B can reactivate in pregnancy and knowledge of status can aid management of the pregnant mother.

Syphilis

Syphilis used to be a rare infection in the UK, but the incidence is now inexorably rising. Untreated syphilis in pregnancy is associated with increased risk of pregnancy loss and intrauterine growth restriction. There is a risk of transmission to the fetus both transplacentally and at the time of vaginal birth if genital lesions are present. Identification and treatment of syphilis can reduce these risks and prevent long-term problems for the mother. A positive screening result does not distinguish between syphilis and other treponemal infections, so specialist input is required if the initial screening test is positive.

Testing for infection in early pregnancy is recommended. Written information should be provided at least 24 h prior to decisions being made. In order for the woman to make an informed choice, the midwife should discuss the following points:

- the infections that are screened for, their routes of transmission and the implications of a positive test
- the benefits, to both mother and baby, to be gained from the identification and management of those with positive results
- the results procedure, including the feedback of results and the possibility of a false-negative or false-positive result
- All pregnant women should be advised that if they develop, or are exposed to, a rash during the pregnancy they should seek professional advice.

Documentation should include the date that the offer was made and the response to the offer. Women who initially decline should be re-offered testing at a later date; usually it is best to do this before 28 weeks. If testing is declined, it is good practice to enquire why and to explore and document the reasons. Women who book late or who arrive untested in labour can be urgently screened with their consent.

Women with a positive result for syphilis, HIV or HBV should be seen and counselled as soon as possible and within 10 days, in the UK. Appropriate referrals should then be made to ensure that the correct care pathway is inducted.

Screening for infectious diseases in pregnancy can be enormously challenging for the mother and for the midwife. The cultural and social stigma that is still attached to a diagnosis of HIV means that some women will be reluctant to consider testing or may be devastated when a positive test is confirmed. Issues such as partner testing need sensitive exploration and should be undertaken by the wider multidisciplinary team that will care for these women. The midwife needs to have enough knowledge to understand the disease, the process following a positive test and the ability to answer questions or direct women to the answers.

Mid-Stream Urine Testing

Screening for asymptomatic bacteriuria is recommended, as in pregnancy progression to pyelonephritis can occur in up to 25% of women. Pyelonephritis can be life-threatening and can lead to miscarriage and premature labour. A mid-stream urine sample should be checked at every antenatal appointment. Findings on urine dip such as nitrites, blood and leucocytes should prompt the sample to be sent to the laboratory for culture, even in the absence of symptoms of urinary tract infection. If bacteriuria is found, treatment is simple and effective with appropriately targeted antibiotics.

Screening for Anaemia

Anaemia is one of the most common complications of pregnancy. The most common reason for iron deficiency anaemia in pregnancy is the increased demands of the fetus for iron. Risk factors for the development of iron deficiency in pregnancy include iron deficiency prior to pregnancy, hyperemesis, vegetarian or vegan diet, multiple pregnancies, pregnancy recurring after a short interval and blood loss.

Pregnant women should be offered screening for anaemia early in pregnancy and at 28 weeks. This allows enough time for treatment if anaemia is detected.

Haemoglobin levels outside the normal UK range for pregnancy (i.e. 110 mg/dL at first contact and 105 mg/dL at 28 weeks) should be investigated. Provided there are no unusual features to suggest another cause for the anaemia, treatment with iron can be started and a blood test for serum ferritin sent at the same time to confirm iron stores are low. The woman should be asked if she is known to have a haemoglobinopathy. These women should be directly referred to an obstetric haematology clinic for assessment. Women who are unable to tolerate oral iron therapy or who are still anaemic despite iron supplementation should be referred to the hospital for further investigation and management.

Screening for Red Cell Antibodies

All pregnant women should be offered antenatal testing at booking and at 28 weeks to assess ABO and rhesus status and to look for red cell antibodies.

Red cell antibodies are antibodies against red cell antigens, and the relevance to pregnancy will vary depending on the type and level of the circulating antibody. Some antibodies occur naturally, without any sensitizing event, but most of the important ones require a sensitizing event such as a previous pregnancy or transfusion. Antibodies to the ABO system tend to be naturally occurring, as does anti-E.

Once an antibody has been identified it is relevant to understand the issues for both the mother and baby.

For the mother with any red cell antibody, the major issue is related to increased difficulty in cross-matching blood. Women with antibodies will not be able to undergo rapid electronic cross-matching and therefore women at increased risk of haemorrhage either intrapartum or postpartum may require cross-matched blood to be requested for them prior to birth.

For the fetus, red cell antibodies are of significance, as IgG antibodies can cross the placenta. If the fetal red blood cells carry the antigen the antibody is directed against, they will be destroyed. This can lead to fetal anaemia and in severe cases cause fetal hydrops. Jaundice and kernicterus (brain damage caused by very high unconjugated bilirubin levels) in the neonatal period are the major neonatal risks (see Chapter 37).

Routine antibody testing in pregnancy aims to:
- identify Rhesus-negative women who will be eligible for anti-D immunoglobulin prophylaxis
- identify women who are difficult to crossmatch so that steps can be taken to minimize risk
- identify women with antibodies that put the fetus at risk of haemolytic disease of the newborn (HDN).

The UK recommends that all women should be tested at booking and again at 28 weeks' gestation (NICE 2008).

There are many red cell antibodies and it is useful to understand which ones are important causes of HDN.
- Antibodies to the Rhesus antigens are the most common to cause problems.
- Rhesus D antibodies are the principal causes of severe HDN.
- Rhesus c can cause HDN, especially if antibodies to Rhesus E are also present.
- Rarely antibodies to Rhesus E, e, C and CW can cause HDN.

Antibodies to non-Rhesus antigens can also cause HDN. Anti-K (Kell) antibodies are an important cause of severe HDN. These antibodies not only destroy the fetal red cells, but inhibit production in the bone marrow, exacerbating any developing anaemia.

Other antibodies known to cause HDN less commonly include anti-Fya (Duffy), anti-Jka (Kidd) and anti-S.

Antibodies to the ABO system may be detected on routine testing. In general, these occur in Group O women and are naturally occurring anti-A and anti-B antibodies. Because these antibodies are IgM antibodies they do not cross the placenta and do not harm the fetus. Occasionally some Group O women produce IgG antibodies when carrying Group A or B infants. These IgG

antibodies can cross the placenta and cause HDN, but this tends to be mild.

How the Results are Presented

Antibody levels are either given as the actual measured amount or as the dilution achieved before there is insufficient antibody to cause red cell clumping.

RhD and Rhc are always measured and the result will be given in IU/mL; hence the higher the result the worse the effects are likely to be.

Other antibody levels are expressed as titres. A titre of 1:2 means that after a single dilution there was no clumping of the red cells. This would be a low level of antibody. A titre of 1:16 states that there were four dilutions before the antibody was too weak to clump cells, implying a much higher level of antibody. It is useful to understand that a jump from 1:2 to 1:4 is a single dilution, as is a jump from 1:16 to 1:32.

What Parents Need to Know

Parents need to understand the purpose of blood group and red cell antibody screening, what is being tested for and what the test involves. This will involve discussion about the nature and effects of red cell antibodies, how and when test results will be available and the meaning of the results.

Management when an Antibody is Detected

When an antibody is detected it is important that the relevance of this is discussed with the mother. The discussion should cover the potential for difficulties in cross-matching blood and the potential for fetal or neonatal problems. If significant antibody titres are found, management needs to be discussed, including the need for surveillance for fetal anaemia and the possibility of intrauterine transfusion – this would usually be done by the obstetrician managing the pregnancy.

Surveillance will depend on the type of antibody found; for some antibodies, the titre (level) of the antibody and the gestation of pregnancy at which it is discovered.

Discussion with the consultant team is usually needed to define the steps that need to be taken. When an antibody is detected that may cause HDN the next steps will usually be:
1. Referral for discussion with an appropriate consultant/haematology team.

2. Partner testing. This is to determine the potential for fetal risk. Only a fetus that is antigen-positive for the antibody found can be at risk. This means that, for instance, if a woman has anti-D antibodies and an RhD-positive partner, there will be a 50–100% risk of producing a baby who is RhD-positive, depending on whether the partner carries one or two RhD-positive genes. It is imperative that the woman understands the importance of partner testing, the need to be honest if there can be any doubt regarding paternity (and for this to be asked about sensitively, without the partner being present). For IVF pregnancies, it is important to ask whether there has been egg donation, as in these cases, it may be the maternal genetic complement that differs and cases of HDN have occurred where this vital fact has not been ascertained.

3. Free fetal DNA testing. Where the fetus is potentially at risk because the partner is positive for the antigen to the detected antibody or where partner testing cannot be undertaken, typing of the fetal red cell status can be performed on a blood test from the woman. The test is usually carried out between 12 and 18 weeks. The results are accurate in 99% of cases but in some cases, a result cannot be given.

4. Confirmatory testing. Invasive testing using CVS or amniocentesis is usually undertaken only where there is a need to establish fetal karyotype for other reasons. In cases where ultrasound suggests developing anaemia, a fetal blood sample prior to intra-uterine transfusion will be tested for fetal blood typing.

Ongoing Surveillance

Once the risk of a pregnancy being affected has been established, the timing and frequency of repeat testing of antibody titres can be determined. The need for assessment of the fetus at risk can also be established.

Surveillance for fetal anaemia is now undertaken primarily using ultrasound measurement of the blood flow velocity within the fetal brain. Measurement of the maximum velocity in the fetal middle cerebral artery has been found to be as accurate as the old-fashioned measurement of bilirubin in amniotic fluid, but is without the attendant risks of serial amniocentesis.

The frequency of surveillance will be determined by the risk of anaemia, which is dependent on the type and level of antibody and the risk of the fetus being antigen-positive.

Non-Invasive Prenatal Testing for Fetal RhD Genotype

A number of studies have now looked at the role of NIPT for assessing fetal Rhesus D status from fetal cell free DNA when the mother is found to be Rhesus D-negative (Yang et al. 2019). As a woman who is Rhesus D-negative will not have any RHD gene present in her blood, the finding of RHD gene on a maternal blood test indicates that the fetus is Rhesus D-positive. The International Blood Group Reference Laboratory in Bristol have developed a polymerase chain reaction (PCR) test, which allows high-throughput testing so that women who are Rhesus D-negative can be screened for the fetal Rhesus status from 11 weeks' gestation. This has been shown to reduce the routine administration of anti-D without causing any significant increase in maternal sensitization. NICE (2016) recommends that NIPT is offered to women who are Rhesus-negative, as this will result in reduced administration of unnecessary blood products and is cost-efficient, providing the sample testing is <£24/test (at time of writing). This blood test would be offered at 16 weeks as part of the routine midwife appointment.

CONDITIONS NOT CURRENTLY SCREENED

Maternal Group B Streptococcus Carriage

Group B Streptococcus (GBS) is carried in the genital tract and gut of many healthy people (between 10% and 40%), and can be detected on a urine sample or vaginal swab. It is estimated that about 25% of pregnant women in the UK carry GBS. In the UK, GBS is either detected opportunistically or by screening in high-risk situations, such as after premature or prolonged rupture of the membranes. Women who are found to be GBS-positive on vaginal swabs or urine samples are offered IV antibiotics in labour to reduce the risk of early-onset GBS infection to the neonate. In 2017, the UK National Screening Committee (PHE 2017) reviewed the evidence and has recommended there is insufficient evidence to support a national screening programme.

Reasons for this include the difficulty predicting which babies are at risk of early onset GBS, and the effects of antibiotics on what could be up to 25% of the pregnant population.

In the USA, screening is offered by vaginal swabs at 35–37 weeks. However, the risk of GBS in the USA is considerably higher, again for reasons that are not entirely understood.

Vasa Praevia

Vasa praevia is a rare but important condition where vessels from the umbilical cord or placenta are present in the membranes close to the cervix. These vessels can sometimes be detected on antenatal ultrasound scanning. There is risk of damage to these vessels at the time of ruptured membranes or labour, leading to fetal blood loss and risk of serious harm or death for the baby. Women who are thought to have vasa praevia are recommended to have a planned caesarean section as the preferred mode of birth to reduce these risks. The National Screening Committee reviewed the evidence in 2017 and did not recommend routine screening for vasa praevia, as it is not clear at present how common the condition is, or how accurate ultrasound scans are for detecting the condition. There is therefore a risk that, until more evidence is available, women may be advised to have caesarean sections later proven to have been unnecessary.

CONCLUSION

Fetal investigations are an integral aspect of antenatal care. Scientists and clinicians have developed a range of new diagnostic and imaging technologies. Some of these have been incorporated into national screening programmes and standards of care. The midwife must therefore ensure that women are informed about the benefits and risks associated with these technologies, so that they can make choices to suit their requirements. Undoubtedly, testing technologies profoundly influence women's experiences of pregnancy and their early attachment to their unborn child. Midwives therefore have a duty to prepare women for tests through sensitive and accurate communications and then to support parents in their assimilation of information and decision-making once the results are known.

Maternal investigations also require careful counselling and thought, as a constellation of unintended consequences can arise if women do not think through their screening choices, or are inadequately counselled.

▋ REFLECTIVE ACTIVITY FOR SELF-ASSESSMENT

1. What is the key difference between an antenatal screening test and an antenatal diagnostic test for fetal anomaly?
2. What is meant by the term 'false-positive' when used in the context of the result relating to an antenatal screening test?
3. How would you explain the limitations and benefits of antenatal screening?

REFERENCES

Abramowicz, J. S. (2013). Benefits and risks of ultrasound in pregnancy. *Seminars in perinatology*, 37(5), 295–300.

Åhman, A., Sarkadi, A., Lindgren, P., et al. (2016). 'It made you think twice' – an interview study of women's perception of a web-based decision aid concerning screening and diagnostic testing for fetal anomalies. *BMC Pregnancy and Childbirth*, 16, 267.

Ahmed, S., Bryant, L. D., & Cole, P. (2013). Midwives' perceptions of their role as facilitators of informed choice in antenatal screening. *Midwifery*, 29(7), 745–750.

Asplin, N., Wessel, H., Marions, L., et al. (2013). Pregnant women's perspectives on decision-making when a fetal malformation is detected by ultrasound examination. *Sexual & Reproductive Healthcare*, 4(2), 79–84.

Berryman, J. C., & Windridge, K. C. (1999). Women's experiences of giving birth after 35. *Birth*, 26(1), 16–23.

Chen, Q. J., Gao, Z. G., Tou, J. F., et al. (2014). Congenital duodenal obstruction in neonates: A decade's experience from one center. *World Journal of Pediatrics*, 10(3), 238–244.

Côté-Arsenault, D., Krowchuk, H., Jenkins Hall, W., et al. (2015). We want what's best for our baby: Prenatal parenting of babies with lethal conditions. *Journal of Prenatal and Perinatal Psychology and Health, 29*(3), 157–176.

ECMUS (European Committee for Medical Ultrasound Safety). (2017). EFSUMB Clinical safety statement for diagnostic ultrasound. Available at: www.efsumb-archive.org/safety/resources/2017-clinical_safety_statement.pdf.

Fisher, J. (2006). Pregnancy loss, breaking bad news and supporting parents. In A. Sullivan, L. Kean, & A. Cryer (Eds.), *Midwife's guide to antenatal investigations* (pp. 31–42). London: Elsevier.

Glenn, O. A., & Barkovich, A. J. (2006). Magnetic resonance imaging of the fetal brain and spine: An increasingly important tool in prenatal diagnosis, Part 1. *American Journal of Neuroradiology, 27*, 1604–1611.

Glover, V. (2014). Maternal depression, anxiety and stress during pregnancy and child outcome; what needs to be done? *Best Practice and Research Clinical Obstetrics and Gynaecology, 28*(1), 25–35.

Green, J. M., Hewison, J., Bekker, H. L., et al. (2004). Psychosocial aspects of genetic screening of pregnant women and newborns: A systematic review. *Health Technology Assessment, 8*(33) Executive summary.

Hothi, D. K., Wade, A. S., Gilbert, R., et al. (2009). Mild fetal renal pelvis dilatation—much ado about nothing? *Clinical Journal of the American Society of Nephrology, 4*(1), 168–177.

Hunt, L. M., de Voogd, B., & Castaneda, H. (2005). The routine and the traumatic in prenatal genetic diagnosis: Does clinical information inform patient decision-making? *Patient Education and Counselling, 56*(3), 302–312.

Hunter, M. (1994). *Counselling in obstetrics and gynaecology.* Leicester: British Psychological Society Books.

Kennard, A., Goodburn, S., Golightly, S., et al. (1995). Serum screening for Down syndrome. *Royal College of Midwives Journal, 108*, 207–210.

Kessler, S., & Levine, E. (1987). Psychological aspects of genetic counselling IV. The subjective assessment of probability. *American Journal of Medical Genetics, 28*, 361–370.

Kingston, H. M. (2002). *ABC of clinical genetics* (3rd ed.). London: BMJ Publishing.

Kleinveld, J. H., Timmermans, D. R., de Smit, D. J., et al. (2006). Does prenatal screening influence anxiety levels of pregnant women? A longitudinal randomised controlled trial. *Prenatal Diagnosis, 26*(4), 354–361.

Kumar, S., & O'Brien, A. (2004). Recent developments in fetal medicine. *British Medical Journal, 328*, 1002–1006.

NICE (National Institute for Health and Care Excellence). (2008). (updated 2015) Antenatal care. *Routine care for the healthy pregnant woman.* Clinical Guideline: CG 62. London: NICE.

NICE (National Institute for Health and Care Excellence). (2016). *High-throughput non-invasive prenatal testing for fetal RHD genotype.* DG25. London: NICE.

Nieuwenhuijze, M. J., Korstjens, I., de Jonge, A., et al. (2014). On speaking terms: A Delphi study on shared decision-making in maternity care. *BMC Pregnancy and Childbirth, 14*, 223.

NSC (National Screening Committee). (2013). What is screening? Available at: www.gov.uk/guidance/nhs-population-screening-explained.

NMC (Nursing and Midwifery Council). (2018a). *Standards of competence for registered midwives.* London: NMC.

NMC (Nursing and Midwifery Council). (2018b). The Code: Professional standards of practice and behaviour for nurses, midwives and nursing associates. Available at: www.nmc.org.uk/standards/code/.

Oliver, S., Rajan, L., Turner, H., et al. (1996). *A pilot study of informed choice leaflets on positions in labour and routine ultrasound.* York: NHS Centre for Reviews and Dissemination.

PHE (Public Health England). (2013). Guidance: Sickle cell and thalassaemia screening: Programme overview. Available at: www.gov.uk/guidance/sickle-cell-and-thalassaemia-screening-programme-overview#thalassaemia.

PHE (Public Health England). (2016). *NHS infectious diseases in pregnancy screening programme standards 2016 to 2017.* Available at: www.gov.uk/government/publications/infectious-diseases-in-pregnancy-screening-programme-standards.

PHE (Public Health England). (2017). Press release: Screening pregnant women for GBS not recommended. Available at: www.gov.uk/government/news/screening-pregnant-women-for-gbs-not-recommended.

PHE (Public Health England). (2018a). Fetal anomaly screening programme service specifications 16 and 17. Available at: www.england.nhs.uk/publication/public-health-national-service-specifications/.

PHE (Public Health England). (2018b). Guidance: Our approach to fetal anomaly screening standards. Available at: www.gov.uk/government/publications/fetal-anomaly-screening-programme-standards/fetal-anomaly-screening-standards-valid-for-data-collected-from-1-april-2018.

PHE (Public Health England). (2018c). *NHS fetal anomaly screening programme handbook valid from August 2018.* Available at: www.gov.uk/government/publications/fetal-anomaly-screening-programme-handbook.

PHE (Public Health England). (2018d). Antenatal and newborn screening key performance indicators. Available at: www.gov.uk/government/publications/nhs-population-screening-reporting-data-definitions/antenatal-and-newborn-screening-kpis-for-2018-to-2019-definitions.

Raphael-Leff, J. (2005). *Psychological processes of childbearing.* London: Anna Freud Centre.

Raynor, M. D., & England, E. (2010). *Psychology for midwives: Pregnancy, childbirth and puerperium.* Open University Maidenhead: Press/McGraw-Hill.

Roberts, J. (2011). 'Wakey wakey baby': Narrating four–dimensional (4D) bonding scans. *Sociology of Health and Illness, 34*(2), 299–314.

Rothman, B. (1986). The tentative pregnancy. *How amniocentesis changes the experience of motherhood.* New York: Norton Paperbacks.

Sebire, N. J., Weber, M. A., Thayyil, S., et al. (2012). Minimally invasive perinatal autopsies using magnetic resonance imaging and endoscopic postmortem examination ('keyhole autopsy'): Feasibility and initial experience. *Journal of Maternal-Fetal & Neonatal Medicine, 25*(5), 513–518.

Sedgman, B., McMahon, C., Cairns, D., et al. (2006). The impact of two-dimensional versus three-dimensional ultrasound exposure on maternal–fetal attachment and maternal health behavior in pregnancy. *Ultrasound in Obstetrics and Gynecology, 27*, 245–251.

Seed, M. (2016). Fetal cardiovascular magnetic resonance. In G. Masselli (Ed.), *MRI of Fetal and Maternal Diseases in Pregnancy.* Cham: Springer.

Seror, V., & Ville, Y. (2009). Prenatal screening for Down syndrome: Women's involvement in Decision–making and their attitudes to screening. *Prenatal Diagnosis, 29*(2), 120–128.

Sjögren, B. (1996). Psychological indications for prenatal diagnosis. *Prenatal Diagnosis, 16*, 449–454.

Stephenson, N., McLeod, K., & Mills, C. (2016). Ambiguous encounters, uncertain foetuses: Women's experiences of obstetric ultrasound. *Feminist Review, 113*(1), 17–33.

Thornton, J. G., Hewison, J., Lilford, R. J., et al. (1995). A randomised trial of three methods of giving information about prenatal testing. *British Medical Journal, 311*, 1127–1130.

Turner, L. (2013). Problems surrounding late prenatal diagnosis. In L. Abramsky, & J. Chapple (Eds.), *Prenatal diagnosis: The human side.* London: Chapman & Hall.

Whitworth, M., Bricker, L., Neilson, J. P., et al. (2010). Ultrasound for fetal assessment in early pregnancy. *Cochrane Database of Systematic Reviews* (4), CD007058.

Yang, H., Llewellyn, A. R., Walker, R. A. E., et al. (2019). High-throughput, non-invasive prenatal testing for fetal rhesus D status in RhD-negative women: A systematic review and meta-analysis. *BMC Medicine, 17*(1), 37.

ANNOTATED FURTHER READING

Carlsson, T., Starke, V., & Mattsson, E. (2017). The emotional process from diagnosis to birth following a prenatal diagnosis of fetal anomaly: A qualitative study of messages in online discussion boards. *Midwifery, 48*, 53–59.

This article explores the range of emotions women experience after the breaking of significant news relating to prenatal diagnosis for fetal anomalies, and provides some insight as to what midwives and other healthcare professionals can do to help.

Lou, S., Nielsen, C. P., Hvidman, L., et al. (2016). Coping with worry while waiting for diagnostic results: A qualitative study of the experiences of pregnant couples following a high-risk prenatal screening result. *BMC Pregnancy and Childbirth, 16*(1), 321.

A useful perspective that highlights the importance of empathetic understanding and effective communication following screen-positive results.

USEFUL WEBSITES

Antenatal Results and Choices: www.arc-uk.org

Health Talk – Patient experiences website: www.health-talk.org

National Childbirth Trust: www.nct.org.uk

National Institute for Health and Care Excellence: www.nice.org.uk/

UK National Screening Committee: www.gov.uk

14

Problems Associated with Early and Advanced Pregnancy

Helen Crafter, Clare Gordon

CHAPTER CONTENTS

Problems of pregnancy range from the mildly irritating, to life-threatening conditions. Due to improvements in general health and social conditions in developed countries, lower parity and effective health care, severe morbidity and mortality are rare. However, as the obesity crisis develops and women delay childbearing, they become more at risk of disorders associated with increasing age such as placenta praevia and problems associated with excessive weight such as diabetes mellitus. Regular antenatal examinations beginning early in pregnancy are undoubtedly valuable. They help to prevent many complications and their ensuing problems, contribute to timely diagnosis and treatment and enable women to form relationships with midwives, obstetricians and the other health professionals who become involved with them in striving to achieve the best possible pregnancy outcomes.

THE CHAPTER AIMS TO

- provide an overview of problems of pregnancy
- describe the role of the midwife in relation to the identification, assessment and management of the more common disorders of pregnancy
- consider the needs of both parents for continuing support when a disorder has been diagnosed.

THE MIDWIFE'S ROLE

The midwife's role in relation to the problems associated with pregnancy is clear. At initial and subsequent encounters with the pregnant woman, it is essential that an accurate health history is obtained. General and specific physical examinations must be carried out and the results meticulously recorded. The examination and recordings enable effective referral and management. Where the midwife detects a deviation from the norm, which is outside her sphere of practice, she must refer the woman to a suitable qualified health professional and respect their skills, expertise and contributions (Nursing and Midwifery Council, NMC 2018a). The midwife will continue to offer the woman care and support throughout her pregnancy and beyond. The woman who develops problems during her pregnancy is no less in need of the midwife's skilled attention; indeed, her condition and psychological state may be considerably improved by the midwife's continued presence and support. It is also the midwife's role in such a situation to ensure that the woman and her family understand the situation; are enabled to take part in decision-making; and are protected from unnecessary fear. As the primary care manager, the midwife must ensure that all the attention the woman receives from different health professionals is balanced and integrated – in short, the woman's needs remain paramount throughout.

ABDOMINAL PAIN IN PREGNANCY

Abdominal pain is a common complaint in pregnancy. It is probably suffered by all women at some stage, and therefore presents a problem for the midwife in how to distinguish between the physiologically normal (e.g. mild indigestion or muscle stretching), the pathological but not dangerous (e.g. degeneration of a fibroid) and the dangerously pathological requiring immediate referral to the appropriate medical practitioner for urgent treatment (e.g. ectopic pregnancy or appendicitis).

The midwife should take a detailed history and perform a physical examination in order to reach a decision about whether to refer the woman. Treatment will depend on the cause (Box 14.1) and the maternal and fetal conditions.

Many of the pregnancy-specific causes of abdominal pain in pregnancy listed in Box 14.1 are dealt with in this and other chapters. For most of these conditions,

abdominal pain is one of many symptoms and not necessarily the overriding one. However, an observant midwife's skills may be crucial in procuring a safe pregnancy outcome for a woman presenting with abdominal pain.

BLEEDING BEFORE THE 24TH WEEK OF PREGNANCY

Any vaginal bleeding in early pregnancy is abnormal and of concern to the woman and her partner, especially if there is a history of previous pregnancy loss. The midwife can come into contact with women at this time, either through the booking clinic or through phone contact. If bleeding in early pregnancy occurs, a woman may contact the midwife, the birthing unit or a triage telephone helpline for advice and support. The midwife should be aware of the local policies pertaining to her employment and how to guide the woman. In some areas of the UK, women are reviewed within the maternity department from early pregnancy, whereas in others, they will be seen by the gynaecology team until 20 weeks' gestation, possibly in an early pregnancy clinic. However, women are often advised to contact their GP in the first instance, and many will visit an accident and emergency department.

In all cases, a history should be obtained to establish the amount and colour of the bleeding, when it occurred and whether there was any associated pain. Fetal wellbeing may be assessed either by ultrasound scan or, in the second trimester, using a handheld Doppler device to hear the fetal heart sounds. Maternal reporting of fetal movements may also be useful in determining the viability of a pregnancy.

There are many causes of vaginal bleeding in early pregnancy, some of which can occasionally lead to life-threatening situations and others of less consequence for the continuance of pregnancy. The midwife should be aware of the different causes of vaginal bleeding in order to advise and support the woman and her family accordingly.

Implantation Bleed

A small vaginal bleed can occur when the blastocyst embeds in the endometrium. This usually occurs 5–7 days after fertilization, and if the timing coincides with the expected menstruation, this may cause confusion over the dating of the pregnancy if the menstrual cycle is used to estimate the date of birth (see Chapter 5).

BOX 14.1 Causes of Abdominal Pain in Pregnancy

Pregnancy-specific causes

Physiological
- heartburn, soreness from vomiting, constipation
- Braxton Hicks contractions
- pressure effects from growing/vigorous/malpresenting fetus
- round ligament pain
- severe uterine torsion (can become pathological).

Pathological
- spontaneous miscarriage
- uterine leiomyoma
- ectopic pregnancy
- hyperemesis gravidarum (vomiting with straining)
- preterm labour
- chorioamnionitis
- ovarian pathology
- placental abruption
- spontaneous uterine rupture
- abdominal pregnancy
- trauma to abdomen (consider undisclosed domestic abuse)

- severe pre-eclampsia
- Acute fatty liver of pregnancy.

Incidental causes

More common pathology
- appendicitis
- acute cholestasis/cholelithiasis
- gastro-oesophageal reflux/peptic ulcer disease
- acute pancreatitis
- urinary tract pathology/pyelonephritis
- inflammatory bowel disease
- intestinal obstruction

Miscellaneous
- rectus haematoma
- sickle cell crisis
- porphyria
- malaria
- arteriovenous haematoma
- tuberculosis
- malignant disease
- psychological causes.

Adapted from Mahomed K. (2011) Abdominal pain. In: D. James (Ed.) High risk pregnancy management options. Philadelphia: Saunders Elsevier, pp. 1013–1026.

Cervical Ectropion

More commonly known as *cervical erosion*. The changes seen in cases of cervical ectropion are as a physical response to hormonal changes that occur in pregnancy. The number of columnar epithelial cells in the cervical canal increase significantly under the influence of oestrogen during pregnancy to such an extent that they extend beyond to the vaginal surface of the cervical os, giving it a dark red appearance. As this area is vascular, and the cells form only a single layer, bleeding may occur either spontaneously or following sexual intercourse. Normally, no treatment is required, and the ectropion reverts back to normal cervical cells during the puerperium.

Cervical Polyps

These are small, vascular, pedunculated growths on the cervix, which consist of squamous or columnar epithelial cells over a core of connective tissue rich with blood vessels. During pregnancy, the polyps may be a cause of bleeding, but require no treatment unless the bleeding is severe or a smear test indicates malignancy.

Carcinoma of the Cervix

Carcinoma of the cervix is the most common gynaecological malignant disease occurring in pregnancy with an estimated incidence of 1–2 per 2000 to 10,000 pregnancies (Salani and Copeland 2017). The most common presentation is vaginal bleeding and increased vaginal discharge, although around one-third of pregnant women diagnosed with cervical cancer are asymptomatic. On speculum examination, the appearance of the cervix may lead to a suspicion of carcinoma, which is diagnosed following colposcopy or a cervical biopsy.

The precursor to cervical cancer is cervical intraepithelial neoplasia (CIN), which can be diagnosed from an abnormal Papanicolaou (Pap) smear. Where this is diagnosed at an early stage, treatment can usually be postponed for the duration of the pregnancy. In the UK, the Pap smear is not routinely carried out during pregnancy, but the midwife should ensure that pregnant women know about the 'National Health Service Cervical Screening Programme' (NHS 2018), recommending a smear 3 months postnatally if one has not been carried out in the previous 3 years.

Treatment for cervical carcinoma in pregnancy will depend on the gestation of the pregnancy and the stage of the disease, and full explanations of treatments and their possible outcomes should be given to the woman and her family. For carcinoma in the early stages, treatment may be delayed until the end of the pregnancy, or a cone biopsy may be performed under general anaesthetic to remove the affected tissue. However, there is a risk of haemorrhage due to the increased vascularity of the cervix in pregnancy, as well as a risk of miscarriage. Where the disease is more advanced, and the diagnosis made in early pregnancy, the woman may be offered a termination of pregnancy in order to receive treatment, as the effects of chemotherapy and radiotherapy on the fetus cannot be accurately predicted at the present time. During the late second and third trimester, the obstetric and oncology teams will consider the optimal time for birth in order to achieve the best outcomes for both mother and baby.

Spontaneous Miscarriage

The term *miscarriage* is used to describe a spontaneous pregnancy loss in preference to the term *abortion*, which is associated with the deliberate ending of a pregnancy. In the UK, a miscarriage is seen as the loss of the products of conception prior to the completion of 24 weeks' gestation, with an early pregnancy loss being one that occurs before the 12th completed week of pregnancy (National Institute for Health and Care Excellence, NICE 2012).

It is estimated that 20% of pregnancies will end in a miscarriage, resulting in 50,000 hospital admissions annually. Approximately 1–2% of second trimester pregnancies will result in a miscarriage (Royal College of Obstetricians and Gynaecologists, RCOG 2011a). Methods of managing pregnancy loss are currently evolving, with more emphasis being placed on medical intervention and/or management.

In all cases of miscarriage, the woman and her family will need guidance and support from those caring for her. In all areas of communication, the language used should be appropriate, avoiding medical terms and should be respectful of the pregnancy loss. Following the miscarriage, the parents may wish to see and hold their baby, and will need to be supported in doing this by those caring for them. Even where there is no recognizable baby, some parents are comforted by being given this opportunity (Stillbirth and Neonatal Death Society,

SANDS 2016). It is also important to create memories for the parents in the form of photographs, and, for pregnancy losses in the second and third trimesters, footprints and handprints may be taken (see Chapter 31).

In the UK, for a pregnancy loss prior to 24 weeks' gestation, there is no legal requirement for a baby's birth to be registered or for a burial or cremation to take place. However, many National Health Service (NHS) facilities now make provision for a service for these babies, or parents may choose to make their own arrangements. In the case of cremation, the parents should be advised that there will be very few ashes.

Following a miscarriage, blood tests may be carried out on the woman, and depending on gestational age, the parents may be offered a postmortem examination of the fetal remains, in an effort to try to establish a reason for the pregnancy loss. However, in many cases, there is no identifiable cause. Should this be the case, the outlook for future pregnancies is generally good. Many early pregnancy losses are due to chromosomal malformations, resulting in a fetus that does not develop. Should a reason for the miscarriage be identified, it may be of some comfort to the woman and her partner to allow medical management to be put in place to enable a subsequent pregnancy to be more successful. A spontaneous miscarriage may present in a number of ways, all associated with a history of bleeding and/or lower abdominal pain.

A *threatened miscarriage* occurs where there is vaginal bleeding in early pregnancy, which may or may not be accompanied by abdominal pain. The cervical os remains closed, and in about 80% of women presenting with these symptoms, a viable pregnancy will continue.

Where the abdominal pain persists and the bleeding increases, the cervix opens and the products of conception will pass into the vagina in an *inevitable miscarriage*. Should some of the products be retained, this is termed an *incomplete miscarriage*. These women will be offered a dose of 600 micrograms (µg) misoprostol as a form of treatment (NICE 2012). Infection is a risk with incomplete miscarriage and therapeutic termination of pregnancy. The signs and symptoms of miscarriage are present, accompanied by uterine tenderness, offensive vaginal discharge and pyrexia. In some cases, this may progress to overwhelming sepsis, with the accompanying symptoms of hypotension, renal failure and disseminated intravascular coagulation (DIC). The remaining products may be passed spontaneously to become a *complete miscarriage.*

Where there is a *missed* or *silent miscarriage*, a pregnancy sac with identifiable fetal parts is seen on ultrasound examination, but there is no fetal heartbeat. There may be some abdominal pain and bleeding but the products of the pregnancy are not always passed spontaneously. Women will be offered a dose of 800 μg misoprostol for the medical treatment of a missed miscarriage (NICE 2012).

The first priority with any woman presenting with vaginal bleeding is to ensure that she is haemodynamically stable. Profuse bleeding may occur where the products of conception are partially expelled through the cervix.

Human chorionic gonadotrophic hormone (hCG) is present in the maternal blood from 9–10 days following conception, and assessing hCG levels may be used as an indication of the pregnancy's viability. Where a woman has persistent bleeding, serial readings can be taken to assess the progress of a pregnancy or distinguish an ectopic pregnancy from a complete miscarriage where the uterus is empty on an ultrasound scan. The levels of hCG double every 48 h in a normal intrauterine pregnancy from 4 to 6 weeks' gestation.

As a pregnancy progresses, transvaginal ultrasound and/or abdominal ultrasound may be used to confirm the presence or absence of a viable pregnancy sac (NICE 2012). A gentle vaginal or speculum examination may also be performed to ascertain if the cervical os is open, and to observe for the presence of any products of conception within the vagina.

In the case of threatened miscarriage where viability of the pregnancy has been confirmed, there is no specific treatment as the likelihood of the pregnancy progressing is usually good. The practice of bed rest to preserve pregnancy is not supported by evidence so women should be neither encouraged nor discouraged from doing this.

For a complete miscarriage, there also is no required treatment if the woman's condition is stable, however the woman should receive expectant management for 7–14 days (NICE 2012) during which time the woman and her family will be offered support and guidance to deal with their loss.

If there are retained products of conception, an incomplete or missed miscarriage, the options for treatment will often depend on gestational age and the condition of the woman. Miscarriages may be managed expectantly, medically or surgically. In many cases, the appropriate management is to wait for the products of the conception to be passed spontaneously. However, women should be aware that this can take several weeks (NICE 2012). Women adopting this option must be given written and oral information regarding the probable sequence of events and be provided with contact details for further advice, with the option of admission to hospital if required (NICE 2012). It is important that women are educated to actively observe for signs of infection and know what to do if they suspect this.

The surgical method, where the uterine cavity is evacuated of the retained products of conception (ERPC) prior to 14 weeks' gestation, is suitable for women who do not want to be managed expectantly and who are not suitable for medical management. Under either a general or local anaesthetic the cervix is dilated and a suction curettage is used to empty the uterus. The use of prostaglandins prior to surgery makes the cervix easier to dilate, thus reducing the risk of cervical damage. Between 1% and 2% of surgical evacuations result in serious morbidity for the woman with the main complications being perforation of the uterus, tears to the cervix and haemorrhage.

Medical management of miscarriages involves the use of prostaglandins, such as misoprostol administered vaginally, however an oral option is a suitable alternative should the woman prefer. Women will often spend time at home between the administration of the first drug and subsequent treatment, so it should be ensured that they have full knowledge of what might happen and a contact number to use at any time. Although the complications include abdominal pain and bleeding, overall the medical management of miscarriage reduces both the number of hospital admissions and the time women spend in hospital. These women should be offered analgesia and antiemetics during this time.

Recurrent Miscarriage

Tests may be carried out on the woman and fetus following a miscarriage to try to establish any underlying cause. This is especially important where there is a history of recurrent miscarriage. Recurrent miscarriage can be defined as the loss of three or more consecutive pregnancies. Following several consecutive pregnancy losses a referral is usually made to a specialist recurrent miscarriage clinic (RCOG 2011a), where appropriate investigations, accurate information and support can be given.

There are several risk factors for recurrent miscarriage: epidemiological factors such as maternal and paternal age and previous reproductive history; antiphospholipid syndrome – which is the most treatable cause of recurrent miscarriage; genetic factors with around 2–5% of couples with recurrent miscarriage carrying some sort of chromosomal anomaly; anatomical factors such as congenital uterine malformation and cervical weakness; endocrine factors such as polycystic ovary syndrome, diabetes and thyroid disease; and inherited thrombophilic defects such as factor V Leiden (RCOG 2011a). It is recommended that all women with recurrent miscarriage are screened before another pregnancy for antiphospholipid antibodies. Where this is confirmed, treatment is with a low-dose aspirin plus low molecular-dose heparin. Genetic reasons for the miscarriage may be identified through karyotyping of the fetal tissue, as well as both parents. All women should also receive a pelvic ultrasound to assess the uterine anatomy and any suspected anomalies would require further investigation. Women with a second trimester miscarriage should be offered screening for inherited thrombophilias. Other treatments depend on the cause, or causes, of the miscarriages being identified.

Ectopic Pregnancy

An ectopic pregnancy occurs when a fertilized ovum implants outside the uterine cavity, often within the fallopian tube. However, implantation can also occur within the abdominal cavity (for instance on the large intestine or in the Pouch of Douglas), the ovary or in the cervical canal. The incidence is 11 per 1000 pregnancies, with approximately 11,000 ectopic pregnancies diagnosed each year (RCOG 2016a). There is a maternal mortality of 0.2 per 1000 associated with ectopic pregnancies (NICE 2012).

The conceptus produces hCG in the same way as for a uterine pregnancy, maintaining the corpus luteum, which leads to the production of oestrogen and progesterone and the preparation of the uterus to receive the fertilized ovum. However, following implantation in an abnormal site, the conceptus continues to grow, and in the more common case of an ectopic pregnancy in the fallopian tube, until the tube ruptures often accompanied by catastrophic bleeding in the woman, or until the embryo dies.

Many ectopic pregnancies occur with no identifiable risk factors. However, it is recognized that damage to the fallopian tube through a previous ectopic pregnancy or previous tubular surgery increases the risk, as do smoking and in vitro fertilization. Further risk factors include a pregnancy that commences with an intrauterine contraceptive device (IUCD) *in situ* or the woman conceives while taking the progestogen-only pill.

Ectopic (tubal) pregnancies most commonly present with vaginal bleeding and a sudden onset of lower abdominal or pelvic pain, which is initially one-sided, but spreads as blood enters the peritoneal cavity. There is referred shoulder tip pain caused by the blood irritating the diaphragm.

In 25% of cases, the presentation will be acute, with hypotension and tachycardia. On abdominal palpation, there is abdominal distension, guarding and tenderness, which assists in confirming the diagnosis. However, in the majority of cases, the presentation is less acute, so there should be a suspicion of ectopic pregnancy in any woman who presents with amenorrhea and lower abdominal pain. In these cases, the presentation may be confused with that of a threatened or incomplete miscarriage or a urinary tract infection, thus delaying appropriate treatment.

A transvaginal ultrasound of the lower abdomen is a useful diagnostic tool in confirming the site of the pregnancy. A single blood test for hCG level may be either positive (where the corpus luteum remains active) or negative, so is of limited diagnostic value. Serial testing is of greater value.

The basis of treatment in the acute, advanced presentation is surgical removal of the conceptus and ruptured fallopian tube, as these threaten the life of the woman if she is not stabilized and treated rapidly. In the majority of cases, surgery is currently by laparoscopy as opposed to a laparotomy, as this reduces blood loss, as well as postoperative pain. The ectopic pregnancy may either be removed through an incision in the tube itself, a salpingotomy or by removing part of the fallopian tube, i.e. a salpingectomy. Although a salpingotomy will enable a higher chance of a uterine pregnancy in the future, it is associated with a higher incidence of subsequent tubal pregnancies (RCOG 2016a).

Where the fetus has died, hCG levels will fall and the ectopic pregnancy may resolve itself, with the products either being reabsorbed or miscarried. Medical management is also a choice where the diagnosis of an ectopic pregnancy is made and the woman is haemodynamically stable. Methotrexate is given in a single dose according to the woman's body weight (RCOG 2016a), and works by interfering with DNA (deoxyribonucleic acid) synthesis, thus preventing the continued growth of the fetus (NHS Choices 2016). Should this be the treatment of choice, the woman should be informed that further treatment may be needed as well as how to access support at any time should it be required (RCOG 2016a).

Women who are Rhesus-negative should be given anti-D immunoglobulin as recommended by national and local guidelines following any form of pregnancy loss (RCOG 2016a).

OTHER PROBLEMS IN EARLY PREGNANCY

Cervical Insufficiency

Formally known as *incompetent cervix, cervical insufficiency* will lead to silent, painless dilatation of the cervix and loss of the products of conception, either as a miscarriage or a preterm birth. The incidence varies between 1:100 and 1:2000, the large variation being due to differences in populations and reporting bias between practitioners (Ludmir et al. 2017).

The cervix consists mainly of connective tissue, collagen, elastin, smooth muscle and blood vessels, and undergoes complex changes during pregnancy. The exact mechanism for an insufficient cervix is unknown, but the risk is increased where there has been trauma to the cervix during surgical procedures such as a dilatation and curettage or cone biopsy, or the weakness may be of congenital origin.

The diagnosis of an insufficient cervix is usually made retrospectively on review of gynaecological and obstetric history and after other causes have been eliminated. There will have been a painless dilatation of the cervix typically followed by premature rupture of the membranes, preterm birth or miscarriage. A formal diagnosis is made using a transvaginal ultrasound when the cervical length will be measured as <25 mm and/or cervical changes will be detected prior to 24 weeks' gestation and spontaneous preterm birth before 37 weeks' gestation will have occurred (Ludmir et al. 2017).

A cervical cerclage may be inserted. This suture is inserted around the cervix and tightened to keep the cervix closed around the end of the first trimester or start of the second trimester and remains *in situ* until 37 weeks' gestation, unless there are earlier signs of labour. The associated risks are that the cervix may dilate with the suture *in situ*, leading to lacerations of the cervix and infection. In 3% of cases, the cervix fails to dilate during labour, resulting in a caesarean section (Ludmir et al. 2017). However, there is a lack of evidence to support the efficacy of this procedure, and both the procedure and the implications should be fully discussed with the woman (NICE 2007).

Gestational Trophoblastic Disease

In this condition, there is abnormal placental development, resulting in either a complete *hydatidiform mole* or a *partial mole* and there is no viable fetus. The grape-like appearance of the mole is due to the over-proliferation of chorionic villi. Usually, this is a benign condition, which becomes apparent in the second trimester, characterized by vaginal bleeding, a larger than expected uterus, hyperemesis gravidarum and often symptoms of pre-eclampsia. However, if a molar pregnancy does not spontaneously miscarry, two associated disorders can occur: *gestational trophoblastic neoplasia* (GTN) where the mole remains *in situ* and is diagnosed by continuing raised hCG levels and ultrasound scanning; and *choriocarcinoma,* which can arise as a malignant variation of the disease. It is thought that 3% of complete hydatidiform moles will progress to choriocarcinoma.

In the UK, gestational trophoblastic disease (GTD) is a rare event, but women of Asian origin are at higher risk. There is an increased risk in women below the age of 16 and above the age of 45. If there has been a previous GTD, the risk of occurrence increases (Seckl et al. 2013). Other risk factors include a previous molar pregnancy and those with blood type Group A or AB. Treatment is by evacuation of the uterus, followed by histology of the tissue to enable accurate diagnosis of molar pregnancy (RCOG 2010).

Due to the risk of carcinoma developing following a molar pregnancy, all cases should be followed up at a trophoblastic screening centre, with serial blood or urine hCG levels being monitored. In the UK, this programme has resulted in 98–100% of cases being successfully treated and only 5–8% requiring chemotherapy (RCOG 2010). Where the hCG levels are within normal limits within 56 days of the end of the pregnancy, follow-up continues for a further 6 months. However, if the hCG levels remain raised at this point, the woman will continue to be assessed until the levels are within normal limits. Following subsequent pregnancies, hCG levels should be monitored for 6–8 weeks to ensure that there is no recurrence of the disease (RCOG 2010).

Following a hydatidiform mole, those women who are Rhesus-negative should be administered anti-D immunoglobulin as recommended by national and local guidelines.

Uterine Fibroid Degeneration

Fibroids (leiomyomas) can degenerate during pregnancy as a result of their diminishing blood supply, resulting in abdominal pain as the tissue becomes ischaemic and necrotic. Suitable analgesia and rest are indicated until the pain subsides, although it can be a recurring problem throughout a pregnancy. Not all fibroids degenerate during pregnancy, as some may receive an increased blood supply, causing enlargement with the consequential impact of obstructing labour.

Induced Abortion/Termination of Pregnancy

In the UK, under the terms of the Abortion Act 1967, amended by the updated Human Fertilisation and Embryology Act 2008, provision is made for a pregnancy to be terminated up to 23 weeks and 6 days of pregnancy for a number of reasons and with the written agreement of two registered medical practitioners. The medical practitioners must agree that, in their opinion, the termination is justified under the terms of the statutory Act (see Box 14.2) In the UK, in 2017, 197,700 terminations of pregnancy were undertaken; the majority of these occurring before 20 weeks' gestation (Department of Health, DH 2018). It should be noted that the law in Northern Ireland and the Republic of Ireland is highly restricted but women have the right to travel to another country for a termination. The UK Government in 2017 agreed to cover the cost of abortion for women who travel from Northern Ireland to England, Wales or Scotland (RCOG 2018).

The majority of terminations in the UK are carried out under clause (a) of the Abortion Act, meaning that continuing the pregnancy would involve a greater mental or physical risk to the woman or her existing family than if the pregnancy were terminated. Prior to any termination of pregnancy, the woman should receive counselling to discuss the options available. Whatever the reason for the termination, support should be offered before, during and following the procedure. In many cases, the care and support provided for women

> ### BOX 14.2   Statutory Grounds for Termination of Pregnancy
>
> - that the pregnancy has not exceeded its 24th week and that the continuance of the pregnancy would involve risk, greater than if the pregnancy were terminated, of injury to the physical or mental health of the pregnant woman or any existing children of her family; or
> - that the termination is necessary to prevent grave permanent injury to the physical or mental health of the pregnant woman; or
> - that the continuance of the pregnancy would involve risk to the life of the pregnant woman, greater than if the pregnancy were terminated; or
> - that there is a substantial risk that if the child were born it would suffer from such physical or mental abnormalities as to be seriously handicapped.

From the Abortion Act (1967). Amended by the Human Fertilisation and Embryology Act (2008).

experiencing a spontaneous miscarriage will also apply to those undergoing an induced termination of pregnancy. The reasons for the termination may include malformations of the fetus that are incompatible with life, or a condition that adversely affects the health of the women such that terminating the pregnancy offers the best option to expedite appropriate and timely treatment.

Before the commencement of the termination, it must be ensured that the HSA1 form, which is a legal requirement of the Abortion Act 1967 has been completed and signed by the two medical personnel agreeing to the termination. In addition, it is also a legal requirement that the Chief Medical Officer is notified of all terminations of pregnancy that take place, within 14 days of their occurrence (Sexual Health Policy Team 2014), by the practitioners completing form HSA4. The data on this form is then used for statistical purposes and monitoring terminations of pregnancies that take place within the UK. Only a medical practitioner can terminate a pregnancy. However, in practice, drugs that are prescribed to induce the termination may be administered by registered nurses and midwives working in this area of clinical practice.

The methods used for terminating the pregnancy will depend on the gestational age. Prior to 14 weeks' gestation, the pregnancy is generally terminated surgically by gradually dilating the cervix with a series of dilators and evacuating the uterus via vacuum aspiration or suction curettes. This may be carried out under general or local anaesthesia.

Terminations in later pregnancy are carried out medically, using a regime of drugs to prepare and dilate the cervix. The actual regime used may vary across healthcare providers. Current practice is to use a combination of mifepristone (a progesterone antagonist) and misoprostol (a synthetic prostaglandin) followed by further doses 24–48 h later, either vaginally or via the sublingual route. The woman may return home in between the administration of the two drugs and must be provided with clear information about what to expect; the contact details of a named healthcare professional; and the reassurance that admission to hospital can be at any time. During the termination, analgesia appropriate to her needs should be available.

A termination of pregnancy should not result in the live birth of the fetus. To this effect, should the procedure take place after 21 weeks and 6 days' gestation, feticide may be performed prior to the commencement of the termination process. This involves an injection of potassium chloride being injected into the fetal heart to prevent the fetus being born alive (RCOG 2011b).

Where nurses and midwives have a conscientious objection to termination of pregnancy, they have the right to refuse to be involved in such procedures. However, they cannot refuse to give life-saving care to a woman, and must always be non-judgemental in any care and contact that they provide (NMC 2018b).

As with other pregnancy losses, those women who undergo a termination of pregnancy and are Rhesus-negative will require anti-D immunoglobulin as recommended by national and local guidelines.

Pregnancy Problems Associated with Assisted Conception

There are a number of techniques available to attempt assisted conception for women and couples who have fertility problems. However, achieving a pregnancy is not always the end of the difficulties that may occur.

A serious condition is that of *ovarian hyperstimulation syndrome*. When fertility drugs have been taken to stimulate the production of follicles, massive enlargement of the ovaries and multiple cysts can develop (RCOG 2016b). Around a quarter of women taking fertility drugs will experience a mild form of this syndrome, but in a considerable percentage

(0.5–5%), this develops to include oliguria, renal failure and hypovolaemic shock (Mahomed and Kumar 2017). This risk increases when pregnancy has been achieved. The condition itself subsides spontaneously, but medical support and treatment is required for those who are severely unwell.

In assisted conception, the risk of miscarriage is approximately 14.7%. This rate is probably associated with the quality and length of freezing of the oocytes or embryos that are used. However, there are no differences in the number of chromosomal malformations when compared with spontaneous pregnancies (Mahomed and Kumar 2017).

The number of multiple pregnancies increases with assisted conception, with rates of 27% for twins and 3% for triplets (Mahomed and Kumar 2017). Assisted reproductive technology accounts for 1% of all births, but 18% of all multiple births; consequently multiple birth in itself is a risk factor for pregnancy (see Chapter 16). With all pregnancies resulting from assisted techniques, there is an increase in the rate of preterm birth, small for gestational age babies, placenta praevia, pregnancy induced hypertension and gestational diabetes. The reasons for these rates are not known, but it is considered that they relate to the original factors leading to the infertility (Mahomed and Kumar 2017).

Nausea, Vomiting and Hyperemesis Gravidarum

Nausea and vomiting are common symptoms of pregnancy, affecting approximately 75% of women (Gregory et al. 2017), with the onset from 4–8 weeks' gestation and lasting until 16–20 weeks (NICE 2010). Very occasionally, the symptoms persist for the whole of the pregnancy. From the woman's point of view, nausea and vomiting is frequently dismissed by others as being a common symptom of physiological pregnancy, so the impact that it may have on her life and that of her family may be ignored (Tiran 2014).

The cause of these symptoms are thought to be as a result of higher levels of hCG that is present when nausea and vomiting is most prevalent, and the relaxation of the smooth muscle of the stomach. However, there is little data to support this (Antony et al. 2017). There is substantial evidence to support the use of raw root ginger to help in reducing the symptoms, as is wrist acupressure or acupuncture, a form of treatment for nausea in pregnancy often chosen by women as it is drug-free (Tiran 2014).

According to Tiran (2014), acupressure or acupuncture on the Nei guan acupuncture point of the wrist has been shown to alleviate symptoms of nausea and vomiting.

Hyperemesis gravidarum is the most severe form of nausea and vomiting and occurs in 0.3–3% of pregnancies (London et al. 2017). The woman presents with a history of vomiting that has led to weight loss and dehydration, which may also be associated with postural hypotension, tachycardia, ketosis and electrolyte imbalance, and this will often require hospitalization (Gregory et al. 2017). Intravenous fluids are given to rehydrate the woman and correct the electrolyte imbalance, with antiemetics being administered to control the vomiting. Very often a combination of drugs will be needed in order to achieve this. It is important to exclude other conditions, such as a urinary tract infection, disorders of the gastrointestinal tract or a molar pregnancy, where vomiting may also be excessive.

The aim of treatment is not only to stabilize the woman's condition, but also to prevent further complications. Continual vomiting during the pregnancy may lead to vitamin deficiencies, and/or hyponatraemia, which can present with confusion and seizures, leading ultimately to respiratory arrest if left untreated (Gregory et al. 2017). For women who are immobilized through the severity of the vomiting, deep vein thrombosis is also a potential complication due to the combination of dehydration and immobility. In cases of hyperemesis gravidarum the fetus may be at risk of being small for gestational age due to a lack of nutrients.

Pelvic Girdle Pain

During pregnancy, the activity of pregnancy hormones, especially relaxin, can cause the ligaments supporting the pelvic joints to relax, allowing for slight movement. The resulting lumbopelvic pain affects 50–70% of women in pregnancy, for which adequate rest, attention to good posture, back massage, a simple support garment and occasional mild analgesia, will allow women to cope effectively. However, pelvic girdle pain (PGP), formerly known as *symphysis pubis dysfunction*, occurs when this relaxation is excessive, allowing the pelvic bones to move asymmetrically when the woman is walking. PGP usually starts from around 28 weeks of pregnancy and for the 14–22% of affected women, the pain will be disabling and lead to severe mobility difficulties. Some women also experience pain and discomfort when lying down in certain positions and on standing (Association of Chartered Physiotherapists in Women's Health, ACPWH 2015).

On suspecting that a woman has PGP, the midwife should explain the condition and the possible causes to the woman and organize a referral to an obstetric physiotherapist. The woman should be advised to rest appropriately and undertake activities that do not cause her further pain. Very often, movement that involves abducting the hips increases the pain and discomfort. A physiotherapist can be helpful in advising on mobility and coping with daily tasks, and in supplying aids such as pelvic girdle support belts and in extreme cases, crutches, so that the pain may be reduced.

A plan for both pregnancy and care in labour should be developed and recorded, so that the midwives caring for the woman during the birth are aware of the PGP and any positions that can be beneficial, such as being upright and kneeling, as well as the woman's analgesia requirements. As there may be a reduction in hip abduction, the midwife should take care when performing vaginal examinations, and the lithotomy position should be avoided. If instrumental birth is advisable, ventouse extraction is preferred with the woman in the left lateral position (ACPWH 2015). However, some women will prefer caesarean birth. Postnatally, the ligaments slowly return to their pre-pregnant condition, but this may take some time and around 7% of women continue to experience severe pelvic pain. Extra support may be required and sometimes physiotherapy may need to be continued beyond the postnatal period.

BLEEDING AFTER THE 24TH WEEK OF PREGNANCY

Antepartum Haemorrhage

Antepartum haemorrhage (APH) is bleeding from the genital tract after the 24th week of pregnancy, and before the onset of labour. It complicates 3–5% of pregnancies and globally, it is a leading cause of perinatal and maternal mortality (RCOG 2011c). As shown in Table 14.1, it is caused by:
- bleeding from local lesions of the genital tract (*incidental causes*)
- placental separation due to *placenta praevia* or *placental abruption*.

Effect on the mother

A small amount of bleeding will not physically affect the woman (unless she is already severely anaemic) but it is

TABLE 14.1 Causes of Bleeding in Late Pregnancy

Cause:
Placenta praevia
Placental abruption
'Unclassified bleeding'
- Show
- Cervicitis
- Trauma
- Vulvovaginal varicosities
- Genital tumours
- Genital infections
- Vasa praevia

Adapted from Navti OB, Konje JC. (2017) Bleeding in late pregnancy. In: D James, PJ Steer, CP Weiner, et al. (Eds) High risk pregnancy management options. Cambridge: Cambridge University Press, pp. 1557–1580.

likely to cause her anxiety. In cases of heavier bleeding, this may be accompanied by medical shock and blood clotting disorders. The midwife will be aware that the woman can die or be left with permanent morbidity if bleeding in pregnancy is not dealt with promptly and effectively.

Effect on the fetus

Fetal mortality and morbidity are increased as a result of severe vaginal bleeding in pregnancy. Stillbirth or neonatal death may occur. Premature placental separation and consequent hypoxia may result in severe neurological damage in the baby.

Initial appraisal of a woman with antepartum haemorrhage

Antepartum haemorrhage is unpredictable and the woman's condition can deteriorate at any time. A rapid decision about the urgency of need for a medical or paramedic presence, or both, must be made, often at the same time as observing and talking to the woman and her partner.

Assessment of maternal condition
- Take a history from the woman.
- Assess basic observations of temperature, pulse rate, respiratory rate and blood pressure, including their documentation.
- Observe for any pallor or restlessness.
- Assess the blood loss (consider retaining soiled sheets and clothes in case a second opinion is required).

- Perform a *gentle* abdominal examination, while assessing for signs of labour.
- **On no account must any vaginal or rectal examination be undertaken, nor should an enema or suppositories be administered to a woman experiencing an APH as these could result in torrential haemorrhage.**

Sometimes, bleeding that the woman had presumed to be from the vagina may be from haemorrhoids or haematuria. The midwife should consider this differential diagnosis and confirm or exclude this as soon as possible by careful questioning and examination.

Assessment of fetal condition
- The woman is asked if the baby has been moving as much as normal.
- An attempt should be made to listen to the fetal heart. An ultrasound apparatus may be used in order to obtain information. However, if the woman is at home and the bleeding is severe, this would not be a priority. The midwife will need to ensure the women is transferred to hospital as soon as her condition is stabilized in order to give the fetus the best chance of survival. Speed of action is vital.

Supportive treatment for moderate or severe blood loss and/or maternal collapse should consist of:
- providing ongoing emotional support for the woman and her partner/relatives
- administering rapid fluid replacement (warmed) with a plasma expander, with whole blood if necessary
- administering appropriate analgesia
- arranging transfer to hospital by the most appropriate means, if the woman is at home.

Management of antepartum haemorrhage depends on the definite diagnosis (see Table 14.2).

Placenta Praevia

In this condition, the placenta is partially or wholly implanted in the lower uterine segment. The lower uterine segment grows and stretches progressively after the 12th week of pregnancy. In later weeks, this may cause the placenta to separate and severe bleeding can occur. The amount of bleeding is not usually associated with any particular type of activity and commonly occurs when the woman is resting. The low placental location allows all of the lost blood to escape unimpeded and a retroplacental clot is not formed. For this reason, pain is not a feature of placenta praevia. Some women with this

TABLE 14.2   Comparison of Clinical Issues in Placental Abruption and Placenta Praevia

Comparison	Placental Abruption	Placenta Praevia
Onset of bleeding	May follow trauma (road traffic accident, domestic violence) but usually unprovoked Amount variable May contain clots	Almost always unprovoked Usually heavy No clots present
Signs	Generalized abdominal pain *if* some blood is trapped behind the placenta (concealed) When acute bleeding ceases, altered (old, brown) blood will continue vaginally for a few hours	Always painless Bleeding is always fresh (bright red)
Initial symptoms for moderate and severe blood loss	Temperature may be raised if there is infection in the uterus (sepsis) Pulse and respirations may be raised due to blood loss and shock Blood pressure low due to blood loss and shock	Temperature normal Pulse and respirations may be raised due to blood loss and shock Blood pressure low due to blood loss and shock
On palpation	Uterus tense and painful *if* there is concealed blood loss If palpation is possible (i.e. not too painful for the woman), fetal presentation and engagement not affected by abruption Fetal heart rate may be normal, erratic or absent	Non-tender uterus Likely fetal malpresentation, as the placenta occupies the pelvis Fetal heart rate may be normal, erratic or absent
On diagnostic ultrasound scan	Normally situated placenta Blood clots may be seen in the cavity of the uterus	Placenta is lying in the lower segment of the uterus

condition have a history of a small repeated blood loss at intervals throughout pregnancy, whereas others may have a sudden single episode of vaginal bleeding after the 20th week. However, severe haemorrhage occurs most frequently after the 34th week of pregnancy. The degree of placenta praevia does not necessarily correspond to the amount of bleeding. A type 4 placenta praevia may never bleed before the onset of spontaneous labour or elective caesarean section in late pregnancy or, conversely, some women with placenta praevia type 1 may experience relatively heavy bleeding from early in their pregnancy.

Degrees of placenta praevia

Type 1 placenta praevia. The majority of the placenta is in the upper uterine segment (Figs 14.1, 14.5). Blood loss is usually mild and the mother and fetus remain in good condition. Vaginal birth is possible.

Type 2 placenta praevia. The placenta is partially located in the lower segment near the internal cervical os (marginal placenta praevia) (Figs 14.2, 14.6). Blood loss is usually moderate, although the conditions of the mother and fetus can vary. Fetal hypoxia is more likely

to be present than maternal shock. Vaginal birth is possible, particularly if the placenta is anterior.

Type 3 placenta praevia. The placenta is located over the internal cervical os but not centrally (Figs 14.3, 14.7). Bleeding is likely to be severe, particularly when the lower segment stretches and the cervix begins to efface and dilate in late pregnancy. Vaginal birth is inappropriate because the placenta precedes the fetus.

Type 4 placenta praevia. The placenta is located centrally over the internal cervical os (Figs 14.4, 14.8) and torrential haemorrhage is very likely. Caesarean section is essential to save the lives of the woman and fetus.

Incidence

Placenta praevia affects 2.8 per 1000 of singleton pregnancies and 3.9 per 1000 of twin pregnancies (Navti and Konje 2017). There is a higher incidence of placenta praevia among women with increasing age and parity, in women who smoke and those who have had a previous caesarean section. Furthermore, it is known that there is also an increased risk of recurrence where there has been a placenta praevia in a previous pregnancy.

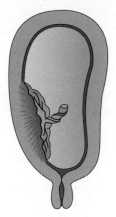

Fig. 14.1 Type 1.

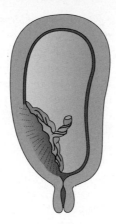

Fig. 14.3 Type 3.

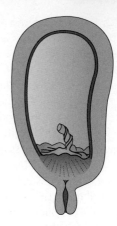

Fig. 14.4 Type 4.

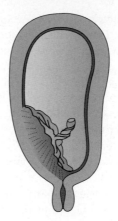

Fig. 14.2 Type 2.

Figs. 14.1–14.4 Types and positions of placenta praevia.

Fig. 14.5 Type 1.

Fig. 14.6 Type 2.

Fig. 14.7 Type 3.

Fig. 14.8 Type 4.

Figs. 14.5–14.8 Relation of placenta praevia to cervical os.

Management

Immediate re localization of the placenta using both abdominal and transvaginal ultrasonic scanning (RCOG 2011c) is a definitive aid to diagnosis, and as well as confirming the existence of placenta praevia it will establish its degree. Relying on an early pregnancy scan at 20 weeks of pregnancy is not very useful when vaginal bleeding starts in later pregnancy, as the placenta tends to migrate up the uterine wall as the uterus grows in a developing pregnancy.

Further management decisions will depend on:

- the amount of bleeding
- the condition of the woman and fetus
- the location of the placenta
- the stage of the pregnancy.

Conservative management. This is appropriate if bleeding is slight and the woman and fetus are well. The woman will be kept in hospital at rest until bleeding has stopped. A speculum examination will have ruled out incidental causes. Further bleeding is almost inevitable

if the placenta encroaches into the lower segment; therefore it is usual for the woman to remain in, or close to hospital for the rest of her pregnancy. A visit to the special care baby unit/neonatal intensive care unit and contact with the neonatal team may also help to prepare the woman and her family for the possibility of preterm birth.

A decision will be made with the woman about how and when the birth will be managed. If there is no further severe bleeding, vaginal birth is highly likely if the placental location allows. The midwife should be aware that, even if vaginal birth is achieved, there remains a danger of postpartum haemorrhage because the placenta has been situated in the lower segment where there are fewer oblique muscle fibres and the action of the *living ligatures* is less effective.

Immediate management of life-threatening bleeding. Severe vaginal bleeding will necessitate immediate birth of the baby by caesarean section regardless of the location of the placenta. This should take place in a maternity unit with facilities for the appropriate care of the newborn, especially if the baby is preterm. During the assessment and preparation for theatre, the woman will be extremely anxious and the midwife must comfort and encourage her, sharing information with her as much as possible. The partner will also need to be supported, whether he/she is in the operating theatre or waits outside.

If the placenta is situated anteriorly in the uterus, this may complicate the surgical approach, as it underlies the site of the normal incision. In major degrees of placenta praevia (types 3 and 4), caesarean section is required even if the fetus has died *in utero*. Such management aims to prevent torrential haemorrhage and possible maternal death.

Complications. Complications include:

- maternal shock, resulting from blood loss and hypovolaemia
- anaesthetic and surgical complications, which are more common in women with major degrees of placenta praevia, and in those for whom preparation for surgery has been suboptimal
- placenta accreta, in up to 15% of women with placenta praevia
- air embolism, an occasional occurrence when the sinuses in the placental bed have been broken
- postpartum haemorrhage: occasionally uncontrolled haemorrhage will continue, despite the administration of uterotonic drugs at the birth, even following the best efforts to control it, and a ligation of the internal iliac artery; a caesarean hysterectomy may be required to save the woman's life
- maternal death is rare in the developed world
- fetal hypoxia and its sequelae due to placental separation
- fetal death, depending on gestation and amount of blood loss.

Placental Abruption

Premature separation of a normally situated placenta occurring after the 24th week of pregnancy is referred to as a placental abruption. The aetiology of this type of haemorrhage is not always clear, but it may be associated with:

- hypertension
- fetal growth restriction
  - non-vertex presentations
  - a sudden reduction in uterine size, for instance when the membranes rupture or after the birth of a first twin or where polyhydramnios is present

- advanced maternal age
- high parity
- low body mass index
- uterine infection
- trauma, for instance external cephalic version of a fetus presenting by the breech, a road traffic accident or domestic violence, as these may partially dislodge the placenta
- smoking and drug misuse.

However, the most predictive risk factor is a history of APH (RCOG 2011d).

Incidence

Placental abruption occurs in 0.49–1.8% of all pregnancies with 20–35% of cases being classed as *concealed* and 65–80% being *revealed* (Navti and Konje 2017), although there is probably a combination of both in many situations (mixed haemorrhage). In any of these situations the blood loss may be mild, moderate or severe, ranging from a few spots to continually soaking clothes and bed linen.

In *revealed* haemorrhage, as blood escapes from the placental site, it separates the membranes from the uterine wall and drains through the vagina. However, in *concealed* haemorrhage blood is retained behind the placenta where it is forced back into the myometrium, infiltrating the space between the muscle fibres of the uterus. This extravasation (seepage outside the normal vascular channels) can cause marked damage and, if observed at operation, the uterus will appear bruised, oedematous and enlarged. This is termed *Couvelaire uterus* or *uterine apoplexy*. In a completely concealed abruption with no vaginal bleeding, the woman will have all the signs and symptoms of hypovolaemic shock and if the blood loss is moderate or severe, she will experience extreme pain. In practice, the midwife cannot rely on visible blood loss as a guide to the severity of the haemorrhage; on the contrary, the most severe haemorrhage is often that which is totally concealed.

As with placenta praevia, the maternal and fetal condition will dictate the management.

Mild separation of the placenta

Most commonly a woman self-admits to the maternity unit with slight vaginal bleeding. On examination, the woman and fetus are in a stable condition and there is no indication of shock. The fetus is alive with normal heart sounds. The consistency of the uterus is normal and there is no tenderness on palpation. The management would include the following plan of care:

- An ultrasound scan can determine the placental localization and identify any degree of concealed bleeding.
- The fetal condition should be assessed by frequent or continuous monitoring of the fetal heart rate while bleeding persists. Subsequently, a cardiotocograph (CTG) should be undertaken once or twice daily.
- If the woman is not in labour and the gestation is <37 weeks, she may be cared for in the antenatal ward for a few days. She may return home if there is no further bleeding and the placenta has been found to be in the upper uterine segment. The woman should be encouraged to return to hospital if there is any further bleeding.
- Women who have passed the 37th week of pregnancy may be offered induction of labour, especially if there has been more than one episode of mild bleeding.
- Further heavy bleeding or evidence of fetal compromise could indicate that a caesarean section is necessary.

The midwife should offer the woman comfort and encouragement by attending to her emotional needs, including her need for information. Physical domestic abuse should be considered by the midwife, which the woman may be frightened to reveal. It should also be noted that if the woman is already severely anaemic, then even an apparently mild abruption may compromise her wellbeing and that of the fetus.

Moderate separation of the placenta

About a quarter of the placenta will have separated and a considerable amount of blood may be lost, although concealed haemorrhage must also be considered. The woman will be shocked and in pain, with uterine tenderness and abdominal guarding. The fetus may be alive, although hypoxic, however intrauterine death is also a possibility.

The priority is to reduce shock and to replace blood loss:

- Fluid replacement should be monitored with the aid of a central venous pressure (CVP) line. Meticulous fluid balance records must be maintained.
- The fetal condition should be continuously assessed by CTG if the fetus is alive, in which case immediate caesarean section would be indicated once the woman's condition is stabilized.

- If the fetus is in good condition or has died, vaginal birth may be considered, as this enables the uterus to contract and control the bleeding. The spontaneous onset of labour frequently accompanies moderately severe placental abruption, but if it does not, then amniotomy is usually sufficient to induce labour. Oxytocics may be used with great care, if necessary. The birth of the baby is often quite sudden after a short labour. The use of drugs to attempt to stop labour is usually inappropriate.

Severe separation of the placenta

This is an **acute and time critical obstetric emergency** where at least two-thirds of the placenta has detached and ≥2000 mL of blood are lost from the circulation. Most or all of the blood may be concealed behind the placenta. The woman will be severely shocked, perhaps far beyond the degree to which would be expected from the visible blood loss (see Chapter 25). The blood pressure will be lowered but if the haemorrhage accompanies pre-eclampsia the reading may lie within the normal range owing to a preceding hypertension. The fetus will almost certainly be dead. The woman will have very severe abdominal pain with excruciating tenderness and the uterus would have a board-like consistency.

Features associated with severe antepartum haemorrhage are:
- coagulation defects
- renal failure
- pituitary failure
- postpartum haemorrhage.

Treatment is the same as for moderate haemorrhage:
- Whole blood should be transfused rapidly and subsequent amounts calculated in accordance with the woman's CVP.
- Labour may begin spontaneously in advance of amniotomy and the midwife should be alert for signs of uterine contraction causing periodic intensifying of the abdominal pain.
- If bleeding continues or a compromised fetal heart rate is present, caesarean section will be required as soon as the woman's condition has been adequately stabilized.

Blood Coagulation Failure
Normal blood coagulation

Haemostasis refers to the arrest of bleeding, preventing loss of blood from the blood vessels. It depends on the mechanism of coagulation. This is counterbalanced by fibrinolysis, which ensures that the blood vessels are reopened in order to maintain the patency of the circulation.

Blood clotting occurs in three main stages:

1. When tissues are damaged and platelets break down, *thromboplastin* is released.
2. Thromboplastin leads to the conversion of *prothrombin* into *thrombin*: a proteolytic (protein-splitting) enzyme.
3. Thrombin converts *fibrinogen* into *fibrin* to form a network of long, sticky strands that entrap blood cells to establish a *clot*. The coagulated material contracts and exudes *serum*, which is plasma depleted of its clotting factors. This is the final part of a complex cascade of coagulation involving a large number of different clotting factors (simply named Factor I, Factor II, etc. in order of their discovery).

It is equally important for a healthy person to maintain the blood as a fluid in order that it can circulate freely. The coagulation mechanism is normally held at bay by the presence of *heparin*, which is produced in the liver.

Fibrinolysis is the breakdown of fibrin and occurs as a response to the presence of clotted blood. Unless fibrinolysis takes place, coagulation will continue. It is achieved by the activation of a series of enzymes culminating in the proteolytic enzyme *plasmin*. This breaks down the fibrin in the clots and produces *fibrin degradation products* (FDPs).

Disseminated intravascular coagulation

The cause of disseminated intravascular coagulation (also known as disseminated intravascular coagulopathy, DIC) is not fully understood. It is a complex pathological reaction to severe tissue trauma, which rarely occurs when the fetus is alive and usually starts to resolve after birth. Inappropriate coagulation occurs within the blood vessels, which leads to the consumption of clotting factors. As a result, clotting fails to occur at the bleeding site. DIC is never a primary disease, as it always occurs as a response to another disease process.

Events that trigger DIC include:

- placental abruption
- intrauterine fetal death, including delayed miscarriage
- amniotic fluid embolism
- intrauterine infection, including septic miscarriage
- pre-eclampsia and eclampsia.

BOX 14.3 Aims of the Management of DIC

- To manage the underlying cause and remove the stimulus provoking DIC
- To ensure maintenance of the circulating blood volume
- To replace the used up clotting factors and destroyed red blood cells.

Management. The aims of the management of DIC are summarized in Box 14.3.

The midwife should be alert to conditions that affect DIC, as well as the signs that clotting is abnormal. The assessment of the nature of the clot should be part of the midwife's routine observation during the third stage of labour. Oozing from a venepuncture site or bleeding from the mucous membrane of the woman's mouth and nose must be noted and reported. Blood tests should include assessing the full blood count and the blood grouping, clotting studies and the levels of platelets, fibrinogen and fibrin degradation products (FDPs).

Treatment involves the replacement of blood cells and clotting factors in order to restore equilibrium. This is usually done by the administration of fresh frozen plasma, fibrinogen and platelet concentrates. Banked red cells will be transfused subsequently. Management is carried out by a team of obstetricians, anaesthetists, haematologists, midwives and other healthcare professionals who must strive to work together harmoniously and effectively to achieve the best possible clinical outcomes for the woman.

Care by the midwife. DIC causes a frightening situation that demands speed both of recognition and of action. The midwife has to maintain her own calmness and clarity of thinking as well as assisting the couple to deal with the situation in which they find themselves. Frequent and accurate observations must be maintained in order to monitor the woman's condition. Blood pressure, respirations, pulse rate and temperature are recorded. The general condition is noted and recorded on a critical or high dependency care chart using a 'track and trigger' scoring system such as Modified Obstetric Early Warning Score (MOEWS, as outlined in Chapter 26). Fluid input and output via a fluid balance chart is documented and monitored with vigilance for any sign of renal failure.

> **BOX 14.4 Hepatic Disorders of Pregnancy**
>
> **Specific to pregnancy**
> - intrahepatic cholestasis of pregnancy
> - acute fatty liver in pregnancy (see Chapter 15)
> - pre-eclampsia and eclampsia (see Chapter 15)
> - severe hyperemesis gravidarum
>
> **Pre- or co-existing in pregnancy**
> - gall bladder disease
> - hepatitis.

> **BOX 14.5 Causes of Jaundice in Pregnancy**
>
> **Not specific to pregnancy**
> - viral hepatitis – A, B, C are the most prevalent
> - hepatitis secondary to infection, usually cytomegalovirus, Epstein–Barr virus, toxoplasmosis or herpes simplex
> - gallstones
> - drug reactions
> - alcohol/drug misuse
> - Budd–Chiari syndrome.
>
> **Pregnancy-specific causes**
> - acute fatty liver
> - HELLP (haemolysis, elevated liver enzymes, low platelets) syndrome
> - intrahepatic cholestasis of pregnancy
> - hyperemesis gravidarum.
>
> *Note*: Jaundice is not an inevitable symptom of liver disease in pregnancy.

The partner in particular is likely to be confused by a sudden turn in events, when previously all seemed to be under control. The midwife must make sure that someone is giving him/her appropriate attention, keeping him/her informed of what is happening. All health professionals need to be aware that the partner may find it impossible to absorb all that he/she is told and may require repeated explanations. The partner may be the best person to help the woman to understand her condition. The death of the woman from organ failure as a result of DIC is a real possibility (Knight et al. 2018).

HEPATIC DISORDERS AND JAUNDICE

Some liver disorders are specific to pregnant women, and some pre-existing or co-existing disorders may complicate the pregnancy, as shown in Box 14.4. Causes of jaundice in pregnancy are listed in Box 14.5.

Obstetric Cholestasis

This is an idiopathic condition that usually begins in the second half of pregnancy. It affects 0.7% of women in multiethnic populations (RCOG 2011e) and resolves spontaneously following birth, but it has up to a high recurrence rate of 45–70% in subsequent pregnancies (Janneke van der Woude et al. 2017). Its cause is unknown, although hormonal, genetic, environmental and dietary factors are considered to be contributory. It is not a life-threatening condition for the woman, but there is an increased risk of preterm labour, fetal compromise and meconium staining, and the stillbirth risk is increased unless there is active management of the pregnancy.

Clinical presentation

The presentation may include:
- pruritus without a rash, usually starting between 25 and 32 weeks of pregnancy

- insomnia and fatigue as a result of the pruritus
- fever, abdominal discomfort, nausea and vomiting
- urine may be darker and stools paler than usual
- a few women develop mild jaundice.

Investigations

The following investigations should be done:
- tests to eliminate differential diagnoses such as eczema, other liver disease or pemphigoid gestationalis (a rare autoimmune disease of late pregnancy that mimics OC)
- an ultrasound scan of the hepatobiliary tract
- blood tests to assess the levels of bile acids, serum alkaline phosphatase, bilirubin and liver transaminases, which are raised.

Management

Management consists of:
- application of topical antipruritic agents
- administration of ursodeoxycholic acid (UDCA) to improve pruritus and improve liver function should be considered for symptomatic cholestasis with a dosage of 10–20 mg/kg per day (Janneke van der Woude et al. 2017)
- vitamin K supplements are administered to the woman, 5–10 mg orally daily, as her absorption will be poor, leading to prothrombinaemia, which predisposes her to obstetric haemorrhage if left untreated

- liver function tests should be repeated weekly until birth
- monitor fetal wellbeing by fetal growth scans and cardiotocography
- consider elective birth when the fetus is mature, or earlier if the fetal condition appears to be compromised by the intrauterine environment, or the bile acids are significantly raised, as this is associated with impending intrauterine death
- provide sensitive psychological care to the woman
- advise the woman that her pruritus should disappear within 3–14 days of the birth
- if the woman chooses to use oral contraception in the future, she should be advised that her liver function should be regularly monitored.

Obstetric cholestasis in pregnancy is increasingly being suspected as a marker for underlying liver and biliary disease in some women (see Chapter 15).

Gall Bladder Disease

Pregnancy appears to increase the likelihood of gallstone formation but not the risk of developing acute cholecystitis. Diagnosis is made by exploring the woman's previous history, with an ultrasound scan of the hepatobiliary tract. The treatment for gall bladder disease is based on providing symptomatic relief of biliary colic by analgesia, hydration, nasogastric suction and antibiotics. If at all possible, surgery in pregnancy should be avoided.

Viral Hepatitis

Viral hepatitis is one of the most commonly diagnosed viral infections of pregnancy (Nuangchamnong and Andrews 2017). See Table 14.3 for information about hepatitis A, B and C in pregnancy. Hepatitis D, E and G have also been described in medical literature elsewhere (see Bothamley and Boyle 2015 for further information).

SKIN DISORDERS

Many women suffer from physiological pruritus in pregnancy, particularly over the abdomen as it grows and stretches. The application of calamine lotion is often helpful. However, pruritus can be a symptom of a disease process, such as OC and pemphigoid gestationalis, an autoimmune disease of pregnancy, where blisters develop over the body as the pregnancy progresses.

Women with pre-existing skin conditions such as eczema and psoriasis should be advised about the use of steroid creams and applications containing nut oil derivatives, which may adversely affect the fetus.

Where the midwife suspects an infectious disease such as chicken pox, rubella, measles or parvovirus, all of which commonly present with skin rash and/or pustules, speedy referral to a medical specialist is essential due to the potential seriousness of these conditions for the fetus.

ABNORMALITIES OF THE AMNIOTIC FLUID

On careful history-taking from the woman and abdominal palpation, the midwife may suspect an abnormal amount of liquor around the fetus, especially as the woman nears term. The amount of liquor present in a pregnancy can also be estimated by measuring 'pools' of liquor around the fetus with ultrasound scanning. There are two abnormalities of amniotic fluid: *polyhydramnios* (or hydramnios) and *oligohydramnios*.

Polyhydramnios

Polyhydramnios is present when there is an excess of amniotic fluid in the amniotic sac. The condition affects 1–2% of pregnancies (Macones 2017). Known causes and predisposing factors include:

- fetal malformation such as oesophageal atresia, open neural tube defect, anencephaly (35%)
- maternal diabetes (25%)
- other very rare causes include fetal anaemia (maternal alloimmunization, syphilis/parvovirus infection), twin-to-twin transfusion syndrome or a fetal tumour.

However, in 40% of cases no causative factors can be isolated.

Types

Chronic polyhydramnios. This is gradual in onset, usually starting from about the 30th week of pregnancy. It is the most common type.

Acute (severe) polyhydramnios. This is very rare. It usually occurs at about 20 weeks and develops very suddenly. The uterine size reaches the xiphisternum in about 3 or 4 days. The acute presentation is frequently associated with monozygotic twins or severe fetal malformation.

TABLE 14.3 Viral Hepatitis in Pregnancy

	Incidence	Clinical Presentation	Mode of Spread	Incubation Period	Mother to Baby (Vertical) Transmission	Diagnosis	Management	Complications	Other
Hepatitis A (HAV)	Endemic worldwide	Fatigue, malaise, fever, nausea, anorexia, weight loss, pruritus, jaundice, hepato-splenomegaly	Contaminated food and water (fecal matter), sexual contact	15–50 days	Possible at birth, but rare	HAV-specific IgM is a serological marker for acute infection Abnormal liver function tests	No specific antiviral treatment available May need to admit to hospital for fluid replacement (barrier nurse)	Usually complete recovery, but can last for 12 months	Vaccination is available for women who travel to high risk areas and is safe in pregnancy Immunoglobulin is available for babies born within 2 weeks of acute maternal infection Hepatitis A is a rare cause of acute hepatitis in pregnancy Breastfeeding is safe
Hepatitis B (HBV)	2 billion infected worldwide In the West 0.5–5% of population are chronic carriers; 600,000 deaths a year worldwide attributable to consequences	All of the above plus arthralgia, rash and myalgia	Body fluids especially blood, semen and saliva	1–6 months	Possible in pregnancy, at birth making baby prone to liver damage in childhood	Woman's history and lifestyle Serological studies useful after antibodies for HBV have formed – serum markers	Caesarean birth not useful in preventing transmission Treat symptoms as they arise Infection control procedures while woman infective Nutrition and sexual advice Monitor long-term liver function if carrier, and baby is infected Vaccinate contacts Vaccinate baby postnatally	Longer-term liver damage can be fatal Danger of being mistaken for pre-eclampsia and HELLP syndrome because of liver pain and coagulopathy	8–10% of those infected become chronic carriers 25–30% of these will die from chronic liver failure years later if they do not receive a liver transplant In 90% of primary carriers symptoms resolve in 1–3 months Routine pregnancy screening enables neonatal prophylaxis Breastfeeding safe in acute disease if mother receives immunoprophylaxis

Continued

TABLE 14.3 Viral Hepatitis in Pregnancy—cont'd

	Incidence	Clinical Presentation	Mode of Spread	Incubation Period	Mother to Baby (Vertical) Transmission	Diagnosis	Management	Complications	Other
Hepatitis C (HCV)	In the USA, 2.3–4.5% in pregnant women No data from other countries	75% have no symptoms, but in 25% same as for Hepatitis A but to a lesser extent	Shared needles, sexual contact (extent unknown) Blood transfusion since 1992 in the USA Sharps injury	30–60 days	Thought to be 2–7% in preliminary studies	Woman's history and lifestyle HCV screening assays currently limited	None available No vaccine available yet	B cell lymphoma Chronic liver disease 75–85% of acutely infected individuals will get chronic liver damage and require a liver transplant	Outcome for baby is not yet known Screening not recommended as there is no known treatment yet HCV infection is often accompanied by HIV infection Transmission rate in breastfeeding not yet known

Diagnosis

General examination. The woman may complain of breathlessness and discomfort. If the polyhydramnios is acute in onset, she may experience severe abdominal pain. The condition may cause exacerbation of symptoms associated with pregnancy, such as indigestion, heartburn and constipation. Oedema and varicosities of the vulva and lower limbs may also be present. The woman may test positive for diabetes mellitus (maternal and concomitant fetal polyuria from high maternal fluid intake lead to excessive amniotic fluid).

Abdominal examination. On inspection, the uterus is larger than expected for the period of gestation and is globular in shape. The abdominal skin appears stretched and shiny, with marked striae gravidarum and superficial blood vessels.

On palpation, the uterus feels tense and it is difficult to feel the fetal parts, but the fetus may be balloted between the two hands. A *fluid thrill* may be elicited by placing a hand on one side of the abdomen and tapping the other side with the fingers.

Ultrasonic scanning is used to confirm the diagnosis of polyhydramnios and may also reveal a multiple pregnancy or fetal malformation. Karyotyping of the fetus may be offered if malformation is suspected or to further enable diagnosis.

Auscultation of the fetal heart may be difficult due to the polyhydramnios.

Complications

These include (Macones 2017):

- An overdistended uterus may lead to preterm prelabour rupture of the membranes (PPROM), preterm labour, maternal respiratory compromise, maternal ureteric obstruction and postpartum haemorrhage.
- Rapid decompression within the uterus as a result of rupture of the membranes may lead to placental abruption and cord prolapse.
- Fetal malpresentation.
- Increased perinatal mortality.

Management

Care will depend on the condition of the woman and fetus, the cause and degree of the polyhydramnios and the stage of pregnancy. The presence of fetal malformation will be taken into consideration in choosing the mode and timing of birth. If there is a gross malformation present, labour may be induced. Should the fetus have an operable condition, such as oesophageal atresia, transfer will be arranged to a neonatal surgical unit.

Mild polyhydramnios is managed expectantly. Regular ultrasound scans will reveal whether or not it is progressive. Some cases of idiopathic polyhydramnios resolve spontaneously as pregnancy progresses.

For a woman with symptomatic polyhydramnios, an upright position will help to relieve any dyspnoea and antacids can be taken to relieve heartburn and nausea. If the discomfort from the swollen uterus is severe, then therapeutic *amniocentesis*, or *amnioreduction*, may be considered. However, the fluid often rapidly reaccumulates and the procedure may need to be repeated.

Labour may need to be induced in late pregnancy if the woman's symptoms become worse. The lie must be corrected if it is not longitudinal and the membranes ruptured cautiously, allowing the amniotic fluid to drain out slowly in order to avoid altering the lie and to prevent cord prolapse (see Chapter 25). In addition, placental abruption is also a risk if the uterus suddenly diminishes in size.

Labour usually progresses physiologically, but the midwife should be prepared for the possibility of postpartum haemorrhage. The baby should be carefully examined for malformations at birth and the patency of the oesophagus is ascertained by passing a nasogastric tube before the first feed.

Oligohydramnios

Oligohydramnios is an abnormally small amount of amniotic fluid. It affects 10% of pregnancies (Macones 2017). When diagnosed in the first half of pregnancy the prognosis for the baby is very poor. Later in pregnancy from around 20 weeks onwards, oligohydramnios may be due to fetal abnormalities, PPROM where amniotic fluid fails to accumulate, maternal dehydration or a placental condition such as pre-eclampsia or post-term insufficiency. The lack of amniotic fluid reduces the intrauterine space and over time and causes compression malformations. Left untreated, at birth the baby will be born with a squashed-looking face, flattening of the nose, micrognathia (a malformation of the jaw) and talipes. The skin is dry and leathery in appearance.

Diagnosis

On inspection, the uterus may appear smaller than expected for the period of gestation. The woman may have noticed a reduction in fetal movements.

On palpation, the uterus is small and compact and fetal parts are easily felt.

Ultrasonic scanning will enable differentiation of oligohydramnios from intrauterine growth restriction (IUGR). Fetal renal malformation (resulting in reduced fetal urine production and therefore liquor) may be visible on the scan. Fetal karyotyping may be discussed with the parents to further enable clarification of suspected malformation and to help decide management of the condition.

Auscultation of the fetal heart should be heard without any undue difficulty.

Management

This will depend on the gestational age, the severity and the cause of the oligohydramnios. In the first trimester, the pregnancy is likely to miscarry. The condition causes the greatest dilemmas in the second trimester but is often associated at this time with fetal death and congenital malformations, in which case the woman may request a termination of pregnancy. Liquor volume will be estimated by ultrasound scan and the woman should be questioned about the possibility of preterm rupture of the membranes. If the woman is dehydrated she should be encouraged to drink plenty of water or offered intravenous hypotonic fluid.

Where fetal anomaly is not considered to be lethal, or the cause of the oligohydramnios is not known, prophylactic transabdominal amnioinfusion may be performed in order to prevent compression malformations and hypoplastic lung disease, and prolong the pregnancy. Little evidence is available to determine the benefits and hazards of this intervention in mid-pregnancy. Management of oligohydramnios due to PPROM is discussed in the next section.

If the oligohydramnios starts in the third trimester the condition is likely to be associated with either PPROM (Macones 2017), in which case induction of labour is indicated to circumvent maternal and fetal infection, or post-term reduction in efficiency of the placenta which is managed by induction of labour or if the woman prefers, close monitoring with ultrasound and CTG until labour intervenes. Regardless of whether labour commences spontaneously or is induced, epidural analgesia

may be indicated because uterine contractions can be unusually painful due to the lack of amniotic fluid. Continuous fetal heart rate monitoring is desirable because of the potential for impairment of placental circulation and cord compression. Furthermore, if meconium is passed *in utero* it will be more concentrated and represent a greater danger to an asphyxiated fetus during birth.

Preterm Prelabour Rupture of the Membranes

Preterm prelabour rupture of the membranes (PPROM) occurs before 37 completed weeks' gestation, where the fetal membranes rupture without the onset of spontaneous uterine activity and the consequential cervical dilatation.

It affects 1–5% of pregnancies and is associated with vaginal infection and inflammation, tobacco use, uteroplacental blood flow disruption (ischaemia or haemorrhage) and uterine distension (multiple pregnancy, polyhydramnios). The condition has a 17–32% recurrence rate in subsequent pregnancies of affected women (Willekes 2017).

Risks of PPROM

Risks associated with PPROM include:
- imminent labour resulting in a preterm birth
- chorioamnionitis, which may be followed by fetal and maternal sepsis if not treated promptly
- oligohydramnios if prolonged PPROM occurs
- cord prolapse
- malpresentation associated with prematurity
- antepartum haemorrhage
- neonatal sepsis
- psychosocial problems resulting from uncertain fetal and neonatal outcome and long-term hospitalization; increased incidence of impaired mother and baby bonding after birth.

Management

If PPROM is suspected, the woman will be admitted to the maternity unit. A careful history is taken and rupture of the membranes confirmed by a sterile speculum examination of any pooling of liquor in the posterior fornix of the vagina. Saturated sanitary towels over a 6-h period will also offer a reasonably conclusive diagnosis if urine leakage has been excluded. In cases of doubt, an insulin-like growth factor binding protein-1 test or placental alpha-microglobulin-1 test of vaginal fluid can be useful (NICE 2015). If these are negative, it is unlikely that the woman has ruptured her membranes.

Digital vaginal examination should be avoided to reduce the risk of introducing infection. Observations are made of the fetal condition from the fetal heart rate, as an infected fetus may have a tachycardia, and also a maternal infection screen, temperature and pulse, uterine tenderness and any purulent or offensively smelling vaginal discharge. An ultrasound scan will be conducted to assess liquor volume, estimated fetal weight, fetal age, any fetal malformation, the presenting part and if indicated, a biophysical profile of the fetus. A decision on future management will then be made.

If the pregnancy is <24 weeks, the woman may be offered an induction/termination of pregnancy, to prevent further trauma from ongoing infection or haemorrhage or because the fetus has a major malformation. The woman and her partner will face difficult decisions requiring ongoing emotional support, however successful pregnancies have been recorded following uncomplicated PPROM in early pregnancy where the membranes have apparently resealed and liquor volume has reaccumulated. From 24–36 weeks, if the fetus appears to be uncompromised and APH and labour have been excluded, the pregnancy will be managed expectantly with a 'watch and wait' approach. The woman can go home to await events and should be advised to take her temperature twice a day and report any pyrexia, flu-like symptoms, purulent or smelly vaginal discharge, abdominal pain, bleeding, contractions or prolapsed cord. She will be offered fortnightly ultrasound scanning to assess fetal wellbeing.

If the woman is >32 weeks pregnant, the fetus appears to be compromised and APH or intervening labour is suspected or confirmed, active management will ensue. The mode of birth will need to be decided and induction of labour or caesarean section performed.

In all cases of continuing pregnancy following PPROM, Willekes (2017) suggests the following considerations:
- antenatal corticosteroids to mature the fetal lungs where preterm birth is considered likely
- prophylactic antibiotics based on individual risk, but not given routinely
- tocolytic agents administered while corticosteroids take effect, although their use is currently controversial as chorioamnionitis may be present
- magnesium sulphate should be considered as it reduces cerebral palsy in preterm infants.

CONCLUSION

Midwives have an important role to play when women experience pathological problems in their pregnancy. The woman is likely to report symptoms first to a midwife, who will then make basic observations that confirm or exclude the likelihood of a deviation from normal. While explaining her findings to the woman and her partner, the midwife must make a decision about possible diagnoses, whether to transfer her to a high-risk obstetric unit and if this warrants transportation by ambulance. The midwife may be required to start managing the woman's condition prior to admission to hospital. In hospital, the midwife is required to ensure the woman's care is coordinated with other healthcare professionals, who must be supplied with appropriate background information; that the woman and her partner receive psychological support; and that contemporaneous records are kept (NMC 2018a). The midwife must report any deterioration in a woman's condition immediately to an appropriate healthcare professional. The midwife is responsible for maintaining continual updating of her professional knowledge and skills in all areas of practice to ensure that every woman receives optimal maternity care throughout her pregnancy.

▌ REFLECTIVE ACTIVITY FOR SELF-ASSESSMENT

1. How would you support a woman in relation to some of the more common disorders of pregnancy?
2. Where a more complex diagnosis is made, what other support networks and advice can be given to women and their families?
3. What role does the midwife take in supporting parents when a disorder in pregnancy has been diagnosed?

REFERENCES

Abortion Act. (1967) c.87. London: HMSO. Available at: www.legislation.gov.uk/ukpga/1967/87.

ACPWH (Association of Chartered Physiotherapists in Women's Health). (2015) Pregnancy-related pelvic girdle pain. Available at: pogp.csp.org.uk.

Antony, K. M., Racusin, D. A., Aagaard, K., & Dildy, G. A., III. (2017). Maternal physiology. In S. Gabbe, J. L. Niebyl, J. Simpson, et al. (Eds.), *Obstetrics: Normal and problem pregnancies* (pp. 39–63). Philadelphia: Elsevier.

DH (Department of Health). (2018). *Abortion Statistics, England and Wales 2017*. Available at: https://assets.publishing.service.gov.uk/government/uploads/system/uploads/attachment_data/file/714183/2017_Abortion_Statistics_Commentary.pdf.

Gregory, K. D., Ramos, D. E., & Jauniaux, E. R. M. (2017). Preconception and prenatal care. In S. Gabbe, J. L. Niebyl, J. Simpson, et al. (Eds.), *Obstetrics: Normal and problem pregnancies* (pp. 102–121). Philadelphia: Elsevier.

Human Fertilisation and Embryology Act. (2008). London: HMSO. Available at: www.legislation.gov.uk/ukpga/2008/22/pdfs/ukpga_20080022_en.pdf.

Janneke van der Woude, C., Kanis, S. L., & De Lima, A. (2017). Gastrointestinal and liver diseases in pregnancy. In D. James, P. J. Steer, C. P. Weiner, et al. (Eds.), *High risk pregnancy management options* (pp. 1236–1272). Cambridge: Cambridge University Press.

Knight, M., Bunch, K., Tuffnell, D., et al. (Eds); on behalf of MBRRACE-UK. (2018). Saving Lives, Improving Mothers' Care – Lessons learned to inform maternity care from the UK and Ireland Confidential Enquiries into Maternal Deaths and Morbidity 2014–2016. Oxford: National Perinatal Epidemiology Unit, University of Oxford.

London, V., Grube, S., Sherer, D. M., & Abulafia, O. (2017). Hyperemesis gravidarum: A review of recent literature. *Pharmacology*, 100(3–4), 161–171.

Ludmir, J., Owen, J., & Berghella, V. (2017). Cervical insufficiency. In S. Gabbe, J. L. Niebyl, J. Simpson, et al. (Eds.), *Obstetrics: Normal and problem pregnancies* (pp. 595–611). Philadelphia: Elsevier.

Macones, G. A. (2017). Disorders of amniotic fluid. In D. James, P. J. Steer, C. P. Weiner, et al. (Eds.), *High risk pregnancy management options* (pp. 269–280). Cambridge: Cambridge University Press.

Mahomed, K. (2011). Abdominal pain. In D. James (Ed.), *High risk pregnancy management options* (pp. 1013–1026). Philadelphia: Saunders Elsevier.

Mahomed, K., & Kumar, S. (2017). Nonmalignant gynecology. In (5th ed.) D. James, P. J. Steers, C. P. Weiner, et al.

(Eds.), *High risk pregnancy management options* (Vol. 2) (pp. 1544–1556). Cambridge: Cambridge University Press.

Navti, O. B., & Konje, J. C. (2017). Bleeding in late pregnancy. In D. James, P. J. Steer, C. P. Weiner, et al. (Eds.), *High risk pregnancy management options* (pp. 1557–1580). Cambridge: Cambridge University Press.

NHS. (2018). National Health Service Cervical Screening Programme. Available at: www.nhs.uk/conditions/cervical-screening/.

NHS Choices. (2016). Ectopic pregnancy. Available at: www.nhs.uk/conditions/ectopic-pregnancy/treatment/.

NICE (National Institute for Health and Care Excellence). (2007). *Laparoscopic cerclage for prevention of recurrent pregnancy loss due to cervical incompetence*. London: NICE. Available at: www.nice.org.uk/guidance/ipg228.

NICE (National Institute for Health and Care Excellence). (2010). *Antenatal care*. CG 62. London: NICE. Available at: www.nice.org.uk/nicemedia/live/11947/40115/40115.pdf.

NICE (National Institute for Health and Care Excellence). (2012). *Ectopic pregnancy and miscarriage: Diagnosis and initial management*. London: NICE. Available at: www.nice.org.uk/guidance/cg154.

NICE (National Institute for Health and Care Excellence). (2015). Preterm labour and birth. Available at: www.nice.org.uk/guidance/ng25.

Nuangchamnong, G. N., & Andrews, J. I. (2017). Hepatitis virus infections in pregnancy. In D. James, P. J. Steer, C. P. Weiner, et al. (Eds.), *High risk pregnancy management options* (pp. 604–621). Cambridge: Cambridge University Press.

NMC (Nursing and Midwifery Council). (2018a). *The Code – Professional standards of practice and behavior for nurses, midwives and nursing associates*. London: NMC. Available at: www.nmc.org.uk/standards/code/.

NMC (Nursing and Midwifery Council). (2018b). Conscientious objection by nurses and midwives. Available at: www.nmc.org.uk/standards/code/conscientious-objection-by-nurses-and-midwives/.

RCOG (Royal College of Obstetricians and Gynaecologists). (2010). *The management of gestational trophoblastic disease. Green-top Guideline No 38*. London: RCOG. Available at: www.rcog.org.uk/files/rcog-corp/GT38ManagementGestational0210.pdf.

RCOG (Royal College of Obstetricians and Gynaecologists). (2011a). *The investigation and treatment of couples with recurrent first-trimester and second-trimester miscarriage. Green-top Guideline No 17*. London: RCOG. Available at: www.rcog.org.uk/globalassets/documents/guidelines/gtg_17.pdf.

RCOG (Royal College of Obstetricians and Gynaecologists). (2011b). *The care of women requesting induced abortion. Evidence-Based Clinical Guideline No. 7.* London: RCOG. Available at: www.rcog.org.uk/en/guidelines-research-services/guidelines/the-care-of-women-requesting-induced-abortion/.

RCOG (Royal College of Obstetricians and Gynaecologists). (2011c). *Placenta praevia, placenta praevia accrete and vasa praevia: Diagnosis and management. Green-top Guideline No 27.* London: RCOG. Available at: www.rcog.org.uk/globalassets/documents/guidelines/gtg_27.pdf.

RCOG (Royal College of Obstetricians and Gynaecologists). (2011d). *Antepartum haemorrhage. Green-top Guideline No 63.* London: RCOG. Available at: www.rcog.org.uk/globalassets/documents/guidelines/gtg_63.pdf.

RCOG (Royal College of Obstetricians and Gynaecologists). (2011e). *Obstetric cholestasis. Green-top Guideline No 43.* London: RCOG. Available at: www.rcog.org.uk/globalassets/documents/guidelines/gtg_43.pdf.

RCOG (Royal College of Obstetricians and Gynaecologists). (2016a). *Diagnosis and management of ectopic pregnancy. Green-top Guideline No 21.* London: RCOG. Available at: https://obgyn.onlinelibrary.wiley.com/doi/epdf/10.1111/1471-0528.14189.

RCOG (Royal College of Obstetricians and Gynaecologists). (2016b). *The management of ovarian hyperstimulations syndrome. Green-top Guideline No 5.* London: RCOG. Available at: www.rcog.org.uk/globalassets/documents/guidelines/green-top-guidelines/gtg_5_ohss.pdf.

RCOG (Royal College of Obstetricians and Gynaecologists). (2018). *Abortion care for women from Northern Ireland.* London: RCOG. Available at: www.rcog.org.uk/en/patients/patient-leaflets/abortion-care/abortion-care-for-women-from-northern-ireland/.

SANDS (Stillbirth and Neonatal Death Society). (2016). *Pregnancy loss and the death of a baby: Guidelines for professionals* (4th ed.). London: SANDS.

Salani, R., & Copeland, L. J. (2017). Malignant diseases and pregnancy. In S. G. Gabbe, J. R. Niebyl, J. L. Simpson, et al. (Eds.), *Obstetrics: Normal and problem pregnancies* (pp. 1057–1075). Philadelphia: Elsevier.

Seckl, M. J., Sebire, N. J., Fisher, R. A., et al. (2013). Gestational trophoblastic disease: EMSO Clinical Practice Guidelines for diagnosis, treatment and follow-up. *Annals of Oncology, 24*(Suppl. 6), vi39–vi50.

Sexual Health Policy Team. (2014). *Guidance in relation to requirements of the Abortion Act 1967.* London: Department of Health. Available at: https://assets.publishing.service.gov.uk/government/uploads/system/uploads/attachment_data/file/313459/20140509_-_Abortion_Guidance_Document.pdf.

Tiran, D. (2014). Nausea and vomiting in pregnancy: An 'alternative' approach to care. *British Journal of Midwifery, 22*(8), 544–550.

Willekes, C. (2017). Prelabour rupture of the membranes. In D. James, P. J. Steer, C. P. Weiner, et al. (Eds.), *High risk pregnancy management options* (pp. 1655–1674). Cambridge: Cambridge University Press.

ANNOTATED FURTHER READING

Bond, D. M., Middleton, P., Levett, K. M., et al. (2017). Planned early birth versus expectant management for women with preterm prelabour rupture of membranes prior to 37 weeks' gestation for improving pregnancy outcome. *Cochrane Database of Systematic Reviews* (3), CD004735.
A useful review of conservative versus interventionalist approach to the management of preterm prelabour rupture of the membranes.

Bothamley, J., & Boyle, M. (2015). *Infections affecting pregnancy and childbirth.* London: Radcliffe Publishing.
This book, aimed at midwives, has a detailed section on viral hepatitis.

Boyle, M. (Ed.). (2017). *Emergencies around childbirth.* Milton Keynes: Radcliffe.
This book has useful sections on antepartum haemorrhage and maternal collapse, written with student and newly qualified midwives in mind.

Kenny, L., & Bickerstaff, H. (2017). *Gynaecology by ten teachers.* London: CRC Press.
A general gynaecology textbook, which will provide students and midwives with useful background information about early pregnancy and pregnancy-related gynaecology conditions.

Raynor, M. D., Marshall, J. E., & Jackson, K. (2012). *Midwifery practice: Critical illness, complications and emergencies case book.* Maidenhead: McGraw–Hill/Open University Press.
Provides a useful case study approach with questions and answers for the reader to enhance their knowledge and understanding in recognizing the critically ill woman, and conditions such as APH, DIC and obstetric cholestasis.

USEFUL WEBSITES

Antenatal Results and Choices: www.arc-uk.org
This charity website aims to offer information and support to parents and families following the diagnosis of a fetal abnormality, which may then lead to difficult decisions having to be made. Information, leaflets and training are also available for professionals.
Ectopic Pregnancy Trust: www.ectopic.org.uk
Website for professionals and women, related to ectopic pregnancy.
ICP Support: www.icpsupport.org

Website offering support and information for women and professionals regarding intrahepatic cholestasis of pregnancy (obstetric cholestasis).

Miscarriage Association: www.miscarriageassociation.org.uk

Offers support and information to parents following the various forms of early pregnancy loss. Information is also available for professionals.

National Institute for Health and Care Excellence: www.nice.org.uk

In the UK, this is an executive non-departmental public body of the Department of Health, which publishes evidence-based guidelines for the public and healthcare professionals.

NHS Cervical Screening Programme: www.cancerscreening.nhs.uk/cervical/

This provides details of the cervical cancer screening programme offered in the UK, as well as information relevant for the public and professionals.

Pelvic Partnership: www.pelvicpartnership.org.uk

This website is run by volunteers who all have personal experience of pelvic girdle pain (PGP). The information provided is mainly provided for women, but provides additional knowledge and guidance for students and midwives alike.

Pregnancy Sickness Support: www.pregnancysicknesssupport.org.uk

A charity website that offers information and support to both women and professionals with regards to nausea and vomiting in pregnancy. There is also guidance regarding hyperemesis gravidarum.

Royal College of Obstetricians and Gynaecologists: www.rcog.org.uk

RCOG website that provides a wealth of information and guidance through the Green-top series on best practice relating to gynaecological and obstetric-related situations.

SANDS (Stillbirth and Neonatal Death Society): www.uk-sands.org

This is a comprehensive website offering information and support for parents and families following the loss of a baby. SANDS also produces guidelines for professionals to help support those caring for bereaved families.

15

Medical Conditions of Significance to Midwifery Practice

Rowena Doughty, Moira McLean, Sarah Coombes

CHAPTER CONTENTS

Medical disorders are of increasing significance in midwifery practice. A few years ago, a student midwife would have learnt about a few medical disorders during education and training, but increasing maternal age and advances in medical treatment have resulted in women who might have previously died, or been advised against pregnancy, now presenting for maternity care and bringing considerable challenges along with them. In addition to using this chapter as a resource, a midwife caring for such women may need to seek additional sources for advancing her knowledge, as not every medical condition or infection can be fully explored within this chapter (Knight et al. 2018, 2019).

THE CHAPTER AIMS TO

- provide an account of the most common medical conditions and their effect on childbearing women
- provide an overview of the less common medical conditions and their significance to the health and wellbeing of the woman and her family
- explain the importance of midwives having an in-depth knowledge of medical conditions in order to recognize women with such conditions and care for them effectively.

HYPERTENSIVE DISORDERS

Blood Pressure Regulation and Measurement

Blood pressure (BP) is the force exerted by blood volume on the blood vessel walls, known as 'peripheral resistance'. This force is generated by contraction of the ventricles of the heart, and in the case of young, healthy adults, blood enters the aorta at 120 mmHg at systole (contraction) and falls to 80 mmHg at diastole (relaxation) (Tortora and Derrickson 2016). As the blood is dispersed through the arterial system, the pressure gradually lowers to 16 mmHg by the time it reaches the capillaries. Blood pressure is never zero (0) unless there is a cardiac arrest (Webster et al. 2013). Blood pressure is determined by the volume of blood in the circulation (the cardiac output), the strength of the heart contractions and the heart rate, the degree of stretch in the vessel walls and the resistance to blood flow, i.e. blood vessel length, blood viscosity and vessel wall smoothness.

Regulation of Blood Pressure

Blood pressure is regulated by neural, chemical and hormonal controls, of which the midwife needs a basic knowledge because drugs to control BP often act on these pathways. Baroreceptors are mechanoreceptors, also known as mechanosensitive nerve endings, located in the carotid sinus and aortic arch that function as arterial blood pressure sensors. They sense pressure changes by responding to alterations in the tension of the arterial wall, in other words they are excited by a stretch of the blood vessels. Increased pressure in these vessels stimulates the baroreceptors to relay this information

to the cardiovascular centre of medulla oblongata in the brain. The cardiovascular centre responds by putting out parasympathetic impulses via the motor (efferent) fibres of the vagus nerve supplying the heart, causing fewer sympathetic impulses reaching the heart. This causes a lowered heart rate, lowered cardiac output and vasodilatation of arterioles giving rise to a fall in BP (Tortora and Derrickson 2016). Conversely, if pressure on the baroreceptors decreases, the feedback to the cardiovascular centre results in increased sympathetic impulses causing accelerated heart rate, increased force of contraction and vasodilatation; BP then rises. Chemoreceptors monitor blood chemicals, in particular hydrogen ions, oxygen and carbon dioxide, and are situated close to the baroreceptors. They also relay information to the cardiovascular centre of the medulla oblongata (Tortora and Derrickson 2016). If there is a deficiency of oxygen (hypoxia) the carbon dioxide level rises and hydrogen ion concentration increases causing acidity, such that the chemoreceptors are stimulated and send responses to the medulla oblongata. In response the cardiovascular centre increases sympathetic nerve stimulation causing vasoconstriction of arterioles and veins, and BP rises.

Certain hormones influence blood pressure

- Epinephrine and norepinephrine from the adrenal medulla increase heart rate and raise BP.
- Antidiuretic hormone (ADH) released from the posterior pituitary gland causes vasoconstriction especially if there is hypovolaemia due to haemorrhage.

Alcohol inhibits release of ADH, leading to vasodilatation, which lowers BP.

- Angiotensin II causes vasoconstriction and stimulates secretion of aldosterone resulting in greater reabsorption of water by the kidneys, both resulting in raised BP.
- Atrial natriuretic peptide (ANP) from cells in the heart's atria causes vasodilatation, and lowers BP.
- Histamine released by mast cells in an inflammatory response is a vasodilator, decreasing BP.
- Progesterone of pregnancy causes vasodilatation and lowers BP (see below).

Blood pressure adaptation in pregnancy

In pregnancy, blood plasma volume increases from approximately 2600 mL to 3800 mL by 32 weeks' gestation and red cell mass from 1400 to 1800 mL; consequently, cardiac output increases by 40%, with the majority of the extra output directed to the uterus and kidneys. This should result in raised BP, however the increasing release of progesterone throughout pregnancy causes vasodilatation, and systolic and diastolic pressures actually fall in the first and second trimesters by about 10 mmHg (Burrow et al. 2004), which can predispose the pregnant woman to fainting due to hypotension. Systolic and diastolic measurements rise slowly to the pre-pregnancy levels in the third trimester.

Measurement of Blood Pressure

Accurate measurement of BP is essential in order to confirm wellness or to diagnose hypotension or hypertension at the earliest possibility. The gold standard method for measuring blood pressure is using a mercury sphygmomanometer and stethoscope, but increasingly anaeroid devices are used (Waugh and Smith 2012). They require regular calibration and need to have been validated for use in pregnancy, but their use does reduce the health and safety concerns surrounding mercury devices. Diastolic BP is determined at Korotkoff Phase V (disappearance of sound) rather than Korotkoff Phase IV (muffling sound) when using manual devices. Box 15.1 outlines recommendations for measuring BP (National Institute for Health and Care Excellence, NICE 2019a). The woman should be at rest; if she is supine she should be placed in a left lateral position (Townsend et al. 2016). The cuff size is an important consideration, as a cuff, and the bladder inside it that is too small will undercuff the woman's upper limb with risk of overestimating the

---

BOX 15.1 Blood Pressure Measurement

- The woman should be seated for at least 5 min, relaxed and not moving or speaking.
- The arm must be supported and outstretched.
- Ensure no tight clothing constricts the arm.
- Place the cuff neatly, with the centre of its bladder over the brachial artery. Use an appropriate cuff size for the person's arm.

Digital devices

- Some monitors allow manual blood pressure setting selection, where you choose the appropriate setting.
- Other monitors will automatically inflate and re-inflate to the next setting if required.
- Repeat three times and record the measurement as displayed.
- Initially test blood pressure in both arms and use the arm with the highest reading for subsequent measurement. Ensure devices are properly maintained as per manufacturer's instructions.

Manual devices

- Estimate the systolic pressure beforehand:
  - palpate the brachial artery
  - inflate cuff until pulsation disappears
  - deflate cuff
  - estimate systolic pressure.
- Then inflate to 30 mmHg above the estimated systolic level needed to occlude the pulse.
- Place the stethoscope diaphragm over the brachial artery and deflate at a rate of 2–3 mm/s until you hear regular tapping sounds.
- Measure systolic (*first sound*) and diastolic (*disappearance*) to the nearest 2 mmHg.

---

blood pressure. About 25% of antenatal women could fall into this category, so both standard and large size cuffs should be available in all maternity clinics and wards (Waugh and Smith 2012). Thigh cuffs can also be used for women with an arm circumference ≥41 cm.

Hypertension in Pregnancy

Hypertension in pregnancy is defined as a blood pressure of ≥140 mmHg systolic or ≥90 mmHg diastolic BP on at least two measurements separated by a period of rest. Severe hypertension is defined as a blood pressure >160–17/110 mmHg, with systolic blood pressures ≥180 being a medical emergency (Townsend et al. 2016). Hypertensive disorders during pregnancy increases the risk of morbidity and mortality for both the mother and fetus. Rates of mortality are falling, but morbidity remains a concern, for instance intrauterine growth restriction (IUGR) and prematurity are common in newborns of pre-eclamptic mothers (National Institute for Health and Care Excellence, NICE 2010a).

Chronic hypertension

Chronic hypertension encompasses hypertension >140/90 mmHg that has existed and was diagnosed before pregnancy (NICE 2019c). This was previously known as benign or essential hypertension. Most women have no underlying cause, but risk factors such as obesity, Black and Minority Ethnic (BaME) groups and a family history of hypertension, plus lifestyle factors such as lack of exercise, alcohol consumption and poor diet with high salt or fat intake may be present. The risk of developing chronic hypertension increases with age and can be primary or secondary in aetiology.

If this condition is known to be present pre-pregnancy, the women should be directed to specialist joint medical-obstetric antenatal clinics. Current medication will be reviewed and the pregnancy closely monitored. Angiotensin-converting-enzyme (ACE) inhibitors and angiotensin II receptor blockers (ARBs) are associated with an increased risk of congenital malformations and women should be offered alternatives during the pre-conception period or as soon as possible antenatally.

The normal vasodilatation and drop in vascular resistance that occurs in early pregnancy will be exaggerated in women with chronic hypertension. However, many women may not know they have chronic hypertension, as they will not have had their blood pressure measured until their antenatal 'booking' appointment, and so will remain undiagnosed until the 6-week postnatal check (Webster et al. 2013). Risks in pregnancy from chronic hypertension include IUGR due to poor implantation, placental abruption that is further compounded if the woman smokes and episodes of severe hypertension, especially if the woman stops her antihypertensive medication, with increased risk of cerebrovascular incidents, i.e. stroke. Women with chronic hypertension are also at increased risk of developing superimposed pre-eclampsia. In these women, the blood pressure profile may be more difficult to interpret as the baseline BP is likely to be higher and exacerbated by the effects of treatment with antihypertensives (Webster et al. 2013).

Additional antenatal appointments may be offered and the aim is to maintain a maternal BP of around 135/85 mmHg. Aspirin 75–150 mg daily from 12 weeks is also recommended, with PlGF testing between 20 and 35 weeks, to detect pre-eclampsia (NICE 2019a). The pregnancy should be monitored through ultrasound fetal growth, amniotic fluid volume assessment and umbilical artery Doppler velocimetry between 28 and 30 weeks and between 32 and 36 weeks. In women with chronic hypertension, it is recommended to only carry out cardiotocography (CTG) if fetal activity is abnormal (NICE 2019c). Induction of labour/elective birth to women with chronic hypertension whose blood pressure is <160/110 mmHg, with or without antihypertensive treatment, before 37 weeks is not recommended (NICE 2019c). Women with chronic hypertension whose blood pressure is <160/110 mmHg after 37 weeks, with or without antihypertensive treatment, timing of birth and maternal and fetal indications for birth should be agreed between them and the senior obstetrician. If severe chronic hypertension is present, a course of corticosteroids (if required) should be completed. Postnatally, maternal blood pressure should be monitored closely, i.e. daily for the first 2 days after birth and at least once between day 3 and day 5 after birth; as clinically indicated. In women with chronic hypertension the aim is to keep her blood pressure <140/90 mmHg. Her longer-term antihypertensive management should be reviewed around 2 weeks postpartum and her BP assessed at the 6–8 weeks postnatal check (NICE 2019c).

Secondary hypertension

Some women develop secondary hypertension as a complication of underlying pathophysiology or disease. These may include renal disease, which results in sodium retention by the kidney leading to water retention, an increased blood volume and thereafter hypertension. This may be classified as renal hypertension (Webster et al. 2013). Phaeochromocytoma is an adrenal gland tumour secreting the hormones dopamine, adrenaline and noradrenaline and results in hypertension. Congenital heart disease may result in hypertension, especially if there is constriction of the aorta. The management is to address the underlying cause; however, substantive treatment might have to wait until the woman has given birth.

BOX 15.2 Definitions of Hypertension in Pregnancy

Hypertension

Diastolic blood pressure 90–109 mmHg; systolic blood pressure 140–159 mmHg.

Severe hypertension

Diastolic blood pressure ≥110 mmHg; systolic blood pressure ≥160 mmHg.

Note the lower measurements for this definition when compared with severe hypertension in the general population.

Chronic hypertension

This is hypertension that is present at the initial visit (booking) or before 20 weeks, or if the woman is already taking antihypertensive medication when referred to maternity services. It can be primary or secondary in aetiology.

Gestational hypertension

This is new hypertension presenting after 20 weeks without significant proteinuria.

Pre-eclampsia

This is new hypertension presenting after 20 weeks with significant proteinuria.

Severe pre-eclampsia

This is pre-eclampsia with severe hypertension and/or with symptoms and/or biochemical and/or haematological impairment.

Adapted from NICE (National Institute for Health and Clinical Excellence). (2010a) (updated 2018). *Hypertension in pregnancy: The management of hypertensive disorders during pregnancy.* CG 107. London: NICE.

HYPERTENSIVE CONDITIONS OF PREGNANCY

Around 10% of women will develop hypertension during pregnancy; 5% will develop gestational hypertension and 3–4% will develop pre-eclampsia, with 1–2% resulting in a serious condition (APEC, Action of Pre-Eclampsia). There are therefore several classifications of hypertension in pregnancy and the midwife is therefore advised to use the definitions in Box 15.2. The following will attempt to clarify how the conditions present and develop and the risks and complications during childbearing.

Gestational Hypertension

Gestational hypertension (previously referred to as pregnancy induced hypertension) is hypertension >140/90 mmHg that presents after the 20th week of pregnancy and without significant proteinuria, and where the BP returns to normal values postnatally. The aetiology is unclear; the predominant cause is thought to be the effect of poor placentation, which results in the release of biochemical markers causing inflammatory responses. Complications are similar to those associated with chronic hypertension.

The management of a woman with gestational hypertension requires a full assessment, which should be carried out in a secondary care setting by a healthcare professional who is trained in the management of hypertensive disorders. Antenatally, the woman should 'book' for consultant-led care coupled with increased and extra antenatal appointments at joint medicine-obstetric or hypertension specialist clinics (NICE 2019c). She may be prescribed low-dose aspirin (75–150 mg once daily). Care will focus around the close surveillance by the multidisciplinary team of the mother's blood pressure and screening for signs of pre-eclampsia, including PIGF testing, plus monitoring of fetal growth and wellbeing. In women with gestational hypertension, NICE (2019c) recommends taking into account the following risk factors that require additional assessment and follow-up:

- nulliparity
- age ≥40 years
- pregnancy interval of >10 years
- family history of pre-eclampsia
- multiple pregnancy
- BMI of ≥35 kg/m^2
- gestational age at presentation
- previous history of pre-eclampsia or gestational hypertension
- pre-existing vascular disease
- pre-existing kidney disease.

Women with gestational hypertension are offered an integrated package of care covering measurement of blood pressure, testing for proteinuria and blood tests (NICE 2019a). Labetalol is the drug of choice and other antihypertensive treatment other than labetalol should only be contemplated after considering side-effect profiles for the woman, fetus and newborn baby. Alternatives include methyldopa and nifedipine. In the UK, NICE (2019c) do not recommend bed rest in hospital as a treatment for gestational hypertension.

It is recommended that fetal wellbeing should be assessed using cardiotocography (CTG), ultrasound fetal growth and amniotic fluid volume assessment, plus umbilical artery Doppler velocimetry from 28 weeks' gestation. These are repeated fortnightly if indicated. (NICE 2019c). In women with mild or moderate gestational hypertension, it is recommended to only carry out CTG if fetal activity is abnormal.

NICE (2019c) recommend that the birth should occur in a consultant-led environment, the timing of which will be determined by the maternal and fetal condition. During labour, measure blood pressure hourly in women with mild or moderate hypertension and every 15–30 minutes in women with severe hypertension. Continued use of antenatal antihypertensive treatment is recommended during labour.

If the woman labours, an epidural can help to stabilize her blood pressure. However, do not preload women who have severe pre-eclampsia with intravenous fluids before establishing low-dose epidural analgesia and combined spinal epidural analgesia (NICE 2019c). Furthermore, the duration of the second stage of labour should not be limited in women with stable mild or moderate hypertension or if blood pressure is controlled within target ranges in women with severe hypertension. NICE (2019c) recommends operative birth or assisted birth in the second stage of labour for women with severe hypertension whose hypertension has not responded to initial treatment. Syntocinon is recommended for use for active management of the third stage, to prevent the vasoconstrictive effects of the ergometrine in Syntometrine (see Chapter 21).

NICE (2019c) recommends close observation of the mother's blood pressure and wellbeing during the postnatal period, with liaison with her GP and adjustment of medication as required. In women with gestational hypertension who have given birth, measure the BP daily for the first 2 days after birth, at least once between day 3 and day 5 after birth and as clinically indicated if antihypertensive treatment is changed after birth. It is also recommended for continued use of antenatal antihypertensive treatment and to consider reducing antihypertensive treatment if the blood pressure falls below 130/80 mmHg. For women with gestational hypertension who did not take antihypertensive treatment and have given birth, NICE (2019c) recommends starting antihypertensive treatment if their blood pressure is >149/99 mmHg.

Pre-Eclampsia

Pre-eclampsia is an idiopathic (= cause unknown) condition of pregnancy. For simplicity, NICE (2019c) states that pre-eclampsia 'is new hypertension presenting after 20 weeks with significant proteinuria'. However, because of the varied clinical presentation or pre-eclampsia, a more up-to-date definition may be *hypertension with any proteinuria, organ dysfunction and fetal growth restriction*. Duhig et al. (2018) acknowledge that despite recent advances in research, the pathophysiology of pre-eclampsia is still not fully understood. They state that pre-eclampsia is characterized by abnormal placentation with subsequent maternal inflammatory and vascular response (Burton et al 2019). To add to its complexity, diagnosis remains a challenge. The clinical presentation of the pre-eclampsia is a progressive disease; it can develop gradually over a few weeks or fulminant within hours. There is no cure, except birth, and management depends on monitoring the condition and balancing the maternal and fetal condition to determine the optimum gestation for birth. Pre-eclampsia occurs in 3–4% of all pregnancies (Hutcheon et al. 2011) and around 10% of women will develop this in their first pregnancy. Black women are three times more likely to develop pre-eclampsia than white women (Action on Pre-Eclampsia, APEC 2019). While most of these women will have a successful outcome to their pregnancy, some will proceed to multisystem complications. See Box 15.3 for the associated factors for developing pre-eclampsia.

Women at high risk of pre-eclampsia should have an ultrasound scan for fetal growth, amniotic fluid volume assessment and umbilical artery doppler velocimetry; these should commence at between 28 and 30 weeks (or at least 2 weeks before previous gestational age of onset if earlier than 28 weeks) and repeating 4 weeks later in women with previous, severe pre-eclampsia, pre-eclampsia that needed birth before 34 weeks, pre-eclampsia with a baby whose birth weight was less than the 10th centile, intrauterine death and placental abruption. As previously stated CTGs are only indicated if fetal activity is abnormal (NICE 2019c).

A plan of care should be written that includes the frequency and type of future fetal monitoring and fetal indications for delivery and when corticosteroids should be administered. Management is generally conservative until 34 weeks' gestation and is dependent on

BOX 15.3 Associated Risk Factors for Developing Pre-eclampsia

Maternal Factors

- Primigravida (Primipaternity; first pregnancy with a new partner)
- Extremes of maternal age (<20 and >40 years)
- Family history of pre-eclampsia
- Pre-eclampsia in a previous pregnancy
- Pregnancy after assisted reproductive technology
- Obesity
- Pre-existing diabetes mellitus type 1
- Pre-existing hypertensive disease
- Pre-existing medical conditions, e.g. renal disease, systemic lupus erythematosus (SLE), rheumatoid arthritis

Pregnancy-Related Factors

- First pregnancy
- Multiple pregnancy
- Developing a medical disorder during pregnancy, e.g. venous thromboembolic disease (VTE), such as anti-phospholipid (Hughes) syndrome (APS), gestational diabetes, gestational hypertension
- Developing infection with inflammatory response
- Hydropic degeneration of the placenta

From NICE (2019a); James et al. (2017).

the maternal biochemical, haematological and clinical thresholds and the fetal thresholds for early planned birth (NICE 2019c). Once pre-eclampsia is diagnosed, labetalol is the first-line treatment (unless the woman has asthma); other antihypertensives such as methyldopa and nifedipine (Box 15.4) might be offered after considering the side-effect profiles for woman and fetus (NICE 2019c).

The clinical manifestation may vary; most cases will present as a maternal condition with hypertension and proteinuria during the antenatal period. However, some women may present as a fetal condition with fetal growth restriction. Others may present with eclampsia or Haemolytic elevated Liver enzymes Low Platelets (HELLP) syndrome with no recorded changes to blood pressure and no proteinuria prior to the onset of seizures or HELLP symptoms. The timing of the presentation may also vary, most cases arise in the third trimester of pregnancy, but some cases present in the postnatal period. The severity can be mild, moderate

or severe and may be pre-eclampsia or eclampsia (see below). Mild pre-eclampsia may present with hypertension and proteinuria in a woman who otherwise feels well, whereas in cases of severe pre-eclampsia the woman will feel unwell.

In the UK, maternal deaths from hypertensive disorders of pregnancy have reduced significantly over the past 60 years (Knight et al. 2019). This is also the case globally, but not as dramatically as in the UK. Globally, it is estimated that pre-eclampsia and eclampsia result in approximately 30,000 maternal deaths annually, mostly in resource-poor countries (Alkema et al. 2016). MBRRACE-UK, produces a triennial report relating to the confidential enquiry into maternal deaths. This is a well established national programme in the UK and Ireland. The 2019 triennial report by MBBRACE-UK reviewed deaths between 2015 and 2017, which were a result of hypertensive disorders (Tuffnell et al. 2019). They reported that the mortality from hypertensive disorders remains low during that period; six women died during this period resulting in a rate of 0.22 per 100,000 maternities. Intracranial haemorrhage and liver failure remains the most common cause of death. This report supports the care and management detailed in the recently updated NICE guideline on hypertension in pregnancy (NG133) (NICE 2019c).

Management of pre-eclampsia

Early recognition of pre-eclampsia is paramount, as the midwife is likely to be the first health professional to notice the clinical signs at an antenatal appointment, and prompt referral to an obstetrician is necessary for investigations, albeit the ultimate responsibility for the diagnosis and management lies within the multidisciplinary team. All pregnant women should be made aware of the signs and symptoms of pre-eclampsia such as severe headache, visual disturbances, e.g. blurring or flashing lights before the eyes, severe pain just under the ribs, vomiting and sudden onset of marked oedema of the face and hands. Women also should be informed about how to see support and advice from a healthcare professional (NICE 2019c).

Routine antenatal care can screen for pre-eclampsia by the measurement of blood pressure, using an

BOX 15.4 Antihypertensive Drugs Used in Pregnancy

Beta-blockers
- Inhibit action of catecholamines on the adrenoreceptors
- Beta-1 affects heart rate and contractility
- Beta-2 affects vascular and smooth muscle
- Associated with neonatal hypoglycaemia and IUGR

Labetalol (first-line treatment)
- Combined alpha- and beta-blocker that can be given orally or IV
- Licensed for use in pregnancy. Used IV for the acute treatment of severe hypertension
- Avoid use with asthmatic women as it causes bronchospasm
- Compatible with breastfeeding

Nifedipine
- Calcium channel-blocker that inhibits transport of calcium across cell membranes
- Causes vasodilatation, which reduces blood pressure
- Not licensed for pregnancy use before 20 weeks' gestation
- Probably compatible with breastfeeding

Methyldopa
- Acts centrally to produce a decrease in vascular resistance

- Has a maximum effect 48 hours after commencement of treatment
- Small amounts are secreted into breastmilk, but it is classified as compatible with breastfeeding

Hydralazine
- Direct-acting vasodilator
- No adverse fetal effects, but many maternal side-effects, including acute hypotension, tachycardia and palpitations
- Initially 25 mg twice/day given orally in the third trimester only
- Compatible with breastfeeding

Diuretics
- Relieve oedema by inhibiting sodium reabsorption in the kidney and increasing urine production, thus lowering blood volume and in turn blood pressure
- Act within 1–2 h of oral administration and last for 12–24 h
- Usually administered in the morning so that diuresis does not interfere with sleep
- Loss of potassium (*hypokalaemia*) is a complication and potassium supplements may be given for long-term treatment of hypertension
- Use in pregnancy is restricted to treating complex disorders, e.g. heart disease or renal disease in combination with other drugs

From Webster et al. (2019).

automated reagent-strip reading device to assess urine for proteinuria and observing for oedema. Ankle oedema is a common phenomenon in pregnancy and tends to diminish overnight. More generalized oedema that pits on pressure on the pre-tibial surface, face, hands, abdomen and sacrum, especially if sudden in onset, warrants further investigation. The severity of the oedema increases with the severity of the pre-eclampsia.

NICE (2019c) recommend the triage PIGF test and Elecsys immunoassay sFlt-1/PIGF ratio alongside the standard clinical assessment to diagnose pre-eclampsia. Other tests include maternal bloods, e.g. full blood count (FBC), urea and electrolytes (U&Es) and liver function tests (LFTs), and a 24-h urine collection to quantify any proteinuria. Assessment of proteinuria should be undertaken using an automated reagent-strip reading device or a spot urinary protein:

creatinine ratio for estimating proteinuria in a secondary care setting. If an automated reagent-strip reading device is used to detect proteinuria and a result of 1+ or more is obtained, use a spot urinary protein: creatinine ratio or 24-h urine collection to quantify proteinuria. NICE (2019c) recognize significant proteinuria if the urinary protein: creatinine ratio is >30 mg/mmol or a validated 24-h urine collection result shows >300 mg protein. Where 24-h urine collection is used to quantify proteinuria, there should be a recognized method of evaluating completeness of the sample (NICE 2019c). See Box 15.5 for determining proteinuria in pregnancy.

NICE (2019c) recommends that if conservative management of severe gestational hypertension or pre-eclampsia is planned, ultrasound fetal growth and amniotic fluid volume assessment umbilical artery Doppler velocimetry should be undertaken. If the

BOX 15.5 Determining Proteinuria in Pregnancy

- If using a dipstick to test the urine, ensure the reagent strips are in date and read according to the stipulated times along the exterior label.
- A mid-stream specimen of urine (MSSU) may be necessary to exclude urinary tract infection (UTI) as a cause of proteinuria.
- If an automated reagent-strip reading device is used to detect proteinuria and a result of 1+ or more is obtained, use a spot urinary protein:creatinine ratio or an albumin:creatinine ratio or 24-h urine collection to quantify proteinuria.
- Significant proteinuria is diagnosed when the urinary protein:creatinine ratio is >30 mg/mmol, or if a 24-h urine collection result shows >300 mg protein.

From NICE (2019c).

results of all fetal monitoring are normal in women with pre-eclampsia, do not routinely repeat CTG more than weekly. In women with severe pre-eclampsia, repeat cardiotocography if any of the following occur:

- the woman reports a change in fetal movement
- vaginal bleeding
- abdominal pain
- deterioration in maternal condition.

In women with severe pre-eclampsia, NICE (2019) recommendation is not to routinely repeat the ultrasound fetal growth, amniotic fluid volume assessment or umbilical artery Doppler velocimetry more than every 2 weeks. However, if the results of any fetal monitoring in women with severe pre-eclampsia are abnormal, referral and consultation with a consultant obstetrician is recommended.

All women with severe pre-eclampsia should have a written care plan that includes all of the following:

- the timing and nature of future fetal monitoring
- fetal indications for birth and if and when corticosteroids should be given
- discussion with neonatologist/paediatrician, obstetrician and anaesthetist should take place, and a clear plan of action based on informed decision-making should be in place.

While drugs will treat the hypertension, the solution for pre-eclampsia is to expedite the birth of the baby and placenta. Timing of birth is determined by the maternal and fetal condition. It tends to be conservative pre-37 weeks, although may be warranted, e.g. if the MDT is unable to control the mother's blood pressure or her oxygen saturation is <90%, there is deterioration of the maternal blood results or an ongoing neurological condition, reversed end-diastolic flow in the umbilical artery Doppler velocimetry or a non-reassuring CTG. Post-37 weeks' gestation, birth is initiated within 24–48 hours (NICE 2019c; Vijgen et al. 2010). The mode of birth is dependent on the maternal or fetal condition and the gestation, with caesarean section being undertaken for urgent clinical situations or if the fetus is very preterm (Webster et al. 2013), ensuring close liaison with neonatal intensive care and anaesthetist teams (NICE 2019c).

Management in labour

Vigilant care by the midwife is paramount in labour, and while this is a high-risk labour, the midwife may facilitate the birth of the baby in the absence of obstetric complications. Intrapartum care is similar to that provided to a woman with chronic hypertension and in particular, there should be continuous fetal monitoring. Hourly blood pressure assessments, as a minimum, should take place during labour and an epidural anaesthetic is encouraged after review of the most recent clotting profile/platelet count and continuation of antenatal antihypertensive drugs and blood tests according to previous results and the clinical picture are also warranted (Webster et al. 2013). Do not pre-load fluids with epidural use. If severe pre-eclampsia, the MDT will consider an operative birth, or an assisted second stage (NICE 2019c). Oxytocin is used to control haemorrhage during the third stage of labour in preference to syntometrine or ergometrine, which are contraindicated for use in cases of hypertensive disorders (see Chapter 21). Blood pressure should be measured hourly, with the midwife being alert for signs of fulminant eclampsia.

Postnatal management

NICE (2019c) recommends that women with pre-eclampsia, who did not take antihypertensives should have their blood pressure measured at least four times a day while an inpatient, at least once between day 3 and day 5 after birth and on alternate days until normal, if blood pressure was abnormal on days 3–5. They should be asked about the presence of severe headache and epigastric pain each time the blood pressure is measured.

In women with pre-eclampsia who did not take antihypertensive treatment and have given birth, antihypertensive treatment is usually commenced if the blood pressure is ≥150/100 mmHg. NICE (2019c) guidelines now place emphasis on keeping systolic blood pressure <150 mmHg and diastolic blood pressure <80–100 mmHg. Globally, it is recognized that in order to reduce morbidity, the judicious treatment of blood pressure is necessary, even though the precise thresholds to treat do differ across the globe (Duhig et al. 2018).

In women with pre-eclampsia who took antihypertensive treatment and have given birth, measure blood pressure at least four times a day, while the woman is hospitalized, every 1–2 days for up to 2 weeks after transfer to community care, until the woman is off treatment and has no residual hypertension remains.

If the woman had taken antihypertensive medications during pregnancy and birth, these are usually continued until the blood pressure falls to <140/90 mmHg; the antihypertensive treatment will be reduced if the blood pressure falls <130/80 mmHg. As before, if a woman has taken methyldopa to treat pre-eclampsia, again this should be stopped within 2 days of birth (NICE 2019c).

In women who have pre-eclampsia with mild or moderate hypertension, or after step-down from critical care, NICE (2019c) advocates measuring platelet count, transaminases and serum creatinine 48–72 h after birth or step-down, but not to repeat platelet count, transaminases or serum creatinine measurements if results were normal at 48–72 h. If biochemical and haematological indices are improving but stay within the abnormal range in women with pre-eclampsia who have given birth, repeat platelet count, transaminases and serum creatinine measurements as clinically indicated and at the postnatal review (6–8 weeks after the birth).

If biochemical and haematological indices are not improving relative to pregnancy ranges in women with pre-eclampsia who have given birth, repeat platelet count, transaminases and serum creatinine measurements as clinically indicated. Women who still have proteinuria (1+ or more) at the postnatal review (6–8 weeks after the birth) require a further review at 3 months after the birth to assess kidney function and may need a referral for specialist kidney assessment.

Transfer home will occur only when the women does not exhibit symptoms of pre-eclampsia, her blood pressure is ≤149/99 and blood results are stable or improving. A plan of care should be written for all women with pre-eclampsia before transfer to primary care. This will include details of who will provide follow-up care, the frequency of blood pressure measurement, thresholds for reducing or stopping treatment, when to refer to primary care for review and the self-monitoring for symptoms (NICE 2019c). There should be a review of hypertensive treatment by the GP at 2 weeks, which includes a dipstick urine test for proteinuria. Women who have had pre-eclampsia and who still need antihypertensive treatment at the postnatal review (6–8 weeks after the birth) should have a specialist assessment of their hypertension (NICE 2019c).

It is important to inform women who have had gestational hypertension or pre-eclampsia that experiencing these conditions during childbearing increases a woman's risk of developing high blood pressure and cardiovascular complications in later life. She should be counselled to adopt a lifestyle that reduces that risk, including achieving and maintaining a healthy BMI (NICE 2019c).

Severe Pre-Eclampsia and Eclampsia

Severe pre-eclampsia encompasses high blood pressure of systole >160 mmHg or diastole >110 mmHg on two occasions and significant proteinuria. Modern definitions also include women with moderate hypertension who have at least two of the features below:
- low blood platelet count $<100 \times 10^6$/L
- abnormal liver function
- liver tenderness
- HELLP syndrome
- clonus (intermittent muscular contractions and relaxations)
- papilloedema
- epigastric pain
- vomiting
- severe headache
- visual disturbance (flashing light similar to migraine).

This condition, unless treated effectively, can lead to eclampsia with risk of mortality and morbidity. The woman must be admitted to a regional obstetric centre for specialist medical treatment to bring her blood pressure under control, reduce the risk of fluid overload and prevent seizures. The treatment of choice in severe pre-eclampsia is magnesium sulfate (Box 15.6) (NICE 2019c). Oral labetalol or nifedipine may be used but if the BP is >170/110 mmHg, intravenous (IV) labetalol or hydralazine are given in bolus doses to lower the BP and then as a continuous IV infusion (IVI). Intravenous magnesium sulfate will also be administered, as this drug can reduce the chance of an eclamptic seizure by 50%. However, its use in clinical practice varies globally (Jana et al. 2018). Fluid restriction and a low salt diet should be initiated and monitored with a fluid balance chart, including regular urinalysis to assess proteinuria. The midwife should also be aware that magnesium toxicity may present with a marked reduction in urine output (<100 ml/4h), reducing respiratory rate (<12/min) and a loss of patellar reflexes. The effects on the fetus are as for pre-eclampsia, but there is an 80-fold increased risk of iatrogenic pre-term birth before 33 weeks, IUGR and consequent admission to neonatal intensive care (Hutcheon et al. 2011).

An acute worsening of symptoms, especially headache, epigastric pain and vomiting accompanied by high blood pressure, indicates that severe pre-eclampsia is potentially developing into eclampsia and that a convulsion is imminent. Consequently, emergency intervention is required.

Eclampsia

Eclampsia is a neurological condition associated with pre-eclampsia, manifesting with tonic clonic convulsions in pregnancy that cannot be attributed to other conditions such as epilepsy (NICE 2019c; Hutcheon et al. 2011). A national study undertaken throughout the UK by the Obstetric Surveillance System (UKOSS) between February 2005 and February 2006 identified 214 cases, indicating an estimated incidence of 26.8 cases per 100,000 births. Rates of eclampsia have actually decreased in the developed world, due to improved antenatal care, timing of birth and use of magnesium sulphate (Burton et al. 2019; Knight 2007; Hutcheon et al. 2011; Knight et al. 2018; Knight et al. 2019).

Eclampsia can develop any time from 20 weeks' gestation up to 6 weeks postpartum and indeed 44% of cases occur postnatally (Shennan and Waugh 2003), with most occurring within 12 h of birth. The UKOSS data revealed that 63% of women in the UK who had eclampsia did not have established pre-eclampsia and over 20% of women had their first convulsion at home (Knight 2007) and were initially admitted to accident and emergency departments. When a woman has an eclamptic seizure, the midwife must summon medical aid immediately, initiate Airway, Breathing, Circulation, Disability and Exposure (ABCDE) principles (see Chapter 26) and then assist the multidisciplinary team with treatment as outlined in Box 15.6.

Intrapartum care

If eclampsia arises during the antenatal or intrapartum period, the woman is likely to require an emergency caesarean section, so the midwife should prepare her for this type of birth and a potentially preterm baby. An epidural or spinal anaesthesia is preferred to reduce the consequences associated with general anaesthesia. If the woman gives birth vaginally, syntometrine and ergometrine should be avoided to manage the third stage of labour and syntocinon used instead. Once the woman's condition is stabilized she should have one-to-one care in either the Intensive Care Unit (ICU) or receive Critical Care/High Dependency Care (HDC) within the labour ward. The aim of the care is to attain a systolic BP <150 and a diastolic BP of between 80 and 100 mmHg (NICE 2019c). The woman will require an electrocardiogram (ECG) for 1 h after the loading dose of magnesium sulfate, and this drug is continued by IVI for at least 24 h. A blood sample to measure serum magnesium should be taken as this drug can reach a toxic level. If the urinary output reduces to <100 mL over 4 h, the magnesium sulfate may be reduced by 50% by the doctor, hence accurate fluid balance recording is essential. Continuous monitoring of the woman's BP is warranted along with hourly monitoring of other vital signs/physiological parameters including pulse, respiration, oxygen saturation, urine output and reflexes using a 'track and trigger' system (as outlined in Chapter 26). Ongoing antihypertensive therapy should be continued and adjusted as determined by the woman's blood pressure readings (Hull and Rucklidge 2009). This monitoring usually continues for 24–48 h, after which, providing the woman's condition improves, she can be transferred to the postnatal ward for a few more days until the medical team considers her condition is satisfactory for transfer home. The baby is likely to be initially cared for on the neonatal unit and the woman should be taken to see her baby as soon as her condition permits. Breastfeeding is to be encouraged and psychological support given by the midwife and neonatal staff.

Haemolysis, Elevated Liver Enzymes and Low Platelets Syndrome

This is a multisystem disorder that represents a severe form of pre-eclampsia and occurs in up to 20% of women with pre-eclampsia (Joshi et al. 2010). HELLP

BOX 15.6 Management of an Eclamptic Seizure

- Do not leave the convulsing woman alone.
- Get help while noting time of onset and duration of the seizure.
- Summon appropriate help: medical and midwifery support in hospital.
- In the community, ambulance and a paramedic team are required.
- Aim to protect the woman from injury, but do not move unnecessarily, e.g. put padding under her head.
- Try to reassure the woman and her relatives.

Once the seizure has stopped: assess Responsiveness and ABC (primary survey):

A: Airway. Is the airway clear? Protect from aspiration by placing the woman in the left lateral position, assisted by a wedge if still pregnant. Use suction for oral secretions.

B: Breathing. Is the woman breathing normally? Consider an oral airway. Anaesthetist should be called for possible intubation. Administer supplementary oxygen by non-rebreathing face mask.

C: Circulation. Observe the pulse, and if cardiac arrest occurs, commence continuous chest compressions (cardiac massage).

- The doctor should site an IVI, cannulate and take blood samples for: full blood count, group and save, clotting factors, uric acid, liver function tests, serum calcium, and urea and electrolytes.
- Accurate records of all fluid given should be maintained.

- A Foley catheter should be inserted in the bladder to ensure accurate recording of the urinary output and regular urine testing for proteinuria.

Drugs:

- *Magnesium sulfate* is the first-line drug of choice in the management of eclamptic seizures; the administration regime, as recommended by NICE (2019c) is:
  - loading dose of 4 g given IV over 5–15 min, followed by an infusion of 1 g/h maintained for 24 h, continued for 24 h after last seizure.
  - recurrent seizures should be treated with a further dose of 2–4 g given over 5–15 min.
- Observe for magnesium toxicity.
- Antidote: Calcium gluconate 10 ml of 10% solution IV over 10 min.

An electrocardiogram (ECG) should be conducted during the loading dose and for 1 hour afterwards.

Do not use diazepam or other anticonvulsants NICE (2019c).

D: Documents. All observations and treatment to be documented in the woman's case notes.

E: Environment. Ensure the woman keeps safe.

F: Fundus. If the woman is still pregnant, the uterus should be displaced by assisting her into the left lateral position, assisted by a wedge. Assess fetal well-being if still pregnant.

From NICE (2019c); Hull and Rucklidge (2009).

syndrome presents antenatally in 70% of cases, most usually in the third trimester and in the postnatal period, it occurs in 30% of cases. If HELLP syndrome occurs before 26 weeks, it is usually associated with antiphospholipid syndrome (APS) (Pawelec et al. 2012). HELLP syndrome is associated with increased maternal and perinatal morbidity and mortality rates (Kongwattanakul et al. 2018; Turgut et al. 2010; Mihu et al. 2007).

In HELLP syndrome, there is activation of the coagulation system causing increased deposits of protein fibrin throughout the body resulting in fragmentation of erythrocytes (Webster et al. 2013). Fibrin deposits on blood vessel walls initiate clumping of platelets resulting in blood clots and lowering of the platelet count. These deposits decrease the diameter of the blood vessels, raising blood pressure and reducing the blood flow to organs (Webster et al. 2013). The liver is especially affected, with destruction of liver cells leading to abnormal liver function and a distended liver with symptoms of epigastric discomfort.

The woman will present with nonspecific symptoms, often malaise, including nausea, vomiting and right upper quadrant or epigastric pain with liver tenderness. In some cases there may be haematuria or jaundice. If there is pre-eclampsia there will be raised blood pressure and proteinuria. These symptoms are similar to acute fatty liver disease (AFLD) and the blood tests define the diagnosis.

Complications can include:

- progressive disseminated intravascular coagulation (DIC)
- liver haematoma and rupture
- placental abruption
- pulmonary oedema and adult respiratory distress
- pleural effusions
- renal failure.

The main treatment is to expedite the birth of the baby with the management and midwifery care being similar to that for severe pre-eclampsia, with emphasis on the administration of magnesium sulphate to prevent convulsions. The condition usually resolves, however, 2 weeks after the baby's birth.

Acute Fatty Liver Disease

Acute fatty liver disease of pregnancy is a rare and serious condition with uncertain aetiology, and current theory implies it is part of the pre-eclampsia spectrum (Doughty and Waugh 2013). Women with a raised body mass index (BMI), primigravidae and women with a multiple pregnancy appear to be at risk.

Five out of the following symptoms denote diagnosis, which usually present after 30 weeks of pregnancy: nausea, vomiting, polyuria, polydipsia, fever, headache, encephalopathy, pruritus, abdominal pain, tiredness, confusion, jaundice, anorexia, ascites, coagulopathy, hypertension, proteinuria, liver failure and hepatic encephalopathy (James et al. 2017). Diagnosis is made on the clinical picture and abnormal LFT results. Ultrasound or MRI would show fatty infiltration of the maternal liver.

The condition of the woman can deteriorate rapidly, especially liver function, affecting both maternal and fetal morbidity and mortality. The woman must be referred promptly to a specialist hepatologist for further investigation and to exclude alternative diagnoses such as HELLP. Management is to hasten the birth of the baby such that the midwife may need to prepare the woman for a preterm birth. Careful fluid balance is required in labour and vigilant observation, as DIC is a significant risk. Following the birth, the woman is likely to be transferred to an ICU/HDCU where her condition is monitored and supportive care measures instigated to correct coagulopathy, treat hypoglycaemia and improve renal function. Improvements are usually seen after 48 h (Doughty and Waugh 2013).

METABOLIC DISORDERS

Obesity

Obesity is considered to be one of the most significant health concerns affecting society, with significant impact on the maternity services (Solmi and Morris 2018). Individual risk of serious morbidity or mortality is related to increasing weight through the development of disease pathways directly attributable to obesity, e.g.

cardiovascular disease, certain cancers and type 2 diabetes mellitus. However, these pathways are unclear as individuals of normal body weight may also develop these conditions.

The increasing prevalence of obesity is commonly called an epidemic (World Health Organization, WHO 2017), although obesity does not resemble an infectious disease; rather, it is used to describe a trend. Using the BMI classification, statistics demonstrate 25% of women over 16 years of age are obese (BMI $\geq$30 kg/m^2). These figures rise to almost 60% when those in the overweight category are included. Currently only around 40% of women have a normal BMI. Severe or morbid obesity (BMI $\geq$40 kg/m^2) is increasing more rapidly and is higher in women at 4% than in men at 2%, which is a tripling of morbid obesity rates since 1993 (Public Health England, PHE 2017) and studies have suggested this will continue to see a steady increase until 2035 (Keaver and Webber 2016). Therefore, globally, obesity and fatness is becoming 'normal', especially in Western societies such as the UK, with the adult BMI distribution curve peaking at a BMI of around 25 for both men and women (NHS Digital 2018). It is estimated that if this trend continues to rise, by 2050, >50% of women will be classed as obese (Butland et al. 2007).

In pregnancy, 21% of women are obese at antenatal 'booking' and 1 in 1000 women during pregnancy have a BMI >50 (National Maternity and Perinatal Audit, NMPA 2017). This increase in the number of obese mothers adds to the resources needed to care for these mothers during childbearing and poses challenges for those professionals who care for them. Overweight and obese mothers are more likely to require extra resources through increased surveillance, investigations and the management of any pregnancy complications, which has been shown to result in significantly higher hospital costs, mainly through operative and preterm births and longer in-hospital stays (Solmi and Morris 2018).

Classifying Size Using Body Mass Index

Obesity is diagnosed using the BMI classification, implemented over 50 years ago as a measure of fatness, being considered a more robust way of assessing a person's level of body fat than measuring solely height and weight (Gard and Wright 2005). Obesity is defined as a BMI $\geq$30 kg/m^2 and can be subdivided into classes I, II and III (Box 15.7). As a screening tool for fatness, BMI is considered accurate in 75% of cases at best, failing to account for variations in body fat distributions, muscle and bone density, ethnic variations, gender specifics or age effect. It is not a good indicator of mortality.

Distribution of Body Fat and Disease

Distribution of body fat is considered a significant indicator of future ill-health, being suggestive of a disordered glucose tolerance (WHO 2017), which often contributes to medical complications such as type 2 diabetes mellitus. In such conditions, visceral fat (fat retained abdominally) is metabolically more active, contributing to metabolic syndrome which is directly associated with cardiovascular disease and type 2 diabetes (Gluckman and Hanson 2012). Waist circumference or waist to hip ratios may be more effective tools, as may be skin-fold thicknesses, computed tomography (CT) and magnetic resonance imaging (MRI) scans of the abdomen (Nuttall 2015; Chan and Woo 2010).

Obesity as a Concept

Being obese is not in itself a disease, although, as the level of obesity increases, so does the individual risk of developing chronic disease (Gluckman and Hanson 2012). Social scientists would agree that obesity is not a disease, but is a social construct defined as a disease, because it is considered abnormal in current Western culture (de Vries 2007). Obese individuals are consequently subject to significant stigma and discrimination directly attributed to their size and shape, even by healthcare professionals (Nyman et al. 2010). This negative attitude probably reflects deeper cultural prejudices that exist towards obesity, reflected in the prevailing ideology of it being caused by the individual. However, the cause of obesity is multifactorial: it is considered a complex interplay of genetics, biology and behaviour on a background of cultural, environmental and social factors, where the individual plays a passive role within an obesogenic society (Butland et al. 2007).

Obesity Demographics

A high incidence of obesity is seen associated with socioeconomic inequalities, where increased rates of obesity are associated with increased parity, age, poverty and social deprivation (Bogaerts 2014). Sellstrom et al. (2009) identified increased rates of obesity in poorer societal groups, especially younger age groups. Children born into lower social class families are likely to become obese, although this trend is seen more in women than in men, probably because of the complexity of the role of women in society (Khlat et al. 2009). The cause of obesity is multifactorial and is clearly more than just 'eating too much' (see section on Causes of obesity, below).

Pathophysiology of Obesity

The main effect obesity has on an individual's health is increasing their risk of developing metabolic syndrome. Obesity, especially central obesity, causes metabolic dysfunction involving primarily lipids and glucose, which eventually results in organ dysfunction within many of the body systems, especially the cardiovascular system. Other risk factors for metabolic syndrome include family history, poor diet and a sedentary lifestyle.

Metabolic syndrome is thought to be caused by visceral adipose tissue causing the release of pro-inflammatory cytokines, known as adipokines, which promote insulin resistance. This causes a systemic inflammatory response, which over time results in microvascular and endothelial dysfunction in all of the body systems. The individual will have atherogenic dyslipidaemia, identified by low high-density lipoprotein (HDL), raised triglycerides, hypertension and raised fasting blood glucose levels. As well as insulin resistance, such individuals develop a prothrombotic state with raised fibrinogen and plasminogen-activator-inhibitor levels (Miller and Mitchell 2006).

In pregnancy, the increased maternal insulin resistance in the obese mother results in hyperinsulinaemia, inflammation and oxidative stress. This contributes to placental dysfunction and results in the increased risk of complications seen throughout the childbearing episode and culminates in poorer pregnancy outcomes (Catalano and Shankar 2017).

Causes of Obesity

The cause of obesity is multifactorial including:

- obesogenic environment
- genetic influences
- diet – refined sugars and processed foods leading to insulin surges
- ethnicity
- psychosocial – hormonal interplay
- socioeconomic factors
- alcohol intake
- lifestyle behaviour
- depression and mental ill-health, including medication
- stress – causing rises in corticosteroids/comfort eating.

Nutritional Needs in Pregnancy

Weight gain is usual at certain times in a female's life, e.g. during infancy, between the ages of 5 and 7 years, adolescence, pregnancy and the menopause (Webb 2008). Schmitt et al. (2007) in their meta-analysis suggest that weight gain in pregnancy is inevitable due to hormonal changes and lifestyle behaviour adaptations, plus the development of the fetal-uterine unit, as the pregnancy develops. Pregnancy itself could therefore be regarded to be a possible risk factor to the development of obesity. Maternal over-nutrition has been shown to have a permanent effect on a fetus, that is, a higher birth weight tends to result in a higher BMI as an adult (Denison et al. 2018). Physiological changes in pregnancy predispose to weight gain, essentially to provide energy for labour and lactation, and this storage is facilitated by the effect that increases in oestrogen, progesterone and human placental lactogen (HPL) have on glucose metabolism (Webb 2008). Women with a raised BMI should be advised and encouraged to lose weight in the pre-conception period to optimize pregnancy outcomes (Modder and Fitzsimons 2010).

A woman's basal metabolic rate (BMR) increases during pregnancy due to the increased metabolic activity of the maternal and fetal tissues. The increased body weight and the increased maternal cardiovascular, renal and respiratory load also influence a rise in the basal metabolic rate (BMR), but in part this is counterbalanced by a general decrease in activity. The resulting increase in required calorie intake is therefore relatively small; an extra 200 kcal/day are required during the third trimester for most women (NICE 2010b).

Weight gain in pregnancy is dependent on factors such as diet, activity and maternal wellbeing (Gardner et al. 2011).

Gestational Weight Gain

There are two types of women with obesity during pregnancy. There are those with pre-pregnancy obesity; this group is in a potentially poorer state of health than a mother who has a BMI within the normal range and may have existing comorbidities. They are at most risk of developing pregnancy complications. There are those who gain excessive weight during pregnancy; these individuals usually have a lower BMI pre-pregnancy, but weight gained in pregnancy can cause birth complications. Excessive gestational weight gain (GWG) is difficult to lose postnatally and is often retained (postpartum weight retention), risking long-term obesity and ill health in later life.

Gestational weight gain, as the term suggests, is defined as weight gained during pregnancy, while excessive GWG is weight gained during pregnancy that is over and above the weight of the fetus and its environment and so is subsequently at risk of being retained by a mother post-birth (Swinburn et al. 2011). Minimizing and controlling excessive GWG is important regardless of pre-pregnancy BMI and excessive GWG has been shown to increase maternal and fetal risks (Poston et al. 2016; Haugen et al. 2014). Reducing GWG reduces the incidence of operative births, macrosomia (Muktabhant et al. 2015) and pre-eclampsia (Thangaratinam et al. 2012). There is increasing emphasis on the role of the midwife in managing GWG during antenatal care encounters.

Antenatal Care

The BMI is routinely calculated at the initial visit with the midwife (booking) and a discussion about the implications of a raised BMI should consequently take place between the midwife and the woman. Depending on local guidelines, women with a raised BMI are often referred to a multiprofessional antenatal clinic, which involves specialist midwives, obstetricians and dieticians (Denison et al. 2018; Modder and Fitzsimons 2010). The role of the midwife when caring for an obese woman during pregnancy is both supportive and facilitative. The midwife should ensure discussions meet individual needs and talk sensitively about the topic of obesity and weight. The midwife should be able to provide advice about healthy eating and moderate exercise. She should also be able to discuss risks associated with obesity and this should be tailored to individual circumstances and risks. Antenatal interventions such as classes to discuss diet, nutrition and activity have been shown to reduce excessive GWG and subsequent postpartum weight retention at 6 weeks post-birth (Shieh et al. 2018; Haby et al. 2015).

Knight et al. (2019) reporting for MBRRACE on maternal mortality in the UK highlight that >34% of the women who died in the triennium 2015–2017 were obese, with 24% being overweight. They also raised concerns around global maternal health and the need to do more as highlighted by the seminal papers in the 2016 *Lancet* series study group on maternal health global health (Lancet 2016).

The subsequent risk of morbidity associated with childbearing of women who have a raised BMI is outlined in Box 15.8 (Denison et al. 2018; Modder and Fitzsimons 2010). However, it is important to note that obesity alone is not associated with poor perinatal outcomes, but that it does increase the risk, which subsequently increases as the BMI increases (Scott-Pillai et al. 2013). Women with obesity might find some disorders of pregnancy, such as back pain and fatigue, are exacerbated (see Chapter 10).

If the woman has a BMI >35, she will be offered increased doses of folic acid (5 mg), oral Vitamin D supplementation 10 mg daily during pregnancy and while breastfeeding, if at high risk of pre-eclampsia low dose Aspirin may be prescribed. The midwife should consider venous thromboembolic (VTE) prophylaxis if two or more other risk factors are present (Royal College of Obstetricians and Gynaecologists, RCOG 2009) and refer the woman to specific consultant-led clinics if complications arise.

If the woman has a BMI >40 she should be referred for anaesthetic review. The midwife should monitor her closely for complications, including pre-eclampsia; and refer her for assessment by 'Manual Handling Team' prior to birth.

During pregnancy, women who are obese may report a range of psychosocial issues related to their increased BMI. For instance, they may feel disappointed at not being recognized as pregnant until later in pregnancy (Nash 2012a) and worry about their weight gain in pregnancy (Nash 2012b).

The maternity services need to ensure suitable equipment and staffing levels are available, e.g. suitable beds and chairs, large BP cuffs, sufficient operating department staff in respect of caring for women with obesity (Denison et al. 2018; Modder and Fitzsimons 2010).

BOX 15.8 Risks Associated with Obesity in Pregnancy

Maternal
- Miscarriage and stillbirth
- Gestational diabetes: offer a glucose tolerance test (GTT) at 24–28 weeks if BMI ≥30
- Hypertension: ensure correct size cuff and increase surveillance if BMI ≥35; increase antenatal appointments to screen for PET to every 3 weeks between 24 and 32 weeks and refer to specialist care if one or more additional risk factors are present, e.g. first baby, raised BP at booking
- Venous thromboembolism: assess risk at every visit; prophylaxis is recommended if two or more risk factors are present
- Prolonged pregnancy: risks associated with induction of labour
- Presence of pre-existing medical conditions, e.g. ischaemic heart disease
- Poorer mental health, e.g. depression

Fetal
- Neural tube defects (NTDs): all women should take 5 mg folic acid daily
- Macrosomia
- Preterm labour
- Lower Apgar scores
- Late stillbirth
- Neonatal mortality

Maternity services
- Increased hospital admissions
- Increased costs associated with managing complications
- Increased length of hospital stay
- Increased neonatal care requirements.

From Denison et al. (2018); Modder and Fitzsimons (2010).

Risk assessments for labour should be undertaken antenatally for each woman, considering moving and handling issues in order to ensure suitable aids are available to assist with movement (Denison et al. 2018; Modder and Fitzsimons 2010; Marshall and Brydon 2012). Furthermore, Royal College of Obstetricians and Gynaecologists (Modder and Fitzsimons 2010) endorse that all maternity units should have documented environmental risk assessments regarding the availability of facilities for pregnant women presenting with a BMI of >30 kg/m² at the initial visit.

BOX 15.9 Intrapartum Risks Associated with Obesity

- Prolonged pregnancy and induction of labour
- Prolonged labour: labour is slower and there is often a delay between 4 and 7 cm with syntocinon use being higher. There should be close observation of progress in labour with one-to-one care for women with a BMI ≥40
- Complications, e.g. shoulder dystocia
- Emergency caesarean birth: if a woman has a BMI >40 the incidence is almost 50%. There is an increased risk of malpresentation, e.g. occipitoposterior (OP) position, and VBAC is less successful
- Primary postpartum haemorrhage: venous access and active management of the third stage of labour is recommended for women with a BMI ≥40.

From Kerrigan and Kingdon (2010); Modder and Fitzsimons (2010).

Intrapartum Care

Obesity is a significant risk factor during labour, as detailed in Box 15.9. For women who have a BMI >35 kg/m^2 it is recommended that the birth should occur in a consultant-led environment (Kerrigan and Kingdon 2010). However, these women will benefit from good-quality midwifery-led care to promote optimal outcomes, e.g. encouraging mobility and an upright position. It could also be argued that these women might benefit from birthing in a midwife-led unit/birth centre alongside an obstetric unit. It is recommended by NICE (2014) that individual discussions with women whose BMI is between 30 and 34 kg/m^2 should take place regarding the local birthplace options available.

It is worth noting that there may be difficulties in assessing maternal and fetal wellbeing during labour, e.g. ensuring a good quality CTG recording, undertaking vaginal examinations and performing manoeuvres in an emergency such as shoulder dystocia (Doughty and Waugh 2013). In addition, there may be difficulties in managing intraoperative complications such as controlling haemorrhage.

Postnatal Care

Obesity has a direct influence on short- and long-term health and wellbeing for the mother and the baby following birth, as indicated in Box 15.10.

Breastfeeding has been shown to reduce the weight a woman has gained in pregnancy more effectively than in

BOX 15.10 Risks Associated with Obesity in the Postnatal Period

Maternal
- Venous thromboembolism: early mobilization following birth encouraged. Prophylaxis considered even following vaginal birth
- Longer postoperative recovery
- Increased postoperative complications, e.g. wound dehiscence and infection
- Tendency to retain pregnancy weight gain
- Lowered rates of breastfeeding duration
- Reduced contraception choices: depending on presence of comorbidities.

Neonatal
- Increased risk of congenital abnormality, e.g. heart defects
- Macrosomia: increased risk of trauma from birth; practical difficulties associated with undertaking the neonatal examination
- Low birth weight: associated with the presence of antenatal maternal comorbidity, with increased risk of possible long-term effects on health, e.g. increased rates of cardiovascular disease and diabetes mellitus in middle age.

From Denison et al. (2018); Modder and Fitzsimons (2010).

those women who choose to artificially feed their babies (Bertz et al. 2015; Baker et al. 2008). Obese women are as likely to initiate breastfeeding as women of a normal weight but tend to breastfeed for a shorter time (Amir and Donath 2007). It is known that obese women have delayed lactogenesis and a lowered response of prolactin to suckling, leading to reduced milk production and premature cessation of breastfeeding. However, the response to prolactin is reduced over time, so extended support from midwives skilled at supporting the continuance of breastfeeding is especially important in this group of women (Jevitt et al. 2007).

Retained excessive gestational weight gained in pregnancy is difficult to lose postnatally due to a number of factors such as the demands of caring for a new baby, eating irregular meals and an inability to exercise as frequently. This may result in higher rates of obesity in later life (Gardner et al. 2011). Excessive GWG and postpartum weight retention increases the risk that the mother may enter a subsequent pregnancy with a BMI ≥30 and may increase the mother's risk of complications in any subsequent pregnancies (Catalano and Shankar 2017; Poston et al. 2016). Postpartum weight retention also increases the chances of her becoming obese in the long term (Nehring et al. 2011). Women who were obese during pregnancy also exhibit a tendency to retain fat centrally following the baby's birth, which may result in increased morbidity and mortality later in life (Catalano and Shankar 2017; Villamor and Cnattingius 2006).

However, interpregnancy weight reduction has been shown to improve outcomes in any subsequent pregnancy (Modder and Fitzsimons 2010). Discussions around weight, activity and healthy lifestyle modification behaviours by healthcare professionals during the 6–8 weeks postnatal examination are recommended by NICE (2010b) and the Department of Health (DH 2016). If comorbidities such as gestational diabetes have been diagnosed during pregnancy, a glucose tolerance test (GTT) should be undertaken at the postnatal examination and the woman should continue to have annual cardiometabolic screening (Modder and Fitzsimons 2010). The Royal College of Midwives (RCM) has collaborated with Slimming World© to develop strategies to positively influence and improve the health of childbearing women (Avery et al. 2010; Pallister et al. 2010).

Obstetric Cholestasis

Obstetric cholestasis (OC) is also known as intrahepatic cholestasis of pregnancy and is a condition specific to pregnancy that denotes a disruption and reduction of bile products by the liver. It is diagnosed by the presence of raised serum bile acids and usually appears after 28 weeks' gestation, resolving a couple of weeks following the birth of the baby. Obstetric cholestasis manifests as intense itching (pruritus) that mainly affects the soles of the feet, hands and body, becoming worse at night, albeit there is no visible rash. The woman often complains of loss of sleep. Urinary tract infections (UTI) are common and jaundice may occur, with the woman stating that her faecal stools are pale.

Treatment is based on the use of topical creams, but medications such as ursodeoxycholic acid and chlorampheniramine may be prescribed. Obstetric cholestasis causes severe liver impairment and increases perinatal morbidity and mortality (Saleh and Abdo 2007). Timing of the birth depends on gestational age and fetal wellbeing, which is monitored through fetal growth and serial ultrasonography, fetal movements and CTG. Birth before 38 weeks is usually advocated (RCOG 2011a). There is also an increased risk of postpartum haemorrhage (PPH) due to coagulation disruption. Oral vitamin K 10 mg is often prescribed to lessen the risk and active management of the third stage of labour is advised. Postnatal care is based on ensuring liver function tests (LFTs) return to normal. Recurrence in a subsequent pregnancy is high, at around 90%.

Endocrine Disorders

Insulin is a polypeptide hormone produced in the pancreas by the beta cells of the islets of Langerhans. It has a pivotal role in the metabolism of carbohydrate, fat and protein and lowers the level of blood glucose. Conversely, the alpha cells produce the hormone glucagon which increases the blood glucose. In healthy individuals, the blood glucose level regulates the secretion of insulin and glucagon on a negative-feedback principle. Hence, if the blood glucose level is high (hyperglycaemia) more insulin is released, whereas if the blood glucose level is low (hypoglycaemia) insulin is inhibited and glucagon is released (Tortora and Derrickson 2016). Excess glucose is stored in the liver where it can be released depending upon metabolic demands. In the longer term, excess glucose is stored as body fat and this is an important issue when considering obesity and also macrosomic babies of mothers with diabetes.

Diabetes Mellitus

Diabetes mellitus is a metabolic disorder due to deficiency or diminished effectiveness of endogenous insulin affecting 5.5% of the adult population in the UK and is the most common pre-existing medical disorder complicating pregnancy in the UK (NICE 2015; James et al. 2017). It is characterized by hyperglycaemia, deranged metabolism and complications mainly affecting blood vessels.

The classic presentation, especially in type 1 diabetes, is of weight loss and the occurrence of the three polys: polydipsia (excess thirst), polyuria (excessive, dilute urine production) and polyphagia (excessive hunger) (Tortora and Derrickson 2016). There may also be lethargy, prolonged infection, boils and pruritis vulvae. Conversely, with type 2 diabetes, individuals are often obese with few or no presenting symptoms.

A random blood glucose result >11.1 mmol/L is highly suggestive of diabetes and the diagnosis is confirmed by a fasting blood glucose test. A GTT entails taking a fasting blood sample, giving a 75 g glucose drink and a taking a further blood test 2 h later to determine the plasma glucose levels. If the plasma level is >7.0 mmol/L following the fasting test, or >7.8 mmol/L following the 2-hour test, a diagnoses of diabetes is made by the physician (NICE 2015). There are several types of diabetes mellitus.

Type 1 Diabetes

Type 1 diabetes (formally insulin-dependent or juvenile onset diabetes) develops as a result of progressive auto-immune destruction of the pancreatic beta cells, most probably initiated by infection, with the result that no, or an inadequate amount of, insulin is produced. Hyperglycaemia occurs leading to glycosuria, dehydration, lipolysis and proteolysis with the classic symptoms listed above. Metabolism of type 1 diabetes mimics starvation. In the absence of insulin, the body cells use fatty acids to produce adenosine triphosphate (ATP). By-products of this process produce organic acids called 'ketones'. As ketones accumulate, they lower the pH of the blood, making it acidic, known as 'ketoacidosis' (Tortora and Derrickson 2016). This can be detected by the presence of ketones in the urine and the breath smelling of pear drop sweets. If untreated, the ketoacidosis will lead to coma and death.

In 85% of cases there is no first-degree family history of the condition; however, if one parent has type 1 diabetes, there is a 2–9% chance of an individual developing it but if both parents have the condition the risk rises to 30%. Diagnosis is confirmed by raised blood glucose results. Complications include nephropathy, neuropathy, retinopathy and cataract formation. Microvascular complications arise if there is chronic hyperglycaemia, leading to secondary complications such as atherosclerosis and gangrene of the feet due to sensory neuropathy and ischaemia. For this reason, individuals with diabetes are discouraged from walking barefooted and may need referral to a diabetic foot clinic.

Treatment is the lifelong administration of insulin, which has to be given by subcutaneous injections 2–5 times a day. This is usually self-administered. Traditionally, animal-derived insulins from beef and pork were used; from the 1980s human insulin was introduced prior to a genetically modified form known as human analogue. All of these can be short and long lasting, as shown in Table 15.1. Treatment is based upon best practice guidelines and is determined for each individual person with diabetes and the specialist diabetes team (NICE 2015; Scottish Intercollegiate Guidelines Network, SIGN 2010). The blood glucose levels aimed for are in the range of a person without diabetes, which are: preprandial (fasting/before a meal) between 3.5 and 5.9 mmol/L, and 1 h postprandial <7.8.00 mmol/L. Insulin dosage is adjusted according to blood glucose levels and the individual needs to test their blood sugar at least twice a day using finger-prick tests and reagent strips read against a colour chart, or with a glucose meter (glucometer). In the home setting, urine is also tested for ketones using dipsticks.

Hypoglycaemia is a potential problem when insulin therapy is used, as insulin will decrease blood glucose levels. When the level is low, adrenergic symptoms of palpitations, perspiration, tremor and hunger alert the individual to take action and resolve this by eating a meal or taking glycogen sweets or gel (de Valk and Visser 2011). If the blood glucose decreases further the individual is likely to experience neuroglycogenic symptoms of altered behaviour and mood swings (de Valk and Visser 2011). If left untreated, convulsions and loss of consciousness can result, leading to coma and death.

Severe hypoglycaemia is associated with loss of consciousness and requires the assistance of another person to administer glucagon intramuscularly, as there is a risk of asphyxiation with oral administration. Individuals who have diabetes should always carry glucagon ready-to-use devices with them for this purpose.

Where diabetes control cannot be achieved by a traditional basal/bolus regime, individuals with diabetes are increasingly being offered the choice of insulin pump therapy. Continuous subcutaneous insulin infusion pumps (CSII) are in common use in the USA and the midwife is increasingly likely to encounter them in the UK. The pump controls the constant administration of insulin as a basal dose, in bursts at 3 min intervals with the individual self-administering a bolus dose via the pump when they consume carbohydrate, or if they need to reduce severely high blood glucose levels. This is not currently a closed loop system, as each individual has to have a good understanding of their own personal carbohydrate to insulin ratios in order to regulate the pump to administer an appropriate bolus dose whenever carbohydrate is consumed and set the pump up to follow their required basal dose profile. There are also some pumps that work in conjunction with a

TABLE 15.1	Types of Insulin According to Origin and Length of Action			
Insulin type	**Rapid action**	**Short action**	**Intermediate action**	**Long action**
Analogue	Apidra Humalog NovoRapid			Lantus Levemir
Human		Actrapid Humulin S Insuman Rapid	Humulin I Insuman Basal Insulatard	
Animal		Hypurin Bovine Neutral Hypurin Porcine Neutral	Hypurin Bovine Isophane Hypurin Porcine Isophane	Hypurin Bovine Lente Hypurin Bovine Protamine Zinc

Note: Pre-mixed insulin can be prescribed, but only when two injections a day are required.
From NICE (2019b).

continuous glucose monitoring sensor which is injected into the skin, with a transmitter clipped to the surface. The transmitter sends readings to the pump once every 5 min. The pump can be set up to sound an alarm if the readings are outside limits defined by the individual and is particularly useful for diabetics who are susceptible to serious hypoglycaemic episodes while asleep. However, as the individual remains responsible for defining appropriate insulin doses based on the information provided by the sensor, they are still required to perform daily blood glucose and urinary ketones tests, which necessitates the mental capacity to cope with the system and calculations.

A fully closed loop system, also known as the artificial pancreas, which mimics normal pancreatic administration of insulin, has also been developed. As with the CSII, there is a pump and a sensor, but there is an additional handheld control device that contains an algorithm to calculate the insulin dose required. This information is transmitted to the pump and the insulin is administered automatically without any intervention from the individual. There is also a suspend insulin command to prevent hypoglycaemic episodes. Results from clinical trials are promising and this treatment may become mainstream in just a few years, with midwives encountering it soon in a research context with childbearing women. Islet cell transplants are now available in the UK for individuals who meet strict criteria, being intended for those unable to recognize severe hypoglycaemia or those who are otherwise healthy renal transplant recipients.

Regular attendance at outpatient clinics is necessary to monitor diabetic control. The glycated or glycosylated haemoglobin (HbA$_{1c}$) test is performed every 2–6 months. This measures the average blood glucose level by analysing the molecule in the haemoglobin in the red blood cell where glucose binds. The higher the HbA$_{1c}$ the poorer is the diabetic control. Treatment aims to keep the HbA$_{1c}$ at <48 mmol/mol (6.5%). However, since 2011, HbA$_{1c}$ has been expressed in mmol/mol to comply with the International Federation of Clinical Chemistry (IFCC) Units.

Type 2 Diabetes

In type 2 diabetes (formally non-insulin-dependent or maturity onset diabetes), there is a gradual resistance to the action of insulin in the liver and muscle. This can also be combined with impaired pancreatic beta cell function leading to a relative insulin deficiency. Type 2 diabetes accounts for 85% of cases of diabetes and tends to cluster in families. All racial groups are affected but it is six times more common in people of South Asian descent and three times more common among people of African and African-Caribbean origin. Traditionally, it was associated with older people but it is increasingly diagnosed in children, young adults and among those with a raised BMI and sedentary lifestyle (Gregory and Todd 2013).

The initial treatment is by strict diet to reduce weight and increased physical activity to improve glucose tolerance and control the diabetes. As the condition progresses, oral diabetic agents such as metformin become necessary, and eventually insulin treatment might be required. Furthermore, ancillary medication such as ACE inhibitors and statins may be prescribed to prevent cardiovascular complications. Diabetic monitoring is the same as for type 1 diabetes.

Secondary Diabetes

This is a type of diabetes that presents secondary to another medical condition such as pancreatic disease or cystic fibrosis (Ali and Dornhorst 2018).

Maturity Onset Diabetes of the Young

In this type of diabetes, there is a genetic defect affecting pancreatic beta cell insulin secretion. Out of all cases presenting, 95% have a first-degree relative affected. However, maturity onset diabetes of the young (MODY) is not associated with obesity and it tends to be diagnosed in the second or third decade of life (Ali and Dornhorst 2018).

Diabetes in Pregnancy

During pregnancy, up to 5% of women have either pre-existing diabetes or gestational diabetes. Within this statistic, it is estimated that approximately 87.5% have gestational diabetes, 7.5% have type 1 diabetes and the remaining 5% have type 2 diabetes. The prevalence of type 1 and type 2 diabetes has increased in recent years. The incidence of all types of diabetes is increasing; the increase in gestational diabetes and type 2 diabetes is associated with higher rates of obesity in the general population and more pregnancies occurring in older women. Women with diabetes in pregnancy are at an increased risk; miscarriage, stillbirth, pre-eclampsia and preterm labour are more common in women with pre-existing diabetes and the baby is at increased risk of congenital malformations, macrosomia, birth injury, perinatal mortality (NICE 2015).

Gestational Diabetes Mellitus

Gestational diabetes mellitus (GDM) is a form of diabetes that arises in the second or third trimester of pregnancy and resolves after the birth of the baby. There is intolerance to glucose, which is attributed to increasing levels of placental hormones, in particular HPL and increasing maternal insulin resistance, especially after 20 weeks' gestation (Gregory and Todd 2013). Gestational diabetes is usually asymptomatic and according to Reece et al. (2009), it is associated with:

- increasing maternal age
- previous or family history of diabetes or GDM
- certain ethnic groups (Asian, African-Caribbean, Latin American, Middle Eastern)
- previous unexplained stillbirth
- previous macrosomic infant ($\geq$4.5 kg)
- obesity (three-fold risk of GDM).

It is diagnosed by a glucose tolerance test (GTT), using a 2-h 75 g oral GTT at 24–28 weeks' gestation. Results showing a fasting plasma glucose level of $\geq$5.6 mmol/L or a 2-h plasma glucose level of $\geq$7.8 mmol/L are diagnostic (NICE 2015). Prompt referral to a joint diabetes and antenatal clinic is required, where the woman will be supported to achieve and maintain good glucose control throughout her pregnancy, which includes advice about nutrition and exercise.

Gestational diabetes should resolve shortly after the birth of the baby. The finite diagnosis is therefore made in retrospect, as it is not possible during pregnancy to differentiate between GDM and types 1 and 2 diabetes that present for the first time in pregnancy (the latter two of which do not resolve following the baby's birth). It is therefore important that observations and outpatient follow-up appointments are undertaken in the postnatal period. The lifetime risk of developing type 2 diabetes after gestational diabetes is seven-fold (Bellamy et al. 2009). The treatment is referral to a dietician with adherence to a diet restricting sugar and fat, encouragement of 30 min exercise a day, self-monitoring of blood glucose and insulin therapy if necessary.

Pre-conception Care

Pre-conception care is essential for any women with diabetes because of the potential pregnancy complications and four-fold increased risk overall of congenital malformations which are associated with hyperglycaemia. Pre-conception advice should be included in all contact that women with diabetes may have with healthcare professionals, including their diabetes care team, throughout their childbearing years (NICE 2015; Hughes et al. 2012).

NICE (2015) recommends that women with diabetes are supported to aim for fasting capillary plasma glucose of 5–7 mmol/L on waking and a capillary plasma glucose of 4–7 mmol/L before meals throughout the day. Keeping their HbA$_{1c}$ to below 48 mmol/mol (6.5%) reduces the risk of fetal congenital malformation; NICE (2015) strongly advise that women with a HbA$_{1c}$ >86 mmol/L (10%) should avoid pregnancy. Good diabetic control before conception is very important to reduce the risk of complications during pregnancy; this includes achieving a BMI within the normal range, taking a daily dose of 5 mg of folic acid prior to conception and for the first 12 weeks of pregnancy (NICE 2015).

Pre-conception care for women with diabetes includes having a thorough medical assessment, as existing complications such as retinopathy and nephropathy can deteriorate during pregnancy (Scanlon and Harcombe 2011; Gregory and Todd 2013). Assess nephropathy risk including albuminuria, i.e. assess the serum creatinine and estimated glomerular filtration rate (eGFR). If serum creatinine is ≥120 μmol/L, the urinary albumin/creatinine ratio is >30 mg/mmol or the eGFR is <45 mL/min per 1.73 m, a referral should be made to a nephrologist before contraception is discontinued (NICE 2015). Medication should also be reviewed; metformin may be continued during pregnancy, but other oral glucose lowering drugs should be discontinued/changed to insulin. Women with type 2 diabetes may also be on statins and ACE inhibitors, which should also be discontinued.

Antenatal Management

The midwife will increasingly encounter women with pre-existing diabetes because of the increased prevalence of diabetes in young people. Furthermore, some multigravidae might silently develop type 2 diabetes, conceive their fourth or fifth child and present late for the initial appointment with the midwife due to being familiar with pregnancy, however they are at risk of developing complications associated with hyperglycaemia.

Existing medical complications can worsen during pregnancy or be recognized for the first time. Furthermore, the midwife will care for women when diabetes presents during pregnancy: indeed, the midwife is likely to be the first health professional to recognize the altered state of health. If diabetes is identified in the first trimester, then this is likely to be pre-existing diabetes diagnosed for the first time in pregnancy rather than GDM. Complications for the pregnancy encompass:

- pre-eclampsia
- macrosomic baby, due to hyperglycaemia, with risk of shoulder dystocia
- IUGR
- polyhydramnios
- exacerbation of diabetic complications in the woman, in particular retinopathy and nephropathy
- risk of iatrogenic preterm birth leading to the baby being admitted to the neonatal unit.

In addition, the risks to the fetus/baby born to a woman with diabetes are that they are:

- five times more likely to be stillborn
- three times more likely to die in the first few months of life
- four times more likely to have a major congenital malformation.

These risks, however, are substantially reduced if there is good blood glucose control before and after pregnancy. The initial visit to the midwife where a detailed medical history is taken should identify those women with pre-existing diabetes for a referral to be made to a specialist endocrine/obstetric clinic. Regular appointments at this clinic are usually at fortnightly (2-week) intervals, where a multidisciplinary team of obstetrician, physician, dietician and specialist nurse/midwife will provide care. As this will be a high-risk pregnancy, the woman should not be assigned to low-risk schemes of care.

Newly diagnosed women will require education in monitoring their blood sugar glucose levels using the necessary equipment and reagent strips, which need prescribing. They will require education in self-administration of insulin and in balancing insulin requirements based on their blood glucose readings. Dietary assessment and advice is essential so that the insulin dose can be adjusted according to a woman's normal eating habits. The midwife's role is to support a woman with diabetes meet the plan of care created by the joint diabetes antenatal clinic team.

Medical management should achieve a delicate balance between preventing both hyperglycaemia and hypoglycaemia (de Valk and Visser 2011). Blood glucose target levels in pregnancy are a fasting blood glucose of around 5.3 mmol/L and 1-h postprandial blood glucose below 7.8 mmol/L (NICE 2015), which may be lower than the woman is used to. Qualitative research has shown that pregnant women are happier if their pre- and postprandial blood glucose levels are between 7 and 10 mmol/L, with no hypoglycaemia (Richmond 2009). Hence, the midwife should stress to the woman the importance of complying with the prescribed levels and give advice to her and her family about recognizing the signs and symptoms of hypoglycaemia. However, the woman should be informed that her blood glucose levels will change throughout pregnancy due to altered hormone levels and the developing fetus having its own metabolic demands. Consequently, it is important that the woman always carries glucose tablets/gel and a ready-to-use intramuscular device in case of hypoglycaemic episodes; glucogan should be prescribed to all women with type 1 diabetes and her partner/family should be instructed on how to give this intramuscular injection. In addition, women should be advised that as most hypoglycaemia occurring during weeks 8–16 is attributed to nausea and vomiting of pregnancy, it is important they seek advice if this becomes a significant problem in maintaining diabetic control. Women with type 1 diabetes may achieve better glucose control using a continuous subcutaneous insulin infusion (CSII). Continuous glucose monitoring may also be beneficial for women at risk of unstable or severe hypoglycaemia (NICE 2015).

Key points to consider relating to the antenatal care of women presenting with/developing diabetes:

- A supplement of 5 mg folic acid should be taken daily for the first 12 weeks of pregnancy to reduce the risk of congenital malformations in the fetus.
- Urinalysis should be undertaken at each visit to test for glucose, ketones as well as the protein.
- Women with type 1 diabetes should be offered ketone testing strips and be advised to test for ketonuria if they have symptoms of hyperglycaemia or become unwell.
- Blood pressure should be recorded at each visit with the midwife being alert for signs of pre-eclampsia, especially with GDM.
- Women should be discouraged from fasting, especially for long periods (e.g. as with religious observances).
- Women should test their blood glucose levels on waking and 1 hour postprandial after every meal during pregnancy.
- If taking insulin, women should also test their blood glucose level before going to bed.
- Women with type 2 diabetes are likely to be started on insulin: if taking metformin pre-pregnancy, some centres may decide to continue its use until 32 weeks due to emerging evidence of its safety (Gregory and Todd 2013).
- An ultrasonic scan is undertaken at 7–9 weeks' gestation to confirm viability and gestational age, followed by a further scan at 18–20 weeks to assess the four chambers of the fetal heart for any anomalies, estimate liquor volume and to ascertain fetal growth.
- Monthly scans from 28–36 weeks are undertaken to assess fetal growth and amniotic fluid volume and their results recorded, observing for signs of macrosomia (dimensions above the 95th centile for the period of gestation).

- Weekly tests of fetal wellbeing, including CTG or biophysical profiles, are offered from 38 weeks until labour commences (may be earlier in cases of fetal growth restriction).

Intrapartum management

NICE (2015) recommends offering induction of labour or caesarean section (if clinically indicated) between 37 and 39 weeks for women with type 1 or type 2 diabetes. An elective birth is recommended before 37 weeks if there are metabolic, maternal or fetal complications (NICE 2015). Women with gestational diabetes should consider an elective birth before 41 completed weeks. Vaginal birth after caesarean section (VBAC) is not contraindicated in women with diabetes.

- If the labour is preterm, steroids are given to the woman to improve fetal lung maturation and additional insulin may be required to control blood glucose levels; betamimetic medicines to slow or stop preterm labour are not recommended.
- If the fetus is macrosomic, the woman should be informed of the risks and benefits of vaginal birth, induction of labour and caesarean section.
- Capillary plasma glucose levels should be monitored hourly through labour and birth, aiming to maintain them between 4 and 7 mmol/L.
- For women with type 1 diabetes, an IVI of insulin and dextrose should be started from the onset of established labour.
- For women with type 2 and GDM, an IVI of insulin and dextrose should be started if capillary plasma blood glucose levels cannot be maintained between 4 and 7 mmol/L.
- The neonatal team should be alerted that the woman is in labour, should their assistance be required when the baby is born.

Care of the baby at birth

- A neonatologist should be present at the birth if the woman is receiving insulin.
- The midwife should be alert for signs of respiratory distress, hypoglycaemia, hypothermia, cardiac decompensation and neonatal encephalopathy (see Chapter 37).
- A baby should be admitted to a neonatal intensive care unit (NICU) only if a significant complication is apparent.
- The woman should hold her baby as soon as is practical after the birth and prior to any transfer to the NICU.

- Capillary plasma blood glucose testing of the baby should be carried out after birth and at intervals according to local protocols.
- The baby should feed within 30 min of birth and then every 2–3 h until pre-feed capillary plasma blood glucose levels are at least 2 mmol/L. If the capillary plasma blood glucose falls <1.5 mmol/L the neonatologist must be called and admission to the NICU is a possibility. (Note: NICUs tend to set a higher baseline for neonatal hypoglycaemia, so local protocols should be consulted.)
- Capillary plasma blood glucose levels should be assessed in babies who show signs of hypoglycaemia (abnormal muscle tone, level of consciousness, apnoea or seizures) with referral to the neonatologist, who is likely to treat with IV dextrose.
- The baby should not be transferred home until at least 24 hours old, is maintaining blood glucose levels and is feeding well.

Postnatal care of the woman with diabetes

- Women with insulin-treated pre-existing diabetes; should have their insulin reduced immediately after birth and blood glucose levels monitored with insulin adjusted until the appropriate dose is obtained.
- The woman should be observed for signs of hypoglycaemia.
- As placental hormone levels fall, the insulin sensitivity improves, such that the insulin infusion rate is likely to need reducing in the early postnatal period.
- The woman will usually return to her pre-pregnancy insulin levels, unless she is breastfeeding, when the insulin requirements are reduced by 30% (Gregory and Todd 2013).
- The woman should be advised that breastfeeding affects glycaemic control and there is the need for continued blood glucose monitoring and insulin adjustment.
- For women with type 2 diabetes: insulin should cease immediately and the doctor should confer with the pharmacist as to which oral diabetic agents the woman may safely take if breastfeeding (otherwise she returns to her pre-pregnancy drug therapy).
- For GDM: insulin ceases immediately and blood glucose monitoring can stop.
- A fasting blood glucose test should be undertaken at 6 weeks and if there is a possibility that would indicate another form of diabetes, a GTT should be performed immediately.
- The woman should be advised of the risk of developing diabetes in future pregnancies and the need for pre-pregnancy screening.
- The woman should be informed of the importance of using contraception to prevent pregnancies in rapid succession and to seek pre-conception care prior to future pregnancies.
- A healthy lifestyle with regular exercise, smoking cessation and maintaining a BMI within normal limits should also be emphasized to the woman.
- A follow-up appointment at 6 weeks with the diabetes team or the local GP is also essential (Gregory and Todd 2013).

THYROID DISEASE

The thyroid gland is a highly vascular organ that is shaped like a butterfly and is situated at the front of the neck. Its main function is to produce the iodine-rich hormones tri-iodothyronine (T3) and thyroxine (T4). These hormones are secreted directly into the blood circulation in response to a negative feedback to the hypothalamus, which secretes thyrotropin releasing hormones (TRH) that stimulate the anterior pituitary gland to secrete thyroid stimulating hormones (TSH) (Tortora and Derrickson 2016). TSH also initiates the uptake of iodine, which combines with an amino acid called 'tyrosine', which enables synthesis of the thyroid hormones within the thyroid follicles (Ali and Dornhorst 2018). Once in the blood circulation, 99% of T3 and T4 are bound to thyroxine-binding globulin (TBG), with the remaining 1% unbound or free: e.g. fT3 and fT4 (James et al. 2017). It is fT3, fT4 and TSH that are measured in thyroid function tests. Excess T4 is converted to the more potent T3 by deionization in the peripheral tissue (Ali and Dornhorst 2018). Most body tissue has receptors for fT3, and once bound to the tissue, metabolic activities result. The thyroid hormones regulate the metabolic rate throughout all body tissue and influence growth and maturity.

In pregnancy, the circulating level of TBG enables increased levels of T3 and T4, so only fT3 and fT4 should be measured by laboratory testing (Ali and Dornhorst 2018). The fetus cannot synthesize T3 and T4 until the 10th week of pregnancy and is dependent upon maternal thyroid hormones from placental transfer (Ali and

TABLE 15.2   Similarities between Clinical Symptoms of Thyroid Disease and Pregnancy

Pregnancy	Hyperthyroidism	Hypothyroidism
Heat intolerance	Yes	
Increased appetite	Yes	
Nausea	Yes	
Palpitations	Yes	
Tachycardia	Yes	
Tremor	Yes	
Sweating	Yes	
Warm palms	Yes	
Goitre	Yes	Yes
Amenorrhoea	Yes	
Weight gain		Yes
Carpal tunnel syndrome		Yes
Fluid retention		Yes
Constipation		Yes
Loss of concentration	Yes	Yes
Tiredness	Yes	Yes

Reproduced from Girling JC. (2006) Thyroid disorders in pregnancy. Current Obstetrics and Gynaecology 16:47–53, with permission from Elsevier.

Dornhorst 2018). Normal development of the fetal brain is dependent upon maternally derived T4, which is converted intracellularly to T3 (Girling 2006).

Thyroid disease is the second most common cause of endocrine dysfunction in pregnancy and is difficult to recognize as the symptoms mimic pregnancy (Girling 2006; James et al. 2017) indicated by Table 15.2. The most common thyroid disorders in pregnancy are hypothyroidism and hyperthyroidism (thyrotoxicosis), being of considerable significance due to their effect on both the woman and fetus.

Hypothyroidism

This is *underactivity* of the thyroid gland with absent or low levels of thyroid hormones T3 and T4 due to malfunctioning thyroid tissue, or secondary to pituitary or hypothalamic disease. The most common cause in pregnancy is autoimmune thyroiditis and goitre may or

may not be present (Gregory and Todd 2013). Lack of dietary iodine can also cause goitre. Goitre is enlarged thyroid tissue due to infiltration of lymphocytes and increase of fibrous tissue; this condition is also known as Hashimoto disease.

Hypothyroidism is familial and may be associated with other autoimmune diseases such as type 1 diabetes (Gregory and Todd 2013). Symptoms include weight gain, intolerance to cold temperature, constipation, alopecia, dry skin, lethargy, hoarse voice, ataxia, bradycardia and cognitive impairment. Menstrual irregularities and infertility are common, because TRH stimulation induces hyperprolactinaemia, which prevents ovulation. Not all women have symptoms and consequently the disease might be first recognized during infertility investigations. The most serious complication of untreated hypothyroidism is myxoedema coma, which presents with hypothermia, hypoventilation and bradycardia, followed by unconsciousness (Gregory and Todd 2013).

Pregnancy complications of hypothyroidism are hypertension and low birth weight and psychomotor retardation in the fetus. Ali and Dornhorst (2018) raise concern of the low Intelligence Quotient (IQ) of children born to mothers with untreated hypothyroidism and cretinism may result from severe maternal iodine deficiency associated with hypothyroidism (James et al. 2017). Pre-conception care is therefore very important and fT4 and thyroxine levels should be measured and the dose of thyroxine adjusted until TSH reaches normal level (Gregory and Todd 2013).

During pregnancy, the woman should be reviewed by an endocrinologist to measure fT4 and TSH levels at the outset in order to obtain a baseline measurement (Gregory and Todd 2013). The TSH level rises in pregnancy causing an increased demand for thyroxine and so the dose of therapeutic thyroxine is adjusted, usually increasing by 25–50% (Gregory and Todd 2013). Iron supplements should be taken at a different time to the thyroxine to maximize absorption (James et al. 2017). Although a large goitre might cause complications for general anaesthesia (James et al. 2017), there are otherwise no specific issues for labour and consequently intrapartum care may be provided by the midwife (Gregory and Todd 2013).

Postnatally, the thyroxine dose is reduced to the pre-pregnancy level and the fT4 and TSH levels should be measured at the 6-week follow-up or postnatal appointment. It is important that the neonatal bloodspot screening test is undertaken, as the condition can be familial and thus the midwife should provide support to the parents, who are likely to be anxious (Gregory and Todd 2013). In addition, the woman needs to be observed for signs of thyroiditis and postnatal depression (James et al. 2017).

Hyperthyroidism (Thyrotoxicosis)

Hyperthyroidism is an *overactivity* of the thyroid gland that affects 0.2% of pregnant women (James et al. 2017). It usually manifests as a clinical syndrome called 'thyrotoxicosis' with signs and symptoms that include weight loss, despite having a good appetite, intolerance to heat, sweating, tachycardia with bouncing pulse, insomnia, agitation, tremor, exophthalmos (protrusion of the eyeballs due to the tissue behind the eye becoming oedematous and fibrous), diarrhoea and menstrual irregularities (Gregory and Todd 2013). Non-pregnancy treatment is with carbimazole and propylthiouracil, which inhibit thyroid hormone synthesis (Ali and Dornhorst 2018). Thyroidectomy is reserved for cases where there is excessively large goitre and drug therapy is ineffective. If radioiodine treatment has been used to destroy thyroid tissue to lower the thyroid levels, the woman should be counselled to delay conception for at least 4 months (James et al. 2017).

The main complication of hyperthyroidism is the medical emergency of thyroid crisis (or thyroid storm), where there are exaggerated features of thyrotoxicosis with additional hyperpyrexia, cardiac dysrhythmias, congestive cardiac failure, altered mental state and ultimately coma. Goitre may also be present. Hyperthyroidism is treated with IV fluids, hydrocortisone, propranolol, oral iodine, carbimazole and propylthiouracil (Ali and Dornhorst 2018). If the thyrotoxicosis is autoimmune, with antibodies to the TSH receptor, it is called Graves disease, which accounts for 95% of hyperthyroidism in pregnancy (James et al. 2017). Although the risk of miscarriage increases in early pregnancy, the disease otherwise tends to improve in pregnancy and women may go into remission in the latter half of pregnancy (Gregory and Todd 2013).

Care in pregnancy aims to normalize thyroid function and carbimazole and propylthiouracil are the drugs of choice with the dose adjusted after monthly measurements of fT4 and TSH. If the control is poor, the fetus is at risk of fetal thyrotoxicosis, which may necessitate cordocentesis to measure fetal fT4 and TSH (Gregory and Todd 2013). This is a high-risk pregnancy and the woman should consequently be referred to a specialist obstetric unit. The midwife should ensure monthly measurements of fT4 and TSH are undertaken and organize serial fetal growth ultrasound scans. There should also be regular assessment of the fetal heart rate to detect fetal tachycardia. As a result, continuous fetal heart monitoring during labour is required and the paediatrician should be informed when labour is established (Gregory and Todd 2013).

Labour can precipitate thyroid crisis/storm so meticulous monitoring and recording of maternal observations and wellbeing is vital. As with hypothyroidism, should goitre be present and is large, there may be complications if general anaesthesia is warranted (James et al. 2017).

Postnatally, the midwife should be alert for signs of thyrotoxicosis flare in the woman and extend the period of undertaking observations with emphasis on maternal pulse. Propylthiouracil is the drug of choice if the woman chooses to breastfeed her baby. The woman's thyroid hormone levels should also be measured 6 weeks following the baby's birth and the drug dose revised accordingly.

When examining the baby, the midwife should be alert for signs of neonatal goitre and thyrotoxicosis such as weight loss, jitteriness, irritability, tachycardia and poor feeding, referring promptly to the paediatrician if these are suspected. The baby might require temporary treatment with antithyroid drugs and propanolol necessitating admission to the NICU (Gregory and Todd 2013).

PROLACTINOMA

The pituitary gland increases in size by 50–70% in pregnancy due to normal lactotroph hyperplasia, which, in rare cases, causes symptoms in pregnancy (Ali and Dornhorst 2018). The presence of an adenoma, called a 'prolactinoma', in the pituitary gland will further increase its size and cause symptoms. This adenoma, or cyst, increases the production of prolactin, which is the hormone that initiates lactation (Gregory and Todd 2013). There are two types of adenoma:

- Microadenoma: accounts for 90% of cases in pregnancy. They are <10 mm in diameter and rarely grow significantly, with some regressing spontaneously.
- Macroadenoma: accounts for 10% of cases in pregnancy. They are >10 mm in diameter and are more likely to expand and cause symptoms of headache and visual disturbance. Occasionally, they may progress to pituitary apoplexy or diabetes insipidus (Ali and Dornhorst 2018).

With both types of adenoma, there is a risk of infertility and treatment is with dopamine agonists, such as Cabergoline, which can cause side-effects of nausea, vomiting, postural hypotension, constipation, nasal congestion and Raynaud phenomenon. Pre-conception care is important and management depends upon the size of the adenoma, which might involve a trial of discontinuing the dopamine agonist or changing to bromocriptine. In some cases, surgery might be attempted prior to conception to reduce the bulk size of the adenoma (Gregory and Todd 2013).

Once pregnant, the woman should be referred to a specialist unit as this is a high-risk pregnancy. Antenatal care, however, can be shared with the community midwife and medical/obstetric team. At the initial visit the midwife should take note of past surgery and current medication when undertaking the woman's history. At each subsequent visit the woman should be asked about headache and visual symptoms. It is the medical team who will determine the type and dose of dopamine agonist and perform monthly visual perimetry to detect early signs of compression on the optic chiasma. If there are indications of adenoma expansion, a magnetic resonance imaging (MRI) scan should be performed urgently and bromocriptine commenced.

In most cases, the intrapartum care can be facilitated by the midwife, however if the adenoma is expanding, the woman is likely to have a preterm induction of labour. The obstetric team may advise an elective instrumental birth to avoid a rise in intracranial pressure during the second stage of labour (Gregory and Todd 2013).

In the postnatal period, the woman is advised to report any symptoms. An MRI scan might be ordered by the medical team and prolactin levels measured after 3 weeks, by which time the values should have returned to their pre-pregnancy levels. Follow-up appointments should be made with the specialist medical team who will evaluate the symptoms when determining the recommencement of pre-pregnancy treatment with dopamine agonists. The midwife should consult with the doctor and pharmacist for suitable alternative medication if the woman wishes to breastfeed her baby as dopamine agonists are usually contraindicated. Furthermore, the woman will require specialist contraception advice as oestrogen contained within the oral contraceptive pill might further increase the size of the adenoma and consequently is contraindicated (Gregory and Todd 2013).

CARDIAC DISEASE

The chance of midwives caring for a woman with pre-existing cardiac disease, or developing cardiac disease in pregnancy, has increased over recent years due to many factors, including the increased age of childbearing women and the association it has with co-existing medical conditions such as diabetes, hypertension, as well as obesity, smoking and previous illicit drug use. Furthermore, improved life expectancy of women born with congenital cardiac disease and increased immigration revealing an increase in rheumatic heart disease adds to the prevalence. However, the majority of pregnancies complicated by maternal cardiac disease are expected to have a favourable outcome for both the woman and fetus.

Risk for morbidity and mortality depends on the nature of the cardiac lesion, its effect on the functional capacity of the heart and the development of pregnancy-related complications such as hypertensive disorders of pregnancy, infection, thrombosis and haemorrhage. Cardiac disease is the commonest indirect cause of maternal death in the UK (Bunch and Knight 2018, Knight et al. 2019). During the triennium 2015–17 the deaths of 82 women from heart disease associated with, or aggravated by, pregnancy were reported. Knight et al. (2019) highlighted that 48 of these deaths occurred in the UK during pregnancy or within 42 days of delivery. This represents a maternal mortality rate from cardiac disease in the UK of 2.10 per 100,000 maternities, which is slightly lower than the rate in the previous triennium. Knight et al. (2019) reported that 24% of women died from ischaemic causes and 27% from myocardial disease/cardiomyopathy. There has been an apparent decrease in the proportion of women dying from sudden arrhythmic cardiac deaths with a morphologically normal heart (SADS/MNH) among those dying from cardiovascular causes. However, there is no statistically significant decrease in the mortality rate from SADS/MNH between 2009–2014 and 2015–2017.

The majority of deaths secondary to cardiac causes occur in women with no previous history, this in itself providing need for midwives to remain vigilant and to be certain of what constitutes normal physiological changes in pregnancy (see Chapter 10) and what may be symptoms of cardiac disease.

It remains vital that a midwife undertakes an accurate history from the woman at the first visit. Should any history of cardiac disease be revealed, a more detailed account should be elicited in order to ensure prompt and appropriate referral to an appropriately skilled and experienced multidisciplinary team, usually in regional centres. These women require an individualized midwifery approach to care to address the psychosocial concerns that may often get subsumed within a medical model of care. The midwife's role involves not only being astute to any deviation that may arise in the course of the woman's pregnancy, but also being supportive of the woman's individual needs as she may have the same pregnancy concerns as any other woman.

In a healthy pregnancy, the haemodynamic profile alters in order to meet the increasing demands of the developing fetoplacental unit. Healthy pregnant women are able to adjust to these physiological changes quite easily; for women with co-existing cardiac disease, however, the added workload can precipitate complications. The three sensitive periods of cardiovascular stress (28–32 weeks of pregnancy, during labour and 12–24 h postpartum) are the most critical and life-threatening for women with cardiac disease (Roberts and Adamson 2013). Understanding the changes in cardiovascular dynamics during pregnancy can support the midwife's recognition of key indicators and when limitations to cardiac function are occurring that require prompt referral (see Chapter 10).

Diagnosis of Cardiac Disease

Along with the signs and symptoms, physical assessment of functional capacity and laboratory tests can assist with the diagnosis of cardiac disease and determine the type of lesion. These may include:

- full cardiovascular examination, including personal history and assessment of lifestyle risk factors
- blood tests: full blood count, clotting studies and cardiac enzymes (Troponin)
- 12-lead electrocardiogram (ECG)
- echocardiogram: an ultrasound examination to examine cardiac structure and function
- chest X-ray to assess cardiac size and outline, pulmonary vasculature and lung fields (always undertaken when clinically indicated, e.g. in women presenting with chest pain)
- other imaging: computerized tomography (CT) scan or magnetic resonance imaging (MRI) scan of the chest

Care of Women with Cardiac Disease
Pre-conception care

This is of great importance given the increase in the number of pregnant women with heart disease and the findings of the confidential enquiries (Knight et al. 2016, 2017, 2019). This document also recommended assessment using the WHO classification system and referral for appropriate pre-conception and pregnancy management based on the WHO Classification (Brennand et al 2016). Women with a pre-existing cardiac problem should receive pre-conception counselling, this should include a visit with a maternal fetal specialist particularly for women at high possibility of complications during pregnancy or birth, to inform them of any potential risks that a pregnancy may have on their health and that of their unborn baby in terms of inheriting any congenital malformations. This will enable them to make informed decisions and plan their pregnancy monitoring more carefully to reduce any subsequent morbidity and mortality. This should include a review of all medications for pregnancy risk as well as laboratory testing, ECG, chest X-ray and assessment of stress or cardiopulmonary exercise test to obtain assessment of functional capacity and determine the presence of exercise induced arrythmias. More advance testing may be recommended in those who have suspected pulmonary hypertension. These assessments will give a current risk potential and help the woman with decision-making as to whether pregnancy should be avoided or determine what treatments or advice may be necessary to reduce the pregnancy risk. Provision of appropriate education around contraception is also an important part of preconception care (Knight et al. 2019).

The risk of inheriting cardiac disease varies between 3% and 50% depending on the type of maternal heart disease. Children of parents with a cardiovascular condition inherited in an autosomal dominant manner (e.g. *Marfan syndrome*, *hypertrophic cardiomyopathy* or *long QT syndrome*) have an inheritance risk of 50%, regardless of gender of the affected parent.

For a steadily increasing number of genetic defects, genetic screening by chorionic villous biopsy (CVS) can be offered in the 12th week of pregnancy. All women with congenital heart disease should be offered fetal echocardiography between the 19th and 22nd week of pregnancy. Measurement of nuchal fold thickness around the 12–13th week of pregnancy is an early screening test for Down syndrome in women over 35 years of age. The sensitivity for the presence of a significant cardiac defect is 40–45%, while the specificity of the method is 99%. The incidence of congenital cardiac disease with normal nuchal fold thickness is 1/1000 (Eleftheriades et al. 2012).

Antenatal care

The symptoms of physiological pregnancy can mimic the signs and symptoms of cardiac disease, e.g. dyspnoea on exertion, orthopnoea, palpitations, dizziness, fainting, a bounding pulse, tachycardia, peripheral oedema, distended jugular veins and alterations in heart sounds. Observations and investigations of the woman's health should be undertaken prior to and at the beginning of pregnancy to obtain baseline referral points. Adapted antenatal records that include triggers such as *shortness of breath, palpitations, pulse rate and rhythm* as well as *auscultation of the heart for any murmur and lung fields for signs of pulmonary oedema* are useful to prompt the midwife into early detection of subtle increases of any worsening symptoms. These observations should be undertaken alongside the usual antenatal examination, but the midwife also needs to be mindful that women with cardiac disease can also develop other complications such as pre-eclampsia or gestational diabetes (RCOG 2011b).

There should be frequent assessment of the woman with a multidisciplinary approach involving midwives, obstetricians, cardiologists and anaesthetists. The aim is to maintain a steady haemodynamic state and prevent complications, as well as promote physical and psychological wellbeing. In addition, the fetal wellbeing is assessed by the following means:

- ultrasound examination to confirm gestational age and any congenital malformation
- clinical assessment of fetal growth and amniotic fluid volume and by ultrasound
- monitoring of the fetal heart rate by CTG
- measurement of fetal and maternal placental blood flow indices by Doppler ultrasonography.

A care plan using a shared decision model should be developed by the multidisciplinary team and the woman for pregnancy, labour and the early postnatal period should be informed by the individual woman's situation, reflecting and acknowledging the woman's own understanding of her condition, with a view to optimizing outcomes for her and her baby (Dawson et al. 2018). Copies being available in woman's own handheld records and those held at a central point.

Potential support interventions, such as attending parent education classes, can help in allaying the woman's general anxieties about motherhood alongside the antenatal care received from the midwife. This may involve advice regarding modifying and adjusting physical activity during pregnancy. More realistically social support from on line source, such as peer mentoring and on line blogs have been identified as being beneficial (Dawson et al. 2018), particularly as some women may need to commence maternity leave earlier than anticipated whereas others may require admission to hospital for rest and close monitoring. In addition, guidance about the constituents of a well-balanced diet with restricted intake of cholesterol, sodium-rich foods and salt should also be provided. Monitoring of weight gain should be undertaken as excess weight gain will place additional strain on the heart. Compliance with taking iron and folic acid supplementation is also important in preventing anaemia.

Antithrombotic therapy

The hypercoagulable state in pregnancy increases the risk of thromboembolic disease in women who have arrhythmias, mitral valve stenosis or who have had mechanical cardiac valve replacements. However, the treatment of women requiring antithrombotic therapy during pregnancy is challenging. *Warfarin* is commonly used as an antithrombotic, but as it is teratogenic to the developing embryo/fetus and associated with a high fetal loss rate, it is not used in pregnancy. Furthermore, warfarin also predisposes the woman and her fetus to haemorrhage when used in the third trimester (D'Souza et al. 2017). Subcutaneous low molecular weight heparins, such as *enoxaparin*, are useful for thromboprophylaxis but may not be suitable for women with mechanical heart valves. As a consequence, the advice of a haematologist should be sought. Full length thromboembolism deterrent (TED) support stockings should be worn if the woman is admitted to hospital for rest and assessment, and should also be worn during labour and in the immediate postnatal period.

Intrapartum care: the first stage of labour

Many women with cardiac disease have an uncomplicated labour but it is good practice that there is effective communication among a dedicated multidisciplinary team of midwife, obstetrician, cardiologist, neonatologist, anaesthetist and the woman and her family to optimize birth outcome. Vaginal birth is preferred unless there is an obstetric indication for caesarean section as haemodynamic stability is greater and there is less chance of postoperative infection and pulmonary complications (RCOG 2011b).

Intrapartum care involves monitoring the maternal condition using the Modified Early Obstetric Warning Scoring (MEOWS) system that triggers any deviation in order to prompt timely intervention and maximize maternal and fetal wellbeing (McLean et al. 2013). Continuous ECG is recommended in nearly all cases and pulse oximetry may be utilized to assess arterial haemoglobin saturation, which may be reduced in women with cardiac disease owing to disruption of normal gas exchange between the lungs and blood. Fluid balance should be recorded, and use of intravenous fluids may be limited. Routine antibiotic prophylaxis is not recommended. Continuous electronic fetal heart rate monitoring is usually recommended (Regitz-Zagrosek et al. 2011).

Labour induction. If induction is indicated and the cervix is favourable, assessed using the Bishop score (see Chapter 22), artificial rupture of the membranes (ARM) is undertaken with an IVI of oxytocin should contractions not establish. A prolonged induction should be avoided. If the cervix is unfavourable, synthetic prostaglandin is used to soften/*ripen* it. While there is no absolute contraindication to *misoprostol* (prostaglandin E_1) or *dinoprostone* (prostaglandin E_2), there is a theoretical risk of coronary vasospasm and a low risk of arrhythmias. In addition, dinoprostone has more profound effects on BP than misoprostol and is therefore contraindicated in active cardiovascular disease. Transcervical Foley catheter ripening is associated with a lower risk of tachysystole (Fox et al. 2011; Zhu et al. 2018) and may be particularly useful when inducing labour in women at increased risk of fetal hypoxaemia such as cardiac disease avoiding the side-effects of synthetic prostaglandins.

Pain relief. The midwife should assist the woman to use the techniques that she has learned for coping with stress. Nitrous oxide and oxygen (Entonox) and opioids such as pethidine are usually considered safe means of intrapartum analgesia for women with cardiac disease, but it is important to review the labour plan with the multidisciplinary team before administration. In some situations, epidural anaesthesia may be the analgesia of choice for its effectiveness in relieving pain and decreasing cardiac output and heart rate (RCOG 2011b). It causes peripheral vasodilatation and decreases venous return, which alleviates pulmonary congestion. Furthermore, an effectively working epidural *in situ* may eliminate the need for emergency general anaesthesia.

Positioning. Cardiac output is influenced by the position of the woman during labour and consequently those with cardiac disease are particularly sensitive to aortocaval compression by the gravid uterus if adopting the supine position. It is recommended that midwives encourage an upright or left lateral position for women to adopt during labour and birth wherever possible (McLean et al. 2013).

The second stage of labour

There is limited evidence related to optimum management of this stage (Cauldwell et al. 2017a); for clinically stable women with complex heart disease a normal labour and birth should be anticipated. Historically, caution has been suggested in use of prolonged pushing with held breath (the *Valsalva manoeuvre*) as it can further compromise the health of the woman with cardiac disease particularly if obstructive lesions, fragility of aorta, pulmonary hypertension venous return and myocardial contractility is compromised (Canobbio et al. 2017). Such a manoeuvre raises the intrathoracic pressure, forces the blood out of the thorax and impedes venous return, resulting in a fall in cardiac output. The midwife should therefore support the woman to breathe as normal and follow her natural desire to bear down giving several short pushes during each contraction.

Epidural analgesia may be recommended allowing prolongation of the passive phase of second stage with the aim to facilitating more spontaneous births avoiding what D'Souza et al. (2017) suggest is the erroneous notion of elective shortening of the active phase with use of forceps or ventouse.

The third stage of labour

Rates of postpartum haemorrhage (PPH) in women with cardiac disease have been reported to be as high as 23%, with uterine atony being the single largest cause (Cauldwell et al. 2017b). While this may be due to restrictive and cautious doses of oxytocics leading to current suggested regimes such as a slow IVI of 2 IU/min oxytocin administered after the birth of the placenta to avoid systemic hypotension and prevent haemorrhage (see Chapter 21), alongside this the active management should include a 10–40 IU oxytocin infusion over 1–4 h. Optimum oxytocin doses remain uncertain. What is clear is that bolus doses should be avoided (D'Souza et al. 2017). Prostaglandin F analogues and Misoprostol can cause cardiac ischaemia and infarction and only be used in life-threatening atonic PPH. *Ergometrine* is contraindicated in women with cardiac disease as it can cause vasoconstriction and hypertension (Kapoor and Wallace 2016).

Postnatal care

The first 48 h following the baby's birth are critical for the woman with significant cardiac disease. The heart must be able to cope with the extra volume of blood (*autotransfusion*) from the uterine circulation as well as the increased venous return following relief of aortocaval compression of the uterus. Conversely, the total blood volume may be diminished by the amount lost at birth and during the postnatal period. Furthermore, the heart will need to compensate should the blood flow be impaired due to PPH. Careful haemodynamic monitoring is recommended for ≥24–72 h, depending on the specific cardiac condition and the midwife should identify early signs of infection, thrombosis or pulmonary oedema. Observation of the condition of the woman's legs, the use of TED stockings and early ambulation are important strategies for the midwife to adopt in order to reduce the risk of thromboembolism.

Breastfeeding should be encouraged, as cardiac output is not affected by lactation, although drug therapy for specific heart conditions may need to be reviewed for safety during breastfeeding (see Table 15.3). The midwife is required to provide the woman with support to successfully breastfeed her baby, emphasizing the importance of adequate rest and a dietary intake containing sufficient calories to sustain breastfeeding.

It is important that *prior* to transfer from hospital, the midwife explores the help and support available in the home for when the woman returns home with her baby. Relatives and friends often fulfil this need but community support services should also be considered if necessary. In addition, the midwife should offer appropriate contraceptive advice and the options available to the woman who has cardiac disease, considering their individual risks need to be balanced against the risk of pregnancy (Govind and De Martino 2018).

Congenital Heart Disease

The most common congenital heart diseases (CHD) found in pregnancy are: atrial septal defect (ASD); ventricular septal defect (VSD); patent ductus arteriosus (PDA); pulmonary stenosis; aortic stenosis and tetralogy of Fallot. The majority of these lesions should have been surgically corrected in childhood, resulting in a growing population of women with CHD achieving a pregnancy. Uncorrected lesions may cause pulmonary hypertension, cyanosis and severe left ventricular failure and therefore present a greater risk in achieving successful pregnancy outcome. In women with aortic stenosis, hypotension should be avoided, as it can cause reduced strength of ventricular contraction, causing difficulty in forcing blood flow through a stenotic aortic valve increasing the risk of left ventricular failure. Congenital heart disease is also associated with increased fetal complications such as fetal loss, IUGR, preterm birth and an increased risk of fetal CHD (Kapoor and Wallace 2016). Particularly high-risk cardiac conditions for pregnancy are listed below.

Eisenmenger syndrome

A large left–right shunt of blood is apparent usually through a VSD, ASD or PDA, which is still patent. This results in an increase in the pulmonary blood flow, which over time leads to fibrosis and the development of pulmonary hypertension and cyanosis (Kapoor and Wallace 2016). When the right-sided heart pressures exceed left heart pressures, the shunt reverses, with worsening cyanosis. Women with this condition are advised against pregnancy as maternal mortality lies in the region of 30–50%. Risk of prematurity contributes to the high perinatal mortality rate.

Marfan syndrome

This syndrome is caused by an autosomal dominant defect on chromosome 15. It is a connective tissue disease affecting the musculoskeletal system, the cardiovascular system and eyes. The cardiovascular malformations are the most life-threatening as the elastic fibres in the media of the blood vessels weaken. Dilatation of the ascending and descending aorta results, followed in some instances by dissection or rupture, or both. Pregnancy poses a significant risk because of the increased stress on the cardiovascular system. There is a 50% chance of a child inheriting Marfan syndrome if one parent is affected. Women who have minimal cardiovascular involvement and normal aortic root dimensions have a better pregnancy outcome. Careful monitoring is required throughout pregnancy, including the use of serial echocardiography to identify progressive aortic root dilatation. Prophylactic antihypertensive therapy using beta-blockers is recommended to reduce blood pressure and the rate of aortic dilatation (Elkayam et al. 2014). Some individuals with Marfan syndrome also present with dural ectasia which, unless mild, presents an increased risk of a spinal cerebrospinal fluid (CSF) leak in the case of accidental dural puncture during epidural; consequently, epidural anaesthesia is not usually recommended. While Marfan syndrome is a genetic condition, approximately 15% of cases are as a result of a new

TABLE 15.3   Cardiovascular Drugs in Pregnancy and Postnatal Period

Drug	Use	Side-effects	Breastfeeding
Adenosine	Maternal and fetal arrhythmias	No reported side-effects; limited first trimester data	Limited data; unlikely passage into milk due to short half-life and acute use
Amiodarone	Maternal arrhythmias	IUGR; congenital goitre; hypo- or hyper-thyroidism; prolonged QT in the newborn	Not recommended
Beta blockers	Maternal hypertension; maternal arrhythmias; mitral stenosis; cardiomyopathy; hyperthyroidism; Marfan syndrome	IUGR; low placental weight; fetal bradycardia	Compatible; consider monitoring newborn heart rate (esp. aten-olol)
Digoxin	Maternal and fetal arrhythmias; heart failure	No fetal side-effects	Compatible
Diuretics (Furose-mide, hydrochlo-rothiazide)	Hypertension; congestive heart failure	Growth restriction; hypona-tremia and hypokalaemia; thiazides can inhibit labour and suppress lactation	Compatible
Flecanide	Maternal and fetal arrhythmias	Limited data; case reports of fetal SVT	Limited data; probably compatible
Hydralazine	Hypertension	None reported	Limited data; probably compatible
Nifedipine	Hypertension; tocolysis	Hypotension	Compatible
Nitrates	Myocardial infarction; ischaemia; hypertension; pulmonary oedema; tocolysis	Limited data; fetal distress	Limited data; unlikely passage into milk due to acute use
Procainamide	Maternal and fetal arrhythmia	Limited data; no reported fetal effects	Compatible
Quinidine	Maternal and fetal arrhythmia	Preterm labour; miscarriage; transient fetal thrombocytope-nia; damage to eighth nerve	Compatible
Sodium nitroprus-side	Hypertension; aortic dissection	Limited data; possible thiocyanate fetal toxicity	No data; possible toxicity
Sotalol	Maternal arrhythmias; hypertension; fetal tachycardia	Limited data; reported cases of fetal death; neurological mor-bidity; newborn bradycardia	Recommended other drugs are used as high passage into breast-milk
Verapamil	Maternal and fetal arrhythmias; hypertension; tocolysis	Limited data; no adverse fetal or newborn effects reported	Compatible

Data derived from https://toxnet.nlm.nih.gov/cgi-bin/sis/htmlgen? LACTMED. Available at: www.sps.nhs.uk/articles/safety-in-lacta-tion-drugs-for-hypertension/

mutation and thus some individuals remain undiagnosed and do not seek any pre-conception counselling. Pregnant women with Marfan syndrome should be referred to the specialist team containing a cardiologist for immediate assessment and investigation (RCOG 2011b).

Aortic dissection (acute)

Aortic dissection (acute) may occur in pregnancy in association with severe hypertension (systolic >160 mmHg) due to pre-eclampsia, coarctation of the aorta or connective tissue disease such as Marfan syndrome.

The woman typically presents with severe chest or intrascapular pain. Early diagnosis using CT chest scan, MRI or transoesophageal echocardiogram is critical, as maternal mortality is high.

Spontaneous coronary artery dissection

Spontaneous coronary artery dissection (SCAD) is an increasingly recognized disorder that can cause acute coronary syndrome (ACS) (Hayes et al. 2018; Adlam et al. 2018). It is defined as an epicardial coronary artery dissection that is not associated with atherosclerosis or trauma, and is not iatrogenic. Tweet et al. (2017) suggest the formation of an intramural haematoma (IMH) or intimal disruption causing coronary artery obstruction is the mechanism of myocardial injury in SCAD, rather than more classical atherosclerotic plaque rupture or intraluminal thrombus formation. The high rate of recurrent SCAD, its association with female sex, pregnancy, peri- and postpartum period, physical and emotional stress triggers and concurrent systemic arteriopathies, particularly fibromuscular dysplasia, highlight the differences in clinical characteristics of SCAD compared with atherosclerotic disease. The causes of pregnancy associated SCAD (P-SCAD) are not fully understood, but one suggestion is that the oestrogen and progesterone receptors present in the coronary arteries may mediate changes, as they do in other connective tissues, weakening the vessel wall, and culminating in arterial wall rupture, IMH, and onset of clinical symptoms (Hayes et al. 2018). The majority of cases of pregnancy associated SCAD occur in the first 4 weeks after birth, but it has been reported during virtually all stages of pregnancy. Given the concerns for possible recurrent SCAD, many clinicians recommend against subsequent pregnancy. There are, however, few data to support this life-changing recommendation and some clinicians have supported women through successful post-SCAD pregnancies using a multidisciplinary team approach. Contraceptive choices may be limited, steering away from hormonal methods and relying on barrier methods and male sterilization (Tweet et al. 2017; Jakes et al. 2018). (Please see Nicki's story in Case Study 15.1, as she is a mother and survivor of SCAD. For further information and resources about the condition, see SCAD websites: https://scad.lcbru.le.ac.uk/ and www.mayoclinic.org/diseases-conditions/spontaneous-coronary-artery-dissection/symptoms-causes/syc-20353711.)

CASE STUDY 15.1 Spontaneous Coronary Artery Dissection (SCAD)

Nicki's story

I was pregnant with my second child, suffering with hyperemesis, early bleeds, the flu and a high heart rate so had already spent some time in hospital. At 29 weeks, I felt a dull pain in my chest. I knew instinctively something was wrong so called an ambulance as the pain edged down my arms and I began to feel lightheaded.

Paramedics did an ECG which was normal, they took me to hospital to 'get checked out'. On the way, the symptoms got worse. I was told I was panicking and 'You're pregnant and full of oestrogen – it won't be your heart'. I vomited, which was also attributed to being pregnant.

After an 8-hour wait in the Accident and Emergency department (A&E) and further ECGs, I was given a bed in the Acute Assessment Unit. The pain was unbearable. The troponin blood test done 6 hours after the pain began was not checked for several hours. When it was checked, doctors queried whether pregnancy could cause a falsely raised troponin, so repeated the test. This showed even higher troponin levels. I was rushed to the cardiac unit and given an MRI scan, which confirmed SCAD, which I have since discovered is often missed or mis-diagnosed.

I had arrived at A&E at 5pm, it was not until 3am the next day that doctors started thinking I might have a problem with my heart.

A multidisciplinary team (cardiologist, obstetrician, neonatologist and midwife) decided to do an elective C-section at 34 weeks. This was then brought forward to 33, then 32 weeks. Four days before the planned date, my waters broke and within an hour my daughter was born – no epidural, no monitoring, just one midwife present – a bit different to the carefully made plans aimed at protecting my heart from the strains of labour!

Although my 3 lb daughter was healthy, I had now been in hospital for 3 weeks when I experienced further chest pains. I was taken back to the cardiac monitoring unit where they diagnosed a second SCAD.

Thankfully both I and my daughter survived. I was extremely lucky not to suffer major heart damage. The dissections were in my LAD (95% blocked) and RCA (50% blocked). I now help a campaign to raise awareness and push for NICE guidelines for SCAD in the UK, so that women in the future with SCAD do not have to go through what I did.

Nicki's story, reproduced with thanks to Beat SCAD, www.beatscad.org.uk.

Acquired Heart Disease

Rheumatic heart disease

Rheumatic heart disease causes inflammation and scarring of the heart valves and results in valve stenosis, with or without regurgitation. The mitral valve is most often affected with stenosis, occurring in two-thirds of cases. This condition is often diagnosed for the first time during pregnancy, presenting as severe breathlessness and tiredness; a diastolic murmur is usually present. It tends to appear in immigrant or refugee women who have not had access to medical care. Most women with valvular heart disease can be treated medically, aiming to reduce the heart's workload. The times of highest risk of developing pulmonary oedema were shown to be times of greatest increased preload, with higher heart rate and stroke volume – the first trimester, labour and the early postpartum period. Blood in the left atrium cannot easily travel across a stenotic mitral valve, leading to back pressure in the pulmonary veins, which can result in pulmonary oedema, possibly causing pulmonary hypertension and right ventricular failure.

During pregnancy, this involves bed rest, oxygen therapy and the use of cardiac drugs, e.g. *diuretics* (to reduce the fluid load); *digoxin* (to reduce and regulate the heart rate); and *heparin* (to reduce the risk of thromboembolic disease) (Kapoor and Wallace 2016). Women with more severe symptomatic disease may require surgical intervention such as *balloon valvuloplasty* or *valve replacement*, although both of these procedures carry a degree of maternal and fetal mortality. Antibiotic prophylaxis is no longer recommended for all women with valvular lesions during labour, although it may still be advisable for those who have mechanical valves (McLean et al. 2013).

Myocardial infarction and ischaemic heart disease

Myocardial infarction (MI) and ischaemic heart disease (IHD) are an increasing cause of maternal death in the UK. Identifiable risk factors include increasing maternal age, obesity, diabetes, pre-existing hypertension, smoking, family history and poor socioeconomic status. A myocardial infarction is most likely to occur in the third trimester of pregnancy and the peripartum period, when haemodynamic changes are at their optimum creating a higher risk of thrombotic events due to the hypercoagulability induced by hormonal changes. In the immediate postpartum period, spontaneous coronary artery dissection is the most common cause of MI. Typically, women present with ischaemic chest pain in the presence of an abnormal ECG and elevated cardiac enzymes, although these signs and symptoms may be masked during labour and birth (McLean et al. 2013). Atypical features include abdominal or epigastric pain and vomiting. *Coronary angioplasty* is the therapy to improve the patency of blocked arteries (Roberts and Adamson 2013).

Peripartum cardiomyopathy

Peripartum cardiomyopathy is relatively rare but is potentially fatal, with mortality rates ranging from 25% to 50%. A number of these deaths occur shortly after the onset of signs and symptoms. The incidence of this type of cardiac disease varies from 1:300 to 1:4000 pregnancies, with heart failure developing very rapidly in some cases. Predisposing factors to peripartum cardiomyopathy comprise of multigravidae, multiple pregnancies, family history, ethnicity, smoking, diabetes, hypertension, pre-eclampsia, malnutrition, pregnant teenagers or older pregnant women and prolonged use of beta-agonists (McLean et al. 2013).

Commonly, women have no previous history of heart disease and diagnosis is usually made within a specific period of time between the last month of pregnancy and the first 5 months postpartum. Inflammation and enlargement of the myocardium (*cardiomegaly*) give rise to left ventricular heart failure and thromboembolic complications. Presenting features include orthopnoea and dyspnoea, chest pain and palpitations, new resurgent murmurs and pulmonary crackles, raised jugular pressure, ankle oedema and fatigue. Management should initially focus on managing the arrhythmia and heart failure and should include the use of oxygen, diuretics, and vasodilators to decrease pulmonary congestion and fluid overload, followed by inotropic agents to improve myometrial contractility and anticoagulation therapy (Regitz-Zagrosek et al. 2011). Birth may be necessary if the condition remains unstable (Kapoor and Wallace 2016). As the cardiomegaly resolves there should be a corresponding improvement in the woman's condition but this process may take up to 6 months and there is a risk of recurrence in a subsequent pregnancy. In some women, left ventricular dysfunction persists and unless a heart transplant is performed mortality can be high (Regitz-Zagrosek et al. 2011).

Arrhythmias

Cardiac arrhythmias may present for the first time in pregnancy possibly because of the physiological changes to the cardiovascular system. Symptoms such as palpitations, dizziness and shortness of breath are common symptoms of pregnancy. It is important that women presenting with these symptoms are not dismissed and are investigated properly. A prior history of arrhythmias or structural heart disease or a family history of sudden death increases the risk of tachyarrhythmias during pregnancy (Laksman et al. 2011). The most common type of sustained arrhythmia presenting in pregnancy is supraventricular tachycardia (SVT). As arrhythmias may be intermittent a 12-lead ECG does not rule them out, and a 24-h ambulatory ECG monitor should be considered. This is especially true if women feel unwell with these symptoms, or symptoms fail to settle. Most SVTs are benign and will respond to vagal stimulation or Valsalva manoeuvre. The three most commonly used antiarrhythmic medications in an acute SVT are adenosine, calcium channel blockers and beta blockers (Bircher et al. 2016).

NEUROLOGICAL DISORDERS

Epilepsy

Epilepsy is the commonest non-communicable neurological disorder characterized by the presence of seizures, with a prevalence of 6–7 per 1000. Epilepsy is one of the most common neurological conditions in pregnancy, with a prevalence of 1 in 200 women in pregnancy receiving treatment for epilepsy (O'Connor et al. 2018), with an estimated 2500 infants born to mothers with epilepsy every year in the UK (Edey et al. 2014). Most cases occur with no identified aetiology, although epileptic-type seizures can be secondary to head trauma and brain tumours for instance (Fiest et al. 2017). However, its presence during childbearing increases the risk of maternal mortality by ten-fold (O'Connor et al. 2018).

Seizures result from a sudden excess of electricity to the brain disrupting the normal message passing between the cortical neurons (brain cells). The messages become mixed or halted, and a seizure results. These seizures can be subcategorized as partial and generalized (McAuliffe et al. 2013), as shown in Table 15.4. Treatment is with antiepileptic drugs (AEDs) with monotherapy (one drug) or polytherapy (two or more) if seizure control is more problematic. In certain cases, surgery or vagus nerve stimulation might be used (McAuliffe et al. 2013).

Epilepsy is an important cause of disability and mortality. Complications associated with epilepsy are:

- trauma occurring during the seizure, including tongue biting and head or limb injury
- status epilepticus: a seizure lasting for >30 min, or a series of seizures without regaining consciousness in between
- sudden unexpected death in epilepsy (SUDEP), of which there is no cause found for the sudden death. This is the most common cause of death associated with epilepsy (O'Connor et al. 2018; Knight et al. 2017; Edey et al. 2014).

Between 2013 and 2015, eight women with epilepsy died during pregnancy or during the immediate postpartum period, and another six mothers died between 6 weeks and 1 year, giving a total of 14 cases, reviewed by MBRRACE-UK (Knight et al. 2017). The team reviewed all the cases and improvements in care were highlighted. It is worth noting that during the triennium 2015–2017, 27 (13%) of maternal deaths in the UK were attributable to epilepsy and stroke (Knight et al. 2019).

Care for women with epilepsy during childbearing is often fragmented and many reports have identified the need for more collaborative working and better communication between obstetricians, midwives and epilepsy specialists during childbearing (Kelso et al. 2017; Thangaratinam et al. 2016). Joint obstetric and epilepsy clinics, shared record-keeping, guidelines for management of epilepsy in pregnancy and shared decision-making between women and their care teams are all recognized as possible improvements (Kelso et al. 2017).

Pre-conception care has been widely recommended, as many AEDs are associated with folate deficiency and fetal malformations such as neural tube defects, congenital heart defects, urinary tract and skeletal malformations and cleft palate. It is a balance between managing the risk and prevalence of maternal seizures versus the risk of congenital malformation; the latter depends on the type of medication and is dose-related. Lamotrigine and carbamazepine monotherapy at lower doses has been shown to present the least risk, while sodium valproate and phenytoin polytherapy have the higher prevalence. However, there is insufficient research evidence of estimated risk for all AEDs. Maternal lamotrigine and carbamazepine monotherapy also do not appear to affect the neurodevelopment of the infant through intrauterine exposure (Thangaratinam et al. 2016). To minimize the risk of congenital malformation to the fetus, all women with epilepsy should be taking the lowest effective dose of the most appropriate AED and to lessen exposure to

TABLE 15.4   **Categories of Epileptic Seizures**

Category	Type	Characteristics
Partial	Simple	Remains conscious
		Experiences an aura (premonition)
		Déjà vu (experienced this previously)
		Pins and needles sensation in arms or legs
		Pallor, or alternatively a flushed face with sweating
		Muscle twitching in limbs with some stiffness
	Complex	Awareness of changes; loses memory of the event
		Rubbing of hands
		Chewing and smacking of lips
		Picking at clothes or fiddling
		Makes random noises
		Exhibits unusual posture
Generalized	Absence	Staring and blinking, day-dreaming, loss of awareness for 5–20 s (*mainly affects children*)
	Myoclonic	Brief muscle jerking in an arm or leg. Lasts for a fraction of a second and individual remains conscious
	Tonic	All body muscles contract for <20 s, but there are no convulsions. The individual falls.
	Tonic–clonic	The whole body contracts, then arms and legs convulse. Incontinence is possible. Lasts 1–2 min and the individual appears tired, wanting to sleep. The most common type of seizure (60% of cases).
	Atonic	All muscle tone is lost momentarily. The individual falls limply and head injury is probable, but gets up immediately with no confusion.

Adapted from McAuliffe F et al. (2013) Neurological disorders. In: SE Robson, J Waugh (Eds) Medical disorders in pregnancy: a manual for midwives (2nd ed.). Oxford: Wiley-Blackwell, pp. 125–52.

sodium valproate and other polytherapy pre-conception care should include a medication review by an epilepsy specialist. In women with an unplanned pregnancy, who has had no pre-conception care, an individualized management plan should be created, which may include a change in dose or type of AED. All women taking AEDs should be provided with written and verbal communication on the risks of AED use and the risks of self-discontinuation of their AED. The latter is considered a significant risk, as research has shown that women often over-estimate the risk of teratogenicity (Williams et al. 2002). All women with epilepsy should also be advised to take 5 mg/day of folic acid prior to conception and continue throughout the first trimester.

Antenatal care should be a joint enterprise shared between a specialist in epilepsy, an obstetrician and a specialist midwife. Knight et al. (2014) recommended that all antenatal services should have an identified liaison epilepsy nurse integrated into routine antenatal services. Most women with epilepsy do not experience a seizure during pregnancy, especially if they were seizure-free for at least 9 months before conception, despite the known reduced blood levels of AEDs due to the changes in absorption, metabolism, haemodilution and excretion during pregnancy. It is not recommended that clinicians monitor serum levels of AEDs, but rather they monitor the effectiveness of the dosage through clinical observation of symptoms. Women with epilepsy and taking AEDs are at risk of depression, often due to worry about the effect of AED use on the fetus and fear of seizures. Midwives need to be aware of this risk and provide support and referral as appropriate. All women with epilepsy should be invited to join the UK Epilepsy and Pregnancy Register, which collects data to inform clinical practice and future research (Thangaratinam et al. 2016).

Women with epilepsy should also be provided with individualized risk assessment prior to making decisions on prenatal screening. Biochemical serum alpha-feto-protein and ultrasonography in the first trimester can detect almost 100% of neural tube defects, and morphology scans at 18–20 weeks' gestation is the optimum method for diagnosing cardiac anomalies. Assessment of fetal growth through serial ultrasound fetal growth screening should commence from 28 weeks' gestation for all women taking AEDs (Thangaratinam et al. 2016).

During pregnancy, there is an increased risk of spontaneous miscarriage, antepartum haemorrhage, hypertensive disorders and fetal growth restriction. In labour, there are increased rates of induction of labour, operative birth, preterm birth and PPH when compared with women without epilepsy. However, studies which compared women not treated with AEDs with those treated with AEDs, found that those women treated with AEDs had increased rates of IUGR and in labour induction of labour and PPH, but no differences in miscarriage, operative birth or preterm birth rates. There is an increased metabolism seen when using prophylactic corticosteroids in cases at risk of preterm birth, which reduces the benefit, but increasing the dose is not recommended due to the known side-effects of high steroid doses (Thangaratinam et al. 2016).

Women with epilepsy with no associated obstetric risk factors, where the seizures are well-controlled, usually labour normally and experience an uncomplicated labour and birth. Induction of labour or operative birth may be considered in cases where there is a decrease in seizure control. Tonic-clonic seizures are uncommon during labour; it is estimated that these occur in 1–2% of mothers during labour and measures should be taken to react speedily should a seizure result (Battino et al. 2013). The management principles for an epileptic seizure are the same as for eclampsia (Box 15.6). If they do occur, there is a risk of fetal hypoxia and acidosis due to uterine hypertonus. AED use should continue during labour and may need to be given parenterally if vomiting occurs. Adequate analgesia and avoiding dehydration will also lessen the risk of a seizure. If the risk of seizure is significant, short-acting benzodiazepines are often prescribed, e.g. clobazam. The neonatal team should be informed in these cases, as there is a risk of neonatal withdrawal syndrome seen in infants of mothers given AEDs and benzodiazepines. If a seizure occurs in labour, prompt management is necessary to reduce maternal and fetal hypoxia (Thangaratinam et al. 2016).

The midwife should discuss a realistic birth plan; birthing in a consultant-led environment with access to facilities for maternal and neonatal resuscitation and control of seizures is advised (NICE 2012). One-to-one care in labour is also recommended to facilitate close monitoring and provide support to minimize stress-induced seizures. The use of water for labour and birth should be decided on an individual basis and is restricted for use by women not taking AEDs who have been seizure-free for a year. The midwives providing care also need to be aware of how to manage a seizure in the pool and be conversant with hoists, etc. Pethidine is contraindicated as it is metabolized to norpethidine, which can also induce seizure, and diamorphine is recommended as a substitute. Trans-electrical nerve stimulation (TENS), Entonox or regional analgesia, e.g. epidural, are safe alternatives. Intermittent fetal monitoring is suitable for women at low risk of seizure, but those women at high risk of seizures should be advised to have continuous fetal monitoring in labour (Thangaratinam et al. 2016).

All babies born to women with epilepsy taking an enzyme-inducing AED, e.g. carbamazepine, phenytoin, should be offered IM vitamin K 1 mg to prevent haemorrhagic disease of the newborn (HDN). There is insufficient research to promote the use of oral vitamin K in these cases. The use of prenatal vitamin K given IM to the mother has not been demonstrated to show any benefits to reducing HND in the neonate or reducing postpartum haemorrhage in the mother (Thangaratinam et al. 2016).

In the first 24 h following the birth, the woman is at risk of a seizure of 1–2% and so women with epilepsy should be advised to remain in hospital, especially if they have a history of a seizure within the last month of pregnancy. There is also a potential high-risk period for seizures in the immediate post-birth period, due to increased stress and sleep deprivation, etc. The mother should continue to take her AED medication. If the dose was increased during pregnancy, then this should be reviewed by the neurological team within 10 days following the birth to avoid postpartum toxicity. Symptoms of AED toxicity include drowsiness, diplopia and unsteadiness (Thangaratinam et al. 2016).

Breastfeeding can be encouraged in women with epilepsy and psychomotor development is enhanced in breastfed babies born to mothers taking AEDs (Davanzo et al. 2013). The rates of transfer of AEDs to the neonate through breastfeeding vary and the medical team and pharmacist should discuss suitable AEDs while lactating. The baby should be carefully observed for adverse effects such as lethargy, poor feeding, excessive sleepiness and withdrawal symptoms, e.g. excessive crying and any concerns should be reported to the paediatrician immediately (Thangaratinam et al. 2016).

Antiepileptic drugs affect hormonal contraceptives and alternative contraception such as barrier methods and IUDs are recommended (see Chapter 28). Women with epilepsy should be offered contraception and pre-conception advice to avoid unplanned pregnancies. Women with epilepsy are also at an increased risk of postpartum depression (see Chapter 30); midwives should encourage mothers to self-monitor for symptoms and refer for early intervention to improve quality of life (Thangaratinam et al. 2016).

Advice should be given about safety when caring for the baby in case of maternal seizure, as seizures can result in accidental trauma such as falls, drowning, burns, etc. The midwife should endeavour to begin preparation for the postnatal period during antenatal care encounters. She should encourage the woman to dress, change and feed the baby on a changing mat on the floor, to prevent falling during a seizure while attending to the baby, plus laying the baby down if the women experiences an aura. It is advisable that the baby is bathed by the mother in shallow water when someone else is around to assist if necessary and a carrycot or baby car seat should be used to carry the baby up and down stairs. When parents choose a pram/buggy for their baby, the midwife should advise them to ensure that they select one with brakes that initiate when the handle is released. Family and friends should be aware of first aid and how to summon help in an emergency (Thangaratinam et al. 2016).

RESPIRATORY DISORDERS

Asthma

Asthma is a chronic inflammatory respiratory disease. It can affect people of any age, but often starts in childhood. Asthma is a variable disease, which can change throughout a person's life, throughout the year and from day to day. It is characterized by attacks (also known as exacerbations) of breathlessness and wheezing, with the severity and frequency of attacks varying from person to person. The attacks are associated with variable airflow obstruction and inflammation within the lungs, which if left untreated can be life-threatening, however with the appropriate treatment, can be reversible (NICE 2017).

> ### BOX 15.11   Triggers for Asthma
>
> - Pollen and house-dust mite allergens
> - Chronic nasal rhinitis
> - Smoking: primary and passive
> - Infection
> - Occupational exposure
> - Pollution
> - Cold air and physical exercise
> - Food additives, e.g. monosodium glutamate, tartrazine and sulphites
> - Drugs, e.g. aspirin
> - Premenstrual conditions and pregnancy.
> - There are 5.4 million people with asthma in the UK, which means asthma affects one in every 11 people and one in five households (NICE 2017).
> - In 2016 (the most recent data available) 1410 people died from asthma (Asthma UK 2018).
> - Of the 10 maternal deaths attributed to respiratory disease in the triennium 2009–12, three died from asthma (Knight et al. 2014).

From Tortora and Derrickson (2016); Scullion et al. (2013).

Inflammatory hyper-responsiveness of the airways to certain triggers (Box 15.11) causes episodic narrowing, resulting in obstruction of the airways and mucous production. Key statistics reveal the extent of the problem in the UK.

Investigations include:

- *peak expiratory flow measurements* using a small handheld device (peak flow meter) to assess the speed by which air is exhaled
- *spirometry* via a spirometer to measure the volume and speed of air exhaled
- allergy testing
- chest X-ray to exclude other conditions
- steroid trial: 2 weeks of oral prednisolone or 6 weeks of an inhaled corticosteroid.

Treatment follows a *stepwise* approach and initial therapy will depend on the severity of the presentation. Some individuals may only require salbutamol for occasional symptoms, whereas others may start on two inhalers (British Thoracic Society/Scottish Intercollegiate Guidelines Network, BTS/SIGN 2016):

- a corticosteroid inhaler (e.g. *betclometasone dipropionate*), twice a day: usually colour-coded brown or orange and described as a *preventer inhaler*

- a bronchodilator inhaler/beta-2 agonist (e.g. *salbutamol*), when required: colour-coded blue and described as a *reliever inhaler*.

Further treatment may involve long acting beta-2 agonists, theophyllines, leukotriene antagonists and, in extreme cases, oral corticosteroids (Holmes and Scullion 2011).

During pregnancy, around one-third of women find their asthma improves. A third experience more symptoms, and a third do not notice any change (Mehita et al. 2015). In general, pregnant women who have asthma should be treated in the same way as anyone else. Midwives have a unique opportunity to investigate women's barriers to adherence (perhaps fear of side-effects for themselves or their baby) and encourage better adherence to asthma medicines, as well as other behaviours that will benefit mother and child for years to come, such as smoking cessation or taking regular exercise.

Mundle (2017) identifies key advice midwives can give to encourage women to help keep their asthma controlled and have a better chance of staying well in their pregnancy. This includes use of a personalized written asthma action plan, which describes what to do: every day; when asthma symptoms get worse; and during an asthma attack. They can encourage the woman to check their symptoms and discuss an action plan regularly with a GP or practice nurse. In addition, midwives can ensure the woman's asthma is recorded on the birth plan so that everyone responsible for her care is aware of it, and of any extra concerns she may have. Women should be encouraged to take their medicines as prescribed. Even women who were adherent before pregnancy may be wary about taking preventer medication. Reassure women that asthma medicines will not harm their baby. This includes reliever inhaler; preventer inhalers; long-acting and combined relievers; theophylline and steroid (prednisolone) tablets. It helps to make sure women are clear about how to recognize an asthma attack and that they and those around them know what to do and where the reliever inhaler is kept (see the toolkit of actions to support a woman during an asthma attack, in Box 15.12). Women may find it helpful to take a photo of their written asthma action plan on their phone, so it is always to hand and can easily be shared. As per PHE (2016) Guidelines, midwives should encourage influenza immunization, as it reduces the likelihood of complications resulting from flu to mother or baby, and protects the baby from flu for the first few months of life (NHS 2018a).

> **BOX 15.12 Actions for a Pregnant Woman Having an Asthmatic Attack**
>
> 1. *Action*: Ask woman to sit upright and keep calm.
>   - *Advise*: Take one puff of reliever inhaler every 30–60 s, up to a maximum of 10 puffs.
> 2. *Action*: If woman feels worse at any point while using the inhaler or she does not feel better after 10 puffs or if she is worried at any time, call 999 for an ambulance.
>   - *Advise*: If the ambulance is taking longer than 15 min to arrive, repeat step 2.

Midwives should discuss asthma treatments at each encounter and if a woman has not been prescribed inhaler treatments before pregnancy, or has not been taking them, refer her to her usual prescriber (PHE 2016). Women who find that their asthma gets worse during pregnancy are likely to see the biggest difference during the second and third trimester, peaking around the 6th month.

In pregnancy, women who are well controlled do not have significantly higher adverse outcomes than women without asthma (Mehita et al. 2015), but those with exacerbations are at increased risk of birthing low birth weight and preterm babies and have a greater tendency to other medical complications such as pre-eclampsia. Women should be referred to a consultant clinic if their asthma is uncontrolled: when she has daytime symptoms, night time awakening due to asthma; the need for rescue medication – women who require add on therapy beyond inhaled short-acting β agonist and inhaled steroids and women with persistent poor control asthma attacks/exacerbations and limitations in daily activity.

Severe acute asthma, also termed *status asthmaticus* or *asthma attack*, occurs when there is spasm of the smooth muscle in the walls of the smaller bronchi and bronchioles leading to partial or complete obstruction of the airways, known as *bronchoconstriction*. This manifests with periods of coughing, wheezing and difficulty with exhalation. Air may become trapped in the alveoli during exhalation. Excessive secretion of mucous may obstruct the bronchioles and worsen the attack. This is a medical emergency and pregnant women should be treated in hospital.

Severe asthma in pregnancy is a medical emergency and should be vigorously treated in hospital in conjunction with the respiratory physicians. Treatment of severe asthma is not different from the non-pregnant patients. Treatment should include the following:

- high flow oxygen to maintain saturation of 94–98%
- β2 agonists administered via nebulizer, which may need to be given repeatedly
- nebulized ipratropium bromide should be added for severe or poorly responding asthma
- corticosteroids (IV hydrocortisone 100 mg) and/or oral (40–50 mg prednisolone for at least 5 days)
- chest radiograph should be performed if there is any clinical suspicion of pneumonia or pneumothorax or if the woman fails to improve.

Management of life-threatening or acute severe asthma that fails to respond to treatment should involve consultation with the critical care team and consideration should be given IV β2 agonists, IV magnesium sulphate and IV aminophylline. High flow oxygen should be administered immediately to maintain saturations between 94% and 98%, a systemic corticosteroid given and inhaled short-acting beta-2 agonists administered via a large volume spacer or nebulizer. Research studies in progress aim to understand further differing approaches to the management of asthma exacerbations (Murphy et al. 2016).

The labour of a woman whose asthma is well controlled may progress physiologically, supported by the midwife. Those women who have been receiving oral steroids may require hydrocortisone during labour. If anaesthesia is required, epidural is preferable to general anaesthesia. If ergometrine and syntometrine are used to control blood loss following the birth of the placenta, extreme caution should be taken to reduce the risk of inducing bronchoconstriction (BTS/SIGN 2016). Breastfeeding should be encouraged and the woman should continue to take all prescribed medication for her asthma during lactation.

THROMBOEMBOLIC DISEASE

Thromboembolic disease is of considerable importance to midwifery practice because of the associated maternal mortality. It remains the leading cause of direct maternal death in the UK, with 39 deaths occurring in the previous triennial report, 2014–16 (Tuffnell 2018; Unger et al. 2018). There is no statistically significant change in the trend for the triennium 2015–17. Thromboembolic disorders remain the leading cause of direct maternal deaths occurring within 42 days of the end of pregnancy (Knight et al. 2019).

Thromboprophylaxis in Pregnancy

Changes to population demographics such as increasing maternal age and obesity and increasing operative mode of birth have continued to see thromboembolism rates remaining significant, despite thromboprophylaxis risk assessments and regimes being part of the midwife's daily role.

There are additional risk factors for VTE in pregnancy and the RCOG (2015a) provides a risk assessment scale, as summarized in Box 15.13.

In the UK, most NHS hospitals will have a risk assessment based on the criteria in Box 15.13. The midwife should perform and document this risk assessment on the following occasions:

- initial meeting with the woman (*antenatal booking visit*)
- any hospital admission
- following the birth of the baby.

If this assessment identifies a woman at risk of developing VTE, the midwife should promptly refer her to a consultant-led maternity unit with an expert in thrombosis in pregnancy (Elliott and Pavord 2013). The woman is likely to be started on subcutaneous injections of low molecular weight heparin (LMWH), as this does not cross the placental barrier with consequential effects on the fetus. The midwife, or specialist nurse, should educate the woman in self-administration of the heparin, alerting her to carry a medical alert card containing such details at all times. The woman should be provided with a sharps bin for safe disposal of the injection devices.

Gradient compression stockings or TED stockings will be prescribed. Such stockings are available in two lengths, below the knee or thigh, and are designed to give a pressure gradient from the ankle to the knee or thigh that mimics the pumping action of the deep leg vein calf muscles, with the highest pressure being at the ankle. It is important that the woman is measured correctly around the ankle and calf or thigh circumference depending upon the type of stocking prescribed (Llewelyn 2013). Midwives should be trained in their use to be able to instruct the woman how to wear them correctly and monitor their use (Elliott and Pavord 2013; Sachdeva et al. 2018). For hygiene purposes, stockings should be removed daily, but this should be for no more than 30 min. The legs should be inspected and measured

BOX 15.13 Risk Factors for Venous Thromboembolism

	Tick	Score
Pre-existing factors		
Previous VTE (except a single event related to major surgery)		4
Previous VTE provoked by major surgery		3
Known high-risk thrombophilia		3
Medical comorbidities, e.g. cancer, heart failure; active systemic lupus erythematosus, inflammatory polyarthropathy or inflammatory bowel disease; nephrotic syndrome; type 1 diabetes mellitus with nephropathy; sickle cell disease; current intravenous drug user		3
Family history of unprovoked or oestrogen-related VTE in first-degree relative		1
Known low-risk thrombophilia (no VTE)		1
Age (>35 years)		1
Obesity		1 or 2
Parity ≥ 3		1
Smoker		1
Gross varicose veins		1
Obstetric factors		
Pre-eclampsia in current pregnancy		1
ART/IVF (antenatal only)		1
Multiple pregnancy		1
Caesarean section in labour		2
Elective caesarean section		1
Mid-cavity or rotational operative delivery		1
Prolonged labour (>24 h)		1
PPH (>1 litre or transfusion)		1
Preterm birth <37+^{0} weeks in current pregnancy		1
Stillbirth in current pregnancy		1
Transient risk factors		
Any surgical procedure in pregnancy or puerperium except immediate repair of the perineum, e.g. appendicectomy, postpartum sterilization		3
Hyperemesis		3
OHSS (first trimester only)		4
Current systemic infection		1
Immobility, dehydration		1

Actions

- If the total score is ≥4 antenatally, consider thromboprophylaxis from the first trimester
- If the total score is 3 antenatally, consider thromboprophylaxis from 28 weeks
- If the total score is ≥2 postnatally, consider thromboprophylaxis for at least 10 days
- If admitted to hospital antenatally, consider thromboprophylaxis
- If prolonged admission (≥3 days) or readmission to hospital within the puerperium, consider thromboprophylaxis.

For patients with an identified bleeding risk, the balance of risks of bleeding and thrombosis should be discussed in consultation with a haematologist with expertise in thrombosis and bleeding in pregnancy.

ART, assisted reproductive technology; *IVF, in vitro* fertilization; *OHSS*, ovarian hyperstimulation syndrome; *VTE* venous thromboembolism. If the known low-risk thrombophilia is in a woman with a family history of *VTE* in a first-degree relative, postpartum thromboprophylaxis should be continued for 6 weeks. BMI ≥30 = 1; BMI ≥40 = 2.
From RCOG (Royal College of Obstetricians and Gynaecologists). (2015a,b).

by the midwife every 3 days to detect any changes in size or tissue damage (Llewelyn 2013).

The woman should be given advice about avoiding dehydration, ceasing smoking and eating a healthy diet (Copple and Coser 2013). If the pregnant woman is expecting to travel long distances, especially by air, she will benefit by wearing loose fitting clothing and flight socks (TED stockings), drinking plenty of water, avoiding alcohol and remaining ambulant for as long as possible/performing leg exercises when at rest (Elliott and Pavord 2013).

During labour, the midwife should encourage mobility with regular changes of position and passive leg exercises when the woman is at rest. It is important that hydration is maintained and regular observations are undertaken, including frequent examination of the woman's legs. If the woman has been prescribed LMWH in pregnancy, this should be omitted at the onset of contractions and regional anaesthesia avoided within 12 h of the last administered dose. There should be active management of the third stage of labour with the oxytocic drug being administered IV. If perineal suturing is required, the midwife should undertake this promptly to avoid the woman being in the lithotomy position (if this is necessary) for a prolonged time, as this further increases the risk for deep vein thrombosis (DVT). If surgery is necessary, intermittent calf compression will be required in theatre.

The postnatal period presents further risk to the woman for both DVT and pulmonary embolism (PE), and early mobilization should be encouraged. Routine postnatal observations are important, especially respiration rate and the development of any leg swelling. If either condition is suspected, the woman must be referred urgently to a haematologist, or if at home she must be re-admitted to hospital.

Deep Vein Thrombosis

A blood clot formed within a blood vessel is termed a *thrombus*, which can become detached and lodge in another blood vessel and partially or wholly occlude it. *Virchow's triad* (Fig. 15.1) outlines predisposing factors for thrombus formation (Bagot and Arya 2008).

In pregnancy, Virchow's triad is affected by the physiological changes to the haematological system (see Chapter 10). Despite pregnancy presenting a state of *hypervolaemia*, by term *hypercoagulability* also develops to compensate for the demands of the

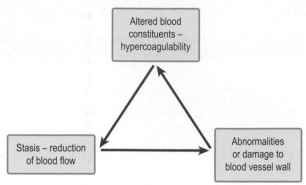

Fig. 15.1 Virchow's triad. (From Bagot CN, Arya R. (2008) Virchow and his triad: a question of attribution. British Journal of Haematology 143(2):180–90.)

forthcoming labour and maintenance of haemostasis. In addition, there is relative venous stasis with a gradual 50% reduction in venous flow velocity, reaching its peak at 36 weeks and declining to pre-pregnancy values by 6 weeks following the baby's birth. Furthermore, the physical effect of the gravid uterus exerts pressure on the pelvic veins and the inferior vena cava, increasing the woman's risk of developing a DVT in the veins of the calf, thigh and pelvis (Elliott and Pavord 2013).

In pregnancy, 90% of DVTs occur in the left leg, compared with 55% in the non-pregnant woman due to compression of the left iliac vein by the left iliac artery in pregnancy (Davis and Pavord 2018). The ileofemoral veins are the most common location, having 70% of pregnancy occurrences versus 9% in the non-pregnant woman, and are more likely to result in pulmonary embolism (Davis and Pavord 2018).

The complications of DVT are *pulmonary embolism* (PE) and *post-thrombotic syndrome* arising from damage to the venous valves that result in a backflow of blood, venous hypertension, oedema and tissue hypoxia (Elliott and Pavord 2013). The midwife needs to be aware of the signs of DVT, as she may be the first person to identify this when undertaking an antenatal or postnatal examination on the woman. Signs include:

- pain in the area of the clot
- swelling (usually one-sided)
- red discoloration
- difficulty in weight-bearing on the affected leg
- low-grade pyrexia
- lower abdominal or back pain.

If the leg appears swollen, a tape measure should be used to assess the circumference of both legs at the affected area for comparison. A DVT is potentially life-threatening and the midwife **must refer the woman immediately** to hospital for medical examination, investigation and treatment (RCOG 2015a). The classic diagnostic use of dorsiflexion of the foot (*Homans sign*) is considered unreliable in pregnancy and the presence of severe lower back pain has greater significance (James et al. 2017). Medical investigations involve Doppler ultrasound and serum investigations might be performed; however, Elliott and Pavord (2013) debate the usefulness of measuring D-dimers levels in pregnancy. Venography is generally avoided in pregnancy due to the small radiation risk to the fetus.

Treatment of DVT in pregnancy is with LMWH administered 12-hourly by subcutaneous injection to sustain the levels, and which should continue for at least 6 months after the diagnosis. Gradient compression stockings should be prescribed and the woman taught how to put them on. The woman will need to wear one on the affected leg for 2 years to reduce the risk of post-thrombotic syndrome (Elliott and Pavord 2013). Anticoagulation therapy should continue for at least 6 months after the diagnosis (RCOG 2015b).

The woman should be seen by the anaesthetist prior to labour to discuss the risks that thromboembolic disorders have on the administration of regional/general anaesthesia. As soon as labour commences, heparin should be omitted and compression stockings should be worn. As regional anaesthesia carries a risk of spinal bleeding, this should be avoided within 12 h of administration of heparin. Although general anaesthetic is itself a thrombotic risk, it may have to be considered for caesarean section. The woman should be encouraged to remain mobile or undertake passive leg exercises and maintain hydration. An IVI should be sited, and drugs given intravenously (IV) instead of intramuscularly (IM). Prolonged use of the lithotomy position should be avoided, as this is a DVT risk. The third stage of labour should be actively managed with the oxytocic drug being administered IV to prompt haemostasis. If perineal suturing is required, it should be undertaken promptly to limit the length of time the woman is in the lithotomy position (RCOG 2015b; Elliott and Pavord 2013).

The midwife should be aware that there is a 25-fold increased risk of DVT and the potential for PE during the postnatal period. As a consequence, the woman who has had a previous DVT is especially at high risk and thus the midwife is required to be particularly vigilant is assessing her condition, encouraging early ambulation and hydration. Heparin is recommenced as directed by the medical team. This is usually 2 h after a vaginal birth or longer if the woman had an epidural and/or caesarean section, and should continue until at least the 6-week postnatal appointment, at which point a decision to change to warfarin may be made (RCOG 2015b; Elliott and Pavord 2013). Oestrogen-based contraceptive pills are contraindicated so Depo-Provera or barrier methods of contraception should be discussed with the woman and her partner.

Pulmonary Embolism

Pulmonary embolism (PE) most commonly occurs when a DVT detaches and becomes mobile, known as an *embolus*. A large embolus might lodge in the pulmonary artery and smaller ones can travel distally to small vessels in the lung periphery, where they may wholly or partially occlude the blood vessel (James et al. 2017; Elliott and Pavord 2013). Initially, the lung tissue is ventilated but not perfused, producing intrapulmonary dead space, and there is impaired gaseous exchange (Kumar and Clarke 2004). After some hours, surfactant production by the affected lung ceases, the alveoli collapse and hypoxaemia results. Pulmonary arterial pressure rises and there is a reduction in cardiac output. The area of the lung affected by the embolism may become infracted, however, in some instances, oxygenation of tissue continues to some extent from the bronchial circulation and airways (Kumar and Clarke 2004).

In the case of a small embolism, there is likely to be dyspnoea, discomfort or pain in the chest, haemoptysis and low-grade pyrexia, all of which can be misdiagnosed as a chest infection. Dyspnoea associated with PE is sudden in onset and can be associated with increased respiratory rate, pleuritic chest pain and haemoptysis. Cardiovascular examination is usually normal (Kumar and Clarke 2004; James et al. 2017).

A larger embolism that occludes a major vessel will result in a more acute presentation, because of sudden obstruction of the right ventricle and its outflow (Kumar and Clarke 2004). There is severe central chest pain due to ischaemia, and pallor with sweating as shock develops. Tachycardia occurs and a *gallop rhythm* of the heart may be heard on examination. Hypotension develops as peripheral shutdown occurs. Syncope may result when cardiac output is suddenly reduced (Kumar and Clarke 2004). Admission to an intensive care unit is highly likely as there is a significant risk of death if treatment is delayed.

Pulmonary embolism is a medical emergency and urgent referral to hospital is indicated. Diagnosis is made from a combination of clinical probability score ECG and radiological imaging including chest X-ray, CT scan or pulmonary angiogram. Arterial blood gases are indicated if oxygen saturation is <96%. Women should be involved in the decision to undergo CTPA or VQ scanning. Informed consent must be obtained before these tests are undertaken as they are associated with reduced radiation to the maternal breasts but increased radiation risks to the fetus, particularly in early pregnancy (Goodacre et al. 2015). Breast tissue is especially sensitive to radiation exposure during pregnancy. In addition, special consideration should be given to women with a family history of breast cancer before iodine-based IV contrast is given during CTPA. The effects of iodine on the fetus is still uncertain (Burton 2018).

Treatment with LMWH should be started prior to diagnosis if high clinical probability or delay in diagnostic imaging, unless there is strong contraindication to subsequent anticoagulation treatment. This should be following discussion with the woman about risk and benefits of commencing treatment. Prior to starting LMWH, it is good practice to ensure renal and hepatic function are normal, this is especially important in women with comorbidities such as diabetic nephropathy. Treatments such as thrombolysis may be considered, particularly if there is severe hypotension or shock but carry risks of bleeding. Management in labour and the postnatal period is similar to that for a woman presenting with DVT (Elliott and Pavord 2013).

Disseminated Intravascular Coagulation

In DIC (also known as disseminated intravascular coagulopathy), damage to the endothelium (lining of blood vessel walls) arising from pre-eclampsia, placental abruption, major haemorrhage, embolism, sepsis, acute fatty liver of pregnancy, amniotic fluid embolism, intrauterine fetal death or retained placenta results in thromboplastins being released from the damaged cells, causing the extrinsic pathway to mount a coagulation cascade. Blood clotting occurs at the original site and then small clots (*micro-thrombi*) disperse throughout the rest of the vascular system. Large quantities of fibrinogen, thrombocytes

(platelets) and clotting factors V and VIII are consumed. The micro-thrombi produced can occlude small blood vessels, resulting in ischaemia, hence some organ tissue dies and releases more thromboplastins and the cycle restarts. All clotting factors and platelets are subsequently consumed and bleeding results. There is simultaneously widespread blood clotting *and* a clotting deficiency. Bleeding occurs, petechiae develop in the skin and, if untreated, major haemorrhage can result (Kumar and Clarke 2004; Watson et al. 2012). Diagnosis is according to clinical examination and history of the woman as well as laboratory tests of platelets, fibrin degradation products, fibrinogen, prothrombin time and activated partial prothrombin time. Serial examination is required and management involves the multidisciplinary team, including haematology and the major haemorrhage protocol should be utilized, alerting laboratories to the need for multiple blood products. The woman will require critical care/high dependency or intensive care and monitoring. The midwives' role would be to carry out care and observations, communicate with the MDT and family.

HAEMATOLOGICAL DISORDERS

Anaemia

Anaemia is a condition in which the number of red blood cells or their oxygen carrying capacity is insufficient to meet the physiological needs of the individual, which consequently will vary by age, sex, altitude, smoking and pregnancy status (WHO 2013). In its severe form, it is associated with fatigue, weakness, dizziness and drowsiness, pregnant women and children being particularly vulnerable (WHO 2013; Daru et al. 2018). Anaemia in pregnancy is normally defined as a haemoglobin (Hb) concentration of <110 g/dL, however considerations accounting for haemodilution or population variance may need to be made (Pavord et al. 2012). Serum ferritin is recommended as a measurement of iron stores alongside haemoglobin to test for iron status, as a low haemoglobin indicates anaemia but not its cause. Iron stores become depleted before a drop in haemoglobin (Walsh et al. 2011). Concurrent testing with C-reactive protein in situations where inflammation or infection is present or suspected is also recommended (Pavord et al. 2012).

Physiological anaemia of pregnancy

The increase of blood plasma in pregnancy causes a state of haemodilution (see Chapter 10). On laboratory

TABLE 15.5 Anaemia Defined by Trimester

Trimester	Serum ferritin concentration	Haemoglobin
1	<30 µg/L	<11 g/dL
2 and 3	<30 µg/L	<10.5 g/dL

testing, the Hb values decline, reaching the lowest in the second trimester followed by a gradual rise in the third trimester. This situation is not pathological unless the Hb reduces to such an extent that iron deficiency anaemia results.

Iron deficiency anaemia

Iron deficiency is thought to be the most common cause of anaemia globally (Bah et al. 2017). The daily iron requirement for a healthy woman is 1.3 mg, which can be acquired through a diet rich in iron and folate. In pregnancy, this requirement rises to 3 mg/day, further increasing to 7 mg/day after 32 weeks (Addo et al. 2013). Prophylactic antenatal iron supplementation is not administered routinely in the UK, unless the woman is at risk of developing iron deficiency anaemia (Table 15.5). However, ongoing research, since the discovery of liver hormone hepcidin, is developing awareness and understanding of the complexities of iron regulation absorption and metabolism of iron, and may lead to changes in practice related to both screening and management with iron therapy (Bah et al. 2017; Schrier 2015).

Iron deficiency is associated with:
- reduced intake of iron due to gastric malabsorption, gastric surgery or dietary deficiency
- short intervals between pregnancies
- chronic infection such as malaria or human immunodeficiency virus (HIV)
- chronic blood loss, e.g. menorrhagia or gastric ulcer
- haemorrhage
- secondary cause to medical disorders
- multiple pregnancy.

Iron deficiency interferes with body functions, leading to:
- tiredness
- irritability and depression
- breathlessness
- poor memory
- muscle aches
- palpitations

- cardiac failure
- maternal exhaustion in labour
- poor recovery from blood loss at birth and during the postnatal period
- impaired maternal infant interaction
- infant brain development
- thyroid hormone metabolism
- breastfeeding
- severe maternal anaemia is associated with low birth weight and IUGR (Walsh et al. 2011; Khambalia et al. 2016).

Routine serum blood samples should be taken from healthy pregnant women at intervals during the antenatal period according to local protocols for the early identification of anaemia. It is recommended that women with known anaemia be screened at every antenatal appointment (Addo et al. 2013). *Borderline anaemia* can be managed in the community setting, however severe or chronic cases should be referred to a consultant-led maternity unit as should those women who are symptomatic (Addo et al. 2013).

Dietary advice about iron-rich foods should be offered, sensitive to the woman's individual needs and documented in the woman's records. The initial treatment with iron tablets, such as Pregaday, one tablet per day for 2 weeks, should be started. The woman should be advised to take the tablet 1 h before food with orange juice, which contains ascorbic acid (vitamin C) to aid absorption of the iron, and to avoid taking tablets with tea and coffee as these reduce the absorption. Unfortunately, many brands of oral iron tablets have unpleasant gastric side-effects, which reduce maternal compliance in taking them. Serum Hb estimation is undertaken after 2 weeks, and if the Hb appears to be rising, the woman should continue taking the iron tablets. However, if the Hb does not rise or there is intolerance or poor compliance, the woman should be referred to a haematology clinic for further management. Additional investigations may be undertaken to determine the cause of the anaemia, and other oral iron, such as ferrous sulphate (200 mg 2–3 times daily) may be prescribed. If there is absolute intolerance or non-compliance with oral iron, IV iron should be considered, providing iron deficiency has been confirmed with a low serum ferritin. Anaphylactic reaction is a risk with iron infusions and the woman should be observed in hospital while undertaking this treatment; oral iron supplements following this should be omitted for 1 week then reviewed. Blood transfusion is used only in extreme cases during pregnancy.

If the anaemia persists, then the woman should be assessed regarding her risk for haemorrhage. An IV cannula should be sited in labour and blood samples taken for full blood count (FBC) and for group and save. The midwife should be alert for signs of maternal exhaustion during labour with active management of the third stage of labour being undertaken, and all perineal trauma should be sutured promptly to minimize the effects of blood loss at the time of the birth.

In the postnatal period, the woman with anaemia is at risk of infection, PPH, depression, poor wound healing and delayed lactation. The midwife should observe and support her accordingly and ensure that an FBC blood sample is taken to identify further treatment requirements. Contraceptive advice should be given for adequate spacing of pregnancies, along with dietary advice and a follow-up appointment. The FBC will also need repeating at the 6-week postnatal examination.

Folic Acid Deficiency

Folic acid is part of the vitamin B complex. In pregnancy, it is necessary for effective cell growth and synthesis of ribonucleic acid (RNA) and deoxyribonucleic acid (DNA) especially for the embryo, and a deficiency is associated with neural tube defects in the fetus. Deficiency can be due to multiple pregnancy, poor diet and adverse social circumstances, which may arise secondary to drug therapy such as antiepileptic drugs (AEDs). The average daily folate requirements rise in pregnancy from 50 to 400 µg/day (Addo et al. 2013). Although this can usually be met through a healthy diet, women are encouraged to take prophylactic folic acid 400 µg/day (0.4 mg) routinely in the first trimester, which should be increased to 5 mg if the woman is also taking AEDs or other drugs affecting folate metabolism. Chronic maternal folate deficiency can lead to megaloblastic anaemia.

Megaloblastic anaemia

Megaloblastic anaemia refers to a malformation of the erythroblasts in the bone marrow in which the maturation of the nucleus is delayed due to defective DNA synthesis, resulting in the production of larger than normal red blood cells (*macrocytosis*). This arises from a deficiency of either of two B vitamins, *folic acid* and *cyanocobalmin* (B12), both of which are necessary for DNA synthesis (Hoffbrand and Moss 2016). A deficiency of

vitamin B12 alone is termed *pernicious anaemia*. One-third of pregnancies worldwide are affected by megaloblastic anaemia, but the UK incidence is low, at 0.5%. Megaloblastic anaemia is secondary to dietary deficiency (especially a vegan diet); alcoholism; gastrointestinal surgery; autoimmune disease; medical disorders, especially sickle cell disease; and drug therapy, e.g. azathioprine (Hoffbrand and Moss 2016; NICE 2019b).

Diagnosis is made through taking a detailed history from the woman, undertaking a physical examination and investigations, including an FBC, blood film and assessing serum concentrations of vitamin B12 and folate. If vitamin B12 deficiency is evident, serum anti-intrinsic factor and antiparietal cell antibodies should be examined. If folate levels are low, tests for antiendomysial or antitransglutaminase antibodies are likely to be performed (NICE 2019b). Treatment is determined according to the identity of the underlying cause. Supplements of *folic acid* and *cyanocobalamin* will be prescribed as necessary, and a referral to a dietician may be necessary.

The midwife has an important role in identifying at-risk women and referring them to appropriate personnel, encouraging compliance with medication and providing dietary advice.

Haemoglobinopathies

Haemoglobinopathies are a group of inherited conditions with malformations of the Hb. Haemoglobin consists of a group of four molecules, each of which as a *haem* unit made up of an iron porphyrin complex and a protein or *globin* chain. A total of 97% of adult Hb (HbA) has two α- and two β-chains and the remaining 3% is composed of two α- and two δ-chains. Fetal Hb (HbF) has two α- and two γ-chains, the latter being gradually replaced by the β-chain by around the age of 6 months. The type of globin chain is genetically determined and defective genes lead to the formation of malformed haemoglobin. This may be as a result of impaired globin synthesis (*thalassaemia syndromes*) or from structural malformation of globin (*haemoglobin variants* such as *sickle cell anaemia*). Haemoglobinopathies mainly affect people from Africa, West Indies, Asia, the Middle East and the Eastern Mediterranean and the theory is that the carrier state offers some protection against malaria (Hoffbrand and Moss 2016). In the UK, antenatal screening is offered for haemoglobinopathies dependent on prevalence in areas and administration of family origins questionnaire (PHE 2018). However, screening programmes differ throughout the world, depending on population needs, culture and/or ethics, and although antenatal diagnosis remains a personal choice, policies are focused on education and counselling (Petrakos et al. 2016).

Thalassaemia

There are different types of thalassaemia depending upon which haemoglobin chain has been affected: α-chains are formed by two genes from each parent whereas β-chains are formed by one gene from each parent. In α-thalassaemia, the production of α-globin is deficient and in β-thalassaemia the production of β-globin is defective. The classifications are:

α-thalassaemia

- *Normal*: genotype = α/α, α/α
- *α+-thalassaemia heterozygous*: genotype = α/−, α/α. One defective α gene. Borderline Hb level and mean corpuscular volume (MCV), low mean corpuscular Hb (MCH): clinically asymptomatic
- *α+-thalassaemia homozygous*: genotype = α/−, α/−. Two defective α genes. Slightly anaemic, low MCV and MCH; clinically asymptomatic. This is known as *thalassaemia trait* and is associated with Africans
- *α0-thalassaemia heterozygous*: genotype = α/α, −/−. Two defective α genes. Slightly anaemic, low MCV and MCH; clinically asymptomatic. This is also known as *thalassaemia trait* and is associated with Asians
- *Haemoglobin H disease (HbH)*: genotype = α/−, −/−. Three defective α genes. Mild to moderate anaemia with very low MCV and MCH; splenomegaly and variable bone changes
- *α-thalassaemia major*: genotype = −/−, −/−. Four defective α genes. This type is also known as Hb Bart's. It presents as severe non-immune intrauterine haemolytic anaemia where the fetus has little circulating haemoglobin that is all tetrametric γ-chains. As a result, the fetus becomes oedematous: known as *hydrops fetalis/Hb Bart's hydrops*, which is usually fatal (Addo et al. 2013; Hoffbrand and Moss 2016).

β-thalassaemia

- *Normal*: genotype = β2, β2
- *β-thalassaemia trait*: genotype = −, β2. One defective β gene is inherited. HbA_2 is >4% and the individual presents with mild anaemia, a low MCV and MCH, but is clinically asymptomatic.

- *β-thalassaemia intermedia*: genotype = −, $β^0$ or $β^+$, $β^+$. Both defective β genes are inherited. This type presents with high levels of HbF which can fluctuate, resulting in anaemia upon which symptoms usually develop when the haemoglobin level remains below 70 g/dL, a very low MCV and MCH, splenomegaly and variable bone changes. The dependency on blood transfusion to improve an individual's wellbeing is variable
- *β-thalassaemia major*: genotype = $−^0/−^0$. In this type, both defective β genes are also inherited, but the Hb is comprised of >90% HbF (untransfused). As a result, the individual presents with severe haemolytic anaemia, a very low MCV and MCH, and hepatosplenomegaly, such that they are chronically dependent on frequent blood transfusions (Addo et al. 2013; Hoffbrand and Moss 2016) resulting in iron overload, and the need for chelation therapy. However, the majority of sufferers will ultimately develop organ damage, in particular, the heart and liver, with reduced life quality and expectancy.

Diagnosis is made by identifying those at high risk and performing the following:

- FBC would reveal a low mean corpuscular haemoglobin (MCH <27 pg) and a low mean cell volume (MCV <75 fl).
- Bone marrow examination would reveal microcytic, hypochromic red blood cells.
- Haemoglobin analysis would reveal elevated HbA_2 levels (Addo et al. 2013).

Pre-conception care is important and genetic counselling may be required, especially if there is inter-marriage of cousins. There is a 1 in 4 chance of a baby inheriting a major condition if both parents are carriers (Fig. 15.2). Preimplantation genetic diagnosis (PGD) may be offered (De Rycke et al. 2001).

In early pregnancy diagnostic tests are offered to the woman, consisting of DNA analysis of chorionic villi and fetal blood sampling (Addo et al. 2013; Petrakos et al. 2016), with termination of pregnancy being discussed should the fetus be adversely affected. Antenatal care should be provided within an obstetric unit where the woman can be assessed within a combined clinic with a haematologist in attendance. The treatment would entail regular assessment of FBC and serum ferritin. Iron is prescribed only if serum ferritin levels are low, as there is a risk of iron overload, which may lead to congestive cardiac failure. Consequently, further investigations may be required to assess

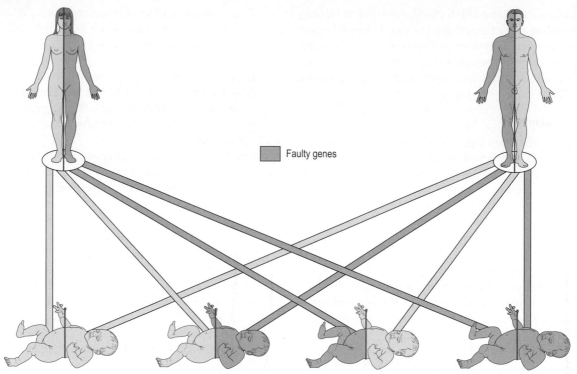

Fig. 15.2 The inheritance of a haemoglobinopathy when both parents are heterozygous.

Faulty genes

cardiac function. Thalassaemic women have an increased risk for thrombosis, as the disease entity is a chronic hypercoagulable state with high incidence of thromboembolic episodes (Petrakos et al. 2016; Lao 2017).

If the woman has *thalassaemia major* she is at risk of preterm labour, which might be iatrogenic, as well as both maternal and fetal hypoxia in labour. If the woman has any bone deformities, caesarean section may be necessary. There should be continuous fetal monitoring in labour and strict monitoring of BP and fluid balance. Due to the risk of haemorrhage, it would be wise for the midwife to facilitate active management of the third stage of labour.

During the postnatal period, the woman should be observed for signs of infection and haemorrhage and any wound should be inspected for signs of poor healing. Furthermore, the anaemia might worsen following the birth if the baby and tiredness could also predispose to depression. The baby will require paediatric assessment prior to transfer home from hospital and any follow-up appointments should be made to monitor growth and development, as well as determine the baby's thalassaemia status.

Sickle cell disease. Sickle cell disease refers to a group of disorders arising from defective genes that produce malformed Hb molecules (HbS). Defective genes produce malformed haemoglobin α- or β-chains resulting in HbS. There are several variations and those of most significance to the midwife are the homozygous sickle cell anaemia/sickle cell disease (*HbSS*) and heterozygous sickle cell trait (*HbAS*).

Other variations can be summarized as follows:
- *Sickle cell HbC disease (HbSC)*: double heterozygote for HbS and HbC with intermediate clinical severity
- *Sickle cell β^0-thalassaemia (HbS/β^0)*: severe double heterozygote for HbS and β^0-thalassaemia with no normal β-chains produced. It is almost clinically indistinguishable from sickle cell anaemia
- *Sickle cell β^+-thalassaemia (HbS/β^+)*: in this type, a reduced amount of chains are made resulting in mild-to-moderate anaemia.

In sickle cell anaemia (HbSS) the erythrocytes are fragile, with a short life span of 17 days, compared with 120 days in a healthy individual. The erythrocytes have a characteristic crescent, or sickle shape, which blocks up the capillaries. This predisposes to clot formation in the capillaries. Diagnosis is by Hb electrophoresis, and identification of the malformed sickle-shaped cells on a blood film. A bone marrow biopsy may also be required. Treatment outside of pregnancy includes the administration of 1 mg/day oral folic acid tablets, prophylactic penicillin, thromboprophylaxis, iron chelation agents and exchange blood transfusion.

A sickle cell crisis arises when the sickle cells form clots in the capillaries resulting in deoxygenation and tissue death as a result of infarction. The crisis presents acutely with severe pain, breathlessness, pallor, fever, joint swelling and pain, and general weakness (Addo et al. 2013). The crisis can be triggered, or exacerbated, by infection, cold temperature, dehydration, stress and exercise. Other complications are chronic anaemia, bone marrow suppression, thromboembolic disease, cardiac failure due to chronic hypoxaemia and aplastic anaemia, as well as sudden death (Addo et al. 2013).

Pre-conception care is important to optimize the health of the woman, during which time the folic acid should be increased to 5 mg/day and iron chelation discontinued 3–6 months prior to conception due to possible teratogenicity (Addo et al. 2013). If the woman has pulmonary hypertension, pregnancy is contraindicated due to the 30–40% maternal mortality (Rogers et al. 2019).

In pregnancy the woman's care should be shared between the obstetric and haematology team, with appointments being made for every 2–4 weeks to assess maternal and fetal wellbeing. The woman presenting with sickle cell anaemia is at risk of experiencing a sickle cell crisis secondary to infection, pre-eclampsia, miscarriage, IUGR, stillbirth and possible maternal death. Investigations include FBC, blood group and antibody screen, reticulocyte count, serum ferritin levels, HIV and hepatitis screening (because of history of blood transfusions) renal and liver function tests. Folic acid should be increased to 5 mg/day if not done pre-conception, and iron supplements only given if indicated by serum ferritin results. Antibiotic therapy may need to be continued and aspirin prophylaxis should be considered in women with SCD without contraindications (Rogers et al. 2019).

During the antenatal booking history, the midwife should review current medications and vaccination history (confirming that hydroxycarbamide, ACE inhibitors and iron chelating have been stopped prior to pregnancy), a surgical history, highlighting joint surgery, splenectomy or cholecystectomy (it is important to assess hip mobility in women, in order to plan

and discuss positions in labour). Sickling crisis type and frequency, and details of how this is self-managed should be discussed as well as details of transfusion history and any alloimmunization (Rogers et al. 2019). A VTE assessment should be performed at 'booking' due to associated risk of thrombosis and thromboprophylaxis considered (RCOG 2015a). All women with SCD should be commenced on LMWH if admitted to hospital, unless contraindicated. Vitamin D supplementation should be advised (10 µg daily) and increased if deficiency is present. Advice to attend for routine whooping cough and flu vaccinations at 28 weeks' gestation should be given. Blood pressure should be monitored at every visit and a baseline oxygen saturation recorded and, if low, investigated with an echocardiogram. Monthly screening for asymptomatic bacteriuria should be performed. In the third trimester, serial growth scans and Doppler blood flow assessment should be undertaken (RCOG 2011c; Rogers et al. 2019).

Acute chest syndrome (ACS) has been reported to occur in 7–20% of pregnancies complicated by SCD. It is a potentially life-threatening complication, characterized by fever, audible lung crackles and respiratory symptoms, accompanied by a new infiltrate on chest X-ray. ACS may mimic pneumonia or pulmonary embolism. If ACS is suspected, close monitoring should be undertaken. Treatment includes antibiotics, oxygen, hydration and transfusion. Urgent exchange transfusion may be required, however in milder cases top-up transfusion may suffice.

In labour an epidural is recommended for pain relief as opiates should be avoided. Blood should be taken for FBC, group and save. Graduated compression stockings are used to reduce the risk of VTE and the woman should be kept warm and hydrated to prevent any sickle cell crisis from occurring. Oxygen therapy might be required to maintain adequate oxygenation and improve cardiac function. Prophylactic antibiotics may be considered to reduce infection. A prolonged labour should be avoided and active management or caesarean section may be advised depending on the woman's health (RCOG 2011c; Addo et al. 2013). Where there is IUGR, continuous fetal monitoring would also be recommended.

During the postnatal period, the midwife should be vigilant in her observations as the woman is at increased risk of sickle cell crisis, thromboembolism and postpartum haemorrhage (Oteng-Ntim et al. 2015). Prophylactic antibiotics and thromboprophylaxis should continue and early mobilization is encouraged. Four-hourly observations should be undertaken, including respiration rate. Breastfeeding can be encouraged but avoidance of hydroxycarbamide is necessary as this passes into breastmilk.

The woman should be advised about subsequent pregnancies and the risk they carry in increasing the frequency of crises. It is therefore important that the woman uses appropriate contraception in order to maximize her health, as intrauterine contraceptive devices (IUCDs) are relatively contraindicated due to the risk of infection. Neonatal screening of babies must be undertaken by obtaining a capillary or venous sample of blood at birth. Those with a positive result require a follow-up appointment and electrophoresis at 6 weeks, including prophylactic antibiotic cover from 3 months of age (Addo et al. 2013).

In sickle cell trait (HbAS) the individual is usually asymptomatic. Although the sickle screening test is positive, the blood appears normal. In pregnancy the woman may present with mild anaemia and so 5 mg/day folic acid is recommended to improve erythropoiesis. Thromboprophylaxis is usually started as there is an increased risk of thromboembolism (Oteng-Ntim et al. 2015).

INFECTION/SEPSIS

Genital Tract Sepsis

Globally, genital tract sepsis remains a cause of maternal morbidity and mortality and accounted for 11 deaths in the most recent MBRRACE – UK report (Knight 2018).

Genital tract sepsis arises from polymicrobial infections, usually from streptococcal bacteria, which can lead to overwhelming septicaemia that can affect not only the wellbeing of the pregnant woman but also the fetus (Wylie and Bryce 2016). Signs and symptoms include pyrexia, swinging pyrexia and hypothermia, abdominal pain, diarrhoea, vomiting, tachycardia and tachypnoea. Midwives should ensure all childbearing women are advised of the possible signs and symptoms of infection at all stages and be encouraged to seek advice promptly, to pay attention to effective hygiene and be aware of the risk from others, particularly anyone who has a bacterial throat infection.

Bacterial Vaginosis

It is estimated that between 10% and 30% of women will experience bacterial vaginosis (BV) during their pregnancy, which is a common cause of abnormal discharge due to an imbalance of normal bacteria that inhabit the vagina. Typical symptoms are an offensive, fishy-smelling discharge. Although BV may regress spontaneously but, even if treated with topical or oral metronidazole or clindamycin, it may recur. While there is evidence that links BV with preterm labour, late miscarriage and preterm prelabour rupture of membranes (PPROM), treatment studies have yielded inconsistent results. Consequently, current guidelines only recommend screening pregnant women identified as high risk of preterm birth (Bothamley and Boyle 2015).

Candida Albicans

Candida albicans is a yeast that causes itching, soreness and swelling of the genital area, producing a creamy-white vaginal discharge. *Candida albicans* is not a sexually transmitted infection (STI) as it commonly occurs during pregnancy, following antibiotic therapy and in individuals who have diabetes or a lowered immune system. It is easily diagnosed by a high vaginal swab (HVS) and treatment in pregnancy is via topical cream and/or vaginal pessaries, rather than via the oral route. Candida does not affect fertility or pregnancy outcome, but the baby may develop oral or genital thrush. This in turn may affect breastfeeding, should candida be transferred to the breast while feeding (Bothamley and Boyle 2015).

Chlamydia Trachomatis

Chlamydia is the most commonly diagnosed STI, especially in under 25-year-olds, and is caused by the bacterium *Chlamydia trachomatis*. Between 70% and 80% of women affected by chlamydia are asymptomatic. Signs and symptoms usually occur from 1 to 3 weeks following infection and include dysuria, vaginal discharge, lower abdominal pain, postcoital and intermenstrual bleeding, anal discharge, conjunctivitis, eye infections and sore throats, following anal or oral sexual practices. If left untreated, chlamydial infection can cause pelvic inflammatory disease (PID), which increases infertility and the risk of miscarriage and ectopic pregnancy. Chlamydia has also been associated with prematurity and stillbirth (Adachi et al. 2016).

Methods of testing are varied and can include urine testing, low vaginal swab (self-testing kits) and cervical swab. In the UK, the NHS National Chlamydia Screening Programme (PHE 2014) recommends annual screening for under 25-year-olds if sexually active. Chlamydia can be transmitted to the neonate during vaginal birth and can result in neonatal eye infections and pneumonia. Treatment entails antibiotics such as azithromycin.

Cytomegalovirus

Cytomegalovirus (CMV) is a common viral infection from the *Herpes* family, contacted sexually or through contact with young children. The virus may lie dormant and recur at a later time. It is estimated that 50% of the adult population has had the infection at some point in their lives. The virus causes a mild flu-like illness and pregnant women have an increased susceptibility to infection during pregnancy, however, primary infection in pregnancy is low, at around 1%. There is a 40% chance of transmission to the fetus causing congenital malformations such as hearing loss, learning difficulties and cerebral palsy (Fowler and Boppanna 2018). Around 5–10% of infected babies are symptomatic at birth and consequently their prognosis is poor. Furthermore, the risk relative to gestation is unclear. Although antiviral drugs have been used to treat CMV, there is currently no screening programme and CMV vaccine is currently unavailable. The midwife should highlight to pregnant women the need to undertake simple hygiene measures and handwashing frequently when caring for young children (Fowler and Boppanna 2018).

Gonorrhoea

Gonorrhoea is a common STI globally, affecting the genital tract (especially the cervix) and rectum. It is transmitted by sexual activity with an infected individual and is caused by the bacterium *Neisseria gonorrhoeae*. Although most individuals are often asymptomatic, signs and symptoms may occur 2–10 days after initial contact (Bothamley and Boyle 2015), such symptoms include painful micturition, yellow/bloodstained vaginal discharge and postcoital bleeding.

If untreated, in women it can cause pelvic inflammatory disease (PID), giving rise to abdominal cramps, fever and intermenstrual bleeding, with an increased risk of ectopic pregnancy. In pregnancy, risks include (PPROM), rupture membranes, chorioamnionitis and postnatal sepsis. Individuals are also at a greater risk of acquiring HIV.

Testing for gonorrhoea is via urine and cervical swabs. More effective screening programmes detect the genes of the bacteria, rather than try to culture the bacteria. Treatment is with antibiotics, but drug resistance

can be problematic. Gonorrhoea can be transmitted to the neonate during vaginal birth and can result in severe eye infections – ophthalmia neonatorum, which presents within 8 h of birth and if not treated effectively, can lead to blindness.

Hepatitis A, B and C

Hepatitis comprises a group of blood-borne viruses that cause hepatocellular inflammation and necrosis. They are found in bodily fluids, e.g. blood, saliva and semen, and are often transmitted via sexual activity, by sharing injecting equipment and via the placenta to the fetus during pregnancy. Vaccinations for hepatitis A and B are available. Hepatitis B and C can lead to liver failure and death and are therefore notifiable diseases in some countries including the UK.

Pregnant women are offered routine screening for hepatitis B during early pregnancy and those at risk, e.g. sex workers, can be tested for hepatitis C. Hepatitis B immunization is safe to give in pregnancy for any woman at risk. Any woman found to have hepatitis B virus (HBV) should have further tests to determine whether she is acutely or chronically infected; the presence of the e-antigen (HBeAg) denotes high infectivity, while the presence of antibodies (antiHBe) suggest a lower infectivity. During pregnancy, women are counselled as to how they can reduce transmission and infants should be given hepatitis B immunization within 24 h of birth and immunoglobulin with their mother's consent, which can reduce vertical transmission by 95% (Watkins et al. 2013). Babies will then receive a further 5 doses of Hep B immunization. Hep B immunization is now part of routine infant immunization schedule (NHS 2018b). Breastfeeding is not contraindicated, although the presence of cracked nipples is a significant transmission risk.

Clinical care for women with Hepatitis C disease has advanced considerably due to an enhanced understanding of the pathophysiology of the disease, and because of developments in diagnostic procedures and improvements in therapy and prevention. However, the difficulty remains that many people do not recognize that they are infected with Hepatitis C (European Association for Study of the Liver, EASL 2018).

Human Immunodeficiency Virus and Acquired Immune Deficiency Syndrome

The human immunodeficiency virus (HIV) is a *retrovirus* that weakens an individual's immune system by invading the T4-helper cells making it difficult to mount an immune response to infection. There are two types of HIV, which belong to the lentivirus subfamily of retroviruses that cause acquired immunodeficiency syndrome (AIDS). HIV-1 is the cause of the world pandemic of acquired immune deficiency syndrome (AIDS), whereas HIV-2 is largely confined to West Africa. HIV is transmitted through unprotected sexual activity with an infected person, contact with infected bodily fluids, e.g. blood, or perinatally via mother-to-fetus-transmission. At 2–6 weeks after exposure to HIV, 50–70% develop a transient nonspecific illness (primary infection or seroconversion illness) with flu-like symptoms, e.g. pyrexia, rash and sore throat. This coincides with the development of serum antibodies to the core and surface proteins of the virus. The illness begins abruptly and usually lasts for 1–2 weeks but may be more protracted.

Diagnosis is through an HIV test, where blood is examined for the presence of antibodies and/or antigens; this is known as the *combined test*. Many woman are now aware of HIV status when approaching antenatal services, though HIV testing in pregnancy continues to be part of antenatal screening (Hamlyn and Barber 2018). The aim of pregnancy care to HIV-positive women is to suppress the HIV viral load, as transmission to the baby can occur in the antenatal, intrapartum or postnatal period. The prevalence of HIV in pregnancy is around 1 in 1000 maternities (Raffe et al. 2017).

For women who are known to be HIV-positive as well as usual antenatal care and bloods at booking, a CD4 count and viral load should be requested and repeated at 36 weeks. Care should be taken to avoid invasive prenatal testing. The success of antiviral retroviral therapy (ART) has meant that for many women, vaginal birth is possible, however if viral load is >400, a planned caesarean section should be recommended (Hamlyn and Barber 2018). Infants require post-exposure zidovudine (AZT) for 4 weeks and to have routine immunizations. While advice to formula-feed is still recommended, for those women who are virally suppressed, it opens up a choice to breastfeed (Raffe et al. 2017).

Infants are followed up with an HIV test at 48 h, 6 weeks and 12 weeks, then again at 18–24 months. For women who have HIV diagnosed in pregnancy, referral should be made for them to be seen by a genitourinary medicine specialist and have specialist HIV screening. Immediate ART should be given regardless of immune status or from at least 24 weeks' pregnancy. Local

guidelines should be followed for triple therapy and women advised to continue antivirals after pregnancy, even if the viral count is reduced. The woman recently diagnosed will have to come to terms emotionally; mental health, relationship, financial and legal issues may all be of concern (Hamlyn and Barber 2018).

Human Papillomavirus

The human papillomavirus (HPV) is attributed to causing the second most common STI in the UK. It has over 100 strains, of which strains 6 and 11 are known to cause genital warts, which are more common in teenagers and young adults. They present as small, fleshy, painless growths, single or in clusters, appearing on the vaginal and anal regions following close genital contact or sexual activity with an affected person. The warts usually appear within 2–3 months of infection, but can take up to a year to become evident.

Active treatment in pregnancy should be weekly cryotherapy and consideration of excision or deferred treatment, if there is no improvement after 4 weeks. Warts often regress spontaneously postpartum (Thwaites et al. 2016). Pregnancy may affect the size and number of warts and there is a small risk that they may affect progress in labour, as well as there being evidence of rare cases of transmissions to the baby during birth. Human papillomavirus strains 16 and 18 are associated with cervical cancer and vaccinations are available to all young women up to the age of 18 years. Emerging evidence would indicate that vaccination is reducing genital wart prevalence in young women (Thwaites et al. 2016).

Streptococcus A and B

Group A streptococcus (GAS) bacteria cause a variety of infections, such as acute pharyngitis, toxic shock syndrome, cellulitis and puerperal sepsis.

Group B streptococcus (GBS) bacteria is commonly found in the vagina and lower bowel of around 20% of healthy adult women (Russell et al. 2017). It usually causes no harm, but if a woman is colonized at the time of labour, around 36% will transmit the bacteria to their newborn child. Crucially, the majority of neonates colonized with GBS remain asymptomatic, but about 3% develop early onset infection. However, GBS infection has been known to pass across the membranes and colonize the fetus *in utero*. Affected neonates present with sepsis, pneumonia and meningitis, and may die as a result. Neurological impairment is reported in some cases who survive infection. The true burden of early onset GBS infection is likely to be higher (Seedat et al. 2019). Currently in the UK, screening is not routinely offered (RCOG 2017; Seedat et al. 2019; NICE 2008).

Women at higher risk of GBS include those in preterm labour, those with PPROM and prolonged rupture of membranes (>18 h). However, those with maternal pyrexia and a previous history of GBS would be offered antibiotics (RCOG 2017). GBS causes invasive disease in the first 6 days of life (early onset GBS infection) in around one of every 2000 live births (O'Sullivan et al. 2019). There are two types of neonatal GBS. The most common type is *early onset GBS*, which is seen in 75% of cases and occurs within the first week of life, usually presenting within 24 h of birth. The other type is *late onset GBS*, which presents in 25% of cases within the first 3 months of life. Signs and symptoms in an affected neonate may be vague and include problems maintaining their temperature, grunting, limpness, poor feeding behaviours and seizures. It is very important that midwives inform women of the signs and symptoms and promptly refer any ill baby.

Syphilis

Syphilis is an STI caused by the spirochete bacterium *Treponema pallidum*. Transmission occurs through contact with a syphilitic sore or chancre. Although the incidence of syphilis is low in the UK, worldwide the incidence in developing countries is 20%. Syphilis in pregnancy is the second leading cause of stillbirth globally and also results in prematurity, low birth weight, neonatal death and infections in newborns (WHO 2017). Most maternal syphilis infections are latent (asymptomatic), but still result in poor pregnancy outcomes in >50% of cases.

There are four stages to the progression of the infection:

- *Primary*: occurring on average 21 days after exposure, where a single painless, firm, non-itchy ulcer or chancre appears
- *Secondary*: occurs between 4 and 10 weeks after exposure, with the appearance of a non-itchy, diffuse rash with fever and sore throat evident. In the latent stage, the individual is generally asymptomatic, but still contagious to others
- *Latent*: can occur between 3 and 30 years after the initial exposure. No signs or symptoms but can be detected serologically.

- *Tertiary*: if the individual does not seek treatment, neurological symptoms such as general paresis and seizures, as well as cardiac symptoms including aneurysms will manifest.

The presence of syphilitic sores increases the transmission risk of HIV (BASHH 2015). Diagnosis is via a blood test and the treatment is penicillin. It is highly likely that transmission of syphilis will occur in pregnancy, causing preterm birth, stillbirth or perinatal death, thus screening for syphilis should be routinely offered to all pregnant women during the early antenatal period (NICE 2008). The baby may be born with *congenital syphilis*, which is asymptomatic during infancy, but later in childhood they may develop multiorgan conditions such as deafness, seizures and cataracts.

Urinary Tract Infection

Urinary tract infection (UTI) is a common problem in pregnancy if pathogenic bacteria colonize the urinary tract. The bacteria originate from the bowel and the most commonly encountered is *Escherichia coli* (*E. coli*) (Johnston et al. 2017). Such an infection may be asymptomatic or present with symptoms of *dysuria*, *frequency*, *suprapubic discomfort* and *haematuria*. If the infection is confined to the bladder it is termed *cystitis*, and in addition to these symptoms there may be *urgency* of micturition.

The infection can ascend to the kidneys and pyelonephritis develops. Acute pyelonephritis may present with nausea and vomiting, pyrexia, rigors and abdominal pain (NICE 2019b). If inadequately treated, septicaemia may result, leading to acute renal failure, multiple organ failure and death (Brunskill and Goodlife 2013).

Asymptomatic bacteriuria

Asymptomatic bacteriuria (ABU), as the name implies, is an infection without symptoms and occurs in 2–10% of pregnancies (NICE 2019b). The presence of 10^5/mL of the same bacterial species in a mid-stream specimen of urine (MSU) in the absence of symptoms confirms the diagnosis. This is of significance in pregnancy, as 25% of women will proceed to develop pyelonephritis and there is also risk of preterm labour (Johnston et al. 2017). All pregnant women should have their urine tested for nitrates (which are produced by most urinary pathogens) at each antenatal visit. A mid-stream specimen of urine (MSU) should be taken early in pregnancy (NICE 2019b), and repeated if there are symptoms of a UTI. Treatment is with antibiotics according to the culture and sensitivity from the MSU results, and the MSU should be repeated following treatment. If the causative organism is group B streptococcus, 7 days antibiotics should be prescribed; the woman may require antibiotics in labour (Johnston et al. 2017). The midwife should encourage the woman to drink at least 2 litres of fluid per day,

comply with antibiotic therapy and report if symptoms do not recede. She should also give advice on personal hygiene, especially following micturition, and recommend cranberry juice, which may reduce infection and its symptoms (Brunskill and Goodlife 2013). A MSU should be taken following treatment. Recurrent urinary tract infections require referral for further investigations (NICE 2019b).

REFLECTIVE ACTIVITY FOR SELF-ASSESSMENT

1. How does knowledge of maternal adaptation/physiological changes in pregnancy, assist the midwife in her understanding of the management of medical conditions explored within this chapter?
2. What are the responsibilities of a midwife when supporting a woman with a medical condition in

the postnatal period who wants to breastfeed her baby?
3. How can the midwife effectively meet the needs of women with obesity during the childbearing period?

REFERENCES

Adachi, K., Nielsen-Saines, K., & Klausner, J. D. (2016). Chlamydia trachomatis infection in pregnancy: The global challenge of preventing adverse pregnancy and infant outcomes in Sub-Saharan Africa and Asia. *BioMed Research International*, *2016*, 9315757.

Addo, A., Oppenheimer, C., & Robson, S. E. (2013). Haematological disorders. In S. E. Robson, & J. Waugh (Eds.), *Medical disorders in pregnancy: A manual for midwives* (2nd ed.) (pp. 255–278). Oxford: Wiley-Blackwell.

Adlam, D., Alfonso, F., Maas, A., et al. (2018). European Society of Cardiology, Acute Cardiovascular Care Association, SCAD study group: A position paper on spontaneous coronary artery dissection. *European Heart Journal*, *39*(36), 3358–3368.

Ali, S. A., & Dornhorst, A. (2018). Diabetes in pregnancy. In D. K. Edmonds, C. Rees, & T. Bourne (Eds.), *Dewhurst's textbook of obstetrics and gynaecology* (9th ed.) (pp. 97–115). Oxford: Wiley-Blackwell.

Alkema, L., Chou, D., Hogan, D., et al. (2016). United Nations maternal mortality estimation inter-Agency group collaborators and technical advisory group. Global, regional, and national levels and trends in maternal mortality between 1990 and 2015, with scenario-based projections to 2030: A systematic analysis by the UN maternal mortality estimation inter-Agency group. *Lancet*, *387*, 462–474.

Amir, L., & Donath, S. (2007). A systematic review of maternal obesity and breastfeeding intention, initiation and duration. *BMC Pregnancy and Childbirth*, *7*, 9.

APEC. (2019). *Action on pre-eclampsia parliamentary briefing for Westminster hall debate on pre-eclampsia 9th May 2019.*

Available at: https://action-on-pre-eclampsia.org.uk/wp-content/uploads/2019/05/APEC-Parliamentary-brief-final.pdf. (Accessed 5th Feb 2020).

Asthma, U. K. (2018). *Annual asthma survey*. Available at: www.asthma.org.uk.

Avery, A., Allan, J., Lavin, J., et al. (2010). Supporting postnatal women to lose weight. *Journal of Human Nutrition and Dietetics*, *23*(4), 439.

Bagot, C. N., & Arya, R. (2008). Virchow and his triad: A question of attribution. *British Journal of Haematology*, *143*(2), 180–190.

Bah, A., Pasricha, S. R., Jallow, M. W., et al. (2017). Serum hepcidin concentrations decline during pregnancy and may identify iron deficiency: Analysis of A Longitudinal Pregnancy Cohort in the Gambia. *Journal of Nutrition*, *147*(6), 1131–1137.

Baker, J., Gamborg, M., Heitmann, B., et al. (2008). Breastfeeding reduces postpartum weight retention. *American Journal of Clinical Nutrition*, *88*, 1543–1551.

BASHH (British Association for Sexual Health and HIV). (2015). *UK National guidelines on Management of syphilis*. Available at: www.bashhguidelines.org/current-guidelines/genital-ulceration/syphilis-2015/.

Battino, D., Tomson, T., Bonizzoni, E., et al. (2013). EURAP study group. Seizure control and treatment changes in pregnancy: Observations from the EURAP epilepsy pregnancy Registry. *Epilepsia*, *54*, 1621–1627.

Bellamy, L., Casas, J. P., Hingorani, A. D., et al. (2009). Type 2 diabetes mellitus after gestational diabetes: A systematic review and meta-analysis. *Lancet*, *373*(9677), 1773–1779.

Bertz, F., Winkvist, A., & Brekke, H. (2015). Sustainable weight loss among overweight and obese lactating women is achieved with an energy-reduced diet in line with dietary recommendations: Results from the Leva Randomised Controlled Trial. *Journal of the Academy of Nutrition and Dietetics, 115*(1), 78–86.

Bircher, C. W., Farrakh, S., & Gada, R. (2016). Supraventricular tachycardia presenting in labour: A case report achieving vaginal birth and review of the Literature. *Obstetric Medicine, 9*(2), 96–97.

Bogaerts, A. (2014). Obesity and pregnancy, an epidemiological and intervention study from a psychosocial perspective. *Facts, Views & Vision in ObGyn, 6*(2), 81–95.

Bothamley, J., & Boyle, M. (2015). *Infections affecting pregnancy and childbirth.* London: Radcliffe Publishing.

Brennand, J., Northridge, R., Scott, H., et al. (2016). *Addressing the heart of the issue: Good clinical practice in the shared obstetric and Cardiology care of women of childbearing age.* Glasgow: Royal College of Physicians and Surgeons of Glasgow.

Brunskill, N. J., & Goodlife, A. (2013). Renal disorders. In S. E. Robson, & J. Waugh (Eds.), *Medical disorders in pregnancy: A manual for midwives* (2nd ed.) (pp. 91–104). Oxford: Wiley-Blackwell.

BTS/SIGN (British Thoracic Society/Scottish Intercollegiate Guidelines Network). (2011, 2016). British guideline on the management of asthma. *BTS/SIGN* .

Bunch, K., & Knight, M. (2018). on behalf of the MBRRACE-UK chapter-writing group. Maternal mortality in the UK 2014–16: Surveillance and epidemiology. In M. K. B. Knight, D. Tuffnell, et al. (Eds.), *(2018); on behalf of MBRRACE-UK. Saving lives, improving mothers' care – lessons learned to inform maternity care from the UK and Ireland confidential enquiries into maternal deaths and morbidity 2014–16* (pp. 5–22). Oxford: National Perinatal Epidemiology Unit, University of Oxford.

Burrow, G. N., Duffey, T. P., & Copel, J. A. (2004). Hypertensive disorders in pregnancy. In *Medical complications during pregnancy* (6th ed.) (pp. 43–67). London: Elsevier.

Burton, K. R. (2018). Risk of early-onset breast cancer among women exposed to thoracic computed tomography in pregnancy or early postpartum. *Journal of Thrombosis and Haemostasis, 16*(5), 876–885.

Burton, G., Redman, C., Roberts, J., Moffett, A. (2019). Pre-eclampsia: pathophysiology and clinical implications. *British Medical Journal, 16*(5), 876–885.

Butland, B., Jebb, S., Kopelman, P., et al. (2007). *Foresight; tackling obesities; future choices project report.* London: Government Office for Science. Available at: www.foresight.gov.uk/obesity.

Canobbio, M., Warnes, C., Aboulhosn, J., et al. (2017). Management of pregnancy in patients with complex congenital heart disease: A scientific statement for healthcare professionals from the. *American Heart Association, 135*(8), e50–e87.

Catalano, P., & Shankar, K. (2017). Obesity and pregnancy: Mechanisms of short term and long term adverse consequences for mother and child. *British Medical Journal, 356*, j1.

Cauldwell, M., Cox, M., Gatzoulis, M., et al. (2017a). The management of labour in women with cardiac disease: Need for more evidence? *British Journal of Obstetrics and Gynaecology, 124*(9), 1307–1309.

Cauldwell, M., Steer, P. J., Swan, L., et al. (2017b). The management of the third stage of labour in women with heart disease. *Heart, 103*(12), 945–951.

Chan, R., & Woo, J. (2010). Prevention of overweight and obesity: How effective is the current public health approach. *International Journal of Environmental Research and Public Health, 7*, 765–783.

Copple, M., & Coser, P. (2013). Stop the clot. *Midwives, 4*, 48–49.

Daru, J., Zamora, J., Fernández-Félix, B. M., et al. (2018). Risk of maternal mortality in women with severe anaemia during pregnancy and postpartum: A multilevel analysis. *Lancet Global Health, 6*(5), e548–e554.

Davanzo, R., Dal Bo, S., Bua, J., et al. (2013). Antiepileptic drugs and breastfeeding. *Italian Journal of Paediatrics, 39*, 50.

Davis, S., & Pavord, S. (2018). Haematological problems in pregnancy. In D. K. Edmonds, C. Lees, & T. Bourne (Eds.), *Dewhurst's Textbook of Obstetrics and Gynaecology* (9th ed.) (pp. 147–160). Oxford: Wiley-Blackwell.

Dawson, A. J., Krastev, Y., Parsonage, W. A., et al. (2018). Experiences of women with cardiac disease in pregnancy: A systematic review and metasynthesis. *BMJ Open, 8*, e022755.

De Rycke, M., Van de Velde, H., Sermon, K., et al. (2001). Preimplantation genetic diagnosis for sickle-cell anemia and for beta-thalassemia. *Prenatal Diagnosis, 21*, 214–222.

Denison, F. C., Aedla, N. R., Keag, O., & on behalf of the Royal College of Obstetricians and Gynaecologists., et al. (2018). *Care of women with obesity in pregnancy. Greentop Guideline No 72.* London: RCOG.

Department of Health), D. H. ((2016). *Physical activity in pregnancy infographic: Guidance.* Available at: https://assets.publishing.service.gov.uk/government/uploads/system/uploads/attachment_data/file/622623/Physical_activity_pregnancy_infographic_guidance.pdf.

Doughty, R., & Waugh, J. (2013). Metabolic disorders. In S. E. Robson, & J. Waugh (Eds.), *Medical disorders in pregnancy: A manual for midwives* (2nd ed.) (pp. 241–254). Oxford: Wiley-Blackwell.

Duhig, K., Vandermolen, B., & Shennan, A. (2018). Recent advances in the diagnosis and management of pre-eclampsia. *F1000Res, 7*, 242.

D'Souza, R., Ostro, J., Shah, P., et al. (2017). Anticoagulation for pregnant women with mechanical heart valves: A systematic review and meta-analysis. *European Heart Journal, 38*(19), 1509–1516.

EASL (European Association for Study of the Liver). (2018). EASL recommendations on the treatment Hepatitis C. *Journal of Hepatology*, *69*(2), 461–511.

Edey, S., Moran, N., & Nashef, L. (2014). SUDEP and epilepsy-related mortality in pregnancy. *Epilepsia*, *55*, e72–e74.

Eleftheriades, M., Tsapakis, E., Sotiriadis, A., et al. (2012). Detection of congenital heart defects throughout pregnancy: Impact of first trimester ultrasound screening for cardiac abnormalities. *Journal of Maternal-Fetal and Neonatal Medicine*, *25*(12), 2546–2550.

Elkayam, U., Jalnapurkar, S., Barakkat, M. N., et al. (2014). Pregnancy-associated acute myocardial infarction: A review of contemporary experience in 150 cases between 2006 and 2011. *Circulation*, *129*, 1695–1702.

Elliott, D., & Pavord, S. (2013). Thrombo-embolic disorders. In S. E. Robson, & J. Waugh (Eds.), *Medical disorders in pregnancy: A manual for midwives* (2nd ed.) (pp. 279–297). Oxford: Wiley-Blackwell.

Fiest, K., Sauro, K., Weibe, S., et al. (2017). Prevalence and incidence of epilepsy: A systematic review and meta-analysis of international studies. *Neurology*, *88*(3), 296–303.

Fowler, K., & Boppanna, S. (2018). Congenital cytomegalovirus infection. *Seminars in Perinatology*, *42*, 149–154.

Fox, N., Saltzman, D., Roman, A., et al. (2011). Intravaginal misoprostol versus Foley catheter for labour induction: A meta–analysis. *British Journal of Obstetrics and Gynaecology*, *118*, 647–654.

Gardner, B., Wardle, J., Poston, L., et al. (2011). Changing diet and physical activity to reduce gestational weight gain: A meta-analysis. *International Association for the Study of Obesity*, *12*, e602–e620.

Gard, M., & Wright, J. (2005). *The obesity epidemic: Science, morality and ideology*. Oxford: Routledge Press.

Girling, J. (2006). Thyroid disorders in pregnancy. *Current Obstetrics and Gynaecology*, *16*, 47–53.

Gluckman, P., & Hanson, M. (2012). *Fat, fate and disease*. Oxford: Oxford University Press.

Goodacre, S., Nelson–Piercy, C., & Hunt, B. (2015). When should we use diagnostic imaging to investigate for pulmonary embolism in pregnant and postpartum women? *Emergency Medical Journal*, *32*, 78–82.

Govind, A., & De Martino, M. (2018). Re: A review of contraceptive methods for women with cardiac disease. *The Obstetrician and Gynaecologist*, *20*(4), 273–274.

Gregory, R., & Todd, D. (2013). Endocrine disorders. In S. E. Robson, & J. Waugh (Eds.), *Medical disorders in pregnancy: A manual for midwives* (2nd ed.) (pp. 105–124). Oxford: Wiley-Blackwell.

Haby, K., Glantz, A., Hanas, R., et al. (2015). Mighty mums – an antenatal health care intervention can reduce gestational weight gain in women with obesity. *Midwifery*, *31*, 685–692.

Hamlyn, E., & Barber, T. J. (2018). Management of HIV in pregnancy. *Obstetrics, Gynaecology and Reproductive Medicine*, *28*(7), 203–207.

Haugen, M., Brantsaeter, A., Winkvist, A., et al. (2014). Associations of pre-pregnancy body mass index and gestational weight gain with pregnancy outcome and postpartum weight retention: A prospective observational cohort study. *BMC Pregnancy and Birth 14, 201*. www.ncbi.nlm.nih.gov/pubmed/24917037.

Hayes, S. N., Kim, E. S. H., Saw, J., et al. (2018). Spontaneous coronary artery dissection: Current state of the science: A scientific statement from the American Heart Association. *Circulation*, *137*, e523– e557.

Hoffbrand, A. V., & Moss, P. A. H. (2016). *Hoffbrand's essential haematology* (7th ed.). Chichester: Wiley-Blackwell.

Holmes, S., & Scullion, J. (2011). Better asthma control could avoid majority of hospital admissions. *Guidelines in Practice*, *14*(7), 1–8.

Hughes, C., Spence, D., Holmes, V. A., et al. (2012). Pre-conception care for women with diabetes: The midwife's role. *British Journal of Midwifery*, *18*(3), 144–149.

Hull, J., & Rucklidge, M. (2009). Management of severe pre-eclampsia and eclampsia. *Update in Anaesthesia*, *25*(2), 49–54.

Hutcheon, J. A., Lisonkova, S., & Joseph, K. (2011). Epidemiology of pre-eclampsia and the other hypertensive disorders of pregnancy. *Best Practice & Research Clinical Obstetrics & Gynaecology*, *25*, 391–403.

Jakes, A. D., Coad, F., & Nelson-Piercy, C. (2018). A review of contraceptive methods for women with cardiac disease. *The Obstetrician and Gynaecologist*, *20*, 21.

James, D. K., Steer, P. J., Weiner, C. P., et al. (Eds.). (2017). *High risk pregnancy management options* (5th ed.) Cambridge: Cambridge University Press.

Jana, N., Barik, S., & Arora, N. (2018). Re: Clinical practice patterns on the use of magnesium sulphate for treatment of pre–eclampsia and eclampsia: A multi–country survey. *BJOG: An International Journal of Obstetrics and Gynaecology*, *125*(7), 909.

Jevitt, C., Hernandez, I., & Groer, M. (2007). Lactation complicated by overweight and obesity: Supporting the mother and newborn. *Journal of Midwifery & Women's Health*, *52*(6), 606–613.

JJS, W., & Smith, M. C. (2012). Hypertensive disorders. In K. Edmonds (Ed.), *Dewhurst's textbook of obstetrics and gynaecology* (8th ed.) (pp. 101–110). Oxford: Wiley-Blackwell.

Johnston, C., Johnston, M., Corke, A., et al. (2017). A likely urinary tract infection in a pregnant woman. *British Medical Journal*, *357*, j1777.

Joshi, D., James, A., Quaglia, A., et al. (2010). Liver disease in pregnancy. *Lancet*, *375*(9714), 594–605.

Kapoor, D., & Wallace, S. (2016). Cardiovascular disease in pregnancy. *Obstetrics, Gynaecology and Reproductive Medicine*, *26*(4), 114–119.

Keaver, L., & Webber, L. (2016). Future trends in morbid obesity in England, Scotland, and Wales: A modelling projection study. *The Lancet388*(2). S63.

Kelso A, Wills A, Knight M; On behalf of the MBRRACE-UK neurology chapter writing group. Lessons on epilepsy and stroke (2017). In: M Knight, M Nair, D Tuffnell et al. (Eds); On behalf of MBRRACE-UK. *Saving lives, improving mothers' care – lessons learned to inform maternity care from the UK and Ireland confidential enquiries into maternal deaths and morbidity 2013–15* (pp. 24–36). Oxford: National Perinatal Epidemiology Unit, University of Oxford.

Kerrigan, A. M., & Kingdon, C. (2010). Maternal obesity and pregnancy: A retrospective study. *Midwifery, 26*, 138–146.

Khambalia, A., Collins, C., Roberts, C., et al. (2016). Iron deficiency in early pregnancy using serum ferritin and soluble transferrin receptor concentrations are associated with pregnancy and birth outcomes. *European Journal of Clinical Nutrition, 70*, 358–363.

Khlat, M., Jusot, F., & Ville, I. (2009). Social origins, early hardship and obesity: A strong association in women, but not in men? *Social Science & Medicine, 68*, 1692–1699.

Knight, M. (2007). Eclampsia in the United Kingdom 2005. *BJOG: An International Journal of Obstetrics and Gynaecology, 114*, 1072–1078.

Knight, M., on behalf of the MBRRACE-UK. (2018). Maternal mortality in the UK 2014–16: Surveillance and epidemiology chapter-writing group. In M. Knight, K. Bunch, D. Tuffnell, et al. (Eds.), *On behalf of MBRRACE-UK. Saving lives, improving mothers' care – lessons learned to inform maternity care from the UK and Ireland confidential enquiries into maternal deaths and morbidity 2014–16*. Oxford: National Perinatal Epidemiology Unit, University of (Oxford).

Knight, M., Bunch, K., Tuffnell D., et al. (Eds.), on behalf of MBRRACE-UK. (2018). *Saving lives, improving mothers' care – lessons learned to inform maternity care from the UK and Ireland confidential enquiries into maternal deaths and morbidity 2014–16*. Oxford: National Perinatal Epidemiology Unit, University of (Oxford).

Knight, M., S. Kenyon, P. Brocklehurst J., et al. (Eds.), on behalf of MBRRACE-UK. (2014). *Saving lives, improving mothers' care – lessons learned to inform future maternity care from the UK and Ireland confidential enquiries into maternal deaths and morbidity 2009–12*. Oxford: National Perinatal Epidemiology Unit, University of (Oxford).

Knight, M. Nair, M. Tuffnell D., et al. (Eds.), on behalf of MBRRACE-UK. (2016). *Saving lives, improving mothers' care: Surveillance of maternal deaths in the UK 2012–14 and lessons learned to inform maternity care from the UK and Ireland confidential enquiries into maternal deaths and morbidity 2009–14*. Oxford: National Perinatal Epidemiology Unit, University of (Oxford).

Knight, M. Nair, M. Tuffnell D., et al. (Eds.), on behalf of MBRRACE-UK. (2016). *Saving lives, improving mothers' care: Lessons learned to inform maternity care from the UK and Ireland confidential enquiries into maternal deaths and morbidity 2013–15*. Oxford: National Perinatal Epidemiology Unit, University of (Oxford).

Knight, M., Bunch, K., Tuffnell, D. et al. (Eds.) on behalf of MBRRACE-UK. (2019). *Saving Lives, Improving Mothers' Care – Lessons learned to inform maternity care from the UK and Ireland Confidential Enquiries into Maternal Deaths and Morbidity 2015–17*. Oxford: National Perinatal Epidemiology Unit, University of Oxford.

Kongwattanakul, K., Saksiriwuttho, P., Chaiyarach, S., et al. (2018). Incidence, characteristics, maternal complications, and perinatal outcomes associated with preeclampsia with severe features and HELLP syndrome. *International Journal of Women's Health, 10*, 371–377.

Kumar, P., & Clarke, M. (2004). *Clinical medicine* (5th ed.). London: Saunders.

Laksman, Z., Harris, I., & Silversides, C. K. (2011). Cardiac arrhythmias during pregnancy: A clinical approach. *Fetal and Maternal Medicine Review, 22*, 23–143.

Lancet. (2016). *Maternal health series study group. Maternal health: An executive summary for the Lancet series*. Available at: www.thelancet.com/pb/assets/raw/Lancet/stories/series/maternal-health-2016/mathealth2016-ex-ec-summ.pdf.

Lao, T. T. (2017). Obstetric care for women with thalassemia. *Best Practice & Research Clinical Obstetrics & Gynaecology, 39*, 89–100.

Llewelyn, C. (2013). We've got it covered! Graduated compression stockings. *The Practising Midwife, 16*(5), 19–22.

Marshall, J. F., & Brydon, S. (2012). Case study 2. Obesity: Risk management issues. In M. D. Raynor, J. E. Marshall, & K. Jackson (Eds.), *Midwifery practice: Critical illness, complications and emergencies case book* (pp. 19–40). Maidenhead: Open University Press.

McAuliffe, F., Burns-Kent, F., Frost, D., et al. (2013). Neurological disorders. In S. E. Robson, & J. Waugh (Eds.), *Medical disorders in pregnancy: A manual for midwives* (2nd ed.) (pp. 125–152). Oxford: Wiley-Blackwell.

McLean, M., Bu'Lock, F. A., & Robson, S. E. (2013). Heart disease. In S. E. Robson, & J. Waugh (Eds.), *Medical disorders in pregnancy: A manual for midwives* (2nd ed.) (pp. 43–74). Oxford: Wiley-Blackwell.

Mehita, N., Chen, K., Hardy, E., et al. (2015). Respiratory disease in pregnancy. *Best Practice and Research in Obstetrics and Gynaecology, 29*, 598–611.

Mihu, D., Costin, N., Mihu, C., et al. (2007). HELLP syndrome – a multisystemic disorder. *Journal of Gastrointestinal and KLiver Diseases, 16*(4), 419–424.

Miller, E., & Mitchell, A. (2006). Metabolic syndrome: Screening, diagnosis and management. *Journal of Midwifery & Women's Health, 51*(3), 141–151.

Modder, J., & Fitzsimons, K. S. (2010). *Management of women with obesity in pregnancy*. Joint Guideline. London: CMACE/RCOG.

Muktabhant, B., Lawrie, T., Lumbiganon, P., et al. (2015). Diet or exercise, or both, for preventing excessive weight gain in pregnancy (review). *Cochrane Database of Systematic Reviews* (6), CD007145.

Mundle, S. (2017). *What do practice nurses need to know about asthma in pregnancy? Nursing in practice.* Available at: www.nursinginpractice.com/article/what-do-practice-nurses-need-know-about-asthma-pregnancy.

Murphy, V. E., Jensen, M. E., Mattes, J., et al. (2016). The breathing for life trial: A randomised controlled trial of fractional exhaled nitric oxide (FENO)-based management of asthma during pregnancy and its impact on perinatal outcomes and infant and childhood respiratory health. *BMC Pregnancy and Childbirth, 16,* 111.

Nash, M. (2012a). Weighty matters: Negotiating 'fatness' and 'in-between-ness' in early pregnancy. *Feminism & Psychology, 22*(3), 307–323.

Nash, M. (2012b). Working out for two: Performance of fitness and feminity in Australian prenatal aerobics classes. *Gender, Place & Culture, 19*(4), 449–471.

Nehring, I., Schmoll, S., Beyerlein, A., et al. (2011). Gestational weight gain and long-term postpartum weight retention: A meta-analysis. *American Journal of Clinical Nutrition, 94,* 1225–1231.

NHS Digital. (2018) Statistics on obesity, physical activity and diet – England, 2018 [PAS]. Available at: https://files.digital.nhs.uk/publication/0/0/obes-phys-acti-diet-eng-2018-rep.pdf.

NHS (National Health Service). (2018a). *Pregnant women urged to have flu vaccine.* Available at: www.england.nhs.uk/south-east/2018/11/15/pregnant-women-urged-to-have-flu-vaccine/.

NHS (National Health Service). (2018b). *Infant immunisation schedule 2018/19.* Available at: www.nhs.uk/conditions/vaccinations/childhood-vaccines-timeline/.

NICE (National Institute for Health and Care Excellence). (2012). *The epilepsies: The diagnosis and management of the epilepsies in adults and children in primary and secondary care* (Vol. 137). London: CG (NICE).

NICE (National Institute for Health and Care Excellence). (2014). *Intrapartum care: Care of healthy women and their babies during childbirth* (Vol. 190). London: CG (NICE).

NICE (National Institute for Health and Care Excellence). (2015). *Diabetes in pregnancy: Management from pre-conception to the Postnatal Period* (Vol. 3). London: NG (NICE).

NICE (National Institute for Health and Care Excellence). (2017). *Asthma: Diagnosis, monitoring and asthma: Diagnosis, monitoring and chronic asthma management chronic asthma management* (Vol. 80). London: NG (NICE).

NICE (National Institute for Health and Care Excellence). (2019a). *Hypertension: Clinical management of primary hypertension in adults* (Vol. 136). London: NG (NICE).

NICE (National Institute for Health and Care Excellence). (2019b). Urinary tract infection (lower) women clinical knowledge summaries. Available at: https://cks.nice.org.uk/urinary-tract-infection-lower-women#!scenario:4.

NICE (National Institute for Health and Care Excellence). (2019c). *Hypertension in Pregnancy: Diagnosis and Management* (NG133). London: NG (NICE).

NICE (National Institute for Health and Clinical Excellence). (2008) (updated 2019). *Antenatal care: Routine care for the healthy pregnant woman.* CG 62. London: NICE.

NICE (National Institute for Health and Clinical Excellence). (2010b) (updated 2018). *Weight management before, during and after pregnancy.* PH 27. London: NICE.

NMPA (National Maternity and Perinatal Audit Project Team). (2017). *National maternity and perinatal Audit: Clinical report 2017.* London: RCOG.

Nuttall, F. (2015). Obesity. BMI and health: A critical review. *Nutrition Research, 50*(3), 117–128.

Nyman, V. M. K., Prebensen, A. K., & Flensner, G. E. M. (2010). Obese women's experiences of encounters with midwives and physicians during pregnancy and childbirth. *Midwifery, 26*(4), 424–429.

Oteng-Ntim, E., Ayensah, B., Knight, M., et al. (2015). Pregnancy outcome in patients with Sickle cell disease in the UK – a national cohort study comparing sickle cell anaemia (HbSS) with HbSC disease. *British Journal of Haematology, 169,* 129–137.

O'Connor, M., Kurinczuk, J. J., & Knight, M. (2018). *UKOSS Annual Report 2018.* Oxford: NPEU.

O'Sullivan, C. P., Lamagni, T., Patel, D., et al. (2019). Group B streptococcal disease in UK and Irish infants younger than 90 days, 2014–2015: A prospective surveillance study. *The Lancet Infectious Diseases, 19,* 83–90.

Pallister, C., Allan, J., Lavin, J., et al. (2010). Changes in well-being, diet and activity habits of pregnant women attending a commercial weight management organization. *Journal of Human Nutrition and Dietetics, 23*(4), 459.

Pavord, S., Myers, B., Robinson, S., et al. (2012). UK guidelines on the management of iron deficiency in pregnancy. *British Journal of Haematology, 156*(5), 588–600.

Pawelec, M., Palczynski, B., & Karmowski (2012). HELLP syndrome in pregnancies below 26th week. *Journal of Maternal-Fetal and Neonatal Medicine, 25*(5), 467–470.

Petrakos, G., Andriopoulos, P., & Tsironi, M. (2016). Pregnancy in women with thalassemia: Challenges and solutions. *International Journal of Women's Health, 8,* 441–451.

PHE (Public Health England). (2016). *Making every contact count. Consensus Statement.* Available at: https://assets.publishing.service.gov.uk/government/uploads/system/uploads/attachment_data/file/515949/Making_Every_Contact_Count_Consensus_Statement.pdf.

PHE (Public Health England). (2018). *Guidance in antenatal screening.* Available at: www.gov.uk/government/publications/handbook-for-sickle-cell-and-thalassaemia-screening/antenatal-screening.

PHE (Public Health England). (2014) (updated 2018). *National chlamydia screening programme standards* (7th ed.). Available at: https://assets.publishing.service.gov.uk/government/uploads/system/uploads/attachment_data/file/759846/NCSP_Standards_7th_edition_update_November_2018.pdf.

Poston, L., Caleyachetty, R., Cnattingius, S., et al. (2016). Preconceptual and maternal obesity: Epidemiology and health consequences. *Lancet Diabetes and Endocrinology, 4*(12), 1025–1036.

PRECOG. (2004). *Precog: The pre-eclampsia community guideline.* Available at: https://action-on-pre-eclampsia.org.uk/wp-content/uploads/2012/07/PRECOG Community-Guideline.pdf.

Raffe, S., Savage, C., Perry, L., et al. (2017). The management of HIV in pregnancy: A 10-year experience. *European Journal of Obstetrics & Gynecology and Reproductive Biology, 210*, 310–313.

RCOG (Royal College of Obstetricians and Gynaecologists). (2009). *Thrombosis and embolism during pregnancy and puerperium: Reducing the risk. Green-top guideline No 37a.* London: RCOG.

RCOG (Royal College of Obstetricians and Gynaecologists). (2011a). *Obstetric cholestasis. Green-top guideline No 13.* London: RCOG.

RCOG (Royal College of Obstetricians and Gynaecologists). (2011b). *Cardiac disease and pregnancy: Good practice guide. Green-top guideline No 13.* London: RCOG.

RCOG (Royal College of Obstetricians and Gynaecologists). (2011c). *Management of sickle cell disease in pregnancy. Green-top Guideline No 61.* London: RCOG.

RCOG (Royal College of Obstetricians and Gynaecologists). (2015a). *Reducing the risk of venous thromboembolism during pregnancy and puerperium. Green-top Guideline No 37a.* London: RCOG. Available at: www.rcog.org.uk/globalassets/documents/guidelines/gtg-37a.pdf.

RCOG (Royal College of Obstetricians and Gynaecologists). (2015b). *Thromboembolic disease in pregnancy and the puerperium: Acute management. Green-top guideline No. 37b.* London: RCOG. Available at: www.rcog.org.uk/globalassets/documents/guidelines/gtg-37b.pdf.

RCOG (Royal College of Obstetricians and Gynaecologists). (2017). *The prevention of early onset neonatal Group B streptococcal disease. Green-top Guideline No 36.* London: RCOG.

Reece, E. A., Leguizamón, G., & Wiznitzer, A. (2009). Gestational diabetes: The need for a common ground. *Lancet, 23*(373), 1789–1797.

Regitz-Zagrosek, V., Blomstrom Lundqvist, C., Borghi, C., et al. (2011). ESC Guidelines on the management of cardiovascular diseases during pregnancy. *European Heart Journal, 32*, 3147–3197.

Richmond, J. (2009). Coping with diabetes in pregnancy. *British Journal of Midwifery, 17*(2), 84–91.

Roberts, W., & Adamson, D. (2013). Cardiovascular disease in pregnancy. *Obstetrics, Gynecology and Reproductive Medicine, 23*(7), 195–201.

Rogers, K., Balachandren, N., Awogbade, M., et al. (2019). Sickle cell disease in pregnancy. *Obstetrics, Gynaecology and Reproductive Medicine, 29*(3), 61–69.

Russell, N. J., Seale, A. C., O'Driscoll, M., et al. (2017). GBS maternal Colonization investigator group). Maternal colonization with group B streptococcus and serotype distribution worldwide: Systematic review and meta-analyses. *Clinical Infectious Diseases, 65*(Suppl. 2), S100–S111.

Sachdeva, A., Dalton, M., & Lees, T. (2018). Graduated compression stockings for prevention of deep vein thrombosis. *Cochrane Database of Systematic Reviews, 11*, CD001484.

Saleh, M. M., & Abdo, K. R. (2007). Consensus on the management of obstetric cholestasis: National UK Survey. *BJOG: An International Journal of Obstetrics and Gynaecology, 114*(1), 99–103.

Scanlon, P., & Harcombe, J. (2011). It's all in the eyes. *Midwives, 5*, 46.

Schmitt, N. M., Nicholson, W. K., & Schmitt, J. (2007). The association of pregnancy and the development of obesity – results of a systematic review and meta-analysis on the natural history of postpartum weight retention. *International Journal of Obesity, 31*, 1642–1651.

Schrier, S. (2015). So you know how to treat iron deficiency anaemia? *Blood, 126*, 1971.

Scott-Pillai, R., Spence, D., Cardwell, C. R., et al. (2013). The impact of body mass index on maternal and neonatal outcomes: A retrospective study in a UK obstetric population, 2004–11. *BJOG: An International Journal of Obstetrics and Gynaecology, 120*(8), 932–939.

Seedat, F., Geppert, J., Stinton, C., et al. (2019). Universal antenatal screening for group B streptococcus may cause more harm than good. *British Medical Journal, 364*, l463.

Sellstrom, E., Arnoldson, G., Alricsson, M., et al. (2009). Obesity: Prevalence in a cohort of women in early pregnancy from a neighbourhood perspective. *BMC Pregnancy and Childbirth, 9*, 37.

Shennan, A. H., & Waugh, J. (2003). *Pre-eclampsia.* London: RCOG Press.

Shieh, C., Cullen, D. L., Pike, C., et al. (2018). Intervention strategies for preventing excessive gestational weight gain: Systematic review and meta-analysis. *Obesity Reviews, 19*, 1093–1109.

SIGN Scottish Intercollegiate Guidelines Network. (2010) (updated 2017) Management of diabetes: National Clinical Guideline 116. Edinburgh: SIGN.

Solmi, F., & Morris, S. (2018). Overweight and obese pre-pregnancy BMI is associated with higher hospital costs of childbirth in England. *BMC Pregnancy and Childbirth, 18*(1), 253.

Swinburn, B., Sacks, G., Hall, K., et al. (2011). The global obesity pandemic: Shaped by global drivers and local environments. *Lancet, 378*(9793), 804–814.

Thangaratinam, S., Frog, F., McCorry, D., et al. (2016). *Epilepsy in pregnancy. Green-top guideline No 68.* London: RCOG.

Thangaratinam, S., Rogozinska, E., Jolly, K., et al. (2012). Effects of interventions in pregnancy on maternal weight and obstetric outcomes: meta-analysis of randomised evidence. *British Medical Journal, 344*, e208801–e208815.

Thwaites, A., Iveson, H., Batta, S., et al. (2016). Non HIV-sexually transmitted infections in pregnancy. *Obstetrics, Gynecology And Reproductive Medicine, 26*(9), 253–258.

Tortora, G., & Derrickson, B. (2016). *Principles of anatomy and physiology* (15th ed.). Chichester: Wiley.

Townsend, R., O'Brien, P., & Khalil, A. (2016). Current best practice in the management of hypertensive disorders in pregnancy. *Integrated Blood Pressure Control, 9*, 79–94.

Tuffnell, D., Bamber, J., Banerjee, A., et al. (2019). On behalf of the Hypertensive Chapter Writing Group "Lessons on Prevention and Treatment of Hypertensive Disorders". In Knight, M., Bunch, K., Tuffnell, D., et al. (2019), on behalf of MBBRACE-UK. *Saving Lives, Improving Mothers Care – Lessons Learned to Inform Maternity Care from the UK and Ireland Confidential Enquiries into Maternal Deaths and Morbidity 2015–2017.* (pp. 54–58). Oxford: National Perinatal Epidemiology Unit, University of Oxford.

Tuffnell, D. (2018). Maternal mortality in the UK 2014–16. In M. K. B. Knight, D. Tuffnell, et al. (Eds.), *On behalf of MBRRACE-UK. Saving lives, improving mothers' care – lessons learned to inform maternity care from the UK and Ireland confidential enquiries into maternal deaths and morbidity 2014–16.* National Perinatal Epidemiology Unit: University of Oxford.

Turgut, A., Demirci, O., Demirci, E., et al. (2010). Comparison of maternal and neonatal outcomes in women with HELLP syndrome and women with severe preeclampsia without HELLP syndrome. *Journal of Prenatal Medicine, 4*(3), 51–58.

Tweet, M. S., Hayes, S. N., Codsi, E., et al. (2017). Spontaneous coronary artery dissection associated with pregnancy. *Journal of the American College of Cardiology, 70*, 426–435.

Unger, H. W., Bhaskar, S., & Mahmood, T. (2018). Venous thromboembolism in pregnancy. *Obstetrics, Gynaecology and Reproductive Medicine, 28*(11–2), 360–365.

de Valk, H. W., & Visser, G. H. A. (2011). Insulin during pregnancy, labour and delivery. *Best Practice & Research Clinical Obstetrics & Gynaecology, 25*, 65–76.

Vijgen, S. M. C., Koopmans, C. M., Opmeer, B. C., et al. (2010). An economic analysis of induction of labour and expectant monitoring in women with gestational hypertension or pre-eclampsia at term (HYPITAT trial). *BJOG: An International Journal of Obstetrics and Gynaecology, 117*(13), 1577–1585.

Villamor, E., & Cnattingius, S. (2006). Interpregnancy weight change and risk of adverse pregnancy outcomes: A population-based study. *Lancet, 368*(9542), 1164–1170.

de Vries, J. (2007). The obesity epidemic: Medical and ethical considerations. *Science and Engineering Ethics, 13*, 55–67.

Walsh, T., O'Broin, S., Cooley, S., et al. (2011). Laboratory assessment of iron status in pregnancy. *Clinical Chemistry and Laboratory Medicine, 49*, 1225–1230.

Watkins, K., Johnson-Roffey, Houghton, J., et al. (2013). Infectious conditions. In S. E. Robson, & J. Waugh (Eds.), *Medical disorders in pregnancy: A manual for midwives* (2nd ed.) (pp. 215–240). Oxford: Wiley Blackwell.

Watson, H. G., Craig, J. I. O., & Manson, L. M. (2012). Blood disease. In B. R. Walker, N.R. College, S. H. Ralston, et al. (Eds.), *Davidson's principles and practice of medicine* (22nd ed.) (pp. 989–1056). Edinburgh: Churchill Livingstone.

Webb, G. (2008). *Nutrition: A health promotion approach* (3rd ed.). London: Hodder Arnold.

Webster, S., Dodd, C., & Waugh, J. (2013). Hypertensive disorders. In S. E. Robson, & J. Waugh (Eds.), *Medical disorders in pregnancy: A manual for midwives* (2nd ed.) (pp. 27–42). Oxford: Wiley-Blackwell.

Webster, K., Fishburn, S., Maresh, M., et al. (2019). Diagnosis and management of hypertension in pregnancy: Summary of updated NICE guidance. *British Medical Journal, 366*, 15119.

WHO (World Health Organization). (2013). *Anaemia.* Geneva: WHO.

WHO (World Health Organization). (2017). *Obesity: Preventing and managing the global epidemic.* Available at: http://www.euro.who.int/en/health-topics/disease-prevention/nutrition/a-healthy-lifestyle/body-mass-index-bmi.

WHO (World Health Organization). (2017). *Syphilis in pregnancy.* Geneva: WHO.

Williams, J., Myson, V., Steward, S., et al. (2002). Self-discontinuation of antiepileptic medication in pregnancy: Detection by hair analysis. *Epilepsia, 43*, 824–833.

Wylie, L., & Bryce, H. (2016). *The midwives' guide to key medical conditions: Pregnancy and childbirth* (2nd ed.). London: Elsevier.

Zhu, L., Zhang, C., Cao, F., et al. (2018). Intracervical Foley catheter balloon versus dinoprostone insert for induction cervical ripening A systematic review and meta-analysis of randomized controlled trials. *Medicine (Baltimore), 97*(48), e13251.

ANNOTATED FURTHER READING

American Heart Association. (2018). *Spontaneous coronary artery dissection: Current state of the science.* A Scientific Statement from the American Heart Association. Available at: www.ncbi.nlm.nih.gov/pmc/articles/PMC5957087.

The US consensus paper on SCAD, not specifically P-SCAD but gives a thorough overview of SCAD.

Control of Hypertension in Pregnancy Study (CHIPS) Trial (NCT01192412).

The results of this research study is awaited. Its key aim is to compare 'tight' (target diastolic blood pressure of 85 mmHg) versus 'less tight' (target diastolic blood pressure of 100 mmHg) control of hypertension in women with non-severe, non-proteinuric maternal hypertension at 14–33 weeks. While awaiting publication of the study, the research protocol is available at: https://clinicaltrials. gov/ct2/show/NCT01192412.

Royal College of Anaesthetists. (2018). *Care of the critically ill woman in childbirth; enhanced maternal care.* Available at: www.rcoa.ac.uk/system/files/EMC-Guidelines2018.pdf.

A useful document that summarizes key recommendations relating to the care of the acutely or chronically unwell childbearing woman, who require critical care from skilled professionals within the multidisciplinary team in the most appropriate hospital setting. Critical care skills required by midwives for the early recognition, escalation and management of a deteriorating woman are also identified.

Spontaneous coronary artery dissection. (2018). *Contemporary aspects of diagnosis and patient management.* Available at: https://academic.oup.com/eurheartj/article-abstract/39/36/3353/4885368?redirectedFrom=fulltext.

Not specifically P-SCAD but gives a thorough overview of the European Position Paper on SCAD.

Taylor, R. N., Roberts, J. M., Cunningham, F. G., & Lindheimer, M. D. (Eds.). (2018). *Chesley's hypertensive disorders in pregnancy* (4th ed.) London: Academic Press/Elsevier.

This is a useful resource/reference guide to strengthen knowledge and understanding of pre-eclampsia and the inherit challenges to management. Available at: https://openheart.bmj.com/content/5/2/e000884.

USEFUL WEBSITES

Action on Pre-eclampsia: www.apec.org.uk

Association for the Study of Obesity: www.aso.org.uk

Asthma UK: www.asthma.org.uk

Asthma Guidelines: https://www.guidelines.co.uk/respiratory/sign-and-bts-management-of-asthma-in-adults-guideline/454878.article

Beat SCAD. Rachel's story: http://beatscad.org.uk/rachels-story/

Beat SCAD. Robyn's story: http://beatscad.org.uk/robyns-story/

Beat SCAD. Victoria's story: http://beatscad.org.uk/victorias-story/

British Heart Foundation: www.bhf.org.uk

British Hypertension Society: www.bhsoc.org

British Society for Haematology: www.b-s-h.org.uk

British Thoracic Society: www.brit-thoracic.org.uk

British Thyroid Foundation: www.btf-thyroid.org.uk

Diabetes UK: www.diabetes.org.uk

Epilepsy Action (British Epilepsy Association): www.epilepsy.org.uk

Group B Strep Support: www.gbss.org.uk

Hepatitis Foundation: www.hepatitisfoundation.org

International Network of Obstetric Survey Systems (INOSS): www.npeu.ox.ac.uk/inoss

International Sepsis Forum: www.sepsisforum.org

National Chlamydia Screening Programme: www.chlamydiascreening.nhs.uk

National Institute for Health and Care (formerly Clinical) Excellence: www.nice.org.uk

Obstetric Cholestasis Support: www.ocsupport.org.uk

Royal College of Obstetricians and Gynaecologists: www.rcplondon.ac.uk/guidelines-policy/acute-care-toolkit-15-managing-acute-medical-problems-pregnancy'

'Royal College of Physicians: https://www.rcplondon.ac.uk/guidelines-policy/acute-care-toolkit-15-managing-acute-medical-problems-pregnancy'

Scottish Intercollegiate Guidelines Network: www.sign.ac.uk

Spontaneous Coronary Artery Dissection (SCAD): https://scad.lcbru.le.ac.uk/ www.mayoclinic.org/diseases-conditions/spontaneous-coronary-artery-dissection/symptoms-causes/syc-20353711

UK National Screening Committee: www.screening.nhs.uk

KEY VIDEOS TO WATCH

It's better to ask: working together to prevent maternal mortality: https://rcpsg.ac.uk/college/influencing-healthcare/policy/maternal-health.

You might die if you have a baby: www.youtube.com/watch?v=jxKiAyGH58w.

*This 8 min video features Dr Abtehale Al-Hussaini who is running a P-SCAD clinic at Chelsea and Westminster hospital in London.*Adapted from NICE (National Institute for Health and Clinical Excellence). (2010a) (updated 2018). Hypertension in pregnancy: The management of hypertensive disorders during pregnancy. CG 107. London: NICE.From NICE (2019a); James et al. (2017).

16

Multiple Pregnancy

Jenny Brewster, Helen Turier

CHAPTER CONTENTS

The term 'multiple pregnancy' is used to describe the development of more than one fetus *in utero* at the same time. Families expecting a multiple birth have different health needs, requiring extra practical support and understanding throughout pregnancy, the postnatal period and the early years. Information and support from well-informed healthcare professionals from the time the multiple pregnancy is diagnosed will help to prepare the parents and avoid potential problems.

THE CHAPTER AIMS TO

- describe how types of multiple pregnancy may be distinguished
- consider the diagnosis and management of twin pregnancy, the labour and the care of the mother and babies after birth
- give an overview of the problems particularly associated with twins and higher order births and the fetal anomalies unique to the twinning process
- explain the special needs of the parents and identify the sources of help available.

INCIDENCE

The incidence of multiple births in England and Wales has stabilized over recent years. In 2016, there were 10,951 multiple births, a rate of 15.9 per 1000 maternities or 1 in 63 with 10,786 twins, 160 triplets and 5 quads or above (Table 16.1, Fig. 16.1) (Office of National Statistics, ONS 2017).

In the 1940s and 1950s, the incidence of twins was 1 in 80 but then fell, with no apparent explanation, to 1 in 104 in 1979. The number of triplets born more than trebled in the 15 years up to 2001 (Blondel and Kaminski 2002). The highest number in any one year was 323 in 1998; this was due to the rise in treatments for infertility such as in vitro fertilization (IVF) and ovulation-stimulating drugs.

TABLE 16.1 Multiple Birth Statistics, England and Wales 1990–2016

Year	Total Maternities	Twins	Triplets	Quads and Above	Twinning Rate/1000 Maternities	Triplet Rate/1000 Maternities	Multiple Birth Rate/1000 Maternities
1990	701,030	7934	201	9	11.3	0.29	11.6
1991	693,857	8160	208	11	11.7	0.3	12.1
1992	683,854	8314	202	9	12.2	0.3	12.5
1993	668511	8302	12	13	12.4	0.35	12.8
1994	659,520	8451	260	8	12.8	0.39	13.2
1995	642,404	8749	282	7	13.6	0.44	14.1
1996	643,862	8615	259	9	13.4	0.4	13.8
1997	636,015	8899	295	7	14	0.46	14.5
1998	629,926	8776	297	7	13.9	0.47	14.4
1999	615,994	8636	267	4	14	0.43	14.46
2000	598,580	8526	262	4	14.2	0.43	14.68
2001	588,868	8484	211	4	14.4	0.35	14.77
2002	590,453	8685	172	4	14.7	0.29	15
2003	615,787	9001	127	3	14.61	0.2	14.82
2004	633,728	9368	148	5	14.78	0.23	15.02
2005	639,627	9396	146	1	14.68	0.22	14.91
2006	662,915	9992	138	7	15.07	0.21	15.29
2007	682,999	10,334	135	2	15.13	0.19	15.3
2008	701,297	10,680	174	1	15.22	0.24	15.5
2009	698,324	11,301	153	5	16.2	0.23	16.4
2010	715,467	11,053	169	6	15.4	0.2	15.7
2011	706,040	11,330	172	3	15.8	0.24	16
2012	729,674	11,228	208	5	15.4	0.29	15.9
2013	690,820	10,593	187	3	15.3	0.27	15.6
2014	687,346	10,839	148	2	15.8	0.21	16
2015	689,251	10,901	169	3	15.8	0.24	16.1
2016	672,172	10,786	160	5	15.7	0.23	15.9

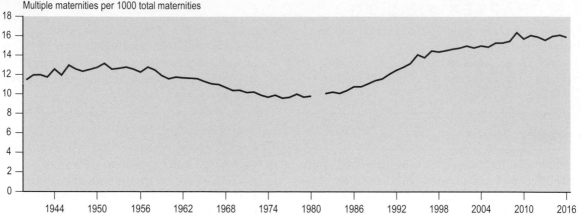

Fig. 16.1 Multiple maternities, 1940–2016. (Data from ONS, Office of National Statistics. (2017) Births characteristics in England and Wales: 2016. Available at: www.ons.gov.uk.)

The single most important reason for the rise in multiple births is assisted conception (Black and Bhattacharya 2010), although women having children when they are older is a contributory factor, though less significant. Multiple birth is the greatest single risk to the health and welfare of babies born after IVF due to the increased rates of stillbirth, preterm birth, neonatal death and disabilities. Maternal complications are also higher with a multiple pregnancy. Concern about the increased morbidity and mortality and high costs for health and social care led the Human Fertilisation and Embryology Authority (HFEA) to commission an expert group to review multiple births after IVF. The report 'One Child at a Time' (Braude 2006) has led to significant changes in practice to reduce iatrogenic multiple births. Elective single embryo transfer in IVF cycles is the normal practice in the UK with spare good-quality embryos frozen for replacement in later cycles (Cutting et al. 2008; Harbottle et al. 2015; HFEA 2016). The One at a Time policy is supported by professional bodies and relevant organizations (Jacklin and Marceniuk n.d.).

TWIN PREGNANCY

Types of Twin Pregnancy

Twins will be either monozygotic (MZ) or dizygotic (DZ). Monozygotic or uniovular twins are also referred to as 'identical twins'. They develop from the fusion of one oocyte and one spermatozoon, which after fertilization splits into two (see Chapter 5). These twins will be of the same sex and have the same genes, blood groups and physical features, such as eye and hair colour, ear shapes

TABLE 16.2	Relationship between Zygosity and Chorionicity
Dichorionic	**Monochorionic**
Two placentae (may be fused)	One placenta
Two chorions	One chorion
Two amnions	Two amnions (one amnion in monoamniotic twins is very rare)
These twins can be either dizygotic or monozygotic	These twins can only be monozygotic

and palm creases. However, they may be of different sizes and often have very different personalities and characters.

Dizygotic or binovular twins develop when two separate oocytes are fertilized by two different spermatozoa; they are often referred to as fraternal or non-identical twins. They are no more alike than any brother or sister and can be of the same or different sex. In any multiple pregnancy, there is a 50:50 chance of a girl or boy, half of dizygotic twins will be boy–girl pairs. A quarter of dizygotic twins will be both boys and a quarter, both girls. Of all twins born in the UK, two-thirds will be dizygotic and one-third monozygotic. Therefore, approximately one-third of twins are girls, one-third boys and one-third girl–boy pairs.

Determination of Zygosity and Chorionicity

Midwives must understand the differences between these two terms (Table 16.2) and why it is important.

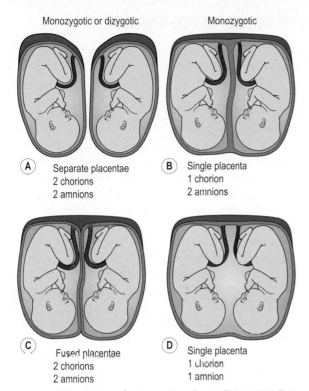

A Separate placentae
2 chorions
2 amnions

B Single placenta
1 chorion
2 amnions

C Fused placentae
2 chorions
2 amnions

D Single placenta
1 chorion
1 amnion

Fig. 16.2 Placentation of twins. (After Bryan EM. (1984) Twins in the family (a parent's guide). London: Constable, with permission of Edward Arnold.)

Determination of *zygosity* means determining whether or not the twins are monozygotic (identical) or dizygotic (non identical). In about one-third of all twins born, it will be obvious as the children will be of a different sex. Of the remaining same-sex twins, zygosity will usually be apparent from physical features by the time the children are 2 years old, although parents are not usually prepared to wait this long. By the age of 2, parents know their children so well and see their differences in character and personalities that they often find it difficult to believe they are identical. At birth, *monochorionic* twins can have a greater weight variation than *dichorionic* twins. In approximately two-thirds of monozygotic twins, a monochorionic diamniotic placenta (MCDA) will confirm *monozygosity*. If the babies have a single outer membrane, the chorion, they must be monochorionic and so monozygotic (Fig. 16.2). In one-third of monozygotic twins, the placenta will have two chorions and two amnions (DCDA), and either fused placentas (Fig. 16.2C) or two separate placentas (dichorionic)

(Fig. 16.2A), which is indistinguishable from the situation in dizygotic twins.

With monozygotic twins, the type of placenta produced is determined by the time at which the fertilized oocyte splits:

- 0–4 days: dichorionic diamniotic placenta DCDA (approx. 33% – one-third of cases) (Fig. 16.2A,C)
- 4–8 days: monochorionic diamniotic placenta MCDA (approx. 66% – two-thirds of cases) (Fig. 16.2B)
- 8–12 days: monochorionic monoamniotic placenta MCMA (approx. 1% of cases) (Fig. 16.2D)
- 12–13 days: (very rare indeed) conjoined twins can develop when the division is incomplete (Bomsel-Helmreich and Al Mufti 2005).

Despite the well-established facts about placentation and zygosity, professionals are still giving couples incorrect information. Same-sex dichorionic twins can be either non-identical or identical and it is only from either an amniocentesis while pregnant or deoxyribonucleic acid (DNA) testing after the birth that accurate zygosity can be known.

Chorionicity: Why is it Important to Know?

This knowledge is important clinically because monochorionic twin pregnancies have a 3–5 times higher risk of perinatal mortality and morbidity than dichorionic twin pregnancies (Pasquini et al. 2004; Kilby and Bricker 2016).

Zygosity Determination After Birth

The most accurate method of determining zygosity is to compare DNA from each baby. The DNA can be extracted from cells taken from a cheek swab from inside the mouth. Specific genetic markers extracted from different chromosomes are compared and the results are up to 99.99% accurate. (For DNA testing, contact the Multiple Births Foundation, MBF.)

Zygosity determination should be routinely offered to all same-sex dichorionic twins for the following reasons:

- Most parents will want to know whether or not their twins are identical, so they can answer the most commonly asked question: 'Are they identical?' Also as the twins get older, they themselves usually want to know.
- If couples are considering further pregnancies, the risk in DZ twin pregnancy increases approximately five-fold: these tend to run in families, usually on the female side. MZ twins do not run in families and the

likelihood does not change (except in rare families who carry a dominant gene for monozygotic twinning). The chance of any fertile woman having MZ twins is approximately 1 in 350–400.

- With the correct parental support around developing and enhancing individuality, the knowledge of zygosity may support the development of their unique sense of self rather than defining themselves solely as a twin or triplet (Twins Trust n.d.).
- The information is important for genetic reasons, not just with monogenic disorders but with any serious illness later in life.
- Twins are frequently asked to be involved in research and for this knowledge of zygosity is essential.

Diagnosis of Twin Pregnancy

This is usually through ultrasound examination. Diagnosis can be made as early as 6 weeks, particularly for women who have had treatment for infertility, but usually at the early scan between 11 weeks and 13 weeks and 6 days (see Chapter 13). If the pregnancy is diagnosed at 6 weeks, the woman should be told about the risk of 'vanishing twin syndrome' (Landy and Keith 1998; Blickstein and Perlman 2013).

The differences between the two types of placenta are more pronounced in the first trimester, so it is important to establish chorionicity at the early scan. The chorions forming the septum between the amniotic sacs can be seen more clearly at this time and the membrane thickness measured, or by studying the septum at its base adjacent to the placenta where a tongue of placental tissue is seen ultrasonically between the two chorions; this is termed the lambda (λ) or T-sign (Wood et al. 1996; Maruotti et al. 2016).

Once a multiple pregnancy has been diagnosed, nomenclature should be assigned to each baby (e.g. A and B, or upper and lower). Recent guidance suggests that this should be carried out by their lateral or vertical orientation, rather than proximity to the cervix. This may be important where there are anomalies or complications, and the twin labelled *in utero* as twin 2 is born first (Dias et al. 2011).

The news that a woman is expecting a multiple pregnancy should be broken to the couple in a sensitive manner, as it may be a huge shock. At diagnosis, the mother must be given relevant information about the pregnancy, be referred to a specialist multiple pregnancy clinic, and given website addresses or telephone numbers of local and national support organizations (see Useful Websites, below).

THE MULTIPLE PREGNANCY

A multiple pregnancy tends to be shorter than a single pregnancy. The average gestation for twins is 37 weeks, triplets 34 weeks and quadruplets 32 weeks.

Antenatal Screening

- A healthcare professional experienced in twin and triplet pregnancies should offer information and counselling before and after every screening test.
- Screening for Down syndrome, Edwards syndrome and Patau syndrome is advocated by NICE (2019) (see Chapter 13). Non-invasive pregnancy tests (NIPT) such as IONA are accurate as a combined test in twins. For monochorionic twins, this is likely to more effective that in a singleton pregnancy, but is not as straightforward for dichorionic pregnancies (Royal College of Obstetricians and Gynecologists, RCOG 2014).
- Amniocentesis can be performed in twin pregnancies, usually between 15 and 20 weeks. It should be performed in a specialist fetal medicine unit. Most obstetricians prefer to do a dual needle insertion, so there is no chance of contamination between the two sacs.
- The role of chorionic villus sampling (CVS) with dichorionic placentas remains controversial because of a relatively high risk of cross-contamination of chorionic tissue, which may lead to false-positive or false-negative results. Such procedures should only be performed after detailed counselling (RCOG 2010).

Ultrasound Examination

- Monochorionic twin pregnancies should be scanned every 2 weeks from 16 weeks' gestation until birth, to check for discordant fetal growth and signs of twin-to-twin transfusion syndrome (TTTS). A detailed cardiac scan should be included with the anomaly scan due to increased incidence of cardiac problems with MZ twins (Khalil et al. 2015; Kilby and Bricker 2016).
- Dichorionic twin pregnancies should be scanned monthly from 16 weeks, with the anomaly scan between $18{+}^0$ to $20{+}^6$ weeks.

Antenatal Care and Preparation

Early diagnosis of a twin pregnancy and of chorionicity is extremely important in order to give parents the specialist support and advice they will need.

Clinical care for women with twin and triplet pregnancies should be provided by a nominated multidisciplinary team consisting of: a core team of named specialist obstetricians, specialist midwives and ultrasonographers, all of whom have experience and knowledge of managing multiple pregnancies.

An enhanced team for referrals should include: a women's physiotherapist, an infant feeding specialist, a dietitian and a perinatal mental health professional. The type of care pathway the woman will follow for her antenatal care will depend on whether she is expecting monochorionic or dichorionic twins. Women expecting an uncomplicated monochorionic diamniotic twin pregnancy should be offered at least 11 antenatal appointments with healthcare professionals from the core team. At least two of these should be with the specialist obstetrician. Women with uncomplicated dichorionic diamniotic twin pregnancies should be offered at least eight antenatal appointments with a healthcare professional from the core team, and two of these with the specialist obstetrician (National Institute for Health and Care Excellence, NICE 2019).

As about 60% of women with multiple pregnancies will give birth before 37 weeks' gestation, NICE (2019) recommend that a discussion is held with the parents regarding the possibility of preterm birth, and this should be held before 24 weeks' gestation. Discussions should also take place regarding the mode of delivery prior to 32 weeks' gestation (NICE 2011, 2019).

Parent Education

Routine parent education classes should be offered earlier for women expecting twins, ideally around 22–24 weeks' gestation. A specialist class for couples expecting a multiple birth would be the ideal, and these are very often provided by individual hospital Trusts, as well as by individual providers (Twins Trust 2018a). When planning these classes, contact with a local twins club can provide a valuable source of practical information. Mothers from twins clubs are usually delighted to participate in the classes and talk on the practical issues such as coping with two or more babies, equipment and breastfeeding (Leonard and Denton 2006). Suggestions for class topics are listed in Box 16.1.

The news a multiple pregnancy is expected can come as a considerable shock and the midwife should give couples the opportunity to discuss any worries or problems they have, as two babies will add a considerable financial burden to any family's income (McKay 2010).

> **BOX 16.1   Topics for Parent Education Classes**
>
> - facts and figures on twins and twinning
> - diet and exercise
> - parental anxieties about obstetric complications
> - labour, pain relief and the birth
> - possibilities of premature labour and the birth outcome
> - visit to the special care baby unit
> - breastfeeding and bottle-feeding
> - zygosity
> - equipment (prams and buggies, car seats, layette, etc.)
> - coping with newborn twins or more
> - development of twins including individuality and identity
> - sources of help.

> **BOX 16.2   Support Needed by the Breastfeeding Mother of Twins or More**
>
> - consistent professional advice
> - reassurance of her ability to produce enough milk to satisfy her babies
> - encouragement from professionals and family in her ability to cope with feeding two or more
> - support from her partner
> - help at home with household chores
> - help with older siblings
> - a high calorie and high protein diet.

Preparation for Breastfeeding

Women will inevitably give a lot of thought to how they are going to feed their babies, not only from the nutritional but also from the practical point of view, as feeding will take up a large amount of their time during the first 6 months. Women should be encouraged right from the beginning that it is not only possible to breastfeed two, and in some cases three babies, but it is the best way for her to feed her babies nutritionally and it can be a very rewarding experience for her (Stagg 2017). However, the mother, as with all new mothers, will need support and guidance both from professionals and their family and friends (Box 16.2). Many sets of twins have been entirely breastfed, some beyond their first birthdays. Very few sets of triplets are totally breastfed (Leonard 2000), but many mothers manage to combine breast and bottle-feeding very successfully.

Early in the antenatal period the woman should be given full information and advice about both breast and bottle-feeding, so she can make an informed choice on how to feed her babies (see Chapter 27). Both parents should have the opportunity to ask questions and be encouraged to meet another mother who is successfully breastfeeding her babies. Introductions can usually be made through a local twins group (Twins Trust 2018b).

Abdominal Examination
Inspection
On inspection, the size of the uterus may be larger than expected for the period of gestation, particularly after the 20th week. The uterus may look broad or round and fetal movements may be seen over a wide area, although the findings are not diagnostic of twins. Fresh striae gravidarum may be apparent. Up to twice the amount of amniotic fluid is normal in a twin pregnancy but polyhydramnios is not an uncommon complication of a twin pregnancy, particularly with monochorionic twins.

Palpation
On palpation, the fundal height may be greater than expected for the period of gestation. The presence of two fetal poles (head or breech) in the fundus of the uterus may be revealed on palpation and multiple fetal limbs may also be palpable. The head may be small in relation to the size of the uterus and may suggest that the fetus is also small and therefore there may be more than one present. Lateral palpation may reveal two fetal backs, or limbs on both sides. Pelvic palpation may give findings similar to those on fundal palpation, although one fetus may lie behind the other and make detection difficult. Location of three poles in total is diagnostic of at least two fetuses.

Auscultation
Hearing two fetal hearts is not diagnostic as one can often be heard over a wide area in a singleton pregnancy. If simultaneous comparison over 1 min of the heart rates reveals a difference of at least 10 bpm, it may be assumed that two hearts are being heard beating.

Effects of the Multiple Pregnancy
Exacerbation of Common Disorders
The presence of more than one fetus *in utero* and the higher levels of circulating hormones often exacerbate the common disorders of pregnancy. Sickness, nausea and heartburn may be more persistent and more troublesome than in a singleton pregnancy.

Anaemia
Iron and folic acid deficiency anaemias are common in twin pregnancies. Early growth and development of the uterus and its contents make greater demands on the maternal iron stores; in later pregnancy (after the 28th week), fetal demands may lead to anaemia. Routine oral iron supplementation remains a controversial issue (Lassi et al. 2013), but a full blood count should be checked at 20–24 weeks' gestation and again at 28 weeks' gestation to screen for anaemia (NICE 2019). All pregnant women are advised to take folic acid daily (NICE 2008/2019).

Polyhydramnios
This is also common and particularly associated with serious complications of monochorionic twins such as twin-to-twin transfusion syndrome (TTTS) and other fetal abnormalities. Polyhydramnios will add to any discomfort that the woman is already experiencing. If acute polyhydramnios occurs, it can lead to miscarriage or preterm labour.

Pressure Symptoms
The increased weight and size of the uterus and its contents may be troublesome. Impaired venous return from the lower limbs increases the tendency to varicose veins and oedema of the legs. Backache is common and the increased uterine size may also lead to marked dyspnoea and indigestion.

There can also be an increase in complications of pregnancy such as obstetric cholestasis, and pelvic girdle pain (PGP) (see Chapters 14 and 15).

LABOUR AND THE BIRTH
Onset
The more fetuses the woman is carrying, the earlier labour is likely to start. Twins are usually born around 37 weeks rather than 40 weeks, and approximately 60% of twins are born spontaneously before 37 weeks' gestation. In addition to being preterm, the babies may be small-for-gestational-age (SFGA) and therefore prone to the associated complications of both conditions. However, research has shown that the use of twin growth charts can provide information regarding the accurate sizing of twins (Stirrup et al. 2014). If spontaneous labour begins before 24 weeks, the chances of survival outside the uterus are very

small, but it is possible the woman can be given drugs to inhibit uterine activity. Causes of preterm labour must, if at all possible, be diagnosed and treated quickly; for example, urinary tract infection should be treated with antibiotics. Antenatal corticosteroids are usually given to all women of multiple pregnancies before 36 weeks' gestation (NICE 2019).

Regarding mode of birth, see NICE (2019; at: https://www.nice.org.uk/guidance/ng137/chapter/Recommendations#mode-of-birth). Evidence shows that after 38 weeks' gestation there is increased risk of higher mortality in babies from multiple pregnancies (Danon et al. 2013). The recommendations from NICE (2011b) and the RCOG (Kilby and Bricker 2016) is that birth should be offered at 36 weeks for MCDA twin pregnancies and at 37 weeks for DCDA twins (see Case Study 16.1). For MCMA twin pregnancies, the risk of fetal demise is greater from an earlier gestation, so birth is recommended between 32 and 34 weeks' gestation. NICE (2018) have endorsed the use of a Multiple Pregnancy Antenatal Care Proforma and Care Pathways, to highlight the chronicity of the pregnancy, document the discussions and plans that are put in place, and provide outlines of the various plans of care (Twins Trust 2018c).

CASE STUDY 16.1

A 34-year-old primigravida was diagnosed with DCDA twins, no family history, so it was a complete shock. At the ultrasound department, a leaflet with local twin clubs and contacts, including details of the Twins Trust, were given to the mother. Through the hospital specialist, the multiple birth midwife and support from the Twins Trust and the local twins club, the mother started to come to terms with the prospect of twins. She knew she was expecting two boys and began to wonder if they were identical or not, but would have to wait until they were born and have DNA tests if they looked alike, and if she wished DNA testing to clarify zygosity. She had a straightforward birth with her first child, so she was keen to have a vaginal birth again. After discussion with her multiples midwife and her consultant she advised that she would like to aim for a vaginal birth. She understood that this was subject to the twin closest to the cervix being in a cephalic position at 37 weeks and there being no complications such as growth restriction in either twin. She understood that there is a 5% risk of needing to deliver twin 2 by emergency C section. The pregnancy progressed normally and with support from the specialist midwife, she wrote her birth plan.

The presenting baby was cephalic, and at 37 weeks labour was induced. The woman had an epidural and progressed to birth both babies vaginally after a short labour. Both babies were put to her breast in the labour suite; twin one sucked well but twin two was not interested. As establishing feeding was more problematic than she had expected and she felt she needed a lot of help from the midwives; the mother stayed in hospital until day 5. Both babies were sucking well on return home, although twin two did occasionally need more feeds than twin one. This did settle over the coming weeks, with support from the local volunteer breastfeeding team and Twins Trust support.

In both uncomplicated monochorionic and dichorionic pregnancies, if the first twin (the twin closest to the cervix) is a cephalic presentation, labour is usually allowed to continue to a vaginal birth, but if the first twin is presenting in any other way, an elective caesarean section (CS) is usually recommended (Fig. 16.3). There is no difference in the neonatal morbidity or mortality between a planned caesarean section and a vaginal birth when the first twin is a cephalic presentation (Barrett et al. 2013). It should also be noted that in 5% of vaginal births, the second twin will need to be born by emergency caesarean section. MCMA twins are generally born by CS and for triplets and above, the mode of birth is almost always by CS.

Management of Labour

During antenatal classes, the couple must be informed that a multiple birth is less common and therefore, for educational purposes in the hospital setting, a number of professionals may ask to observe the birth. If the woman has any objection to this, her wishes must be respected and a record made in her notes that she wants only those concerned with her care to be present. The couple should also be informed that care for women with a twin or triplet pregnancy is usually provided by a multidisciplinary team of midwives and obstetricians who have experience and knowledge of managing twin and triplet pregnancies during the intrapartum period (NICE 2019). Home births are not usually advisable with a multiple pregnancy, but some women may still request one, in which case every effort should be made to support her choice and decision with an uncomplicated pregnancy. This will require meticulous risk assessment and planning, including the involvement of consultant

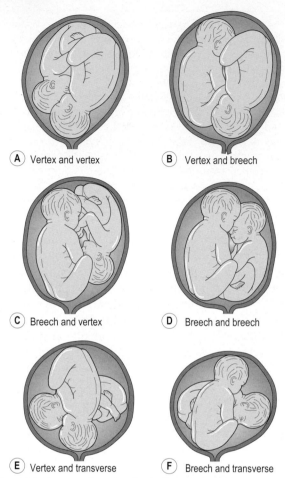

(A) Vertex and vertex   (B) Vertex and breech

(C) Breech and vertex   (D) Breech and breech

(E) Vertex and transverse   (F) Breech and transverse

Fig. 16.3 Presentation of twins before birth. (After Bryan EM, 1984. Twins in the family (a parent's guide). London: Constable, with permission of Edward Arnold.)

midwives and/or senior midwives, in order that a plan of care for labour is clearly articulated and documented in the woman's records. A skilled team of midwives with confidence to deliver intrapartum care to women with twin pregnancies at home will need to be identified to be on-call. It is good practice for the midwifery team to liaise with and communicate the plan of care to the paramedic team and local consultant-led unit. Evidence suggests that the birth mortality for twins at home is 1 in 7 (Bastian et al. 1998), although it is noted that this is now dated research and is included here to provide an historical context, given that birthing twins at home is now a rare phenomenon.

The majority of women expecting twins will go into labour spontaneously. Theoretically, the duration of the first stage of labour should be no different from that of a single pregnancy. However, there is an increased incidence of dysfunctional labour in twin pregnancies, possibly because of overdistension of the uterus. The presence of complications such as pregnancy-induced hypertension, obstetric cholestasis, intrauterine growth restriction (IUGR) or twin-to-twin transfusion syndrome may be reasons for earlier induction of labour.

Labour for women expecting twins must be recognized as high risk and continuous electronic fetal heart monitoring (EFM) of both fetuses is advocated. This can be achieved either with two external transducers or, once the membranes are ruptured, a scalp electrode on the presenting twin and an external transducer on the second for births in a hospital setting. The gold standard for practice is to use a twin monitor, with hourly 'Fresh Eyes' and 'Fresh Ears' (RCOG 2017) (see Chapter 19) and review of the cardiotocograph (CTG) tracing is as for all labours. For more detailed information about intrapartum monitoring, see NICE (2019; at: https://www.nice.org.uk/guidance/ng137/chapter/Recommendations#fetal-monitoring-during-labour-in-twin-pregnancy). Uterine activity will also need to be monitored. An ultrasound scan should be performed at the onset of labour to confirm the presentation and position of the twins, but also to aid with locating the fetal heart.

In the exceptional cases where CTG monitoring is not available, such as at a home birth, use of hand-held Dopplers may be more pragmatic for structured intermittent fetal heart rates (FHRs) auscultation than a Pinard's stethoscope. If the latter has to be used, two people must auscultate simultaneously, so that the two distinct FHRs are counted over the same minute.

While in labour, the woman should be encouraged to adopt whichever position she finds most comfortable. A foam rubber wedge under the side of the mattress will help to prevent supine hypotensive syndrome by giving a lateral tilt. It may be preferable for her to adopt a left lateral position, well supported by pillows or a beanbag. A birthing chair or a reclining chair, if available, may be more comfortable than a conventional labour suite birthing bed.

Regional epidural block provides excellent analgesia, and if necessary, allows easier instrumental births, manipulation of the second twin and is in place and effective, should an emergency caesarean section be required. The use of Entonox analgesia may be helpful, either before the epidural is *in situ* or during the second stage, if the effect of the epidural is wearing off.

The woman should be encouraged to use whatever form of relaxation she finds helpful. If she chooses to use pharmacological means of analgesia only after non-pharmacological methods are no longer effective, her wishes should be respected. The midwife should explain that, if complications arise, intervention and the use of pharmacological analgesia might be necessary. Ideally, this should be discussed with the woman antenatally so that the physiology of labour is not disturbed with new information (see Chapters 9 and 19). NICE (2011b) recommend that this occurs by 32 weeks' gestation. IV access should be obtained at the onset of labour in case an emergency caesarean section be required for fetal compromise or any other concern arises.

If uterine activity is poor, the use of intravenous oxytocin may be required once the membranes have been ruptured. Artificial rupture of the membranes (ARM) may be sufficient to stimulate good uterine activity but it may need to be used in conjunction with intravenous oxytocin. The CTG will give a good indication of the pattern of uterine activity, whether the labour is induced or spontaneous. The response of the fetal hearts to uterine contractions can be observed on the CTG.

If the babies are expected to be preterm, low birth weight, or known to have any other problems, the neonatal intensive care unit (NICU) must be informed that the woman is in labour so they can make the necessary preparations to receive the babies. When birth is imminent, the neonatal team should be summoned.

Throughout labour, the emotional and general physical condition of the woman must be considered. She requires the presence of her birthing partner and one-to-one care from the midwife.

Management of the Birth

The onset of the second stage of labour should be confirmed by a vaginal examination. In the hospital setting, the obstetrician, neonatal team and anaesthetist should be present for the birth, as there is a risk of complications occurring, especially after the birth of the first twin.

Epidural analgesia may need to be 'topped up' prior to the birth. The possibility of emergency CS is ever present and the operating theatre should be ready to receive the mother at short notice. Monitoring of both FHRs should continue until birth. Provided that the first twin is presenting by the vertex, the birth can be expected to proceed normally, as with a singleton pregnancy. When the first twin is born, the time of birth and the sex are noted. This baby and cord must be labelled as 'twin one' immediately. The identity tags should be checked with the mother or father before they are applied to the baby in accordance with local policy. The baby may be given to the mother for skin-to-skin contact and encouraged to go to the breast as sucking stimulates uterine contractions (see Chapter 27).

After the birth of the first twin, abdominal palpation is made to ascertain the lie, presentation (in the event of doubt a portable ultrasound machine should be available) and position of the second twin and to auscultate the FHR to ensure continuous EFM. An assistant may need to stabilize the lie of the second twin. If the lie is not longitudinal, an attempt may be made to correct it by external cephalic version (ECV) (see Chapter 20) or internal podalic version. ECV is less invasive than internal podalic version, and will often be the default manoeuvre employed by obstetricians (Paterson-Brown and Howell 2014). In preparation for the possibility of either of these manoeuvres, epidural anaesthesia is the recommended choice for analgesia for twin births.

If the lie of the second twin is longitudinal, a vaginal examination is made to confirm the presentation. Should the presenting part not be engaged, it should be gently guided into the pelvis and kept in place until it firmly engages. ARM must not be performed on the second sac of membranes until the presenting part engages, as risk of cord prolapse is ever present. The FHR must be auscultated again; a scalp electrode might be required following ARM if external monitoring of the FHR is of poor quality. If uterine activity does not recommence, intravenous oxytocin may be used, and should be prepared prior to the birth in readiness.

When the presenting part becomes visible, the mother should be encouraged to birth her second twin with contractions. The midwife should always be aware there is a risk the placenta may start to separate before the birth of the second twin, causing oxygen deprivation. The birth will proceed as normal if the presentation is vertex, but if the fetus presents by the breech and the midwife is not experienced in breech births, she will need a doctor's assistance. It is ideal to have experienced obstetricians present for the birth of twins in case of delay with the second twin, or to assist with a more complex birth, as the death of the second twin is more common than that of the first in labour.

The birth of the second twin should ideally be completed within 45 min of the first twin but, as long as there are no signs of fetal compromise in the second twin, it may be allowed to continue longer. If there are signs of compromise, the birth must be expedited and the second twin may need to be born by CS. A uterotonic drug (syntometrine or oxytocin) is usually given intramuscularly or intravenously, depending on local policy, after the birth of the anterior shoulder of the second twin as with a singleton pregnancy (see Chapter 21). This baby and cord are labelled as 'twin two'. The time of birth and sex of child must be noted. If either twin needs to be transferred to the NICU for observation, the mother should have a chance to see and hold the baby whenever possible.

Once the uterotonic drug has taken effect, controlled cord traction is applied to both cords simultaneously to aid the birth of the placentas without delay. There is an increased risk of postpartum haemorrhage (PPH) with twin births due to the increased size of the placental site, and also the potential overstretching of the myometrium during pregnancy. Active management of the third stage is recommended, and a Syntocinon infusion (40 IU in 500 mL normal saline, or according to local policy) should be prepared in the room in case of excessive bleeding.

The placenta(s) should be examined not only to check completion but the number of amniotic sacs, chorions and placentas noted (Fig. 16.2). If the babies are of different sexes, they are dizygotic. If the placenta is monochorionic (MCDA), they must be monozygotic. If they are of the same sex and the placenta is dichorionic (DCDA), then further tests will be needed. There may also be what appears to be one large, fused placenta. This may be monozygotic or dizygotic. If it is not easy to determine the number of chorions, further testing in the form of DNA analysis may be recommended. The umbilical cords should also be examined and the number of cord vessels and the presence of any abnormalities noted.

COMPLICATIONS ASSOCIATED WITH MULTIPLE PREGNANCY

The higher perinatal mortality associated with twinning is largely due to complications of pregnancy, such as the preterm onset of labour, IUGR and complications at birth. There is a six-fold increase in perinatal mortality comparing twins to singletons. However, both the stillbirth and neonatal death rates showed significant decreases in the period 2014–16 (Draper et al. 2018). The management of multiple pregnancy is concerned with the prevention, early detection and treatment of these complications.

Polyhydramnios

Mentioned earlier in the chapter, acute polyhydramnios may occur as early as 16 weeks. It may be associated with fetal malformations but is more likely to be due to twin-to-twin transfusion syndrome (TTTS).

Twin-to-Twin Transfusion Syndrome

Twin-to-twin transfusion syndrome can be acute or chronic. The acute form usually occurs during labour and is the result of blood transfusing from one fetus (donor) to the other (recipient) through vascular anastomosis in a monochorionic placenta. Both fetuses may die of cardiac failure if not treated urgently.

Chronic TTTS occurs in about 15% of monochorionic twin pregnancies (Kilby and Bricker 2016) and occurs when the placenta transfuses blood from one twin fetus to the other. This occurs due to a shared placenta and vascular placental anastomoses, which connect the fetal circulation of both of the twins. This results in anaemia and growth restriction in the donor twin (stuck twin) and polycythaemia with circulatory overload in the recipient twin (hydrops). Generally, this occurs before 24 weeks' gestation (Fraser n.d.). The fetal and neonatal

---

CASE STUDY 16.2

A 26-year-old primigravida's early scan showed MCDA twins. The core team of sonographer, midwife and consultant who were all experienced in multiple birth pregnancies supported the mother with information on TTS including signs and symptoms to be aware of and actions to take if these occurred, including contacting the unit immediately for assessment. The mother also read about parent experiences of TTTS on the Twins Trust website.

From 16 weeks, she had 2-weekly scans for signs of discordance of amniotic fluid levels and growth discordance. At 20 weeks, she noticed a rapid increase in abdominal size and her tummy was hard and uncomfortable. Her local hospital immediately referred her to the regional fetal medicine centre for assessment by a fetal medicine subspecialist with expertise in TTTS at a tertiary level hospital. Stage 2 TTTS was diagnosed and immediate treatment was amnio-reduction of over 2 litres and laser ablation of connecting blood vessels. Her care was transferred to this unit for weekly scans. Here she was cared for by the multiples team for that unit so was

mortality is high but infants may be saved by early diagnosis and prenatal treatment. Ultrasound scans should be performed every 2 weeks, looking at liquor volumes as well as fetal bladders. The recommended treatment is fetoscopic laser ablation of the connecting vessels in a specialist centre, followed by close monitoring (Kilby and Bricker 2016) with the optimum time for birth being 34–36 weeks' gestation (see Case Study 16.2).

The midwife should always be alert to the woman who complains of a rapid increase in her abdominal girth in the second trimester and related breathlessness, as well as a uterus that feels hard and uncomfortable continuously. The skin over the uterus may look shiny and tight; this is usually due to polyhydramnios and if not treated urgently can cause preterm labour.

Twin Anaemia-Polycythaemia Sequence

Although this may occur spontaneously in monochorionic twins, TAPS is seen more often following laser ablation for TTTS, with an incidence of about 13%. It is where there is a significant difference in the haemoglobin levels of the fetuses without the associated increase in amniotic fluid, due to there being a few small vessels that are linked, allowing a slow transfusion of blood from the donor to the recipient. There is debate about the optimal treatment of TAPS (Kilby and Bricker 2016).

Selective Growth Restriction

SGR is diagnosed by a difference of 20% in the estimated fetal weight of both twins, and can be found in 15% of monochorionic twins without TTTS, and over 50% where TTTs is a complication of the pregnancy (Kilby

and Bricker 2016). The twins should be monitored by ultrasound scanning and Dopplers every 2 weeks, with plans in place for early delivery at 32–24 weeks' gestation.

Fetal Malformations

This is particularly associated with monochorionic twins.

Conjoined Twins

This extremely rare malformation of monozygotic twinning results from the incomplete division of the fertilized oocyte. The incidence is one in 90,000 to 100,000 pregnancies, with many fetuses dying *in utero*, or the parents opting for the pregnancy to be terminated (Kilby and Bricker 2016). Birth has to be by CS. The site and extent of fusion of the fetuses are infinitely variable. Thoracopagus (conjoined twins united at the thorax) is the commonest form of fusion (over 70% of cases). The feasibility of separating conjoined twins depends on the site and extent of fusion and the degree to which organs are shared. Many conjoined twins can now be successfully separated. Others pose major ethical dilemmas – particularly if one can be saved at the expense of the other (Faulkner 2006).

Twin Reversed Arterial Perfusion

Twin reversed arterial perfusion (TRAP) occurs in about 1 in 30,000 births. In TRAP, one twin presents without a well-defined cardiac structure, but demonstrates no cardiac function. It is kept alive through placental anastomoses to the circulatory system of the viable fetus (Kilby and Bricker 2016).

Fetus in Fetu

In fetus in fetu (endoparasite), parts of a fetus may be lodged within another fetus; this can happen only in MZ twins (Ji et al. 2014; Harigovind et al. 2018; Karaman).

Malpresentations

Although the uterus is large and distended, the fetuses are less mobile than may be supposed. They can restrict each other's movements, which may result in malpresentations (see Chapter 23), particularly of the second twin. After the birth of the first twin, the presentation of the second twin may change.

Preterm Rupture of the Membranes

Malpresentations due to polyhydramnios may predispose to preterm rupture of the membranes.

Cord Prolapse

This too is associated with malpresentations and poly-hydramnios and is more likely if there is a poorly fitting presenting part. The second twin is particularly at risk of cord prolapse (see Chapter 25).

Prolonged Labour

Malpresentations are a poor stimulus to good uterine action and a distended uterus is likely to lead to poor uterine activity and consequently prolonged labour (see Chapter 22).

Monoamniotic Twins

Approximately 1% of MZ twins share the same amniotic sac. Monoamniotic (MCMA) twins have an increased risk of fetal death, and there is almost always cord entanglement with occlusion of the blood supply through the umbilical cords to one or both fetuses. In some centres, this is treated with Sulindac to reduce the amniotic fluid levels, although the evidence for the effectiveness of this drug is poor (Kilby and Bricker 2016). The birth should be planned for 32–34 weeks and by elective CS.

Locked Twins

This is a very rare but serious complication of twin pregnancy. There are two types. One occurs when the first twin presents by the breech and the second by the vertex; the other when both are vertex presentations (Fig. 16.4). In both instances, the head of the second twin prevents the continued descent of the first. Primigravidae are more at risk than multiparous women.

Delay in the Birth of the Second Twin

After the birth of the first twin, uterine activity should recommence within 5 min. Ideally, as stated previously, the birth of the second twin should be completed within 45 min of the first twin being born but with close monitoring, can be extended if there are no signs of fetal compromise. Poor uterine action as a result of malpresentation may be the cause of delay. The risks of such delay are intrauterine hypoxia, birth asphyxia following premature separation of the placenta and sepsis as a result of ascending infection from the first umbilical cord, which lies outside the vulva. After the birth of the first twin the lower uterine segment begins to reform and the cervical canal may have to dilate fully again.

The midwife may need to 'rub up' a contraction and put the first twin to the breast to stimulate

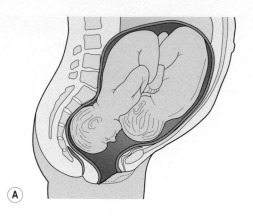

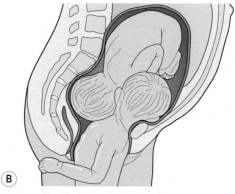

Fig. 16.4 Locked twins.

uterine activity. If there appears to be an obstruction, medical aid is summoned and a CS may be necessary. If there is no obstruction, oxytocin infusion may be commenced or an instrumental birth (see Chapter 24) considered.

Premature Expulsion of the Placenta

The placenta may be expelled before the birth of the second twin. In dichorionic twins with separate placentas, expulsion of one placenta may be separate; in monochorionic twins the shared placenta may be expelled. The risks of severe asphyxia and death of the second twin are very high. Haemorrhage is also likely if one twin is retained *in utero* as this prevents adequate retraction of the placental site.

Postpartum Haemorrhage

Poor uterine tone as a result of overdistension or hypotonic activity is likely to lead to postpartum haemorrhage (see Chapters 21 and 25). There is also a much larger placental site to contract down.

Undiagnosed Twins

The possibility of an unexpected, undiagnosed second baby (in the UK this is unlikely with ultrasound scanning) should be considered if the uterus appears larger than expected after the birth of the first baby or if the baby is surprisingly smaller than expected. If an uterotonic drug has been given after the birth of the anterior shoulder of the first baby, the second twin is in great danger of birth asphyxia and birth should be expedited. The midwife must break the news of undiagnosed twins gently to the parents. These parents will require special support and guidance during the postnatal period.

Delayed Interval Birth of the Second Twin

There have been several reported cases where the first twin has been born, often very prematurely, and then a long gap before labour recommences; it can be days or even weeks before the second twin is born (Tran et al. 2015). This opportunity can be used to give antenatal corticosteroids to the mother to help mature the lungs of the second twin. Careful observations of the mother's condition must be made during this time for signs of infection and fetal compromise. The mother will need additional support from the midwives to cope with her anxieties for her preterm baby on the NICU, which may not survive, or time to grieve if the baby has died, as well as still being pregnant and her concerns for the outcome of her pregnancy.

POSTNATAL PERIOD

Care of the Babies

Immediate care after the birth is the same as for a single baby. Maintenance of body temperature is vital, particularly if the babies are small; use of overhead heaters will help to prevent heat loss. Identification of the babies should be clear and the parents given the opportunity to check the identity bracelets and cuddle the babies. The babies may need to be admitted to the NICU from the labour suite, otherwise they can be encouraged to have skin-to-skin contact, and go to the breast if they are to be breastfed before being transferred to the postnatal ward with their mother.

Temperature Control

Maintenance of a thermoneutral environment is essential, particularly for babies in the NICU. A systematic review (Lai et al. 2017) has shown that twins benefit in several ways from sharing the environment with their twin, mimicking the *in utero* environment. Not only does this help with maintenance of temperature, but also with levels of stress and neurodevelopment. Clothing should be light but warm, and allow air to circulate.

Feeding

The mother may choose to feed her babies by breast or with formula milk, but whatever her choice, the midwife must support her in her decision. With breastfeeding, both babies may be breastfed separately or simultaneously. In the initial postnatal days, it is recommended she breastfeeds her twins separately, as this gives her time to get to know each baby individually and to feel confident in her ability to cope. If the babies are SFGA or preterm, the neonatologists may recommend that the babies be 'topped up' after a breastfeed. Expressed breastmilk is best for these babies. If the babies are not able to suck adequately at the breast, the mother should be encouraged to express her milk regularly. Expressing should be initiated ideally within 6 h of birth, then regularly every 2–3 h during the day and once at night or on average 8 times per 24 h. In some NICUs with a Milk bank, donor milk may be offered to preterm babies, this reduces the risk of necrotizing enterocolitis (NEC) (Huston et al. 2014). As twin babies are more likely to be preterm or SFGA, their ability to coordinate the sucking and swallowing reflexes may be poor. If so, they may need to be fed intravenously or by nasogastric tube, depending on their size and general condition. The mother should be encouraged to participate in whatever method is used. Careful monitoring of weight gain is required. Hypoglycaemia may occur and regular capillary blood glucose estimations may be needed.

In the early postnatal days, mothers often worry that their milk supply is inadequate for two babies. The midwife should reassure her that lactation responds to the demands made by the babies sucking at the breast or expressing. The more stimulation the breasts are given, the more milk she will produce. At feeding times, the midwife must be with the mother to offer support and advice on positioning and fixing the babies (Fig. 16.5), as well as encouraging her in her ability to cope with breastfeeding two babies.

Breastfeeding

The advantages of breastfeeding twins are the same as for singletons (see Chapter 27), but as twins have

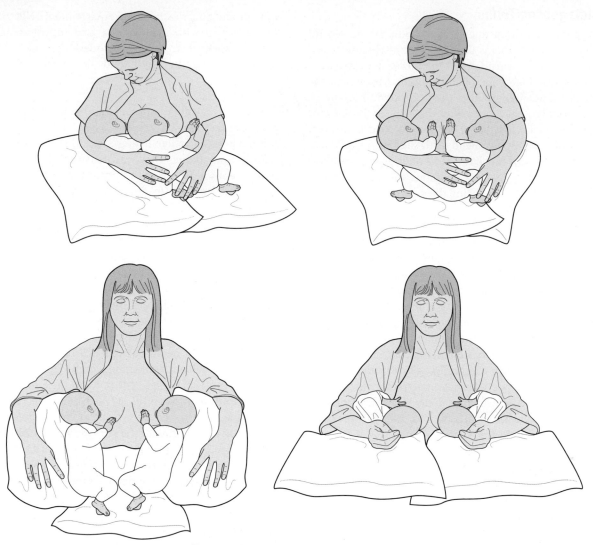

Fig. 16.5 Breastfeeding positions for twins.

a higher tendency to be born preterm and SFGA, it is even more important that they should be breastfed. As well as the medical and nutritional advantages, there are practical reasons too, many of which are outlined in Chapter 27. Additionally, as time is limited for a mother of twins in the early days, twins can be breast-fed together, when the feeds will take only a little longer than with a single baby. Some mothers will, however, prefer to feed separately.

Separate feeding

- It allows her to give one-to-one attention to each baby, something mothers of twins feel they have very little time for.

- It is easier for the mother, as she has both hands free to position and attach one baby at a time.

- If she does feed separately, it is recommended that she adopts a routine where whichever baby wakes first is fed and the second one is woken straight after-wards, so keeping her feeds together.

Simultaneous feeding

- It saves time as both babies are feeding together, though the mother will need to be organized, and will need help in the early days to get both babies attached to the breast.

- If the mother does want to feed the babies together, it is advisable to try this before going home from

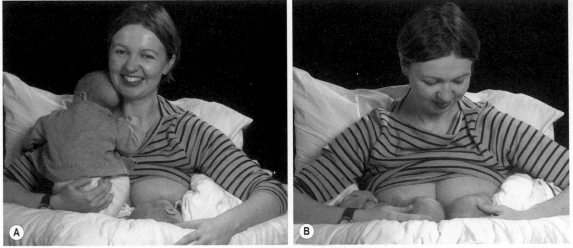

Fig. 16.6 Simultaneous feeding can be a very rewarding experience for the mother.

hospital, where a midwife can stay with her throughout the entire feed, providing advice, support and an extra pair of hands.

- The woman will need additional pillows to support her back and take the weight of the babies, to avoid putting strain on her arms and back (Figs 16.5, 16.6). Routine is the key to coping with two or more babies. It may take 4–6 weeks for a feeding routine to get established (Twins Trust 2018d).

Safe Sleeping

Twins, triplets or more can sleep in the same cot, with their feet at the foot of the cot, until they learn to roll or become more mobile (Twins Trust 2018f). This could be with the babies side by side, where it is recommended they have individual blankets tucked in, or one or more babies at each end of the cot. Always ensure there is plenty of room, so a Moses basket would not be recommended for co-sleeping.

Mother–Baby Relationships

Mothers with a multiple birth often worry they will find it more difficult to bond with each baby equally. This is a common concern and reassurance that their feelings are not unusual should be given. Once the mother gets to know her babies these feelings usually disappear. If, for example, they are of markedly different sizes, a mother may favour one over the other, or if one baby is in the NICU while the other is on the postnatal ward with her, she may find she bonds with the one on the ward much more quickly. In such cases, the mother should be encouraged to spend as much time as possible with the baby on the NICU and to visit as soon after the birth as she feels able. If she has had an operative birth, she may find it difficult to care for two babies and extreme tiredness or anaemia will exacerbate the situation. She may have feelings of guilt if the birth and immediate postnatal period have not gone as she had planned. The midwife should be alert for such circumstances and help the mother to divide her attention between both babies and to give plenty of reassurance that she is not the first mother to feel the same way.

Mother–Partner Relationships

A mother who has had twins or more will inevitably turn to her partner for help with the care of the babies, and many families work well together in the care and upbringing of their children, despite the added strains and stresses a multiple birth puts on a family. In some cases, her partner may feel that she is devoting too much time to the babies and not enough to him, thus making him feel excluded, especially if when he comes home from work she is too exhausted to take any interest in him. The strain on any relationship when a new baby is born can be quite difficult for the couple to adjust to, but with a multiple birth it is even worse. The midwife should always encourage the partner to be involved in the daily care of the babies, either in hospital or at home.

Care of the Mother

Involution of the uterus will be slower because of its increased bulk. 'After pains' may be more troublesome and analgesia should be offered. A good diet is essential and if the mother is breastfeeding, she requires a high protein, high calorie diet. It is quite common for breast-feeding mothers to feel hungry between meals and they should be encouraged to keep sensible snacks to hand for such times. A dietician may be able to offer help. The physiotherapist or midwife should instruct the mother in her postnatal exercises.

The midwife must give the mother of twins extra support. Teaching her simple parenting skills and encouraging her to carry them out with increasing assurance will build up her confidence.

The mother may feel 'in the way' if her babies are in the NICU and require a lot of intensive care. She may have feelings of guilt because of their prematurity and feel it was something she did or did not do that caused them to be born early. She should be given the opportunity to talk her feelings through. On the NICU she should always be kept up-to-date with the care and condition of her infants. Most NICUs now have a named nurse caring for each baby so parents know who to talk to. If one infant is very ill or dies, the parents will experience additional psychological problems. Some NICUs have psychologists as part of the team and parents can be referred to them.

Most units have a rooming-in policy so mothers can stay in the hospital with their babies for 2 or 3 nights before they are transferred home, to give them a chance to take over their total care and prepare them for coping at home.

Best practice is that twins or more should all be transferred home together from the NICU but this is not always possible. If they go home at different intervals, greater demands are placed on the mother, as she has to care for one baby at home and still visit the sick baby in hospital.

It is advisable for a mother of twins to organize help at home for the first 3–4 weeks after transfer. Initially, this may be in the form of her partner taking time off work. If relations or friends have offered to help, the mother should be sure to let them know what kind of help she is expecting from them before it is needed. (See Box 16.3 for comments made by grandparents on supporting a family with twins, triplets or more babies.)

BOX 16.3 Comments from Grandparents on Supporting Parents with Twins, Triplets or More

'The initial support is very important, more so than after having just singletons'.

'Offer as much help as you can to the new parents, making the odd meal, taking older siblings for sleepovers so mum/dad can spend time with the twins to get a routine sorted, and let them have the odd lie in at weekends'.

'If I had that time again I would have gone down to stay and help out more often, and for longer, in order to try and stave off the "emergencies". In my case, I was afraid to be seen as an interfering mother-in-law even though my daughter-in-law never ever made me feel that way. Perhaps having a good discussion well before the birth would have ensured that that didn't happen and more appropriate help would have been provided sooner'.

(The **Twins Trust 2018g**)

Reproduced with kind permission of Twins Trust (2018g) Being a grandparent to twins, triplets or more. Available at: https://twinstrust.org/.

If the parents are fortunate enough to be able to afford paid help, then they can say exactly what it is they expect to be done. There is no statutory help available for twins or triplets in England and Wales.

The community midwife will contact the mother after transfer home from hospital to arrange visits. The health visitor will also arrange to see the mother and her babies after the community midwife has transferred care to the health visitor.

At home, the mother must be encouraged to rest and catch up on her sleep, especially during the day, and eat a well-balanced diet. A good routine is the only way of coping with new babies and all mothers should be encouraged to establish one as soon as possible. Her partner should be encouraged to help as much as possible.

Visitors can be tiring, but also a help. Those that visit may be encouraged to help with the meals, shopping or household chores, but a family should not be afraid to say no if they feel they need rest and time alone.

Isolation can be a real problem for new mothers. The thought of getting two babies ready to go out can be quite fearful. Studies have shown the incidence of postnatal depression to be significantly higher in mothers of twins (Thorpe et al. 1991). Stress, isolation and exhaustion are all significant precipitants of depression (see Chapter 30); mothers of twins are therefore more vulnerable (Twins Trust 2018e).

DEVELOPMENT OF TWINS

Twins in most respects will do as well as a single baby, but the one area they can fall behind in, is language development. With twins, the mother tends to talk to both of them together, so there is less one-to-one communication. Inevitably, she will be much busier and the temptation to leave the twins to amuse themselves is much greater. Talking to each other, the twins act as each other's role model for language (unlike the singleton baby, who has his or her mother). If one child speaks a word incorrectly, the twin will copy it, reinforcing the mistake. This is how the so-called 'secret language' of twins develops, otherwise known as 'cryptophasia' or 'idioglossia'. It is essential that each twin is spoken to individually as much as possible. Eye contact is vital in any relationship but especially for language development. If one twin is more responsive and makes eye contact more easily than the other, the mother may respond much more readily to this twin without realizing it.

Identity and Individuality

Parents of twins should be encouraged to think of their children as individuals. The distinction between twins can start in the postnatal ward with different outfits from day 1, differently coloured blankets, or different small soft toys. As they grow up, dressing them in different style of clothes, giving them different hairstyles can make children individual. People should be encouraged to refer to the children by name, or 'the girls' or 'boys' and not 'the twins'. At birthdays or Christmas, separate cards and different presents help to retain individuality. The infants should be given the opportunity to spend time apart. This can start in the early days with one parent taking one of the twins out for a walk, leaving the other parent at home with the other baby or babies. This can be helpful in the parents connecting individually with each child, as well as supporting the development of their individuality.

Siblings of Multiples

An elder brother or sister of twins may find their arrival very difficult, especially if they have had a number of years of undivided parental attention. Parents must be alert to the feelings of their other children and include them as much as possible in all activities with the twins. A single older sibling may see the parents as a pair, the twins as a pair, while he or she feels isolated. It can be very helpful to find a 'special friend' for the older child, for instance a godparent, or other friend. A good idea is for the parents to arrange not only for the twins to have a present for the older child but for the older child to choose a present for each of the twins. Two different small cuddly toys as the first presents the twins receive can become very special gifts.

TRIPLETS AND HIGHER ORDER BIRTHS

In recent years, the numbers of triplet and higher order births has stabilized (see Table 16.1) following the guidance for IVF discussed earlier in this chapter (HFEA 2016). However, parents of triplets and the higher order multiple births will require special advice and support from healthcare workers. A woman expecting three or more babies is at risk of all the same complications as one expecting twins, but magnified. She is more likely to have a period in hospital resting before the triplets' birth and they will almost certainly be born preterm. Perinatal mortality rates are higher for triplets than twins and the incidence of cerebral palsy is also increased (Pharoah et al. 2002; Draper et al. 2018).

Triplets or more are almost always born by CS. The midwives must be prepared to receive several small babies within a very short time span. It is essential the neonatal team are present as specialist care may be required. The dangers associated with these births are asphyxia, intracranial injury and perinatal death.

The main difficulties these families experience are insufficient practical and financial help and the lack of awareness of their problems by professionals. The emotional stress and anxiety of the birth, having babies in the NICU and the worries of coping with the babies when they go home will seem overwhelming if no arrangements for extra help have been made before the babies are born. A mother should never be expected to

TABLE 16.3	**Stillbirth rates, 2014–2016**		
	2014	**2015**	**2016**
Singleton	3.96	3.72	3.86
Twins	11.07	8.36	6.16
Triplets and higher	9.98	21.81	11.75

(Data from MBRRACE: Draper ES, Gallimore ID, Kurinczuk JJ, et al.; on behalf of the MBRRACE-UK Collaboration. (2018) MBRRACE-UK Perinatal Mortality Surveillance Report, UK Perinatal Deaths for Births from January to December 2016. Leicester: The Infant Mortality and Morbidity Studies, Department of Health Sciences, University of Leicester.)

TABLE 16.4	**Infant mortality, 2014–2016**		
	2014	**2015**	**2016**
Singleton	1.59	1.64	1.60
Twins	7.81	5.26	5.34
Triplets and higher	8.40	22.30	11.93

(Data from MBRRACE: Draper ES, Gallimore ID, Kurinczuk JJ, et al.; on behalf of the MBRRACE-UK Collaboration. (2018) MBRRACE-UK Perinatal Mortality Surveillance Report, UK Perinatal Deaths for Births from January to December 2016. Leicester: The Infant Mortality and Morbidity Studies, Department of Health Sciences, University of Leicester.)

manage by herself. Taking triplets out for a walk or any expedition can need major organization, even without the parents having to cope with uninvited comments from passers-by. Some of these can be insensitive and hurtful, making inferences about fertility and the parents bringing extra work on themselves.

The midwife must ensure that the mother's health visitor and, if necessary, a social worker are involved in her care. If the family needs extra outside help, this must be organized before the babies are born. Applications to the council for rehousing may also be needed.

DISABILITY AND BEREAVEMENT

Perinatal mortality and long-term morbidity are both more common among multiple births than singletons. The perinatal mortality rate for twins is about four times that of singletons, and for triplets, 12 times (Tables 16.3, 16.4).

The grief of parents following the death of one of a multiple set is often underestimated. The specific problems they face are not understood and their needs poorly met. It often feels 'easier' to concentrate on the survivor(s), thus denying the parents essential time and space to grieve. All too often people say that they are lucky because they still have one healthy child (or more). No one ever says that to parents who lose one of their two or three singleton children (Bryan 1986). The conflicting emotions the parents will feel and the need to grieve for the child who has died, while wanting to rejoice at the birth of the healthy twin, can be confusing. Birthdays and anniversaries and the constant presence of the survivor(s) are all reminders of the dead child. The parents may need help in relating to the survivor(s). Addresses of organizations that offer support should be made available to the parents. Where one or more of a multiple set has a disability, it is often the healthy child who needs additional special attention. He or she may feel guilt that it was something they did that caused the twin's disability and may be resentful of the attention the other one needs, or of the loss of twinship. Any of these may lead to emotional and behavioural problems if not addressed early on.

MULTIFETAL PREGNANCY REDUCTION

MFPR is the reduction of an apparently healthy higher-order multiple pregnancy down to two or even one embryo, so the chances of survival are much higher. It may be offered to parents who have conceived triplets or more, whether spontaneously or as a result of assisted reproduction.

The procedure is usually carried out between the 10th and 12th week of the pregnancy. Various techniques may be used, either inserting a needle under ultrasound guidance via the vagina or, more commonly, through the abdominal wall into the fetal thorax. Potassium chloride is usually used, although some doctors prefer saline. Whichever technique is used, all embryos remain in the uterus until birth. Usually, the pregnancy is reduced to two embryos, but in some cases to three or even one (Kilby and Bricker 2016). Any parents who have been offered this treatment must be given counselling, which should include:

- the advantages and disadvantages of reducing the pregnancy
- the risks of continuing with a higher multiple pregnancy
- the risks of MFPR
- the effects on the surviving children
- how the parents may feel afterwards
- help for the parents to reach the right decision for them

- organizations who can help them
- the offer of long-term support if and when required.

Selective Feticide

This may be offered to parents with a multiple pregnancy, where one of the babies has a serious abnormality. The affected fetus is injected as described in MFPR, but this is not usually performed until much later in the pregnancy, so allowing the healthy fetus time to grow and develop normally. Counselling must again be offered to the parents. The full impact of either of these procedures and their bereavement will often not be felt until the birth of all their babies (including the dead baby), often many weeks later. Moreover, unlike the termination of a single pregnancy, the parents will be more aware of what could have been as they watch the survivor(s) grow up. When it comes to the labour, midwives must be ready to offer the appropriate care and understanding of the parents' bereavement. The bereavement should be clearly indicated in the notes so it is not forgotten when the mother comes back for her postnatal check and for future pregnancies.

SOURCES OF HELP

This will vary from country to country. In the UK for example, there is at present no statutory obligation to provide any extra help for families with twins, triplets or more. The support provided by social services varies greatly, so it is always advisable for families with triplets to apply. Healthcare workers should be prepared to write letters supporting any applications these families have made. In the UK, child benefit is paid to all children whose parents have an individual income of less than £50,000. The firstborn child receives a higher allowance than subsequent children. In multiple pregnancies, it is only the firstborn child that receives the higher allowance.

Parents should be advised to contact organizations such as Home Start (see Useful Websites, below), or local colleges with nursery training courses, both of which may be able to offer assistance.

The Multiple Births Foundation

The MBF offers advice and support to families as soon as their multiple pregnancy is diagnosed, as well as to couples considering treatment for infertility. It offers information through its antenatal meetings for couples and professionals. The MBF also provides information and support to professionals through its education programme – study days, courses, lectures and publications.

Multiple births and their impact on families is a series of publications for professionals. It comprises a set of five books, which can be bought together or individually:
- Facts about multiple births
- Multiple pregnancy
- Bereavement
- Special needs in twins
- Twins and triplets: the first five years and beyond.

See the MBF website for a complete list of the publications available.

Twins Trust

- The charity Twins Trust is a UK-wide charity supporting and campaigning for multiple birth families.
- Twins Trust provide a Helpline, a crisis team, online parenting courses both during pregnancy and throughout childhood on multiple specific challenges such a sleep, weaning behaviour and individuality. They provide a wealth of resources including parent voice videos and also free continuous professional development for health professionals.
- They also support research to help improve the outcomes for the vulnerable community.
- A list of local registered twins clubs is available and there is a very generous discount scheme for members.
- Twins Trust provides information and support to both families and health professionals, including bereavement support. Further information can be found at: https://twinstrust.org

■ REFLECTIVE ACTIVITY FOR SELF-ASSESSMENT

Multiple pregnancies are a greater risk for the mother and fetuses.

1. Why is it important to establish chorionicity when the multiple pregnancy is confirmed?
2. What support, resources and education are available in your area for parents with a multiple pregnancy?

3. Consider the role of the midwife as the lead professional for multiple pregnancies, how can she/he ensure continuity of both care and information, especially where there may be other complications to be considered.

REFERENCES

Barrett, J. F., Hannah, M. E., Hutton, E. K., & for the Twin Birth Study Collaborative Group., et al. (2013). A randomized trial of planned caesarean or vaginal delivery for twin pregnancy. *New England Journal of Medicine, 369*, 1295–1305.

Bastian, H., Keirse, M. J., & Lancaster, P. A. (1998). Perinatal death associated with planned home birth in Australia: Population based study. *British Medical Journal, 317*, 384–388.

Black, M., & Bhattacharya, S. (2010). Epidemiology of multiple pregnancy and the effect of assisted conception. *Seminars in Fetal and Neonatal Medicine, 15*(6), 306–312.

Blickstein, I., & Perlman, S. (2013). Single fetal death in twin gestations. *Journal of Perinatal Medicine, 41*(1), 65–69.

Blondel, B., & Kaminski, M. (2002). Trends in the occurrence, determinants, and consequences of multiple births. *Seminars in Perinatology, 26*(4), 239–249.

Bomsel-Helmreich, O., & Al Mufti, W. (2005). *Multiple pregnancy: Epidemiology, gestation and perinatal outcome.* New York: Informa Healthcare, 94–100.

Braude, P. (2006). *One child at a time: Reducing multiple births after IVF.* London: Human Fertilisation & Embryology Authority.

Bryan, E. M. (1986). The death of a newborn twin. How can support for parents be improved? *Acta Geneticae Medicae et Gemellologiae, 5*, 166–170.

Cutting, R., Morroll, D., Stephen, A., et al. (2008). Elective single embryo transfer: Guidelines for practice. *British Fertility Society and Association of Clinical Embryologists Human Fertility, 11*(3), 131–146.

Danon, D., Renuka, S., Hack, K. E., & Fisk, N. M. (2013). Increased stillbirth in uncomplicated monochorionic twin pregnancies: A systematic review and meta-analysis. *Obstetrics and Gynecology, 121*(6), 1318–1326.

Dias, T., Mahsid-Dornan, S., Bhide, A., et al. (2011). Systematic labeling of twin pregnancies on ultrasound. *Ultrasound in Obstetrics and Gynecology, 38*(2), 130–133.

Draper, E. S., Gallimore, I. D., Kurinczuk, J. J., & On behalf of the MBRRACE-UK Collaboration, et al. (2018). *MBRRACE-UK Perinatal Mortality Surveillance Report, UK Perinatal Deaths for Births from January to December 2016.* Leicester: The Infant Mortality and Morbidity Studies, Department of Health Sciences, University of Leicester.

Faulkner, J. (2006). *Conjoined twins: The ethics of separation.* Midwives Magazine. March 2006. Available at: www.rcm.org.

Fraser EM. (n.d.). Twin-to-twin transfusion syndrome: A guide for parents. Aldershot: Twins Trust.

Harbottle, S., Hughes, C., Cutting, R., et al. (2015). On Behalf of the Association of Clinical Embryologists & The (ACE) British Fertility Society (BFS). Elective single embryo transfer: An update to UK Best Practice Guidelines. *Human Fertility, 18*(3), 165–183.

Harigovind, D., Babu, S. H., Nair, S. V., & Sangram, N. (2018). Fetus in fetu – a rare developmental anomaly. *Radiology Case Reports, 14*(3), 333–336.

HFEA (Human Fertilisation and Embryology Authority). (2016). *Fertility treatment 2014: Trends and figures.* London: HFEA.

Huston, R. K., Markell, A. M., McCulley, E. A., et al. (2014). Decreasing necrotizing enterocolitis and gastrointestinal bleeding in the neonatal intensive care unit: The role of donor human milk and exclusive human milk diets in infants ≤1500 g birth weight. *Childhood Obesity and Nutrition, 6*(2), 86–93.

Jacklin P, Marceniuk G. (n.d.). A report by the National Guideline Alliance about twin pregnancy costing. London: Royal College of Obstetricians and Gynaecologists.

Ji, Y., Chen, S., Zhong, L., et al. (2014). Fetus in fetu: Two case reports and literature review. *BMC Pediatrics, 14*, 88.

Khalil, A., Rodgers, M., Baschat, A., et al. (2015). ISUOG Practice Guidelines: Role of ultrasound in twin pregnancy. *Ultrasound in Obstetrics and Gynecology, 47*(2), 247–263.

Kilby, M. D., & Bricker, L. (2016). On behalf of the Royal College of Obstetricians and Gynaecologists. Management of monochorionic twin pregnancy. *BJOG, 124*, e1–e45.

Lai, N. M., Foong, S. C., Foong, W. C., & Tan, K. (2017). Co-bedding in neonatal nursery for promoting growth and neurodevelopment in stable preterm twins. *Cochrane Database of Systematic Reviews* (4), CD008313.

Landy, H. J., & Keith, L. G. (1998). The vanishing twin. A review. *Human Reproduction, 4*, 177.

Lassi, Z. S., Salam, R. A., Haider, B. A., et al. (2013). Folic acid supplementation during pregnancy for maternal health and pregnancy outcomes. *Cochrane Database of Systematic Reviews* (3), CD006896.

Leonard, L. G. (2000). Breastfeeding triplets: The at-home experience. *Public Health Nursing, 17*(3), 211–221.

Leonard, L. G., & Denton, J. (2006). Preparation for parenting multiple birth children. *Early Human Development, 82*, 371–378.

Maruotti, G. M., Saccone, G., & Martinelli, P. (2016). First-trimester ultrasound determination of chorionicity in twin gestations using the lambda sign: A systematic review and meta-analysis. *European Journal of Obstetrics, Gynecology and Reproductive Biology, 202*, 66–70.

McKay, S. (2010). *The effects of twins and multiple births on families and their living standards*. Aldershot: Twins Trust.

NICE (National Institute for Health and Care Excellence). (2008/2019). *Antenatal care: Routine care for the healthy pregnant woman. CG 62*. London: NICE.

NICE (National Institute for Health and Care Excellence). (2011). *Caesarean Section CG 132*. London: NICE.

NICE (National Institute for Health and Care Excellence). (2018). *Endorsed resource – multiple antenatal care pathway*. Available at: www.NICE.org.uk.

NICE (National Institute for Health and Care Excellence). (2019). *Twins and triplet pregnancy. NG 137*. London: NICE.

ONS (Office of National Statistics). (2017). *Births Characteristics in England and Wales*. 2016. Available at www.ons.gov.uk.

Pasquini, L., Wimalasundera, R. C., & Fisk, N. M. (2004). Management of other complications specific to monochorionic twin pregnancies. *Best Practice and Research in Clinical Obstetrics and Gynaecology, 18*(4), 577–599.

Paterson-Brown, S., & Howell, C. (2014). *Managing obstetric emergencies and trauma*. Cambridge: Cambridge University Press.

Pharoah, P. O., Price, T. S., & Plomin, R. (2002). Cerebral palsy in twins: A national study. *Archives of Disease in Childhood Fetal Neonatal Edition, 87*(2), F122–F124.

RCOG (Royal College of Obstetricians and Gynaecologists). (2010). Amniocentesis and chorionic villus sampling. *Greentop Guideline No 8*. London: RCOG.

RCOG (Royal College of Obstetricians and Gynaecologists). (2014). Non-invasive prenatal testing for chromosomal abnormality using maternal plasma DNA. *Scientific Impact Paper No 15*. London: RCOG.

RCOG (Royal College of Obstetricians and Gynaecologists). (2017). *Each baby counts report*. Available at: www.rcog.org.uk/globalassets/documents/guidelines/research–audit/each-baby-counts-2015-full-report.pdf.

Stagg, K. (2017). Breastfeeding twins – and more! *AIMS Journal, 29*, 4.

Stirrup, O. T., Khalil, A., D'Antonio, F., & Thilaganathan, B. (2014). Fetal growth reference ranges in twin pregnancy: Analysis of the Southwest Thames Obstetric Research Collaborative (STORK) multiple pregnancy cohort. *Ultrasound in Obstetrics and Gynecology, 45*(3), 301–307.

Thorpe, K., Golding, J., MacGillivray, I., et al. (1991). Comparisons of prevalence of depression in mothers of twins and mothers of singletons. *British Medical Journal, 302*, 875–878.

Tran, P. L., Desveaux, C., Barau, G., et al. (2015). Delayed-interval delivery in multifetal pregnancy: A review and guidelines for management. *Gynecology and Obstetrics (Sunnyvale), 5*, 333.

Twins Trust. (n.d.). Enhancing individuality in multiples. Available at: https://twinstrust.org.

Twins Trust. (2018a). *Twins Trust courses*. Available at: https://twinstrust.org/Courses.

Twins Trust. (2018b). *Twins and multiples clubs*. Available at: https://twinstrust.org/clubs.

Twins Trust. (2018c). *Multiple pregnancy antenatal care proforma and care pathways*. Available at: www.nice.org.uk/guidance/cg129/resources/endorsed-resource-multiple-antenatal-care-pathway-4844249677.

Twins Trust. (2018d). *How do I feed my twins, triplets or more?* Available at: https://twinstrust.org.

Twins Trust. (2018e). *Postnatal depression (PND)*. Available at: https://twinstrust.org.

Twins Trust. (2018f). *Safer sleeping*. Available at: https://twinstrust.org.

Twins Trust. (2018g). *Being a grandparent to twins, triplets or more*. Available at: https://twinstrust.org.

Wood, S. L., Onge, R. S., Connors, G., et al. (1996). Evaluation of the twin peak or lambda sign in determining chorionicity in multiple pregnancy. *Obstetrics and Gynecology, 88*(1), 6–9.

ANNOTATED FURTHER READING

Cooper, C. (2004). *Twins and multiple births*. London: Vermilion.

A GP and mother of twins gives practical advice on coping with twins and more. Suitable for parents and professionals alike.

Karaman, I., Erdogan, D., Ozalevli, S., et al. (2008). Fetus in fetu: A report of two cases. *Journal of Indian Association of Pediatric Surgeons, 13*(1), 30–32.

An interesting read of a rare phenomenon.

RCOG (Royal College of Obstetricians and Gynaecologists). (2016). *Multiple pregnancy: Having more than one baby*. London: RCOG Press.

Written by specialists in multiple pregnancy.

USEFUL WEBSITES

Homestart UK: www.home-start.org.uk

Multiple Births Foundation: www.multiplebirths.org.uk

Contact details: Tel: 020 3313 3519; e-mail: imperial.mbf@nhs.net

Twins Trust: https://twinstrust.org

Contact details: Tel: 01252 332 344; e-mail: enquiries@twinstrust.org; Twins Trust, Manor House, Church Hill, Aldershot, Hants, GU12 4JU, UK.

Labour

17

Care of the Perineum, Repair and Female Genital Mutilation

Ranee Thakar, Abdul H. Sultan, Maureen D. Raynor, Carol McCormick, Michael R. B. Keighley

CHAPTER CONTENTS

In the UK, approximately 85% of women sustain some degree of perineal trauma following vaginal birth and it can be extrapolated that millions of women will be affected worldwide. The prevalence of perineal trauma is dependent on variations in midwifery and obstetric practice, including rates and types of episiotomy, which vary not only between countries but also between individual practitioners within hospitals. The Euro-Peristat project, which included 20 European countries showed a wide variation in the episiotomy rates ranging from 3.7% in Denmark to 75% in Cyprus. Morbidity in the short and long term following trauma and repair can lead to major physical, psychological, sexual and social problems affecting the woman's ability to care for her newborn baby and other members of the family. Midwives should be aware that suturing is a major and sometimes traumatic event for women. The repair of the perineum is an important part of the continuing care of a woman during labour and birth. The permanent presence of midwives who are trained and continually developing expertise in perineal repair, minimizes the problems associated with the rotation of inexperienced junior medical staff and provides continuity of care for women. This chapter presents an overview of key issues relating to perineal care during labour and childbirth. It is important that the reader has knowledge and understanding of the anatomy and physiology of the pelvic floor (see Chapter 3) prior to engaging with this chapter (Blondel et al. 2016; Green et al. 1998; Kettle 2012; Draper and Newell 1996).

THE CHAPTER AIMS TO

- draw on the evidence base to identify some of the factors associated with a reduced incidence of perineal trauma during the second stage of labour
- examine the standard classification used to describe the different types of perineal trauma
- discuss the systematic assessment necessary in order to accurately diagnose perineal trauma

- highlight the significance of female genital mutilation and the inherent consequences for birth and women's psychosexual wellbeing and health more broadly
- consider the basic principles involved in repairing perineal trauma
- examine the midwife's role and medicolegal considerations involved in perineal trauma.

PREVENTION OF PERINEAL TRAUMA

Proven strategies to reduce perineal trauma include: the practice of perineal massage in the antenatal period (Beckmann and Stock 2013); use of warm perineal compresses in the second stage of labour (Aasheim et al. 2017); restrictive use of episiotomy (Jiang et al. 2017); preference of a correctly performed mediolateral over a midline episiotomy (Coats et al. 1980); and the use of a vacuum extractor instead of forceps for instrumental birth (Gurol-Urganci et al. 2013). Recent years have witnessed a growing interest in the technique of manual perineal protection (Laine et al. 2012) as a means to reduce anal sphincter trauma. It is possible that one intervention on its own may not be as beneficial as a combination of interventions and therefore 'care bundles' have been suggested. Such a health improvement project involving an 'OASI care bundle' is currently underway in the UK. It must be acknowledged that certain antenatal risk factors such as maternal nutritional status, body mass index, ethnicity, infant birth weight, race, length of the perineal body, previous perineal trauma and age cannot be altered at the time of birth, but awareness of these factors might prompt modifications in the care pathway. Box 17.1 provides a summary of some the arsenal of measures the midwife can employ to minimize perineal trauma.

DEFINITION OF PERINEAL TRAUMA

Perineal trauma may occur spontaneously during vaginal birth or when a surgical incision (episiotomy) is intentionally made to facilitate birth. It is possible to have an episiotomy and a spontaneous tear (e.g. extension of an episiotomy). Anterior perineal trauma is defined as injury to the labia, anterior vaginal wall,

BOX 17.1 Strategies to Prevent/Minimize Perineal Trauma during Labour

Influencing Factors	The Evidence
Antenatal perineal massage but not perineal massage during the second stage of labour	Beckmann and Stock (2013)
Use of warm perineal compresses during the second stage of labour	Aasheim et al. (2017)
Restricted use of episiotomy	Jiang et al. (2017)
Upright birth positions – freedom of woman to choose	Gupta et al. (2017)
Non-directed pushing (woman using her own urges to bear down without coaching from the midwife or doctor)	NICE (2014)

urethra or clitoris. Posterior perineal trauma is defined as any injury to the posterior vaginal wall or perineal muscles and may include disruption of the anal sphincters.

In order to standardize definitions of perineal tears, the classification outlined in Table 17.1 is recommended (Royal College of Obstetricians and Gynaecologists, RCOG 2015a; National Institute for Health and Care Excellence, NICE 2014). (See Chapter 3 for details of pelvic floor anatomy; see also Fig. 17.1).

EPISIOTOMY

The traditional teaching that episiotomy is protective against more severe perineal lacerations has not been substantiated and therefore the liberal use of 'prophylactic' episiotomy is no longer recommended (Jiang et al. 2017). However, there are still valid reasons to perform

TABLE 17.1	**Classification of Perineal Trauma**
First degree	Injury to perineal skin only
Second degree	Injury to perineum involving perineal muscles but not involving the anal sphincter
Third degree	Injury to perineum involving the anal sphincter complex: 3a. <50% of external anal sphincter (EAS) thickness torn 3b. >50% of external anal sphincter thickness torn 3c. Both external anal sphincter and internal anal sphincter (IAS) torn
Fourth degree	Injury to perineum involving the anal sphincter complex and anal epithelium
Isolated button hole injury of rectum	Injury to the rectal mucosa without injury to the anal sphincters

NICE (National Institute for Health and Care Excellence). (2014) Intrapartum care: care of healthy women and their babies: CG 190. Available at: www.nice.org.uk/guidance/cg190; RCOG (Royal College of Obstetricians and Gynaecologists. (2015a) Management of third and fourth degree tears. Green-top Guideline No 29. Available at: www.rcog.org.uk/globalassets/documents/guidelines/gtg-29.pdf.

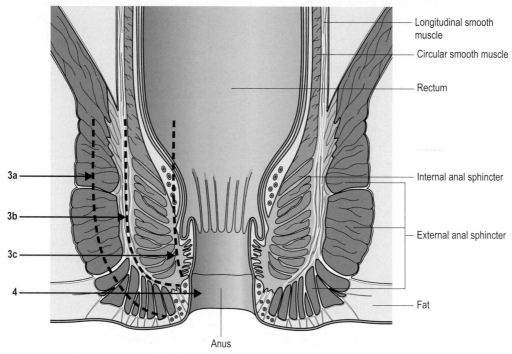

Fig. 17.1 Classification of perineal trauma depicted in a schematic representation of the anal sphincters. (Modified from Sultan AH, Kettle C. (2007) Diagnosis of perineal trauma. In: AH Sultan, R Thakar, D Fenner (Eds) Perineal and anal sphincter trauma. London: Springer-Verlag.)

an episiotomy. A variety of episiotomy techniques are described in the literature (Kalis et al. 2012), but two types of episiotomy are most frequently used:

- *Midline episiotomy.* Advantages of the midline episiotomy are that it does not cut through muscle, the two sides of the incised area are anatomically

balanced, making surgical repair easier, and blood loss is less than with mediolateral episiotomy. A major drawback is that extension through the external anal sphincter and into the rectum can occur. For this reason midline episiotomy is not recommended in the UK.

- *Mediolateral episiotomy.* The right mediolateral episiotomy is the technique approved for use by midwives in the UK. The incision is made starting at the midline of the posterior fourchette and aimed towards the ischial tuberosity to avoid the anal sphincter. In addition to the skin and subcutaneous tissues, the bulbospongiosus and the transverse perineal muscles are cut.

Angle of a Mediolateral Episiotomy

A mediolateral episiotomy is defined as one that is performed between 40 and 60 degrees from the midline. However, in a prospective study of women having their first vaginal birth, Andrews et al. (2006) demonstrated that no midwife and only 13 (22%) doctors performed a truly mediolateral episiotomy and that the majority of the incisions were in fact directed closer to the midline, indicating a need for improved training in the art of performing an episiotomy. The incidence of obstetric anal sphincter injuries (OASIS) appears to be related to the angle of episiotomies as episiotomies angled closer to the midline were associated with a higher incidence of OASIS (Andrews et al. 2006). Eogan et al. (2006) demonstrated that there was a 50% reduction in OASIS for every 6 degrees away from the midline. However, if the episiotomy angle becomes nearly horizontal (90 degrees), the pressure on the perineum is not relieved and OASIS incidence increases nine-fold (Stedenfeldt et al. 2012). In a prospective study, an incision angle of mediolateral episiotomy of 60 degrees resulted in a low incidence of anal sphincter tearing, anal incontinence and perineal pain (Kalis et al. 2011). When episiotomy is indicated, the mediolateral technique should be used on the distended perineum, with careful attention to ensure that the angle is 60 degrees away from the midline (RCOG 2015a).

DIAGNOSIS OF PERINEAL TRAUMA

Following every vaginal birth a thorough assessment should be performed to exclude genital trauma. The healthcare professional should explain to the woman what they plan to do and why, obtain consent, offer inhalational analgesia and ensure that, if there is pre-existing epidural analgesia, it is effective. There must be good lighting and the woman should be positioned so that she is comfortable and the genital structures can be seen clearly. If this is not possible then it is vital to explain to the woman the rationale for the examination and why it is necessary to place her in a comfortable position, i.e. lithotomy (NICE 2014). In the UK, modern birthing beds in the hospital setting mean that the use of lithotomy poles in midwifery practice to support women's legs during examination of the genital tract or to repair perineal trauma is not always warranted. However, supported lithotomy (i.e. use of poles) is necessary to aid the diagnosis and repair of complex trauma to the genital tract. When a supported lithotomy position is to be employed, clear explanation should be provided to the woman in a sensitive manner. The midwife should be mindful that use of lithotomy poles may conjure up images associated with previous sexual abuse or female genital mutilation/female cutting (Kettle and Raynor 2010). Visualization, effective analgesia and systematic assessment of perineal trauma can be even more challenging at a homebirth, not least because of poor lighting and the use of settees or low bedroom furniture. When faced with such complexities, it is perfectly acceptable for midwives attending home births to transfer women into the hospital setting for thorough assessment, especially if the repair is judged not to be straightforward or the midwife does not have the requisite skills/competence to perform the repair.

Importance of Anorectal Examination

Informed consent must be obtained for a vaginal and rectal examination. If the digital assessment is restricted because of pain, adequate analgesia must be given prior to examination. Following inspection of the genitalia, the labia should be parted and a vaginal examination performed to establish the full extent of the vaginal tear. When multiple or deep tears are present it is best to examine and repair in the supported lithotomy position, as previously stated.

A rectal examination should then be performed to exclude anal sphincter trauma. Fig. 17.2 shows a partial tear along the external anal sphincter, which would have been missed if a rectal examination was not performed. Every woman should have a rectal examination prior to suturing in order to avoid missing isolated tears such as a 'button hole' of the rectal mucosa (NICE 2014). Furthermore, a third- or fourth-degree tear may be present beneath apparently intact perineal skin, highlighting the need to perform a rectal examination in order to exclude OASIS following every vaginal birth (Sultan and Kettle 2007) (Fig. 17.3). Following diagnosis of the

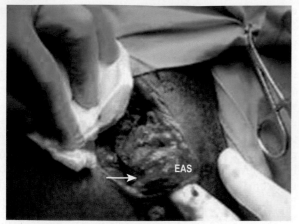

Fig. 17.2 A partial tear (arrow) along the external anal sphincter (EAS), which would have been missed if a rectal examination was not performed. (Sultan AH, Kettle C. (2007) Diagnosis of perineal trauma. In: AH Sultan, R Thakar, D Fenner (Eds) Perineal and anal sphincter trauma. London: Springer-Verlag.)

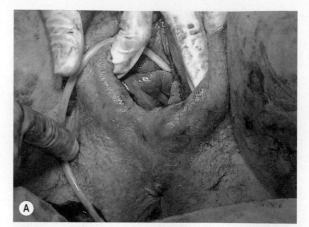

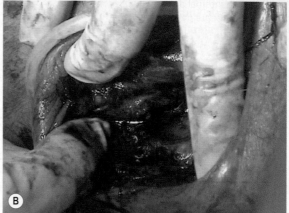

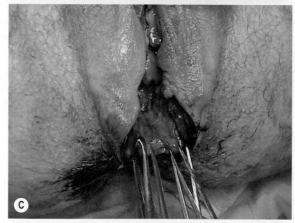

Fig. 17.3 A third- or fourth-degree tear may be present beneath apparently intact perineal skin highlighting the need to perform a rectal examination in order to exclude obstetric anal sphincter injuries (OASIS) following every vaginal delivery. (A) An apparent intact perineum. (B) A 'bucket handle tear' is demonstrated behind the intact perineal skin. (C) The torn external anal sphincter. (Sultan AH, Kettle C. (2007) Diagnosis of perineal trauma. In: AH Sultan, R Thakar, D Fenner (Eds) Perineal and anal sphincter trauma. London: Springer-Verlag.)

tear it should be graded according to the recommended classification (NICE 2014; RCOG 2015a), as delineated earlier in Table 17.1.

In order to diagnose OASIS, clear visualization is necessary and the injury should be confirmed by palpation. By inserting the gloved index finger in the anal canal and the thumb in the vagina, the anal sphincter can be palpated by performing a pill-rolling motion. If there is still uncertainty, the woman should be asked to contract her anal sphincter (in the absence of an epidural) and if the anal sphincter is disrupted, there will be a distinct gap felt anteriorly. If the perineal skin is intact there will be an absence of puckering on the perianal skin anteriorly. This may not be evident under regional or general anaesthesia. As the external anal sphincter (EAS) is normally in a state of tonic contraction, disruption results in retraction of the sphincter ends. The internal anal sphincter (IAS) is a circular smooth muscle that appears paler (similar to raw fish) (Fig. 17.4) than the striated EAS (similar to raw red meat) (Sultan and Kettle 2007) (Fig. 17.5).

FEMALE GENITAL MUTILATION/GENITAL CUTTING/FEMALE CIRCUMCISION

Background

Partly as a result of immigration and refugee movements, women who have undergone female

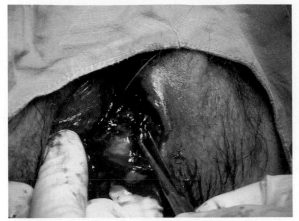

Fig. 17.4 The internal anal sphincter (IAS) is a circular smooth muscle that appears pale (similar to raw fish).

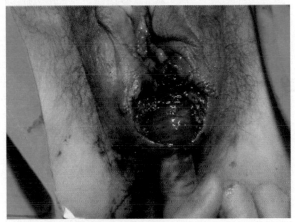

Fig. 17.5 The external anal sphincter (EAS) is striated muscle and appears red in colour (similar to raw red meat).

genital mutilation (FGM) now present all over the world. Therefore healthcare professionals in all countries need to be familiar with the practice of genital cutting and its implications, particularly for childbirth and safeguarding of the next generation, as well as to be proactive in eradicating this harmful cultural practice altogether.

The language used by midwives and doctors when dealing with genital cutting is important, as parents understandably resent the suggestion that they have mutilated their daughters. As a result, the word 'cutting' has increasingly come to be used to avoid alienating communities (World Health Organization, WHO 2018a,b).

TABLE 17.2	**Classification of FGM**
Type I	Partial or total removal of the clitoris and/or the prepuce (clitoridectomy)
Type II	Partial or total removal of the clitoris and labia minora, with or without excision of the labia majora
Type III	Also referred to as infibulation this is narrowing of the vaginal orifice with creation of a covering seal by cutting and appositioning the labia minora and/or the labia majora, with or without excision of the clitoris
Type IV	All other harmful procedures to the female genitalia for non-medical purposes, for example: pricking, piercing, incising, scraping and cauterization.

WHO (World Health Organization). (2001) Management of pregnancy, childbirth and postpartum period in the presence of female genital mutilation. Geneva: WHO.

There has been great debate among holy men as to whether, particularly *type I* genital cutting (sometimes referred to as *Sunna* circumcision), is required in the Muslim faith, but it is clear that female genital cutting is not linked to the *Bible* or the *Koran*. It is in fact condemned by many Islamic scholars. Genital cutting predates both the *Koran* and the *Bible*, appearing in the 2nd century BC. It is a cultural practice, not a religious one. In countries when there is a mixture of Christians and Muslims it is practiced by both faiths (WHO 2001, 2008, 2018b).

What actually happens to the girls and women varies from ritualistic herbs rubbed into the genitalia to complete removal of the clitoris and labia minora, and stitching (or closing by other means, usually thorns) of the labia majora. The WHO (2001) define FGM (Table 17.2) as any procedure that intentionally alters or causes injury to the external female genital organs for non-medical reasons and describes four types, as depicted in Fig. 17.6.

In practice, however, it is often difficult to be clear about the classification. Uneven cutting, scarring and defects in suture lines are very common findings, therefore every woman who has undergone genital cutting should be assessed by an experienced practitioner. Ideally this should be done in the antenatal period in order that an individualized care plan can be

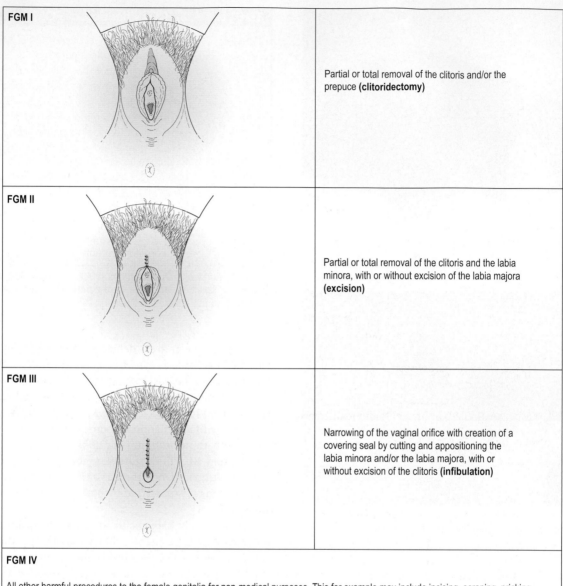

FGM I	Partial or total removal of the clitoris and/or the prepuce (**clitoridectomy**)
FGM II	Partial or total removal of the clitoris and the labia minora, with or without excision of the labia majora (**excision**)
FGM III	Narrowing of the vaginal orifice with creation of a covering seal by cutting and appositioning the labia minora and/or the labia majora, with or without excision of the clitoris (**infibulation**)

FGM IV

All other harmful procedures to the female genitalia for non-medical purposes. This for example may include incising, scraping, pricking, piercing or other mutilating procedure.
Source: (UNICEF 2005)

Fig. 17.6 Types of female genital mutilation (FGM).

formulated in conjunction with the woman in advance of labour.

The age at which girls undergo genital cutting varies enormously according to their community. The procedure may be carried out when the girl is a newborn, during childhood, adolescence, at marriage or during the first pregnancy. Most commonly it is performed on girls between 4 and 8 years of age (WHO 2001, 2008).

Girls are usually compliant when they have the procedure carried out as they believe they will be outcasts if they are not cut. Mothers and other family members believe they are doing the best for their children, as women are thought to be unclean and immoral unless they had been cut. In most cultures that are steeped in patriarchy and the practice of FGM the girls/women would be unmarriageable if uncut. So deep-rooted is this cultural tradition that it is the opinion of some that a woman will not be promiscuous or unfaithful if she derives little or no pleasure from sexual intercourse (Elnashar and Abdelhady 2007). Despite being aware of the dangers associated with genital cutting, it is this very strong belief that makes parents ensure their daughters are cut in accordance with their cultural custom and tradition.

Anaesthetics and antiseptic treatment are not generally used and the practice is usually carried out using basic tools such as circumcision knives, scissors, scalpels, pieces of glass and razor blades. Often iodine or a mixture of herbs is placed on the wound to tighten the vagina and stop the bleeding.

Immediate complications include severe pain, shock, haemorrhage, tetanus, sepsis and urinary retention. Women who are inexperienced or very old cutters may inadvertently cause injury to adjacent tissue. Late complications include sexual dysfunction with anorgasmia, keloid scar formation, dermoid cysts and psychological issues. There is an increasing trend for medically trained personnel to perform FGM in hospitals and institutions (Hassanin et al. 2008). There are no known health benefits associated with FGM.

In the UK, the Prohibition of Female Circumcision Act 1985 (Home Office 1985) makes it an offence to carry out FGM or to aid, abet or procure the service of another person. The Female Genital Mutilation amendment to the Act 2003 makes it against the law for FGM to be performed anywhere in the world on UK permanent residents of any age and carries a maximum sentence of 14 years' imprisonment (Home Office 2004). In an effort to eradicate the anachronistic practice of FGM, Europe and many other countries also have laws against FGM. England and Wales now have enshrined in legislation a mandatory reporting duty that was enforced in 2015 (Home Office 2015). This requires all regulated health and social care professionals and teachers to report known cases of FGM in girls under the age of 18 years old to the police. Further information about mandatory reporting in the aforementioned countries can be accessed at: www.gov.uk/government/publications/

mandatory-reporting-of-female-genital-mutilation-procedural-information.

The Role of the Midwife

In order to have a robust plan of care during labour, identification of women from countries where FGM is a traditional practice, is essential antenatally. NICE (2008) highlights the importance of antenatal screening of these women. This should be performed in a timely manner so that referral and consultation with a practitioner who can address both the physical needs of the woman plus the safeguarding and legal issues for the unborn child in a sensitive manner can take place.

Antenatally, physical examination is necessary to assess the extent of genital cutting and make a birth plan, also to identify whether antenatal surgery (deinfibulation) would be beneficial before 20 weeks of pregnancy. Most women would prefer a deinfibulation in labour but a plan to deinfibulate during labour means all staff must have adequate training and experience in performing the procedure, which in most hospitals is an unrealistic expectation. Even women who have given birth before or have had a previous deinfibulation should be examined, as they may have suffered trauma at the last birth and some women will have undergone a reinfibulation (being 'closed' again), usually in their country of origin.

There is contradicting evidence as to whether FGM is associated with prolonged or obstructed labour (De Silva 1989; Al-Hussaini 2003; Millogo-Traore et al. 2007). However, during the second stage of labour the reduced labia and inelastic anterior tissue may be scarred and adherent to the labial vault and/or urethra, and therefore the birth process can cause significant anterior trauma to these structures. A low threshold for a right mediolateral episiotomy should be discussed with the woman antenatally, particularly if the type of cutting has left scar tissue that may prevent progress or cause additional trauma in the form of an anterior tear in the second stage of labour (RCOG 2015b).

A proforma including a predrawn diagram, akin to that outlined in the RCOG (2015b) guideline, should be completed for the identification of the type of FGM and the agreed birth plan as part of good note-keeping. The impact of FGM is very profound, as captured by the personal story of Kinsi (Case Study 17.1).

CASE STUDY 17.1 Kinsi's Story of FGM

When I was asked if I minded sharing a short personal account about my experience of having undergone FGM, I was only too happy to oblige with the proviso that FGM affects every girl and woman differently.

I was born in a country where the practice of FGM was, and still is, very prevalent where approximately 95–98% of young girls/women have experienced FGM. There was never any doubt or question that I, along with all my sisters, would undergo FGM. It was always a matter of when, not if.

I was about 8 years old when the day arrived. A few days earlier I was told that I would be made clean, proper and a real girl going into womanhood. I was shown a little bag, containing a present for me, a new dress, which I would be allowed to wear on the day. The day before it happened, my mum said I would not need to do any household chores the following day and I could sleep longer in the morning, and enjoy a special breakfast, just for me. I was getting really excited about all these special treats – little did I know what it all meant.

It must have been approaching midday when a strange looking old woman arrived with dusty and dirty looking sack of unknown contents. My mum, my aunty and a neighbour were already present. We lived in a small hut made of straw and twigs in the middle of the open land, 20 miles away from the nearest town. There was no running water, no hygienic environment, and no sanitized equipment. I was told to sit in the middle of the four ladies. The first thing I remember seeing was a razor blade. I remember the old lady showing it to my mum, presumably reassuring her that it was clean and not too rusty. I remember feeling alarmed and frightened by the sight of the razor blade, and mum reassuring me and telling me to be brave and to fill my mouth with my dress and keep gripping it with my teeth.

Things became rather too blurred too quickly. I can't say how long it lasted. I think I might have fainted or was paralysed by the pain but I do not remember struggling too long. I had type III FGM.

Recovery was very painful. I was 'stitched-up' using 16 long thorns, eight in each direction in an alternate pattern. My legs were tied together from hips to toes and I was told to lie only on my side to aid the process of the two edges sealing together. I was not allowed much food, just a very small amount of porridge and milk every other day. Passing water was unbearable and I remember how much I dreaded it and tried to avoid it by not drinking anything. I was told if I didn't pee my bladder would eventually burst and I would have to go through the whole thing all over again, a terrifying prospect.

Eight days later, the old lady came back, inspected her handiwork and declared it a success. She took the thorns out and told me to start walking with very little steps. She also loosened the rope that was tied around my legs. That was the first time in days that I slept a full night's sleep. A week later, I was allowed to remove the rope around my legs.

As I said at the start, FGM affects women and girls differently. I heard many horror stories of girls dying in rural Africa while undergoing FGM. I have been lucky to the extent that I am alive and well.

Nonetheless, in my case, I would say the effects have been more psychological than physical. Of course, I have a mutilated genitalia, which is a daily reminder of the brutal way my clitoris and other parts were removed. It still takes me a lot longer to pass water than the average 'intact' woman, despite being fully 'opened-up' for over 25 years. However, the greatest impact has been the loss of my childhood and the loss of my womanhood. Loss of a childhood because FGM ended who I was: a happy, carefree, playful and a popular child who was full of excitement and of the possibilities of what the future might bring. I emerged as traumatized, subdued, passive, docile, quiet and indifferent young person who was neither a child nor a woman. I do not remember playing or behaving like a child after that day. Nor was I expected to be one. This was the passage to womanhood, to prosperity, to a good marriage and motherhood.

The irony, for me, is that what should have completed me as a woman deprived me of the very thing.

I would have done anything to have my body left intact as it was and to have experienced a normal sex life. For most women sex is probably a pleasurable part of a fulfilled life, but, for me, this was something I never had the chance to find out. It is difficult to quantify or to explain how FGM affected me; it has been a life-long physical and psychological pain which will remain with me for as long as I live.

REPAIR OF PERINEAL TRAUMA

Basic Principles Prior to Repairing Perineal Trauma

The skills and knowledge of the operator are important factors in achieving a successful repair (Sultan and Thakar 2007). Ideally, the repair should be conducted in a timely manner by the same midwife who attended the woman in labour. This ensures seamless continuity of care, as the midwife would have established a good rapport and trust with the woman. The woman should be referred to a more experienced healthcare professional if uncertainty exists as to the nature or extent of trauma sustained. Having fully informed the woman why a detailed examination is required and to gain her consent, an initial systematic assessment of the perineal trauma must be performed including a sensitive rectal examination to exclude any trauma to the IAS/EAS is not missed (NICE 2014).

In order to reduce maternal morbidity, repair of the perineum should be undertaken as soon as possible to minimize the risk of bleeding and oedema of the perineum as this makes it more difficult to recognize tissue structures and planes when the repair eventually takes place. Perineal trauma should be repaired using aseptic techniques. Equipment should be checked and swabs and needles counted before and after the procedure.

A repair undertaken on a non-cooperative woman, due to pain, is likely to result in a poor repair and distress for the woman. Ensure that the wound is adequately anaesthetized prior to commencing the repair. It is recommended that 10–20 mL of lidocaine 1% (maximum dose 3 mg/kg) is injected evenly into the perineal wound. If the woman has an epidural it may be 'topped-up' instead of injecting local anaesthetic.

The issue of obstetric anal sphincter injuries is addressed in more detail later in the chapter, but it is worth noting here that repair of such trauma should be undertaken in theatre, under general or regional anaesthesia. In addition to providing pain relief, this provides the added advantage of relaxing the muscles, enabling the operator to retrieve the ends of the torn sphincter and identify the full length of the anal sphincter prior to repair. An indwelling catheter should be inserted for at least 12 h to avoid urinary retention.

In the case of FGM, if a woman undergoes a deliberate traumatic deinfibulation in labour without antenatal preparation she may ask to be reinfibulated (closed again), but any repair carried out after birth, whether following spontaneous laceration or deliberate defibulation, should be sufficient to repair the raw edges of the perineal trauma and control bleeding. It is important that the raw edges of the wound are not brought back together to reform a seal, i.e. reinfibulate as this is illegal. Refer to earlier comments about mandatory reporting in countries where this is now a legal requirement. Further, the repair must not result in a vaginal opening that makes intercourse difficult or impossible, as this would be in breach of the law.

First-Degree Tears and Labial Lacerations

Women should be advised that, in the case of first-degree trauma, the wound should be sutured in order to improve healing, unless the skin edges are well opposed (NICE 2014). If the tear is left unsutured, the midwife or doctor must discuss the implications with the woman and obtain her informed consent. Details regarding the discussion and consent must be fully documented in the woman's case notes.

Labial lacerations are usually very superficial but may be very painful. Some practitioners do not recommend suturing, but if the trauma is bilateral the lacerations can sometimes adhere together over the urethra and the woman may present with voiding difficulties. It is important to advise the woman to part the labia daily during bathing to prevent adhesions forming. This is particularly important when caring for women with type III FGM.

Episiotomy and Second-Degree Tears

Although the repair of these tears was previously carried out using the interrupted technique, the continuous suturing technique for perineal skin closure has been shown to be associated with less short-term pain. Moreover, if the continuous technique is used for all layers (vagina, perineal muscles and skin), the reduction in pain is even greater (Kettle et al. 2012). The perineal muscles should be repaired using absorbable polyglactin material, which is available in standard and rapidly absorbable forms. A Cochrane review has shown that there are few differences in short-term and long-term pain, between standard and rapidly absorbing synthetic sutures, but more women need standard sutures to be removed (Kettle et al. 2010).

Technique for Perineal Repair

Technique is important, as is the suturing material used (Kettle and Fenner 2007).

Suturing the Vagina

Using 2/0 absorbable polyglactin 910 material (*Vicryl rapide*), the first stitch is inserted above the apex of the vaginal skin laceration to secure any bleeding points (Fig. 17.7A). The vaginal laceration is closed using a loose, continuous, non-locking technique ensuring that each stitch is inserted not more than 1 cm apart to avoid vaginal narrowing. Suturing is continued down to the hymenal remnants and the needle is inserted through the skin at the fourchette to emerge in the centre of the perineal wound.

Suturing the Muscle Layer

The muscle layer is then approximated after assessing the depth of the trauma and the perineal muscles (deep and superficial) are approximated with continuous non-locking stitches (Fig. 17.7B). If the trauma is deep, two layers of continuous stitches can be inserted through the perineal muscles.

Suturing the Perineal Skin

To suture the perineal skin the needle is brought out at the inferior end of the wound, just under the skin surface (Fig. 17.7C). The skin sutures are placed below the skin surface in the subcutaneous tissue, thus avoiding the profusion of nerve endings. Bites of tissue are taken from each side of the wound edges until the hymenal remnants are reached. A loop or Aberdeen knot is placed in the vagina behind the hymenal remnants.

A vaginal examination is carried out to ensure that the vagina is not narrowed and a rectal examination carried out to ensure that sutures have not been inadvertently placed through the anorectal epithelium.

OBSTETRIC ANAL SPHINCTER INJURIES

Obstetric anal sphincter injuries (OASIS) are reported to occur in 2.9% (6.1% in primiparae) of woman in centres where mediolateral episiotomies are practiced (Thiagamoorthy et al. 2014), compared with 12% (Coats et al. 1980) (19% in primiparae) (Fenner et al. 2003) in centres practicing midline episiotomy. However, rates as

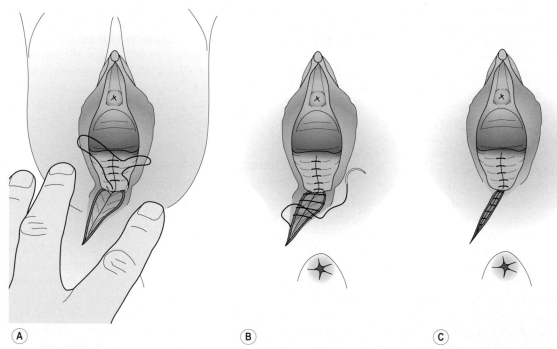

Fig. 17.7 Continuous suturing technique for mediolateral episiotomy: (A) loose continuous non-locking stitch to the vaginal wall; (B) loose, continuous non-locking stitch to the perineal muscle; (C) closure of skin using a loose subcutaneous stitch. (Kettle C, Fenner D. (2007) Repair of episiotomy, first and second degree tears. In: AH Sultan, R Thakar, D Fenner (Eds) Perineal and anal sphincter trauma. London: Springer.)

high as 7.5% have been reported in centres practicing mediolateral episiotomy, suggesting increased awareness, training and improvement in recognition of OASIS (Nordenstam et al. 2008; Ekeus et al. 2008). However, despite recognition and primary repair of acute OASIS, 39% of those diagnosed have symptoms of anal incontinence and persistent anal sphincter defects have been identified on ultrasound in 34–91% within 3 months of delivery (Sultan and Thakar 2007).

Technique for OASIS Repair

In the presence of a fourth-degree tear, the torn anorectal epithelium is sutured with a continuous 3/0 Vicryl suture (Sultan and Thakar 2007). When torn (Grade 3c tear/fourth-degree), the internal anal sphincter tends to retract and can be identified lateral to the torn anal epithelium. It should be repaired with mattress sutures using 3-0 PDS (Polydioxanone) or modern braided sutures such as 2/0 Vicryl (polyglactin – Vicryl). To repair a torn external anal sphincter, the ends are grasped using Allis forceps and the muscle is mobilized. When the EAS is only partially torn (Grade 3a and some 3b) then an end-to-end repair should be performed using two or three mattress sutures. Haemostatic 'figure of 8' sutures must not be used to repair the mucosa or sphincter muscle. If there is a full-thickness EAS tear (some 3b, 3c or fourth-degree), either an overlapping or end-to-end method can be used with equivalent outcome. A Cochrane review (Fernando et al. 2013) including six randomized studies showed that, at 1-year follow-up, immediate primary overlap repair of the external anal sphincter compared with immediate primary end-to-end repair appeared to be associated with lower risks of developing faecal urgency and anal incontinence symptoms. At the end of 36 months, there appeared to be no difference in flatus or faecal incontinence between the two techniques. However, since this evidence was based on only two small trials, more research evidence is needed in order to confirm or refute these findings. After either technique of repairing the external sphincter the remainder of the tear is closed using the same principles and suture material outlined in the repair of episiotomy.

Basic Principles After Repair of Perineal Tears

After repair, complete haemostasis should be achieved (NICE 2014; Sultan and Thakar 2007). A rectal and vaginal examination should be performed to confirm adequate repair, to ensure that no other tears have been missed and that a suture is not inadvertently placed through the rectal mucosa. Confirm that all tampons (if used) or swabs have been removed.

Detailed notes should be made of the findings and repair. Completion of a pre-designed proforma and a pictorial representation of the tears can prove very useful when notes are being reviewed following complications, audit or litigation. An accurate detailed account of the repair should be documented in the woman's case notes following completion of the procedure, including details of suture method and materials used.

The woman should be informed regarding the use of appropriate analgesia, hygiene and the importance of a good diet and daily pelvic floor exercises. It is important that the woman is given a full explanation of the injury sustained and contact details if she has any problems during the postnatal period. In presence of OASIS women should be advised that the prognosis following EAS repair is good, with 60–80% being asymptomatic at 12 months (RCOG 2015a). In the case of FGM, the woman and her partner must be advised about the legalities regarding reinfibulation and safeguarding issues if the baby is female.

POSTOPERATIVE CARE AFTER OASIS

Broad-spectrum antibiotics should be given intraoperatively (intravenously) and continued orally for 3 days. Severe perineal discomfort, particularly following instrumental delivery, is a known cause of urinary retention, and following regional anaesthesia it can take up to 12 h before bladder sensation returns. A Foley catheter should be inserted for at least 12 h unless medical staff can ensure that spontaneous voiding occurs at least every 3–4 h without undue overdistension of the bladder.

The degree of pain following perineal trauma is related to the extent of the injury and OASIS is frequently associated with other more extensive injuries, such as paravaginal tears. In a systematic review, Hedayati et al. (2003) found that rectal analgesia such as diclofenac is effective in reducing pain from perineal trauma within the first 24 h after birth and women used less additional analgesia within the first 48 h after birth. Diclofenac is almost completely protein-bound and therefore excretion in breastmilk is negligible. In women who had a repair of a fourth-degree tear, diclofenac should be administered orally as insertion of suppositories may be uncomfortable and there is a theoretical risk of poor healing associated with local anti-inflammatory agents. Codeine-based preparations are best avoided as they may cause constipation leading to excessive straining and possible disruption of the repair. It is of utmost importance that constipation is avoided as passage of constipated stool or indeed faecal impaction may disrupt the repair. Stool softeners (Lactulose) should be prescribed for the first 10–14 days postpartum and the dose titrated to keep the stools soft. The addition of ispaghula husk (Fybogel) should be avoided as it has been shown to be non-beneficial (Eogan et al. 2007). It is recommended that women with OASIS be contacted by a healthcare provider 24 or 48 h after hospital discharge to ensure bowel evacuation has occurred (Sultan and Thakar 2007).

FOLLOW-UP

Special designated multidisciplinary clinics should be available for women with perineal problems to ensure that they receive appropriate, sensitive and effective management. All women who sustain OASIS should be assessed by a senior obstetrician at 6–12 weeks after birth (RCOG 2015a). If facilities are available, follow-up of women with OASIS should be in a dedicated clinic with access to endoanal ultrasonography and anal manometry, as this can aid decision on future mode of birth (RCOG 2015a; Jordan et al. 2018).

In the clinic, a genital examination is performed looking specifically for scarring, residual granulation tissue and tenderness. Where facilities are available, women may undergo anal manometry and endosonography. The women are assessed by the physiotherapists and advised to continue pelvic floor exercises while others with minimal sphincter contractility may need electrical nerve stimulation.

If a perineal clinic is not available, women with OASIS should be given clear instructions, preferably in writing, before leaving the hospital. In the first 6 weeks following birth, they should look for signs of infection or wound dehiscence and call with any increase in pain or swelling, rectal bleeding or purulent discharge. Any incontinence of stool or flatus should also be reported. Under such circumstances, referral to a specialist gynaecologist or colorectal surgeon for endoanal ultrasound and manometry should be considered (RCOG 2015a).

Consequences of OASIS – Colorectal Surgeon's Perspective

Midwives often do not have first-hand experience of caring for women with long-term consequences of OASIS following childbirth because their interface with women is usually confined to the first few weeks postpartum.

Mothers with anal sphincter injuries are at risk of urinary incontinence, pelvic floor prolapse and various forms of anal incontinence. Sometimes these complications occur soon after the birth but for many these symptoms may not manifest until the mother is perimenopausal, this being particularly the case with genital prolapse. Early symptoms are usually devastating to women who have to cope both with their newborn baby and the indignity of incontinence, which they usually hide because they feel so ashamed (Keighley et al. 2016; Tucker et al. 2014). In fact, anal incontinence is a hidden taboo causing social isolation, a fear of travel and participating in normal daily activities (see Geeta's story in Case Study 17.2). Many mothers are afraid to re-engage in sexual intercourse because of the fear of leakage, pain and because of the psychological scars of the sphincter injury. A small number of mothers who have had a fourth-degree tear may develop a recto-vaginal fistula, which is devastating to a young mother. These are difficult to treat and about two-thirds require a temporary colostomy.

CASE STUDY 17.2 Geeta's Story of OASIS

It is still hard for me to accept that the injuries I sustained during the birth of my first child continue to dominate my life. Over the last decade it has however sadly become very apparent just how common my story is. I was 30, at the height of my legal career that I loved and had worked very hard to achieve. I had recently got married and was expecting my first child;

life was good. However, the events that took place changed my life forever.

In brief, I was admitted to a busy teaching hospital at 4 cm dilated. I was under the care of a lovely midwife, however the ward was short staffed and my labour was not progressing as expected. I had been in a prone position for hours, had stopped dilating at 7 cm and Syntoci-

CASE STUDY 17.2 Geeta's Story of OASIS—cont'd

non was therefore administered. There then followed a 7pm changeover of staff and unfortunately that is where things started to go wrong. The trace became suspicious and despite both myself and my mother asking for a plan if things deteriorated, our concerns were dismissed. Out of the many excellent midwives and obstetricians practising, I unfortunately had both a midwife and obstetrician who were very uncommunicative and seemed determined to avoid the possibility of a C-section at all costs. I was at no point transferred to theatre and sadly the situation continued to deteriorate, and panic then ensued when eventually there was marked fetal distress. There were multiple failed attempts at ventouse and consequently an extremely traumatic forceps delivery that has left my daughter with permanent facial injuries. I sustained a 3c tear that involved most of the length of the external sphincter and the entire length of the internal sphincter. Unfortunately, it was only recognized as a 3b tear at the time and the same obstetrician then poorly attempted to repair the external sphincter. The repair very quickly broke down, and I experienced my first episode of faecal incontinence the very next day.

From this first episode of incontinence to date, I have been incontinent of faeces and flatus, have marked faecal urgency, passive faecal incontinence, urinary stress incontinence and dyspareunia. This is only getting worse with age, and I have been advised will continue to deteriorate.

I was in complete shock at the traumatic delivery I had been through and was solely focussed on the injuries to my daughter at that time, so had no idea how severe my injuries were. I was simply discharged home the next day and, despite knowing I had sustained a tear and had been incontinent, was only told to do pelvic floor exercises. Had I been properly examined and a referral made to a perineal trauma clinic at that stage and it was recognized how traumatized I was, it would have made a huge difference. I would have understood the nature and the extent of my injuries and why I was experiencing such terrible symptoms.

As it was, those first few days, weeks and months were as far apart from how I had envisaged them as possible. I was having regular and severe episodes of incontinence, was pretty much house bound and was suffering from what I now know was postnatal posttraumatic stress disorder (PTSD).

Nearly all the women I have met, through MASIC (Mothers with Anal Sphincters Injuries in Childbirth) who have sustained similar injuries also have suffered from PTSD or depression. The psychological sequelae is complex, compounded with horrendous physical injuries. I went from being a resilient, social, independent, young woman to needing nearly constant help from my husband and mother, which compounded my feelings of guilt and horror at what had taken place and the injuries my daughter and I had sustained. I went over and over the delivery minute by minute; surely there was something I could have done to prevent this, why did no-one listen to us and take action earlier. These major psychological symptoms are in fact a huge barrier in terms of facing, dealing or accepting the physical injuries, which is why early psychological intervention is so important.

My GP was equally shocked at my injuries and symptoms but never had any answers, and sadly never once suggested referring me on to an appropriate perineal trauma clinic, nor did the urogynaecologist I saw.

Six months after the birth of my daughter the situation became so dire that we went to stay with my parents. It was only once my mother who is a doctor, managed to get an appropriate referral to a perineal trauma clinic that I was told for the first time how serious my injuries were, involving complete disruption of the external anal sphincter, pudendal neuropathy and excessive scar tissue in the pelvic floor, perineum and anterior aspect of the sphincters. It was horrifying to hear but also a huge relief to understand why my symptoms were so bad. At this point I was also referred to a colorectal surgeon who advised a secondary repair. This was undertaken a few months after, but sadly the repair failed as the quality of the remaining tissue was so poor.

That was in 2009. Since then I have tried many different management techniques, but there has been no real change in my symptoms, I have simply had to adjust the way I live to cope. My husband now works from home so that he can help with the children in the morning, as I am occupied with my bowels. I have lost my career, which I worked so hard to achieve, my social life has greatly suffered, my confidence, my zest for life. Everything that defined me as me has been affected. It's really hard to try to get that back. And I am one of the lucky ones. I have an amazingly supportive patient husband and family. Yet this has left no-one unscathed.

Through my involvement in MASIC, I have met so many women with such similar stories and symptoms. It has been greatly supportive but also so very sad that women from all over the country, from different backgrounds and ethnicities, have experienced such similar tragedy that have impacted on their lives so profoundly.

I have lost so much because of what I strongly believe stemmed from a lack of training on issues such as manual perineum protection, how to avoid tears and how to correctly repair them. Even with the best intentions, a lack of knowledge and training can have devastating consequences. Relationships breakdown, careers are lost and families suffer.

The incidence of some impairment of continence after having a baby is reported in 20–40% of cases (Brown et al. 2012). Often the symptoms are subtle such as urgency to defaecate and not making it in time to the bathroom. Other distressing symptoms may include having little or no control over flatus or leaking urine uncontrollably, all of which are extremely embarrassing and lead to anxiety, depression in some cases and PTSD (Williams et al. 2005).

As discussed earlier in the chapter, the risk factors for these injuries and symptoms are manifold. There is growing evidence that careful control of the head during crowning, as well as avoiding any force during an assisted birth, reduces the risk of OASIS. Fortunately, provided these injuries are properly identified at birth and are repaired in the way this chapter has already described, the outcome in terms of preventing incontinence is good and about 65–80% become completely asymptomatic (Hayes et al. 2006).

One of the problems sadly is that even today, some of these injuries are missed as not all practitioners are keen to perform a rectal examination following a vaginal birth. There needs to be a consistent and standardized approach to anorectal examination following all vaginal births, regardless if the practitioner is a midwife or doctor. The use of a perineal examination proforma that accounts for an anorectal check following all vaginal births will ensure a consistent approach as the examination will not be overlooked. Midwives must be mindful that women with missed tears become incontinent, because if complex perineal trauma is not recognized and classified as OASIS, they are not given the special follow-up described in the earlier section of this chapter. Consequently, these mothers do not know where to go to find help and advice because they are too ashamed to talk about it. This is why an anorectal examination following vaginal births is recommended. Slowly there is an increasing awareness of this problem and various websites are able to provide information, support and advice to mothers about coping strategies such as: www.masic.org.uk

MEDICOLEGAL CONSIDERATIONS

Although creating a third- or fourth-degree tear is seldom found to be culpable, missing a tear is considered to be negligent. It is essential that a rectal examination is performed before and after any perineal repair and findings must be carefully documented in the notes. Common issues raised at litigation include: delay in repairing in theatre; poor note-keeping; repair by untrained personnel; poor lighting and inadequate exposure; inadequate anaesthesia; failure to recognize extent of the tear; use of wrong suture material; forgotten swab in the vagina; deviation from recommended safe practice; failure to inform and counsel the woman; failure to inform the GP; inappropriate follow-up; and advice regarding subsequent pregnancy. In the UK, a report by the National Health Service Litigation Authority (NHSLA 2012) demonstrated that during the review period, from 1 April 2000 to 31 March 2010, the NHSLA received 441 claims, in which allegations of negligence were made arising out of perineal damage (principally third- and fourth-degree tears) caused during labour. The total value of those claims, including both damages and legal costs, was estimated to be £31.2 million. Allegations of negligence included failure to consider a caesarean section or perform or extend the episiotomy, and failure to diagnose the true extent and grade of the injury, including failure to perform a rectal examination. Failure to perform the repair and the adequacy of the repair itself were also raised as allegations in this cohort of claims (NHSLA 2012).

TRAINING

Throughout the centuries, midwives have received very little formal training in the art of perineal suturing. In June 1967, midwives working in the UK were permitted by their then regulatory body, the Central Midwives Board (CMB), to perform episiotomies, but they were not allowed to suture perineal trauma. In June 1970, the Chairman of the CMB issued a statement that midwives who were working in 'remote areas overseas' may be authorized by the doctor concerned to repair episiotomies, provided they have been taught the technique and were judged to be competent, but the final responsibility lay with the doctor. It was not until 1983, however, that perineal repair was included in the midwifery curriculum in the UK, when the European Community Midwives Directives came into force and the CMB issued the statement that midwives may undertake repair of the perineum provided they received the necessary instruction and are deemed competent to undertake the procedure (Thakar and Kettle 2010). Tohill and Kettle (2013) have provided evidence-based guidelines for midwives on how to suture correctly.

However, it has been reported that there is a lack of general knowledge on the agreed classification of perineal trauma and that midwives feel inadequately prepared to assess or repair perineal trauma (Mutema 2007). It has also been demonstrated that practitioners require more focussed training relating to performing mediolateral episiotomies. Andrews et al. (2005) carried out a prospective study over a 12-month period of women having their first vaginal birth to assess positioning of mediolateral episiotomies. The depth, length, distance from the midline, the shortest distance from the midpoint of the anal canal, and the angle subtended from the sagittal or parasagittal plane were measured following suturing of the episiotomy. Results of the study demonstrated that no midwife and only 13 (22%) doctors performed a truly mediolateral episiotomy and that the majority of the incisions were in fact directed closer to the midline (Andrews et al. 2005). All relevant healthcare professionals should attend training in perineal/genital assessment and repair, and ensure that they maintain these skills.

REFLECTIVE ACTIVITY FOR SELF-ASSESSMENT

1. In accordance with the evidence base, what strategies might be helpful in minimizing perineal trauma?
2. What is the significance of performing an anorectal examination following vaginal births?

3. List the consequences of FGM/female genital cutting and discuss the medicolegal responsibilities of the midwife when caring for this group of women during the antepartum, intrapartum and postpartum periods.

REFERENCES

Aasheim, V., Nilsen, A. B. V., Reinar, L. M., & Lukasse, M. (2017). Perineal techniques during the second stage of labour for reducing perineal trauma. *Cochrane Database of Systematic Reviews*, (6), CD006672.

Al-Hussaini, T. K. (2003). Female genital cutting: Types, motives and perineal damage in laboring Egyptian women. *Medical Principles and Practice*, 12(2), 123–128.

Andrews, V., Thakar, R., Sultan, A. H., & Jones, P. W. (2005). Are mediolateral episiotomies actually mediolateral. *International Journal of Obstetrics and Gynaecology*, 112(8), 1156–1158.

Andrews, V., Thakar, R., & Sultan, A. H. (2006). Occult anal sphincter injuries – myth or reality? *International Journal of Obstetrics and Gynaecology*, 113(2), 195–200.

Beckmann, M. M., & Stock, O. M. (2013). Antenatal perineal massage for reducing perineal trauma. *Cochrane Database of Systematic Reviews*, (4), CD005123.

Blondel, B., Alexander, S., Bjarnadóttir, R. I., et al. (2016). Euro-Peristat Scientific Committee - Variations in rates of severe perineal tears and episiotomies in 20 European countries: A study based on routine national data in Euro-Peristat Project. *Acta Obstetricia et Gynecologica Scandinavica*, 95, 746–754.

Brown, S., Gartland, D., Donath, S., & MacArthur, C. (2012). Faecal incontinence during the first 12 months postpartum. *Obstetrics and Gynecology*, 119(11), 240–249.

Coats, P. M., Chan, K. K., Wilkins, M., & Beard, R. J. (1980). A comparison between midline and mediolateral episiotomies. *British Journal of Obstetrics and Gynaecology*, 87, 408–412.

De Silva, S. (1989). Obstetric sequelae of female circumcision. *European Journal of Obstetrics, Gynecology and Reproductive Biology*, 32, 233–240.

Draper, J., & Newell, R. (1996). A discussion of some of the literature relating to history, repair and consequences of perineal trauma. *Midwifery*, 12(3), 140–145.

Elnashar, A., & Abdelhady, R. (2007). The impact of female genital cutting on health of newly married women. *International Journal of Gynaecology and Obstetrics*, 97, 238–244.

Ekeus, C., Nilsson, E., & Gottvallm, K. (2008). Increasing incidence of anal sphincter tears among primiparas in Sweden: A population-based register study. *Acta Obstetricia et Gynecologica Scandinavica*, 87, 564–573.

Eogan, M., Daly, L., O'Connell, P., & O'Herlihy, C. (2006). Does the angle of episiotomy affect the incidence of anal sphincter injury? *International Journal of Obstetrics and Gynaecology*, 113(2), 190–194.

Eogan, M., Daly, L., Behan, M., et al. (2007). Randomised clinical trial of a laxative alone versus a laxative and a bulking agent after primary repair of obstetric anal sphincter injury. *International Journal of Obstetrics and Gynaecology*, 114, 736–740.

Fenner, D. E., Genberg, B., Brahma, P., et al. (2003). Fecal and urinary incontinence after vaginal delivery with anal sphincter disruption in an obstetrics unit in the United States. *American Journal of Obstetrics and Gynecology*, 189(6), 1543–1549.

Fernando, R. J., Sultan, A. H., Kettle, C., & Thakar, R. (2013). Methods of repair for obstetric anal sphincter injury. *Cochrane Database of Systematic Reviews, 12*, CD002866.

Green, J., Coupland, V., & Kitzinger, J. (1998). *Great expectations: A prospective study of women's expectations and experiences of childbirth*. Hale, Cheshire: Books for Midwives Press.

Gupta, J. K., Sood, A., Hofmeyr, G. J., & Vogel, J. P. (2017). Position in the second stage of labour for women without epidural anaesthesia. *Cochrane Database of Systematic Reviews,* (5), CD002006.

Gurol-Urganci, I., Cromwell, D., Edozien, L., et al. (2013). Third-and fourth-degree perineal tears among primiparous women in England between 2000 and 2012: Time trends and risk factors. *International Journal of Obstetrics and Gynaecology, 120*(12), 1516–1525.

Hassanin, I. M., Saleh, R., Bedaiwy, A. A., et al. (2008). Prevalence of female genital cutting in Upper Egypt: 6 Years after enforcement of prohibition law. *Reproductive Biomedicine.* Available at: www.rbmonline.com.

Hayes, J., Shatari, T., Toozs-Hobson, P., et al. (2006). Early results of immediate repair of obstetric third degree tears, 65% are completely asymptomatic despite persistent sphincter defects in 61%. *Colorectal Disease, 9*, 332–336.

Hedayati, H., Parsons, J., & Crowther, C. (2003). Rectal analgesia for pain from perineal trauma following childbirth. *Cochrane Database of Systematic Reviews,* (1), CD004223.

Home Office. (1985). *Prohibition of Female Circumcision Act 1985*. London: HMSO. Available at: www.legislation.gov.uk/ukpga/1985/38/pdfs/ukpga_19850038_en.pdf.

Home Office. (2004). *Circular 10/2004: The Female Genital Mutilation Act 2003*. London: HMSO. Available at: www.legislation.gov.uk/ukpga/2003/31/pdfs/ukpga_20030031_en.pdf.

Home Office. (2015). *Mandatory Reporting of Female Genital Mutilation – procedural information*. Available at: www.gov.uk/government/publications/mandatory-reporting-of-female-genital-mutilation-procedural-information.

Jiang, H., Qian, X., Carroli, G., & Garner, P. (2017). Selective versus routine use of episiotomy for vaginal birth. *Cochrane Database of Systematic Reviews,* (2), CD000081.

Jordan, P. A., Naidu, M., Thakar, R., et al. (2018). Effect of subsequent vaginal delivery on bowel symptoms and anorectal function in women who sustained a previous obstetric anal sphincter injury. *International Urogynecology Journal, 29*(11), 1579–1588.

Kalis, A., Landsmanova, J., Bednarova, B., et al. (2011). Evaluation of the incision angle of mediolateral episiotomy at 60 degrees. *International Journal of Gynecology and Obstetrics, 112*(3), 220–224.

Kalis, V., Laine, K., de Leeuw, J. W., et al. (2012). Classification of episiotomy: Towards a standardisation of terminology. *International Journal of Obstetrics and Gynaecology, 119*(5), 522–526.

Keighley, M., Perston, Y., Bradshaw, E., et al. (2016). The social, psychological, emotional morbidity and adjustment techniques for women with anal incontinence following obstetric anal sphincter injury: Use of a word picture to identify a hidden syndrome. *BMC Pregnancy and Childbirth, 16*, 275.

Kettle, C., Dowswell, T., & Ismail, K. (2010). Absorbable suture materials for primary repair of episiotomy and second degree tears. *Cochrane Database of Systematic Reviews,* (6), CD000006.

Kettle, C., Dowswell, T., & Ismail, K. M. (2012). Continuous and interrupted suturing techniques for repair of episiotomy or second degree tears. *Cochrane Database of Systematic Reviews,* (11), CD000947.

Kettle, C., & Fenner, D. (2007). Repair of episiotomy, first and second degree tears. In A. H. Sultan, R. Thakar, & D. Fenner (Eds.), *Perineal and anal sphincter trauma* (pp. 20–32). London: Springer.

Kettle, C., & Raynor, M. D. (2010). Perineal management and repair. In J. E. M. Marshall, & M. D. Raynor (Eds.), *Advancing skills in midwifery practice* (pp. 104–120). Edinburgh: Churchill Livingstone.

Kettle, C. (2012). *Evidence based guidelines for midwifery-led care in labour: Suturing the perineum*. London: Royal College of Midwives.

Laine, K., Skjeldestad, F. E., Sandvik, L., et al. (2012). Incidence of obstetric anal sphincter injuries after training to protect the perineum: Cohort study. *BMJ Open, 2*, e001649.

Millogo-Traore, F., Kaba, S. T., Thieba, B., et al. (2007). [Maternal and foetal prognostic in excised women delivery.]. *Journal de Gynecologie, Obstetrique et Biologie de la Reproduction, 36*, 393–408.

Mutema, E. K. (2007). 'A tale of two cities': Auditing midwifery practice and perineal trauma. *British Journal of Midwifery, 15*(8), 511–513.

NHSLA (National Health Service Litigation Authority). (2012). *Ten years of maternity claims: An analysis of NHS Litigation Authority data*. London: NHSLA, 49–60.

NICE (National Institute for Health and Care Excellence). (2014). *Intrapartum care: Care of healthy women and their babies* CG 190. Available at: www.nice.org.uk/guidance/cg190.

NICE (National Institute for Health and Care Excellence). (2008). *Antenatal care. Routine care for the healthy pregnant women* CG 62. Available at: www.nice.org.uk/Guidance/CG62.

Nordenstam, J., Mellgren, A., Altman, D., et al. (2008). Immediate or delayed repair of obstetric anal sphincter tears—a randomised controlled trial. *International Journal of Obstetrics and Gynaecology, 115*(7), 857–865.

RCOG (Royal College of Obstetricians and Gynaecologists). (2015a). Management of third and fourth degree tears. Green-top Guideline No 29. Available at: www.rcog.org.uk/globalassets/documents/guidelines/gtg-29.pdf.

RCOG (Royal College of Obstetricians and Gynaecologists). (2015b). *Female genital mutilation and its management. Guideline No 53*. London: RCOG.

Stedenfeldt, M., Pirhonen, J., Blix, E., et al. (2012). Episiotomy characteristics and risks for obstetric anal sphincter injuries: A case–control study. *International Journal of Obstetrics and Gynaecology, 119*(6), 724–730.

Sultan, A. H., & Kettle, C. (2007). Diagnosis of perineal trauma. In A. H. Sultan, R. Thakars, & D. Fenner (Eds.), *Perineal and anal sphincter trauma* (pp. 13–19). London: Springer-Verlag.

Sultan, A. H., & Thakar, R. (2007). Third and fourth degree tears. In A. H. Sultan, R. Thakar, & D. Fenner (Eds.), *Perineal and anal sphincter trauma* (pp. 33–51). London: Springer-Verlag.

Thakar, R., & Kettle, C. (2010). Episiotomy and perineal repair. In L. Cardozo, & D. Staskin (Eds.), *Textbook of female urology and urogynecology* (3rd ed.) (pp. 875–882). Hampshire: Martin Dunitz.

Thiagamoorthy, G., Johnson, A., Thakar, R., & Sultan, A. H. (2014). National survey of perineal trauma and its subsequent management in the United Kingdom. *The International Urogynecology Journal, 25*(12), 1621–1627.

Tohill, S., & Kettle, C. (2013). How to suture correctly. *Midwives, 1*, 31. Available at: www.rcm.org.

Tucker, J., Clifton, V., & Wilson, A. (2014). Teetering near the edge, women's experiences of anal incontinence following obstetric anal sphincter injury: An interpretive phenomenological research study. *Australian and New Zealand Journal of Obstetrics and Gynaecology, 54*, 377–381.

Williams, A., Lavender, T., Richmond, D., et al. (2005). Women's experiences after a third degree obstetric anal sphincter tear: A qualitative study. *Birth, 32*(2), 129.

WHO (World Health Organization). (2001). *Management of pregnancy, childbirth and postpartum period in the presence of female genital mutilation*. Geneva: WHO.

WHO (World Health Organization). (2008). *Eliminating female genital mutilation. An interagency statement – OHCHR, UNAIDS, UNDP, UNECA, UNESCO, UNFPA, UNHCR, UNICEF, UNIFEM, WHO*. Geneva: WHO.

WHO (World Health Organization). (2018a). Female genital mutilation. Fact sheet. Available at: www.who.int/en/news-room/fact-sheets/detail/female-genital-mutilation.

WHO (World Health Organization). (2018b). *Care of girls and women living with female genital mutilation. A clinical handbook*. Geneva: WHO.

ANNOTATED FURTHER READING

Bidwell, P., Thakar, R., Sevdalis, N., et al. (2018). A multi-centre quality improvement project to reduce the incidence of obstetric anal sphincter injury (OASI): Study protocol. *BMC Pregnancy and Childbirth, 18*, 331.

OASI project registration number: ISCTRN12143325. This protocol outlines the evaluation of a quality improvement project focussing on the prevention of OASI using a bundle of evidence-based interventions that are each widely used in practice.

Kapoor, D. S., Thakar, R., & Sultan, A. H. (2015). Obstetric anal sphincter injuries: Review of anatomical factors and modifiable second stage interventions. *International Urogynecology Journal, 26*(12), 1725–1734.

This article explores how the modification of various risk factors in relation to anatomical considerations can help to reduce the rate of OASIS, including the use of warm compresses in the second stage of labour and the correct angle for performing an episiotomy.

Ness, W. (2017). Obstetric anal sphincter injury: Causes, effects and management. *Nursing Times (online), 113*(5), 28–32.

A useful article written by a colorectal nurse specialist that explores the functions of the anal sphincter complex in a readily accessible way. It also explores the risks and sequelae of complex anal sphincter injuries and their management.

USEFUL WEBSITES/VIDEO RESOURCES

Birth Trauma Association: www.birthtraumaassociation.org.uk

Department of Health: www.gov.uk; www.gov.uk/government/publications/female-genital-mutilation-resource-pack/female-genital-mutilation-resource-pack

Provides useful video and resources on FGM.

Female Genital Mutilation Clinical Group: www.fgmnationalgroup.org

Foundation for Women's Health Research and Development: www.forwarduk.org.uk

Mothers with Anal Sphincter Injuries in Childbirth: www.masic.org.uk

National Patient Safety Agency: www.npsa.nhs.uk

National Society for the Prevention of Cruelty to Children: www.nspcc.org.uk

Ongoing OASI Project: www.rcog.org.uk/OASICareBundle

Royal College of Midwives: www.rcm.org.uk; www.rcm.org.uk/sites/default/files/Care%20of%20the%20Perineum.pdf; iLearn PEARLS: www.ilearn.rcm.org.uk/enrol/index.php?id=203

Provides evidence-based guidelines and a training video on episiotomy and the procedure for perineal repair

Royal College of Obstetricians and Gynaecologists: www.rcog.org.uk/en/guidelines-research-services/audit-quality-improvement/oasi-care-bundle/oasi-videos/; www.rcog.org.uk/OASICareBundle

OASIS Bundle Information and videos.

The FGM National Clinical Group is a registered charity in England & Wales no. 1125319: www.fgmresource.com

Provides a useful video for midwives and doctors about FGM and the issue of deinfibulation.

World Health Organization: www.who.int

18

Fear of Childbirth (Tocophobia)

Liz Snapes

CHAPTER CONTENTS

This chapter offers a review of the morbid fear of childbirth (tocophobia) and explores the psychological impact that childbearing women may experience. The psychological wellbeing of women throughout the childbirth continuum is at least as important as physiological wellbeing, with studies indicating that the two are inextricably linked. To experience fear, a well-known emotional phenomenon, casts a shadow over the pregnancy and can greatly reduce the joy of welcoming a new baby into the family. Whatever the mode of birth and its outcome, childbirth *is* a profound experience and represents a significant transition in the woman and her family's life. The midwife's role within public health, highlights the responsibility for meeting the needs of women's mental health. Responding to the woman's beliefs and attitudes is the main focus of individualized woman-centred care. A key informant of attitude is knowledge and information. Information about childbirth is widely available and accessible through many different sources of media, including internet and television and is part of culture. It may be that the medicalization of childbirth has decreased women's confidence to give birth, while also producing a normative frame of reference. However, this complex cognitive process can combine with knowledge and compassion from professional staff and change behaviour positively. In order to provide further context to the content and enhance the reader's understanding, quotations from women's experiences of childbirth that the author has collected following a request to the *Birth Trauma Association*, have been included: each with a pseudonym to preserve anonymity (Thomson and Downe 2013; Gomez and Chilvers 2017; Hogg and Vaughan 2018).

THE CHAPTER AIMS TO

- examine the risk factors and causes of tocophobia
- explore the relationship between the psychology and physiology of birth
- discuss the importance of the midwife's role during the childbirth continuum and the long-term psychological consequences of the experience of pregnancy and birth on the woman

DEFINITION AND PREVALENCE

The term *tocophobia* is derived from the Greek word *tokos* meaning 'childbirth' and *phobos* meaning 'fear' and is defined as an extreme fear of childbirth (Billert 2007). Considerable heterogeneity within different studies has made it difficult to ascertain the prevalence of fear of childbirth, however a recent study by O'Connell et al. (2017) has cautiously estimated it to be around 14% worldwide with a small proportion of this number of women developing tocophobia.

The paradox remains that while maternity care today is relatively safe, fear of childbirth may cause sufficient stress symptoms that can influence a woman in fundamentally negative ways, including wishing to avoid a natural birth or even pregnancy itself (Nilsson and Lundgren 2009).

HISTORY

Fear of childbirth is not a new phenomenon and was documented as early the 18th century by the German, Dr Osiander (1797) (O'Connell et al. 2015), who noted some women as being suicidal due to the fear of giving birth and also by French psychiatrist, Marcé (1858) (Hofberg and Brockington 2000), who cited pain as the main fear for women. Dick-Read (1960) also believed that pain was the predominant reason for fear of childbirth and was particularly curious about the thoughts of women embarking on pregnancy for the first time, wondering what the outcome would be and how they would see it through. A couple of decades earlier, a documented understanding of the physiological consequences of fear on labour was illustrated by Johnstone (1945), acknowledging that fear was probably the most frequent and most important cause of primary uterine inertia. As fear is often suppressed, to the point of being subconscious, the phenomenon has tended to be perceived as being insignificant.

PSYCHOLOGY AND PHYSIOLOGY

While many women and their partners feel excitement and joy during pregnancy and labour, it is also true that for some, the experience brings anxieties, both practical and emotional, with a degree of uncertainty. Women are able to recount their birth stories for the rest of their lives and the effects of the birth experience leave lifelong positive or negative memories (Aune et al. 2015). Signs and symptoms of fear of childbirth include: women delaying their pregnancies; not enjoying their pregnancy; experiencing episodes of crying; nervousness and sleeplessness; as well as fear and denial.

Physiologically, a small degree of anxiety in women may be advantageous, allowing them to adjust and prepare for changes. However, psychological factors have an impact on hormonal responses such as cortisol, endogenous opioids, the hypothalamic pituitary adrenal axis (HPA axis) and oxytocin (Ayers and De Visser 2018). Furthermore, a continuous anxiety leading to fear and emotional distress has been associated with significant negative physiological symptoms affecting fetal development and growth as well as the development of pre-eclampsia in the mother (Monk 2001). In addition, women are also more likely to have babies who are at risk of developing emotional, cognitive and behavioural difficulties in childhood (Lee et al. 2007). Wilkins et al. (2009) affirm the importance of psychological wellbeing during pregnancy and reiterate comprehensive consequences of antenatal fear and anxiety for public health. Principally, these include a potentially increased risk of longer labour, instrumental birth or elective caesarean section, leading to an increased risk of thromboembolism, infection, bladder trauma, uterine rupture, placenta praevia and placenta abruption in subsequent pregnancies (Royal College of Obstetricians and Gynaecologists, RCOG 2015). Effects on the health and wellbeing of the baby include reduced birth weight, reduced bonding and attachment and long-term emotional effects on the infant.

RISK FACTORS

Tocophobia may be *primary*, describing nulliparous women who have not experienced childbirth, or *secondary*, which defines those women who have previously experienced pregnancy, labour and have given birth (Hofberg and Brockington 2000). The associated risk factors for fear of childbirth are multifactorial and complex and are shown in Table 18.1. Hertzman (2006) has claimed that the socioeconomic gradient in health status is parallelled in cognitive and behavioural development, which indicates that social status may also be a key factor for women experiencing fear of childbirth. As an important public health issue, it is worth taking into consideration that clinical outcomes for women are often linked to underlying social factors, including housing conditions, nutrition, cultural influences and emotional support.

TABLE 18.1 **Associated Risk Factors for Tocophobia**	
Nulliparous	History of Poor Mental Health
Younger age	Low self-efficacy
Lower education achievement	Poor economic status
Lack of communication	Lack of social support

Adapted from Rouhe H, Salmela-Aro K, Halmesmaki E, Saisto T. (2009) Fear of childbirth according to parity, gestational age and obstetric history. BJOG 116(7):67–73.

CAUSES

A feminist perspective from Reiger and Dempsey (2006) contends that women face a cultural crisis fearing that birth and breastfeeding are too difficult to undertake. Indeed, a study in Northern Ireland (Gould 2012) found that 89% of women aspired to having a normal birth but 68% feared that they would not be capable of achieving this goal safely, without the need for intervention. Greer et al. (2014) contends that this is, in part, due to the *language of risk* that is presented to women when discussing birth choices.

One of the experiences that are seldom mentioned is a woman's fear of being '*intruded upon*' or '*exposed and naked*'. It is taken for granted that as it is a part of the birthing process that it is normal to be regularly examined by healthcare professionals. When women were given an opportunity in a national survey to express their concerns about feeling embarrassed during childbirth, more than 10% felt very worried (Redshaw et al. 2007). Shepherd and Cheyne (2012) state, although there are other ways of assessing progress in labour, such as observing the woman's behaviour, palpating the frequency, length and strength of contractions and assessing the descent of the fetal head by abdominal palpation, vaginal examinations have become regarded as an essential measure of the progress of labour. This may be, in part, due to the use of the partogram that requires the midwife to record the dilatation of the cervix against time in labour (see Case Study 18.1). There is evidence, however, that vaginal examinations can be associated with emotional trauma, embarrassment and discomfort and that assessment of the cervix is very subjective and not always reliable.

CASE STUDY 18.1 **Nadia's Birth Experience**

There can be no 'one size fits all' approach to caring for women in labour. The midwives stuck to their fixed ideas about how long the labour would be and when I would need pain relief. All they needed to do was look at me and listen to me, as all the clues of how to care for me were there in what my body was doing and the things I was saying.

TABLE 18.2 **Prediction Tools for Tocophobia**	
Wijma Delivery Expectancy-Experience Questionnaire	W-DEQ
Cambridge Worry Scale	CWS
Edinburgh Postnatal Depression Scale	EPDS
Generalized Anxiety Disorder 2	GAD-2

Ryding et al. (2009) purports that cultural influences as being, in part, a cause of engendering fear of childbirth in women with horror stories about birth being disseminated by family, friends and the media, reframing birth as a frightening experience. Gaskin (2011), affirms that cultural blindness from highly industrialized countries has prevented women from observing natural birth behaviours. It is therefore vital that each midwife reviews their practice, so as not to perpetuate further anxiety and fear in the woman.

PREDICTION TOOLS

A useful indicator of fear of childbirth may be through the use of prediction tools as summarized in Table 18.2. Although they are not widely used in the UK, the most commonly used measure of fear of childbirth, in countries that have extensive research in this area, was developed by Wijma et al. (1998) and is known as the *Wijma Delivery Expectancy-Experience Questionnaire* (W-DEQ). The questionnaire consists of 33 questions that are measured using a 6-point Likert scale and include questions such as '*How do you think you will feel in general during labour and delivery*', with a choice of opposing experience extremes. The higher the score, the more severe would be the woman's fear of childbirth. A review of the W-DEQ, carried out by Garthus-Niegel et al. (2011) found that this scale could detect differences in the measurement of fear. One part of the scale detected the presence of, and nonspecific, fear of childbirth, whereas another part could measure self-efficacy and the ability to cope with the fear of childbirth.

Assessment tools in the UK tend to focus on establishing the presence of mental ill-health and in the absence of dedicated services may be a barrier between the woman and her midwife should she not wish to disclose her fears. *The Cambridge Worry Scale* (CWS) and the *Edinburgh Postnatal Depression scale* (EPDS) have both been utilized antenatally. While the CWS was found to be a valuable psychometric tool, the EPDS was found lacking in detecting anxiety. The National Institute for Health and Care Excellence (NICE 2018) guidelines focus on antenatal depression and advise that an accurate history should be taken at the *first* antenatal appointment with the midwife/healthcare professional and recommend the following two questions:

> *During the past month have you often been bothered by feeling down, depressed or hopeless?*

and

> *During the past month have you been bothered by having little interest or pleasure in doing things?*

Using the Generalized Anxiety Disorder 2 item (GAD-2) scale or the EPDS it is recommended that women who may fit the mental *ill-health* criteria are referred to the General Practitioner (GP) and perinatal mental health services where available. However, a national online survey of UK maternity units discovered that care pathways for women who have a fear of childbirth were not widely available and where support was apparent, the service provision varied considerably (Richens et al. 2015), often necessitating women to seek their own counselling support.

RESEARCH

While there may be a dearth of research and resources around the fear of childbirth in the UK, Nordic countries have been studying the subject for much longer and, as a result, have established clinics that explore women's fears, provide reassurance and work closely with them to create comprehensive birth plans. The teams within the clinics include obstetricians, midwife counsellors and occasionally a psychologist, psychiatrist or social worker (Waldenstrom et al. 2006). As these countries have already acquired a profound understanding of tocophobia, the care pathways are designed to maintain normality, where possible, working with the woman to maintain mental and physical wellbeing, as opposed to being assigned into a mental *ill-health* pathway (see Chapter 30).

Because tocophobia is a complex, multifaceted subject, it may be useful to broadly categorize available studies into the four main themes of: **Control**, **Information**, **Experience** and **Support**. These areas may each present in isolation or be a combination of any, or all, of the themes.

Control as part of the process of childbirth, control may refer to a number of concepts including access to **information**, choices, physical functioning and personal security. A key informant of empowerment as part of maintaining control is knowledge and information. Hogg and Vaughan (2018) contend that this complex cognitive process of combining an individual's existing knowledge with knowledge and compassion from professional staff can positively change behaviour. It is essential that midwives and members of the multidisciplinary team collaborate with women as equals in this process, in order to develop a framework that promotes self-empowerment, such that the woman has the capacity to problem-solve and make decisions that ultimately enhances positive mental health.

Within this context, the dichotomy between the social and medical models of midwifery care means that although the physiological process of childbirth has broadly remained the same, over recent decades increased hospitalization of women along with advances in technology, has inevitably promoted the medical model, resulting in the woman taking on the role of patient/consumer of maternity services (Kirkham 2010). While some women and midwives may feel safer in a medical technologically advanced environment, others may feel that there is more control in a birth centre or at home. Hospitalization inevitably removes the woman out of her normal environment and places her into one that may interfere with the physiological, sociological and psychological components of birth (Walsh 2017).

One of the consequences of a woman giving birth in a hospital environment is a perceived shifting of control. Stevenson (2010) defines *control* as the power to direct people's behaviour or the course of events. When referring to childbirth, this may allude to a number of concepts such as: access to information, decision-making, physical functioning and personal security. Helk et al. (2008) postulate that increased communication using birth plans, as shown in Case Study 18.2, can give women greater control over decision-making and therefore more satisfaction with their birth experience.

CASE STUDY 18.2 Jane's Birth Plan Experience

I was overcome with fear and anxiety about the birth of my second child and had a strong desire to have a clear birth plan in place right from the start. However, neither my midwife nor the consultant wanted to discuss my birth options until the later stages of pregnancy 'because things could change'. What I needed from them was to be heard, have my worries acknowledged, to be given options and to form a plan.

The professional discourse between medical and social models of maternity care, resonate with the subject of control, support, information and experience. The social model prevails in birth centres, which evolved as a result of the closure of smaller obstetric facilities. The midwife-led, woman-centred culture of midwifery is able to thrive in this environment with safety embedded within the concept of trust between mother and midwife. A UK study of 64,538 healthy women with low risk pregnancies showed that only 58% of women who gave birth in hospitals had a *normal birth*: which was defined as a birth *without* induction of labour, epidural or spinal analgesia, general anaesthesia, forceps or ventouse birth, caesarean section or episiotomy (Brocklehurst et al. 2011).

Walsh (2002) contends that perceiving the fear of childbirth to be pathological and therefore a mental illness, deflects attention from maternity care provision and conceptualizes the problem with the individual woman. The diagnosis of tocophobia was endorsed in the NICE (2011) guidelines as an indication for planned caesarean section, which seems contrary to current trends within maternity provision to promote normality. However, a study by Adams et al. (2012) found that although the duration of labour was longer in women who feared childbirth, the emergency caesarean section rate was comparable with those women who had no fear. This would suggest that women with tocophobia, should **not** be offered an elective caesarean section simply to avoid an emergency caesarean section.

It must be acknowledged that both **knowledge** as well as a lack of knowledge can create fear of childbirth for some women. Therefore, professional **support** becomes important in respect of listening and alleviating or dispelling fears (Melender 2002) and as the detail in Case Study 18.3 illustrates. Information is widely available

through many sources of media including the internet and television and it is now possible to view graphic videos and documentaries of women giving birth, usually in a highly medicalized environment 24 h a day. In addition, information and communication should be a two-way process, which may prove challenging for midwives to elicit details from women who are from different ethnic backgrounds and/or those who may have difficulty accessing services.

CASE STUDY 18.3 Maryam's Plea for Midwives to Listen

*Though we may just be one patient, during one shift, of one day … for us that event will be remembered for the rest of our lives. I'd like them [the midwives] to think about how the woman and her family still feel about the **birth experience** in years to come. I'd like them to listen to women intently, even if she [the woman] is saying something that doesn't fit what the midwife would expect to be happening because nobody knows her [the woman's] body like the woman does.*

Support from the birthing partner or the midwife is frequently cited by women as a key factor when reflecting on their positive or negative **birth experiences.** Women are more likely to express a negative experience if they feel ill-informed, inadequately cared for or not listened to (McKenzie-Harg et al. 2015) and as shown by the voice of Katie in Case Study 18.4.

CASE STUDY 18.4 Katie's Need of a Supportive Midwife

Please help mums to feel empowered and to understand what is happening to them. Reassure them and encourage them, don't make them feel powerless and useless. We are humans, laugh with us, have fun with us and help us enjoy the most monumental day of our lives. My son's birth was the best and worst day of my life and all I needed was a positive, friendly midwife who stuck up for me when she needed to. Birth should be exciting, it's a normal event and should not cause fear in women.

The consequences of a reduction in both antenatal and postnatal appointments in some areas of the UK in recent years has resulted in less opportunity for women to express fear and anxiety to the midwife both prior to and following their birth experience. A midwife's role is vital to ensuring the quality and safety of care the woman receives throughout the whole childbirth continuum. This is especially pertinent when caring for multigravidae, who are five times more likely to report fear of childbirth in a second pregnancy and cite previous traumatic birth or a negative previous birth experience as the primary cause (Storksen et al. 2012). The Care Quality Commission (CQC 2018) report, stated where continuity of care had been experienced, women felt they had received compassionate care; a significant point in terms of where women with secondary tocophobia felt the care to have been lacking in previous pregnancies (Hofberg and Brockington 2000).

POLICY CONTEXT

Past and current research and policy reiterates that women should be put at the centre of care. The National Maternity Review *Better Births* in England (National Health Service, NHS England 2016) proposed personalized care to improve women's access to unbiased information and improve choice and individualized care. Continuity of care has also been shown to foster trust between women, midwives and the wider multi-professional team and has been widely documented as a priority for maternity services over the past 25 years in a number of key initiatives including *Changing Childbirth* (Department of Health, DH 1993) and *Maternity Matters* (DH 2007). Choice, control and continuity of carer were recommended in both reports, with the main focus being understanding and responding to the woman's beliefs and attitudes.

NHS England (2016) also recommends that deficits in perinatal mental health care and postnatal care provision should be strengthened. This would enable women with fear of childbirth to be identified early in order that appropriate information and any specialized care can be provided in a timely fashion. Although this is a positive step forward for current service provision, there remains much work to do to ensure this becomes a reality in **all** maternity services.

REFLECTIVE ACTIVITY FOR SELF-ASSESSMENT

1. How do women communicate their experiences to midwives when they are feeling vulnerable or fearful about childbirth?
2. What contributing factors inhibit or enhance interactions between mothers and midwives to facilitate an admission of fear of childbirth?
3. How can midwifery practice make appropriate antenatal care provision for mothers with fear of childbirth?
4. What are the barriers and facilitators for midwives caring for women with tocophobia within current practice?

REFERENCES

Adams, S. S., Eberhard-Gran, M., & Eskild, A. (2012). Fear of childbirth and duration of labour: A study of 2206 women with intended vaginal delivery. *British Journal of Obstetrics and Gynaecology, 119*(10), 1238–1246.

Ayers, S., & De Visser, R. (2018). *Psychology for medicine and healthcare* (2nd ed.) (pp. 58–62). London: Sage Publications Ltd.

Aune, I., Marit Torvik, H., Selboe, S. T., et al. (2015). promoting a normal birth and a positive birth experience – Norwegian women's perspectives. *Midwifery, 31*(7), 721–727.

Billert, H. (2007). Tokophobia – a multidisciplinary problem. *Ginekologia Polska, 78*(10), 807–811.

Brocklehurst, P., Hardy, P., Hollowell, J., et al. (2011). Perinatal and maternal outcomes by planned place of birth for healthy women with low risk pregnancies: The Birthplace in England national prospective cohort study. *British Medical Journal, 343*, d7400.

CQC (Care Quality Commission). (2018). *2017 Survey of Women's Experiences of Maternity Care: Statistical Release*. Available at: www.cqc.org.uk/sites/default/files/20180130_mat17_statisticalrelease.pdf.

DH (Department of Health). (1993). *Changing Childbirth: report of the Expert Maternity Group, Part 1*. London: The Stationery Office.

DH (Department of Health). (2007). *Maternity matters: choice, access and continuity of care in a safe service*. London: DH. Available at: https://webarchive.nationalarchives.gov.uk/20130103035958/www.dh.gov.uk/prod_consum_dh/groups/dh_digitalassets/@dh/@en/documents/digitalasset/dh_074199.pdf.

Dick-Read, G. (1960). The retreat of fear. *Childbirth without fear* (pp. 79–96). London: Whitefriars Press Ltd.

Garthus-Niegel, S., Storksen, H. T., Torgersen, L., et al. (2011). The Wijma delivery expectancy/experience questionnaire – a factor analytic study. *Journal of Psychosomatic Obstetrics and Gynecology, 32*(3), 16–163.

Gaskin, I. M. (2011). The importance of birth and birth stories. *Birth matters: A midwife's manifesta* (pp. 1–15). London: Pinter and Martin Ltd.

Gomez, E., & Chilvers, R. (2017). *Stepping up to public health: A new maternity model for women and families, midwives and maternity support workers.* Available at: www.rcm.org.uk/media/3165/stepping-up-to-public-health.pdf.

Greer, J., Lazenbatt, A., & Dunne, L. (2014). Fear of childbirth and ways of coping for pregnant women and their partners during the birthing process: A salutogenic analysis. *Evidence Based Midwifery, 12*(3), 95–100.

Gould, D. (2012). Synchronicity: Why women choose caesarean section without medical reason. *British Journal of Midwifery, 20*(1), 5.

Helk, A., Spilling, H., & Smeby, N. (2008). Psychological support by midwives of women with a fear of childbirth: A study of 80 Women. *Vård i Norden, 28*(2), 47–49.

Hertzman, C. (2006). The biological embedding of early experience and its effects on health in adulthood. *Annals of the New York Academy of Sciences* (896), 85–95.

Hofberg, K., & Brockington, I. (2000). Tokophobia: An unreasoning dread of childbirth: A series of 26 cases. *British Journal of Psychiatry, 176*, 83–85.

Hogg, M. A., & Vaughan, G. M. (2018). Attitudes. *Social psychology* (8th ed.) (pp. 152–193). Harlow: Pearson Education, 152–193.

Johnstone, R. W. (1945). Section VI pathology of labour: faults in the powers. *A text book of midwifery for students and practitioners* (12th ed.) (pp. 317–318). London: Adam and Charles Black.

Kirkham, M. (2010). The maternity services context. *The midwife–mother relationship* (2nd ed.) (pp. 1–16). Basingstoke: Palgrave Macmillan.

Lee, A. M., Lam, S. K., Sze Mun Lau, S. M., et al. (2007). Prevalence, course and risk factors for antenatal anxiety and depression. *Obstetrics and Gynecology, 110*(5), 1102–1125.

McKenzie-Harg, K., Ayers, S., Ford, E., et al. (2015). Post-traumatic stress disorder following childbirth: an update of current issues and recommendations for future research. *Journal of Reproductive and Infant Psychology, 33*(3), 219–237.

Melender, H. L. (2002). Experiences of fear associated with pregnancy and childbirth. *Birth, 29*, 101–109.

Monk, C. (2001). Stress and mood disorders during pregnancy: implications for child development. *Psychiatric Quarterly, 72*(4), 347–357.

NICE National Institute of Health and Clinical Excellence. (2011). *Caesarean Section: (CG 132).* London: NICE.

NICE National Institute of Health and Clinical Excellence. (2018). *Antenatal and Postnatal Mental Health: Clinical Management and Service Guidance. (CG 192).* London: NICE.

NHS England. (2016). *National Maternity Review. Better births: improving outcomes of maternity services in England: a five year forward view for maternity care.* London: NHS England. Available at: www.england.nhs.uk/wp-content/uploads/2016/02/national-maternity-review-report.pdf.

Nilsson, N., & Lundgren, I. (2009). Women's lived experience of fear of childbirth. *Midwifery, 25*(2), E1–E9.

O'Connell, M., Leahy-Warren, P., Khashan, A. S., et al. (2015). Tocophobia – the new hysteria? *Obstetrics, Gynaecology and Reproductive Medicine, 25*(6), 175–177.

O'Connell, M. A., Leahy-Warren, P., Khashan, A. S., et al. (2017). Worldwide prevalence of tocophobia in pregnant women: systematic review and meta-analysis. *Nordic Federation of Societies of Obstetrics and Gynecology, 96*, 907–920.

Redshaw, M., Rowe, R., Hockley, C., & Brocklehurst, P. (2007). *Recorded delivery: a national survey of women's experience of maternity care 2006.* Oxford: National Perinatal Epidemiology Unit (NPEU). Available at: https://npeu.ox.ac.uk/downloads/files/reports/Maternity-Survey-Report.pdf.

Reiger, K., & Dempsey, R. (2006). Performing birth in a culture of fear: an embodied crisis of late modernity. *Heath Sociology Review, 15*(4), 364–373.

Richens, Y., Hindley, C., & Lavender, T. (2015). A national online survey of UK maternity unit service provision for women with fear of birth. *British Journal of Midwifery, 23*(8), 574–579.

RCOG (Royal College of Obstetricians and Gynaecologists). (2015) *Birth after previous caesarean birth. Green-top Guideline No 45.* London: RCOG.

Rouhe, H., Salmela-Aro, K., Halmesmaki, E., & Saisto T. (2009). Fear of childbirth according to parity, gestational age and obstetric history. *BJOG, 116*(7), 67–73.

Ryding, E., Nieminen, K., & Stephansson, O. (2009). Swedish women's fear of childbirth and preference for caesarean section in 2006. *International Journal of Obstetrics and Gynecology, 107*(Suppl. 2), S425.

Shepherd, A., & Cheyne, H. (2012). The frequency and reasons for vaginal examinations in labour. *Women and Birth, 26*, 49–54.

Stevenson, A. (2010). *Oxford Dictionary of English* (3rd ed.). Oxford: University Press.

Storksen, H. T., Garthus-Niegel, S., Vangen, S., & Eberhard-Gran, M. (2012). The impact of previous birth experiences on maternal fear of childbirth. *Acta Obstetrica et Gynecologica Scandinavica, 92*(3), 318–324.

Thomson, G., & Downe, S. (2013). A hero's tale of childbirth. *Midwifery, 29*(7), 765–771.

Waldenstrom, U., Hildingsson, I., & Ryding, E. L. (2006). Antenatal fear of childbirth and its association with subsequent caesarean section and experience of childbirth. *BJOG, 113*(6), 638–646.

Walsh, D. (2002). Fear of labour and birth. *British Journal of Midwifery, 10*(2), 78.

Walsh, D. (2017). *Care in the first stage of labour, Mayes' Midwifery* (15th ed.) (pp. 586–613). London: Elsevier.

Wijma, K., Wijma, B., & Zar, M. (1998). Psychometric aspects of the W-DEQ: A new questionnaire for the fear of childbirth. *Journal of Psychometric Obstetrics and Gynecology, 19*(2), 84–98.

Wilkins, C., Baker, R., & Bick, D. (2009). Emotional processing in childbirth: A predictor of postnatal depression? *British Journal of Midwifery, 17*(3), 154–159.

ANNOTATED FURTHER READING

Dahlen, H. G., & Gillman, L. J. (2019). Facilitating safety in midwifery education and practice. In J. Marshall, & E. Myles (Eds.), *Professional studies in midwifery education and practice: concepts and challenges* (pp. 141–157). Edinburgh: Elsevier.

This is a useful chapter that explores the concepts of risk and safety and how managing risk is not the same as facilitating safety. The fears that women and healthcare professionals may have about childbirth are discussed along with determination of how midwives can empower women to trust in their ability to give birth and be mothers. The existing research that supports physiological birth, including ways of instilling confidence about normal birth in both women and midwives is also examined.

Dick-Read, G. (2013). *Childbirth without fear: The principles and practice of natural childbirth.* Cornwall: TJ International Ltd.

As one of the most influential birthing books of all time, this book is essential reading for women and midwives alike. The book unpicks the root causes of women's fears and anxieties about pregnancy, childbirth and breastfeeding, with sensitivity and empathy.

National Institute for Health and Care Excellence. (2018). *Antenatal and Postnatal Mental Health: Clinical management and service guidance: (CG 192).* London: NICE.

These clinical guidelines provide recommendations for referral and interventions throughout the childbirth continuum to support and optimize women's mental health. They are particularly useful for midwives in terms of recognizing and treating specific mental health problems in pregnancy.

O'Connell, M., Leahy-Warren, P., Khashan, A. S., & Kenny, L. C. (2015). Tocophobia – the new hysteria? *Obstetrics, Gynaecology and Reproductive Medicine, 25*(6), 175–177.

A useful article from a practising midwife's viewpoint that recognizes the adverse effects that tocophobia can have on both the woman and baby, which can be long term. The importance of all maternity caregivers being aware of presentation, symptoms and predisposing characteristics of women with tocophobia is stressed so that plans can be put in place to support women through their childbirth experience, such as developing an appropriate birth plan: the overall aim being to ensure a safe birth outcome for mother and baby.

USEFUL WEBSITES

Birth Trauma Association: https://birthtraumaassociation.org.uk/

Mind: www.mind.org.uk/

National Institute of Health and Care Excellence: www.nice.org.uk/

National Perinatal Epidemiological Unit: National Perinatal Epidemiology Unit (NPEU) Birthplace in England Research Programme: www.npeu.ox.ac.uk/birthplace

Royal College of Midwives: www.rcm.org.uk/

Royal College of Obstetricians and Gynaecologists: www.rcog.org.uk/

Physiology and Care During the First Stage of Labour

Karen Jackson, Michelle Anderson, Jayne E. Marshall

CHAPTER CONTENTS

Birth is a dynamic and transforming experience, both on an individual and a societal level, and has the power to profoundly affect the lives of those involved. It is a physiological process characterized by non-intervention, a supportive environment and empowerment of the woman. The midwife is a key figure in this process, supporting and assisting women safely through childbirth, recognizing the *woman's needs and wellbeing are the focus* rather than the needs of the maternity service. Consequently, the midwife is required to be a caring supporter, advocate, skilled practitioner, vigilant observer and an accurate recorder of facts. Women have differing needs and the way they approach and experience birth is unique and will depend on a number of factors, including cultural background, education, sexuality, personal beliefs and previous life experience. In order to meet these varying needs, the midwife should possess wide-ranging skills and knowledge and have the willingness to place the woman at the centre of the care that is provided for her. Women and their chosen birth companion(s) should have an equal partnership with health professionals in all decision-making processes, so that they can make informed choices about their own labours and births (Davison et al. 2018; Walsh 2012, Walsh et al. 2018).

THE CHAPTER AIMS TO

- describe the physical changes taking place as labour progresses
- explore the factors that contribute to a positive birth experience for the woman, including communication, environment, support, assessment and monitoring
- reflect on the care and support that can optimize the wellbeing of the woman and her fetus during the course of labour
- consider the various ways in which midwives can support women to work with/relieve the pain of labour
- provide an overview of fetal physiology discussing the factors that influence fetal heart responses when affected by mechanical or iatrogenic stress

- discuss 'intelligent' intermittent auscultation and applied fetal pathophysiology
- discuss the background to CTG interpretation and the introduction of NICE and FIGO Guidelines
- consider the types of hypoxia and offer pathophysiological reasoning for why specific states of hypoxic episodes may manifest during labour
- describe the principles in the assessment and care of labours presenting by breech
- reflect on the midwife's role in caring for women who present with pre-labour rupture of the fetal membranes.

DEFINING LABOUR

A human pregnancy is considered to last approximately 40 weeks, with labour usually occurring between 37 and 42 weeks' gestation (National Institute for Health and Care Excellence, NICE 2017) Complex physiological and psychological changes occur during the last few weeks of pregnancy, and also during the onset of labour, that prepare the woman for the process of labour and birth (Howie and Watson 2017a; McNabb 2017; Walsh 2012) (see Chapter 10).

Labour, purely in the physical sense, may be described as the process by which the fetus, placenta and membranes are expelled through the birth canal; however, labour is much more than a purely physical event. What happens during labour can affect the relationship between the mother and baby and can

influence the likelihood and/or experience of future pregnancies.

Definitions of normal birth in high income countries can be contentious, due to the inclusion of some common but nonetheless interventionist practices. The World Health Organization (WHO) continues to define *normal* labour as one that is low risk throughout, spontaneous in onset with the fetus presenting by the vertex, culminating in the mother and infant being in good condition following birth (WHO 1999). However, a labour where the fetus is presenting by the *breech* with no other risk factors should also be considered *normal* (Evans 2017). Furthermore, most definitions of labour appear to be purely physiological and do not encompass the psychological, spiritual and emotional wellbeing of the woman.

Traditionally, three stages of labour are described: the *first*, *second* and *third stage*, but this is a rather pedantic, medically ascribed view, as labour is obviously a continuous process and many midwives would prefer normal labour to be recognized as such (Walsh 2017). It has also been acknowledged that there are more than three stages of labour, namely the *latent*, *active* and *transitional phases*, and these not only encompass specific physical changes but should also account for the emotional effects observed in women during this time.

Labour for each woman has its own unique ebbs and flows. Walsh (2010a, 2017) describes this as *labour rhythms*. However, as labour tends to be described and recognized traditionally as having distinct *stages* of labour, this approach will be adopted for the purposes of this text. The *first stage of labour* is usually recognized by the onset of regular uterine contractions, an accompanying effacement and at least 4 cm dilatation of the cervix and finally culminates in full dilatation of the cervix (NICE 2017; Howie and Watson 2017b). Some researchers feel that the active first stage of labour should be characterized as commencing at cervical dilatation of 6 cm (Zhang et al. 2010; American College of Obstetricians and Gynecologists, ACOG 2014).

THE ONSET OF SPONTANEOUS PHYSIOLOGICAL LABOUR

The onset of labour is determined by a complex interaction of maternal and fetal hormones and is not fully understood. It would appear to be multifactorial in origin, being a combination of hormonal and mechanical factors. Levels of maternal oestrogen rise sharply during the last weeks of pregnancy, resulting in changes that overcome the inhibiting effects of progesterone. High levels of oestrogens cause uterine muscle fibres to display oxytocic receptors and form gap junctions with each other. Oestrogen also stimulates the placenta to release prostaglandins that induce a production of enzymes that will digest collagen in the cervix, helping it to soften (Tortora and Derrickson 2017). The process is unclear but it is thought that both fetal and placental factors are involved. There is no clear evidence that concentrations of oestrogens and progesterone alter at the onset of labour, but the balance between them does facilitate myometrial activity. Uterine activity may also result from mechanical stimulation of the uterus and cervix. This may be brought about by overstretching, as in the case of a multiple pregnancy, or pressure from a presenting part that is well applied to the cervix (Impey and Child 2017).

Recognition of the Onset of Labour

The onset of labour is a process, not an event; therefore it is very difficult to identify exactly when the painless (sometimes painful) contractions of pre-labour develop into the progressive rhythmic contractions of established labour. Diagnosing the onset of labour is extremely important, since it is on the basis of this finding that decisions are made that will affect the intrapartum care and support subsequently provided (NICE 2017; Zhang et al. 2010).

It is part of the role of the midwife to ensure that women have sufficient information to assist them in recognizing the onset of established labour. This information is also needed to enable women to make informed choices based on current and unbiased evidence. The complex physical, psychological and emotional experience of labour affects every woman differently and midwives must have sound knowledge and experience to enable the woman to maintain control over the birth of her baby. Women in labour should be encouraged to trust their own instincts, listen to their own body and verbalize feelings in order to receive the help and support they require. Anxiety can increase the production of adrenaline (epinephrine), which inhibits uterine activity and may in turn prolong labour (Simkin et al. 2017).

Irrespective of whether they have given birth before, many women experience contractions before the onset of labour, which may be painful and regular for a time, causing them to think that labour has started. Furthermore, some women's lived experiences of early labour report *prolonged contractions* or being *in labour for days* and thus it is important to note that the discomfort or even pain that the woman is conscious of is *genuine to her*. Although the contractions that the woman is experiencing are real, they have yet to settle into the rhythmic pattern of *established* labour, resulting in *effacement and dilatation of the cervix*. Using terminology such as *'spurious'* or *'false labour'* is unhelpful and typically negative in terms of women's genuine experiences of early labour (Walsh 2012). Reassurance should be given, and discussion of this potential situation earlier in the pregnancy can enable the woman and her partner to prepare for labour more effectively. Contact with the midwife should be made when **regular, rhythmic, uterine contractions are experienced** and these are **perceived by the woman as uncomfortable or painful.**

Latent Phase of Labour or Early Labour

The *latent phase* of labour (increasingly being referred to as early labour) is *prior* to the active phase stage of labour and may last 6–8 h in primigravidae when the cervix dilates from 0 cm to 4 cm dilated (Howie and Watson 2017b), but again this is rather a restrictive description and McDonald (2010) argues that the latent phase of labour is so subjective and poorly understood that a normal range is difficult to measure. According to Nirmal and Fraser (2016), the cervical canal shortens from 3 cm long to <0.5 cm in length during this time.

A woman may believe herself to be labouring, whereas sound midwifery judgement and understanding of the physiology of the first stage of labour may lead the midwife to the diagnosis of the *latent phase* of labour. Both the woman and midwife being aware of the latent phase of labour, and allowing this time to pass with no intervention, can prevent the medical diagnosis of *poor progress* or *failure to progress* later in labour. In a hospital setting, it is good practice not to commence the partogram until *active labour* has commenced. Assessing the active phase of labour has been highlighted as essential in reducing interventions in normal labour (Lauzon and Hodnett 2009).

Active Phase of Labour

The *active phase* within the first stage of labour is the time when the cervix usually undergoes more rapid dilatation. This begins when the cervix is at least 4 cm dilated and, in the presence of rhythmic contractions, progressively dilates to 10 cm or full dilatation. However, the parameters of the first stage of labour, in terms of cervical dilatation have been questioned. Zhang et al. (2010) in their large, multicentre trial, concluded that childbearing women may not enter *active* labour until cervical dilatation of at least 5–6 cm. The ACOG (2014) have attempted to stem the rising caesarean section rate by recommending that active labour is not considered until the cervix is at least 6 cm dilated.

When in labour, contractions will often be accompanied or preceded by a bloodstained mucoid *show*: that is, the release of the *operculum* from the cervical canal as effacement and dilatation progresses. Occasionally, the membranes will rupture, at which stage the midwife

may seek assurance that there are no significant changes in the fetal heart rate due to the rare complication of cord prolapse and that meconium is not present in the liquor, indicating fetal compromise.

Transitional Phase of Labour

It is interesting that many women (but not all) experience a transition from the first to second stage of labour but little is found in the midwifery and childbirth literature about transition and it is not mentioned at all in the NICE (2017) guidelines. The *transitional phase* of the first stage of labour is from when the cervix is around 8 cm dilated until it is fully dilated or until expulsive contractions associated with the second stage of labour are felt by the woman. There is often a brief lull in the intensity of uterine activity at this time. Many women may feel the urge to push during transition. In addition to physiological responses, women can experience a range of experiences and emotions. Woods (2006) describes this as being from *inner calm* to *acute distress*. Downe (2017) describes a range of behaviours that women can display during transition such as feeling a loss of control, expressing that they 'cannot do it', nausea, shouting and screaming, a demand for pain relief, among others. The woman may verbalize her distress and direct it at her birth partner(s), or even sometimes at her caregivers, alternatively they may be quiet and contemplative going inside themselves, sometimes referred to as the 'rest and be thankful' phase.

PHYSIOLOGY OF THE FIRST STAGE OF LABOUR

Duration

The length of labour varies widely and is influenced by parity, birth interval, psychological state, presentation and position of the fetus. Maternal pelvic shape and size and the character of uterine contractions also affect timescale.

By far the greatest part of labour is taken up by the first stage and it is common to expect *the active phase* to be completed within 6–12 h (Tortora and Derrickson 2017). Over the years, there has been much debate surrounding the length of physiological active labour in low-risk populations of childbearing women to refute the original claim of Friedman (1954) that cervical dilatation occurred at the rate of 1 cm per hour (Albers 1999; Lavender et al. 2018; Zhang et al. 2010). A cervical

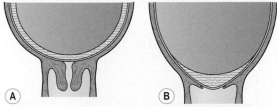

Fig. 19.1 (A) The cervix before effacement. (B) The cervix after effacement. The cervical canal is now part of the lower uterine segment.

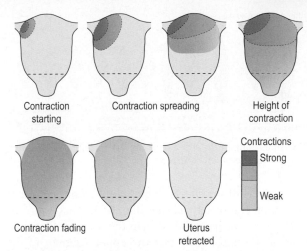

Fig. 19.2 Series of diagrams to show fundal dominance during uterine contractions.

dilatation rate of 0.5 cm per hour, however, has now been incorporated into the NICE (2017) intrapartum guidelines as being within the parameters of *normal* labour.

Cervical Effacement

Effacement refers to the inclusion (*taking up*) of the cervical canal into the lower uterine segment. It is believed that this process takes place from above downwards, meaning that the muscle fibres surrounding the internal os are drawn upwards by the retracted upper segment and the cervix merges into the lower uterine segment. The cervical canal widens at the level of the internal os, whereas the state of the external os remains unchanged (Cunningham et al. 2018) (Fig. 19.1).

Effacement may occur late in pregnancy, or it may not take place until labour begins. In the nulliparous woman, the cervix will not usually dilate until effacement is complete, whereas in the multiparous woman, effacement and dilatation usually occurs simultaneously and a small canal may be felt in early labour. This is often referred to by midwives as a *multips os* (Howie and Watson 2017a).

Cervical Dilatation

Dilatation of the cervix is the process of enlargement of the os uteri from a tightly closed aperture to an opening large enough to permit passage of the fetus. Dilatation is assessed in centimetres and *full dilatation* at term equates to about 10 cm. However, acknowledging that all women are different sizes and shapes means that full cervical dilatation may be between 9 and 11 cm in individual women (Walsh 2012).

Dilatation occurs as a result of uterine action and the counter-pressure applied by either the intact bag of membranes or the presenting part, or both. A well-flexed fetal head closely applied to the cervix favours efficient dilatation. Pressure applied evenly to the cervix

causes the uterine fundus to respond by contraction and retraction, often referred to as the *Ferguson reflex* (Howie and Watson 2017b).

Uterine Action
Fundal dominance (Fig. 19.2)

Each uterine contraction commences in the fundus near one of the cornua and spreads across and downwards. The contraction lasts longest in the fundus, where it is also most intense, but the peak is reached simultaneously over the whole uterus and the contraction fades from all parts together. This pattern permits the cervix to dilate and the strongly contracting fundus to eventually expel the fetus at the end of labour (Howie and Watson 2017b).

Polarity

Polarity is the term used to describe the neuromuscular harmony that prevails between the two poles or segments of the uterus throughout labour. During each uterine contraction, these two poles act harmoniously. The upper pole contracts strongly and retracts to expel the fetus; the lower pole contracts slightly and dilates to allow expulsion to take place. If polarity is disorganized then the progress of labour is inhibited (Bernal and Norwitz 2018).

Contraction and retraction

Uterine muscle has a unique property. During labour the contraction does not pass off entirely, as muscle fibres

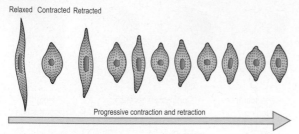

Fig. 19.3 Diagram to show how uterine muscle retains some shortening after each contraction.

retain some of the shortening of contraction instead of becoming completely relaxed (Fig. 19.3). This is termed *retraction*. This process assists in the progressive expulsion of the fetus, such that the upper segment of the uterus becomes gradually shorter and thicker and its cavity diminishes.

Intensity and resting tone

Each labour is individual and does not always conform to expectations, but generally before labour becomes established, uterine contractions may occur every 15–20 min, lasting for about 30 seconds. They are often fairly weak and may even be imperceptible to the woman. The contractions usually occur with rhythmic regularity and the intervals between them where the muscle relaxes (*resting tone*) gradually lessen while the length and strength gradually intensifies through the latent phase and into the active phase of the first stage of labour. By the end of the first stage, the contractions may occur at 2–3 min intervals, last for 50–60 seconds and are very powerful (Cunningham et al. 2018).

Formation of upper and lower uterine segments

By the end of pregnancy, the body of the uterus is described as having divided into two segments, which are anatomically distinct (Fig. 19.4). The upper uterine segment, having been formed from the body of the fundus, is mainly concerned with contraction and retraction, and is thick and muscular. The lower uterine segment is formed of the isthmus and the cervix, and is about 8–10 cm in length. The lower segment is prepared for distension and dilatation. Although there is no clear and strict division of these two segments, the muscle content reduces from the fundus to the cervix, where it is thinner. When labour begins, the retracted longitudinal fibres in the upper segment pull on the lower segment causing it to stretch. This is aided by the force

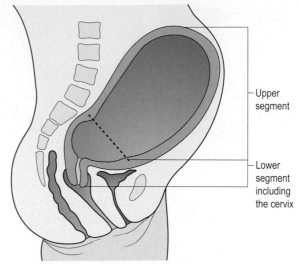

Fig. 19.4 Birth canal before labour begins.

applied by the descending presenting part (Howie and Watson 2017b; Impey and Child 2017).

The retraction ring

A ridge develops between the upper and lower uterine segments, known as the *retraction ring* (Fig. 19.5). The physiological retraction ring gradually rises as the upper uterine segment contracts and retracts and the lower uterine segment thins out to accommodate the descending fetus. Once the cervix is fully dilated and the fetus can leave the uterus, the retraction ring rises no further. However, in extreme cases of *mechanically obstructed labour*, this physiological retraction ring becomes visible above the symphysis pubis and is described as *Bandl's ring*. A Bandl's ring may consequently be associated with fetal compromise (Lauria et al. 2007).

Show. As a result of the dilatation of the cervix, the operculum, which formed the cervical plug during pregnancy, is released. The woman may observe a bloodstained mucoid discharge a few hours before, or within a few hours after labour commences. The blood comes from ruptured capillaries in the parietal decidua where the chorion has become detached from the dilating cervix and should only be a staining (Impey and Child 2017). Frank, fresh bleeding is atypical at this stage, although during the transitional phase and as the first stage ends, there is often a *small* loss of bright red blood that heralds the second stage of labour. Both occurrences may be referred to as a *show*.

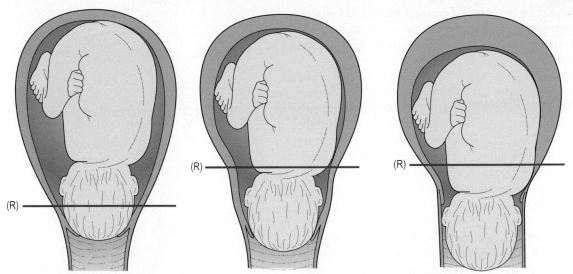

Fig. 19.5 Diagram showing the retraction ring (*R*) between the upper and lower uterine segments.

Mechanical Factors

Formation of the forewaters and hindwaters

As the lower uterine segment forms and stretches, the chorion becomes detached from it and the increased intrauterine pressure causes this loosened part of the sac of fluid to bulge downwards into the internal os, to the depth of 6–12 mm. The well-flexed fetal head fits snugly into the cervix and cuts off the amniotic fluid in front of the head from that which surrounds the body, forming two separate pools of fluid. The former is known as the *forewaters* and the latter, the *hindwaters*. In early labour it is often possible to feel intact forewaters bulging even when the hindwaters have ruptured, making ruptured membranes a difficult diagnosis at times.

The effect of separation of the forewaters prevents the pressure that is applied to the hindwaters during uterine contractions from being applied to the forewaters. This may help to keep the membranes intact during the first stage of labour and be a natural defence against ascending infection (Bernal and Norwitz 2018).

General fluid pressure

While the membranes remain intact, the pressure of the uterine contractions is exerted on the amniotic fluid and, as fluid is not compressible, the pressure is equalized throughout the uterus and over the fetal body, known as *general fluid pressure* (Fig. 19.6). When the membranes rupture and a quantity of fluid emerges, the fetal head, the placenta and umbilical cord are compressed between

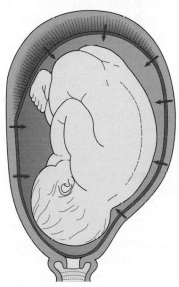

Fig. 19.6 General fluid pressure.

the uterine wall and the fetus during contractions with a consequential reduction in the oxygen supply to the fetus. Preserving the integrity of the membranes, therefore, optimizes the oxygen supply to the fetus and also helps to prevent intrauterine and fetal infection (Howie and Watson 2017b).

Rupture of the membranes

The optimum physiological time for the membranes to rupture spontaneously is at the *end of the first stage of labour,* after the cervix becomes fully dilated and no longer supports the bag of forewaters. The uterine contractions are also applying increasing expulsive force at this time.

The membranes may sometimes rupture days before labour begins or during the first stage. If for any reason there is a suboptimal fitting of the presenting part and the forewaters are not separated effectively then the membranes may rupture early. However, in most cases there is no apparent reason for early spontaneous membrane rupture. Occasionally the membranes do not rupture even in the second stage and appear at the vulva as a bulging sac covering the fetal head as it is born; this is known as the *caul.*

Early rupture of membranes may lead to an increased incidence of variable decelerations on cardiotocography (CTG), resulting in an increase in caesarean sections if fetal blood sampling is not available (Alfirevic et al. 2017). A systematic review found that routine artificial rupture of membranes (ARM) does not significantly reduce the length of labour and thus routine amniotomy should not be performed (Smyth et al. 2013). However, there was some evidence that ARM increased the rate of caesarean section but this finding did not reach significance. All women are required to give consent for this intervention and the midwife should have a clear indication for performing an ARM; details of which should be recorded in the woman's labour records (Nursing and Midwifery Council, NMC 2018).

Fetal axis pressure

During each contraction, the uterus rises forward and the force of the fundal contraction is transmitted to the upper pole of the fetus, down the long axis of the fetus and applied by the presenting part to the cervix. This is known as *fetal axis pressure* (Fig. 19.7) and becomes much more significant after rupture of the membranes and during the second stage of labour.

RECOGNITION OF THE FIRST STAGE OF LABOUR

It is the woman herself who usually diagnoses the onset of physiological labour and many women and their partners are apprehensive in case the labour is very quick, resulting in an unattended birth. Education during pregnancy is important to enable the woman to recognize the beginning of labour and understand the latent

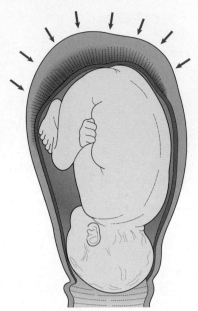

Fig. 19.7 Fetal axis pressure.

phase in order to consider possible strategies she may use for labour and birth.

Women should appreciate that in late pregnancy, vaginal secretions *without* any blood-staining increase. In addition, they should be aware that a *show*, which is usually a pink or bloodstained jelly-like loss, prior to the onset of labour or in early labour, is quite common. If a woman is examined vaginally in late pregnancy they should also be informed that there may be some slight blood loss after the procedure.

Braxton Hicks contractions are more noticeable in late pregnancy and some women experience them as painful. They are usually irregular or their regularity is not maintained for long spells of time, seldom lasting more than 1 min. In active labour, contractions exhibit a pattern of rhythm and regularity, usually increasing in length, strength and frequency as time goes on. When the woman first feels contractions she may be aware only of backache, but if she places a hand on her abdomen she may perceive simultaneous hardening of the uterus. If the pregnancy has been problem-free, with a vaginal birth anticipated, the midwife may advise the woman to stay in her own surroundings, continue with her normal activities, to eat, be active and upright, recognizing her unique needs and that further assessment may be required.

It is sometimes difficult to be certain whether or not the membranes have ruptured spontaneously prior to labour or in early labour. The woman may be experiencing some degree of stress incontinence, so she may be unsure if it is liquor or urine that she is passing. If there is any doubt, the woman should contact her midwife who may decide to insert a speculum into the vagina to observe for any amniotic fluid. Digital examination should be avoided if the woman is not in labour as it can increase the risk of ascending infection (Shepherd et al. 2010).

INITIAL MEETING WITH THE MIDWIFE

Ideally, the woman should know the midwife (or a small team of midwives) who will be providing the intrapartum care ahead of labour commencing to make direct contact when labour actually starts (NHS England 2016). Where this is not possible, it is crucial that the first meeting between the midwife, the labouring woman and her partner establishes a rapport, which sets the scene for the remainder of labour. If the woman is planning to birth in hospital, they may worry about the reception she and her companion will receive and the attitude of the people attending her. In addition, an unfamiliar environment may provoke feelings of vulnerability and undermine their confidence. Comfortable surroundings, a welcoming manner and a midwife who greets the woman as an equal in a partnership will engender feelings of mutual respect, thus enabling the woman to relax and respond positively to the amazing forces of labour and to her baby after it is born (Berry 2006; Fisher et al. 2006; Raynor and England 2010).

The Language of Childbirth

It has been recognized that some of the childbirth terminology used when communicating with women appears medical, paternalistic and negative (Mobbs et al. 2018). The terms *pain* and *labour* are suggestive of *difficulty* and *trouble*. It is therefore vital the midwife uses appropriate and adapted language, which is woman-friendly when they speak to women during childbirth. The word *delivery* has been replaced by the term *birthing* or *birth* as these appear more suitable when discussing the concept and practice of normality within midwifery.

Communication

The key issues for women relate to achieving a safe birth, feeling in control within the birth environment, developing supportive relationships with their carers, and being treated with kindness, respect, dignity and cultural sensitivity if they are to realize a positive experience of birth (Helman 2007; Main and Bingham 2008; Redshaw and Heikkila 2010). Effective communication between the midwife and the woman and her partner, and with other clinicians in the multidisciplinary team, is essential to providing effective safe supportive care in labour and achieving the woman's objectives (NHS England 2016; Royal College of Obstetricians and Gynaecologists, RCOG 2016). Communication does not consist only of the content of what is said, but also includes non-verbal communication and written records, such as the woman's birth plan.

Poor communication is the commonest cause of preventable adverse outcomes in hospitals and remains a significant cause of written complaints (NHS Digital 2018). An inquiry conducted by the Kings Fund into the safety of birth in England concluded that the overwhelming majority of births are safe but when there are increased risks to the woman or baby, that render some births *less safe*, *functioning teams* are key to improving the outcome for the woman and baby (Kings Fund 2008).

Interpreting Services

If the woman and midwife are unable to understand each other because of language differences, communication will be ineffective and it is essential that adequate interpretation services are available when necessary. Although there is a tendency to rely on family members or friends to provide interpreting services, the use of such interpreters is deemed inappropriate when the midwife wishes to discuss sensitive issues such as past history, domestic abuse or the need for interventions. Wherever possible, professional interpretation services should be provided for all non-English-speaking women (Knight et al. 2017). If a face-to-face interpreter cannot be obtained, then the use of a telephone or internet interpretation service should be considered.

Birth Plan

Regardless of where the woman plans to give birth, a birth plan is a valuable tool for midwives to observe and use to facilitate the provision of holistic, individualized care. This is especially so in situations where the maternity care is fragmented and the woman first encounters the midwife who will be caring for her in labour when she attends the hospital to give birth. The birth plan therefore provides the opportunity for the midwife to discuss with each woman and their partner any plans about the type of birth they would like and that they may have already prepared with support from their community midwife. An outline may be present in the case notes, or the couple may bring a birth plan with them. Frequently, the partner is involved in this forward planning, which should be a flexible proposal that can be reviewed and revised as labour progresses (Divall et al. 2017). Some women, however, may not have prepared a birth plan and so the midwife should encourage them to consider any preferences that they may have, for example:

- their choice of birth companion(s)
- their choice of clothes for labour
- ambulation and fetal monitoring (intermittent, electronic or a combination)
- strategies for labour (water immersion, massage, pharmacological pain relief)
- position for labour and birth
- expectant or actively managed third stage of labour
- cutting of the umbilical cord
- skin-to-skin contact and feeding the baby after birth.

Having the opportunity to discuss such issues in early labour enables the establishment of a trusting relationship between the woman and the midwife to develop where the woman feels valued and involved in intrapartum decision-making; all details of which should be clearly documented in the intrapartum records (NMC 2018).

Emotional and Psychological Care

When a woman begins to labour, she may have a mixture of emotions. Most women anticipate labour with a degree of excitement, anxiety, fear and hope. Many other emotions are influenced by cultural expectations and previous life experiences. The state of the woman's knowledge, her fears and expectations are also influenced by her companions during labour, including the attitude and behaviour of the caregiver.

By the time labour starts, a decision will already have been reached about where the woman plans to give birth. Some women may choose to give birth at home, some in a midwife-led unit/birthing centre and others in hospital. Some women may also wish to labour as long as possible at home but give birth in hospital. Whatever choice the woman makes, they must always be the focus of the care, able to feel they are in control of what is happening and contributing to the decisions made about their care (Sinivaara et al. 2004; Department of Health, DH 2007). Hodnett et al. (2012) assert that there is a powerful effect on maternal birth satisfaction and labour progress where women feel in control and involved in decision-making.

Providing that there are no complications and labour is not well advanced, the woman may remain at home as long as she feels comfortable and confident. If labour commences prior to term, however, admission to hospital is always advised (see Chapter 14).

Companion in Labour

The fact that women should be encouraged to have support by birth partners of their choice is well recognized (NICE 2017; National Childbirth Trust, NCT 2019). Each woman is *central* to all the decisions made about care during labour and their chosen companion, whether sexual partner, friend or family member, should understand this. Ideally the companion should be involved in pre-labour preparation and decision-making, have participated in compiling the birth plan and be aware of all the available options.

If the woman is giving birth in hospital, admission to a labour ward can be an alienating experience and the company of a supportive companion can help reduce anxiety. During labour, the companion should be made to feel useful and part of the team by the midwife, as they too may be feeling anxious (Longworth and Kingdon 2010). Such activities may include massaging the woman's back, offering drinks, assisting with breathing and relaxation awareness and supporting their decisions regarding strategies they can use for working with, or controlling, pain.

In some cases, a midwife will be able to remain with one woman through her entire labour, but due to the unpredictable workloads and staffing levels, this is not always possible. This can leave the woman feeling unsupported and processed, rather than cared for and can have profound negative effects on their satisfaction and memory of the birth (Kirkham 2011). Despite such constraints it is not appropriate to use the birth partner as a substitute for close observation and attendance by the midwife. Equally so, the midwife should also recognize the need for the couple to have some personal space and leave them alone, albeit with the means to summon assistance should it be required. This would not be acceptable, however, when labour is well advanced, as being left alone could prove very frightening for the woman and her partner.

It would be a mistake to consider that all women have the same requirements as they have varying needs, with some preferring presence and others preferring complete privacy. The task for the midwife is to provide the individualized service that ensures that the woman feels safe and supported. Despite the aim to provide a good outcome for the woman, there is no doubt that a proportion of women are dissatisfied with the birthing experience and some are positively traumatized by their experience (Gribbin 2017).

It is also important to ensure that support is available to the partner when it is needed if the woman is in significant pain or a sudden emergency develops, and they are encouraged to take short breaks during a prolonged labour. If a caesarean section becomes necessary, the midwife should delegate someone to keep the partner informed, so they are not left feeling abandoned or uncared for.

The concept of continuous support in labour

There is evidence that the presence of the midwife and one-to-one personal attention is positively associated with a woman's satisfaction with her care. Kennedy et al. (2010) describe that the presence and demeanour of the midwife can enhance the woman's trust in her own ability to cope. In a systematic review by Bohren et al. (2017), the value of continuous support during labour and birth is clearly evident. The review, consisting of 27 clinical trials, involving almost 16,000 women, showed evidence that women who laboured *with* continuous support had shorter labours and were less likely to experience intrapartum interventions. These women were also less likely to have an epidural or other forms of pain medication, give birth by caesarean section, ventouse or forceps and consequently appeared more satisfied with their overall experience of childbirth. Babies were less likely to have low 5-min Apgar scores (Bohren et al. 2017).

Similar positive results have been reported in a Cochrane systematic review by Sandall et al. (2016), who collected data from 15 trials culminating in the birth outcomes of 17,674 women. It was found that where women received midwife-led care throughout pregnancy and birth from a small group of midwives they were less likely to give birth prematurely or require interventions in labour such as regional analgesia, instrumental birth, or amniotomy than those women who received care based on a shared care model or medical model. Childbearing women were more likely to achieve spontaneous vaginal birth and for the birth to be attended by a midwife known to them and report higher rates of satisfaction if the service was midwife-led. Consequently, Sandall et al. (2016) affirm that all women should be offered *midwife-led continuity of care* unless they have serious medical or obstetric complications, and women should be encouraged to ask for this option.

The essence of midwifery is to be *with woman*, providing comfort and support to women in labour. Although the midwife has an important role to play in providing support and care, there is evidence that a birth partner who is neither from the woman's social network or a member of the midwifery team, such as a doula, can provide the most effective continuous support during labour, resulting in less interventions and pain medication and an increase in positive childbirth experiences (Bohren et al. 2017).

The Physical Environment

In mid- to high-income countries, most births occur in hospital and therefore the atmosphere and environment of hospital birthing rooms are important (Walsh 2017). The clinical appearance of hospital birthing rooms, coupled with associated clinical regimes and loss of privacy, can alienate women and lead to feelings of loss of control (Marshall et al. 2011). In turn, this loss of control can interfere with the normal physiological process of labour (Walsh 2010a,b).

Less clinical environments and the addition of equipment to enhance relaxation, mobility and calm have a positive effect on women and care providers according to Hodnett et al. (2009). It is important that the philosophy of woman-centred-care accompanies any change in environment, such as compassionate, kind and supportive care. A change in environment alone will not be sufficient to fulfil labouring women's needs, or improve birth outcomes or the birthing experience.

Reducing the Risk of Infection

Since the last triennial report into maternal deaths, there has been a considerable reduction in women dying from sepsis. However, sepsis remains an important and significant cause of maternal deaths (Knight et al. 2019). In the latest MBRRACE report, between 2015 and 2017, there were 20 maternal deaths/100,000 maternities attributed to sepsis in the UK and Ireland (Knight et al. 2019). The message to *think sepsis* in childbearing women who become unwell is still emphasized by the latest MBRRACE report.

With the introduction of a national strategy to reduce the rates of methicillin-resistant *Staphylococcus aureus* (MRSA) and *Clostridium difficile* (*C. difficile*), there is evidence that the rates of both types of infection have reduced dramatically (British Standards Institution, BSI 2014; NICE 2014a).

Hand hygiene, the combination of processes including handwashing, the use of alcohol handrub and carefully drying and caring for the skin and nails, is considered to be the single most important measure in preventing the spread of infection. Handwashing will remove transient microorganisms and render the hands socially clean, however, evidence suggests that the process of handwashing is poorly performed and therefore less effective than it otherwise could be. Prior to and immediately following any direct contact with the woman or baby and their immediate surroundings or after an exposure risk to any body fluids, effective hand hygiene practices, as determined by the WHO (2017), should be followed.

A clean environment is essential if infection rates are to be kept to a minimum and the midwife has an important role to play in ensuring that all equipment is cleaned according to local Trust guidelines and that there is adherence to all infection control measures. Rooms, birthing pools, beds and any equipment used by the midwife should be effectively cleaned before use.

When a woman is admitted to hospital, invasive procedures should be kept to a minimum as an intact skin provides an excellent barrier to organisms. Ideally, women should spend as little time in hospital as determined by their individual needs to minimize their exposure risk to infection. The fetal membranes should also be preserved intact unless there is a positive indication for their rupture that would outweigh the advantage of their protective functions (NICE 2017).

Certain invasive techniques, such as the performance of vaginal examinations, may be deemed necessary during labour, however the midwife should ensure that they have a sound reason before embarking on any procedure. Women whose labour is prolonged are at particular risk of infection, often being subjected to a number of invasive procedures including the administration of intravenous fluids, repeated vaginal examinations, epidural analgesia and fetal blood sampling, all of which will increase the risk of infection. By adhering to infection control policies and minimizing interventions when required, the midwife should reduce the potential risk of infection to the woman and promote safety.

The midwife is encouraged to use personal protective equipment if they assess that there is a risk of transmission of microorganisms to the woman, or the risk of contamination of their clothing and skin by the woman's body fluids (NICE 2017). This poses a difficulty for the midwife, as every birth presents a risk of cross-contamination, but wearing a full gown, face masks and eye goggles can create an artificial barrier between themselves and the labouring woman at a time when a relationship of trust is vital. Furthermore, face masks and eye goggles provide limited protection from spills or inhalation of spray. In most instances, appropriate hand hygiene and the use of single-use sterile gloves will be sufficient to reduce cross-contamination (NICE 2017).

The Midwife's Initial Physical Examination of the Woman

The initial examination should include a discussion with the woman about when labour commenced, whether the membranes have ruptured and the frequency and strength of the contractions. The midwife should be aware that the woman will be very conscious of their body and may be unable to concentrate on the conversation or respond while experiencing a contraction. Since the woman has embarked on an intensely energy-demanding process, enquiry should be made about her ability to sleep and her most recent intake of food. If in early labour and there are no concerns about the pregnancy, the woman should be advised that they can eat and drink as they wish, remain mobile and maybe bathe if they would find this relaxing. Consideration should be given to the woman's social circumstances, including the care of other children and whether a birthing partner is available and has been contacted.

Past history

Of particular relevance at the onset of a woman's labour are:
- the contents of the birth plan
- their parity and age
- the gestational age and outcomes of previous labours
- the weights and condition of previous babies
- their blood results including grouping, Rhesus factor and haemoglobin
- their attendance at any specialist clinics
- evidence of any known problems: social or physical.

Consent

Prior to touching the woman, a sound explanation of the proposed examination and their significance should be given. Verbal consent should be obtained and recorded in the notes (NMC 2018). The midwife must be aware that a competent woman, with a capacity to make decisions, is within her rights to refuse any treatment regardless of the consequences to them and their unborn baby and she does *not* have to give a reason (DH 2009). Should the midwife be providing care to a pregnant teenager under the age of 16 years, it is important to carefully assess whether there is evidence that she has sufficient understanding in order to give valid consent, i.e. complies with the Fraser guidelines, previously referred to as being *Gillick competent* (*Gillick v West Norfolk and Wisbech AHA* 1986; General Medical Council, GMC 2018).

General assessment

Initial observations form a baseline for further examinations carried out throughout labour. Basic observations, including pulse rate, temperature and blood pressure, are assessed and recorded. The woman's hands and feet are usually examined for signs of oedema. Slight swelling of the feet and ankles is physiological, but pretibial oedema or puffiness of the fingers or face is not.

A detailed *abdominal examination* including symphysis fundal height and optimum position for auscultation of the fetal heart, as described in Chapter 11, should be undertaken and recorded. The abdominal examination may be repeated at intervals in order to assess descent of the presenting part, whether it be cephalic or breech. This is measured by the number of fifths palpable above the pelvic brim and should be recorded on the partogram and in the labour records.

The fetal heart rate should be auscultated for a minimum of *1 minute* immediately after a contraction using a Pinard stethoscope and the rate should be recorded as an average, in a single figure. The maternal pulse should be palpated to differentiate between maternal and fetal heart rates (NICE 2017). Although the Pinard stethoscope is recommended for the initial assessment of the fetal heart, this may not be suitable for use in women who are markedly obese or unable to remain still during auscultation. In such circumstances, a handheld Doppler may be used.

A *vaginal examination* (VE) may also be undertaken to help confirm the onset of labour and determine the

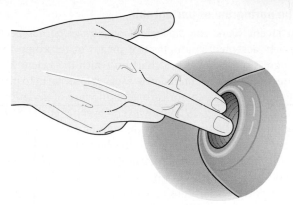

Fig. 19.8 Cervix 4 cm dilated.

extent of cervical effacement and dilatation (Fig. 19.8), with some women requesting it when seeking reassurance about the status of their labour. The procedure, however, is invasive, can be uncomfortable and also poses an infection risk.

Records

The midwife's record of labour is a legal document and must be clear, accurate and relevant to their sphere of practice. The records may be examined by any court for up to 25 years, or the Nursing and Midwifery Council's Fitness to Practise Committee or on behalf of the Clinical Negligence Scheme for Trusts (CNST; see NHS Resolution 2018) monitoring process. A summary of good record-keeping is provided below (NMC 2018):

- Complete records at the time or as soon as possible after an event, recording if the notes are written some time after the event.
- Identify any risks or problems that have arisen and the steps taken to deal with them, so that colleagues who use the records have all the information they need.
- Complete records accurately and without any falsification, taking immediate and appropriate action if you become aware that someone has not kept to these requirements.
- Attribute any entries you make in any paper or electronic records to yourself, making sure they are clearly written, dated and timed, and do not include unnecessary abbreviations, jargon or speculation.
- Take all steps to make sure that records are kept securely.
- Collect, treat and store all data and research findings appropriately.

The partogram or partograph

In recent years, the *partogram* or *partograph* has been widely accepted as an effective means of recording the progress of labour. It is a chart on which the salient features of labour are entered in a visual graphic form to provide the opportunity for early identification of deviations from normal (Fig. 19.9). However, Lavender et al. (2018) found no evidence to support the routine use of the partogram in women who commenced labour spontaneously at term with regards to maternal and fetal outcomes in those labours where a partogram was used against those where there was no partogram. Nonetheless, the partogram remains an integral part of intrapartum record-keeping. The charts are usually designed to allow for recordings at 15-min to 4-hourly intervals and include:

- fetal heart rate
- maternal temperature, pulse and blood pressure
- frequency and strength of contractions
- descent of the presenting part
- cervical effacement and dilatation
- colour of the amniotic fluid/liquor
- degree of caput succedaneum/moulding
- fluid balance
- urine analysis
- any medication administered.

The cervicograph is the diagrammatic representation of the dilatation of the cervix charted against the hours in labour. Some initial studies (Friedman 1954; Pearson 1981) demonstrated that the cervical dilatation time of normal labour has a characteristic sigmoid curve. This curve can be divided into two distinct parts: the latent phase and the active phase. Women's progress in labour, however, does not fit neatly into predetermined criteria, therefore rigid parameters of *normal* progress should not be adopted (Albers 1999; Lavender et al. 2018). The rate of progress in labour must be considered in the context of the woman's total wellbeing and choice.

SUBSEQUENT CARE IN THE FIRST STAGE OF LABOUR

Assessing Progress

Physical examination of the cervix is not the only way to assess labour. Midwives can use a range of skills, including visualization of the purple line, appearing from the woman's anal margin gradually extending to the nape of the buttocks (Hobbs 1998; Shepherd et al. 2010), and observing the Rhombus of Michaelis, a kite-shaped area between the sacrum and ilea, which becomes increasing visible as the fetal head descends in the pelvis (Shepherd et al. 2010). In addition, the midwife should be vigilant in observing for changes in the woman's breathing, behaviour, noises, movements and posture, alongside changes in the nature of the contractions.

Abdominal Examination

An abdominal examination should be repeated by the midwife at intervals throughout labour in order to assess the length, strength and frequency of contractions and the descent of the presenting part. Palpation is of benefit prior to undertaking a vaginal examination, as the findings will assist the midwife to be accurate when defining the position and station of the head/breech. It is also useful to record the position of the fetus contemporaneously during the labour, as this can assist with the analysis of events should a shoulder dystocia occur (Brydon and Raynor 2012).

Contractions

The frequency, length and strength of the contractions should be noted and recorded on the partogram, usually at 30-min intervals. The uterus should always feel softer between contractions and if it does not relax between contractions, it is evidence of hypertonicity: defined as a contraction lasting more than 2 min (NICE 2017). The contraction rate is usually assessed manually with the midwife placing their hand on the fundus of the uterus and by counting the number of contractions in 10 min, over a 20-min period. Evidence of five contractions or more in 10 min is evidence of *tachysystole* in spontaneous labour, or *hyperstimulation* in induced labour (see Chapter 22).

An excessive number of contractions or hypertonicity can result in fetal compromise as a result of prolonged cord compression or reduction in placental perfusion with consequent reduction in blood supply to the fetus. In such circumstances, continuous fetal monitoring (CFM) would be undertaken that includes monitoring the uterine contractions. An abdominal transducer (*toco*) is placed on the mother's abdomen over the fundus of the uterus to monitor the frequency and length of contractions (Stevenson and Chandraharan 2017). The abdominal transducer is effectively a pressure sensor, which picks up the changes in shape and tone of the maternal abdomen during a contraction. It responds to any change in pressure, including coughing or vomiting and because of this, it is essential that a conversation is had with the

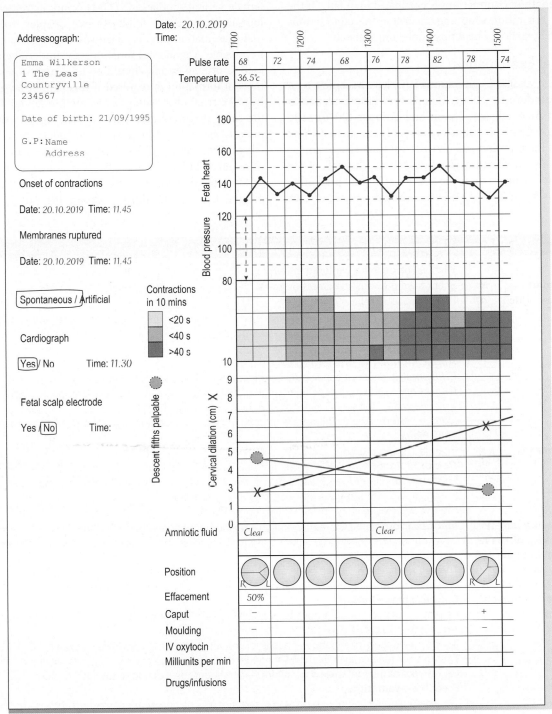

Fig. 19.9 Example of a partogram.

woman about the intensity of her contractions and that the strength of contractions are palpated manually. If the toco is not monitoring and recording the contractions effectively, it should be repositioned immediately.

Vaginal Examination

Although vaginal examinations (VE) have become a routine procedure in labour there is very little evidence to support their efficacy. Dixon and Foureur (2010) state that vaginal examinations are arguably considered to be both an intervention and an essential clinical assessment tool in labour. VEs only give a *snapshot* of the state of the cervix at one given moment and are of limited predictive value (Jackson 2017). Midwives should remember that

to women who have survived sexual abuse, experienced female genital mutilation (FGM) or are extremely anxious and have fear of childbirth (see Chapter 18), a vaginal examination can be very distressing and sometimes impossible. Vaginal examinations are undertaken using aseptic principles and should be used judiciously when more information is required if this cannot be gleaned from external observations of women in labour. Ideally, the same person should perform the vaginal examinations to be in a better position to judge any changes. Observations and findings, as detailed in Box 19.1, should be noted and recorded accordingly by the midwife.

Despite there being little evidence to support the routine use of VEs during labour, the NICE (2017)

BOX 19.1 Vaginal Examination Observation and Findings

Labia	Varicosities/oedema/warts/other lesions
Perineum	Scars from previous tears/episiotomies
Vaginal orifice	Discharge/liquor/'show'/bleeding
Rectum	Loaded rectum may be felt on vaginal examination (*can impede descent of presenting part*)
Cervix	***Position of cervix***: central/posterior/anterior/lateral
	Consistency: hard, soft
	Application to the presenting part: loose/well applied
	Effacement: length of canal; may be effaced but closed in a primigravida
	Dilatation: Approximate assessment (Fig. 19.8); 10 cm equates to full dilatation or when no cervix can be felt (*ensure no lips of cervix remain*, Fig. 19.12)
	Note in preterm labour, the smaller presenting part may pass through at a smaller cervical diameter
Membranes	Intact/bulging/ruptured
	Colour of liquor: clear/bloodstained/offensive smell (indicating infection)/meconium staining
	Following rupture of membranes, the midwife needs to check that the cord has not prolapsed and should listen to the fetal heart through contractions
	Hindwaters may leak while forewaters remain intact
Presenting part (PP): the part of the fetus lying over the cervical os (96% are cephalic)	***Identification***: cephalic/breech/footling/knee/compound (see Figs 19.31–19.34)
	Level of bony part of PP in relation to the ischial spines, in cm *above*, *below* or *at the level* of the ischial spines (Fig. 19.10)
	The fetus follows the curve of carus, therefore it is impossible to judge the station precisely
	Presence of *caput succedaneum/moulding/meconium* (in a breech presentation)
Position of presenting part	***Cephalic presentation***:
	Sagittal suture: left or right oblique or transverse should rotate to anteroposterior diameter of the maternal pelvis (Fig. 19.11)
	If *well flexed* the small triangular posterior fontanelle is felt; it has three sutures leaving it
	The anterior fontanelle is diamond-shaped, has a membrane and four sutures leaving it
	Landmarks of the fontanelles give information about the location of the fetal occiput
	Breech presentation:
	The sacrum is the diagnostic point in respect of its position with the maternal pelvis and the ischial spines

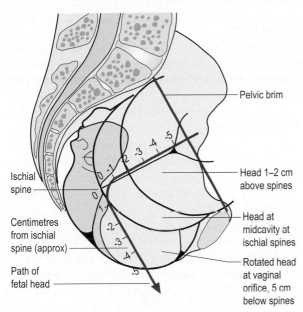

Fig. 19.10 Diagram to show stations of the fetal head in relation to the pelvic canal

guidelines recommend offering labouring women 4-hourly VEs. However, in practice, generally, the trend has moved away from conducting routine 4-hourly VEs in normal labour and justification for each examination should always be recorded. An explanation of the procedure, obtaining of verbal consent from the woman and an abdominal examination should always precede the VE (DH 2009). The woman's bladder should be empty as the presenting part may be displaced by a full bladder as well as being very uncomfortable for the woman. In order to obtain the most information, the woman is usually asked to lie on her back but the technique can be easily adapted to accommodate other positions that suit the woman better. During the examination the woman's dignity and privacy need to be considered. In order to avoid unnecessary exposure, the woman can be asked to move and uncover herself when the midwife is ready to commence the examination. Tap water may be used to cleanse the vagina for this procedure (NICE 2017). With the combination of external and internal findings, the skilled midwife should gain a detailed account of the labour and its subsequent progress.

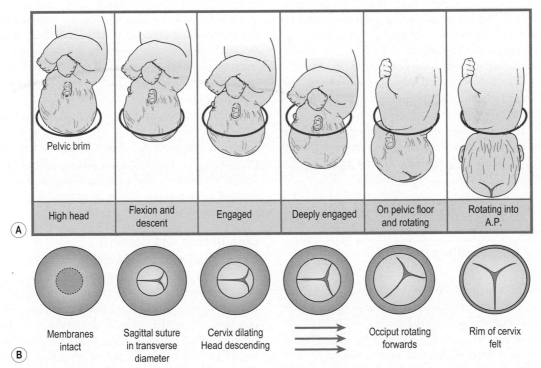

Fig. 19.11 (A) Diagrams showing descent of the fetal head through the pelvic brim. A.P., anteroposterior (B) Diagram showing dilatation of the cervix and rotation of the fetal head as felt on vaginal examination.

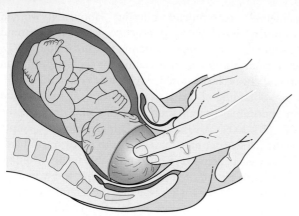

Fig. 19.12 Cervix fully dilated.

Indications for Vaginal Examination

There should always be valid reasons to undertake a VE in labour, which are to:

- make a positive identification of the presentation
- determine whether the head is engaged in case of doubt
- ascertain whether the forewaters have ruptured, or to rupture them artificially
- exclude cord prolapse after rupture of the forewaters, especially if there is an ill-fitting presenting part or there are fetal heart rate changes
- assess progress or slow labour
- confirm full dilatation of the cervix (see Fig. 19.12)
- confirm the axis of the fetus and presentation of the second twin in a multiple pregnancy in order to rupture the second amniotic sac, if necessary.

Under no circumstances should a midwife undertake a vaginal examination if there is any frank bleeding unless the placenta is positively known to be in the upper uterine segment.

ASSESSING THE WELLBEING OF THE WOMAN

Maternal Observations

Pulse rate

A tachycardia can indicate pain or anxiety and is also associated with pyrexia, exhaustion and shock. The pulse rate should be recorded hourly (NICE 2017). If the rate increases to >100 bpm it may be indicative of anxiety, pain, infection, ketosis or haemorrhage. The pulse should also be assessed and recorded at any time that there is concern about fetal wellbeing or if there is

uncertainty about whether the maternal rather than the fetal pulse is being recorded (NICE 2017).

Temperature

A rise in temperature can be indicative of infection or dehydration. The temperature should be recorded 4-hourly (NICE 2017) and additionally when there is a clinical indication.

Blood pressure

Hypotension may be caused by the woman being in the supine position, by shock or as a result of vasodilation associated with epidural anaesthesia. *Hypertension* is an indicator of pre-eclampsia and in cases where a woman has pre-eclampsia or essential hypertension during pregnancy, labour may further elevate the blood pressure. Blood pressure should be assessed every 4 h (NICE 2017) and additionally when there is a clinical indication. It is usual practice to monitor the blood pressure at 5-min intervals for 20 min following the administration of an epidural anaesthetic and following the administration of any subsequent bolus dose.

Fluid balance and urinalysis

A record should be kept of all urine passed in order to ensure that the bladder is being emptied. If an intravenous infusion is in progress, the fluids administered must be recorded accurately. It is particularly important to note how much fluid remains if a bag is changed when only partially used.

A trace of protein may be a contaminant following rupture of the membranes or a sign of a urinary tract infection, but more significant proteinuria may indicate pre-eclampsia. Urine passed during labour should be tested for ketones and protein. Ketones may occur in normal labour and a low level is very common and is not usually thought to be significant.

Cleanliness and Comfort

Enemas and perineal shaving

There is no evidence to support the routine procedure of administering enemas or undertaking a perineal shave to women in labour. However, if a woman reports constipation, or the midwife detects that the rectum is full on vaginal examination, or if the woman feels there would be benefit, an enema or glycerine suppositories can be offered. Sometimes for cultural reasons, women will shave their own genital/perineal areas.

Bath or shower

Immersion in a warm bath or birthing pool can be an effective form of pain relief for labouring women that facilitates increased mobility with no increased incidence of adverse outcome for the woman or fetus (Cluett and Burns 2018). The midwife should invite the woman who is mobile to have a bath or shower whenever she wishes during labour.

Clothing

It is entirely up to the individual woman what she wears in labour. If in hospital she may prefer to wear the loose gown offered or she may feel more comfortable wearing her own choice of clothing. As long as she is aware that the garment may become wet and bloodstained and that she may require more than one, there is no reason to restrict her choice.

Position and Mobility

There are physical benefits if the woman maintains an upright position, including: a shorter labour; reducing the risk of caesarean section; a reduction in the need for analgesia (Lawrence et al. 2013); fewer episiotomies; and fewer instrumental deliveries. However, there is an apparent increased risk of blood loss >500 mL (Gupta et al. 2017). Other benefits include increasing the woman's sense of control (Lawrence et al. 2013), thus contributing to a positive birth experience. Lying on the bed during labour or birth does little to enhance the physiological birth process and has disadvantages, including a risk of aorto-caval compression and reduced interspinous diameter of the pelvic outlet, increased pain and slower descent of the presenting part (Fig. 19.13).

The need to provide a continuous tracing of the fetal heart can inhibit maternal mobility and in some cases, such as with women who are significantly obese, have pre-existing mobility problems or have an epidural *in situ*, this cannot be avoided. Despite this, the majority of women, including some obese women, will be able to maintain an upright position, retain a degree of mobility and achieve birth away from a birthing bed if supported in doing so. A key factor in encouraging different labour positions and mobility is the environment. The birthing room should contain equipment such as beanbags, birthing balls and chairs (Albers 2007) and the midwife should be proactive in encouraging the woman to remain active and to change her position. Although women should be encouraged to move and adopt whatever position they find most comfortable (NICE 2017), the midwife should be aware that the woman's choice of birth position may be influenced by what she thinks is expected of her rather than what is actually more comfortable.

Cultures where women are constrained and limited in their posture and positioning during labour appear to be the exception rather than the rule. Many cultures use movement, dance, physical contact and massage to encourage and sustain the process of labour. Henley-Einion (2007) discusses the value of the *Five Rhythms method*. Movements described as *flowing*, *staccato*, *chaos*, *lyrical* and *stillness*, which are a combination of expressive movements rather than a set of routine exercises, are employed to provide dance, and the music defines, guides, inspires and prompts the body. Such a strategy is a fitting one to use during the birthing process.

Pressure ulcer prevention

A pressure ulcer (*decubitus ulcer*) is a localized injury to the skin and underlying tissue that arises when an area of skin is placed under pressure. Where women have pre-existing mobility problems or an epidural in progress, they will be at increased risk of developing pressure ulcers during labour. In the 5 years between 2001 and 2018, 96 women submitted litigation claims after developing pressure sores while in labour (NHS Resolution 2018). Of these, 87 were successful in being awarded compensation, costing the NHS £2,473,244. It is important to note that all of these women had epidurals and no risk assessment was recorded on these women prior to epidural insertion (NHS Resolution 2018). All maternity areas should therefore have guidelines for the prevention of pressure ulcers and the midwife must take great care to ensure that the condition of the woman's skin is observed and specific details documented in the records at 2-hourly intervals.

Nutrition in Labour

It has been estimated that in established labour, a woman requires a calorie intake of 121 kcal/h and that 47 kcal/h is required to prevent ketosis (Hall Moran and Dykes 2013). Most women will be able to draw on glucose stores to provide energy but if insufficient carbohydrate is available energy will be obtained from body fat and this will release ketones, resulting in ketoacidosis.

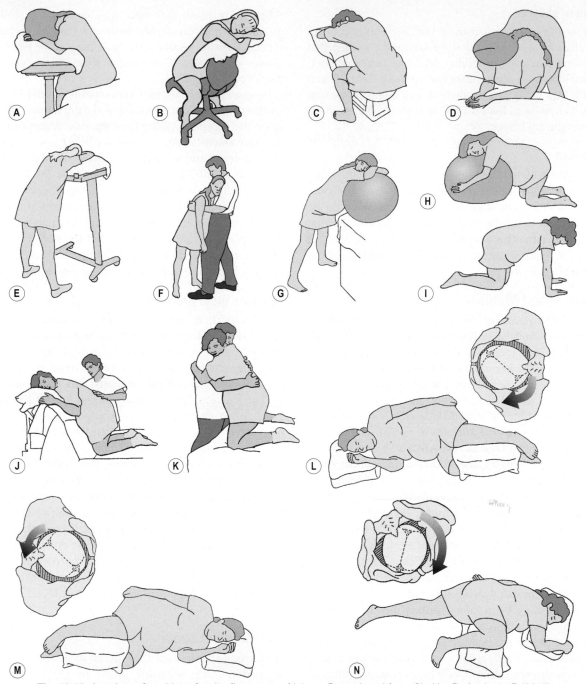

Fig. 19.13 A variety of positions for the first stage of labour. Reproduced from Simkin, P., Ancheta, R (2017) The labour progress handbook. Oxford: Blackwell Science.

Dietary care in labour is a controversial issue due to the dearth of good-quality evidence and as a result, there is no universal consensus on management. Hospital policies are usually based on the need to restrict food intake in order to prevent gastric aspiration. However, the number of women experiencing gastric aspiration is extremely low and there is no evidence to support the view that starvation will guarantee an empty stomach or prevent gastric acidity (NICE 2017). Starvation in labour can also have psychosocial effects as the provision of food and drink can provide comfort and reassurance, while the denial can be seen as authoritarian, stressful and intimidating, which can increase feelings of apprehension. For many women in physiological labour, a low residue, low fat diet and freely available fluids will be appropriate. As there is evidence that the desire to eat is more common in women in early labour (Singata et al. 2013) – and most women do not want to eat in active labour, it is important that the woman is not encouraged to eat if she has no desire to do so.

Bladder Care

Although frequent bladder emptying during labour is recommended, there is no evidence to support any particular regime of intervention. It is therefore reasonable to consider that the bladder should be emptied at least 4-hourly or more frequently if it is palpable abdominally. There is some evidence that infrequent bladder emptying in labour is associated with an increased risk of urinary incontinence in the postpartum period (Birch et al. 2009). A full bladder may increase pain, reduce efficiency of uterine contractions and delay descent of the presenting part (Simkin et al. 2017).

The woman's sensation to micturate during labour may be reduced by pressure of the presenting part during its descent through the pelvis, or by an effective epidural block. In all cases of delay in labour, the midwife should ascertain whether the bladder is full and encourage the woman to void regularly. Where possible, the woman should be encouraged to use the toilet, and if this is not possible, the midwife should provide privacy and ensure maximum comfort by placing the bedpan on the chair, stool or bed and encouraging the woman to adopt a leaning forward position. The sound or feel of water can also help to trigger the micturition reflex. If the bladder is incompletely emptied or the woman is unable to void for some hours, it may become necessary to introduce a catheter into the bladder. As the risk of infection is increased with the use of retaining catheters, it is generally recommended that an 'in-out' catheter is used.

Medicine Records

Midwives have an exemption from requiring a prescription for specific medicines used in the care of women in physiological labour. In the UK, NHS Trusts also have locally agreed patient group directions (PGDs) to which the midwife should adhere, providing guidance as to which medicines are preferred and what doses and frequency should be used within that Trust. PGDs are only used where midwives exemptions do not apply. If the midwife is in any doubt regarding any matters relating to the supply, administration, storage or surrender of controlled drugs or medicines, she can refer to the local pharmacology department (NMC 2018).

As well as being entered on the partogram, doses of drugs are recorded on the prescription sheet, in the summary of labour and, in the case of controlled drugs, in the Controlled Drugs Register.

ASSESSING THE WELLBEING OF THE FETUS

Assessing fetal wellbeing during labour, whether it be via intermittent auscultation (IA) or continuous (electronic) fetal monitoring (C[E]FM) using a cardiotograph (CTG), is an important aspect of intrapartum care. Understanding fetal physiology and applying this to fetal surveillance is crucial to ensure robust standards of care for the mother and her baby. This is primarily to detect suspected fetal hypoxia, prevent the onset of metabolic acidosis and offer timely and appropriate intervention when required. Despite the widespread practice of both intermittent and continuous fetal monitoring, there are no statistical differences in the rates of cerebral palsy, infant mortality or other standard measures of neonatal wellbeing with either form of monitoring (Alfirevic et al. 2017).

NICE (2017) recommend that in all low-risk established labours, *intermittent auscultation* should be practised. The midwife should discuss the recommendations for fetal monitoring and the available evidence with the woman in order that she can make an informed decision about how her baby's wellbeing will be monitored during labour. It is the responsibility of the midwife to ensure they have a thorough understanding of fetal physiology so that this can be applied to the care that they provide during the intrapartum period.

Fetal Heart Physiology

The intrinsic fetal heart rate is under the complex influence of many physiological factors and is modulated by the central nervous system, specifically the autonomic element (ANS), which consists of sympathetic and parasympathetic branches (Wood and Dobbie 1989). Interplay between the sympathetic and parasympathetic branches of the ANS have a crucial role in regulating the fetal heart when required.

In the event of mechanical stress, such as cord compression, an increase in arterial pressure will cause the fetal blood pressure to rise. A rise in arterial pressure will stimulate a baroreflex response (Chapleau 2012). Baroreceptors are located in the aortic arch and the carotid sinus. They are stretch receptors and sensitive to changes in arterial pressure. A rise in blood pressure will usually increase activity of the afferent pathway, which conducts via the glossopharyngeal and vagus nerves (Chawia 2016), to inhibit sympathetic activity and/or activate parasympathetic activity. This mechanism will slow the fetal heart in order to lower the fetal blood pressure. Decelerations mediated through a baroreceptor response usually have a rapid drop below the baseline and a rapid recovery (Chandraharan 2017) and are not usually indicative of hypoxaemia/hypoxia (International Federation of Gynecology and Obstetrics, FIGO 2018).

Fetuses exposed to ongoing stress may go on to develop hypoxaemia, resulting in hypercarbia (carbon dioxide [CO_2] retention) and developing acidosis (Perez-Bonfils and Chandraharan 2017). Hypoxaemia occurs when the oxygen (O_2) saturation in the blood falls but the function of cells and organs are usually not affected. Hypoxia occurs when hypoxaemia is not corrected leading to a state of reduced oxygen tension in the tissue and subsequent anaerobic metabolism (Rainaldi et al. 2017).

Hypoxaemia will stimulate a chemoreceptor response (Chandraharan 2017). Peripheral chemoreceptors are situated, like baroreceptors, in the aortic arch and carotid sinus, while central chemoreceptors are located in the medulla oblongata (Shimokawa et al. 2006). In response to hypoxic stress, fetal adrenal glands secrete catecholamine (adrenaline and noroadrenaline) (Lagercrantz and Bistoletti 1977), which progressively increase the fetal heart and causes peripheral vasoconstriction in order to divert blood flow to the central organs (Joho 2017; Perez-Bonfils and Chandraharan 2017; Iaizzo and Fitzgerald 2015). The chemoreceptor-mediated deceleration will usually manifest on the CTG trace as late decelerations, due to the placental venous sinuses refilling with fresh oxygenated blood leading to a gradual removal of CO_2 (Aghoja 2014). In summary, if the fetus is exposed to stress, either mechanical or iatrogenic, decelerations will be observed on the CTG trace. This would usually be followed by a lack of accelerations and a loss of cycling. Circulating catecholamines in response to stress will cause a progressive increase in the fetal heart and peripheral vasoconstriction in order to divert blood to the vital organs (myocardium and brain). This is considered a *compensatory* response to hypoxia (Chandraharan 2017).

During a developing hypoxia, the fetal pCO_2 rises increasing the level of hydrogen ions (H_2) resulting in a respiratory acidosis and a fall in pH (Aghoja 2014). If the hypoxic insult continues, the myocardium will revert from aerobic metabolism to anaerobic metabolism, which is not energy efficient and leads to an accumulation of lactic acid and reduced cellular function. The time at which the fetus can sustain anaerobic metabolism will depend on glycogen reserves, which is why a preterm or growth restricted fetus is less likely to compensate effectively in the event of hypoxaemia/hypoxia (Aghoja 2014). As the acidosis worsens cardiac function becomes impaired and eventually the fetus will die. During this stage of hypoxia, the fetus has moved to a *decompensatory* stage (FIGO 2018). The features of decompensation follow the compensatory stage of a gradually evolving hypoxia. At this point fetal heart rate variability will reduce due to decreased oxygenation to the fetal brain and if this is not rectified the myocardium will fail (Perez-Bonfils and Chandraharan 2017).

Intermittent Auscultation

Intermittent auscultation (IA) is the primary method of fetal surveillance in the labours of those women who have experienced no complications during pregnancy. Intermittent auscultation helps to facilitate normal physiology of labour by allowing freedom of movement (Lowe and Archer, 2017). Randomized control trials comparing CEFM and IA between 1975 and 2008 found no evidence of improved outcomes to the baby by using CEFM for low-risk pregnancies (NICE 2017). In fact, there is some evidence to suggest that offering low-risk women CEFM on admission may increase the caesarean section rate by 20% (Davane et al. 2017).

Intermittent auscultation involves listening to the fetal heart rate at intervals using a Pinard stethoscope or a handheld Doppler. During the first stage of labour, auscultation should take place every 15 min for a minimum of 60 s immediately following a contraction (NICE 2017). The maternal pulse should be palpated on admission and every hour thereafter to differentiate it from the fetal heart rate (NICE 2017). The Pinard stethoscope will simply amplify the actual heart sound so that it can be heard and counted. However, it may be difficult to use when the woman is in certain positions, such as all-fours or squatting, and as the sound cannot be heard by the woman, this method may be less reassuring for her.

The handheld Doppler uses ultrasound to detect movement, either of the fetal heart muscle or valves, which are converted into a sound that can be heard and counted, such that the woman and her partner can also hear the fetal heart. It should be recognized that as the Doppler converts movement into sound, it is possible for the maternal pulse to be detected and be mistaken for the fetal pulse. For this reason, it is recommended that the Pinard stethoscope should be used to check the fetal heart when any concerns arise (Medicines and Healthcare Products Regulatory Agency, MHPRA 2010) and that the maternal pulse is also counted (NICE 2017).

It is important to consider the whole clinical picture when undertaking IA and to record any accelerations and decelerations that may be heard that are outside normal parameters (NICE 2017). If fetal movement is felt during auscultation, it is important to document that also. If a rise in the fetal heart baseline is heard through auscultation, then the midwife should consider whether there are signs of maternal dehydration, pyrexia or tachycardia. If decelerations become apparent, carrying out IA more frequently is recommended, usually over three consecutive contractions (NICE 2017; FIGO 2018).

If the baseline rises or decelerations are confirmed, assistance should be summoned. Timely intervention is crucial and in the case of midwifery-led settings, such as a free standing birth centre or in the woman's home, a paramedic ambulance should be summoned. The use of the SBAR tool (situation, background, assessment and recommendation) as discussed in Chapter 26, should be used to clearly communicate the details to members of the multidisciplinary team. If the woman is in a midwifery-led setting, an assessment of whether or not it is safe to transfer to an obstetric unit should be undertaken by the midwife. If birth is imminent then it is usually safer to expedite the birth rather than moving the woman. Midwives who work in low-risk settings should be competent with neonatal life support (NLS) in case the newborn requires resuscitation (see Chapter 33).

The *Each Baby Counts* 2015 Report (RCOG 2016) highlights key learning points from serious incident reviews to improve care during labour when IA is the most appropriate method of fetal surveillance. Contributory factors that led to babies requiring therapeutic cooling and hypoxic ischaemic encephalopathy (HIE) were assigning mothers to a low-risk pathway when not appropriate, errors of interpretation or failure to detect pathology and failure to act upon suspicious findings (RCOG 2016).

The term *intermittent **intelligent** auscultation* is widely used to describe facilitating IA of the fetal heart while understanding the pathophysiology and hypoxic processes that may manifest during labour (NICE 2014b; Lowe and Archer 2017).

NICE (2017) recommends that if the following are found then cardiotocography should be commenced:

- maternal pulse over 120 beats/minute on two occasions 30 min apart
- temperature of 38°C or above on a single reading, or 37.5°C or above on two consecutive occasions 1 h apart
- suspected chorioamnionitis or sepsis
- pain reported by the woman that differs from the pain normally associated with contractions
- the presence of significant meconium
- fresh vaginal bleeding that develops in labour
- severe hypertension: a single reading of either systolic blood pressure of ≥160 mmHg or diastolic blood pressure of >110 mmHg, measured between contractions
- hypertension: either systolic blood pressure of ≥140 mmHg or diastolic blood pressure of ≥90 mmHg on two consecutive readings taken 30 min apart, measured between contractions
- a reading of 2+ of protein on urinalysis and a single reading of either raised systolic blood pressure (≥140 mmHg) or raised diastolic blood pressure (≥90 mmHg)
- confirmed delay in the first or second stage of labour
- contractions that last longer than 60 s (hypertonus), or >5 contractions in 10 min (tachysystole).

Cardiotocography

Cardiotocography (CTG) was first introduced in the 1960s and since then has been a central feature in the care provided to women during labour. All women who are assessed as having a pregnancy with a risk of complications developing in labour, which may lead to hypoxic stress in the fetus should be offered continuous fetal monitoring (CFM) (NICE 2017; FIGO 2018). Although CTG interpretation is common practice, it is not without flaws (Chandraharan 2017). Interestingly, CTGs were introduced without robust clinical trials and a lack of clinical guidance on how to interpret the fetal heart trace (Chandraharan 2017). Consequently, this led to an increase in operative interventions such as emergency caesarean sections and operative vaginal births (Nelson et al. 2016). Many experts agree that these problems have evolved because of inter- and intra-observer variation (Kundu et al. 2017). This has led to misinterpretation of CTG traces, due to clinicians making decisions based on declarative patterns rather than an understanding of fetal physiology, failing to take the whole clinical picture into account and not acting upon an abnormal CTG trace in a timely fashion (Berglund 2011). The CTG itself is not diagnostic and should be more accurately described as a *screening tool* to aid the clinician's decision-making when fetal hypoxia/acidosis is suspected.

In recent years, there has been a paradigm shift in the approach towards CTG interpretation from pattern recognition to an applied understanding of fetal physiology. FIGO presents a consensus towards a more physiological approach when analysing the fetal heart trace (Ayres-de-Campos et al. 2015) and NICE has recently updated its fetal heart monitoring guidelines, advocating that decisions about the woman's care should not be made solely on the basis of CTG findings (RCOG 2016). As a consequence NICE and/or FIGO guidance have been incorporated into local CTG guidelines in many maternity units. However, it is important that the midwife develops secure knowledge in fetal heart physiology so as to apply this awareness to intrapartum CTG interpretation. This is to ensure a high standard of *safe* and competent care is given to all women requiring CEFM in labour.

Interpretation of the cardiotocograph

Understanding how physiological changes in response to fetal hypoxia may manifest on the CTG trace is important so as to be able offer timely intervention, if appropriate to do so. The CTG trace is categorized by systematically analysing four main features of the fetal heart rate (*baseline heart rate, baseline variability, decelerations* and *accelerations*) as to whether they are *reassuring, non-reassuring* or *abnormal* in conjunction with uterine contractions and the immediate clinical picture, as shown in Box 19.2.

An overall classification of **normal**, **suspicious** or **pathological** as identified in Box 19.3 is then applied to the trace according to how many of its features are described as *reassuring, non-reassuring* or *abnormal* (NICE 2017). It is important to record the classification of the trace at *each assessment* in order to inform appropriate actions. FIGO (2018) have produced an example of a CTG assessment tool (as a form) to assist midwives

and obstetricians in interpreting traces and determining subsequent actions, which is illustrated in Box 19.4.

This section discusses the features of CTG analysis and how the physiological responses to labour and hypoxia may become apparent on the CTG trace.

Baseline heart rate. A baseline heart rate is the mean fetal heart rate visible on the CTG trace rounded to increments of 5 beats per minute (bpm) in 10 min segments. To be considered a stable baseline, the fetal heart should spend a minimum of 2 min on a stable baseline in a 10 min segment, otherwise the baseline for that segment is defined as indeterminate (FIGO 2018). It is important that good contact is maintained throughout the trace in order to accurately clarify the fetal heart baseline.

A normal baseline is considered to be between 110–160 bpm (NICE 2017), however it is widely accepted that preterm fetuses may have a slightly higher baseline, usually at the upper end of normal, and post-term fetuses may have a baseline on the lower end of normal (Ayres-de-Campos et al. 2015).

Tachycardia is a baseline of >160 bpm for more than 10 min. Maternal infection is the most frequent cause of tachycardia, but it can also be attributed to a variety of aetiologies such as maternal medication or indicate a non-acute fetal hypoxia (Ayres-de-Campos et al. 2015; Abernathy et al. 2017). A rising baseline that remains within normal parameters should be viewed with suspicion, as it may indicate subclinical chorioamnionitis (FIGO 2018). Bradycardia is a baseline of <110 bpm for more than 10 min. Maternal hypotension is commonly associated with fetal bradycardia especially after epidural administration or top-up (Reynolds et al. 2002; Ayres-de-Campos et al. 2015).

It is important to note that if the maternal pulse and the fetal heart are similar in rate, pulse-oximetry should be applied to the mother and a fetal scalp electrode should be considered to ensure there is clear distinction between maternal pulse and fetal pulse.

Baseline variability. This refers to oscillations in the fetal heart rate signal and is the degree to which the baseline varies over the period of a minute and appears as an irregular jagged pattern on the CTG trace. Normal variability is considered to be between 5 and 25 bpm and is reflective of a well-oxygenated central nervous system (FIGO 2018; NICE 2017).

Reduced variability can be observed as <5 bpm for more than 50 min or for >3 min during decelerations (Ayres-de-Campos et al. 2015). Decreased variability

BOX 19.2 Description of Cardiotocograph Trace Features

Description			Feature
	Baseline (beats/min)	Baseline variability (beats/min)	Decelerations
Reassuring	110 to 160	5 to 25	None or early Variable decelerations with no concerning characteristics[a] for less than 90 min
Non-reassuring	100 to 109[b] or 161 to 180	Less than 5 for 30 to 50 min or More than 25 for 15 to 25 min	Variable decelerations with no concerning characteristics[a] for 90 min or more or Variable decelerations with any concerning characteristics[a] in up to 50% of contractions for 30 min or more or Variable decelerations with any concerning characteristics[a] in over 50% of contractions for less than 30 min or Late decelerations in over 50% of contractions for less than 30 min, with no maternal or fetal clinical risk factors such as vaginal bleeding or significant meconium
Abnormal	Below 100 or Above 180	Less than 5 for more than 50 min or More than 25 for more than 25 min or Sinusoidal	Variable decelerations with any concerning characteristics[a] in over 50% of contractions for 30 min (or less if any maternal or fetal clinical risk factors, see above) or Late decelerations for 30 min (or less if any maternal or fetal clinical risk factors) or Acute bradycardia, or a single prolonged deceleration lasting 3 min or more

[a]Regard the following as concerning characteristics of variable decelerations: lasting >60 s; reduced baseline variability within the deceleration; failure to return to baseline; biphasic (W) shape; no shouldering.

[b]Although a baseline fetal heart rate between 100 and 109 beats/min is a non-reassuring feature, continue usual care if there is normal baseline variability and no variable or late decelerations.

The presence of fetal heart rate accelerations, even with reduced baseline variability, is generally a sign that the baby is healthy.

NICE (National Institute for Health and Care Excellence). (2017). Intrapartum Care: Management and Delivery of care to Women in Labour CG190. London: NICE. Available at: www.nice.org.uk/guidance/cg190/resources/intrapartum-care-for-healthy-women-and-babies-pdf-35109866447557.

for >50 min can be indicative of central nervous system hypoxia/acidosis resulting in decreased autonomic nervous system activity (Ayres-de-Campos et al. 2015; NICE 2017; Schneider et al. 2018) and therefore should be escalated for review by the obstetric team.

Just as reduced variability can occur, so can increased variability. This can be observed as a band-width value exceeding 25 bpm lasting for >30 min (FIGO 2018; Ayres-de-Campos et al. 2015) and is classified as a *saltatory* pattern. The pathophysiology of this pattern is not completely understood but is thought to be caused by fetal autonomic instability/hyperactivity and associated with recurrent decelerations when hypoxia/acidosis is evolving very rapidly (FIGO 2018; Nunes et al. 2014).

The *saltatory* pattern should not be confused with the *sinusoidal* pattern. The sinusoidal pattern is a smooth, undulating signal, resembling a sine wave with an amplitude of 5–15 bpm (FIGO 2018). Similarly, this pattern is also not completely understood but it tends to occur in association with severe fetal

---

BOX 19.3   Overall Classification of a Cardiotocograph Trace

Category	Definition	Management
Normal	All **four** features are classified as **reassuring**	• Continue CTG (unless it was started because of concerns arising from intermittent auscultation and there are no ongoing risk factors; usual care • Talk to the woman and her birth companion(s) about what is happening
Non-reassuring	1 **non-reassuring** feature *and* 2 **reassuring** features	• Correct any underlying causes, such as hypotension or uterine hyperstimulation • Perform a full set of maternal observations • Start 1 or more conservative measures • Inform an obstetrician *or* a senior midwife • Document a plan for reviewing the whole clinical picture and the CTG findings • Talk to the woman and her birth companion(s) about what is happening and take her preferences into account

Abnormal	1 **abnormal** feature *or* 2 **non-reassuring** features	• Obtain a review by an obstetrician **and** a senior midwife
		• Exclude acute events (e.g. cord prolapsed, suspected placental abruption or suspected uterine rupture
		• Correct any underlying causes, such as hypotension or uterine hyper stimulation
		• Start 1 or more conservative measures
		• Talk to the woman and her birth companion(s) about what is happening and take her preferences into account
		• If the cardiotocograph is still pathological after implementing conservative measures:
		  • obtain a further review by an obstetrician **and** a senior midwife
		  • offer digital fetal scalp stimulation and document the outcome
		• If the cardiotocograph is still pathological after fetal scalp stimulation:
		  • consider fetal blood sampling
		  • consider expediting the birth
		  • take the woman's preferences into account

Adapted from: NICE (National Institute for Health and Care Excellence). (2017) Intrapartum care: management and delivery of care to women in labour: CG 190. London: NICE. Available at: www.nice.org.uk/guidance/cg190/resources/intrapartum-care-for-healthy-women-and-babies-pdf-35109866447557.

---

anaemia and is found in anti-D alloimmunization, fetal-maternal haemorrhage, twin-to-twin transfusion syndrome and ruptured vasa praevia (FIGO 2018). A sinusoidal pattern that continues for >30 min must be escalated to the obstetric team (Ayres-de-Campos et al. 2015).

A pseudo-sinusoidal pattern is said to resemble a shark-tooth type of pattern and is thought to be caused by fetal-hypotension occurring secondary to fetal–maternal haemorrhage (Yanamandra and Chandraharan 2014). The administration of remifentanil during labour may also be associated with sinusoidal fetal heart patterns, which do not appear to have an adverse effect on neonatal outcomes (Boterenbrood et al. 2018). A true sinusoidal and a pseudo-sinusoidal can sometimes be difficult to distinguish between therefore, if any such pattern is suspected, urgent review by a senior obstetrician is required.

Accelerations. Accelerations refer to an abrupt increase in the fetal heart rate at least 15 bpm above the baseline lasting more than 15 seconds (FIGO 2018). Most accelerations coincide with fetal movement (Schneider et al. 2018) and are thought to be a sign of a neurologically responsive fetus and integrity of the somatic nervous system (Ayres-de-Campos et al. 2015; Perez-Bonfils and Chandraharan 2017) as shown in the trace classified as normal in Fig. 19.14.

It has been suggested that the absence of accelerations during labour, when all other features of the CTG are normal, is unlikely to indicate fetal hypoxia/acidosis (Ayres-de-Campos et al. 2015; NICE 2017). During the later stage of labour, accelerations after a

BOX 19.4 Example of CTG Assessment Tool

Baseline: Variability:	Accelerations: Decelerations:
Rise in baseline (≥10%):	Yes / No
Inter-contraction interval >90 s:	Yes / No
Maintained cycling:	Yes / No
Abnormal variability (<5 or 25):	Yes / No
Features of hypoxia:	Yes / No
Type: _____	
Central organs well oxygenated:	Yes / No
Other risk factors noted: _____	
Recommended management: _____	

Adapted from: FIGO (International Federation of Gynecology and Obstetrics). (2018) *Physiological CTG Interpretation: Intrapartum Fetal Monitoring Guideline*. Available at: https://www.icarectg.com/wp-content/uploads/2018/03/Intrapartum-Fetal-Monitoring-Guideline.pdf.
The coloured text is to flag up warning signs.

contraction are less likely and probably more related to an *overshoot* following a deceleration. An overshoot is an exaggerated compensatory response to fetal hypotension secondary to sustained compression of the umbilical cord and would require further investigation (Lowe and Archer 2017). However, if accelerations occur with contractions during the second stage of labour, it may suggest erroneous recording of the maternal heart rate, as the fetal heart more commonly decelerates due to head compression (Ayres-de-Campos et al. 2015). If this is observed, it is important to quickly distinguish between the maternal and fetal pulse. This can be done by manually palpating the maternal pulse and/or applying pulse-oximetry as well as applying a scalp electrode to the fetus.

Decelerations. Decelerations present during CTG monitoring, as decreases below the fetal heart baseline of >15 bpm and last more than 15 seconds (FIGO 2018). Terminology in relation to how decelerations are interpreted can vary, for example *early* and *late* are more commonly used to describe the *types* of decelerations. It is suggested that the terms *'typical'* and *'atypical'* should

not be used as they can cause confusion (NICE 2017). It is important to understand the differences between types of deceleration so that the fetal heart trace can be analysed correctly.

Early decelerations. Early declarations usually occur with head compression, coincide with contractions and demonstrate normal variability within the main body of the deceleration (FIGO 2018; NICE 2017). They are generally seen in the late first stage and second stage of labour (Ayres-de-Campos et al. 2015). They are relatively uncommon (NICE 2017) and they are not thought to be indicative of fetal hypoxia (Ayres-de-Campos et al. 2015).

Variable decelerations. Variable decelerations (Fig. 19.15) are the most common type of deceleration seen throughout labour and are usually mediated though a baroreceptor response to increased arterial pressure as seen with cord compression (FIGO 2018). They are typically V-shaped and exhibit a rapid fall followed by a rapid recovery to baseline (FIGO 2018). These decelerations usually display variation in size, shape and relationship to uterine contractions (FIGO 2018). They do not usually indicate fetal hypoxia/acidosis, unless they evolve to exhibit a U-shape component and demonstrate a staggered recovery back to baseline, they meet the **60s criteria**: that is 60 beats below the baseline lasting for 60s, and/or their individual duration exceeds 3 min (FIGO 2018; NICE 2017).

Late decelerations. Late decelerations as shown in Fig. 19.16, exhibit a gradual onset and/or a gradual return to baseline and/or reduced variability within the main body of the deceleration (FIGO 2018). Late decelerations with a nadir >20 s after the peak of the contraction and recovery at the end of the contraction (RCOG 2001) are indicative of a chemoreceptor mediated response to hypoxaemia (FIGO 2018). The slow to recover element of the deceleration is an important component of detecting hypoxaemia in the fetus as it usually indicates a 'buffering' response in an attempt to remove the build-up of CO_2. It is important to be aware that, in a trace showing no accelerations and reduced variability, shallow decelerations are also considered worrying and defined as *late* (FIGO 2018).

Prolonged decelerations. Decelerations lasting for >3 min are likely to indicate hypoxaemia and are usually mediated through a chemoreceptor response, therefore

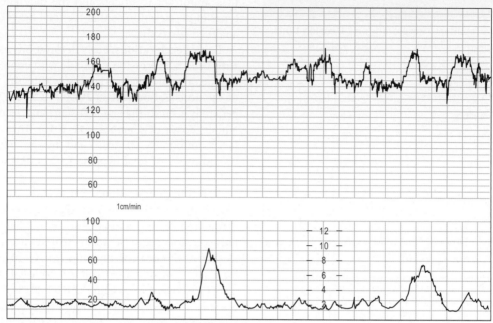

Fig. 19.14 Image of a normal CTG trace with reassuring features: baseline variability, presence of accelerations and *no* decelerations. (Courtesy Dr Maggie Blott.)

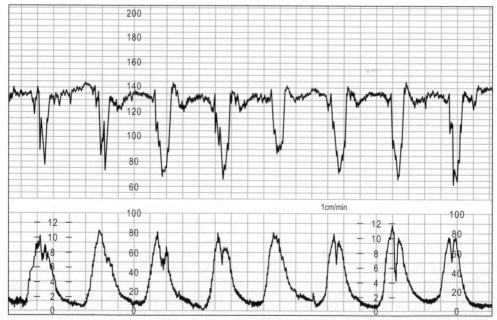

Fig. 19.15 Image of variable decelerations mediated through a baroreceptor response usually due to cord compression; note the rapid fall and rapid recovery to the baseline. (Courtesy Dr Maggie Blott.)

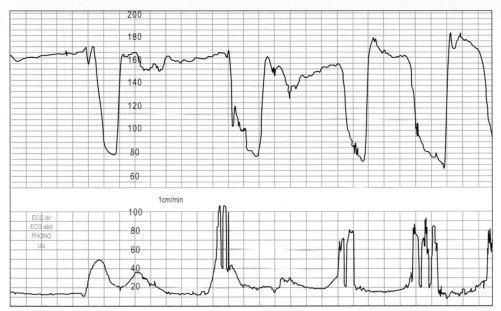

Fig. 19.16 Image of late decelerations mediated through a chemoreceptor response due to hypoxemia; note the wider appearance of the deceleration, the reduction of variability and, in this case, an unstable baseline. (Courtesy Dr Maggie Blott.)

immediate escalation is required (FIGO 2018; NICE 2017). Single prolonged decelerations of 3 min that do not recover are associated with an acute episode of hypoxia and require urgent intervention (FIGO 2018).

Fetal Defence Against Intrapartum Hypoxic Ischaemic Injury

Fetal hypoxia can occur when maternal oxygenation is compromised, maternal perfusion of the placenta is reduced or delivery of oxygenated blood to the fetus is impeded (Aghoja 2014). Both iatrogenic and mechanical factors can cause the development of hypoxia in the fetus, as can labour itself. Uterine contractions cause transient disruptions to placental oxygenation through the compression of branches of the uterine artery (Perez-Bonfils and Chandraharan 2017); therefore observing an adequate inter-contraction interval during labour is important to ensure effective oxygenation of the fetus. Most healthy fetuses cope with the ongoing stress of labour without sustaining any hypoxic injury (Muhunthan and Arulkumaran 2017). However, fetuses with additional risk factors, such as growth restriction or prematurity, are more at risk of hypoxic injury as they have less compensatory reserves (Aghoja 2014). It is important to remember that the main aim of the fetus

is to protect the myocardium first, and second the brain, and it does so by following a predicted pathway of compensatory responses to hypoxic stress (Chandraharan 2017).

Types of hypoxia

Understanding the type of hypoxia in relation to fetal heart rate patterns is important when assessing the CTG and communicating with the multidisciplinary team. Dependent on the type of hypoxic insult will depend on how the pathophysiology manifests on the CTG trace. However, experts agree that adaptive mechanisms in response to hypoxia usually follow one of three pathways as outlined in this section (FIGO 2018).

Acute hypoxia. Acute hypoxia (Fig. 19.17) presents with a prolonged deceleration of usually <80 bpm lasting ≥3 min (Muhunthan and Arulkumaran 2017; NICE 2017). Acute hypoxia may be due to cord prolapse, placental abruption or uterine rupture (FIGO 2018). Iatrogenic causes may be due to maternal hypotension (usually post-epidural top up or supine hypotension) or uterine hyperstimulation (FIGO 2018). When the fetal heart falls to such a low rate there is a significant reduction in CO_2 expulsion, which leads to respiratory acidosis. If this continues due to a reduction in O_2 intake, it

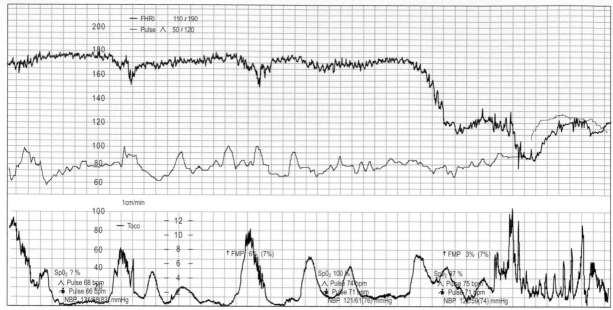

Fig. 19.17 Image of an acute episode of hypoxia with prolonged deceleration due to uterine rupture. (Courtesy Dr Maggie Blott.)

results in anaerobic metabolism and consequently metabolic acidosis (Muhunthan and Arulkumaran 2017). The fetal pH can fall at a rate of approximately 0.01/min. Therefore, a pH of 7.25 can fall to 7.15 in 10 min (Chandraharan 2017), which is why it is important to expedite the birth, if the fetal heart rate does not recover.

If the prolonged deceleration has not recovered by 3 min, help should be summoned immediately. It is important that the midwife communicates with the mother and her partner to offer reassurance in what is usually a frightening situation for the family. An attempt to reverse the cause of the incident should be made, for example by changing position and discontinuing any intravenous oxytocin infusion (NICE 2017; FIGO 2018). In the event of maternal hypotension, IV fluids should be commenced and consideration to the use of maternal vasoconstrictors if the hypotension is secondary to a regional anaesthesia. The following *3–6–9–12 minute rule* is recommended by FIGO (2018) as a guide to subsequent management:

- **0–3:** If a deceleration is noted for more than 3 min, with no signs of recovery, the emergency alarm must be raised to summon the on-call team.
- **3–6:** Attempt to diagnose the cause of the deceleration. If an accident is found, such as the cord prolapsed, the aim would be for immediate birth as

soon as safely possible by the fastest route possible (assisted vaginal birth/caesarean section). If an iatrogenic cause is diagnosed, immediate measures to correct the situation should be commenced. This includes avoiding the supine position, discontinuing uterine stimulants, commencing IV fluids (if appropriate) and administering tocolytics.

- **6–9:** Signs of recovery should be noted (return of variability and improvement in heart rate). If no signs of recovery are noted, preparation for immediate birth **MUST** be started.
- **9–12:** By this point in time, the deceleration has either recovered, or preparation for an assisted vaginal birth/caesarean section is in progress aiming for the birth of the baby by 12–15 min.

Subacute hypoxia. Subacute hypoxia usually presents as a fetal heart rate that is below the baseline fetal heart and is usually caused by uterine hyperstimulation (FIGO 2018). During a subacute episode, the accumulation of CO_2 increases and O_2 intake decreases, which results in a build-up of hydrogen ions (H+) leading to acidosis (Muhunthan and Arulkumaran 2017).

The nature of the uterine contractibility is important, as it is vital the uterus relaxes for at least 60 s in between contractions in order that the blood flow from the placenta can oxygenate the baby adequately.

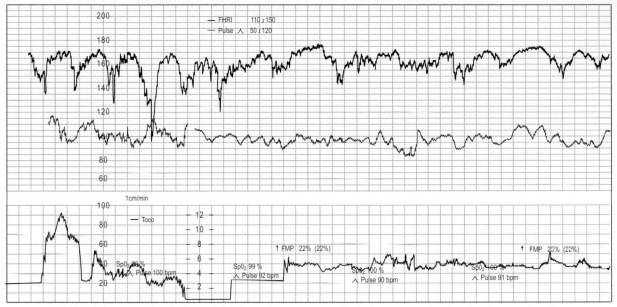

Fig. 19.18 Image of gradually evolving hypoxia compensated response, note decelerations, loss of cycling and rise in baseline. (Courtesy Dr Maggie Blott.)

There are two types of uterine contractile anomalies the midwife should be aware of that can lead to fetal heart rate changes such as subacute hypoxia:

- **Tachysystole:** more than 5 contractions in 10 min
- **Hyperstimulation:** an increase in the frequency of uterine contractions, strength of contraction and an increased uterine tone between contractions and/or prolonged contractions for over 2 min (FIGO 2018).

It is important to escalate this type of trace immediately to a senior midwife or obstetrician (NICE 2017) and to reverse the potential related cause. The woman should be asked to change position, oxytocin infusions (if being administered) should be reduced or discontinued, prostaglandin delivery systems should be removed and IV fluids should be considered (FIGO 2018; NICE 2017). If hyperstimulation is the cause and reducing oxytocin or removing the prostaglandin does not resolve the situation, tocolytics such as terbutaline, should be considered (FIGO 2018; NICE 2018). Tocolytics, are beta adrenergic receptor agonists and work by relaxing the muscles of the uterus.

There is some suggestion that if subacute hypoxia is detected in the second stage of labour when the woman is pushing, then encouraging her to stop pushing for 10 min to allow placental reoxygenation may be effective in improving the fetal heart rate (FIGO 2018).

Gradually evolving hypoxia. Gradually evolving hypoxia is the most common type of hypoxia seen during labour (FIGO 2018) (Figs 19.18, 19.19). Typically, the CTG will appear normal and will gradually show signs suggestive of hypoxic stress (decelerations). If the stress is not resolved then a loss of accelerations and cycling become apparent. The decelerations will become wider and deeper. A catecholamine release in response to stress will be seen in the form of a progressively rising baseline in an attempt to centralise blood flow to the heart and brain. At this point the fetus is in a *compensatory* stage. If the suspected hypoxia is not reversed, the fetus will start to decompensate and a loss of variability will manifest on the trace because of further vasoconstriction affecting the brain. Finally terminal heart failure will result in an unstable decline/falling baseline (FIGO 2018).

Key features to look out for on the CTG in a gradually evolving hypoxic fetus:

- decelerations
- a loss of accelerations and cycling
- decelerations that become wider and deeper with a slower recovery back to baseline
- a progressive rise in the baseline.

Detection of gradually evolving hypoxia will be dependent on accurate and systematic reviews of the fetal

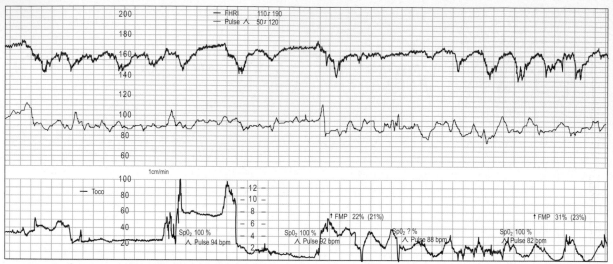

Fig. 19.19 Gradually evolving hypoxia-decompensated response, noting the reduced variability. (Courtesy Dr Maggie Blott.)

heart trace. It is recommended that a *'buddy'/'fresh eyes'* approach, as part of the systematic analysis of the CTG, should be undertaken to ensure features that may indicate fetal hypoxia are not missed (RCOG 2016). A summary of *good practice points before and during CTG monitoring* are provided in Box 19.5.

Fetal Blood Sampling

Fetal blood sampling (FBS) is used to predict metabolic acidosis in a fetus suspected of developing hypoxia. NICE (2017) recommend that, before carrying out fetal blood sampling, conservative measures should first be implemented and consideration should be given as to whether or not the fetus has responded to digital fetal scalp stimulation (NICE 2017). If accelerations are noted on the CTG in response to digital scalp stimulation, it is usually a sign that the fetus is healthy (NICE 2017). Fetal blood sampling is usually carried out after gaining consent from the woman. It is undertaken with the woman in a left lateral position and involves a small sample of blood being taken from the scalp of the fetal head as shown in Fig. 19.20. The blood is analysed for pH and lactate levels. Levels are shown in Box 19.6.

A *normal* fetal blood sample should be repeated no longer than an hour later, should there be no accelerations during a vaginal examination and hypoxic features remain on the CTG trace, whereas a *borderline* result should be repeated in 30 min, if there are still signs of hypoxia (NICE 2017).

NICE (2017) recommends that if the fetal blood sample result is *abnormal* then this should be explained to the woman and her preferences taken into account. The result should be interpreted by taking into account any previous result and the clinical features of the woman and baby, such as progress in labour in order to determine the most appropriate mode to expedite the birth (NICE 2017).

WOMEN'S CONTROL OF PAIN DURING LABOUR

The relationship between the woman and the midwife is important and can also impact on how the woman perceives the pain of labour. The idea of patience and supporting the woman on her journey, giving meaning and sense to the pain of labour, is paramount.

The issue of pain during labour should be woman-centred, not medically-oriented. A clear differentiation must be made between the traditional goal of pain relief and the control of pain in labour. Leap and Anderson (2008) proposed that midwives adopt one of two paradigms: *the pain relief* model and *the working with pain* model. In the *pain relief* model, midwives present a menu of pain-relieving options to the woman, but while this approach has the best of intentions, it inevitably undermines the woman's confidence in herself and her body to give birth without the aid of medication. However, in the *working with pain* model, it is expected that

BOX 19.5 Good Practice Points Before and During Continuous (Electronic) Fetal Monitoring (C[E]FM)

- On admission, an explanation of why CEFM is the most appropriate form of fetal surveillance should be given to the woman and her birth partner.
- CEFM should *not* be offered to women who are low risk.
- A full assessment of the woman should be carried out on admission, including documentation of the risk factors present, which require CTG monitoring.
- The time and paper speed of the CTG should be checked to ensure it is correct.
- Abdominal palpation should be performed to detect the position of the baby so that the cardiotocograph can be placed in the correct area. This is usually over the fetus' anterior shoulder (Stevenson and Chandraharan 2017).
- An initial auscultation of the fetal heart using a Pinard stethoscope or handheld Doppler should be carried out before CTG monitoring is commenced.
- The maternal pulse should be documented to ensure distinguishable differences with the fetal heart rate.
- The midwife should ensure that the woman has passed urine before commencing the CTG and that she is in a comfortable position. All women who require CEFM should be offered telemetry monitoring if available (NICE 2017).
- During labour, the woman should be encouraged to change position and mobilize (if able) during CTG monitoring. There is no reason why women cannot use a birthing ball and adopt upright positions, but quality of the trace must be good.
- The trace should be systematically assessed at least hourly by two clinicians using a *fresh eyes approach* (RCOG 2016; FIGO 2018; NICE 2017).
- Significant events should be recorded on the CTG, such as vaginal examinations and time and date of birth.
- When assessing the trace, the findings should be explained to the mother and her birth partner avoiding terms such as *fetal distress* as it may cause anxiety in the mother (NICE 2017).
- All staff involved in interpreting CTG traces should receive up-to-date training at least annually (RCOG 2016).
- The focus of the care should always remain the mother and *not* the CTG trace (NICE 2017).

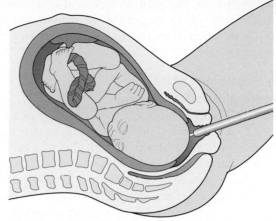

Fig. 19.20 Fetal blood sampling. Access to the fetal scalp via an amnioscope passed through the cervix.

BOX 19.6 Fetal Blood Sampling: pH and Lactate Levels

	pH	Lactate
Normal	≥7.25	≤4.1 mmol/L
Borderline	7.21–7.24	4.2–4.8 mmol/L
Abnormal	<7.20	≤4.9 mmol/L

most women in labour will experience some degree of pain that is fundamental to a physiological labour. Pain of normal labour is *positive* and has a purpose, and if this philosophy is embraced, midwives and women can work together to ensure labour is an enabling and ultimately uplifting experience.

It is appreciated that emotions such as fear, confidence and also cognition affect the person's perception of pain (Leap and Anderson 2008; Mander 2011). More than any other type of sensation, pain can be modified by past experience, anxiety, emotion and suggestion. Lack of food, rest and sleep also impact on the woman's perception of pain. The midwife must take into account not only the level or extent of the woman's pain, but also all other subjective or perceptive aspects that may be contributing to the experience, and also to realize the importance of her own attitude to intrapartum *pain relief*, as this may be informed by the medical model.

The role of pain in labour is an important one. For some women, it provides the dominant negative memory of the birth, while for others, it is viewed as empowering, bestowing a sense of triumphant achievement. As the pain of labour affects women in different ways, so then must the response of the midwife be tailored to the individual needs of the woman.

The Physiology of Pain

Pain stimulus and pain sensation

Unlike most pain, the pain experienced in labour is not caused by a pathological process or trauma and instead is the result of an interaction between physiological and psychological factors (Abushaikha and Oweis 2005). The discomfort or pain of labour is caused by the descent of the fetal head further into the pelvis. It is also caused by pressure on the cervix and the stretching of the vaginal walls and pelvic floor muscles, as descent of the presenting part occurs. The large uterine muscle contracts more strongly, more frequently and for a longer duration as labour progresses. This also increases the discomfort felt by the woman. It is not suitable to use the pain-relieving measures used in other medical circumstances, as the purpose is not to stop or impair the birth process (or contractions), but to facilitate the labour progress physiologically, with the descent and rotation of the presenting part.

Pain is caused by a stimulus that may cause, or be on the verge of causing, tissue damage. Pain sensation may therefore be distinguished from other sensations, although emotions such as fear and anxiety are also experienced at the same time, thereby affecting the person's perception of pain. It must also be remembered that a painful stimulus may also induce such changes by the sympathetic nervous system as increased heart rate, a rise in blood pressure, release of adrenaline (epinephrine) into the bloodstream and an increase in blood glucose levels. There is also a decrease in gastric motility and a reduction in the blood supply to the skin, causing sweating. Thus, stimuli that cause pain result in a *sensory* incident or occurrence.

Pain transmission

The pain pathway or *ascending sensory tract* originates in the sensory nerve endings at the site of trauma. The impulse travels along the sensory nerves to the dorsal root ganglion of the relevant spinal nerve and into the posterior horn of the spinal cord. This is known as the *first neuron*. The *second neuron* arises in the posterior horn, crosses over within the spinal cord (the *sensory decussation*) and transmits the impulse via the *medulla* *oblongata*, *pons varolii* and the *midbrain* to the *thalamus*. From here, it travels along the *third neuron* to the *sensory cortex* (Fig. 19.21).

In cases of *acute pain*, sensations are transmitted along *Aδ fibres*, which are large diameter nerve fibres. This type of pain is perceived as being a pricking pain that is readily localized by the sufferer. The pathway for *chronic pain* is slightly different as the nerve fibres involved are of smaller diameter and are called *C fibres*. Chronic pain is often described as a burning pain that is difficult to localize.

Somatosensory function

Somatic sensation refers to the sensory function of the skin and body walls. This is moderated by a variety of somatic receptors of which there are particular receptors for each sensation, such as heat, cold, touch, pressure, etc. On entering the central nervous system, the afferent nerve fibres from somatic receptors form synapses with interneurons that comprise the specific ascending pathways going to the somatosensory cortex via the brain stem and the thalamus.

An *afferent neuron*, with its receptor, makes up a sensory unit. Usually the peripheral end of an afferent neuron branches into many receptors. The receptors whose stimulation gives rise to pain are situated in the peripheries of small unmyelinated or slightly myelinated afferent neurons. These receptors are known as *nociceptors* because they detect injury (*noci*, being the Latin word for 'harm/injury'). The primary afferents coming from nociceptors form synapses with interneurons after entering the central nervous system. *Substance P* is a *neurotransmitter* that is liberated at some of these synapses when there is a pain impulse that facilitates information about pain, which is then transmitted to the higher centres.

The stretching of the muscles and ligaments of the pelvic cavity and the pressure of the descending fetus during the birthing process causes pain in labour to varying degrees (Fig. 19.22). This sensation is transmitted by afferent or *visceral sensory neurons*, visceral pain being caused by the stretching or irritation of the viscera. Afferent neurons convey both autonomic sympathetic and parasympathetic fibres. Pain fibres from the skin and the viscera run adjacent to each other in the *spinothalamic tract*. Therefore pain from an internal organ may be perceived or felt as if it was coming from a skin area supplied by the same section or part of the

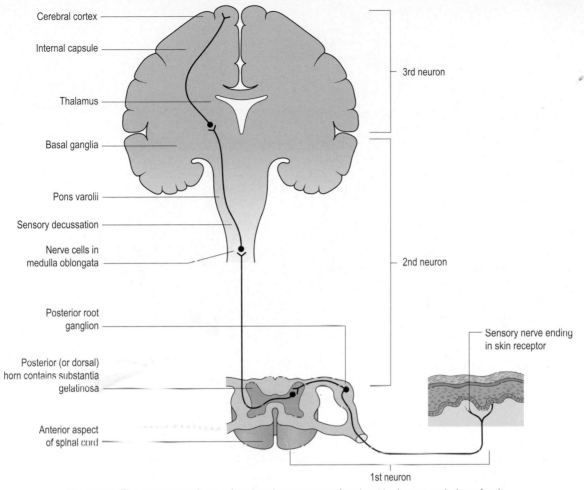

Cerebral cortex

Internal capsule

3rd neuron

Thalamus

Basal ganglia

Pons varolii

Sensory decussation

Nerve cells in
medulla oblongata

2nd neuron

Posterior root
ganglion

Sensory nerve ending
in skin receptor

Posterior (or dorsal)
horn contains substantia
gelatinosa

Anterior aspect
of spinal cord

1st neuron

Fig. 19.21 The sensory pathway showing the structures involved in the appreciation of pain.

spinal cord: for example, pain from the uterus may be perceived or felt by the woman as being in her back or labia. When this sort of pain occurs or is experienced, it is commonly called *referred pain*.

Martini et al. (2018) suggest that the level of pain experienced can be disproportionate to the amount of painful stimuli due to the facilitation resulting from glutamate and substance P release. This effect can be one reason why women's perception of pain associated with childbirth differs so widely.

Endorphins and enkephalins

Endorphins are described as being opiate-like peptides, or *neuropeptides*, which are produced naturally by the body at neural synapses at various points in the central nervous system pathways. They modulate

the transmission of pain perception in these areas. Endorphins are found in the limbic system, hypothalamus and reticular formation (Martini et al. 2018). They bind to the presynaptic membrane, inhibiting the release of substance P, and therefore inhibit the transmission of pain. *Enkephalins* are also neuropeptides that have the ability to inhibit neurotransmitters along the pathway of pain transmission, thereby reducing it. These act like a natural pain relieving substance.

Theories of Pain

Theories of pain include specificity, pattern, affect and psychological/behavioural theory (Mander 2011), however these are not always applicable to the pain experienced in childbirth. The most widely used and

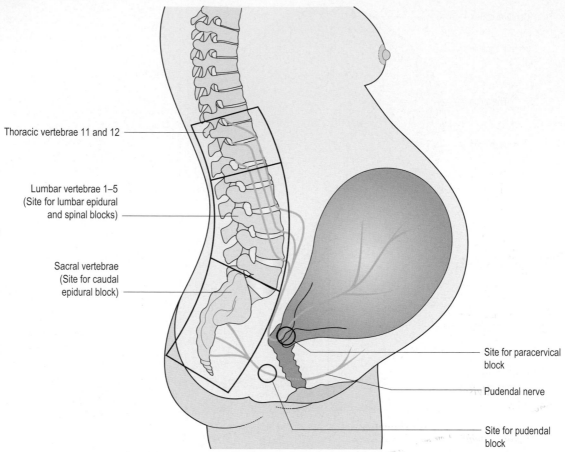

Thoracic vertebrae 11 and 12

Lumbar vertebrae 1–5
(Site for lumbar epidural
and spinal blocks)

Sacral vertebrae
(Site for caudal
epidural block)

Site for paracervical
block

Pudendal nerve

Site for pudendal
block

Fig. 19.22 Pain pathways in labour showing the sites at which pain may be intercepted by local anaesthetic techniques.

accepted theory is the *gate-control theory* of Melzack and Wall (1965), who established that gentle stimulation actually inhibits the sensation of pain. The *gate-control theory* declares that a neural or spinal gating mechanism occurs in the *substantia gelatinosa* of the dorsal horns of the spinal cord. The nerve impulses received by nociceptors, the receptors for pain in the skin and tissue of the body, are affected by the gating mechanism. It is the position of the gate that determines whether or not the nerve impulses travel freely to the medulla and the thalamus, thereby transmitting the sensory impulse or message to the sensory cortex. If the gate is closed, pain is blocked and does not become part of the conscious thought. If the gate is open, the impulses and messages pass through and are transmitted freely (Fig. 19.22), resulting in pain being experienced.

Physiological Responses to Pain of Labour

Pain of labour is associated with an *increased respiratory rate*. This may cause a decrease in the $PaCO_2$ level, with a corresponding increase in the pH and a subsequent fall in the fetal $PaCO_2$ ensues. This may be suspected by the presence of late decelerations on the CTG trace if continuous monitoring is being employed during labour. The acid–base equilibrium of the system may be altered by hyperventilation and breathing exercises. Alkalosis may then affect the diffusion of oxygen across the placenta, leading to a degree of fetal hypoxia.

Cardiac output increases during the first and second stages of labour up to an extent of 20% and 50%, respectively. This increase is caused by the return of uterine blood to the maternal circulation, which constitutes about 250–300 mL with each contraction.

Pain, apprehension and fear may also cause a sympathetic response, thereby producing a greater cardiac output.

Both the respiratory and cardiac systems are affected by catecholamine release. Adrenaline (epinephrine), which comprises about 80% of this release, has the effect of reducing the uterine blood flow, leading to a potential reduction in uterine activity.

Non-Pharmacological Methods for Pain Control in Labour

Increasingly, non-pharmacological methods are being used by women during labour. In addition to the methods described below, there is evidence that hypnosis, massage, acupuncture and acupressure reduce pain or decrease the need for pharmacological analgesia during labour (Tiran 2018). However, in the case of administering medicines including complementary therapies, the *NMC Code* (NMC 2018: 16) clearly states this has to be within the limits of the individual midwife's training and competence, the law, and professional and other relevant policies, guidance and regulations such that they:

> *can prescribe, advise on or provide medicines or treatment, including repeat prescriptions (**only if suitably qualified**) if they have enough knowledge of that person's health and are satisfied that the medicines or treatment serve that person's health needs.*

Aromatherapy

Aromatherapy is the use of essential oils for a range of purposes, for example to induce relaxation, or reduce pain, nausea and vomiting. These oils may be massaged into the skin, inhaled through diffusers or oil burners, or used in conjunction with hydrotherapy. This particular complementary therapy has become popular among childbearing women and midwives, with many maternity units in the UK providing this service for women during labour and birth (Smith et al. 2011). Zahra and Leila (2013) conducted a randomized controlled trial (RCT) in Iran with women randomly assigned to either massage only or aromatherapy massage with lavender oil. Pain intensity was significantly lower in the aromatherapy massage group and first and second stages of labour were shorter. There were, however, only 30 women assigned to each group. Furthermore, the systematic review conducted by Smith et al. (2011) on the efficacy of aromatherapy for pain management was also too small to draw any significant conclusions and thus there remains a need for more research in this area.

Homeopathy

Homeopathy uses small doses of natural medicines to stimulate the body's own physiological response to heal itself (Idarius 2010). Homeopathic remedies are prepared from plant extracts and from minerals. Professional advice is recommended during pregnancy as the holistic approach of this method entails a consideration of all the facets and the requirements of the individual. *Aconite* may be used to relieve fear and anxiety and *Kali Carbonate* to alleviate back pain during labour (Steen and Calvert 2006).

Hydrotherapy

Immersion in water during labour as a means of analgesia has been used for many years. Cluett and Burns (2018) cite that the effectiveness of hydrotherapy is due to heat-relieving muscle spasm, and therefore pain, and *hydrokinesis* eliminates the effects of gravity and also the discomfort and strain on the pelvis. Two studies comparing immersion in water during labour with land labour found that those immersed in water had significantly reduced duration of labour (Zanetti-Dallenbach et al. 2007; Thoni et al. 2010). Cluett and Burns (2018) also found that immersion in water in the first stage of labour reduces the use of epidural/spinal analgesia with no evidence of an increase in adverse effects on fetus/neonate or the woman. Water immersion is usually highly rated by both women and midwives, and the calming atmosphere of a pool room can benefit everyone as the woman appears less anxious and therefore feels less pain (Benjoya Miller and Magill-Cuerden 2006).

Music therapy

As well as at home, many birthing rooms are equipped with a radio or CD apparatus and this is often a useful means to help women relax, be entertained and find some distraction during the early stages of labour. Many types of music are available for relaxation, some of which are specifically for childbirth. Henley-Einion (2007) recounts that music can have a positive effect on the woman's body, mind and spirit by providing empowerment and creating an enabling effect.

Transcutaneous electrical nerve stimulation

Transcutaneous electrical nerve stimulation (TENS) is a widely used and well-appreciated method of pain relief. TENS stimulates the production of natural endorphins and enkephalins and impedes incoming pain stimuli. It consists of a small device that distributes low intensity electrical charges across the skin which is thought to prevent pain signals from the uterus, vagina and cervix arriving at the brain (de Ferrer 2006). The body's own pain relievers, the *endorphins*, are then released. TENS works by stimulating low threshold afferent fibres, such as the fibres of touch receptors, which inhibit neurons in the pain pathways. As pathways activated by the touch receptors add a synaptic input into the pain pathways, the individual may massage a painful area to relieve the pain, which is how TENS functions.

The apparatus consists of four electrodes and four flexes that connect these to the TENS unit, which has controls to alter the frequency and the intensity of the impulse (Fig. 19.23). The electrodes are positioned at the level of T10 and L1 on the woman's back and have been found to be effective in reducing pain during the first stage of labour. The remaining electrodes are placed between S2 and S4 and provide control of pain during the second stage of labour. The woman can use a boost control button to convey high intensity and high frequency patterns of stimulation of the dermatomes during the uterine contraction to provide additional relief, thus enhancing control over the birth process.

TENS is considered to be more effective when started in early labour (Juman Blincoe 2007). However, while some studies have found the use of TENs to be effective as a method of pain relief (Shahoei et al. 2017), Dowswell et al. (2009) found that women using TENs were less likely to rate their pain as severe and overall they did not find any overwhelming evidence that TENs significantly reduces pain in labour.

Pharmacological Methods for Pain Control

Inhalation analgesia

A premixed gas made up of 50% nitrous oxide (N$_2$O) and 50% oxygen (O$_2$) administered via the Entonox apparatus is the most commonly used inhalation analgesia in labour. Nitrous oxide (also known as *laughing gas*), like many other forms of analgesia, acts by limiting the neuronal and synaptic transmission within the central nervous system. Evidence shows that N$_2$O induces opioid peptide release in *the periaqueductal* grey area of the midbrain leading to the activation of the descending inhibitory pathways, resulting in modulation of the pain/nociceptive processing in the spinal cord (Fujinaga and Maze 2002). The mixture of gases is stable at normal temperature, but separates below −7°C. In many large obstetric units the gas is stored in a bank and piped to each birthing room or is available in cylinders. Midwives attending women at home births are responsible for the safe storage of the gas cylinders, which should be on their side, rather than upright. This is because nitrous oxide is heavier than oxygen and the horizontal position reduces the risk of administering a severely hypoxic mixture. The cylinders must be brought into a warm room if they have been exposed to cold temperatures, and the gases remixed by inverting the cylinder at least three times before use.

Entonox apparatus is usually manufactured by the British Oxygen Company (BOC). Both the apparatus and the cylinder are made so that they do not fit on to other equipment. These fit together by a pin index system. The cylinder is blue with a blue and white shoulder. The one-way valve opens on inspiration and the woman

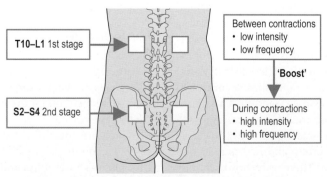

Fig. 19.23 TENS electrode positioning for use during labour.

should be advised that optimal analgesia is obtained by closely applying the lips around the mouthpiece or firmly applying the mask to the face. The gases take effect within 20 s and it is important that the woman uses it before a contraction commences. The maximum efficacy of the gases occurs after about 45–50 s, which should coincide with the height of the contraction, providing maximum relief for the woman. This method of pain control is useful in that the woman is able to administer it herself, but its effectiveness is determined by the woman's ability to use the equipment as advised. A study by Teimoori et al. (2011) showed that nitrous oxide and oxygen provided better analgesia and had more beneficial effects when compared with pethidine.

Exposure to high levels of nitrous oxide can cause teratogenic and other side-effects such as infertility among midwives and other staff. It is important that scavenging equipment to extract expired gases is installed in all birthing rooms to reduce such effects on staff.

Opiate drugs

Opiate drugs are frequently used during childbirth because of their powerful analgesic properties. The action of these drugs lies in their ability to bind with receptor sites, which are mainly found in the *substantia gelatinosa* of the dorsal horn of the spinal cord (Anderson 2011). Others are located in the midbrain, thalamus and hypothalamus.

In the UK, three systemic opioids are commonly used for pain relief in labour:

- pethidine (meperidine in the USA)
- diamorphine
- meptazinol (Meptid).

All have similar pain-relieving properties, but little evidence exists in relation to their effectiveness, maternal satisfaction of their use or their effect on the fetus/neonate in labour (Smith et al. 2018). There are numerous side-effects of opiate drugs and the extent to which they are experienced is influenced by the woman's metabolism of the drug, the degree and speed of transfer of the drug and metabolites from maternal to fetal circulation and the ability of the fetus to process and excrete both. Common side-effects of opiate drugs include:

- nausea and vomiting
- delayed emptying of the stomach
- drowsiness or sedation in the woman, which may impair decision-making

- reduction in fetal heart rate variability and depression of the baby's respiratory centre at birth
- a sleepy baby affecting the establishment of breast-feeding.

An antiemetic agent is sometimes given to the woman at the same time to reduce the feeling of nausea. It is therefore important to ensure that the woman is fully informed during pregnancy of the effects of the drugs so that she can make informed decisions about methods of pain control.

Pethidine. Pethidine is a synthetic compound acting on the receptors in the body and is the most frequently used systemic narcotic analgesic in the UK. It is usually administered intramuscularly in doses of 50–100 mg, depending on the woman's size, and takes about 20 min to have an effect. Pethidine can be administered intravenously for a faster effect and some maternity units use a machine to enable the woman to control the administration: known as *patient-controlled analgesia* (PCA). Some reports show that opiates, especially pethidine, slow down the process of labour and are not significantly effective in relieving labour pain, as often sedation is confused with analgesia (Anderson 2011).

Diamorphine. Diamorphine has been found to provide effective analgesia for up to 4 h in labour with the usual dose being 5 mg. It is more rapidly metabolized, accounting for its greater speed of effectiveness and consequently, it is eliminated more readily from maternal and neonatal plasma (Setty and Fernando 2019). Diamorphine is used far less commonly than other opiates in labour, even though some claim it gives better pain relief and hence more comparative studies are needed (Jones et al. 2012). It is possible that the lack of use of diamorphine in labour might be due to fears of its potentially addictive nature.

Meptazinol. Meptazinol is usually given in doses of 100–150 mg intramuscularly. It is fast-acting and is effective for about 4 h. This opiate provides similar pain relief to pethidine and like other opiates, meptazinol is also associated with an increased incidence of nausea and vomiting (Smith et al. 2018).

Regional (epidural) analgesia

Epidurals are effective in relieving pain in labour and may be requested by women at any point during the first stage of labour. Women who have used other methods of pain relief on experiencing strong contractions may decide to request an epidural when labour is well advanced. This makes explanation of the benefits and risks of epidural analgesia *during pregnancy* even more important. The pain relief from an epidural is obtained by blocking the conduction of impulses along sensory nerves as they enter the spinal cord. It is an invasive procedure that requires informed consent from the woman and an experienced (obstetric) anaesthetist to initiate under strict aseptic conditions.

An intravenous infusion of crystalloid fluids is commenced prior to siting the epidural. The need for *preloading* has reduced since *low-dose epidural blockades* have been used, reducing the risk of hypotension (NICE 2017). The woman either adopts the left lateral position to reduce the risk of supine hypotension or a sitting position to flex the spine, in an effort to separate the vertebrae, thus facilitating the management of the procedure. The fetal heart rate and the woman's blood pressure must be recorded throughout the procedure.

The skin is first cleansed followed by administration of local anaesthetic into the epidural space of the lumbar region, usually between L2 and L3, before the anaesthetist cautiously inserts a Tuohy needle (usually 16G) that has centimetre marking and a bevelled end to aid the insertion and positioning of a fine catheter, into the epidural space (Fig. 19.24). To locate the epidural space, the needle is first advanced until resistance of the *ligamentum flavum* is encountered. At this point, a syringe is attached to the Tuohy needle and inserted further until it enters the epidural space. This is recognized by the loss of resistance when pressure is applied to the plunger of the syringe or loss of resistance to saline (Hawkins 2010). It is particularly important that the woman remains still at this stage as the subarachnoid space is only a few millimetres deeper and any slight movement could result in the Tuohy needle puncturing the meninges and causing a *dural tap*. Smaller gauge needles are used for spinal anaesthesia reducing the risk of dural tap and have the advantage of relieving pain rapidly (Hawkins 2010).

Once the Tuohy needle is in the epidural space and there is no evidence of any leakage of blood or cerebrospinal fluid (CSF), a fine catheter is threaded through the needle and left *in situ* to facilitate bolus injections or continuous infusion of the local anaesthetic bupivacaine (Marcaine). The injection of bupivacaine into the epidural space bathes the nerves of the *corda equina*, blocking the autonomic nerve pathways supplying the uterus. The first dose is given by the anaesthetist to test for effect and observe for any adverse reactions. The needle is subsequently removed and an antibacterial filter is attached to the end of the catheter. The catheter is then secured to the woman's back with strapping and a syringe pump commenced if there is to be a continuous infusion.

Continuous infusion of dilute bupivacaine and opioids (usually fentanyl) has resulted in significant reductions in the amount of local anaesthetic used while ensuring rapid analgesia. In addition, because of the minimal motor block effect with this regime, the woman is able to move about more freely and bear down more effectively in the second stage of labour (Anim-Somuah et al. 2011). The Comparative Obstetric Mobile Epidural

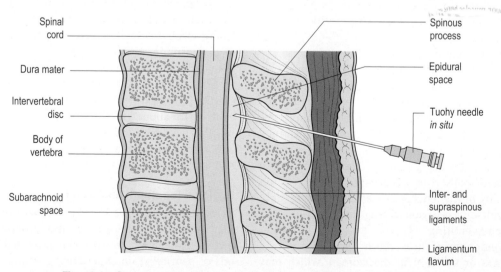

Fig. 19.24 Sagittal section of the lumbar spine with Tuohy needle in position.

Trial (COMET) Study Group UK (COMET 2001) found that low-dose infusion epidurals resulted in a lower incidence of instrumental vaginal births compared with traditional bolus epidurals.

Observations and epidural care by the midwife

Each midwife is personally responsible for ensuring that they are competent to care for women who have epidural analgesia, including topping up the epidural block as specifically prescribed by the anaesthetist, being aware of the possible complications and their immediate treatment.

After the administration of the first dose of bupivacaine and subsequent top-up doses of local anaesthetic the blood pressure and pulse should be measured and recorded every 5 min for 15 min and then every 30 min (NICE 2017). The temperature should also be recorded regularly. The woman may adopt any position she finds comfortable, avoiding aorto-caval compression, and encouraged to change position regularly to avoid soft tissue damage. The fetal heart is usually monitored electronically.

The spread of the block should be assessed hourly by the midwife using a cold object or ethyl chloride spray (NICE 2017). The sensation to void urine may be reduced so the midwife must ensure that the woman is encouraged to empty her bladder regularly to avoid postnatal urinary retention. Similarly, the woman may not be as sensitive to feeling uterine contractions or the desire to bear down in the second stage of labour. This is due to the pelvic floor muscles being relaxed and affecting rotation of the fetal presenting part. The midwife therefore needs to be observant of these physiological changes.

Complications of epidural analgesia. The use of low-dose bupivacaine solutions for analgesia in labour has limited the risks of hypotension and local anaesthetic toxicity. Nevertheless, potential complications of epidurals still exist and these with their treatment are detailed in Box 19.7.

FIRST STAGE OF LABOUR: VAGINAL BREECH AT TERM

This section considers the physiology and intrapartum care in the first stage of labour of those term pregnancies presenting by the breech. In addition, the controversies surrounding the evidence of breech birth and the effect on women's choice for labour and birth are explored.

Incidence of Breech Presentation

Breech presentation involves a longitudinal lie of the fetus, with the buttocks in the lower pole of the maternal uterus. The presenting diameter is the *bitrochanteric* (10 cm) and the denominator is the *sacrum*. As pregnancy progresses, the incidence of breech presentation reduces: being around 15% at 28–32 weeks to around 3–4% by term, as a result of spontaneous version (Chadwick 2002). It is worth considering, therefore, that a breech presentation at term is ***not*** an abnormality, it is just ***unusual*** and so a normal labour and spontaneous vaginal birth should not be excluded. Although in Western childbirth culture a breech birth has the status of an ***emergency***, in many parts of the world a vaginal breech birth is part of normal practice (Burvill 2005). This used to be the case in the UK for most community midwives during the last century (Allison 1996). However, following the Peel Report (Maternity Advisory Committee 1970) that gave rise to the transfer of childbirth from the home to the hospital environment, such skills of the midwife regarding vaginal breech births have been eroded, as midwifery became subsumed into a medico-technocratic model, where obstetric intervention prevails.

There has been much sociopolitical influence in the UK over the past couple of decades, aimed at improving childbirth choices and quality of maternity services for women. This has provided the opportunity for midwives to re-examine their role in providing a more holistic model of maternity care (DH 1993, 2004a,b, 2007, 2008a,b, 2010a,b; NHS England 2016). The consequential reduction in junior doctors' hours (DH et al. 2002) provided further opportunities for NHS Trusts to embrace collaborative working between health professionals (DH 2001; NHS England 2016), leading to a redefining of roles and responsibilities for midwives and their medical colleagues.

The clearly documented accounts from Cronk (1998a,b), Reed (1999, 2003) and Evans (2007, 2012a,b, 2017) provide first-hand detail of how midwives can support women with a breech presentation to give birth naturally other than by caesarean section and are an inspiration to other midwives seeking to develop or re-establish skills in this area. However, the authors above acknowledge that not all breeches can, or should, be born vaginally.

BOX 19.7   Complications of Epidural Analgesia

Complication	Cause	Treatment
Hypotensive incident	Affects the sympathetic nervous system by causing vasodilation and a fall in blood pressure	Assist woman into left lateral position, administer oxygen, call anaesthetist, rapidly infuse Hartmann's solution intra-venously. Epinephrine, a vasopressor, may be given to raise the blood pressure
Dural puncture and consequent headache	Lowering of pressure/leakage of cerebrospinal fluid causing a stretching of brain tissue	Epidural injection of 10–20 mL of maternal blood (*a blood patch*), to seal the puncture and relieve the headache
Loss of bladder sensation	Poor intrapartum bladder care	Catheterization of the bladder
Total spinal leading to respiratory arrest	Induction of a high nerve block/injection of bupivacaine into a vein	Stop epidural and employ immediate resuscitation procedures
Local anaesthetic toxicity leading to cardiac arrest	Over infusion of local anaesthetic or too rapid administration	Stop epidural and employ immediate resuscitation procedures
Fetal compromise	Maternal hypotension or local analgesic toxicity	Stop epidural and assist woman into left lateral position
Increase in assisted vaginal births	Reduced muscle tone of the pelvic floor	Consider low-dose infusion epidural. Delay pushing if fetal condition is satisfactory
Neurological sequelae	Any of the above causes	Serious damage extremely rare; weakness/sensory loss is uncommon and soon resolves
Long-term backache	Common problem throughout childbirth due to the hormones of pregnancy softening the ligaments, *but* no evidence to suggest that epidurals cause long-term backache	Encourage mobility during labour so that pressure on the back is given relief

For further details, see: Hawkins 2010; Anim-Somuah et al. (2011) and NICE (2017).

Types of Breech Presentation and Position

There are six positions for a breech presentation, as illustrated in Figs 19.25–19.30.

Breech with extended legs (Frank breech)

The breech presents with the hips flexed and legs extended on the abdomen (Fig. 19.31). This type is particularly common in primigravidae, whose efficient uterine muscle tone inhibits flexion of the legs and free turning of the mobile fetus. Consequently, this type of breech constitutes 70% of all breech presentations.

Complete breech

The fetal attitude is one of complete flexion (Fig. 19.32) with hips and knees both flexed and the feet tucked in beside the buttocks.

Footling breech

One or both feet present due to the fact that neither hip is fully flexed (Fig. 19.33). The feet are lower than the buttocks, distinguishing it from the complete breech. This type of breech is rare.

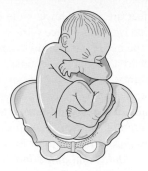

Fig. 19.25 Right sacroposterior.

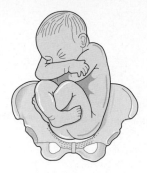

Fig. 19.26 Left sacroposterior.

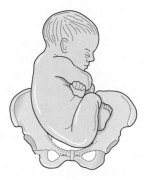

Fig. 19.27 Right sacrolateral.

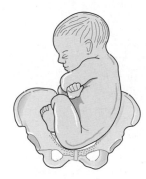

Fig. 19.28 Left sacrolateral.

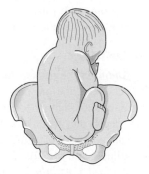

Fig. 19.29 Right sacroanterior.

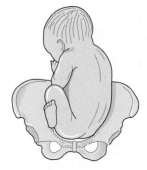

Fig. 19.29 Left sacroanterior.

Figs. 19.25–19.30 Six positions in a breech presentation.

Knee presentation

This breech type is particularly rare and presents with one or both hips extended, with the knees flexed (Fig. 19.34).

Causes of Breech Presentation

Often there is no identifiable cause, but the following situations favour breech presentation:

- extended legs
- preterm labour
- multiple pregnancy
- polyhydramnios
- hydrocephaly
- uterine abnormalities such as a *septum* or a *fibroid*
- placenta praevia.

Diagnosis of Breech Presentation
During pregnancy

The woman may inform the midwife that she can feel something very hard and uncomfortable under her ribs that makes breathing uncomfortable at times. If the fetal

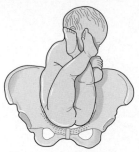

Fig. 19.31 Frank breech.

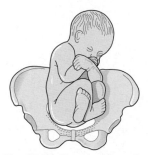

Fig. 19.32 Complete breech.

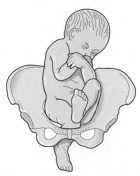

Fig. 19.33 Footling breech.

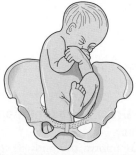

Fig. 19.34 Knee presentation.

feet are in the lower pole of the uterus, the woman is likely to experience some very hard kicks on her bladder. The use of ultrasound examination may be used to confirm a breech presentation where there is some uncertainty, however a decision on subsequent care, such as undertaking an external cephalic version (ECV), is usually deferred until nearer term. Some women may also attempt the use of moxibustion from 34 weeks' gestation to reduce the need for ECV (Tiran 2018; Smith 2013).

Abdominal palpation. In primigravidae, diagnosis is more difficult because of the woman's firm abdominal muscles. The lie will be longitudinal with a *soft* presenting part felt in the lower part of the uterus. The head can usually be felt in the fundus as a round hard mass, which the midwife may be able to move independently of the back by balloting it with one or both hands. If the legs are extended, the feet may prevent such movement of the head. When the breech is anterior and the fetus well flexed, it may be difficult to locate the head. However, the woman may complain of discomfort under her ribs, especially at night, owing to pressure of the head on the diaphragm, thus contributing to the diagnosis.

Auscultation. Prior to the breech passing through the pelvic brim, the fetal heart will be heard most clearly above the umbilicus. When the legs are extended, the breech descends into the pelvis easily such that the fetal heart is heard at a lower level.

During labour

Abdominal examination. A previously unsuspected breech presentation may not be diagnosed until the woman is in established labour. If the legs are extended, the breech may feel like a head on abdominal palpation and also on vaginal examination should the cervix be <3 cm dilated and the breech is high.

Vaginal examination. The breech feels soft and irregular with no sutures palpable. On occasion, the sacrum may be mistaken for a hard head and the buttocks for caput succedaneum. In addition, the anus may be felt and should the membranes have already ruptured, fresh meconium on the examining finger is diagnostic. If the legs are extended (Fig. 19.35) the external genitalia are very obvious, however, as these become oedematous, a swollen vulva can be mistaken for a scrotum.

If a foot is felt (Fig. 19.36), the midwife should differentiate it from the hand. Toes are all the same length, are shorter than fingers and the big toe cannot be opposed to other toes. The foot is at right-angles to the leg and the heel has no equivalent in the hand.

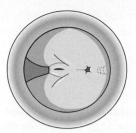

Fig. 19.35 No feet felt: the legs are extended.

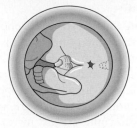

Fig. 19.36 Feet felt: complete breech presentation.

Figs. 19.35–Fig. 19.36 Vaginal touch pictures of left sacrolateral position.

Mode of Birth: the Evidence

The evidence regarding the safest mode for breech babies to be born has been somewhat controversial and misleading, with the randomized multicentre Term Breech Trial conducted by Hannah et al. (2000) concluding the safest way to give birth was by planned caesarean section. This had a major impact on the birth choices offered to women who may be presenting with a breech at the end of their pregnancy, leading to a consequential increase in planned caesarean sections. By 2004, doubts had been cast on Hannah et al.'s (2000) research, with questions being raised over the validity and ethical basis of using a RCT for such a study and further research distrusting the results and recommendations (Alarab et al. 2004; Háheim et al. 2004; Kotaska 2004; Ulander et al. 2004; Pradham et al. 2005; Glezerman 2006; Fahy 2011). Furthermore, the 2-year follow-up study by Whyte et al. (2004) and Hannah et al. (2004) did not show any differences in long-term outcomes between planned caesarean section or planned vaginal breech births.

Two further prospective trials undertaken by Goffinet et al. (2006) and Maier et al. (2011) clearly found that where planned vaginal breech birth is common practice and when strict criteria are met before and during labour, vaginal breech birth at term can still be a *safe* option. For a successful outcome, the evidence indicates that the most important factor is the presence of *an experienced health professional*, be it a midwife or obstetrician, facilitating the birth. As approximately one-third of all breech presentations are undiagnosed until labour and there is no evidence to support a caesarean section at this late stage, unless there is another clinical indication, it is important that midwives and obstetricians are competent to support vaginal breech birth. The RCOG (2017) recommend that the most experienced available practitioner should be present at a vaginal breech birth and that all maternity units have guidelines in place, including structured simulated training for all staff who may encounter vaginal breech births.

Place of Birth

Vaginal birth should be presented to the woman as the norm for breech presentation, provided there are no contraindications or complications. The woman should also be informed that there is an increase in the risk to the mother associated with caesarean section births (Chapter 24). If a vaginal breech birth is planned for the home environment, it is important that the midwife is competent to facilitate the birth and has clear lines of communication and support from her colleagues, with a second midwife being present for the birth itself (NMC 2018). Midwife Clinical Supervisors or Professional Midwifery Advocates (PMA) (NHS England 2017) may provide support and advice in this scenario. However, according to NICE (2017), a breech is considered to be a *malpresentation* indicative of risk, and recommends the labour and birth should be planned to take place in an obstetric unit.

Outside of the hospital environment, any decision to transfer the woman from the home should be made promptly taking into consideration the time it would take to complete. An action plan for the labour and birth should be made with the woman that includes specifying those situations where midwives would make the decision to transfer to hospital, namely where there is a lack of progress or fetal compromise.

Posture for Labour and Birth

When women labour instinctively, without interruption or direction, they rarely choose to labour in a semi-recumbent position. Evans (2017) endorses an upright position or all fours for breech labour and birth, which aids descent of the presenting part and assists the normal physiology of labour. The study by Louwen et al. (2017) found that upright vaginal breech birth was associated with a shorter second stage of labour, less manoeuvres required, fewer maternal/neonatal injuries, and a lower caesarean rate than vaginal birth in the dorsal position (Chapter 20). However, the RCOG (2017) still recommends the woman to be in a dorsal position for the actual birth when obstetric intervention is required.

Care in Labour

Basic care during the first stage of labour is the same as those labours where the presentation is cephalic: minimizing intervention and enabling the normal physiology to progress. The breech with extended legs fits the cervix quite well, but with a less well applied presenting part as in the complete breech, there is a tendency for the membranes to rupture early, increasing the risk of cord prolapse (Chapter 25). Should this occur, the midwife must undertake a vaginal examination to exclude cord prolapse and assess the fetal heart rate. It is not uncommon to find meconium staining of the amniotic fluid liquor with a breech presentation due to the compression of the fetal abdomen, and for this reason is *not* always indicative of fetal compromise.

PRELABOUR RUPTURE OF THE MEMBRANES AT TERM

Prelabour rupture of membranes (PROM) at term (after 37 weeks) complicates between 8% and 10% of all pregnancies and most women with PROM will labour spontaneously within 24 h (NICE 2017). Following PROM with no signs of labour, regardless of whether or not liquor is draining, digital examination should be avoided owing to an increased risk of ascending infection (NICE 2013; NICE 2017). If there is doubt about whether the membranes have ruptured, a sterile speculum examination can be performed in order to observe whether there is pooling of liquor in the posterior fornix of the vagina (NICE 2013). If there are no facilities for this, the woman can be encouraged to wear a sanitary pad for an hour or two in order for the midwife to reassess for signs of any liquor before a definite diagnosis can be made. The taking of low vaginal swabs is not recommended (NICE 2017). Initial assessment of the woman should include observation of her pulse, respiration rate, blood pressure, temperature, oxygen saturation and urinalysis. An abdominal examination should be undertaken and the fetal heart auscultated.

Following PROM, the risk of serious neonatal infection is increased from 0.5% to 1%, compared with women whose membranes remain intact, and the woman should be advised of this (NICE 2017). In view of this, and in the absence of any clinical indication for immediate induction, such as Group B *Streptococcus*, maternal infection or meconium staining of the liquor, it is usual practice to advise the woman that if she does not go into spontaneous labour within 24 h, labour should be induced after PROM (NICE 2017) (see Chapter 22). Women should be given adequate information to decide between expectant management and active management of labour following PROM. Hospital admission, in the absence of any other concerns, is not required while waiting for induction to take place.

Until the induction is commenced or if expectant management beyond 24 h is chosen by the woman, the following recommendations regarding advice to women and subsequent care should be followed (NICE 2017):

- Bathing or showering are *not* associated with an increase in infection, but having sexual intercourse may be.
- Body temperature should be recorded every 4 h during waking hours and any change in the colour or smell of the vaginal loss should be reported to the midwife immediately.
- Fetal movements should be observed.
- In the absence of any risk indicators and with satisfactory evidence of fetal movements and a normal fetal heart rate, there is no reason for a CTG to be performed.
- Low vaginal swabs and blood samples to assess maternal C-reactive protein should not be taken.

PRETERM PRELABOUR RUPTURE OF THE MEMBRANES

Preterm prelabour rupture of the membranes (PPROM) occurs before 37 completed weeks' gestation, where the fetal membranes rupture without the onset of spontaneous uterine activity and the consequential cervical dilatation. It is discussed in Chapter 14.

THE RESPONSIBILITIES OF THE MIDWIFE

The midwife has an important enabling and facilitating role to support the woman during childbirth. It is vital that shared decision-making takes place between women and their caregivers at all times (Hodnett et al. 2012). Careful assessment of the wellbeing of the woman and fetus with accurate and detailed records of *all care* given during the first stage of labour, including the careful administration and monitoring of any medicines, is essential to the provision of quality care. These in turn will provide a good basis from which appropriate decisions may be made concerning the progress and the needs of the woman to optimize her labour experience and eventual birth outcome.

REFLECTIVE ACTIVITY FOR SELF-ASSESSMENT

1. Within your place of work, how can childbearing women in the latent phase of labour, be best supported using an evidence-based but individualized approach?

2. What is the local practice of undertaking vaginal examinations in labour and is it supportive of woman's choice? How would you facilitate a woman's choice to decline being examined vaginally during labour?

3. Consider your approach to pain in labour. Do you feel that you use a *pain relief* approach or a *working with pain* approach? What measures can you take to ensure pain relief in labour is entirely woman-centred and not led by the organization?

4. Describe the physiology behind fetal heart rate control and regulation. When caring for an otherwise healthy woman within a midwifery led setting, explain the actions you would take if you heard a prolonged deceleration during intermittent auscultation.

5. How can childbearing women with a breech presentation, be supported to make an informed decision about the mode of birth for their baby? If a choice of vaginal birth is chosen how can this be best facilitated?

REFERENCES

Abernathy, A., Alsina, L., Greer, J., & Egerman, R. (2017). Transient fetal tachycardia after intravenous diphenhydramine administration. *Obstetrics and Gynaecology*, 130(2) 374–37.

Abushaikha, L., & Oweis, A. (2005). Labour pain experience and intensity: A Jordanian experience. *International Journal of Nursing Practice*, 11(1), 33–38.

ACOG (American College of Obstetricians and Gynecologists). (2014). Obstetric care consensus No. 1: Safe prevention of the primary cesarean delivery. *Obstetrics & Gynecology*, 123(3), 693–711.

Aghoja, L. O. (2014). Maternal and fetal acid-base chemistry: A major determinant of perinatal outcome. *Annals of Medical and Health Science Research*, 4(1), 8–17.

Alarab, M., Regan, C., O'Connell, M. P., et al. (2004). Singleton breech delivery at term: Still a safe option. *Obstetrics & Gynecology*, 103(3), 407–412.

Albers, L. (1999). The duration of labor in healthy women. *Journal of Perinatology*, 19(2), 114–119.

Albers, L. (2007). The evidence for physiologic management of the active phase of the first stage of labour. *Journal of Midwifery & Women's Health*, 52, 207–215.

Alfirevic, Z., Devane, D., Gyte, G., & Cuthbert, A. (2017). Continuous cardiotocography (CTG) as a form of electronic fetal monitoring (EFM) for fetal assessment during labour. *Cochrane Database of Systematic Reviews* (2), CD006066.

Allison, J. (1996). *Delivered at home*. London: Chapman and Hall.

Anderson, D. (2011). A review of systemic opioids commonly used for labor pain relief. *Journal of Midwifery & Women's Health*, 56(4), 222–239.

Anim-Somuah, M., Smyth, R., & Jones, L. (2011). Epidural versus non epidural or no analgesia in labour. *Cochrane Database of Systematic Reviews Issue*, 12, CD000331.

Ayres-de-Campos, D., Spong, C. Y., & Chandaraharan, E. (2015). FIGO consensus guidelines on intrapartum fetal monitoring: Cardiotocography. *International Journal of Gynecology & Obstetrics*, 131, 13–24.

Benjoya Miller, J., & Magill-Cuerden, J. (2006). All women in labour should have the choice of waterbirth. *British Journal of Midwifery*, 14(8), 484–485.

Berglund, S. (2011). 'Every case of asphyxia can be used as a learning example': Conclusions from an analysis of substandard obstetrical care. *Journal of Perinatal Medicine*, 40(1), 9–18.

Bernal, A., & Norwitz, E. (2018). The normal mechanism of labour. In K. Edmonds (Ed.), *Dewhurst's textbook of obstetrics and gynaecology* (9th ed.) (pp. 247–268). Chichester: Wiley-Blackwell.

Berry, D. (2006). *Health communication: Theory and practice*. Maidenhead: Open University Press.

Birch, L., Doyle, P., Ellis, R., & Hogard, E. (2009). Failure to void in labour: Postnatal urinary and anal incontinence. *British Journal of Midwifery*, 17, 562–566.

Bohren, M., Hofmeyr, G., Sakala, C., et al. (2017). Continuous support for women during childbirth. *Cochrane Database of Systematic Reviews* (7), CD003766.

Boterenbrood, D., Wassen, M. M., Visser, G. H. A., & Nijhuis, J. G. (2018). Retrospective study of the effect of remifentanil use during labor on fetal heart rate patterns. *International Journal of Gynecology & Obstetrics*, 140(1), 60–64.

Brydon, S., & Raynor, M. (2012). Case study 14: Shoulder dystocia. In M. Raynor, J. Marshall, & K. Jackson (Eds.), *Midwifery practice: Critical illness, complications and emergencies case book* (pp. 227–246). Maidenhead: McGraw Hill/Open University Press.

BSI (British Standards Institution). (2014). *Specification for the planning, Application, Measurement and review of Cleanliness services in hospital (PAS 5748:2014)*. London: DH. Available at: http://qna.files.parliament.uk/qna-attachments/175888/original/PAS5748%20Specification%-20for%20the%20planning,%20application,%20measurement%20and%20review%20of%20cleanliness%20services%20in%20hospitals.pdf.

Burvill, S. (2005). Managing breech presentation in the absence of obstetric assistance. In K. B. V Woodward, & N. Young (Eds.), *Managing childbirth emergencies in community settings* (pp. 111–139). Houndsmill: Palgrave Macmillan.

Chadwick, J. (2002). Malpresentations and malpositions. In M. Boyle (Ed.), *Emergencies around childbirth* (pp. 63–81). Oxon: Radcliffe Medical Press.

Chandraharan, E. (2017). 'An eye opener': Perils of CTG misinterpretation: Lessons from confidential enquiries and medico-legal cases. In E. Chandraharan (Ed.), *Handbook of CTG interpretation from patterns to physiology* (pp. 1–5). Cambridge: Cambridge University Press.

Chapleau, M. W. (2012). Baroreceptor reflexes. In D. Robertson, I. Biagioni, G. Burnstock, et al. (Eds.), *Primer on the autonomic nervous system* (3rd ed.) (pp. 161–165). Amsterdam: Academic Press/Elsevier.

Chawia, J. (2016). Autonomic nervous system anatomy. *Medscape*. Available at: https://emedicine.medscape.com/article/1922943-overview.

Cluett, E., & Burns, E. (2018). Immersion in water in labour and birth. *Cochrane Database of Systematic Reviews*, 5, CD000111.

COMET. Comparative Obstetric Mobile Epidural Trial (COMET) Study Group UK. (2001). Effect of low-dose mobile versus traditional epidural techniques on mode of delivery: A randomised controlled trial. *Lancet*, 358, 19–23.

Cronk, M. (1998a). Midwives and breech births. *The Practising Midwife*, 1(7/8), 44–45.

Cronk, M. (1998b). Hands off the breech. *The Practising Midwife*, 1(6), 13–15.

Cunningham, F. G., Leveno, K. J., Bloom, S. L., et al. (2018). *Williams obstetrics* (25th ed.). New York: McGraw-Hill.

Davane, D., Lalor, J. G., Daly, S., et al. (2017). Cardiotocography versus intermittent auscultation of fetal heart on admission to labour ward for assessment of fetal wellbeing. *Cochrane Database of Systematic Reviews* (1), CD005122.

Davison, C., Geraghty, S., & Morris, S. (2018). Midwifery students' knowledge of normal birth before 'delivery' of curriculum. *Midwifery*, 58(13), 77–82.

de Ferrer, G. (2006). Tens: Non-invasive pain relief for the early stages of labour. *British Journal of Midwifery*, 14(8), 480–482.

DH (Department of Health). (1993). *Changing childbirth, Part 1: Report of the expert maternity group*. London: HMSO.

DH (Department of Health). (2001). *Working together, learning together: A framework for lifelong learning in the NHS*. London: TSO.

DH (Department of Health), & the National Assembly for Wales, the NHS Confederation and the British Medical Association. (2002). *Guidance on working patterns for junior doctors*. London: TSO.

DH (Department of Health). (2004a). *National service framework for children young people and maternity services*. London: TSO.

DH (Department of Health). (2004b). *The NHS Knowledge and Skills Framework (NHS KSF) and the development review process*. London: TSO.

DH (Department of Health). (2007). *Maternity matters: Choice access and continuity of care in a safe service*. London: TSO.

DH (Department of Health). (2008a). *High quality care for all: NHS Next stage review final report (Darzi report)*. London: TSO.

DH (Department of Health). (2008b). *Framing the nursing and midwifery contribution: Driving up the quality of care*. London: TSO.

DH (Department of Health). (2009). *Reference guide to consent for examination or treatment* (2nd ed.). London: TSO.

DH (Department of Health). (2010a). *Equity and excellence: Liberating the NHS*. London: TSO.

DH (Department of Health). (2010b). *Midwifery 2020: Delivering expectations*. London: TSO.

Divall, B., Spiby, H., Nolan, M., & Slade, P. (2017). Plans, preferences or going with the flow: An online exploration of women's views and experiences of birth plans. *Midwifery*, 54, 29–34.

Dixon, L., & Foureur, M. (2010). The vaginal examination during labour: Is it of benefit or harm? *New Zealand College of Midwives Journal*, 42, 21–26.

Downe, S. (2017). Care in the second stage of labour. In S. Macdonald, & G. Johnson (Eds.), *Mayes midwifery* (15th ed.) (pp. 614–627). Edinburgh: Elsevier.

Dowswell, T., Bedwell, C., Lavender, T., & Neilson, J. (2009). TENS (transcutaneous nerve stimulation) for pain management in labour. *Cochrane Database of Systematic Reviews* (2), CD007214.

Evans, J. (2007). First do no harm. *The Practising Midwife*, 10(8), 22–23.

Evans, J. (2012a). The final piece of the breech jigsaw puzzle? *Essentially MIDIRS*, 3(3), 46–49.

Evans, J. (2012b). Understanding physiological breech birth. *Essentially MIDIRS*, 3(2), 17–21.

Evans, J. (2017). Breech birth. In K. Jackson, & H. Wightman (Eds.), *Normalising challenging or complex childbirth.* (pp. 112–131). London: Open University Press.

Fahy, K. (2011). Is breech birth really unsafe? Treatment validity in the term breech trial. *Essentially MIDIRS, 2*(10), 17–21.

FIGO (International Federation of Gynecology and Obstetrics). (2018). *Physiological CTG Interpretation: Intrapartum fetal monitoring guideline.* Available at: https://physiological-ctg.com/guideline/Intrapartum%20Fetal%20Monitoring%20Guideline.pdf.

Fisher, C., Hauck, Y., & Fenwick, J. (2006). How social context impacts on women's fears of childbirth: A Western Australian example. *Social Science & Medicine, 63*(1), 64–75.

Friedman, E. (1954). The graphic analysis of labour. *American Journal of Obstetrics and Gynaecology, 68,* 1568–1575.

Fujinaga, M., & Maze, M. (2002). Neurobiology of nitrous oxide-induced antinociceptive effects. *Molecular Neurobiology, 25*(2), 167–189.

Gillick v West Norfolk and Wisbech AHA [1986] AC 112.

Glezerman, M. (2006). Five years to the term breech trial: The rise and fall of a randomized controlled trial. *American Journal of Obstetrics and Gynecology, 194*(1), 20–25.

GMC (General Medical Council). (2018). *0–18 years: Guidance for all doctors (2007 updated).* London: GMC. Available at: www.gmc-uk.org/-/media/documents/0_18_years_english_0418pdf_48903188.pdf.

Goffinet, F., Carayol, M., Foidart, J., et al. & PREMODA Study Group. (2006). Is planned vaginal delivery of breech presentation at term still an option? Results of an observational prospective survey in France and Belgium. *American Journal of Obstetrics and Gynecology, 194*(4), 1002–1011.

Gribbin, C. (2017). Fear of childbirth: The impact of tocophobia (including post-traumatic stress disorder) on normal birth. In K. Jackson, & H. Wightman (Eds.), *Normalising challenging or complex childbirth.* (pp. 64–81). London: Open University Press.

Gupta, J., Sood, A., Hofmeyr, G., & Vogel, J. (2017). Position in the second stage of labour for women without epidural anaesthesia. *Cochrane Database of Systematic Reviews* (5), CD002006.

Háheim, L. L., Albrechtsen, S., Nordbó Berge, L., et al. (2004). Breech birth at term: Vaginal delivery or elective caesarean section? A systematic review of the literature by a Norwegian review team. *Acta Obstetrica et Gynecologica Scandinavica, 83*(2), 126–130.

Hall Moran, V., & Dykes, F. (Eds.). (2013). *Maternal and infant nutrition and nurture. Controversies and challenges* (2nd ed.) Salisbury: Quay Books.

Hannah, M. E., Hannah, W. J., Hewson, S. A., et al. (2000). Term breech trial collaborative group. Planned caesarean section versus planned vaginal birth for breech presentation at term: A randomized multicentre trial. *Lancet, 356*(9239), 1375–1383.

Hannah, M. E., Whyte, H. D., Hannah, W. J., et al. (2004). Term breech trial collaborative group. Maternal outcomes at two years after planned caesarean section versus planned vaginal birth for breech presentation at term: The international randomized multi-centre trial. *American Journal of Obstetrics and Gynecology, 191*(3), 917–927.

Hawkins, J. (2010). Epidural analgesia for labor and delivery. *New England Journal of Medicine, 362*(16), 1503–1510.

Helman, G. (2007). *Culture health and illness* (5th ed.). London: Hodder Arnold.

Henley-Einion, A. (2007). The ecstasy of the spirit: Five rhythms for healing. *British Journal of Midwifery, 10*(3), 20–23.

Hobbs, L. (1998). Assessing cervical dilatation without VEs. *The Practising Midwife, 1*(11), 34–35.

Hodnett, E., Downe, S., & Walsh, D. (2012). Alternative versus conventional institutional settings for birth. *Cochrane Database* (8), CD000012.

Hodnett, E., Stremler, R., Weston, J., & McKeever, P. (2009). Re-conceptualizing the hospital labor room: The PLACE (pregnant and labouring in an ambient clinical environment) pilot trial. *Birth, 36*(2), 159–166.

Howie, L., & Watson, J. (2017a). The onset of labour. In J. Rankin (Ed.), *Physiology in childbearing* (4th ed.) (pp. 373–380). London: Elsevier.

Howie, L., & Watson, J. (2017b). The first stage of labour. In J. Rankin (Ed.), *Physiology in childbearing* (4th ed.) (pp. 381–398). London: Elsevier.

Iaizzo, P. A., & Fitzgerald, K. (2015). Autonomic nervous system. In P. A. Iaizzo (Ed.), *Handbook of cardiac anatomy physiology and devices* (3rd ed.) (pp. 235–250). Switzerland: Springer.

Idarius, B. (2010). *The homeopathic childbirth manual: A practical guide for labor, birth and the immediate postpartum period* (2nd ed.). Ukiah, CA: Idarius Press.

Impey, L., & Child, T. (2017). *Obstetrics and Gynaecology* (5th ed.). Chichester: Wiley–Blackwell.

Jackson, K. (2017). When labour stops or slows. In K. Jackson, & H. Wightman (Eds.), *Normalising challenging or complex childbirth.* (pp. 172–193). London: Open University Press.

Joho, S. (2017). Muscle sympathetic nerve activity and cardiovascular disease. In S. Iwase, J. Hayano, & S. Orimo (Eds.), *Clinical assessment of the autonomic nervous system* (pp. 31–46). Japan: Springer.

Jones, L., Othman, M., Dowswell, T., et al. (2012). Pain management for women in labour: An overview of systematic reviews. *Cochrane Database of Systematic Reviews* (3), CD009234.

Juman Blincoe, A. (2007). TENS machines and their use in managing labour pain. *British Journal of Midwifery, 15*(8), 516–519.

Kennedy, H. P., Grant, J., Walton, C., et al. (2010). Normalizing birth in England: A qualitative study. *Journal of Midwifery & Women's Health, 55*(3), 262–269.

King's Fund (2008). *Safe births: everybody's business. An independent inquiry into the safety of maternity services in England.* London: Kings Fund.

Kirkham, M. (2011). The role of the midwife with the woman in labour: To be with, to monitor or to wait on the landing. *MIDIRS Midwifery Digest, 21*(4), 469–470.

Knight, M., Bunch K., Tuffnell, D., & on behalf of MBRRACE-UK. (2019). *Saving lives, improving mothers' care – Lessons learned to inform maternity care from the UK and Ireland Confidential Enquiries into maternal deaths and Morbidity 2015–2017.* Oxford: National Perinatal Epidemiology Unit, University of Oxford.

Knight, M., Nair, M., Tuffnell, D., & on behalf of MBRRACE-UK. (2017). *Saving lives, improving mothers' care – Lessons learned to inform maternity care from the UK and Ireland Confidential Enquiries into maternal deaths and Morbidity 2013–2015.* Oxford: National Perinatal Epidemiology Unit, University of Oxford.

Kotaska, A. (2004). Inappropriate use of randomized trials to evaluate complex phenomena: Case study of vaginal breech delivery. *British Medical Journal, 329*(7473), 1039–1042.

Kundu, S., Kuehnle, E., Schippert, C., et al. (2017). Estimation of neonatal outcome artery pH value according to CTG interpretation of the last 60 min before delivery: A retrospective study. Can the outcome pH value be predicted? *Archives of Gynecology and Obstetrics, 296*(5), 897–905.

Lagercrantz, H., & Bistoletti, P. (1977). Catecholamine release in the newborn infant at birth. *Pediatric Research, 11*(8), 889–893.

Lauria, M. R., Barthold, J., Zimmerman, R., et al. (2007). Pathologic uterine ring associated with fetal head trauma and subsequent cerebral palsy. *Obstetrics & Gynecology, 109*(2), 495–497.

Lauzon, L., & Hodnett, E. (2009). Antenatal education for the self diagnosis of the onset of active labour at term. *Cochrane Database of Systematic Reviews, 1*, CD000935.

Lavender, T., Cuthbert, A., & Smyth, R. (2018). Effect of partogram use on outcomes for women in spontaneous labour at term and their babies. *Cochrane Database of Systematic Reviews* (8), CD005461.

Lawrence, A., Lewis, L., Hofmeyr, G., et al. (2013). Maternal positions and mobility during the first stage of labour. *Cochrane Database of Systematic Reviews, 10*, CD003934.

Leap, N., & Anderson, P. (2008). The role of pain in normal birth and empowerment of women. In S. Downe (Ed.), *Normal childbirth evidence and debate* (2nd ed.) (pp. 29–46). London: Churchill Livingstone.

Longworth, H., & Kingdon, C. (2010). Fathers in the birth room: What are they expecting and experiencing? A phenomenological study. *Midwifery, 27*(5), 588–594.

Louwen, F., Daviss, B., Johnson, K., & Reitter, A. (2017). Does breech delivery in an upright position instead of on the back improve outcomes and avoid caesareans? *International Journal of Gynaecology & Obstetrics, 136*, 151–161.

Lowe, V., & Archer, A. (2017). Intermittent (intelligent) auscultation in the low-risk setting. In E. Chandraharan (Ed.), *Handbook of CTG interpretation: From patterns to physiology* (pp. 55–58). Cambridge: Cambridge University Press.

Maier, B., Georgoulopoulos, A., Jaeger, T., et al. (2011). Fetal outcome for infants in breech by method of delivery experiences with a stand-by service system of senior obstetricians and women's choices of mode of delivery. *Journal of Perinatal Medicine, 39*(4), 385–390.

Main, E., & Bingham, D. (2008). Quality improvement in maternity care: Promising approaches from the medical and public health perspectives. *Current Opinions in Obstetrics and Gynecology, 20*(6), 574–580.

Mander, R. (2011). *Pain in childbearing and its control* (2nd ed.). London: Blackwell Science.

Marshall, J., Fraser, D., & Baker, P. (2011). An observational study to explore the power and effect of the labour ward culture on consent to intrapartum procedures. *International Journal of Childbirth, 1*(2), 82–99.

Martini, F., Nath, J., & Bartholomew, E. (2018). *Fundamentals of anatomy and physiology* (Global edn.). Harlow: Pearson.

Maternity Advisory Committee. (1970). *Domiciliary and maternity bed needs Chairman Sir John Peel.* London: HMSO.

McDonald, G. (2010). Diagnosing the latent phase of labour: Use of the partogram. *British Journal of Midwifery, 18*(10), 630–637.

McNabb, M. (2017). Physiological changes from late pregnancy until the onset of lactation: From nesting to suckling-lactation and parent infant attachment. In S. Macdonald, & G. Johnson (Eds.), *Mayes Midwifery* (15th ed.) (pp. 562–585). Edinburgh: Elsevier.

Melzack, R., & Wall, P. D. (1965). Pain mechanisms: A new theory. *Science, 150*, 971–979.

MHPRA (Medicines and Healthcare Products Regulatory Agency). (2010). *Medical device Alert (MDA/2010/054) fetal monitor/cardiotocograph (CTG).* Available at: https://assets.publishing.service.gov.uk/media/5485ac34e5274a428d00028f/con085077.pdf.

Mobbs, N., Williams, C., & Weeks, A. D. (2018). Humanising birth: Does the language we use matter? *The BMJ Opinion.* Available at: https://blogs.bmj.com/bmj/2018/02/08/humanising-birth-does-the-language-we-use-matter/.

Muhunthan, K., & Arulkumaran, S. (2017). Medico-legal issues with CTG. In E. Chandraharan (Ed.), *Handbook of CTG interpretation from patterns to physiology* (pp. 171–179). Cambridge: Cambridge University Press.

NCT (National Childbirth Trust). (2019). *Choosing your birth partner.* London: NCT. Available at: www.nct.org.uk/labour-birth/dads-and-partners/choosing-your-birth-partners.

Nelson, K. B., Sartwelle, T. P., & Rouse, D. J. (2016). Electronic fetal monitoring, cerebral palsy, and caesarean section: Assumptions versus evidence. *British Medical Journal, 355,* i6405.

NHS Digital. (2018). *Data on written complaints in the NHS 2017–8.1–2012.* London: Health and Social care Information Centre (NHS Digital). Available at: https://files.digital.nhs.uk/5B/D86467/Data%20on%20Written%-20Complaints%20in%20the%20NHS%202017–uk/5B/D86467/Data%20on%20Written%20Complaints%20in%20the%218%20Report.pdf.

NHS England. (2016). *National maternity review. Better births: Improving outcomes of maternity services in England: A five year forward view for maternity care.* London: NHS England. Available at: www.england.nhs.uk/wp-content/uploads/2016/02/national-maternity-review-report.pdf.

NHS England. (2017). *A-EQUIP (Advocating & Educating for QUality ImProvement): A model of clinical midwifery supervision.* London: NHS England. Available at: www.england.nhs.uk/wp-content/uploads/2017/04/a-equip-midwifery-supervision-model.pdf.

NHS Resolution. (2018). *Did you know? Maternity pressure ulcers.* Available at: https://resolution.nhs.uk/wp-content/uploads/2018/10/Did-you-know-Maternity-Pressure-Ulcers.pdf.

NICE (National Institute for Health and Care Excellence). (2013). *Vision amniotic leak detector to assess unexplained vaginal wetness in pregnancy. Medical Technology Guidance (MTG 15).* London: NICE. Available at: www.fdanews.com/ext/resources/files/archives/10113-01/08–com/ext/resources/files/archives13-Pregnancy.pdf.

NICE (National Institute for Health and Care Excellence). (2014a). *Infection prevention and control: (QS61).* London: NICE. Available at: www.nice.org.uk/guidance/qs61/resources/infection-prevention-and-control-pdf-2098782603205.

NICE (National Institute for Health and Care Excellence). (2014b). *Intelligent auscultation – 'listen' for fetal wellbeing. Shared Learning Database.* Available at: www.nice.org.uk/sharedlearning/intelligent-auscultation-listen-for-fetal-wellbeing.

NICE (National Institute for Health and Care Excellence). (2017). *Intrapartum care: Management and delivery of care to women in labour: (CG 190).* London: NICE. Available at: www.nice.org.uk/guidance/cg190/re-

sources/intrapartum-care-for-healthy-women-and-babies-pdf-35109866447557.

NICE (National Institute for Health and Care Excellence). (2018). *Terbutaline sulfate.* London: NICE. Available at: https://bnf.nice.org.uk/drug/terbutaline-sulfate.html.

Nirmal, D., & Fraser, D. (2016). The first stage of labour. In R. Warren, & S. Arulkumaran (Eds.), *Best practice in labour and delivery* (2nd ed.) (pp. 14–27). Cambridge: Cambridge University Press.

NMC (Nursing and Midwifery Council). (2018). *The Code: Professional standards of practice and behaviour for nurses midwives and nursing associates.* London: NMC.

Nunes, I., Ayres-de-Campos, D., Kwee, A., et al. (2014). Prolonged saltatory fetal heart rate pattern leading to newborn metabolic acidosis. *Clinical and Experimental Obstetrics and Gynaecology, 41*(5), 507–511.

Pearson, J. (1981). Partography. *Nursing Mirror, 153*(2), xxv–xxix.

Perez-Bonfils, A. G., & Chandraharan, E. (2017). Physiology of fetal heart rate control and types of hypoxia. In E. Chandraharan (Ed.), *Handbook of CTG interpretation from patterns to physiology* (pp. 13–25). Cambridge: Cambridge University Press.

Pradham, P., Mohajer, M., & Deshpande, S. (2005). Outcome of term breech births: 10 year experience at a district general hospital. *BJOG: An International Journal of Obstetrics and Gynaecology, 112*(2), 218–222.

Rainaldi, M. A., Jeffery, M., & Perlman, M. B. (2017). Pathophysiology of birth asphyxia. *Clinics in Perinatology, 43*(3), 409–422.

Raynor, M., & England, C. (2010). *Psychology for midwives.* Maidenhead: Open University Press.

RCOG (Royal College of Obstetricians and Gynaecologists). (2001). *The use of electronic fetal monitoring: The use and interpretation of cardiotocography in intrapartum fetal surveillance. Evidence based Clinical Guideline No 8.* London: RCOG Press. Available at: http://ctgutbildning.se/images/Referenser/RCOG-2001.pdf.

RCOG (Royal College of Obstetricians and Gynaecologists). (2016). *Each baby counts: Key messages from 2015.* London: RCOG.

RCOG (Royal College of Obstetricians and Gynaecologists). (2017). *The management of breech presentation. Green-top guideline No 20b.* London: Rcog. Available at: https://obgyn.onlinelibrary.wiley.com/doi/epdf/10.1111/1471-0528.14465.

Redshaw, M., & Heikkila, K. (2010). *Delivered with care: National survey of women's experience of maternity care.* Oxford: National Perinatal Epidemiology Unit, University of Oxford.

Reed, B. (1999). Knee deep at a home birth. *The Practising Midwife, 2*(8), 46.

Reed, B. (2003). A disappearing art: Vaginal breech birth. *The Practising Midwife*, 6(9), 6–18.

Reynolds, F., Sharma, S. K., & Seed, P. T. (2002). Analgesia in labour and fetal acid-base balance: A meta-analysis comparing epidural with systemic opioid analgesia. *BJOG: An International Journal of Obstetrics and Gynaecology*, 109(12), 1344–1353.

Sandall, J., Soltani, H., Gates, S., et al. (2016). Midwife-led continuity models versus other models of care for child-bearing women. *Cochrane Database of Systematic Reviews* (4), CD004667.

Schneider, U., Bode, F., Schmidt, A., et al. (2018). Developmental milestones of the autonomic nervous system revealed via longitudinal monitoring of fetal heart rate variability. *PLoS One*, 13(8), e0202611.

Setty, T., Fernando, R. (2019). Systemic analgesia: parenteral and inhalational agents. In D. H. Chestnut C. A. Wong L. C. Tsen, et al. (Ed.), *Chestnut's obstetric anaesthesia: principles and practice (pp. 453–473)* Philadelphia: Elsevier.

Shahoei, R., Shahghebi, S., Rezaei, M., & Naqshbandi, S. (2017). The effect of transcutaneous electrical nerve stimulation on the severity of labor pain among nulliparous women: A clinical trial. *Complementary Therapies in Clinical Practice*, 28, 176–180.

Shepherd, A., Cheyne, H., Kennedy, S., et al. (2010). The purple line as a measure of labour progress: A longitudinal study. *BMC Pregnancy and Childbirth*, 10, 54.

Shimokawa, N., Londono, M., & Koibuchi, N. (2006). Gene expression and signalling pathways by extracellular acidification. In Y. Hayashida, C. Gonzalalez, & H. Kondo (Eds.), *The arterial chemoreceptors: Advances in experimental medicine and biology* (Vol. 580).

Simkin, P., Ancheta, R., & Hanson, L. (2017). *The labor progress handbook: Early interventions to prevent and treat dystocia* (4th ed.). Chichester: Wiley–Blackwell.

Singata, M., Tranmer, J., & Gyte, G. (2013). Restricting oral fluid and food intake during labour. *Cochrane Database of Systematic Reviews* (8), CD003930.

Sinivaara, M., Suominen, T., Routasolo, P., et al. (2004). How delivery ward staff exercise power over women in communication. *Journal of Advanced Nursing*, 46(1), 33–34.

Smith, C. A. (2013). Moxibustion for breech presentation: Significant new evidence. *Acupuncture in Medicine*, 31(1), 5–6.

Smith, C., Collins, C., & Crowther, C. (2011). Aromatherapy for pain management in labour. *Cochrane Database of Systematic Reviews*, 12, CD009514.

Smith, L., Burns, E., & Cuthbert, A. (2018). Parenteral opioids for maternal pain management in labour. *Cochrane Database of Systematic Reviews*, 6, CD007396.

Smyth, R., Markham, C., & Dowswell, T. (2013). Amniotomy to shorten spontaneous labour. *Cochrane Database of Systematic Reviews* (6), CD006167.

Steen, M., & Calvert, J. (2006). Homeopathy for childbirth: Remedies and research. *Midwives*, 9(11), 438–440.

Stevenson, H., & Chandraharan, E. (2017). Understanding the CTG: Technical aspects. In E. Chandraharan (Ed.), *Handbook of CTG interpretation: From patterns to physiology* (pp. 26–31). Cambridge: Cambridge University Press.

Teimoori, B., Sakhavar, N., Mirteimoori, M., et al. (2011). Nitrous oxide versus pethidine with promethesine for reducing labor pain. *Gynaecology and Obstetrics*, 1(1), 1–4.

Thoni, A., Mussner, K., & Ploner, F. (2010). Water birthing: Retrospective review of 2625 water births. Contamination of birth pool water and risk of microbial cross infection. *Minerva Ginecologica*, 62(3), 203–211.

Tiran, D. (2018). *Complementary therapies in maternity care: An evidence based approach*. London: Singing Dragon.

Tortora, G., & Derrickson, B. (2017). *Principles of anatomy and physiology* (15th ed.). New York: John Wiley.

Ulander, V. M., Gissler, M., Nuutila, M., et al. (2004). Are health expectations of term breech infants unrealistically high? *Acta Obstetrica et Gynecologica Scandinavica*, 83(2), 180–186.

Walsh, D. (2010a). Labour rhythms. In D. Walsh, & S. Downe (Eds.), *Essential midwifery practice: Intrapartum care* (pp. 63–80). Chichester: Wiley–Blackwell.

Walsh, D. (2010b). Birth environment. In D. Walsh, & S. Downe (Eds.), *Essential midwifery practice: Intrapartum care* (pp. 45–62). Chichester: Wiley–Blackwell.

Walsh, D. (2012). *Normal labour and birth: A guide for midwives* (2nd ed.). London: Routledge.

Walsh, D. (2017). Care in the first stage of labour. In S. Macdonald, & G. Johnson (Eds.), *Mayes Midwifery* (15th ed.) (pp. 586–627). Edinburgh: Elsevier.

Walsh, D., Spiby, H., Grigg, C., et al. (2018). Mapping midwifery and obstetric units in the UK. *Midwifery*, 56, 9–16.

WHO (World Health Organization). (2017). *Save lives: Clean your hands: WHO's global annual call to action for health workers*. Geneva: WHO.

WHO (World Health Organization), Department of Reproductive Health and Research. (1999). *Care in normal labour: A practical guide*. Geneva: WHO.

Whyte, H. D., Hannah, M., Saigal, S., et al. (2004). Infant follow-up term breech trial collaborative group: Outcomes of children at two years after planned caesarean birth versus planned vaginal birth for breech presentation at term: The international randomized term breech trial. *American Journal of Obstetrics and Gynecology*, 191(3), 864–871.

Wood, P. L., & Dobbie, H. G. (1989). *Electronic fetal heart monitoring*. London: Palgrave.

Woods, T. (2006). The transitional stage of labour. *MIDIRS Midwifery Digest*, 16(2), 225–228.

Yanamandra, N., & Chandraharan, E. (2014). Saltatory and sinusoidal fetal heart rate (FHR) patterns and significance of FHR 'overshoots'. *Current Women's Health Reviews*, *9*(3), 175–182.

Zahra, A., & Leila, M. (2013). Lavender aromatherapy massages in reducing labor pain and duration of labor. *African Journal of Pharmacy and Pharmacology*, *7*(8), 426–430.

Zanetti-Dallenbach, R., Tschudin, S., Zhong, X., et al. (2007). Maternal and neonatal infections and obstetrical outcome in water birth. *European Journal of Obstetrics & Gynecology and Reproductive Biology*, *134*(2), 37–43.

Zhang, J., Landy, H., & Branch, W. (2010). Contemporary patterns of spontaneous labor with normal neonatal outcomes. *Obstetrics and Gynaecology*, *116*(6), 1281–1287.

ANNOTATED FURTHER READING

Downe, S. (Ed.). (2008). *Normal childbirth: Evidence and debate* (2nd ed.) London: Churchill Livingstone.

This text explores contemporary issues in maternity care. It includes thought-provoking chapters on the role of pain in normal birth, rethinking risk and safety in maternity care and on the early pushing urge.

Evans, J. (2017). Breech birth. In K. Jackson, & H. Wightman (Eds.), *Normalising challenging or complex childbirth.* (pp. 112–131). London: Open University Press.

This chapter comprehensively covers breech presentation. It uses the most up-to-date evidence to underpin practice and also describes both straightforward breech births and those that are a little more challenging. The accompanying illustrations are extremely useful to bring breech birth to life.

McCormick, C., & Cairns, A. (2010). Reducing unnecessary caesarean section by external cephalic version. In J. E. Marshall, & M. D. Raynor (Eds.), *Advancing skills in midwifery practice* (pp. 47–55). Edinburgh: Elsevier, Churchill Livingstone.

This chapter examines the rationale for the procedure of external cephalic version (ECV). It discusses why and how midwives and obstetricians should acquire competency in such a skill to improve a woman's choice in achieving a vaginal birth should their baby be presenting by the breech.

National Institute for Health and Care Excellence. (2017). *Intrapartum care: Management and delivery of care to women in labour. CG 190.* London: NICE.

This document contains evidence-based information for intrapartum care of women with uncomplicated pregnancies. The intention of the guidelines is to standardize practices among maternity units across the UK.

Walsh, D. (Ed.). (2012). *Normal labour and birth: A guide for midwives* (2nd ed.) London: Routledge.

This textbook examines care during normal labour and birth, including excellent evidence-based guidance to normalize childbirth.

USEFUL WEBSITES

Association of Radical Midwives: www.midwifery.org.uk

Cochrane Reviews: www.cochranelibrary.com/cdsr/reviews

Department of Health (and social care) England: www.gov.uk/government/organisations/department-of-health-and-social-care

FIGO (International Federation of Gynecology and Obstetrics): www.figo.org/

International Confederation of Midwives: www.internationalmidwives.org/

Midwifery Action: YouTube: www.youtube.com/user/midwiferyaction

Midwives Information and Resource Service: www.midirs.org/

National Childbirth Trust: www.nct.org.uk/

National Health Service (NHS) Resolution/Clinical Negligence Scheme for Trusts: https://resolution.nhs.uk/

National Institute for Health and Care Excellence: www.nice.org.uk/

National Perinatal Epidemiology Unit (NPEU) Birthplace in England Research Programme: www.npeu.ox.ac.uk/birthplace

Royal College of Midwives: www.rcm.org.uk/

Royal College of Obstetricians and Gynaecologists: www.rcog.org.uk/

The Lancet Series on Midwifery: www.thelancet.com/series/midwifery

World Health Organization: www.who.int/

20

Physiology and Care During the Transition and Second Stage Phases of Labour

Soo Downe, Jayne E. Marshall

CHAPTER CONTENTS

When labour moves to the phase of active maternal pushing, the whole tempo of activity changes. Women who have adjusted to the rhythm of labour as the baby descends and rotates can be thrown off balance as they experience alterations in neurohormonal signals and the consequent physical sensations that signal a shift towards active bearing down. Intense physical effort and exertion is needed as the baby is finally pushed towards its birth. The woman, her supporting companions and her midwife all require stamina and courage. Excitement and expectation mount as the birth becomes imminent. A positive outcome will depend upon mutual respect and trust with the labouring woman and her companions, and between all the professional groups who may be involved. A woman will never forget a midwife who positively supports her capacity to give birth to her baby, as shown in Diane's story (see Case Study 20.1).

THE CHAPTER AIMS TO

- consider the nature of the transition and second stage phases of labour
- describe the usual sequence of events during these stages
- summarize the signs of transition and the following expulsive phase of labour

- discuss the care of the mother, father and birth companions during these stages
- review the observations that should be undertaken by the midwife at this time
- discuss the physiology of birth and the role of the midwife when the term fetus is presenting by breech.

The first section of this chapter is focused on labour where the presentation is cephalic. The specific situation of the breech presentation at term and its subsequent vaginal birth is described in the second half of the chapter.

THE NATURE OF THE TRANSITION AND SECOND STAGE PHASES OF LABOUR

Traditionally, the second stage of labour has been regarded as the phase between full dilatation of the cervical os, and the birth of the baby. However, the physiological reality of stages and phases of labour, particularly as defined by cervical dilatation, has been questioned (Walsh 2010; Zhang et al. 2010; Downe et al. 2013; Buckley 2015; Oladapo et al. 2018; Souza et al. 2018). Women are more likely to describe it as a continuous process, marked by changes in sensations, and in psychological responses (Dixon et al. 2013a, 2014; Olza et al. 2018). (Box 20.1 gives examples of other controversial issues at this point in labour.) Most midwives and labouring women are aware of a transitional period between the period of cervical dilatation, and the time when active maternal pushing efforts begin. This is can be characterized by a lull in contractions – the so-called 'resting' phase. In other cases, women may feel restless and have discomfort, a desire for pain relief and a sense that the process is never-ending. Some women demand that attendants end the whole process by whatever means possible; others may fall asleep. These sensations are triggered by the degree to which either endorphin or adrenalin production is dominant at this stage in the labour process (Dixon et al. 2013b; Buckley 2015). If women are supported and encouraged over this phase, most will regain neurohormonal balance, and will move into the active pushing stage of labour with heightened alertness and concentration. Appropriate midwifery care encompasses both knowledge of the usual physiological

processes of this phase and of the mechanism of birth, with insight into the needs and choices of each individual

---

BOX 20.1 Examples of Areas of Controversy in Labour Transition and Second Stage

Discussion about the nature of normal physiological labour and birth has taken place for at least the last 60 years, with an increase in publications in this area over the last decade (Montgomery 1958; Crawford 1983; Downe 1994, 2004, 2006, 2008; Gould 2000; Anderson 2003; Downe et al. 2013, Oladapo et al. 2018; Downe and Byrom 2019). These debates include:

- The utility of dividing labour into standard 'phases' or 'stages'
- The nature and optimal response to transition
- The extent to which findings about second stage outcomes from studies that include many women who are not mobile and upright in labour and birth apply to those who are able to move around freely (e.g. hands on the perineum and Obstetric Anal Sphincter Injury (OASI) outcomes)
- How to help women who have induced labours and/ or epidural analgesia to achieve a birth that is as straightforward as possible
- The need or otherwise for regular vaginal examinations to assess the progress of labour, and the effectiveness of any alternatives (such as maternal behavioural cues, or the anal cleft/'purple' line)
- Frequency of intermittent auscultation of the fetal heart in the active second stage of labour
- The best way to support women who have the early pushing urge
- Pushing techniques in the context of epidural analgesia
- The physiological limits to the length of the second stage of labour
- Long-term outcome for the neonate relating to childbirth interventions, such as instrumental birth, antibiotics or caesarean section.

labouring woman. Explaining the physiology and anatomy of what is happening to women, in simple and direct terms between contractions, can also help them to regain confidence in their bodies, and in their abilities to give birth to their babies. Fig. 20.1 demonstrates the link between neurohormonal responses, maternal feelings and maternal behaviours. Keeping this in mind can help the midwife to 'read' and understand the progress of labour through maternal behaviour.

As Fig. 20.1 shows, the physiological changes in the transition and the second stage phases of labour are a continuation of the same forces that occurred in the earlier hours of labour. The pace of labour as women move towards active pushing is not predictable for each individual. Some women may experience an urge to push before the cervical os is fully dilated, and in some women, this seems to be a physiological response, especially when it occurs later in labour (Downe et al. 2008; Borrelli et al. 2013). As noted above, others may experience a lull in labour sensations before the onset of strong expulsive second stage contractions. The formal onset of the second stage of labour is traditionally confirmed with a vaginal examination to assess for full dilatation of the cervical os. However, a finding of full cervical dilatation may occur some time after this stage has in fact been reached, and maternal behavioural changes may be

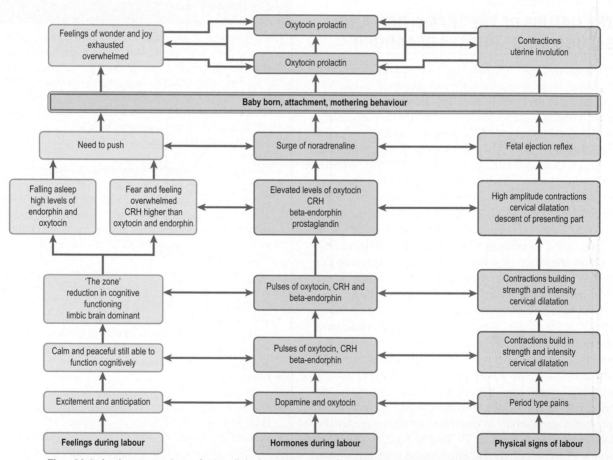

Fig. 20.1 A demonstration of the link between neurohormonal responses, maternal feelings and maternal behaviours. (Reproduced with permission from the New Zealand College of Midwives Journal. Available at: www.researchgate.net/publication/259714461_The_Emotional_and_Hormonal_Pathways_of_Labour_and_Birth_Integrating_Mind_Body_and_Behaviour)

a good indication that expulsive contractions are occurring in the absence of other signs (Baker and Kenner 1993; Dahlen et al. 2013; Downe et al. 2013; Dixon et al. 2013b; Olza et al. 2018).

Uterine Action

Contractions become stronger and longer but may be less frequent, allowing both mother and fetus regular recovery periods. The membranes often rupture spontaneously towards the end of the first stage or during transition to the second stage. The consequent drainage of liquor allows the presenting part, either the hard, round fetal head or the buttocks, to be directly applied to the vaginal tissues. This pressure aids distension. Fetal axis pressure increases flexion of the presenting part, resulting in smaller presenting diameters, more rapid progress and less trauma to both mother and fetus. If the mother is upright and leaning forward during this time, these processes are optimized.

The contractions become expulsive as the fetus descends further into the vagina. Pressure from the presenting part stimulates nerve receptors in the pelvic floor. This phenomenon is termed the *Ferguson reflex*. As a consequence, the woman experiences the need to push. This reflex may initially be controlled to a limited extent but becomes increasingly compulsive, overwhelming and involuntary. The mother's response is to employ her secondary powers of expulsion by contracting her abdominal muscles and diaphragm.

Soft Tissue Displacement

As the fetal head descends, the soft tissues of the pelvis become displaced. Anteriorly, the bladder is pushed upwards into the abdomen, where it is at less risk of injury during fetal descent. This results in the stretching and thinning of the urethra so that its lumen is reduced. Posteriorly, the rectum becomes flattened into the sacral curve and the pressure of the advancing head expels any residual faecal matter. The levator ani muscles dilate, thin out and are displaced laterally, and the perineal body is flattened, stretched and thinned. The fetal head becomes visible at the vulva, advancing with each contraction and receding between contractions until crowning takes place. The head is then born. The shoulders and body follow with the next contraction, accompanied by a gush of amniotic fluid and sometimes of blood. The second stage culminates in the birth of the baby.

RECOGNITION OF THE COMMENCEMENT OF THE EXPULSIVE PHASE OF LABOUR

Presumptive Evidence

Expulsive Uterine Contractions

As noted above, some women feel a strong desire to push before full dilatation of the cervical os occurs. Traditionally, it has been assumed that an early urge to push will lead to maternal exhaustion and/or cervical oedema or trauma. Ongoing research over the past few decades indicates that the early pushing urge may in fact be experienced by a significant minority of women, and that, in certain circumstances, spontaneous early pushing may be physiological (Petersen and Besuner 1997; Roberts and Hanson 2007; Downe et al. 2008; Borrelli et al. 2013). It is not clear whether these findings are influenced by factors such as maternal or fetal position or parity, or whether the labour is induced or spontaneous, and there is not enough evidence to date to determine the optimum response to the early pushing urge. The midwife needs to work with each individual woman in the context of their labour to determine the best approach in that specific case.

Rupture of the Forewaters

Rupture of the forewaters may occur at any time during labour. Very rarely (approximately 1:80,000 births), the baby is born still encased in the amnion. If this occurs, it is important for the midwife to remove the membranes as soon as possible, to ensure the airways are not occluded as the baby is born.

Dilatation and Gaping of the Anus

Deep engagement of the presenting part may produce this sign during the latter part of the first stage of labour.

Anal Cleft Line

Some midwives have reported observing this line (also called *the purple line*) as a pigmented mark in the cleft of the buttocks, which gradually ascends the anal cleft as the labour progresses. There is observational evidence from several studies that this sign appears in the majority of women during labour, and that it is somewhat correlated to both cervical dilatation and position of the fetal head (Hobbs 1998; Wickham 2007; Shepherd et al. 2010; Irani et al. 2018). The efficacy of the purple line as an alternative, or adjunct to vaginal examination for assessing labour progress in routine practice however, remains to be tested formally.

Appearance of the Rhomboid of Michaelis

This is sometimes noted when a woman is in a position where her back is visible. It presents as a dome-shaped curve in the lower back, and is held to indicate the posterior displacement of the sacrum and coccyx as the fetal occiput moves into the maternal sacral curve (Sutton and Scott 1996). This seems to lead the labouring woman to arch her back, push her buttocks forward and throw her arms back to grasp any fixed object she can find. Sutton and Scott (1996) hypothesize that this is a physiological response, since it causes a lengthening and straightening of the curve of Carus, optimizing the fetal passage through the birth canal.

Upper Abdominal Pressure and Epidural Analgesia

It has been observed anecdotally that women who have an epidural *in situ* often have a sense of discomfort under the ribs towards the end of the first stage of labour. This seems to coincide with full cervical os dilatation. The efficacy of these observations in predicting the onset of the anatomical second stage of labour still remains to be researched.

Show

This is the loss of bloodstained mucus which often accompanies rapid dilatation of the cervical os towards the end of the first stage of labour. It must be distinguished from frank fresh blood loss caused by partial separation of the placenta or a ruptured vasa praevia (see Chapter 25).

Appearance of the Presenting Part

Excessive moulding of the fetal head may result in the formation of a large *caput succedaneum*, which can protrude through the cervix prior to full dilatation of the os. Very occasionally, a baby presenting by the vertex may be visible at the perineum at the same time as the remaining cervix. This is more common in women of high parity. Similarly, a breech presentation may be visible at the vulva when the cervical os is only 7–8 cm dilated.

Confirmatory Evidence

In many maternity care settings, guidelines (or even protocols) state that a vaginal examination should be undertaken to confirm full dilatation of the cervical os, assuming the labouring woman gives her consent. The stated rationale is usually that pushing when the cervical os is not fully dilated could result in damage. Having a benchmark for the onset of the active pushing stage also provides a baseline for timing, for the purposes of labour management and of standardized record-keeping. However, in some maternity settings, midwives are more likely to respond on the basis of maternal behaviour (and particularly active bearing down efforts) than on routine assessment of cervical dilation at this stage of labour (Downe et al. 2008; Borrelli et al. 2013). Enkin et al. (2000) noted that vaginal assessment of cervical dilatation is largely unevaluated, and the most recent Cochrane review in this area concludes that this lack of evidence persists (Downe et al. 2013). Recent evidence from two hospital sites in Africa also concluded that vaginal examination alone is a poor predictor of labour progress (Oladapo et al. 2018). Despite this, vaginal examinations are undertaken by most midwives and obstetricians to confirm full dilation of the cervical os, and are expected by many women. Whether the midwife undertakes an examination or not, they should record all the signs she observes and all the measurements she takes, and she should advise and support the labouring woman on the basis of accurate observation and assessment of progress.

PHASES AND DURATION OF THE SECOND STAGE

It has been recognized that there are two distinct phases in the progress of the second stage after full dilatation of the cervical os. These have been termed *the latent phase*, during which descent and rotation continue to occur, and when women have no specific urge to push, and *the active phase*, when women have a strong urge to bear down.

The Latent Phase

In some women, full dilatation of the cervical os is recorded, but the presenting part may not yet have reached the pelvic outlet. Women in this situation may not experience a strong expulsive urge until the head has descended sufficiently to exert pressure on the rectum and perineal tissues. There is evidence from a study undertaken over six decades ago that active pushing during the latent phase in the absence of the bearing down urge for women does not achieve much, apart from exhausting and discouraging them (Benyon 1957).

More recent concerns over the impact of epidural analgesia on spontaneous birth have led to an increasing interest in the so-called passive second stage of labour, in which active pushing efforts are delayed until fetal descent and rotation have occurred. This is based on the hypothesis that the prolongation of second stage progress when epidural analgesia is used is due to the relaxation effect of epidural analgesia on the pelvic floor muscles. Consequently, the fetal presenting part does not encounter the necessary resistant force from the pelvic floor to bring about the normal rotation process. Some aspects of this phenomenon have indeed been observed in ultrasound examinations during labour (Pizzicaroli et al. 2018). However, a recent trial has found that, for nulliparous women with an epidural *in situ*, immediate versus delayed pushing in the second stage labour did not affect type of birth, or neonatal morbidity (Cahill et al. 2018). There is currently no agreement on best practice in this area and most of the current evidence does not apply to multiparous women who have an epidural *in situ* and who are also more likely to progress well in labour.

Apart from the timing of pushing in the context of an epidural, there has also been debate about the best position for women during the latent phase when they are using epidural analgesia. The Cochrane review undertaken by Walker et al. (2018a) concluded that there was no strong evidence across all the included studies for adopting any specific position in the passive second stage of labour for women with epidural analgesia *in situ*. However, subanalysis of the best quality studies in the review does suggest that the *lateral position* could be beneficial in terms of clinical outcomes and women's experiences.

The evidence on timing of pushing and position during the latent phase does not, however, apply to women without an epidural *in situ*. These women will generally progress well if they are supported in resting when they have no urge to push, then in actively pushing when they feel the urge to do so, in whatever position they spontaneously adopt, assuming in both cases that there is no cause for concern for mother and/or baby. For women who are not using epidural analgesia, passive descent of the fetus can continue with good midwifery support until the head is visible at the vulva, or until they feel a spontaneous desire to push.

The Active Phase

Most women without epidural analgesia will experience a compulsive urge to push, or bear down, once the fetal head has rotated and started to descend.

Duration of the Second Stage

There is no good evidence about the absolute time limits of physiological labour (Albers 1999; Downe 2004; Allen et al. 2009; Zhang et al. 2010; American College of Obstetricians and Gynaecologists, ACOG 2014; Oladapo et al. 2018). The National Institute for Health and Care Excellence (NICE 2017) suggests that obstetric advice should be sought if the active (pushing) second stage is longer than 2 h in a nulliparous woman, or 1 h in a multiparous woman and the birth is not imminent. However, Oladapo et al. (2018) have shown that setting time limits is less effective than paying attention to steady progress, and to maternal and fetal wellbeing, with intervention dictated by signs of slowing progress and/or fetal or maternal pathology or distress. This is also the position of ACOG (2014).

MATERNAL RESPONSE TO TRANSITION AND THE SECOND STAGE

Pushing

In the first observational study that was undertaken in this area by Bergstrom et al. (1997), women reported intense pain and discomfort when asked not to push against strong urges to do so. Some of the study participants reported an inability to bear down when finally '*allowed*' to do so, after a period of being told by their birth attendants to resist strong pushing urges because they did not have a fully dilated cervical os. When the woman and fetus appear well and labour has progressed spontaneously, an increasing number of midwives have adopted the practice of supporting the woman's overwhelming urge to bear down without confirming full dilatation of the cervical os. This is accompanied with close attention to the maternal and fetal condition, anticipating the rapid appearance of the fetal presenting part externally, and acting if this does not occur within a few bearing down contractions (Downe et al. 2008; Borrelli et al. 2013). However, if a decision is taken, with the woman, that it is better to avoid active pushing for a while, there are a number of techniques that could be offered. These include position change, often to the left lateral, using controlled breathing, inhalation analgesia or even narcotic or epidural pain relief (Downe et al. 2008; Borrelli et al. 2013). As stated above, the optimum response in this situation has not yet been established.

There has been evidence from observational studies for more than two decades that managed active pushing in the second stage of labour accompanied by breath holding *(the Valsalva manoeuvre)* has adverse consequences (Thomson 1993; Aldrich et al. 1995; Enkin et al. 2000; Yildirim and Beji 2008; Prins et al. 2011). The Cochrane review conducted by Lemos et al. (2017), based on randomized trial evidence, concluded that practice in this situation should be based on the woman's preferences and the individual clinical situation. NICE (2017) guidelines advise the following:

- *Inform the woman that in the second stage she should be guided by her own urge to push* (NICE 2017: 1.13.10).
- *If pushing is ineffective or if requested by the woman, offer strategies to assist birth, such as support, change of position, emptying of the bladder and encouragement* (NICE 2017: 1.13.11).

Spontaneous pushing efforts usually result in maximum pressure being exerted at the height of a contraction. In turn, this allows the vaginal muscles to become taut and prevents bladder supports and the transverse cervical ligaments from being pushed down in front of the baby's head. This may help to prevent prolapse and urinary incontinence in later life, although this belief has still not been formally tested with longitudinal follow-up studies. Most studies conducted in this area have been undertaken with women who are giving birth on a bed, in either a semi-recumbent or sitting position. There is little evidence to date relating to typical pushing behaviours or outcomes, in the short or longer term, when women are upright or on all fours during the active pushing stage.

Some women vocalize loudly as they push. This may aid in them coping with the contractions, so they should feel free to express themselves in this way. Reassurance and praise will also help to boost a woman's confidence, enabling them to assert their own control over events. The atmosphere should be calm and the pace unhurried.

Position
Supine or Supported Sitting Position
If the woman lies flat on her back, vena caval compression is increased, resulting in hypotension. This can lead to reduced placental perfusion and diminished fetal oxygenation (Humphrey et al. 1974; Kurz et al. 1982). The efficiency of uterine contractions may also be reduced. The semi-recumbent or supported sitting position, with the thighs abducted, is the posture most commonly used in maternity units (Fig. 20.2). While this may afford the midwife good access and a clear view of the perineum, the woman's weight is on her sacrum, which directs the coccyx forwards and reduces the pelvic outlet. In addition, the midwife needs to bend forward and laterally to support the birth, which may lead to injury.

Lithotomy
In some settings, lithotomy is routinely used during the active pushing stage of labour, and there are anecdotal reports that this technique is becoming more common even where an instrumental birth is not anticipated (Care Quality Commission, CQC 2019). There is no evidence of benefit of this position for women in spontaneous labour, and it is associated with the same constraints on physiology as for the supported sitting position above.

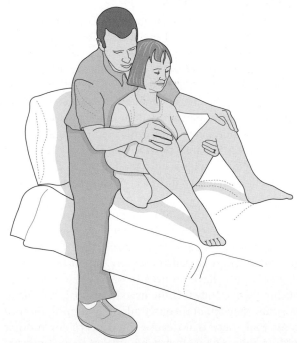

Fig. 20.2 Supported sitting position. (After Simkin P, Ancheta R. (2006) The labor progress handbook (2nd ed.). Oxford: Blackwell, with permission from Blackwell Science.)

Elvander et al. (2015) found in their observational study an increased risk of obstetric anal sphincter injury (OASI) in women using lithotomy position. The degree of abduction of the thighs in lithotomy could also be associated with other iatrogenic injuries, especially if the woman is in the position for a long time. It is also a very exposing position that some women could find traumatic. In the absence of evidence for any clear benefit of lithotomy for an individual woman and/or baby, it should not be used routinely for women giving birth spontaneously.

Lateral Position

This position was widely used in the UK in the 20th century, although it has been less common in current practice. The perineum can be clearly viewed and uterine action is effective, but an assistant may be required to support the woman's uppermost thigh during the birth, which may not be ergonomic. It provides an alternative for women who find it difficult to abduct their hips. As noted above, it may also aid fetal rotation, especially in the context of epidural analgesia (Downe et al. 2004; Bick et al. 2017).

Upright Positions: Squatting, Kneeling, All-Fours, Standing, Using a Birthing Ball

There is good evidence that women who are pregnant or not who adopt an upright kneeling squat position increase the diameter of the pelvis significantly (Reitter et al. 2014). A review of studies examining upright versus recumbent positions during the second stage of labour showed there were advantages for labouring women who adopt any position that was not supine or in lithotomy, as shown in Figs 20.2, 20.3 (Gupta et al. 2017). These included reduced duration of second stage labour, fewer assisted births, fewer episiotomies, reduced severe pain in second stage labour, and fewer abnormal heart rate patterns. There was no difference in the rates of third- or fourth-degree tears. However, increased rates of second-degree tears and of estimated blood loss >500 mL were noted. The experimental group included women who used birthing chairs, a technique known to be associated with increased blood loss (Stewart and Spiby 1989; Turner et al. 1988). It is not clear if this risk accrues to all upright positions. The *upright position* group in this review also included women who were in supported sitting positions on a bed, and in the lateral position. There are a number of studies relating to positions and mobility for women using so-called *walking/mobile epidurals*, but recent data on the physiology of labour and birth for women in spontaneous labour who have not been induced or augmented, and who mobilize without the use of pharmacological pain relief, do not seem to exist.

Radiological evidence demonstrates an average increase of 1 cm in the transverse diameter and 2 cm in the anteroposterior diameter of the pelvic outlet when the squatting position is adopted. This produces an average 28% increase in the overall area of the outlet compared with the supine position (Russell 1969). Some women find the all-fours position to be the optimum approach for all or part of their labours, especially in the case of an occipitoposterior position, due to relief of backache (Stremler et al. 2005). In the case of a breech presentation, anecdotal evidence suggests that most women will spontaneously adopt an all-fours or forward-leaning position (see discussion below). It can, however, be tiring to maintain for a long period of time. A wide range of other standing and leaning positions

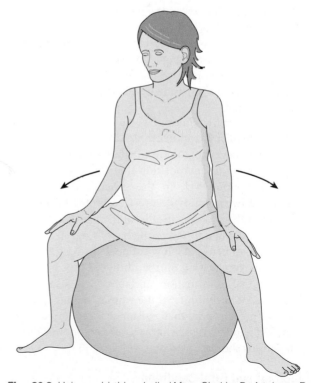

Fig. 20.3 Using a birthing ball. (After Simkin P, Ancheta R. (2006) The labor progress handbook (2nd ed.). Oxford: Blackwell, with permission from Blackwell Science.)

can be experimented with to help the woman cope with her labour (Simkin and Ancheta 2006; Simkin 2010; Royal College of Midwives, RCM 2018). It is important not to insist on any position as the *'right'* one. Positive and dramatic effects on labour progress can be achieved by encouraging the woman to change and adapt her position in response to the way her body feels, as she is likely to be responding to the rotation and descent of her fetus, and the changes in posture may well be helping this process to happen.

The position the woman may choose to adopt is dictated by several factors:

- *The woman's instinctive preference.*
- *The environment*, which should not act as a constraint through lack of privacy or lack of supports such as cushions and chairs. In a hospital setting, it may help to move the labour bed from the middle of the room, and to provide other supports such as cushions and birthing balls, so that the woman can roam from one to another as the labour dictates. Low lighting and music of her choice, or even biophilic moving scenes of nature (Aburas et al. 2017), may help the woman to respond instinctively to the room as a safe and secure place. This is likely to result in increased secretion of endorphins and a reduction in adrenaline production, reducing the sensation of pain, and helping her to cope with labour. To optimize this *'eustress'* state, minimizing unnecessary intrusion by other members of staff is also essential.
- *The midwife's confidence.* A full understanding of the mechanisms and neurophysiology of labour and birth should enable the midwife to adapt their care and support to any position that the woman wishes to adopt. However, in the process, the postures adopted by the midwife must be protective of their own health (and, specifically, of their back). One way of minimizing damage to the back is to refrain from the woman being in a low supported sitting position with her feet resting on the midwife's hip. Minimizing vaginal examinations in labour will also reduce the risk of back injury. If the woman has an epidural *in situ* it is essential that assistance is requested when the woman needs to be moved, and ergonomic lifting positions should be used.

Maternal and Fetal Condition

If the woman has had analgesia, or if there is any concern about her wellbeing or that of her baby, then more frequent or continuous monitoring may limit the choices available to her. However, there are often creative solutions to these situations, and good midwifery care involves finding these solutions where possible.

THE MECHANISM OF NORMAL LABOUR (CEPHALIC PRESENTATION)

As the fetus descends, soft tissue and bony structures exert pressures that lead to descent through the birth canal by a series of movements. Collectively, these movements are called the *mechanism of labour*. There is a mechanism for every fetal presentation and position that can lead to a vaginal birth. Knowledge and recognition of the normal physiological mechanism enables the midwife to anticipate the next step in the process of descent. Understanding and close observation of these movements can help to ensure that physiological progress is recognized, that the woman gives birth safely and positively, or that early assistance can be sought should any problems occur. The fetal presentation, position, and size relative to that of the woman will govern the exact mechanism as the fetus responds to external pressures. Principles common to all mechanisms are:

- descent takes place
- whichever part leads and first meets the resistance of the pelvic floor will rotate forwards until it comes under the symphysis pubis
- whatever emerges from the pelvis will pivot around the pubic bone.

It should be noted that, while the mechanism set out below is the most common, it is not an invariant blueprint, but a guide; each labour is unique.

During the mechanism of normal labour, the fetus turns slightly to take advantage of the widest available space in each plane of the pelvis. The widest diameter of the pelvic brim is the transverse; at the pelvic outlet, the greatest space lies in the anteroposterior diameter.

At the onset of labour, the most common presentation is the vertex and the most common position either left or right occipitoanterior; therefore it is this mechanism which will be described. In this instance:

- the lie is longitudinal
- the presentation is cephalic
- the position is right or left occipitoanterior
- the attitude is one of good flexion
- the denominator is the occiput
- the presenting part is the posterior part of the anterior parietal bone.

Main Movements of the Fetus
Descent
Descent of the fetal head into the pelvis often begins before the onset of labour. For a primigravid woman this usually occurs during the latter weeks of pregnancy. In multigravid women, muscle tone is often more lax and therefore descent and engagement of the fetal head may not occur until labour actually begins. Throughout the first stage of labour the contraction and retraction of the uterine muscles reduces the capacity in the uterus, exerting pressure on the fetus to descend further. Following rupture of the forewaters and the exertion of maternal effort, progress speeds up.

Flexion
This increases throughout labour. The fetal spine is attached nearer the posterior part of the skull; pressure exerted down the fetal axis will be more forcibly transmitted to the occiput than the sinciput. The effect is to increase flexion, which results in smaller presenting diameters that will negotiate the pelvis more easily. At the onset of labour, the suboccipito-frontal diameter, which is approximately 10 cm on average, is presenting. With greater flexion, the suboccipito-bregmatic diameter, that is, approximately 9.5 cm, presents. The occiput becomes the leading part.

Internal Rotation of the Head
During a contraction, the leading part is pushed downwards onto the pelvic floor. The resistance of this muscular diaphragm brings about rotation. As the contraction fades, the pelvic floor rebounds, causing the occiput to glide forwards. As discussed above, resistance is an important determinant of rotation, as Fig. 20.4 demonstrates. This explains why rotation is often delayed following epidural analgesia, which causes relaxation of pelvic floor muscles. The slope of the pelvic floor determines the direction of rotation. The muscles are hammock-shaped and slope down anteriorly, so whichever part of the fetus first meets the lateral half of this slope will be directed forwards and towards the centre. In a well-flexed vertex presentation the occiput leads, and rotates anteriorly through ⅛ of a circle when it meets the pelvic floor. This causes a slight twist in the neck as the head is no longer in direct alignment with the shoulders. The anteroposterior diameter of the head now lies in the widest (anteroposterior) diameter of the pelvic outlet. The occiput slips beneath the sub-pubic arch and crowning occurs when the head no longer recedes between contractions and the widest transverse

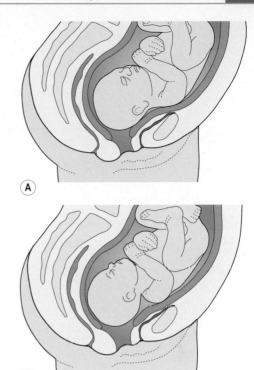

Fig. 20.4 In a standing position: (A) Internal rotation of the head begins and (B) upon completion, the occiput lies under the symphysis pubis.

diameter (biparietal) is born. If flexion is maintained, the suboccipito-bregmatic diameter, approximately 9.5 cm, distends the vaginal orifice.

Extension of the Head
Once crowning has occurred, the fetal head can extend, pivoting on the suboccipital region around the pubic bone. This releases the sinciput, face and chin, which sweep the perineum, and then are born by a movement of extension, as shown in Fig. 20.5.

Restitution
The twist in the neck of the fetus which resulted from internal rotation is now corrected by a slight untwisting movement. The occiput moves ⅛ of a circle towards the side from which it started.

Internal Rotation of the Shoulders
The shoulders undergo a similar rotation to that of the head to lie in the widest diameter of the pelvic outlet, namely anteroposterior. The anterior shoulder is the first to reach the levator ani muscle and it therefore rotates

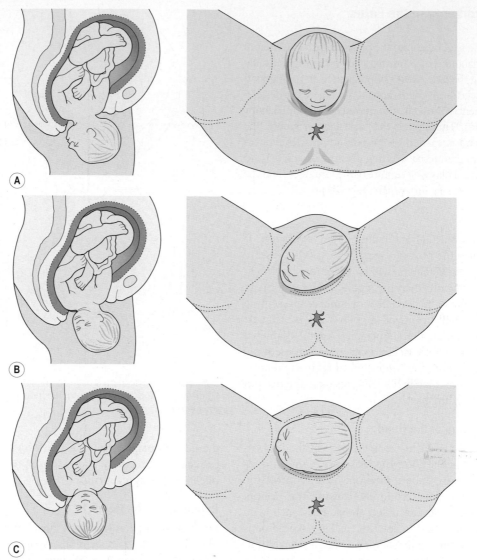

Fig. 20.5 In standing and semi-recumbent positions: (A) Birth of the head; (B) restitution; (C) external rotation.

anteriorly to lie under the symphysis pubis. This movement can be clearly seen as the head turns at the same time (external rotation of the head). It occurs in the same direction as restitution, and the occiput of the fetal head now lies laterally.

Lateral Flexion

The shoulders are usually born sequentially. When the woman is in a supported sitting position, the anterior shoulder is usually born first, although midwives who encourage women to adopt an upright or kneeling position have observed that the posterior shoulder is commonly seen first. In the former case, the anterior shoulder slips beneath the subpubic arch and the posterior shoulder passes over the perineum. In the latter, the mechanism is reversed. This enables a smaller diameter to distend the vaginal orifice than if both shoulders were born simultaneously. The remainder of the body is born by lateral flexion as the spine bends sideways through the curved birth canal.

MIDWIFERY CARE IN TRANSITION AND THE SECOND STAGE

Care of the Parents

The woman and her companions will now realize that the birth of the baby is imminent. They may feel excited and elated but at the same time anxious and frightened by the dramatic change in pace. They will need frequent explanations of events. The midwife's calm approach and information about what is happening can ensure the woman stays in control, and is confident. This is critical at the time of transition, when events can result in a sensation of panic. The midwife should praise and congratulate the woman on her hard work, recognizing that she is probably undertaking the most extreme physical activity she will ever encounter. Birth is an intimate act, which often takes place in a public setting. The midwife should also ensure that privacy and the woman's dignity are maintained.

Crucially, it is at the time of transition that the woman may request analgesia, even if she had originally intended to avoid any pain relief in labour. Such a request will need to be carefully assessed by the attending midwife. This is especially true when a supportive companion is not present. On the basis of her knowledge of the woman, the midwife may be able to help her over this transient phase with good midwifery support, and without utilizing pharmacological analgesia. The decision for or against pain relief at this stage must be made in partnership with the woman, recognizing that, particularly for a nulliparous woman, a demand for pain relief may often be an unconscious proxy for a demand for labour support. In order to achieve the kind of supportive care that can help a woman over the uncertainties and distress of transition, it is eminently preferable that the woman should have continuous support throughout labour (Bohren et al. 2017). Ideally, the same midwife or small group of known midwives should attend the woman throughout (Sandall et al. 2016). Alternatives to pharmacological analgesia include praise and reassurance about progress, changes in position and scenery, massage and appropriate nutrition. Complementary therapies and optimal fetal positioning may also be offered if the midwife is competent to undertake them. Leg cramp is a common occurrence whichever posture is adopted. It can be relieved by massaging the calf muscle, extending the leg and dorsiflexing the foot. These measures may be crucial in re-energizing a labour that is beginning to flag in the second stage.

The midwife should also have regard to the wellbeing of the woman's partner and other companions as far as possible. Witnessing labour and birth is a very positive experience for most birth companions. However, for others it can have long-term negative psychological consequences. In a few cases, being a companion to a woman who experienced a traumatic birth can be associated with symptoms similar to those of post-traumatic stress in the birth companion(s) for years after the birth (White 2007; Steen et al. 2012). The attitude of the midwife to the labour, to the woman, and to the partner/birth companions will have a significant effect on the labour (Halldorsdottir and Karlsdottir 1996; Lundgren 2004; El-Nemer et al. 2006; Thomson and Downe 2008, 2010; Elmir et al. 2010; Berg et al. 2012), with possible consequences for the mother, her partner and the family after the birth (Thomson and Downe 2010). It is crucial to respect the woman and her partner/birth companions, and to respect the meaning that this birth will have for them, both on the day, and in the future.

Observations during the Second Stage

Four factors determine whether the second stage is continuing safely, and these must be carefully monitored:

- uterine contractions
- descent, rotation and flexion of the presenting part
- fetal condition: suspicious or pathological changes in the fetal heart
- maternal condition.

Uterine Contractions

The strength, length and frequency of contractions should be assessed regularly by observation of maternal responses, and by uterine palpation during the second stage of labour. They are usually stronger and longer than during the first stage of labour, with a shorter resting phase. The posture and position adopted by the woman may influence the contractions.

Descent, Rotation and Flexion

Initially, descent may occur slowly, especially in primigravid women, but it usually accelerates during the active phase. It may occur very rapidly in multigravid women. If there is a delay in descent on abdominal palpation, despite regular strong contractions and active maternal pushing, a vaginal examination may be performed with maternal permission. The purpose is to confirm whether or not internal rotation of the head has taken place, to assess the station of the presenting part and to determine whether a caput succedaneum has formed. If the occiput has rotated anteriorly, the head is well flexed and caput succedaneum is not excessive it is likely that progress will continue. In the absence of good rotation and flexion, and/or a weakening of uterine contractions, change of position, nutrition and hydration, or use of optimal fetal positioning techniques dynamically in response to maternal impulses as labour progresses maybe helpful (Simkin and Ancheta 2006). However, enforcing any particular position at a population level (as in randomized controlled trial protocols) does not seem to be effective (Le Ray et al. 2016). Consultation with a more experienced midwife may provide further suggestions to reorientate the labour. For women who are overwhelmed by labour sensations, and pain, pharmacological pain relief may also help in reducing maternal production of adrenaline, and, therefore, in increasing oxytocin levels and consequent fetal descent and rotation. High levels of maternal distress might be associated with pharmacological induction of labour, or indicate underlying pathology. If there is evidence that either fetal or maternal condition is compromised, an experienced obstetrician should be consulted.

Fetal Condition/Suspicious or Pathological Changes of the Fetal Heart

If the membranes are ruptured, the liquor amnii is observed to ensure that it is clear. While thin old meconium staining is not always regarded as a sign of fetal compromise, NICE (2017) guidelines (recommendation 1.5.2) advise action (e.g. transfer if required and/or expedite the birth) after discussion with the mother when *'significant meconium'* is present. This is defined as *'dark green or black amniotic fluid that is thick or tenacious, or any meconium-stained amniotic fluid containing lumps of meconium'* (NICE 2017). The attending midwife should bear in mind that this could also be an indication of an undiagnosed breech presentation.

As the fetus descends, fetal oxygenation may be less efficient owing to either cord or head compression or to reduced perfusion at the placental site. A well-grown healthy baby will not be compromised by this transitory hypoxia. If the woman is labouring normally, NICE (2017) recommend that the fetal heart should be auscultated intermittently, with either a Pinard stethoscope or Doppler ultrasound. During the second stage of labour, this is usually undertaken immediately after a contraction. If continuous electronic fetal monitoring is being undertaken due to risk factors in the woman or baby, it is not unusual at this stage to see early decelerations of the fetal heart, with a swift return to the normal baseline after a contraction, and good beat-to-beat variation throughout. The midwife should learn to recognize the normal changes in fetal heart rate patterns during the second stage of labour, both when monitored intermittently (which should be the norm in healthy pregnancies) and when monitored continuously (where there are specific concerns for the baby). This will minimize the risk of iatrogenic intervention, and maximize a timely response to fetal compromise if it occurs.

Late decelerations, and a lack of return to the normal baseline, a rising baseline or diminishing beat-to-beat variation, are signs of concern. While it is generally acknowledged that beat-to-beat variation is hard to identify in intermittent monitoring, the other characteristics can be identified. If these are heard for the first time in the second stage of labour, they may be due to cord or head compression, which may be helped by a change in maternal position. However, if they persist, experienced aid must be sought. If the labour is taking place in a setting that is distant from a hospital maternity unit, an episiotomy may be considered (see Box 20.2) – with maternal consent – if the birth is imminent, or if trained and experienced in ventouse birth, the midwife may consider expediting the birth using such means. Otherwise, with maternal consent and if the condition of the woman and baby permit, transfer to a hospital unit should take place.

BOX 20.2 Indications for Episiotomy by the Midwife in the Second Stage of Labour

- suspicious or pathological fetal heart rate
- malpresentation or malposition of the fetal head and consequential wider presenting diameters/lack of moulding (face presentation)
- rigid, thick and inelastic perineum that will not stretch, causing delay
- women affected by Female Genital Mutilation (FGM) (Type III)
- excessive vaginal and perineal scar tissue after reconstructive vaginal surgery
- *button holing* of the perineum
- to assist with shoulder dystocia for internal manoeuvres if necessary.

Maternal Condition

The midwife's observation includes an appraisal of the woman's ability to cope emotionally as well as an assessment of her physical wellbeing. This includes close attention to what she says, as well as how she behaves, and a swift supportive response to any indication that she is losing belief in herself to accomplish the birth of her baby.

Maternal pulse rate is usually taken and recorded every 15 min, and blood pressure every hour, provided that these remain within normal limits. Recording the woman's pulse also ensures that the fetal heart sounds are not being confused with the maternal pulse. If the second stage is longer than usual, or if the woman's condition warrants, her temperature could also be assessed. If the woman has an epidural in situ, blood pressure will be monitored more frequently, and continuous electronic fetal monitoring will probably be in use.

Maternal Comfort

As a result of her exertions the woman usually feels very hot and sticky, and she will find it soothing to have her face and neck sponged with a cool flannel. Her mouth and lips may become very dry. Sips of iced water or other fluids are refreshing and a moisturizing cream can be applied to her lips. Her partner may help with these tasks as a positive contribution to ease her discomfort.

The bladder is vulnerable to damage, due to compression of the bladder base between the pelvic brim and the fetal head. The risk is increased if the bladder is distended. The woman should be encouraged to pass urine at the beginning of the second stage unless she has recently done so.

Preparation for the Birth

Once active pushing commences, the midwife should prepare for the birth. There is usually little urgency if the woman is primigravid, but multigravid women may progress very rapidly.

The room in which the birth is to take place should be warm with a spotlight available so that the perineum can be easily observed if necessary. A clean area should be prepared to receive the baby, and waterproof covers provided to protect the bed and floor. Sterile cord clamps, a clean apron, and sterile gloves are placed to hand. In some settings, sterile gowns are also used. An oxytocic agent may be prepared, either for the active management of the third stage if this is acceptable to the woman, or for use during an emergency. A warm cot and clothes should be prepared for the baby. Neonatal resuscitation equipment must be thoroughly checked and readily accessible.

Considerations for Episiotomy

An episiotomy must only be performed when it is required for the immediate protection of the baby and/or the woman. It must never be undertaken routinely during spontaneous vaginal birth (NICE 2017; Jiang et al. 2017). The situations in which a midwife may perform an episiotomy should be restricted to those identified in Box 20.2. An episiotomy is a surgical operation where an incision is made in the perineum to extend the vulval orifice. If an episiotomy is to be performed, the woman must give her consent. It is best to discuss this possibility early in the labour, or preferably, antenatally, as the kinds of situations when episiotomy become necessary are often emergencies, when the woman is highly anxious, and often in pain, and so explanations at that stage are not a good basis for informed consent. Any theoretical agreement to an episiotomy prior to labour should be reconfirmed as soon as the need for one becomes apparent in labour. It is important to ensure the comfort and psychological wellbeing of the woman as much as possible when informing her as to why an episiotomy is being recommended at this point in her labour.

Recommended Technique and Indications for an Episiotomy

The following recommendations are from the NICE (2017) guidelines on intrapartum care:

- *If an episiotomy is performed, the recommended technique is a mediolateral episiotomy originating at the vaginal fourchette and usually directed to the right side. The angle to the vertical axis should be between 45 and 60 degrees at the time of the episiotomy* (NICE 2017: 1.13.20).
- *Perform an episiotomy if there is a clinical need, such as instrumental birth or suspected fetal compromise* (NICE 2017: 1.13.21).
- *Provide tested effective analgesia before carrying out an episiotomy, except in an emergency because of acute fetal compromise* (NICE 2017: 1.13.22).

These guidelines also specifically recommend that women who have had previous third- or fourth-degree tears should not be given a routine episiotomy (NICE 2017: 1.13.17), but, instead, should be offered the opportunity to discuss their hopes, fears and expectations about perineal management (NICE 2017: 1.13.18) before coming to an individualized decision about what is best for them.

Assessment of the Episiotomy Wound, and Suturing

Suturing of an episiotomy should only be undertaken by a practitioner with skills in this technique. If observation indicates that the episiotomy has extended to the anal sphincter, or if there are complex associated tears, the suturing must be undertaken by a practitioner with expertise in identifying and suturing complex perineal damage. It is essential to ensure that adequate lighting is available, that the perineum can be clearly visualized, that the woman is in a comfortable position, and that she has effective pain relief throughout the procedure. More details about optimal suturing techniques and materials are provided in Chapter 17.

Birth of the Baby

The midwife's skill and judgement are crucial factors in minimizing maternal trauma and ensuring an optimal birth for both the woman and her baby. These qualities are refined by experience but certain basic principles should be applied. They are:

- observation of progress
- prevention of infection
- emotional and physical comfort of the woman, and reassurance that she is coping well
- anticipation of the range of potential physiological events, and support for physiological processes of labour
- recognition of abnormal developments and appropriate response to them.

During the birth, both the woman and baby are particularly vulnerable to infection. While evidence indicates that strict antisepsis is unnecessary if the birth is straightforward (Keane and Thornton 1998; Lumbiganon et al. 2014), meticulous aseptic technique must be observed when preparing sterile surgical equipment that could be used for invasive techniques, such as episiotomy scissors. Surgical gloves should be worn during the birth for the protection of both the woman and midwife. Goggles or plain glasses should be available to avoid the risk of ocular contamination with blood or amniotic fluid.

The equipment that is used during the birth of the baby includes the following items:

- warm swabbing solution or tap water
- cotton wool and pads
- sterile cord scissors and clamps
- sterile episiotomy scissors (these should be available in case they are needed).

Birth of the Head

Once the birth is imminent, the perineum may be swabbed with water should this be indicated and a clean pad is placed under the woman to absorb any faeces or fluids. If she is not in an upright position, a pad is placed over the rectum on the perineum (but not covering the fourchette) and a clean towel is placed on or near the woman for receipt of the baby. Throughout these preparations, the midwife observes the progress of the fetus. With each contraction the head descends. As it does so the superficial muscles of the pelvic floor can be seen to stretch, especially the transverse perineal muscles. The head recedes between contractions, which enables these muscles to thin gradually. The skill of the midwife in ensuring that the active phase is unhurried helps to safeguard the perineum from trauma, either observing the gradual advancement of the fetal head or controlling it with light support from her hand. One large study, the HOOP (Hands-On Hands-Poised) trial, indicated that, compared with guarding the perineum, a hands-poised technique was associated with a lower risk of episiotomy, but slightly more maternal discomfort at 10 days postnatally, and a higher risk of manual removal of placenta (McCandlish et al. 1998). More recently, OASI prevention care bundles have included a Hands-On element (Royal College of Obstetricians and Gynaecologists, RCOG 2014; Rasmussen et al. 2016). A series of observational studies have suggested that implementation of the care bundle reduces OASI cases. However, most also indicate an increased use of episiotomy, and none include longer term follow up, or women's views and experiences. Since most studies are conducted in hospital where bed birth is the norm, it is not clear if the findings of any of the studies in this area apply to other birth positions. To date, there is no evidence of the effect of the care bundle from randomized trials, and the Cochrane review in this area finds no strong evidence for either the hands on or poised approach (Aasheim et al. 2017). The midwife should therefore consider the best approach to take in the context of each individual woman/baby dyad, and especially, with relation to the position in which the woman is giving birth (Petrocnik and Marshall 2015). If women are giving birth in a semi-recumbent or sitting position, many midwives place their fingers lightly on the advancing head to monitor descent and prevent very rapid crowning and extension (Fig. 20.6). Excessive pressure on the head, however, may be associated with vaginal lacerations. Whatever technique the midwife adopts, it should be based on the assumption that it is the woman who is giving birth to her baby, and the midwife is there to add the *minimum* physical help necessary at any given time.

Once the head has crowned, the woman can achieve control by gently blowing or 'sighing' out each breath in order to minimize active pushing. Birth of the head in this way may take two or three contractions but may avoid unnecessary maternal trauma. The head is born by extension as the face appears at the perineum.

During the resting phase before the next contraction, and especially if the head is not advancing as expected, the midwife may check descent is not being impeded by a tight nuchal cord. If found, it is usual to slacken it to form a loop through which the shoulders may pass, though in some cases, the usual practice has been to sever a tight nuchal cord (Jackson et al. 2007). This is now **not** recommended as a routine solution, as it deprives the baby of the blood that then becomes trapped on the

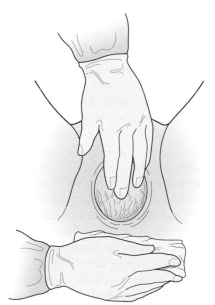

Fig. 20.6 Supporting the head in a semi-recumbent position.

placental side of the umbilical cord divide, and, once the cord is cut the baby has no access to oxygen until it takes its first breath. Unless, rarely, the condition of the baby or woman dictates otherwise, *the cord should not be cut for at least 3 min after birth, and, ideally, until it has stopped pulsating* (Mercer et al. 2005, 2007; Hutton and Hassan 2007; McDonald and Middleton 2008; McDonald et al. 2013). The preferred approach to the finding of a tight nuchal cord is to perform the so-called 'somersault manoeuvre', as shown in Fig. 20.7. If the immediate risk of compromise does not allow for this manoeuvre, two artery forceps can be applied to the umbilical cord approximately 3 cm apart, and the cord can be severed, and unwound from the fetal neck. The baby should then be born very soon afterwards, so that it can breathe, and regain access to oxygen, or be resuscitated if it is severely compromised.

If the cord is clamped, great care must be taken that maternal tissues are not damaged. Holding a swab over the cord as it is incised will reduce the risk of the attendants being sprayed with blood during the procedure.

Birth of the Shoulders

Restitution and external rotation of the head maximizes the smooth birth of the shoulders and minimizes the risk of perineal laceration. However, it is not uncommon for small babies, or for babies of multiparous women, to be born with the shoulders in the transverse, or even to have a twist in the neck opposite to that expected. If the position is upright, it is more common for the shoulders to be left to birth spontaneously with the help of gravity.

During a water birth, it is important not to touch the emerging fetus to avoid stimulating it to gasp underwater. If there is a problem with the birth in this circumstance, the woman should be asked to stand up out of the water before any manoeuvres are attempted.

If the midwife does physically aid the birth of the shoulders and trunk, she should be absolutely sure that restitution has occurred prior to trying to flex the trunk laterally. One shoulder is released at a time to avoid overstretching the perineum. A hand is placed on each side of the baby's head, over the ears, and gentle downward traction is applied (Fig. 20.8). This allows the anterior shoulder to slip beneath the symphysis pubis while the posterior shoulder remains in the vagina. If the third stage of labour is to be actively managed, the assistant will now administer an oxytocic

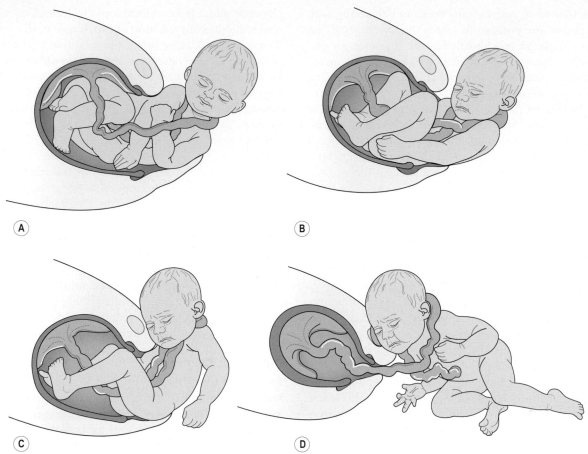

Fig. 20.7 The somersault manoeuvre. (From Mercer J, Skovgaard R, Peareara-Eaves J, et al. (2005) Nuchal cord management and nurse midwifery practice. Journal of Midwifery and Women's Health 50(5):373–379.)

drug to the woman. This is usually administered intra-muscularly. When the axillary crease is seen, the baby's head and trunk are guided in an upward curve to allow the posterior shoulder to escape over the perineum. These manoeuvres are reversed if the mother is in a forward-facing position such as *all-fours*. The midwife or woman may now grasp the baby around the chest to aid the birth of the trunk and lift the baby towards the woman's abdomen. This allows the woman immediate sighting of her baby and close skin contact, removing the baby from the gush of liquor which accompanies the release of the baby's body. If the midwife does not actively assist, she should be ready to support the head and trunk as the baby emerges. The time of birth is noted and recorded.

If this has not already been done, the cord is severed between two cord clamps placed close to the umbilicus.

As noted above, current research suggests that this should not take place before 3 min, and ideally after the cord has stopped pulsating (turned white), unless the fetal or maternal condition dictate otherwise. A cord clamp is applied. The baby is dried and placed in the skin-to-skin position with the mother if she is happy with this (Moore et al. 2016). A warm cover is placed over the baby. Swabbing of the eyes and aspiration of mucus during and immediately following birth are not considered necessary providing the baby's condition is satisfactory. Oral mucus extractors should not be used because of the risks of mucus that is contaminated with a virus such as hepatitis or human immunodeficiency virus (HIV) entering the operator's mouth.

The moment of birth is both joyous and beautiful. The midwife is privileged to share this unique and intimate experience with the parents.

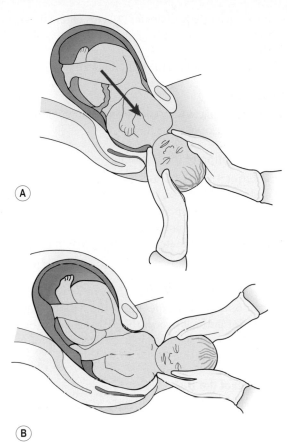

Fig. 20.8 (A) Downward traction releases the anterior shoulder and (B) an upward curve allows the posterior shoulder to escape.

Water Birth

The latest Cochrane review on water birth concluded that it may reduce the need for additional analgesia, and there is no good quality evidence of adverse effects for either the woman or the neonate (Cluett et al. 2018). If a woman has decided that she would like a water birth, and these facilities are available, it is important that the attending staff are able to support her in this choice. The RCM (2012) has produced guidelines for the conduct of water birth.

The RCM (2012) guidelines note that narcotic analgesia should not be used in the pool, though women may find nitrous oxide (Entonox: gas and air) useful. Though women are sometimes advised not to use the pool in early labour, there is no evidence to support a particular time after which women will get most benefit. Local protocols should include checks on the quality of the water supply,

how and when pools should be cleaned, how women should be lifted from the pool in an emergency if they are not mobile, and infection control procedures. Disposable bath linings and thorough cleaning and drying of the bath after use will help to minimize the risk of cross-infection.

It is advised that midwives pay attention to women's comfort. The temperature of the woman and the water should be monitored hourly to ensure that she is comfortable and not becoming pyrexial. It is generally agreed that the temperature of the water should not be above 37.5°C (RCM 2012). Too high a temperature not only will be uncomfortable for the woman, but may cause fetal tachycardia.

The midwife must be aware of the possibility of perineal trauma as with any birth, although the counter-pressure of the water on the perineum is known to steady the emergence of the baby from the birth canal. The midwife can provide encouraging verbal support to the woman to help ease the birth of the head and shoulders.

Once the baby has been born into the water, they should be brought to the surface immediately by the woman, the birth partner or the midwife. As discussed earlier, the cord should not be clamped and cut for at least 3 min and not while the baby is still under water. This is due to the sudden reduction in placental-fetal blood flow being a stimulant to initiate respiration and consequential water inhalation.

VAGINAL BREECH BIRTH AT TERM

This section follows on from Chapter 19, regarding the physiology and management of the first stage of labour for women with term pregnancies where the fetus is presenting by the breech. The main aim for both chapters is to examine the knowledge and skills required to effectively facilitate planned vaginal breech births at term in both home and hospital settings. It is important that midwives are conversant with the controversies surrounding the Term Breech Trial (Hannah et al. 2000) and the subsequent studies and guidance that are available to inform a woman's choice in mode of breech birth (Goffinet et al. 2006; Maier et al. 2011; RCOG 2017; NICE 2019) (see also Chapter 19). The systematic review by Berhan and Haileamlak (2015) found that perinatal mortality and morbidity in the planned vaginal breech birth were significantly higher than with planned caesarean section birth. However, the review showed low absolute risk for vaginal breech birth which substantiates the practice of individualized choice and informed decision-making on the mode of birth in a term breech presentation, which is further emphasized in the recommendations by RCOG (2017) and NICE (2019).

However, many midwives will occasionally find themselves in the situation of diagnosing a breech presentation in transition or the second stage of labour, sometimes while attending an out-of-hospital birth. For this reason, all midwives need to have the knowledge and skills to support the woman in this situation, to make decisions, work with the normal physiology of the labour if the birth is proceeding spontaneously, to know how to recognize impending or actual problems, when to undertake manoeuvres, and/or to transfer the woman to obstetric care in a hospital setting. The RCOG (2017) advocate the presence of a skilled birth attendant being essential for safe vaginal breech birth and that all maternity units must be able to provide skilled supervision for vaginal breech birth where a woman is admitted in advanced labour with protocols being developed for such a situation: elements that resonate with the findings of the study by Fischbein and Freeze (2018) that compared the outcomes of breech and cephalic planned home and birth centre births. Walker et al. (2018b) concluded in their small study of breech skill acquisition among midwives and obstetricians that specialist breech teams may facilitate the development of expertise within maternity care settings in order to rebuild and sustain the skills in breech labour and birth that have become elusive over the past couple of decades.

Mechanism of Right Sacroanterior Position

Similar to cephalic presentations that favour the left occipitoanterior position, breech presentations more commonly adopt the right sacroanterior position, the mechanism of which is described below:

- The lie is longitudinal.
- The attitude is one of complete flexion.
- The presentation is breech.
- The position is right sacroanterior.
- The denominator is the sacrum.
- The presenting part is the anterior (right) buttock.

- The bitrochanteric diameter (10 cm) enters the pelvis in the right oblique diameter of the maternal pelvic brim.
- The sacrum points to the right iliopectineal eminence.

Compaction

Descent takes place with increasing compaction owing to increased flexion of the limbs.

Internal Rotation of the Buttocks

The anterior (right) buttock reaches the pelvic floor first and rotates forward ⅛ of a circle along the left side of the maternal pelvis to lie underneath the symphysis pubis. The bitrochanteric diameter is now in the anterioposterior diameter of the maternal pelvic outlet (Fig. 20.9A).

Lateral Flexion of the Body

The anterior buttock escapes under the symphysis pubis, the posterior buttock sweeps the perineum and the buttocks are born by a movement of lateral flexion: also known as *rumping* (Fig 20.9B, C).

Restitution of the Buttocks

The anterior buttock turns slightly to the mother's left side.

Internal Rotation of the Shoulders

The shoulders enter the brim of the pelvis in the same oblique diameter as the buttocks: namely the right oblique diameter. The anterior shoulder rotates forward 1/8th of a circle along the left side of the maternal pelvis and escapes under the symphysis pubis; the posterior shoulder sweeps the perineum and the shoulders are born (Fig. 20.10).

Internal Rotation of the Head

The fetal head enters the maternal pelvis with the sagittal suture in the transverse diameter of the pelvic brim. The occiput rotates forwards ⅛ of a circle along the left side of the maternal pelvis and the suboccipital region (nape of the neck) impinges on the under-surface of the symphysis pubis (Fig. 20.11).

External Rotation of the Head

At the same time, the baby's body turns so that it lies parallel with the maternal body.

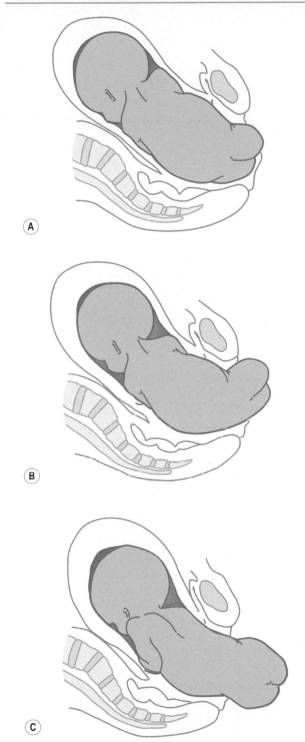

Fig. 20.9 A–C: Birth of the buttocks. (With permission from MacDonald S, Johnson G. (Eds). (2017) Mayes Midwifery (15th ed.). Edinburgh: Elsevier.)

Birth of the Fetal Head

The chin, face and sinciput sweep the perineum, and the baby's head is born in a flexed attitude.

Undiagnosed Breech Presentation

It is still not uncommon for a breech presentation to be discovered for the first time during labour, often towards the end of labour, as the presenting part becomes more easily identified, or in the presence of fresh meconium. If the midwife attends a woman in labour at home with a breech presentation where a hospital birth had initially been planned, it is important to remain calm while undertaking a careful assessment of the risk to the woman and baby taking into consideration the parent's wishes before a decision to transfer to hospital is made. This will depend on the stage of labour, the fetal position and the maternal medical and obstetric history. If the woman is nearing the second stage of labour and the labour is progressing well, assistance should be promptly summoned while supporting her to give birth at home. Should a decision be made to transfer to hospital, the midwife must alert the hospital of the transfer and ensure that the paramedics are equipped for neonatal resuscitation. The fetal heart and maternal condition should be monitored and recorded throughout the journey to hospital. The midwife must always be prepared for the birth in transit as it may progress more rapidly than initially anticipated. In such a situation, the driver should be asked to stop the ambulance in order for the midwife to assist the birth, undertaking any necessary manoeuvres safely. If the baby is likely to be born in transit, it is useful to take a number of towels/blankets to wrap the baby, encouraging skin-to-skin contact and early breastfeeding to maintain thermoregulation, i.e. warmth, and reducing the likelihood of hypoglycaemia and hypothermia.

Types of Breech Birth

Box 20.3 highlights the three types of vaginal breech birth.

Position for Breech Birth

The woman's position can significantly affect the physiological labour and birth process and the one that is adopted should ideally be her choice. Many texts have described vaginal breech births with the assumption the woman should give birth in the hospital environment on

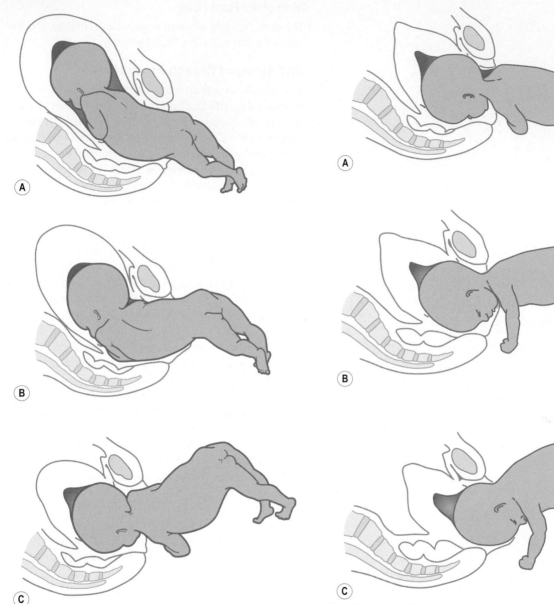

Fig. 20.10 A–C: Birth of the shoulders. (With permission from MacDonald S, Johnson G. (Eds). (2017) Mayes Midwifery (15th ed.). Edinburgh: Elsevier.)

Fig. 20.11 A–C: Birth of the head. (With permission from MacDonald S, Johnson G. (Eds). (2017) Mayes Midwifery (15th ed.). Edinburgh: Elsevier.)

the bed in a semi-recumbent, adapted lithotomy position (Chadwick 2002; Ndala 2005; Coates 2017). Such a position affects the normal physiological process of labour, and may lead to malposition due to the reduction in gravitational force on the fetal mechanisms, consequently increasing the need for the midwife to undertake manoeuvres to assist the birth.

While gravity helps to expel the fetus, it is the expulsive contractions and angle of the pelvis that assist in facilitating a physiological breech birth if the woman adopts an upright forward-leaning position. Little assistance from the midwife is needed if these mechanisms are achieved spontaneously, except in the case of care with the birth of the after-coming head. Use of the birth pool is generally not advised, as the buoyancy of the water may work

BOX 20.3	**Types of Breech Birth**
Spontaneous	The birth occurs with little assistance from the attendant.
Assisted breech	The buttocks are born spontaneously, but some assistance is necessary for the birth of extended legs, arms and the head.
Breech extraction	This birth involves manipulating the fetal body by an experienced attendant (usually an obstetrician) in order to hasten the birth of the baby in an emergency situation, such as fetal compromise.

against gravity and thus impede the physiological mechanisms that affect a spontaneous breech birth. A 'hands off the breech' approach is optimal when the woman either adopts an upright standing or an 'all-fours'/leaning forwards position (Cronk 1998a, 1998b; Reed 2003; Burvill 2005; Evans 2012a; Walker 2015; Louwen et al. 2017). However, the position that is ultimately adopted should be based on the woman's preference and the experience of the attendant (RCOG 2017).

Where the mother is on all-fours or leans upon the bed/settee or on her birth partner (Fig. 20.12), the baby's trunk descends through the pelvis at 45 degrees and is able to move more freely around the curve of Carus of the maternal pelvis. This position provides an excellent view of the birth process and access to the baby's face as it is born over the perineum, as well as ample space for the midwife to undertake any manoeuvres should they be necessary to assist the birth of the baby.

Facilitating a Vaginal Breech Birth in an Upright/Kneeling Position

Breech births can be as physiological as any other vaginal birth and a woman who has chosen to birth vaginally, or discovers in labour that her baby is presenting by the breech, requires calm support from skilled and confident midwives (Marshall 2010). The importance of not pushing until the cervix has been confirmed as fully dilated should be explained to the woman. In addition, the woman should be aware that other skilled attendants may need to be called to the birth.

At the start of the expulsive part of the second stage of labour, the woman tends to make pelvic rocking movements which facilitates the descent of the fetus and corrects positioning for further progress. As the woman

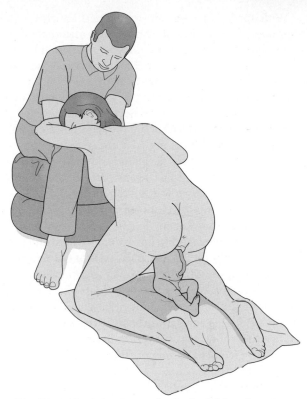

Fig. 20.12 The baby descending in the 'all-fours' position.

commences pushing spontaneously, gradually the anterior buttock should descend, becoming visible at the introitus of the vagina, followed by the baby's anus, genitalia and posterior buttock. The bitrochanteric diameter is then born with lateral flexion, known as *rumping*. While this is occurring, the baby's shoulders are entering the oblique diameter of the maternal pelvis.

Descent continues, the baby's thighs, popliteal fossa (back of the knee) and lower legs become visible and the pelvis is eventually born. The baby is then observed to arch its spine backwards, extending its pelvis causing its lower body to curl round the maternal symphysis pubis. As a result, the tension that this places on the baby's legs assists in their spontaneous release from the introitus, especially when the woman is in an upright, kneeling position, and the baby is born as far as the umbilicus. At this point, the woman may spontaneously lower her body so that the baby is sitting on the floor, further encouraging flexion of the baby. It is no longer common practice to pull down a loop of cord to avoid traction of the umbilicus unless there appears to be constriction of the blood vessels as manipulating the cord or stretching it can induce spasm of the vessels.

With further descent and continued anticlockwise rotation, the head enters the brim of the maternal pelvis as the shoulders rotate in the mid-cavity assisted by the pelvic floor muscles. Evans (2012b) emphasizes that this continued rotation of the baby's body assists in bringing the arms down using the pelvic floor muscles in a way that is very similar to the Løvset manoeuvre (used when the birth is delayed should the arms be extended). The anterior shoulder is released under the symphysis pubis and the posterior shoulder and arm pass over the perineum. At this point, Evans (2012a) refers to the baby flexing its legs up towards its abdomen and its arms up towards its shoulders, similar to a sit-up or tummy scrunch. Such a movement, results in the baby flexing its head by bringing its chin down onto its chest and pivoting the occiput on the internal aspect of the symphysis pubis. This stimulates the woman to lower her body from an upright kneeling position to an all-fours or a knee–chest position, moving her pelvis round the baby's flexing head. This enables the baby's chin, face, sinciput and head to smoothly pass over the perineum. The midwife is only required to support the baby as the head is spontaneously born.

If a uterotonic is to be administered to the woman as part of the third stage of labour management, it should be *withheld* until the baby's head is completely born.

The Birth of the After-Coming Head

To avoid any sudden change in fetal intracranial pressure and subsequent cerebral haemorrhage, it is vital the midwife ensures the head is born in a steady and gradual fashion and often some assistance is given at this point. There are three methods used.

Burns Marshall manoeuvre. This particular manoeuvre facilitates movement of the baby's head through the maternal pelvic outlet, but is only possible when the woman is in a semi-recumbent, adapted lithotomy position. The baby is allowed to *'hang'* until the head descends onto the perineum, when after about 1–2 min, the nape of the neck becomes visible and the suboccipital region is born. The baby's ankles are grasped with forefinger between the two, maintaining sufficient traction to prevent the neck from extending and resulting in possible cervical spine fracture (Fig. 20.13A). The feet are taken up through a 180-degree arc until the mouth and nose are free of the vulva. This should be undertaken slowly to prevent sudden changes in pressure to

the baby's head and undue stretching of the perineum. The perineum can be guarded to prevent sudden escape of the head (Fig. 20.13B). It is imperative that the midwife observes the baby has descended sufficiently to ensure that it is the suboccipital region that pivots under the pubic arch and not the neck to avoid fracture of the cervical vertebra and crushing of the spinal cord.

Mauriceau–Smellie–Veit manoeuvre. Whilst the baby's head is facilitated through the same 180° arc as in the Burns Marshall manoeuvre, the Mauriceau–Smellie–Veit manoeuvre provides more control with the birth of the head and places less strain on the baby's back. This particular manoeuvre can be undertaken in a variety of positions that the woman may adopt for the birth: semi-recumbent, sitting, the adopted lithotomy position or the all-fours position. As this manoeuvre facilitates maximum flexion of the baby's head, it can be used to advantage when the head is extended and descent is delayed. Furthermore, it allows for slow birthing of the baby's head and thus reduces the risk of intracranial haemorrhage.

In an ***all-fours position***, the midwife supports the baby's back over her right arm and flexes the baby's head by tipping the occiput *forwards* with the middle finger

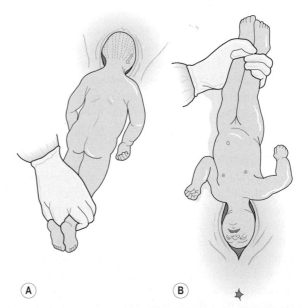

Fig. 20.13 Burns Marshall manoeuvre for the after coming head. (A) Correct grasp around the fetal ankles and (B) The suboccipital region pivots 180 degrees under the pubic arch; the mouth and nose are free of the vulva.

of the right hand and by gentle pressure on the baby's malar bones (cheek bones) with the first and ring fingers of the left hand (Fig. 20.14A,B). It is important that the midwife avoids placing her finger in the baby's mouth to prevent fracture to the jaw or trauma to the mouth and gums, which can result in the baby having difficulties with feeding. The vault of the baby's head should be born slowly and gently to facilitate gradual adaptation of the head to the changing pressures imposed by the birth process. This should be in a *downwards* direction following the pelvic curve of Carus.

In the **semi-recumbent position**, the midwife should support the baby on one of her arms, with her first and ring fingers placed on the baby's malar bones, pulling the jaw down and increasing flexion. The other hand is placed across the baby's shoulders with the midwife's middle finger on the occiput to increase flexion. The outer fingers can apply gentle traction on the baby's shoulders. Maintaining flexion, the head is drawn out of the vagina until the suboccipital region appears and then the baby's head is slowly pivoted gently and slowly *upwards* around the symphysis pubis following the curve of Carus, delivering the chin and face first (Fig. 20.14C).

Forceps birth. If an obstetrician is facilitating the vaginal breech birth, forceps may be applied to the after-coming head to ensure the birth is controlled.

Manoeuvres to Assist the Breech Birth

If the midwife uses her professional judgement and decides to undertake a manoeuvre to assist the breech birth, as this will involve making some contact with the woman, she must obtain the woman's consent in order to avoid the legal tort of trespass to the person (Dimond 2013; Nursing and Midwifery Council, NMC 2018). If the fact that the baby is presenting by the breech is known before the onset of labour, it is recommended that the midwife discusses the reasons for any possible manoeuvres, including their benefit and risks with the woman and seek her consent to undertake any of them, if they become necessary.

The following manoeuvres were originally developed to facilitate a breech birth with the woman positioned on the bed, but can be utilized when the woman is on all fours or standing. With the benefits of gravity encouraging descent of the fetus in the latter positions, the likelihood of the midwife needing to adopt such measures is reduced. Nevertheless, as noted above, unexpected breech presentations in late labour still arise, so it is important that the midwife is

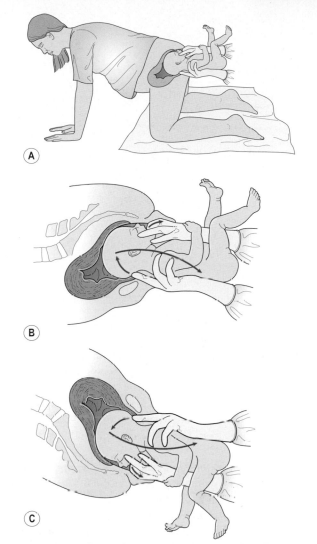

Fig. 20.14 Mauriceau–Smellie–Veit to assist the after coming head manoeuvre in a breech presentation (A,B) 'All fours' position demonstrating how the occiput is tipped *forwards* to achieve flexion, pivoting *downwards* under the symphysis pubis to facilitate birth of the head. (C) In a semi-recumbent/sitting/adapted lithotomy position, showing position of hands and *downward* direction of flexion while pivoting *upwards* through a 180 degrees arc under the pubic arch.

both aware of, and skilled in, these manoeuvres and maintains her proficiency in their practice.

The birth of extended legs. If the fetal legs are not born spontaneously, it is likely they are extended, splinting the baby's body, which impedes lateral flexion of the spine and ultimately delays the birth. Gentle pressure, as shown in Fig. 20.15, can be applied in the popliteal

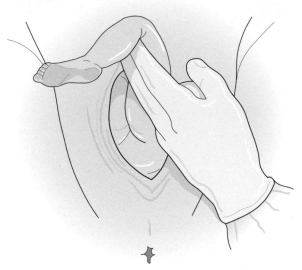

Fig. 20.15 Assisting the birth of an extended leg by applying pressure in the popliteal fossa.

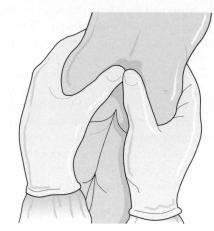

Fig. 20.16 Correct grasp for the Løvset manoeuvre for extended arms.

fossa of one of the legs to encourage knee flexion. This assists in the birth of the leg by sweeping it to the side of the abdomen through abducting the hip. This can be repeated for the other leg if necessary. The knee is a hinge joint which bends in one direction only. If the knee is pulled forwards from the abdomen, severe injury to the joint can result.

The birth of extended arms: the Løvset manoeuvre. This manoeuvre, which is a combination of rotation and downward traction, is used when the arms fail to appear during the birth of the baby's trunk and chest as a result of them being extended above the head. If the arms are not released then the birth will be delayed with increasing risk of hypoxia to the baby.

The baby is held at the iliac crests with thumbs over the sacrum and downward traction is applied while the baby is rotated 180 degrees (Fig. 20.16). Care must be taken to always keep the **baby's back towards the woman's front**, i.e. the baby's *abdomen* must be *uppermost* in an all-fours position or the baby's *back* is *uppermost* in a semi-recumbent position. It is important that the baby is not grasped by the flanks or abdomen as this may cause intra-abdominal trauma resulting in kidney, liver or spleen injury.

To keep the baby's *abdomen* uppermost should the woman have adopted the all-fours position, if the baby's right arm is extended the baby should be rotated to the

right by applying downward traction on the pelvic girdle in order to release the arm. This process is then repeated for the left arm if necessary.

The Løvset manoeuvre creates friction of the baby's posterior arm lying in the sacral curve against the pubic bone as the shoulder becomes anterior, sweeping the arm in front of the face (Fig. 20.17). The movement enables the shoulders to enter the maternal pelvis in the transverse diameter. The anterior arm is then born and the baby can be rotated back in the opposite direction in order for the other arm to be born. If the arm is not born spontaneously, it is usual to splint the humerus with two fingers, flex the elbow and sweep the arm across the face and downwards across the baby's chest (*cat-lick manoeuvre*).

Delay in the birth of the head. If the head is trapped in an incompletely dilated cervix, an air channel can be created to enable the baby to breathe pending intervention. This is done by inserting two fingers or a Sim's speculum in front of the baby's face and holding the vaginal wall away from the nose. Any mucus is wiped away and the airways are cleared. Attempts to release the head from the cervix result in high perinatal morbidity and mortality. Shushan and Younis (1992) have suggested the McRoberts manoeuvre as a method to facilitate the release of the fetal head. This requires the woman to lie flat on her back, bringing her knees up to her abdomen, and abducting the hips. More commonly, this manoeuvre is used to relieve shoulder dystocia and is described in detail in Chapter 25.

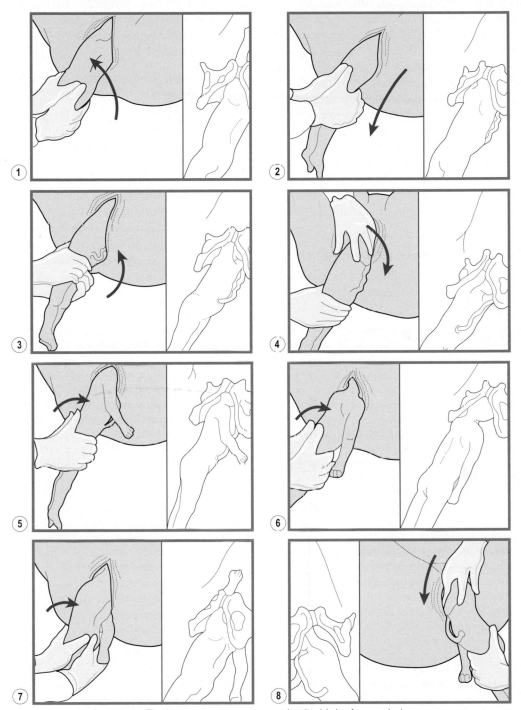

Fig. 20.17 The Løvset manoeuvre to assist the birth of extended arms.

Posterior rotation of the occiput is rare and usually results from mismanagement. If the woman is in a semi-recumbent position, the baby's back should always remain *uppermost* after the shoulders are born. To assist the birth, the head should be in the occipitoposterior position, the baby's chin and face may pass under the symphysis pubis as far as the root of the nose and the baby is then lifted up towards the mother's abdomen to enable the occiput to sweep the perineum.

When facilitating the birth of a woman presenting with a breech at term, there are some important issues for the midwife to consider that are pertinent to the breech scenario. These have been summarized in the Second Stage of Labour Checklist, as detailed in Box 20.4.

Potential Complications of a Breech Birth

It is important that midwives are fully aware of the potential complications associated specifically with vaginal breech births at term, which are listed in Box 20.5. Many of these can be avoided by having an experienced and skilled attendant assisting at the birth that may enable planned vaginal breech birth to be nearly as safe as planned vaginal cephalic birth (RCOG 2017).

Professional Responsibilities and Term Breech Birth

As an autonomous, accountable practitioner, the midwife has responsibility to maintain skills in normal physiological birth in relation to breech presentations at term in order to offer women real choice regarding mode of birth (NMC 2018). This includes being familiar with the current evidence and re-developing the skills midwives once had to facilitate vaginal breech births at term where there are no contraindications. It is therefore essential that these skills are seen as part of the normal physiological birth process rather than viewed as a rare maternity *'emergency'*.

BOX 20.4   Second Stage of Labour Checklist for Vaginal Breech Birth at Term

- **Regular fetal heart monitoring undertaken and documented:** Continuous electronic fetal heart monitoring *in hospital.* Pinard or sonicaid auscultation following every contraction in the second stage *at home* (NICE 2017 recommendations).
- **Check for cord prolapse if membranes rupture and buttocks are not engaged.**
- **Check for full dilatation before encouraging the woman to push:** The woman may experience a premature urge to push as the fetal body can pass through the cervix prior to full dilatation: the fetal head could become entrapped causing asphyxia increasing perinatal morbidity and mortality.
- **The umbilical cord may be loosened gently (*rarely required*):** This may be undertaken to prevent constriction of blood vessels as the baby's body is born. In the all-fours position, the condition of the baby can be easily monitored by observing the chest movements.
- **Encourage a physiological birth with minimum handling (*hands off the breech*):** To allow the baby to be born by gravity and propulsion and reduce trauma to the baby once the buttocks are distending the vulva.
- **Vault of the fetal skull should be born slowly:** To avoid rapid decompression resulting in intracranial haemorrhage.
- **Be aware and skilled in manoeuvres:** To assist the birth of the breech if problems arise with fetal descent and to control the birth of the baby's head.
- **DO NOT PERFORM BREECH EXTRACTION (routine use of manoeuvres/interventions to expedite birth):** This can cause delay and obstruction, e.g. fetal arms pulled upwards, head extended backwards.
- **Care of the baby following birth should include:** Appropriate resuscitation including suction of the oropharynx and inspection of the vocal cords (if thick meconium), maintaining the baby's body temperature, early feeding and paediatric assessment for signs of birth trauma. A follow-up appointment for a hip scan should be made to assess the baby for hip dysplasia (Chapter 32).
- **Postnatal examination of the mother:** To assess the physical condition, including any birth trauma and discuss the birth and its outcome whilst assessing psychological wellbeing.
- **Documentation:** Is vitally important throughout the labour and birth, to include specific details of all discussions and referrals and the time they were initiated. As the breech is born, the time that each stage is reached and any manoeuvres undertaken should also be recorded. Additionally documentation should account for immediate condition of the baby, including any resuscitation measures taken, and the condition of the mother following the birth.

BOX 20.5   Potential Complications of Breech Birth

Potential Fetal/Neonatal Complication	Associated Cause
• Congenital abnormality, e.g. hydrocephaly	• A cause for the presentation • Mechanism of the birth itself poses risks
• Congenital dislocation of the hip (↑ frank/extended breech)	• Usually a complication of the presentation and *not* the birth process
• Fetal asphyxia	• Umbilical cord prolapse (↑ preterm labour/footling breech/ill-fitting presenting part) • Cord compression • Premature placental separation due to uterine retraction once the baby's body has been born
• Intracranial haemorrhage	• Rapid decompression of the fetal skull causing tearing of the dura mater lining the brain and other major blood vessels
• Superficial tissue damage/bruising and oedema of baby's genitalia, feet	• Pressure on the cervix/prolapsed foot that lies in the vagina or at the vulva for some time
• Fractures of the femur, humerus, clavicle and spine/spinal cord damage • Dislocation of the hip, shoulder, neck • Brachial nerve paralysis (Erb's palsy)	• Incorrect or excessive handling during the birth
• Soft tissue damage/rupture to baby's liver, kidneys, spleen and adrenal glands	• Abdominal area is roughly squeezed
• Dislocation of baby's jaw/soft tissue damage to mouth and gums/feeding difficulties	• Baby's mouth incorrectly being used to create traction rather than the malar bones (cheekbones) in the Mauriceau–Smellie–Veit manoeuvre
• Cold injury/thermal shock and hypoglycaemia	• Ambient temperature too cool and baby loses heat during completion of the birth process

Potential Maternal Complication	Associated Cause
• Urethral, vaginal and perineal trauma	• Rapid birth of the baby's head
• Effects of anaesthesia (local, regional, general), infection, haemorrhage, thromboembolic disorders, etc.	• Risks of operative procedures
• Psychological distress, affecting attachment to baby, feeding difficulties and traumatic stress disorder	• Unexpected vaginal breech birth with lack of time to discuss options

---

RECORD-KEEPING

It is the responsibility of the midwife assisting the birth to complete the relevant records. This should include details of any drugs administered, of the duration and progress of labour, of the reason for performing an episiotomy and of perineal repair if they have undertaken it. This information is recorded in the women's notes (paper and/or electronic computerized) as well as in the birth register in some sites. Details of the baby's condition, including Apgar score, are also recorded. In some areas, extra charts and monitoring processes are introduced to respond to a range of imperatives. It is the professional responsibility of the midwife to remember that the primary purpose of record-keeping is to ensure effective delivery and handover of care for each mother and baby, not to protect staff or the organization from the risk of litigation. The *NMC* (2018: 6) Code states:

> *You put the interests of people using or needing nursing or midwifery services first. You make their care and safety your main concern and make sure that their dignity is preserved and their needs are recognised, assessed and responded to.*

Midwives need to balance the requirement for complete and accurate record-keeping with the need to maintain a focus on the woman and her fetus and birth companions. If demands to complete duplicate or unnecessary records hinder this central activity, the midwife should bring the situation to the attention of her line manager and/or Professional Midwifery Advocate (PMA)/clinical supervisor. See Box 20.6 for other current dilemmas in practice, as midwives negotiate around the various requirements of undertaking their vocation, being a professional, being an employee and practising proficiently and ethically. All data in the UK are subject to the Data Protection Act 2018.

Babies born in England, Wales and the Isle of Man are registered on the Personal Demographics Service (PDS) as soon after birth as possible, which fulfils the legal requirement to notify a birth within 36 hours. This ensures that each baby is issued with a unique National Health Service (NHS) Number, which then goes on to form their lifelong electronic patient record. Once the baby's birth has been registered, the PDS notifies the child health services, the NHS newborn hearing screening service and the Office for National Statistics (ONS) about the birth. The NHS number assists healthcare staff and service providers to identify and match patients to their health records should information need to be shared between health and care organizations.

CONCLUSION

The processes of transition and of second stage of labour are likely to be very physically and emotionally intense, particularly for the woman, but also for her partner and other birth companions. If maternal behaviour and instinct are respected, in the context of skilled and watchful waiting, the vast majority of labours will progress physiologically. The skill of the midwife is to support the woman effectively, to guide her when her spirits or the labour are flagging, and to enable her to accomplish her birth safely and in triumph. Diane's story in Case Study 20.1 provides a personal account of how important this is for women.

Clear, comprehensive, proportionate record-keeping is essential. While much practice in this area is still not based on formal evidence (Box 20.7), new observations about normal birth are beginning to be recorded, which will form the basis for future research.

Key issues in the management of the second stage of labour are summarized in Box 20.8.

BOX 20.6 Dilemmas of Practice

- The contrast between the current evidence base and actual practices.
- The contrast between knowledge gained from experience *(empirical knowledge)* and that gained from evidence *(authoritative knowledge)*.
- The problem of using guidelines and clinical risk assessments based on population evidence for individual women/babies
- Balancing maternal choice, institutional demands, and midwifery expertise.

BOX 20.7 Examples of Areas in Need of Research in the Transition and Second Stages of Labour

- The areas of controversy, as set out in Box 20.1.
- The nature of physiological fetal heart patterns, and variation and significance of variation in normal fetal heart tones and rhythms as heard with a Pinard stethoscope.
- The physiological variation in mechanisms and patterns of labour in settings where no restrictions on positioning or length of labour are imposed as a matter of routine.
- Evaluation of maternal behaviours and other non-invasive techniques to assess progress in labour.
- The short-, medium- and long-term epigenetic consequences of physiological labour and birth for the woman and her baby.
- The optimum approach to supporting women who experience the early pushing urge.
- Tools and technologies (including e- and m-technologies) to enhance personalized approaches to tailoring maternity care provision for the specific needs and choices of individual women.
- How to optimize normal birth for women who are experiencing induced labour and/or epidural analgesia.

BOX 20.8   Key Issues in the Management of the Second Stage of Labour

- The transition and second stage phases of labour are emotionally intense and physically hard.
- The majority of labours will progress physiologically.
- Maternal behaviour is usually a good indication of progress and wellbeing for mother and/or baby during this time.
- Unusual and/or persistent maternal distress is an indication for lack of progress and potential pathology for mother and/or baby, and should trigger closer attention to clinical signs of emerging pathology in mother and/or baby.

- Given the importance of *'reading'* maternal behaviour, the core midwifery skill is to be actively present with each labouring woman, to be consciously tuned in to her unique response to labour, and to support her in the context of a sound knowledge of the physiology and the mechanisms of this phase of labour.
- Support should be unobtrusive.
- The woman is the central player.
- Clear, comprehensive record-keeping is essential.
- There are many gaps in the research evidence in this area.

CASE STUDY 20.1   Diane's Birth Story

The birth of my first baby should have been one of the happiest days of my life. Instead I felt I had failed; I was mentally and physically traumatized. Five years on, when I was eventually pregnant again, my fears started creeping back, and I considered having a caesarean section. I was referred to the local caseload midwifery team. When my midwife came to visit I told her that my first birth had left me traumatized, confused and scared about everything. This was my big turnaround; after talking to her I realized I did not want a caesarean section, and I started to feel confident about giving birth naturally.

The big day arrived. I was over the moon that I had started my labour naturally. After a few hours my midwife came to my house, just to check how everything was going. Eventually, we decided it was time to go to the hospital. When I arrived they organized an epidural for me, which I had discussed, and which was in my birth plan. I was getting excited, knowing I was

going to meet my baby soon. My midwife supported me and encouraged me on everything I decided. She was there for me all the time, keeping me focused and positive about my birth. After about 3 hours, I started pushing hard with contractions. The epidural wore off enough for me to turn around on to my knees with my body upright, and I could feel the baby drop down. I gave it my all for two pushes, and out popped the head. I controlled my breathing, pushing slowly, and my beautiful baby girl came out. The midwife brought her through my legs so I could see her and that's when my husband cut her cord, which was memorable and overwhelming for him. I was the happiest person, I had the biggest smile on my face; to me this was a beautiful birth. Thanks to the wonderful midwives – it goes to show that with the right help and guidance you can overcome your fears and anxieties with positive thinking.

REFLECTIVE ACTIVITY FOR SELF-ASSESSMENT

1. How often do you support women to mobilize freely in labour and for their birth? If this is infrequent, how could you increase the opportunity for you to be able to do this?

2. When working within a birthing unit or labour ward, consider how much of each labour you usually stay in the room with a woman in labour, and how much of that time you are actually in physical contact with her (i.e. **not** filling in notes, taking measurements, entering data on the computer, checking stock, etc.). How often do you use therapeutic touch, or take account of her behavioural cues (dilation of her pupils, tone of her skin, the sounds she makes) to support her progress through the stages of labour?

3. Why is it important to develop the skill of using a Pinard stethoscope and how often do you use this tool to assess the fetal heart rate in labour? If this is not your usual practice, try using it for the next few labours. Is what you can hear different from the sounds you hear using a sonicaid or from a CTG machine? If so, what else can you hear, and what (if anything) does it tell you?

4. Considering the evidence taking into account the physiology and anatomy of the pelvis and soft tissues, as well as the neurohormones of labour, what would be your response to a woman who feels a strong need to push before you are certain her cervical os is fully dilated?

5. What are the key factors that you would need to consider when a healthy woman presents nearing the second stage of labour with a breech presentation at term in order to optimize maternal and fetal outcome?

REFERENCES

Aasheim, V., Nilsen, A. B. V., Reinar, L. M., & Lukasse, M. (2017). Perineal techniques during the second stage of labour for reducing perineal trauma. *Cochrane Database of Systematic Reviews* (6), CD006672.

Aburas, R., Pati, D., Casanova, R., & Adams, N. G. (2017). The influence of nature stimulus in enhancing the birth experience. *Health Environments Research and Design Journal*, *10*(2), 81–100.

ACOG (American College of Obstetricians and Gynaecologists). (2014). *Safe prevention of the primary cesarean section.* Available at: www.acog.org/Clinical-Guidance-and-Publications/Obstetric-Care-Consensus-Series/Safe-Prevention-of-the-Primary-Cesarean-Delivery-?IsMobileSet=false.

Albers, L. L. (1999). The duration of labor in healthy women. *Journal of Perinatology*, *19*(2), 114–119.

Aldrich, C. J., D'Antona, D., Spencer, J. A., et al. (1995). The effect of maternal pushing on fetal cerebral oxygenation and blood volume during the second stage of labour. *British Journal of Obstetrics and Gynaecology*, *102*(6), 448–453.

Allen, V. M., Baskett, T. F., O'Connell, C. M., et al. (2009). Maternal and perinatal outcomes with increasing duration of the second stage of labor. *Obstetrics and Gynecology*, *113*(6), 1248–1258.

Anderson, G. (2003). A concept analysis of 'normal birth'. *Evidence Based Midwifery*, *1*(2), 48–54.

Baker, A., & Kenner, A. N. (1993). Communication of pain: Vocalisation as an indicator of stage of labour. *New Zealand Journal of Obstetrics and Gynaecology*, *33*(4), 384–385.

Benyon, C. (1957). The normal second stage of labor: A plea for reform in its conduct. *BJOG*, *64*(6), 815–820.

Berg, M., Asta Ólafsdóttir, O., & Lundgren, I. (2012). A midwifery model of woman-centred childbirth care in Swedish and Icelandic settings. *Sexual and Reproductive Healthcare* (2), 79–87.

Bergstrom, L., Seidel, J., Skillman-Hull, L., et al. (1997). 'I gotta push. Please let me push!' Social interactions during the change from first to second stage labor. *Birth*, *24*(3), 173–180.

Berhan, Y., & Haileamlak, A. (2015). The risks of planned vaginal breech delivery versus planned caesarean section for term breech birth: A meta-analysis including observational studies. *BJOG*, *123*, 49–57.

Bick, D., Briley, A., Brocklehurst, P., et al. (2017). A multi-centre, randomised controlled trial of position during the late stages of labour in nulliparous women with an epidural: Clinical effectiveness and an economic evaluation (BUMPES). *Health Technology Assessment*, *21*(65), 1–176.

Bohren, M. A., Hofmeyr, G. J., Sakala, C., et al. (2017). Continuous support for women during childbirth. *Cochrane Database of Systematic Reviews* (7), CD003766.

Borrelli, S. E., Locatelli, A., & Nespoli, A. (2013). Early pushing urge in labour and midwifery practice: A prospective observational study at an Italian maternity hospital. *Midwifery*, *29*(8), 871–875.

Buckley, S. (2015). *Hormonal physiology of childbearing: Evidence and implications for women, babies, and maternity care.* Available at: www.nationalpartnership.org/our-work/resources/health-care/maternity/hormonal-physiology-of-childbearing.pdf.

Burvill, S. (2005). Managing breech presentation in the absence of obstetric assistance. In V. Woodward, K. Bates, & N. Young (Eds.), *Managing childbirth emergencies in community settings* (pp. 111–139). Houndsmill: Palgrave Macmillan.

Cahill, A. G., Srinivas, S. K., Tita, A. T. N., et al. (2018). Effect of immediate vs delayed pushing on rates of spontaneous vaginal delivery among nulliparous women receiving neuraxial analgesia: A randomized clinical trial. *Journal of the American Medical Association*, *320*(14), 1444–1454.

CQC (Care Quality Commission). (2019). *2018 survey of women's experiences of maternity care: Statistical release.* Available at: www.cqc.org.uk/sites/default/files/20190129_mat18_outliers.pdf.

Chadwick, J. (2002). Malpresentations and malpositions. In M. Boyle (Ed.), *Emergencies around childbirth: A handbook for midwives* (pp. 63–81). Oxford: Radcliffe Medical Press.

Cluett, E. R., Burns, E., & Cuthbert, A. (2018). Immersion in water during labour and birth. *Cochrane Database of Systematic Reviews* (5), CD000111.

Coates, T. (2017). Malpositions and malpresentations. In S. MacDonald, & G. Johnson (Eds.), *Mayes Midwifery* (15th edn.) (pp. 1023–1051). Edinburgh: Elsevier.

Crawford, J. S. (1983). The stages and phases of labour: Outworn nomenclature that invites hazard. *Lancet*, *2*, 271–272.

Cronk, M. (1998a). Midwives and breech births. *The Practising Midwife*, *1*(7/8), 44–45.

Cronk, M. (1998b). Hands off the breech. *The Practising Midwife*, *1*(6), 13–15.

Dahlen, H., Downe, S., Duff, M., & Gyte, G. M. (2013). Vaginal examination during normal labour: Routine examination or routine intervention? *International Journal of Childbirth*, *3*(3), 142–152.

Data Protection Act. (2018) Available at: www.legislation.gov.uk/ukpga/2018/12/contents/enacted?view=plain.

Dimond, B. (2013). *Legal aspects of midwifery* (4th ed.). London: Quay Books.

Dixon, L., Skinner, J., & Foureur, M. (2013a). Women's perspectives of the stages and phases of labour. *Midwifery*, *29*(1), 10–17.

Dixon, L., Skinner, J., & Foureur, M. (2013b). The emotional and hormonal pathways of labour and birth: Integrating mind, body and behaviour. *New Zealand College of Midwives Journal*, *48*, 15–23.

Dixon, L., Skinner, J., & Foureur, M. (2014). The emotional journey of labour-women's perspectives of the experience of labour moving towards birth. *Midwifery*, *30*(3), 371–377.

Downe, S. (1994). How average is normality? *British Journal of Midwifery*, *2*(7), 303–304.

Downe, S. (2004). Risk and normality in the maternity services: Application and consequences. In L. Frith (Ed.), *Ethics and midwifery: Issues in contemporary practice* (2nd ed.) (pp. 91–109). Oxford: Butterworth Heinemann.

Downe, S. (2006). Engaging with the concept of unique normality in childbirth. *British Journal of Midwifery*, *14*(6), 352–356.

Downe, S. (2008). *Normal birth, evidence and debate* (2nd ed.). Oxford: Elsevier.

Downe, S., & Byrom, S. (2019). *Squaring the circle: Normal birth research, theory and practice in a technological age*. London: Pinter and Martin Ltd.

Downe, S., Gerrett, D., & Renfrew, M. J. (2004). A prospective randomised trial on the effect of position in the passive second stage of labour on birth outcome in nulliparous women using epidural analgesia. *Midwifery*, *20*(2), 157–168.

Downe, S., Gyte, G. M. L., Dahlen, H. G., & Singata, M. (2013). Routine vaginal examinations for assessing progress of labour to improve outcomes for women and babies at term. *Cochrane Database of Systematic Reviews* (7), CD010088.

Downe, S., Young, C., & Hall-Moran, V. (2008). The early pushing urge: Practice and discourse. In S. Downe (Ed.), *Normal childbirth, evidence and debate* (2nd ed.) (pp. 129–148). Edinburgh: Churchill Livingstone.

Elmir, R., Schmied, V., Wilkes, L., et al. (2010). Women's perceptions and experiences of a traumatic birth: A meta-ethnography. *Journal of Advanced Nursing*, *66*(10), 2142–2153.

El-Nemer, A., Downe, S., & Small, N. (2006). 'She would help me from the heart': An ethnography of Egyptian women in labour. *Social Science and Medicine*, *62*(1), 81–92.

Elvander, C., Ahlberg, M., Thies-Lagergren, L., et al. (2015). Birth position and obstetric anal sphincter injury: A population-based study of 113 000 spontaneous births. *BMC Pregnancy Childbirth*, *15*, 252.

Enkin, M., Keirse, M., Neilson, J., et al. (2000). *A guide to effective care in pregnancy and childbirth* (3rd ed.). Oxford: Oxford University Press.

Evans, J. (2012a). The final piece of the breech jigsaw puzzle? *Essentially MIDIRS*, *3*(3), 46–49.

Evans, J. (2012b). Understanding physiological breech birth. *Essentially MIDIRS*, *3*(2), 17–21.

Fischbein, S. J., & Freeze, R. (2018). Breech birth at home: outcomes of 60 breech and 109 cephalic planned home and birth centre births. *BMC Pregnancy and Childbirth*, *18*, 397.

Goffinet, F., Carayol, M., Foidart, J. M., & PREMODA Study Group. (2006). Is planned vaginal delivery of breech presentation at term still an option? Results of an observational prospective survey in France and Belgium. *American Journal of Obstetrics and Gynecology*, *194*(4), 1002–1011.

Gould, D. (2000). Normal labour: A concept analysis. *Journal of Advanced Nursing*, *31*(2), 418–427.

Gupta, J. K., Sood, A., Hofmeyr, G. J., et al. (2017). Position in the second stage of labour for women without epidural anaesthesia. *Cochrane Database of Systematic Reviews* (5), CD002006.

Halldorsdottir, S., & Karlsdottir, S. I. (1996). Empowerment or discouragement: Women's experience of caring and uncaring encounters during childbirth. *Health Care for Women International*, *17*(4), 361–379.

Hannah, M. E., Hannah, W. J., Hewson, S. A., et al. (2000). Term Breech Trial Collaborative Group. Planned caesarean section versus planned vaginal birth for breech presentation at term: A randomized multi-centre trial. *Lancet*, *356*, 1375–1383.

Hobbs, L. (1998). Assessing cervical dilatation without VEs: Watching the purple line. *The Practising Midwife*, *1*(11), 34–35.

Humphrey, M. D., Chang, A., Wood, E. C., et al. (1974). A decrease in fetal pH during the second stage of labour when conducted in the dorsal position. *Journal of Obstetrics and Gynaecology of the British Commonwealth*, *81*, 600–602.

Hutton, E. K., & Hassan, E. S. (2007). Late vs early clamping of the umbilical cord in full-term neonates: Systematic review and meta-analysis of controlled trials. *Journal of the American Medical Association*, *297*(11), 1241–1252.

Irani, M., Kordi, M., & Esmaily, H. (2018). Relationship between length and width of the purple line and foetal head descent in active phase of labour. *Journal of Obstetrics and Gynaecology*, *38*(1), 10–15.

Jackson, H., Melvin, C., & Downe, S. (2007). Midwives and the fetal nuchal cord: A survey of practices and perceptions. *Journal of Midwifery and Women's Health*, *52*, 49–55.

Jiang, H., Qian, X., Carroli, G., et al. (2017). Selective versus routine use of episiotomy for vaginal birth. *Cochrane Database of Systematic Reviews* (2), CD000081.

Keane, H. E., & Thornton, J. G. (1998). A trial of cetrimide/chlorhexidine or tap water for perineal cleaning. *British Journal of Midwifery*, *6*(1), 34–37.

Kurz, C. S., Schneider, H., Hutch, R., et al. (1982). The influence of maternal position on the fetal transcutaneous oxygen pressure. *Journal of Perinatal Medicine, 10*(Suppl 2), 74–75.

Lemos, A., Amorim, M. M., Dornelas de Andrade, A., et al. (2017). Pushing/bearing down methods for the second stage of labour. *Cochrane Database of Systematic Reviews* (3), CD009124.

Le Ray, C., Lepleux, F., De La Calle, A., et al. (2016). Lateral asymmetric decubitus position for the rotation of occipito-posterior positions: Multicenter randomized controlled trial EVADELA. *American Journal of Obstetrics and Gynecology, 215*(4), 511.e1–e7.

Louwen, F., Daviss, B., Johnson, K.C. & Reitter, A. (2017). Does breech delivery in an upright position instead of on the back improve outcomes and avoid cesareans? *International Journal of Gynaecology and Obstetrics, 136*(2), 151–161.

Lumbiganon, P., Thinkhamrop, J., Thinkhamrop, B., et al. (2014). Vaginal chlorhexidine during labour for preventing maternal and neonatal infections (excluding Group B Streptococcal and HIV). *Cochrane Database of Systematic Reviews* (9), CD004070.

Lundgren, I. (2004). Releasing and relieving encounters: Experiences of pregnancy and childbirth. *Scandinavian Journal of Caring Sciences, 18*(4), 368–375.

Maier, B., Georgoulopoulos, A., Zajc, M., et al. (2011). Fetal outcome for infants in breech by method of delivery experiences with a stand-by service system of senior obstetricians and women's choices of mode of delivery. *Journal of Perinatal Medicine, 39*(4), 385–390.

Marshall, J. E. (2010). Facilitating vaginal breech at term. In J. E. Marshall, & M. D. Raynor (Eds.), *Advancing skills in midwifery practice* (pp. 89–102). Edinburgh: Churchill Livingstone/Elsevier.

McCandlish, R., Bowler, U., van Asten, H., et al. (1998). A randomised controlled trial of care of the perineum during second stage of normal labour. *British Journal of Obstetrics and Gynaecology, 105*(12), 1262–1272.

McDonald, S. J., & Middleton, P. (2008). Effect of timing of umbilical cord clamping of term infants on maternal and neonatal outcomes. *Cochrane Database of Systematic Reviews* (2), CD004074.

McDonald, S. J., Middleton, P., Dowswell, T., & Morris, P. S. (2013). Effect of timing of umbilical cord clamping of term infants on maternal and neonatal outcomes. *Cochrane Database of Systematic Reviews* (7), CD004074.

Mercer, J., Skovgaard, R., Peareara-Eaves, J., et al. (2005). Nuchal cord management and nurse midwifery practice. *Journal of Midwifery and Women's Health, 50*(5), 373–379.

Mercer, J. S., Erickson-Owens, D. A., Graves, B., et al. (2007). Evidence-based practices for the fetal to newborn transition. *Journal of Midwifery and Women's Health, 52*(3), 262–272.

Montgomery, T. (1958). Physiologic considerations in labor and the puerperium. *American Journal of Obstetrics and Gynecology, 76*(4), 706–715.

Moore, E. R., Bergman, N., Anderson, G. C., et al. (2016). Early skin–to–skin contact for mothers and their healthy newborn infants. *Cochrane Database of Systematic Reviews, 11*, CD003519.

Ndala, R. (2005). Breech presentation. In D. Stables, & J. Rankin (Eds.), *Physiology of childbearing with anatomy and related biosciences* (pp. 541–551). Edinburgh: Elsevier.

NICE (National Institute for Health and Care Excellence). (2017). *Intrapartum care: Management and delivery of care to women in labour.* London: NICE. Available at: www.nice.org.uk/guidance/cg190/resources/intrapartum-care-for-healthy-women-and-babies-pdf-35109866447557.

NICE (National Institute for Health and Care Excellence). (2019). *Intrapartum care for women with existing medical conditions or obstetric complications and their babies.* London: NICE. Available at: www.nice.org.uk/guidance/ng121/resources/intrapartum-care-for-women-with-existing-medical-conditions-or-obstetric-complications-and-their-babies-pdf-66141653845957.

NMC (Nursing and Midwifery Council). (2018). *The Code: Professional standards of practice and behaviour for nurses, midwives and nursing associates.* London: NMC.

Oladapo, O. T., Sousa, J. P., Fawole, B., et al. (2018). Progression of the first stage of spontaneous labour: A prospective cohort study in two sub-Saharan African countries. *PLoS Med, 15*(1), e1002492.

Olza, I., Leahy-Warren, P., Benyamini, Y., et al. (2018). Women's psychological experiences of physiological childbirth: A meta-synthesis. *BMJ Open, 18*(8), e020347.

Petersen, L., & Besuner, P. (1997). Pushing techniques during labor: Issues and controversies. *Journal of Obstetric, Gynecologic and Neonatal Nursing, 26*(6), 719–726.

Petrocnik, P., & Marshall, J. E. (2015). Hands-poised technique: The future technique for perineal management of second stage of labour? A modified systematic literature review. *Midwifery, 31*(2), 274–279.

Pizzicaroli, C., Montagnoli, C., Simonelli, I., et al. (2018). Ultrasonographic evaluation of the second stage of labor. Predictive parameters for a successful vaginal delivery with or without neuraxial analgesia: A pilot study. *Journal of Ultrasound, 21*(1), 41–52.

Prins, M., Boxem, J., Lucas, C., et al. (2011). Effect of spontaneous pushing versus Valsalva pushing in the second stage of labour on mother and fetus: A systematic review of randomised trials. *BJOG, 118*(6), 662–670.

Rasmussen, O. B., Yding, A., Anh Ø, J., et al. (2016). Reducing the incidence of Obstetric Sphincter Injuries using a hands-on technique: An interventional quality improvement project. *BMJ Quality Improvement Report, 5*(1) pii, u217936.w7106.

Reed, B. (2003). A disappearing art: Vaginal breech birth. *The Practising Midwife, 69*, 16–18.

Reitter, A., Daviss, B. A., Bisits, A., et al. (2014). Does pregnancy and/or shifting positions create more room in a woman's pelvis? *American Journal of Obstetrics and Gynecology, 211*(662), e1–e9.

Roberts, J., & Hanson, L. (2007). Best practices in second stage labor care: Maternal bearing down and positioning. *Journal of Midwifery and Women's Health, 52*(3), 238–245.

RCM (Royal College of Midwives). (2012). *Evidence based guidelines for midwifery-led care in labour; immersion in water for labour and birth.* Available at: www.rcm.org.uk/sites/default/files/Immersion%20in%20Water%20for%20Labour%20and%20Birth_0.pdf.

RCM (Royal College of Midwives). (2018). *Midwifery care in labour guidance for all women in all settings (RCM Midwifery Blue-top Guidance).* London: RCM. Available at: www.rcm.org.uk/media/2539/professionals-blue-top-guidance.pdf.

RCOG (Royal College of Obstetricians and Gynaecologists). (2017). *Clinical Green-top Guidelines for Management of Breech Presentation No 20b.* London: RCOG.

RCOG (Royal College of Obstetricians and Gynaecologists). (2014). *OASI Care Bundle Project: Background.* Available at: www.rcog.org.uk/en/guidelines-research-services/audit-quality-improvement/oasi-care-bundle/oasi-background/.

Russell, J. G. B. (1969). Moulding of the pelvic outlet. *Journal of Obstetrics and Gynaecology, 76*, 817–820.

Sandall, J., Soltani, H., Gates, S., et al. (2016). Midwife–led continuity models versus other models of care for childbearing women. *Cochrane Database of Systematic Reviews* (4), CD004667.

Shepherd, A., Cheyne, H., Kennedy, S., et al. (2010). The purple line as a measure of labour progress: A longitudinal study. *BMC Pregnancy and Childbirth, 10*, 54.

Shushan, A., & Younis, J. S. (1992). McRoberts maneuver for the management of the aftercoming head in breech delivery. *Gynecologic and Obstetric Investigation, 34*(3), 188–189.

Simkin, P. (2010). The fetal occiput posterior position: State of the science and a new perspective. *Birth, 37*(1), 61–71.

Simkin, P., & Ancheta, R. (2006). *The labor progress handbook* (2nd ed.). Oxford: Blackwell.

Souza, J. P., Oladapo, O. T., Fawole, B., et al. (2018). Cervical dilatation over time is a poor predictor of severe adverse birth outcomes: A diagnostic accuracy study. *BJOG, 125*(8), 991–1000.

Steen, M., Downe, S., Bamford, N., et al. (2012). Not-patient and not-visitor: A metasynthesis of fathers' encounters with pregnancy, birth and maternity care. *Midwifery, 28*(4), 362–371.

Stewart, P., & Spiby, H. (1989). A randomized study of the sitting position for delivery using a newly designed obstetric chair. *British Journal of Obstetrics and Gynaecology, 96*(3), 327–333.

Stremler, R., Hodnett, E., Petryshen, P., et al. (2005). Randomized controlled trial of hands-and-knees positioning for occipito-posterior position in labor. *Birth, 32*(4), 243–251.

Sutton, J., & Scott, P. (1996). *Understanding and teaching optimal fetal positioning* (2nd ed.). Tauranga: Birth Concepts.

Thomson, A. M. (1993). Pushing techniques in the second stage of labour. *Journal of Advanced Nursing, 18*(2), 171–177.

Thomson, G., & Downe, S. (2008). Widening the trauma discourse: The link between childbirth and experiences of abuse. *Journal of Psychosomatic Obstetrics and Gynaecology, 29*(4), 268–273.

Thomson, G., & Downe, S. (2010). Changing the future to change the past: Women's experiences of a positive birth following a traumatic birth experience. *Journal of Reproductive and Infant Psychology, 28*(1), 102–112.

Turner, M. J., Sil, J. M., Alagesan, K., et al. (1988). Epidural bupivacaine concentration and forceps birth in primiparae. *Journal of Obstetrics and Gynecology, 9*(2), 122–125.

Walker, K. F., Kibuka, M., Thornton, J. G., et al. (2018a). Maternal position in the second stage of labour for women with epidural anaesthesia. *Cochrane Database of Systematic Reviews, 11*, CD008070.

Walker, S. (2015). Turning breech upside down: Upright breech birth. *MIDIRS Midwifery Digest, 25*(3), 325–330.

Walker, S., Scamell, M., & Parker, P. (2018b). Deliberate acquisition of competence in physiological breech birth: A grounded theory study. *Women and Birth, 31*(3), e170–e177.

Walsh, D. (2010). Labour rhythms. In D. Walsh, & S. Downe (Eds.), *Essential midwifery practice: Intrapartum care* (pp. 63–80). Chichester: Wiley–Blackwell.

White, G. (2007). You cope by breaking down in private: Fathers and PTSD following childbirth. *British Journal of Midwifery, 15*(1), 39–45.

Wickham, S. (2007). Assessing cervical dilatation without VEs: Watching the purple line. *The Practising Midwife, 10*(1), 26–27.

Yildirim, G., & Beji, N. K. (2008). Effects of pushing techniques in birth on mother and fetus: A randomized study. *Birth, 35*(1), 25–30.

Zhang, J., Landy, H. J., Branch, D. W., et al. Consortium on Safe Labor. (2010). Contemporary patterns of spontaneous labor with normal neonatal outcomes. *Obstetrics and Gynecology, 116*(6), 1281–1287.

ANNOTATED FURTHER READING

Buckley, S. (2015). *Hormonal physiology of childbearing: Evidence and implications for women, babies, and maternity care.* Available at: www.nationalpartnership.org/our-work/resources/health-care/maternity/hormonal-physiology-of-childbearing.pdf.

This is a clear and comprehensive account of the complex interaction between neurohormones in labour and childbirth, maternal behaviours and the impact on outcomes.

Byrom, S., & Downe, S. (2015). *The Roar Behind the Silence: Why kindness, compassion and respect matter in maternity care.* London: Pinter and Martin.

The Roar Behind the Silence presents a series of short accounts from various professional and service user perspectives as to why kind, respectful childbirth care is essential for the short- and longer-term wellbeing of mothers, partners, babies, families, and for those providing maternity care. Details are provided as to how this can be achieved, even in the most difficult of circumstances.

Davis, E. (2012). *Heart and hands: A midwife's guide to pregnancy and birth* (5th ed.). New York: Ten Speed Press.

This is a manual of midwifery, based on the skills and experiences gained by lay midwives working in America. It offers unique tips and insights.

Evans, J. (2005). *Breech birth: What are my options?* Taunton: AIMS

An informative and empowering text that discusses the major issues surrounding breech birth and explains the options for women and midwives to consider that are reinforced by the inclusion of poignant personal birth stories.

Floyd-Davis, R., & Sargent, C. F. (1997). *Childbirth and authoritative knowledge: Cross-cultural perspectives.* Berkeley: University of California Press.

A seminal work, which explores how authority is given to certain kinds of knowledge, and how the knowledge and expertise of women and of less dominant cultures is not privileged, even in the area of childbirth, and even in the face of the evidence.

Louwen, F., Daviss, B., Johnson, K.C., & Reitter, A. (2017). Does breech delivery in an upright position instead of on the back improve outcomes and avoid cesareans? *International Journal of Gynaecology and Obstetrics, 136*(2), 151–161.

This German retrospective cohort study of 750 women with a term breech presentation, revealed that upright vaginal breech birth was associated with reductions in duration of the second stage of labour, manouevres required, maternal/neonatal injuries and caesarean sections rates, when compared with vaginal birth in the dorsal position.

Marshall, J. E. (2010). Facilitating vaginal breech at term. In J. E. Marshall, & M. D. Raynor (Eds.), *Advancing skills in midwifery practice* (pp. 89–102). Edinburgh: Churchill Livingstone/Elsevier.

This chapter considers the midwife's professional, legal and ethical responsibilities in facilitating vaginal breech births at term within both the hospital and home environment.

Uvnas Moberg, K. (2011). *The oxytocin factor: Tapping the hormone of calm, love and healing.* London: Pinter and Martin.

The author provides insights into the many functions and impacts of the powerful hormone oxytocin that is involved in bonding, sex and childbirth as well as in relaxation and feelings of calm.

USEFUL WEBSITES

All4Maternity Birth Repository: www.all4birth.com/birth-repository/

This site provides a range of material related to pregnancy, birth and the postnatal period, from research to educational programmes and stories. It includes abstracts, videos, guidelines and a range of other information. Some material is free, whereas others are pay-to-view.

Blood2 baby: www.bloodtobaby.com/

A location with extensive information and resources to support practitioners in carrying out physiological transition of the newborn with optimal cord clamping.

The Breech Birth Network: https://breechbirth.org.uk/

This website is a valuable resource to support practitioner training in facilitating vaginal breech birth in the light of best evidence and woman's choice.

International Childbirth Initiative 2018 Mother-Baby Family Friendly 12 Steps: www.internationalchildbirth.com/

The ICI supports the implementation of the 12 steps and self-initiated quality improvement mechanisms that can be used to monitor process, effect and engagement in safe and respectful maternity services. The site includes inspirational material and updates from demonstration sites across the world.

21

Physiology and Care During the Third Stage of Labour

Cecily Begley

CHAPTER CONTENTS

The third stage of labour is a time of profound relief for most women, following the exertions of labour and birth. During this stage, mother, baby and father come together as a family unit for the first time; parents explore and become familiar with their newborn, marvel at their baby's behaviour and relax. The physical mechanisms of birth continue almost unnoticed, and the placenta and membranes are expelled. Until the third stage is complete, continued vigilance on the part of the midwife is essential to ensure that postpartum haemorrhage (PPH) is prevented or treated early, and that the placenta and membranes are born intact. PPH is ranked among the top five major causes of maternal death globally. Although the majority (99%) of deaths reported occur in low-income countries, the incidence of PPH should not be underestimated for any birth, and PPH is currently the seventh leading cause of direct maternal death in the UK. Maternal mortality rates in high resource countries are relatively low when compared with low resource countries; however, maternal morbidity is similar in significance and rates of PPH are increasing worldwide. To facilitate a healthy, enjoyable outcome for mother and baby, good antenatal health plus preparation, coupled with skilled, evidence-based practice of the midwife remain crucial (World Health Organization, WHO 2018a; Ford et al. 2015; Knight et al. 2019).

THE CHAPTER AIMS TO

- describe the normal physiological mechanism of placental separation, descent and expulsion, including factors that facilitate haemostasis
- present evidence on the types, use and side-effects of uterotonic drugs in active management of the third stage of labour
- discuss the evidence relating to the timing of clamping the umbilical cord, and controlled cord traction

- describe the factors most commonly associated with PPH and discuss the current evidence-based management strategies for prevention and treatment
- discuss the midwife's care of the mother and family unit, during and immediately following separation and expulsion of the placenta and membranes.

PHYSIOLOGICAL PROCESSES

The third stage of labour can be defined as the period from the birth of the baby to complete expulsion of the placenta and membranes. It involves the development of the relationship between mother, baby and father, the separation, descent and expulsion of the placenta and membranes, the control of haemorrhage from the placental site and the initiation of skin-to skin contact/ breastfeeding. Although traditionally, labour is divided into three distinct component parts to aid comprehension, it should be viewed as one continuous process. With this in mind, it is important to understand that the physiology of the third stage depends, in part, on what has happened during pregnancy as well as during the first and second stages of labour, and on the woman's basic level of health and wellbeing. The midwife's knowledge and evidence-based skills play a crucial role in ensuring that the care received by the woman works in harmony with, not against, the physiological processes.

The placenta may shear off during the final expulsive contractions accompanying the birth of the baby or remain adherent for some time. The third stage usually lasts between 5 and 15 min, but any period up to 1 h may be considered normal.

Separation and Descent of the Placenta
Mechanical Factors

The unique characteristic of uterine muscle lies in its power of retraction. During the second stage of labour, the uterine cavity progressively empties as the baby moves down, enabling the retraction process to accelerate and the myometrium in the upper segment to thicken (Patwardhan et al. 2015). Thus, by the beginning of the third stage, the placental site has already diminished in area by about 75%. As this occurs, the placenta becomes compressed and the blood in the intervillous spaces is forced back into the spongy layer

of the decidua basalis. Retraction of the oblique uterine muscle fibres exerts pressure on the blood vessels so that blood does not drain back into the maternal system. The vessels during this process become tense and congested. With the next contraction the distended veins burst and a small amount of blood seeps in between the thin septa of the spongy layer and the placental surface, stripping

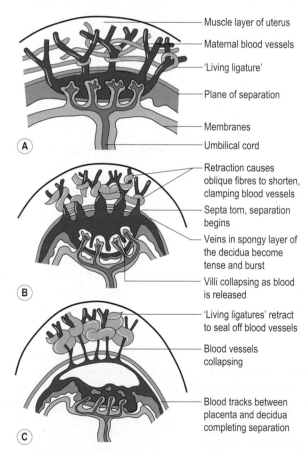

Fig. 21.1 The placental site during separation. (A) Uterus and placenta before separation. (B) Separation begins. (C) Separation is almost complete.

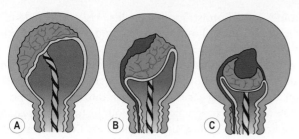

Fig. 21.2 The mechanism of placental separation. (A) Uterine wall is partially retracted, but not sufficiently to cause placental separation. (B) Further contraction and retraction thicken the uterine wall, reduce the placental site and aid placental separation. (C) Complete separation and formation of the retroplacental clot. *Note*: The thin lower segment has collapsed like a concertina following the birth of the baby.

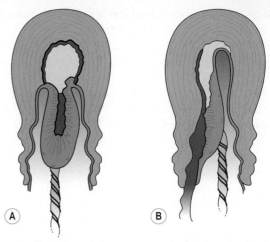

Fig. 21.3 Expulsion of the placenta. (A) Schultze method. (B) Matthews Duncan method.

it from its attachment (Fig. 21.1). As the surface area for placental attachment reduces, the relatively non-elastic placenta begins to detach from the uterine wall.

The majority of placentas are situated on the anterior or posterior wall of the uterus, and separation usually starts from the lower pole of the placenta and moves gradually upwards (Herman et al. 2002). Fundal placentas separate first at both poles, followed by the fundal part. The length of the third stage may be approximately 2 min shorter when the placenta is located at the fundus (Altay et al. 2007) and longer if it is anterior (Torricelli et al. 2015). If separation begins centrally, a retroplacental clot is formed (Fig. 21.2). This further aids separation by exerting pressure at the midpoint of placental attachment so that the increased weight helps to strip the adherent lateral borders and peel the membranes off the uterine wall so that the clot thus formed becomes enclosed in a membranous bag as the placenta descends, with the fetal surface presenting first. This process of separation (first described by Schultze) is associated with more complete shearing of both placenta and membranes and less fluid blood loss (Fig. 21.3A). If the placenta begins to detach unevenly at one of its lateral borders, the blood escapes so that separation is unaided as there is no formation of a retroplacental clot. The placenta descends, slipping sideways with the maternal surface presenting first. This process (first described by Matthews Duncan in the 19th century) takes longer and is associated with ragged, incomplete expulsion of the membranes and a higher fluid blood loss (Fig. 21.3B).

Once separation has occurred the uterus contracts strongly, forcing the placenta and membranes to fall into the lower uterine segment (Fig. 21.4), and finally, into the vagina.

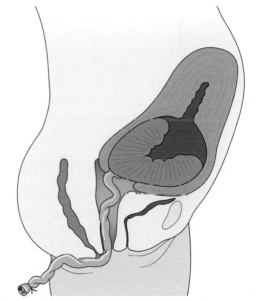

Fig. 21.4 Third stage: placenta in lower uterine segment.

Haemostasis

The normal volume of blood flow through the placental site is 500–800 mL/min, but this is considerably reduced once the baby is born and the placental site on the uterine wall has diminished. At placental separation, blood flow has to be arrested swiftly, or serious haemorrhage can occur. The interplay of four factors within the normal physiological processes that control bleeding are critical in minimizing blood loss and preventing maternal morbidity or mortality. They are:

1. Retraction of the oblique uterine muscle fibres in the upper uterine segment through which the tortuous blood vessels intertwine: the resultant thickening of the muscles exerts pressure on the torn vessels, acting as clamps, and preventing haemorrhage (Fig. 21.1). It is the absence of oblique fibres in the lower uterine segment that explains the greatly increased blood loss usually accompanying placental separation in placenta praevia.

2. The presence of vigorous uterine contraction following separation: this brings the walls into apposition so that further pressure is exerted on the placental site.

3. The achievement of haemostasis: there is a transitory activation of the coagulation and fibrinolytic systems during, and immediately following, placental separation. It is believed that this protective response is especially active at the placental site so that clot formation in the torn vessels is intensified. Following separation, the placental site is rapidly covered by a fibrin mesh utilizing 5–10% of circulating fibrinogen (Blackburn 2013).

4. Breastfeeding: the release of oxytocin from the posterior pituitary in response to skin-to-skin contact between mother and baby, and the baby's nuzzling at the breast, causes uterine contractions, which may assist in birthing the placenta, although it appears to have no difference on blood loss (Abedi et al. 2016).

CARING FOR A WOMAN IN THE THIRD STAGE OF LABOUR

Two methods of care may be used during the third stage, expectant (physiological) care or active management. It is ultimately the woman's decision as to how she would, ideally, prefer her birth plan to be followed in the third stage. She may have philosophical, religious or cultural beliefs that influence her decision. The attending midwife may also have views, based on evidence, as to the ideal method of care for the individual woman. Midwives should ensure that, in order to facilitate informed decision-making by the woman, adequate time for deliberation and questions is made available, during the course of routine antenatal consultations. The best available research information on care during the third stage of labour should be offered in an objective manner (Begley et al. 2019), supported by written information on the available care options for the woman in-keeping with the setting in which she intends to birth. Information on types of uterotonics, explanation of their different routes of administration, benefits, risks and side-effects involved and timing and method of placental birth should be given.

The midwife's care of the mother should be based on an understanding of the normal physiological processes including having access to as much information as possible about her pregnancy and labour history. Progress of the first and second stages of labour are likely to impact on management of the third stage of labour and should not be reviewed in isolation. The midwife's actions can make the third stage a wonderful, relaxing time of birth and can reduce the incidence of haemorrhage, infection, retained placenta and shock; any of which may increase maternal morbidity and even result in death. A mother's ability to withstand complications in the third stage of labour depends, to a large degree, upon her general health and the avoidance of debilitating, predisposing problems, such as anaemia, ketosis, exhaustion and prolonged hypotonic uterine action. Factors that may influence the incidence of haemorrhage are discussed in more detail later.

Detailed, accurate, contemporaneously written documentation is extremely important in all aspects of care, particularly in areas where evidence-based information is relied upon to assess whether due care has been delivered. In the case of third stage management, two examples might be: where a woman requests *expectant* (physiological) management of the third stage of labour (EMTSL), the midwife should clarify the circumstances in which this decision may be reversed (e.g. if severe bleeding should occur); where a woman requests *active* management (AMTSL), the midwife should clarify the circumstances in which this decision may be reversed (e.g. if the baby requires attention and the placenta separates before a uterotonic has been given). The woman's preference for care must be recorded in her notes antenatally, and a record of the discussion may be signed by the woman. It would be prudent for midwives to notify a senior colleague such as the Professional Midwife Advocate (PMA)/clinical supervisor, clinical manager or the attending medical practitioner if any of the woman's requests are contrary to local guidelines.

Expectant (or Physiological) Care during the Third Stage of Labour

In expectant management (EMTSL), the normal, physiological mechanisms of labour are supported and no routine actions (such as administration of a uterotonic drug, or clamping of the umbilical cord) are carried out.

A study of the reported actions of 27 expert midwives (who used EMTSL in at least 30% of births, and had recorded PPH rates of <4%) identified the key actions that they believed led to success when using EMTSL (Begley et al. 2012). A synthesis of these actions, some of which are supported by other research also, provides the following instructions for best practice when using EMTSL:

1. Maintain a calm, quiet, warm environment. Use warmed sheets or blankets to wrap mother and baby together, skin-to-skin. This close contact, and the baby's eventual nuzzling at the breast, will stimulate oxytocin release, which may shorten the third stage of labour and increase long-term breastfeeding rates (Moore et al. 2016).

2. Encourage the woman to adopt a comfortable, semi-upright position (at least a 45 degree angle) to assist placental separation by maintaining a gentle downward weight.

3. Facilitate this time of parent–baby discovery and attachment by minimizing noise and limiting conversation, observing from a distance and not interfering with the physiological processes.

4. Watch and wait. Take cues from the woman's behaviour; if she is alert and happy, examining the baby and talking, she is not bleeding excessively or in need of any intervention. Reassurance can also be obtained by discretely assessing the woman's pulse until there are signs of placental separation.

5. Signs of placental separation:
   • The woman may fidget, facially grimace, or state that she has a contraction.
   • A large 'gush' of blood may follow, indicating partial or complete separation of the placenta. It usually ceases after 10–20 s, especially if the placenta has separated completely and the uterus has contracted well. This gush is larger than that seen when a uterotonic is given routinely, and midwives need to develop an understanding of this physiological blood loss and not rush to administer oxytocic treatment unnecessarily.

6. Signs of placental descent:
   • The woman may wriggle, change position, or complain of pressure or a pain in her lower back or bottom.
   • The cord may lengthen and/or the walls of the vulva may bulge as the placenta descends.

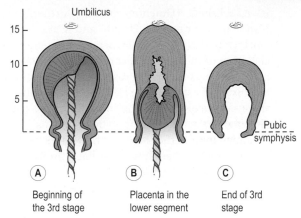

Fig. 21.5 Fundal height relative to the umbilicus and symphysis pubis.

• The uterus becomes hard, round and mobile (Fig. 21.5). This can be seen visually, or by the fact that the baby, resting on the mother's abdomen, has moved downwards. It is inadvisable to touch or manipulate the uterus at this stage, as this can prevent full contraction, disturb the fibrin mesh, and cause excessive bleeding. If there is concern that the uterus may be filling up with blood (a concealed haemorrhage), a gentle hand placed on the fundus will detect if there is a large, soft, uncontracted uterus.

7. Birthing the placenta:
   • Gravity should be used during the birth of the placenta by encouraging a truly upright position: sitting on a birthing stool, standing up in the birthing pool or on the birthing mat, walking out to the toilet, sitting on the toilet, kneeling upright or squatting over a bedpan. A basin, bin bag or disposable sheet can be placed strategically over, or in, the pan of the toilet to receive the placenta. It should be noted that such positions increase visible blood loss (Gupta et al. 2017), more so in women who have perineal damage (de-Jonge et al. 2007).
   • Maternal effort can be used to expedite expulsion, and as soon as they feel pressure, most women will push the placenta out with little effort.
   • The cord should be left unclamped until pulsation ceases (McDonald et al. 2013), or until after the birth of the placenta, unless the mother wishes it to be cut earlier. At a minimum, the cord should be left unclamped for 3–4 min after respiration

is established (Hutchon 2013). Furthermore, National Institute for Health and Care Excellence (NICE 2017a,b) guidance recommend that clamping of the umbilical cord should be delayed between 1 and 5 min, unless the heart rate of the baby is <60 beats per min and is not increasing or there is concern about the integrity of the cord. Any low intervention resuscitation of the baby can be undertaken at the site of birth, with the benefit of continued oxygen flow to the baby through the umbilical cord (Hutchon 2013).

- If the placenta is definitely separated and is situated just inside the vagina (i.e. the insertion of the cord can be seen at the vulva, or the cord has lengthened and the vulval walls are bulging) the midwife may ease gently on the cord to help lift out the placenta (Begley et al. 2012). **This is NOT controlled cord traction as no force is used.** The placenta is separated and has left the uterus, therefore no counter-pressure is required on the abdomen as there is no risk of uterine inversion. **Controlled cord traction should NEVER be used in the absence of a well-contracted uterus following uterotonic administration.**

- Any trailing membranes should be teased out gently, by turning the placenta around and twisting them into a 'rope', thus stripping the ends gently from the uterine wall.

8. At any time, a uterotonic may be administered to control haemorrhage, or if uterine tone is poor following placental birth. It is preferable to withhold administration until the birth of the placenta has occurred to avoid the incidence of a retained placenta when the uterus contracts strongly in response to the treatment. This spontaneous process can take from 10 min to 1 h to complete, with a median of 13 min (Begley 1990). The longer the placenta remains in the uterus, the greater the incidence of bleeding becomes because the uterus cannot contract down fully while the bulk of the placenta is *in situ*. Magann et al. (2005) found that the incidence of PPH increased after 18 min following the birth of the baby. However, patience and confidence not to interfere unnecessarily are required on the part of the midwife to secure a successful conclusion.

Active Management of the Third Stage of Labour

Active management in the third stage (AMTSL) is the policy of third stage of labour management most widely practised throughout the developed world. In the past, an active management policy included the routine prophylactic administration of a uterotonic agent, either intravenously, intramuscularly or (occasionally) orally, as a precautionary measure aimed at reducing the incidence of postpartum haemorrhage. It was often applied regardless of the assessed obstetric risk status of the woman, and was usually undertaken in conjunction with clamping of the umbilical cord shortly after birth of the baby and the placenta and membranes are born by controlled cord traction (CCT). In situations where women are assessed as being more susceptible to PPH (e.g. multiple birth), a prophylactic infusion of larger doses of uterotonics diluted in intravenous solutions may be administered over several hours following the birth. This would also be considered to be part of an active management policy, as would routine uterine massage following birth of the placenta in some countries (Jangsten et al. 2011), although there is no evidence to support this practice once an oxytocic has been given (Hofmeyr et al. 2013) and no reduction in postpartum haemorrhage has been shown (Saccone et al. 2018). Uterine massage is no longer recommended to prevent PPH (Mavrides et al. 2016).

Like all interventions performed, skill in assisting the birth of the placenta and membranes is extremely important to prevent complications. Whether women should routinely receive uterotonic drugs, have the umbilical cord clamped or be given assistance with the birth of the placenta, has been the subject of a great deal of debate and many research trials. These three aspects are considered separately here.

Administration of Uterotonics

Uterotonics (also known as oxytocics or ecbolics), are drugs (e.g. Syntometrine, Syntocinon, ergometrine and prostaglandins) that stimulate the smooth muscle of the uterus to contract. They may be administered with crowning of the baby's head (Soltani et al. 2010), at the birth of the anterior shoulder of the baby, or immediately after the birth of the baby and before the cord is clamped and cut (NICE 2017a), or following the birth of the baby, or after the placenta and membranes have been born. **Administration at crowning of the baby's head is seldom used now in high-income countries except in very exceptional circumstances (e.g. a woman with very low haemoglobin or a bleeding disorder), when the birth of a singleton baby is definitely imminent.**

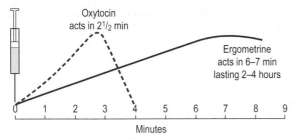

Fig. 21.6 The rapid action of oxytocin in comparison with ergometrine.

In practice, one of the following uterotonic drugs is usually used.

Intravenous ergometrine (0.25–0.5 mg). This drug acts within 45 s of administration, and is particularly useful in securing a rapid contraction where hypotonic uterine action results in haemorrhage. If a doctor is not present in such an emergency, a midwife may give the injection, if it is within their scope of practice. There is no evidence for the continued *routine* use of intravenous ergometrine, which is associated with an increased incidence of retained placenta (Begley 1990), so this drug is more often used to treat a PPH rather than as a prophylactic drug. Ergometrine can cause headache, nausea, vomiting and an increase in blood pressure (Begley 1990) and it is contraindicated where there is a history of hypertensive disorder or cardiac disease (Gallos et al. 2018). To decrease the incidence of nausea and vomiting when the woman has had a caesarean section under epidural, it is advisable not to use ergometrine on its own (Balki and Carvalho 2005).

Combined ergometrine and oxytocin (commonly syntometrine). A 1 mL ampoule of Syntometrine contains 5 IU of oxytocin and 0.5 mg ergometrine and is administered by intramuscular injection. The oxytocin acts within 2.5 min and the ergometrine within 6–7 min (Fig. 21.6). Their combined action results in a rapid uterine contraction enhanced by a stronger, more sustained contraction lasting several hours. It can be administered as the anterior shoulder of the baby is born, or after the birth of the baby. The use of combined ergometrine/oxytocin or any ergometrine-based drug is associated with side-effects such as elevation of blood pressure, nausea and vomiting (Begley 1990). Consequently, the report from the Centre for Maternal and Child Enquiries (CMACE) relating to maternal deaths in the UK advocated that Syntometrine should be completely avoided as a routine drug (CMACE 2011).

CAUTION: No more than two doses of ergometrine 0.5 mg should be given, due to its side-effects.

Oxytocin. Oxytocin (Syntocinon being a common brand) is a synthetic form of the natural oxytocin produced in the posterior pituitary, and is safe to use in a wider context than combined ergometrine/oxytocin agents. It can be administered as an intravenous and/or intramuscular injection, but is usually given as an intramuscular dose of 10 IU, in most high-income countries. No clear difference has yet been shown when comparing benefits and risks of giving oxytocin by the intravenous or intramuscular route, to prevent PPH after vaginal birth (Oladapo et al. 2018). However, an intravenous bolus of oxytocin can cause profound, fatal hypotension, especially in the presence of cardiovascular compromise. The recommendation of the Confidential Enquiry in Maternal Deaths (Lewis and Drife 2001) to slowly administer the drug intravenously in a dose of not more than 5 IU, still remains the best practice principle.

Carbetocin. Carbetocin, originally developed for veterinary use and, until recently, not widely employed for prophylactic use in management of the third stage of labour, is a long-acting synthetic oxytocin analogue, which can be administered as a single-dose 100 mg injection. It requires refrigeration for stability, and is cheaper than other uterotonics (Luni et al. 2017).

Prostaglandins. The use of prostaglandins for the third stage of labour management has up until now, been associated more with the treatment of postpartum haemorrhage than with prophylaxis. This may be partly due to prostaglandin agents being more expensive and associated with side-effects, such as diarrhoea (Gallos et al. 2018) and cardiovascular complications of increased stroke volume and heart rate (Van-Selm et al. 1995).

Misoprostol (a prostaglandin E1 analogue) was first used to treat gastric ulcers, but when its potential as a uterotonic agent was discovered, optimism regarding its suitability in low resource settings was high. It is cheap, not prone to loss of potency, does not need to be sterile or refrigerated and can be administered vaginally, orally or rectally, negating the need for syringes. Misoprostol orally or sublingually (400–600 μg) appears to be a useful drug to prevent PPH, but is not as effective on its own as Syntocinon (Ng et al. 2007; Tunçalp et al. 2012) and has unpleasant side-effects, such as severe shivering and higher temperature, both of which are transient but unacceptable to some women. Its use appears to be no more likely than Syntocinon to necessitate manual removal of the placenta, so it may be useful in circumstances where nothing else is available (Tunçalp et al. 2012).

A Cochrane network analysis compared all available uterotonics and found that three drugs, or drug combinations, were more effective than oxytocin at preventing postpartum haemorrhage of >500 mL: ergometrine plus oxytocin, Carbetocin, and misoprostol plus oxytocin. None of the drugs tested were better at preventing postpartum haemorrhage of >1000 mL than oxytocin. Carbetocin had the least side-effects of all uterotonics (Gallos et al. 2018).

Clamping of the Umbilical Cord

This may be carried out following the birth of the baby's head, as a necessity if the cord is tightly around the neck; however, it is preferable, and often possible, to loosen the loop of cord and slip it over the baby's head, then allow the baby's body to move out beside the loop. If the cord is looped several times around the neck it will be possible to gently tighten one, or more, of the loops of cord and then ease a looser loop over the baby's head. In this way, the baby's oxygen supply is not cut off prematurely, which would be very detrimental to their condition. If this is not successful, the midwife should be ready to clamp and cut the cord just as the woman experiences the next contraction, so that the oxygen supply is only cut off just before the baby is born.

Early clamping of the cord, as part of active management of the third stage of labour (AMTSL), was usually applied in the first 30 s to 3 min after the baby was born, regardless of whether or not cord pulsation had ceased. However, this is no longer recommended as it may have the following effects:

- It may reduce the volume of blood returning to the fetus by an amount between 75 and 125 mL (van-Rheenen and Brabin 2004; Farrar et al. 2011), which is 30–40% of total potential blood volume (Farrar et al. 2011).
- It may prematurely interrupt the respiratory function of the placenta in maintaining O_2 levels and combating acidosis in the early moments of life. This may be of particular importance in a baby who is slow to breathe (Hutchon 2013).
- It may result in lower neonatal bilirubin levels, although the effect on the incidence of clinical jaundice is unclear (McDonald et al. 2013) and some studies show no difference (Mercer et al. 2017).

- It may increase the likelihood of fetomaternal transfusion as a larger volume of blood remains in the placenta (Mercer et al. 2017). Venous pressure is further increased as retraction continues and may be sufficiently high to rupture surface placental vessels, thus facilitating the transfer of fetal cells into the maternal system; this may be a critical factor where the mother's blood group is Rhesus negative (see Chapter 11).
- It results in the truncated umbilical vessels containing a quantity of clotted blood, which provides an ideal medium for bacterial growth; as this is near to, and has a patent opening into the baby's abdomen there is potential for systemic infection (Mercer et al. 2006).
- Heavier placental weight has also been associated with early cord clamping (Newton et al. 1961), which may cause difficulty with birth of the placenta, particularly when the cervix has contracted following administration of a uterotonic.

Proponents of **late** clamping suggest that no action be taken until cord pulsation ceases or the placenta has been completely expelled, thus allowing the physiological processes to take place without intervention. Suggested advantages of late clamping include:

- The route to the low resistance placental circulation remains patent, which provides the baby with a safety valve for any raised systemic blood pressure. This may be critical when the baby is preterm or asphyxiated, as raised pulmonary and central venous pressures may exacerbate the difficulties in initiating respiration and accompanying circulatory adaptation (Dunn 1985).
- The transfusion of the full quota of placental blood to the baby. This may constitute as much as 30–40% of the circulating volume (Farrar et al. 2011), depending on when the cord is clamped and at what level the baby is held prior to clamping and may therefore be important in maintaining haematocrit levels.
- The neonatal effects associated with increased placental transfusion include higher mean birth weight by 87–116 g (Farrar et al. 2011), increased blood pressure and cerebral oxygenation at 12 h (Katheria et al. 2017) and higher neonatal haematocrit accompanied by an increase in the incidence of jaundice in term (McDonald et al. 2013) and preterm babies (Rabe et al. 2012). There is growing evidence that delaying cord clamping confers improved iron status in infants up to 6 months post-birth (Hutton and

Hassan 2007; Andersson et al. 2011; McDonald et al. 2013; Ashish et al. 2017).

- Delayed cord clamping in preterm babies (until at least 30–120 s) is associated with babies requiring fewer transfusions, and having a lower chance of developing necrotizing enterocolitis or intraventricular haemorrhage (Rabe et al. 2012), and improves overall outcomes (Duley et al. 2018).
- Delayed cord clamping may decrease the chance of fetomaternal transfusion, which is important in women with Rhesus-negative blood (Wiberg et al. 2008).

Given the benefits of delayed cord clamping and the documented harms caused by early clamping, many centres have now stopped using early cord clamping as part of their active management package (Afaifel and Weeks 2012). Clamping between 1 and 5 min is recommended (NICE 2017b), despite growing evidence that delaying cord clamping until it turns white: i.e. *'Wait for White'*, is beneficial for the baby.

The actual action to take when clamping the cord early is to place one clamp (usually a disposable plastic one) close to the baby's navel end. Care should be taken to apply the clamp 3–4 cm clear of the abdominal wall, to avoid pinching the skin or clamping a portion of gut, which, in rare instances, may be in the cord. A greater length of cord is left when umbilical vessels are needed for transfusion, for example in preterm babies and cases of Rhesus haemolytic disease. The second clamp is placed closer to the placental end of the cord, with approximately 2–4 cm between them. The cord between the two clamps is then cut, while shielding personnel from blood spurts with a gloved hand. There is very little evidence concerning how much, if any, of a uterotonic agent the baby receives through an intact cord following birth. In five documented cases of accidental administration of an adult dose of Syntometrine to a newborn infant, no long-term adverse effects were reported (Whitfield and Salfield 1980). However, prudence would suggest that the uterotonic should be withheld until after the cord is clamped and cut. If the cord is clamped and cut soon after birth, the midwife should release the second clamp and drain blood from the maternal end of the cord to simulate placental–fetal transfusion, as this may reduce maternal blood loss up to 77 mL and shorten the third stage by up to 3 min (Soltani et al. 2011).

The Birth of the Placenta and Membranes

Controlled cord traction. Continuing research has shown that CCT has no effect on severe haemorrhage (>1000 mL) and little, if any, effect on mild PPH (>500 mL) in both high- (Deneux-Tharaux et al. 2013) and low-income countries (Gülmezoglu et al. 2012). It does, however, shorten the third stage of labour by 6 min. This means that, particularly in low-income countries, oxytocin can be given by healthcare workers, without the need to train them in safe utilization of CCT (Gülmezoglu et al. 2012; Hofmeyr et al. 2015), providing that they are taught to avoid manipulating the uterus or pulling on the cord.

If CCT is to be used successfully, the principles of placental separation described at the beginning of this chapter should be clearly understood. Before proceeding, the midwife should check:

- that a uterotonic drug has been administered
- that it has been given time to act
- that the uterus is well contracted
- that counter-traction is applied
- that signs of placental separation and descent are present.

At the beginning of the third stage, a strong uterine contraction results in the fundus being palpable below the umbilicus (Fig. 21.5). It feels broad as the placenta is still in the upper segment. As the placenta separates and falls into the lower uterine segment, there is a small fresh blood loss, the cord lengthens and the fundus becomes rounder, smaller and more mobile as it rises in the abdomen above the level of the placenta.

It is important not to manipulate the uterus in any way as this may precipitate incoordinate action. No further step should be taken until a strong contraction is palpable. If tension is applied to the umbilical cord without this contraction, uterine inversion may occur. This is an acute obstetric emergency with life-threatening implications for the mother (see Chapter 25) that can result in death.

Once the uterus is found to be contracted, one hand is placed above the level of the symphysis pubis with the palm facing towards the umbilicus, exerting pressure in an upwards direction. This is counter-traction. The other hand, firmly grasping the cord, applies traction in a downward and backward direction following the line of the birth canal (Fig. 21.7). Some resistance may be felt but it is important to apply steady tension by pulling the cord firmly and maintaining the pressure. Jerky movements and force should be avoided. The aim is to complete the action as one continuous, smooth, controlled movement. However, it is only possible to exert

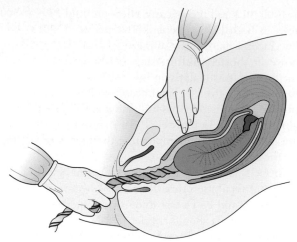

Fig. 21.7 Controlled cord traction (CCT).

this tension for a short time, as it may be an uncomfortable procedure for the mother, and the midwife's hand will tire.

Downward traction on the cord must be released before uterine counter-traction is relaxed, as sudden withdrawal of counter-traction while tension is still being applied to the cord may also facilitate uterine inversion. If the manoeuvre is not immediately successful there should be a pause before the contractibility of the uterus is reassessed and a further attempt is made. Should the uterus relax, tension is temporarily released until a further contraction is palpable. Once the placenta is visible, it may be cupped in the hands to ease pressure on the friable membranes. A gentle upward and downward movement or twisting action will help to coax out the membranes and increase the chances of them being expelled intact. Artery forceps may be applied to gradually ease the membranes out of the vagina. This process should not be hurried; great care should be taken to avoid tearing the membranes, as this can increase the incidence of PPH (Keating et al. 2018).

The Timing of Uterotonic Administration, Cord Clamping and/or CCT
The impact on the incidence of PPH
Although active management of the third stage of labour leads to a reduced incidence of PPH, it is important to establish which of the components of this package contribute(s) to this reduction. Given the difficulties of adhering to an active management policy, the absence of uterotonics in low-resource countries, and the

preferences of some women for physiological management, it is important to explore practice behaviours to clarify whether or not the policy, as it is currently practised, should continue.

Whether oxytocin is administered before or after the placenta is expelled does not appear to make any significant difference to the incidence of PPH, maternal hypotension, retained placenta, length of the third stage of labour, mean blood loss, maternal haemoglobin, need for maternal blood transfusion or therapeutic uterotonics (Soltani et al. 2010).

Similarly, CCT has no effect on severe haemorrhage and little, if any, effect on mild PPH (Gülmezoglu et al. 2012). Given the emerging evidence on the benefits of delaying cord clamping (McDonald et al. 2013), it is now reasonable to suggest an active management package that includes cord clamping after 3 min, waiting for the cord to turn white, followed by administration of oxytocin (either before or after the birth of the placenta) and either maternal effort or controlled cord traction to expel the placenta once separation occurs. If AMTSL has not been implemented in the first 3 or more minutes, the principles of care described for expectant care during the third stage of labour should be followed during that period.

Evidence for Active Versus Expectant Management
There is an increasing amount of appropriate, rigorously conducted research evidence available that suggests that the prophylactic administration of a uterotonic significantly reduces the incidence of PPH, results in a lower mean blood loss, fewer blood transfusions and a reduced need for therapeutic uterotonics (Begley et al. 2019). It has also been highlighted by the widely ranging 'risk status' of women included in several studies that it is in fact very difficult to define a group of women who are not at risk for PPH. However, women truly at 'low risk' for PPH do not appear to suffer undue harm from EMTSL (Dixon et al. 2011; Begley et al. 2019), and this should remain an option for care (NICE 2017a). Student midwives should be provided with the opportunity to experience births where EMTSL is practised, to learn and develop such skills, as the International Confederation of Midwives (ICM 2017) consider knowledge of physiological (expectant) care and management of the third stage of labour is a basic midwifery competency.

It should be noted that the care pathway, whether active or expectant, is reliant on all components of the pathway being carried out as recommended. For example, if management is expectant, then the introduction of a uterotonic drug, cord clamping or pulling on the cord will disrupt the intended sequence of the entire process leading to what is often described as a fragmented approach. Once the sequence of the process is altered, the midwife should commit to completing the process. That is, if the protocol for expectant management is interrupted, the midwife should proceed to completing the process with an active management approach. This practice has been shown to significantly reduce the incidence of PPH in a birth centre setting (Patterson 2005).

Asepsis

The need for asepsis is even greater in the third stage of labour than in the preceding stages of labour. Any laceration and bruising of the cervix, vagina, perineum and vulva will provide a route for the entry of microorganisms. At the placental site, a raw surface provides an ideal medium for infection. Strict attention to the prevention of infection is therefore vital.

Cord Blood Sampling

This may be required for a variety of conditions:

- when the mother's blood group is Rhesus-negative or as a precautionary measure if the mother's Rhesus type is unknown;
- when atypical maternal antibodies have been found during an antenatal screening test;
- where a haemoglobinopathy is suspected (e.g. sickle cell disease);
- when there has been any concern about the baby in labour or immediately after birth.

The sample should be taken as soon as possible from the fetal surface of the placenta where the blood vessels are congested and easily visible. If the cord has not been clamped prior to placental birth the fetal vessels will not be congested, but a sample of sufficient volume may still be easily obtained, or can be taken by syringe prior to the birth of the placenta. In the case of paired cord blood sampling being required for reasons outlined by NICE (2017a), blood will be obtained from the umbilical cord. To achieve this, an additional clamp will need to be applied resulting in double-clamping of the cord. The appropriate containers should be used for any investigations requested. These may include the baby's blood group, Rhesus type, haemoglobin estimation, serum bilirubin level, cord blood analysis for acid base status, Coombs' test or electrophoresis. Maternal blood for Kleihauer testing can be taken upon completion of the third stage of labour.

COMPLETION OF THE THIRD STAGE OF LABOUR

Once the placenta has spontaneously birthed, or has been delivered, the midwife must first assess that the uterus is well contracted and fresh blood loss is minimal. Careful inspection of the perineum and lower vagina is important. A strong light is directed onto the perineum in order to assess trauma accurately prior to instigating repair. This should be carried out as gently as possible as the tissues are often bruised and oedematous. If perineal suturing (see Chapter 17) is required it should be carried out as expediently as possible to prevent unnecessary blood loss, increased risk of oedema at the site of trauma and unnecessary re-infiltration of additional local anaesthetics.

Blood Loss Estimation

Blood loss is difficult to measure and is frequently underestimated (Prasertcharoensuk et al. 2000; Hancock et al. 2015). Account must be taken of any blood that has soaked into linen and swabs as well as measurable fluid loss and clot formation. The site of the blood loss does not necessarily alter the impact in terms of potential debility for affected women. Brandt (1966) believes that most women can withstand around a 1000–1500 mL blood loss. However, any further blood loss may not be tolerated so readily. Women who undergo elective caesarean section should for the most part have been adequately prepared, but those who undergo emergency caesarean section or a vaginal birth who are dehydrated or anaemic are less likely to withstand sudden large volumes of blood loss.

In his study of the importance and difficulties of precise estimation of PPH, Brandt (1967) calculated that 20% of women lose >500 mL of blood after a vaginal birth. Furthermore, it was estimated that 3940 mL of circulating blood volume were required to maintain the central venous pressure at 10 cm H_2O. Most measurement techniques are not sufficiently sensitive to detect a rapid volume change in the immediate setting when decisions need to be made.

Note: It should also be remembered that any amount of blood loss, however small, that causes a physical deterioration in the woman's condition, such as feeling faint, sudden onset of tachycardia, altered respirations or fall in blood pressure, should always be immediately investigated.

Examination of the Placenta and Membranes

The placenta and membranes should be examined as soon after birth as practicable so that, if there is doubt about their completeness, further action may be taken before the woman leaves the birth room or the midwife leaves the home. A thorough inspection must be carried out in order to ensure that no part of the placenta or membranes has been retained. The membranes are the most difficult to examine, as they can become torn during the birth or delivery and may be ragged. Every attempt should be made to piece them together to give an overall picture of completeness. This is easier to see if the placenta is held by the cord, allowing the membranes to hang. The hole through which the baby was born can then usually be identified and a hand can be spread out inside the membranes to aid inspection (Fig. 21.8). The placenta should then be laid on a flat surface and both placental surfaces examined in a good light. The amnion should be peeled from the chorion right up to the umbilical cord, which allows the chorion to be fully viewed.

Any clots on the maternal surface need to be removed and kept for measuring. Broken fragments of cotyledon must be carefully replaced before an accurate assessment is possible.

The lobes of a complete placenta fit neatly together without any gaps, the edges forming a uniform circle. Blood vessels should not radiate beyond the placental edge. If they do, this denotes the presence of a succenturiate lobe, which has developed separately from the main placenta (see Chapter 6). When such a lobe is visible there is no cause for concern, but if the tissue has been retained the vessels will end abruptly at a hole in the membrane. If there is any suspicion that the placenta or membranes are incomplete, they must be kept for inspection and a doctor informed immediately in case a PPH occurs or there is the possibility that a surgical intervention may be required.

Upon completion of the examination, the midwife should return her attention to the mother. The empty uterus should be firmly contracted and below the level

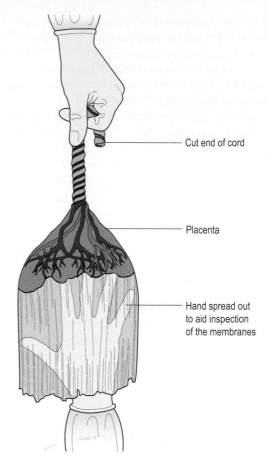

Fig. 21.8 Examination of the membranes.

of the umbilicus. If the fundus has risen in the abdomen, a blood clot may be present. This should be expelled while the uterus is in a state of contraction by pressing the fundus gently in a downward and backward direction – with due regard to the risk of inversion and acute discomfort to the woman. Force should never be used.

Immediate Care

It is advisable for mother and baby to remain in the midwife's care for at least 1 h after birth, regardless of the birth setting. Much of this time will be spent in clearing up and completion of records but careful observation of mother and baby is very important. If an epidural catheter is *in situ* it is usually removed and checked for completeness at this time. Early physiological observations including ensuring a well-contracted uterus, assessment of vaginal blood loss and a gentle inspection of the genital tract to inspect for trauma should be undertaken (NICE 2017a).

The woman should be encouraged to pass urine because a full bladder may impede uterine contraction. She may not actually feel an urge to do so, especially if she has passed urine immediately prior to giving birth or an effective epidural has been in progress, but she should be encouraged to try. Uterine contraction and blood loss should be continually assessed during this first hour. Once basic procedures to ensure the mother's and baby's safety and comfort have been completed, the mother may be offered a light meal such as tea and toast.

Most women intending to breastfeed will put their babies to the breast during these early moments following the birth. This is especially advantageous, as babies are usually very alert at this time and their sucking reflex is particularly strong. There is also evidence to suggest that women who experience early skin-to-skin contact with their babies, successfully breastfeed for a longer period of time (Moore et al. 2016). An additional benefit lies in the reflex release of oxytocin from the posterior lobe of the pituitary gland, which stimulates the uterus to contract. This may result in the mother experiencing a sudden fresh blood loss as the uterus empties and she should be pre-warned and reassured that it is a normal response. The desire to feed a newborn baby is a warm, loving and instinctive response. While early skin-to-skin contact should be encouraged to assist newborn babies in maintaining their own body temperature, midwives must respect the mother's choice of feeding and that some may have decided not to breast feed.

Record-Keeping

A complete and accurate account of the labour, including the documentation of the administration of all medicines, physical examination and observations, is the midwife's responsibility. This should also include details of the examination of the placenta, membranes and umbilical cord, with attention drawn to any abnormalities. The volume of blood loss is particularly important. This record not only provides information that may be critical in the future care of both mother and baby but is a legal document that may be used as evidence of the care given. Signatures are therefore essential, with co-signatories where necessary. In the UK, the majority of women carry their own notes relating to pregnancy with details of the birth. The completed records are a vital communication link between the midwife responsible for the birth and other caregivers, particularly those who take over care and provide ongoing community support services once the woman returns home.

It is usually the midwife who completes the birth notification form. Timely notification and referral may prevent delay in a woman receiving appropriate assistance should she require it.

Transfer from the Birth Room

The midwife is responsible for seeing that all observations are made and recorded prior to transfer of mother and baby to the postnatal ward, or home, or before the midwife leaves the home following the birth. The postnatal ward midwife should verify these details prior to the transfer of mother and baby. Following a home birth, the midwife should leave details of a telephone number where she may be contacted should the parents feel any cause for concern before the next planned home visit.

COMPLICATIONS OF THE THIRD STAGE OF LABOUR

Postpartum Haemorrhage

Primary postpartum haemorrhage is defined as a blood loss of ≥500 mL that occurs within 24 h after birth (WHO 2012). A loss of 500–999 mL in a healthy woman is considered a mild PPH, and severe haemorrhage is deemed to be a loss of >1000 mL (Begley et al. 2019).

Postpartum haemorrhage (PPH) is one of the most alarming and serious emergencies a midwife may face and can occur following both traumatic and straightforward births. It is always a stressful experience for the woman and those supporting her at the birth and may undermine her confidence, influence her attitude to future childbearing and lead to a variety of physical and emotional problems (Carroll et al. 2016). Although the maternal mortality rate (MMR) in high-income countries such as those of Germany, Australia, USA and Japan is quoted as approximately 6, 6, 14 and 5 per 100,000 live births, respectively (WHO 2018b), the reported MMR for lower-income countries is much higher; for example, Afghanistan with 396 per 100,000 live births, and Nigeria with 814 per 100,000 live births (WHO 2018b). A significant number of the deaths recorded in low-income countries were due to PPH, often in the absence of a trained health professional. The midwife is often the first, and may be the only, professional person present when a haemorrhage occurs, so her prompt, competent action will be crucial in controlling blood loss and reducing the risk of maternal morbidity or even death.

Primary Postpartum Haemorrhage

Fluid loss is extremely difficult to measure with any degree of accuracy, especially when a mixture of blood and fluid has soaked into the bed linen and may have also spilled onto the floor. It should also be remembered that measurable solidified clots represent only about half the total fluid loss. With these factors in mind, the best yardstick is that any blood loss, however small, that adversely affects the mother's condition constitutes a PPH. Much will therefore depend upon the woman's general wellbeing. In addition, if the measured loss reaches 500 mL, it must be treated as a PPH, irrespective of maternal condition; however, it should be noted that in high-income countries, and in a woman who is otherwise healthy with a high haemoglobin level, a blood loss of 500 mL is the equivalent of a routine blood donation and usually causes no ill-effects.

Causes

There are several reasons why a PPH may occur, including atonic uterus, retained placenta, trauma and blood coagulation disorder.

Atonic uterus. This is a failure of the myometrium at the placental site to contract and retract and to compress torn blood vessels and control blood loss by a living ligature action (Fig. 21.9). When the placenta is attached, the volume of blood flow at the placental site is approximately 500–800 mL/min. Upon separation, the efficient contraction and retraction of uterine muscle will staunch the flow and prevent a haemorrhage, which can otherwise ensue with horrifying speed (Box 21.1).

Incomplete placental separation. If the placenta remains fully adherent to the uterine wall, it is unlikely to cause bleeding. However, once separation has begun, maternal vessels are torn. If placental tissue remains partially embedded in the spongy decidua, the contraction and retraction mechanism is interrupted.

Retained placenta, cotyledon, placental fragment or membranes. These will similarly impede efficient uterine action (Sosa et al. 2009; Keating et al. 2018).

Precipitate labour. When the uterus has contracted vigorously and frequently, resulting in a duration of labour that is <1 h, then the muscle may have insufficient opportunity to retract.

Prolonged labour. In a labour where the active phase lasts >12 h, uterine inertia (sluggishness) may result from muscle exhaustion (see Chapter 22).

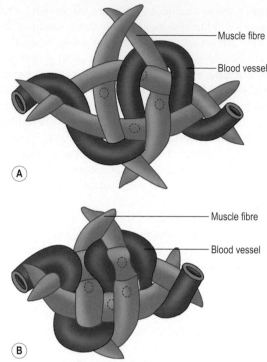

Fig. 21.9 Living ligatures – How the blood vessels run between the interlacing muscle fibres of the uterus (A) relaxed, (B) contracted. (With permission from S MacDonald, G Johnson (Eds) Mayes Midwifery. Edinburgh: Elsevier 2017.)

> ### BOX 21.1 Causes of Atonic Uterine Action
>
> - Incomplete separation of the placenta
> - Retained cotyledon, placental fragment or membranes
> - Precipitate labour
> - Prolonged labour resulting in uterine inertia
> - Polyhydramnios or multiple pregnancy causing overdistension of the uterine muscles
> - Placenta praevia
> - Placental abruption
> - General anaesthesia especially halothane or cyclopropane
> - Episiotomy or perineal trauma
> - Induction or augmentation of labour with oxytocin
> - A full bladder
> - Aetiology unknown.

Polyhydramnios, macrosomia or multiple pregnancy. The myometrium becomes excessively stretched and its contractibility is therefore less efficient (Sosa et al. 2009).

Placenta praevia. The placental site is partly or wholly in the lower segment where the thinner muscle layer contains few oblique fibres, resulting in poor control of bleeding. In the 2017 UK Maternal Mortality Report, there were nine deaths attributed to placenta praevia or accreta (Knight et al. 2017).

Placental abruption. Blood may have seeped between the muscle fibres, interfering with effective action. At its most severe, this results in a Couvelaire uterus/uterine apoplexy (see Chapter 14).

Induction or augmentation of labour with oxytocin. In some circumstances, the use of oxytocin during labour may result in hyperstimulation of the uterus and cause a precipitate, expulsive birth of the baby (Sosa et al. 2009; Grotegut et al. 2011). In this instance, the uterus may still be responding in a stimulated, but ineffective manner in terms of contracting the empty uterus. Hyperstimulation remains a notable cause of postpartum haemorrhage resulting in cases of maternal mortality/morbidity (Knight et al. 2019). In the case of induction or augmentation of labour that continues over a prolonged period there is increased incidence of severe postpartum haemorrhage (Belghiti et al. 2011).

Episiotomy, and need for perineal suturing. Blood loss from perineal trauma, in addition to even a normal blood loss from the uterus, can together equal a mild PPH (Sosa et al. 2009). Shmueli et al. (2016) have shown that an episiotomy is associated with a 70% increased incidence of a postpartum haemorrhage.

General anaesthesia. Anaesthetic agents may cause uterine relaxation, in particular the volatile inhalational agents, for example halothane.

Mismanagement of the third stage of labour. 'Fundus fiddling' or manipulation of the uterus may precipitate arrhythmic contractions so that the placenta only partially separates and retraction is lost.

A full bladder. If the bladder is full, its proximity to the uterus in the abdomen on completion of the second stage of labour may interfere with uterine action in terms of its powers to contract. This would constitute mismanagement on the part of the attending health professional, should a PPH result.

> **BOX 21.2 Predisposing Factors that Might Increase the Incidence of Postpartum Haemorrhage**
>
> - Previous history of postpartum haemorrhage or retained placenta
> - Presence of fibroids
> - Maternal anaemia
> - Ketoacidosis
> - Multiple pregnancy
> - HIV/AIDS
> - Caesarean section.

Aetiology unknown. A precipitating cause may never be discovered.

There is in addition a number of factors that do not directly cause a PPH, but do increase the likelihood of excessive bleeding (Box 21.2).

Previous history of PPH or retained placenta. There may be a chance of recurrence in subsequent pregnancies, depending on the cause of the PPH in the previous birth. A detailed obstetric history taken at the first antenatal visit will ensure that optimum care can be given.

Fibroids (fibromyomata). These are normally benign tumours consisting of muscle and fibrous tissue, which may impede efficient uterine action.

Anaemia. Women who commence labour with a reduced haemoglobin concentration (<10 g/dL) may feel a greater effect of any subsequent blood loss, however small. Moderate to severe anaemia (<9 g/dL) is associated with an increase in blood loss during the third stage of labour with the risk of postpartum haemorrhage (Soltan et al. 2012).

HIV/AIDS. Women who have HIV/AIDS are often in a state of severe immunosuppression, which lowers the platelet count to such a degree that even a relatively minor blood loss may cause severe morbidity or death.

Ketosis. The influence of ketosis upon uterine action is still unclear and there is little research in this area. Foulkes and Dumoulin (1983) demonstrated that, in a series of 3500 women, 40% had ketonuria at some time during labour. They reported that if labour progressed well, this did not appear to jeopardize either the fetal or maternal condition. However, there was a significant relationship between ketosis and the need for oxytocin augmentation, instrumental birth and PPH when labour lasted >12 h. Prevention of ketosis is therefore advisable and can be facilitated by encouraging an adequate intake of fluids and light solid food throughout labour, depending on how much the woman can tolerate. There is **no** evidence to suggest restriction of food or fluids is necessary during the physiological process of labour (Singata et al. 2013).

Caesarean section. Green et al. (2016) highlight that in 1 year in the UK, a total of 181 women required more than 8 units of red blood cells within 24 h of giving birth, and of these, 69% had undergone a caesarean section birth. Furthermore, CMACE (2011) detail that during the period 2006–08, there were five women who died of postpartum haemorrhage, four of whom had undergone a caesarean section. The report noted that in three of the four women (75%), a lack of routine observation of vital signs in the postoperative period, or failure on the part of staff to notice that bleeding was occurring, were key failures in care. It is essential that postoperative observations following caesarean section are recorded regularly, using a modified early obstetric warning score (MEOWS) chart, and any abnormal findings promptly acted upon (CMACE 2011).

Signs of PPH

Signs may be obvious, such as:
- visible bleeding
- maternal collapse.

However, more subtle signs may present, such as:
- pallor
- rising pulse rate
- falling blood pressure
- altered level of consciousness; the mother may become restless or drowsy
- an enlarged uterus as it fills with blood or blood clot; it feels 'boggy' on palpation (i.e. soft and distended and lacking tone); there may be little or no visible loss of blood.

Prophylaxis

By using the above list, the midwife is in a position to recognize causative factors and identify women who may be more susceptible to PPH and thus attempt to reduce/prevent excessive bleeding following the birth of the baby. During the antenatal period, a thorough and accurate history of previous obstetric experiences will identify vulnerable women. Arrangements for the birth can be discussed with the woman, and the necessity for the baby to be born in a unit where facilities to respond to emergencies are available can be explained. The early

detection and treatment of anaemia will help to improve the woman's haemoglobin level, ideally, in excess of 10 g/dL, prior to the onset of labour. Women more prone to anaemia should be closely monitored, e.g. those with multiple pregnancies.

During labour, good management practices within the first and second stages of labour are important to prevent prolonged labour and ketoacidosis. A woman should be regularly encouraged to empty her bladder throughout the entire labour process to avoid interference with the physiological contractibility processes. AMTSL is recommended for all women susceptible to PPH, and will reduce blood loss for women of mixed risk (Begley et al. 2019). Two units of cross-matched blood should be kept available for any woman known to have a placenta praevia or other major predisposing factors for PPH.

Treatment of PPH

Whatever the stage of labour or crisis that may occur, the midwife should adhere to the underlying principle of always reassuring the woman and the persons supporting her by continually relaying appropriate information and involving them in decision-making.

Three basic principles of care should be applied immediately upon observation of excessive bleeding, using the mnemonic **ABC**:
1. Call for appropriate **A**id.
2. Stop the **B**leeding by rubbing up a contraction, giving a uterotonic and emptying the uterus.
3. Resus**C**itate the mother as necessary.

Call for medical aid. This is an important initial step so that help is on the way whatever transpires. If the bleeding is brought under control before appropriate assistance arrives (e.g. doctor, paramedic), then no action by the healthcare professional will be required. However, the mother's condition can deteriorate very rapidly, in which case medical assistance will be required urgently. If the mother is at home or in a stand-alone midwife-led birthing unit, the emergency department of the closest obstetric unit should be contacted and a paramedic/obstetric emergency team summoned and ambulance transfer arranged.

Stop the bleeding. The initial action is always the same regardless of whether bleeding occurs with the placenta *in situ* or not.

Rub up a contraction. Assist the woman to lie flat, with one pillow. The fundus is first felt gently with the fingertips to assess its consistency. If it is soft and relaxed, the fundus is massaged with a smooth, circular motion, applying no undue pressure. When a contraction occurs, the hand is held still.

Administer a uterotonic to sustain the contraction. In many instances, oxytocin 5 units or 10 units, or combined ergometrine/oxytocin 1 mL, will have already been administered and this may be repeated. Alternatively, ergometrine 0.25–0.5 mg may be injected intravenously (in the absence of contraindications), and will be effective within 45 s; vomiting may occur immediately. No more than two doses of ergometrine should be given (including any dose of combined ergometrine/oxytocin), as it may cause pulmonary hypertension. Several reports have described the dramatic haemostatic effects of prostaglandins used in cases of uterine atony. Misoprostol (Cytotec) or carboprost (Hemabate) are the most common prostaglandin drugs used to increase uterine contractility for the treatment of PPH. However, the side-effects (nausea, vomiting, pyrexia, hypertension, diarrhoea) associated with these drugs can make their use limited (Gallos et al. 2018).

The baby may be put to the breast to enhance the physiological secretion of oxytocin from the posterior lobe of the pituitary gland, thus stimulating a contraction. A warm blanket covering the mother will help maintain body heat.

Empty the uterus. Once the midwife is satisfied that the uterus is well contracted, they should ensure that it is emptied. If the placenta is still in the uterus, it should be delivered; if it has been expelled, any clots should be expressed by firm but gentle pressure on the fundus.

Resuscitate the mother. An intravenous infusion should be started while peripheral veins are easily negotiated. This will provide a route for an oxytocin infusion or fluid replacement with warmed crystalloid infusion. At the same time, a 20 mL blood sample should be taken for group and screen, full blood count and coagulation screen, including fibrinogen (Mavrides et al. 2016). As an emergency measure, the woman's legs may be raised in order to allow blood to drain from them into the central circulation. However, the foot of the bed should not be raised as this encourages pooling of blood in the uterus, which prevents the uterus contracting.

It is usually expedient to catheterize the bladder to ensure that a full bladder is not impeding uterine contraction and thus precipitating further bleeding, and to minimize trauma should an operative procedure be necessary. Observations of pulse, blood pressure and respiratory rate should be undertaken and recorded at 15-min intervals until the woman's condition has stabilized.

On no account must a woman in a collapsed condition be moved prior to resuscitation and stabilization.

The flowchart in Fig. 21.10 briefly sets out the possible courses of action that may be taken depending on whether or not bleeding persists. If the above measures are successful in controlling any further loss, administration of oxytocin, 40 units in 1 litre of intravenous solution (e.g. Hartmann's or saline) infused slowly over 8–12 h, will ensure sustained uterine contraction. This will help to minimize the incidence of any recurrence. If bleeding continues uncontrolled, the major obstetric haemorrhage policy of the unit should be instituted. The choice of further action will depend largely upon whether the placenta remains in situ.

Placenta has delivered. If the uterus is atonic following birth of the placenta, light fundal pressure may be used to expel residual clots while a contraction is present. If an effective contraction is not maintained, 40 units of Syntocinon in 1 litre of intravenous fluid should be started. The placenta and membranes must be re-examined for completeness because retained fragments are often responsible for uterine atony (Keating et al. 2018) and may need to be removed manually, under anaesthetic.

Bimanual compression. If bleeding continues, bimanual compression of the uterus may be necessary in order to apply pressure to the placental site. It is desirable for an intravenous infusion to be in progress. Following explanation to, and permission from the woman, the gloved fingers of one hand are inserted into the vagina like a cone; the hand is formed into a fist and placed into the anterior vaginal fornix, the elbow resting on the bed. The other hand is placed behind the uterus abdominally, the fingers pointing towards the cervix. The uterus is brought forwards and compressed between the palm of the hand positioned abdominally and the fist in the vagina (Fig. 21.11). If bleeding persists, a clotting disorder must be excluded before exploration of the vagina and uterus is performed under a general anaesthetic. Compression balloons may also be used to provide pressure on the placental site (Anderson et al. 2017) and if bleeding continues, ligation of the uterine arteries or hysterectomy may be considered.

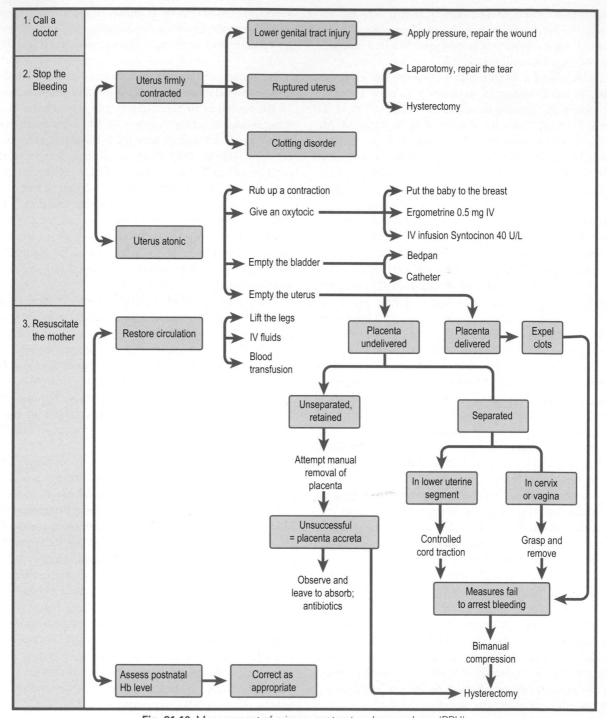

Fig. 21.10 Management of primary postpartum haemorrhage (PPH).

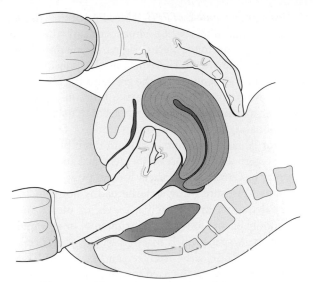

Fig. 21.11 Bimanual compression of the uterus.

Placenta is undelivered. The placenta may be partially or wholly adherent.

Partially adherent. When the uterus is well contracted, an attempt should be made to deliver the placenta by applying CCT. If this is unsuccessful a doctor will be required to remove it manually.

Wholly adherent. Bleeding does not usually occur if the placenta is completely adherent. However, the longer the placenta remains in the uterus the greater is the incidence of partial separation, which may give rise to profuse haemorrhage.

Retained placenta. This diagnosis is reached when the placenta fails to birth after a specified period of time (usually 1 h following the baby's birth). The conventional treatment is to separate the placenta from the uterine wall digitally, effecting a manual removal under epidural or general anaesthetic.

Breaking of the cord. This is not an unusual occurrence during completion of the third stage of labour. Before further action, it is crucial to assess that the uterus remains firmly contracted. If the placenta remains adherent, no further action should be taken before a doctor is notified. It is possible that manual removal may be indicated. If the placenta is palpable in the vagina, it is probable that separation has occurred and when the uterus is well contracted then maternal effort, with a fully upright posture, may be encouraged (see expectant management, above). If there is any doubt, the midwife applies fresh sterile gloves before performing a vaginal examination to ascertain whether this is so. As a last resort, if the woman is unable to push effectively, then gentle fundal pressure may be used, following permission from the woman, administration of a uterotonic drug and pain relief such as self-administered nitrous oxide and oxygen. Great care is exercised to ensure that placental separation has already occurred and the uterus is well contracted. The woman should be relaxed as the midwife exerts gentle downward and backward pressure on the firmly contracted fundus. This method, if abused, can cause considerable pain and distress to the woman and result in the stretching and bruising of supportive uterine ligaments. If it is performed without good uterine contraction, acute uterine inversion may ensue. This is an extremely dangerous procedure in unskilled hands and is not advocated in everyday practice when alternative, safer methods may be employed. It is highly unlikely that this would be practised in the UK.

Manual removal of the placenta. This should be carried out by a skilled practitioner/doctor. An intravenous infusion must first be sited and an effective anaesthetic in progress. The choice of anaesthesia will depend upon the woman's general condition. If an effective epidural anaesthetic is already in progress, a top-up may be given in order to avoid the hazards of general anaesthesia. A spinal anaesthetic offers an alternative but where time is an urgent factor a general anaesthetic will be initiated.

Management. Manual removal is performed with full aseptic precautions and, unless in a dire emergency situation, should not be undertaken until the woman has received adequate analgesia. With the left hand, the umbilical cord is held taut while the right hand is coned and inserted into the vagina and uterus following the direction of the cord. Once the placenta is located the cord is released so that the left hand may be used to support the fundus abdominally, to prevent rupture of the lower uterine segment (Fig. 21.12). The operator will feel for a separated edge of the placenta. The fingers of the right hand are then extended and the border of the hand is gently eased between the placenta and the uterine wall, with the palm facing the placenta. The placenta is carefully detached with a sideways slicing movement. When it is completely separated, the left hand rubs up a contraction and expels the right hand with the placenta in its grasp. The placenta should be checked immediately for completeness, so that any further exploration of the uterus may be carried out without delay. A uterotonic drug is given upon completion.

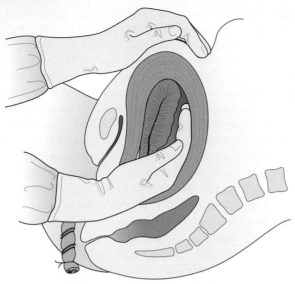

Fig. 21.12 Manual removal of the placenta.

In very exceptional circumstances, when no doctor is available to be called, a midwife would be expected to carry out a manual removal of the placenta. Once they have diagnosed a retained placenta as the cause of PPH, the midwife must act swiftly to reduce the incidence of onset of shock and exsanguination. It must be remembered that the incidence of inducing shock by performing a manual removal of the placenta is greater when no anaesthetic is given. In a mid- to high-income country, midwives are **unlikely** to find themselves dealing with this situation.

At home. If the placenta is retained following a home birth, emergency obstetric help must be summoned. **Under no circumstances should a woman be transferred to hospital until an intravenous infusion is in progress and her condition stabilized**. It is best if the placenta is born without moving the woman but if this is not possible, or if further treatment is needed, she should be transferred to a consultant-led unit, with her baby.

Morbid adherence of the placenta. Very rarely, the placenta remains morbidly adherent; this is known as *placenta accreta*. If it is totally adherent, then bleeding is unlikely to occur and it may be left *in situ* to absorb during the puerperium (Jauniaux et al. 2018). If, however, only part of the placenta remains embedded, then the incidence of fatal haemorrhage are high and an emergency hysterectomy may be unavoidable.

Trauma as a cause of PPH. If bleeding occurs, despite a well-contracted uterus, it is almost certainly the consequence of trauma to the uterus, vagina, perineum or labia, or a combination of these. Predictably, the longer the wait before repair is commenced, the greater is the blood loss.

The woman is assisted into the lithotomy position in order to identify the source of bleeding using a good directional light. An episiotomy wound or tears to the anterior labia, clitoris and perineum often bleed freely. These external injuries are easily identified and torn vessels may be clamped with artery forceps prior to ligation, if manual pressure using a sterile pad is not sufficient. Internal trauma to the vagina, cervix or uterus more commonly occurs following instrumental or manipulative birth. A speculum is inserted to enable the cervix and vagina to be clearly visualized and examined. Tissue or artery forceps may be used to apply pressure prior to suturing under general anaesthesia.

If bleeding persists when the uterus is well contracted and no evidence of trauma can be found, uterine rupture must be suspected. Following a laparotomy this is repaired, but if bleeding remains uncontrolled a hysterectomy may become inevitable.

Blood coagulation disorders causing PPH. As well as the causes already listed above, PPH may be the result of coagulation failure (see Chapters 14 and 15). The failure of the blood to clot is such an obvious sign that it can be overlooked in the midst of the frantic activity that accompanies torrential bleeding. It can occur following severe pre-eclampsia, antepartum haemorrhage, massive PPH, amniotic fluid embolus, intrauterine death or sepsis. Evaluation should include coagulation status and replacing appropriate blood components (Mavrides et al. 2016). Fresh blood is usually the best treatment, as this will contain platelets and the coagulation factors V and VIII. After 4 units of red cells, specific replacement products such as fresh frozen plasma and fibrinogen, to maintain a plasma fibrinogen level of >2 g/L throughout the time of PPH management, may be required (Mavrides et al. 2016).

Maternal Observation Following Postpartum Haemorrhage

Once bleeding is controlled, the total volume lost must be measured and/or estimated as accurately as possible. Large amounts appear less than they are in reality. A MEOWS chart should be maintained postpartum and abnormal scores should be reported and prompt action taken (CMACE 2011). Continuous monitoring of maternal pulse, blood pressure and respiratory rate is required (using oximeter, electrocardiogram and automated blood pressure recording) and the temperature should be taken every 4 h (Mavrides et al. 2016). The uterus should be palpated gently and frequently to ensure that it remains well contracted and lochia lost must be observed. Intravenous fluid replacement should be carefully calculated to avoid circulatory overload. Monitoring the central venous pressure (see Chapter 25) will provide an accurate assessment of the volume required, especially if blood loss has been severe. Fluid intake and urinary output (via indwelling urinary catheter) are recorded hourly as indicators of renal function.

The woman may need high dependency care if closer monitoring is required until her condition becomes stable (see Chapter 26). All records should be meticulously completed and signed contemporaneously. Continued vigilance will be important for 24–48 h. As this woman will need a period of recovery, she will not be suitable for early transfer home.

Secondary Postpartum Haemorrhage

Secondary postpartum haemorrhage is any abnormal or excessive bleeding from the genital tract occurring between 24 hours and 12 weeks postnatally. In high-income countries, 2% of women are admitted to hospital in the postnatal period with this condition, half of them undergoing surgical evacuation of the uterus (Alexander et al. 2007). Secondary PPH is most likely to occur between 10 and 14 days after birth, typically occurring during the second week. Bleeding is usually due to retention of a fragment of the placenta or membranes, or the presence of a large uterine blood clot. The lochia is heavier than normal and will have changed from a serous pink or brownish loss to a bright red blood loss. The lochia may also be offensive if infection is a contributory factor. Subinvolution of the uterus, pyrexia and tachycardia are usually present. As this is an event that is most likely to occur at home, midwives should alert women to the possible signs of secondary PPH prior to discharging them from midwifery care.

Management

The following steps should be taken:
- Call for medical assistance
- Reassure the woman and those supporting her
- Rub up a contraction by massaging the uterus if it is still palpable

- Express any clots from the uterus
- Encourage the woman to empty her bladder
- Give a uterotonic drug either by the intravenous or intramuscular route
- Keep all sanitary pads and linen to assess the volume of blood lost
- If bleeding persists, discuss a range of treatment options with the woman and, if appropriate, prepare her for theatre.

If the bleeding occurs at home and the woman has telephoned the hospital, midwife or her GP, she should be told to lie down flat until professional assistance arrives (the front door should be left unlocked if the woman is alone). On arrival, the doctor, midwife or paramedic will assess the amount of blood loss and the woman's condition and attempt to arrest the haemorrhage. If the loss is severe or uncontrolled, the nearest emergency obstetric unit will be called and the mother and baby prepared for transfer to hospital. The doctor, midwife or paramedic who attends should commence an intravenous infusion and ensure that the mother's condition is stable before transferring her from the home.

Careful assessment is usually undertaken prior to the uterus being explored under general anaesthetic. The use of ultrasound as a diagnostic tool is invaluable in minimizing the number of women who have operative intervention. If retained products of conception cannot be seen on a scan, the woman may be treated conservatively with antibiotic therapy and oral ergometrine. The haemoglobin should be estimated prior to discharge. If it is below 9 g/dL, options for iron replacement should be discussed with the woman. The severity of the anaemia will assist in determining the most appropriate care, which may be dependent on whether or not the woman is symptomatic (e.g. feeling faint, dizzy, short of breath). Management may vary from increased intake of iron-rich foods, iron supplements or, in extreme cases, blood transfusion. It is also important to discuss the common symptoms that may be experienced as a result of anaemia following PPH, including extreme tiredness and general malaise. The woman should be encouraged to seek assistance and contact her GP to assess her general health and haemoglobin levels.

Haematoma Formation

PPH may also be concealed as the result of progressive haematoma formation. This may be obvious at such sites as the perineum or lower vagina, but it is more difficult to diagnose if it occurs into the broad ligament or vault of the vagina. A large volume of blood may collect insidiously (up to 1 L). Involution and lochia are usually normal, the main symptom being increasingly severe maternal pain. This is often so acute that the haematoma has to be drained in theatre under a general anaesthetic. There is a strong possibility of the woman experiencing secondary infection.

Care After a Postpartum Haemorrhage

Whatever the cause of the haemorrhage, the woman will need the continued support of her midwife until she regains her confidence. Her partner may also be fearful of a recurrence and also requires much reassurance. Of women who have had a PPH between the third and sixth postnatal month, 6% report that their health status was worse than a year earlier, indicating that the sequelae of a haemorrhage can be long-lasting (Carroll et al. 2016). If the mother is breastfeeding, lactation may be impaired but this will only be temporary and she should be reassured that persevering will result in a return to normal lactation.

> **BOX 21.3   Key Issues in the Management of the Third Stage of Labour**
>
> - Implementation of well-documented research evidence into practice (e.g. delayed cord clamping particularly in neonates requiring resuscitation, avoidance of routine CCT, using EMTSL for women less susceptible to PPH) needs to be facilitated.
> - Care during the third stage of labour should not be viewed in isolation from what has occurred during the first and second stages of labour.
> - The development of the mother–baby–father relationship should be given priority.
> - The global PPH rate has not reduced significantly in the past decade, regardless of interventions applied.

CONCLUSION

Key issues in the management of the third stage of labour are summarized in Box 21.3.

REFLECTIVE ACTIVITY FOR SELF-ASSESSMENT

1. Consider what you have observed in practice in relation to the third stage of labour management. What are the significant issues you would raise with a woman when discussing expectant and active management of the third stage of labour? What evidence would you use to support your claims?

2. How confident are you in practising expectant management of the third stage of labour? Draw up an action plan that will support you to develop the knowledge and skill if your experience in expectant management is limited.

3. What are the benefits of delayed cord clamping? How does the policy and practice in your maternity unit compare with the current evidence and national guidance?

4. What would be your action should a woman for whom you have provided care in labour, proceeds to have a primary postpartum haemorrhage in the following settings:
   a. The home
   b. A stand-alone birthing unit
   c. A hospital birthing unit

REFERENCES

Abedi, P., Jahanfar, S., Namvar, F., et al. (2016). Breastfeeding or nipple stimulation for reducing postpartum haemorrhage in the third stage of labour. *Cochrane Database of Systematic Reviews* (1), CD010845.

Afaifel, N., & Weeks, A. (2012). Editorial: Active management of the third stage of labour: Oxytocin is all you need. *British Medical Journal, 345*, e4546.

Alexander, J., Thomas, P., & Sanghera, J. (2007). Treatments for secondary postpartum haemorrhage. *Cochrane Database of Systematic Reviews* (2), CD002867.

Altay, M. M., Ilhan, A. K., & Haberal, A. (2007). Length of the third stage of labor at term pregnancies is shorter if placenta is located at fundus: Prospective study. *Journal of Obstetrics and Gynaecology Research, 33*, 641–644.

Anderson, L., St Marie, P., Yadav, P., et al. (2017). The impact of Bakri balloon tamponade on the rate of postpartum hysterectomy for uterine atony. *Journal of Maternal-Fetal and Neonatal Medicine, 30*(10), 1163–1166.

Andersson, O., Hellström-Westas, L., & Andersson, D. (2011). Effect of delayed versus early umbilical cord clamping on neonatal outcomes and iron status at 4 months: A randomised controlled trial. *British Medical Journal, 343*, d7157.

Ashish, K. C., Rana, N., Malqvist, M., et al. (2017). Effects of delayed umbilical cord clamping vs early clamping on anemia in infants at 8 and 12 months: A randomized clinical trial. *Journal of the American Medical Association Pediatrics, 171*(3), 264–270.

Balki, M., & Carvalho, J. C. (2005). Intraoperative nausea and vomiting during cesarean section under regional anesthesia. *International Journal of Obstetric Anesthesia, 14*, 230–241.

Begley, C. M. (1990). A comparison of 'active' and physiological management of the third stage of labour. *Midwifery, 6*, 3–17.

Begley, C. M., Guilliland, K., Dixon, L., et al. (2012). Irish and New Zealand midwives' expertise in expectant management of the third stage of labour: The 'MEET' study. *Midwifery, 28*, 733–739.

Begley, C. M., Gyte, G. M., Devane, D., et al. (2019). Active versus expectant management for women in the third stage of labour. *Cochrane Database of Systematic Reviews* (2), CD007412.

Belghiti, J., Kayem, G., Dupont, C., et al. (2011). Oxytocin during labour and risk of severe postpartum haemorrhage: A population-based, cohort-nested case control study. *BMJ Open, 1*, e000514.

Blackburn, S. (2013). *Maternal fetal and neonatal physiology.* Missouri: Elsevier/Saunders.

Brandt, H. A. (1966). Blood loss at caesarean section. *Journal of Obstetrics and Gynaecology of the British Commonwealth, 73*, 456–459.

Brandt, H. A. (1967). Precise estimation of postpartum haemorrhage: Difficulties and importance. *British Medical Journal, 1*, 398–400.

Carroll, M., Daly, D., & Begley, C. M. (2016). The prevalence of women's emotional and physical health problems following a postpartum haemorrhage: A systematic review. *BMC Pregnancy and Childbirth, 16*, 261–271.

CMACE (Centre for Maternal and Child Enquiries). (2011). Saving Mothers' Lives: Reviewing maternal deaths to make motherhood safer 2006–2008. The Eighth Report on Confidential Enquiries into Maternal Deaths in the United Kingdom. *BJOG: An International Journal of Obstetrics and Gynaecology, 118*(Suppl. 1), 1–203.

de-Jonge, A., van Diem, M. T., Scheepers, P. L., et al. (2007). Increased blood loss in upright birthing positions originates from perineal damage. *British Journal of Obstetrics and Gynaecology, 114*(3), 349–355.

Deneux-Tharaux, C., Sentilhes, L., Maillard, F., et al. (2013). Effect of routine controlled cord traction as part of the active management of the third stage of labour on postpartum haemorrhage: Multicentre randomised controlled trial (TRACOR). *British Medical Journal, 346*, f1541.

Dixon, L., Fullerton, J., Begley, C., et al. (2011). Systematic review: The clinical effectiveness of physiological (expectant) management of the third stage of labour following a physiological labour and birth. *International Journal of Childbirth, 1*, 179–195.

Duley L, Dorling J, Pushpa-Rajah A, et al. (2018) Randomised trial of cord clamping and initial stabilisation at very preterm birth. *Archives of Disease in Childhood. Fetal and Neonatal Edition 103*:F14.

Dunn, P. M. (1985). Management of childbirth in normal women: The third stage and fetal adaptation. In *Perinatal medicine. Proceedings of the IX European Congress on Perinatal Medicine* (pp. 47–54). Dublin: MTP Press.

Farrar, D., Airey, R., Law, G. R., et al. (2011). Measuring placental transfusion for term births: Weighing babies with cord intact. *BJOG: An International Journal of Obstetrics and Gynaecology, 11*(8), 70–75.

Ford, J. B., Patterson, J. A., Seeho, S. K., et al. (2015). Trends and outcomes of postpartum haemorrhage, 2003–11. *BMC Pregnancy and Childbirth, 15*, 334.

Foulkes, J., & Dumoulin, J. G. (1983). Ketosis in labour. *British Journal of Hospital Medicine, 29*, 562–564.

Gallos, I. D., Papadopoulou, A., Man, R., et al. (2018). Uterotonic agents for preventing postpartum haemorrhage: A network meta-analysis. *Cochrane Database of Systematic Reviews, 12*, CD011689.

Green, L., Knight, M., & Seeney, F. M. (2016). The epidemiology and outcomes of women with postpartum haemorrhage requiring massive transfusion with eight or more units of red cells: A national cross-sectional study. *British Journal of Obstetrics and Gynaecology, 123*, 2164–2170.

Grotegut, C. A., Paglia, M. J., Johnson, L. N., et al. (2011). Oxytocin exposure in women with postpartum hemorrhage secondary to uterine atony. *American Journal of Obstetrics and Gynecology, 204*(1), 56.e1–56.e6.

Gülmezoglu, A. M., Lumbiganon, P., Landoulsi, S., et al. (2012). Active management of the third stage of labour with and without controlled cord traction: A randomised, controlled, non-inferiority trial. *Lancet, 379*, 1721–1727.

Gupta, J. K., Sood, A., Hofmeyr, G. J., & Vogel, J. P. (2017). Position in the second stage of labour for women without epidural anaesthesia. *Cochrane Database of Systematic Reviews* (5), CD002006.

Hancock, A., Weeks, A. D., & Lavender, T. (2015). Is accurate and reliable blood loss estimation the 'crucial step' in early detection of postpartum haemorrhage: An integrative review of the literature. *BMC Pregnancy and Childbirth, 15*, 230.

Herman, A., Zimerman, A., Arieli, S., et al. (2002). Down–up sequential separation of the placenta. *Ultrasound in Obstetrics and Gynecology, 19*, 278–281.

Hofmeyr, G. J., Abdel-Aleem, H., & Abdel-Aleem, M. A. (2013). Uterine massage for preventing postpartum haemorrhage. *Cochrane Database of Systematic Reviews* (7), CD006431.

Hofmeyr, G. J., Mshweshwe, N. T., & Gülmezoglu, A. M. (2015). Controlled cord traction for the third stage of labour. *Cochrane Database of Systematic Reviews, 1,* CD008020.

Hutchon, D. J. (2013). Early versus delayed cord clamping at birth; in sickness and in health. *Fetal and Maternal Medicine Review, 24,* 185–193.

Hutton, E. K., & Hassan, E. S. (2007). Late vs early clamping of the umbilical cord in full-term neonates: Systematic review and meta-analysis of controlled trials. *Journal of the American Medical Association, 297,* 1241–1252.

ICM (International Confederation of Midwives). (2017). *Role of the midwife in physiological third stage of labour.* The Hague: ICM.

Jangsten, E., Mattsson, L., Lyckestam, I., et al. (2011). A comparison of active management and expectant management of the third stage of labour: A Swedish randomised controlled trial. *BJOG: An International Journal of Obstetrics and Gynaecology, 118,* 362–369.

Jauniaux, E., Alfirevic, Z., Bhide, A. G., et al. On behalf of the Royal College of Obstetricians and Gynaecologists (2018). *Placenta praevia and placenta accreta: Diagnosis and management. Green-top Guideline No 27a.* London: RCOG.

Katheria, A. C., Brown, M. K., Faksh, A., et al. (2017). Delayed cord clamping in newborns born at term at risk for resuscitation: A feasibility randomized clinical trial. *Journal of Pediatrics, 187,* 313–317.e1.

Keating, J., Barnett, M., Watkins, V., et al. (2018). The association between ragged or incomplete membranes and postpartum haemorrhage: A retrospective cohort study. *The Australian and New Zealand Journal of Obstetrics and Gynaecology.* Available at: https://doi.org/10.1111/ajo.12775.

Knight, M., Nair, M., Tuffnell D., et al., Eds. On behalf of MBRRACE-UK. (2019). *Saving Lives, Improving Mothers' Care – Lessons learned to inform maternity care from the UK and Ireland Confidential Enquiries into Maternal Deaths and Morbidity 2013–2015.* Oxford: National Perinatal Epidemiology Unit, University of Oxford. Available at: https://www.npeu.ox.ac.uk/downloads/files/mbrrace-uk/reports/MBRRACE-UK%20Maternal%20Report%202017%20-%20Web.pdf.

Knight, M., Bunch, K., Tuffnell D., et al., Eds. On behalf of MBRRACE-UK. (2019). *Saving Lives, Improving Mothers' Care – Lessons learned to inform maternity care from the UK and Ireland Confidential Enquiries into Maternal Deaths and Morbidity 2015–2017.* Oxford: National Perinatal Epidemiology Unit, University of Oxford. Available at: https://www.npeu.ox.ac.uk/downloads/files/mbrrace-uk/reports/MBRRACE-UK%20Maternal%20Report%202019%20-%20WEB%20VERSION.pdf.

Lewis, G., & Drife, J. (Eds.). (2001). Why Mothers Die 1997–1999. *The Fifth Report of the Confidential Enquiries into Maternal Deaths in the United Kingdom.* London: RCOG Press.

Luni, Y., Borakati, A., Matah, A., et al. (2017). A prospective cohort study evaluating the cost-effectiveness of carbetocin for prevention of postpartum haemorrhage in caesarean sections. *Journal of Obstetrics and Gynaecology, 37*(5), 601–604.

Magann, F., Evans, S., Chauhan, S. P., et al. (2005). The length of the third stage of labor and the risk of postpartum hemorrhage. *Obstetrics and Gynecology, 105*(2), 290–293.

Mavrides, E., Allard, S., Chandraharan, E., & on behalf of the Royal College of Obstetricians and Gynaecologists., et al. (2016). Prevention and management of postpartum haemorrhage. *British Journal of Obstetrics and Gynaecology, 124,* e106–e149.

McDonald, S. J., Middleton, P., Dowswell, T., et al. (2013). Effect of timing of umbilical cord clamping of term infants on maternal and neonatal outcomes. *Cochrane Database of Systematic Reviews* (7), CD004074.

Mercer, J. S., Vohr, B. R., McGrath, M. M., et al. (2006). Delayed cord clamping in very preterm infants reduces the incidence of intraventricular hemorrhage and late-onset sepsis: A randomized, controlled trial. *Pediatrics, 117,* 1235–1242.

Mercer, J. S., Erickson-Owens, D. A., Collins, J., et al. (2017). Effects of delayed cord clamping on residual placental blood volume, hemoglobin and bilirubin levels in term infants: A randomized controlled trial. *Journal of Perinatology, 37,* 260–264.

Moore, E. R., Bergman, N., Anderson, G. C., et al. (2016). Early skin–to–skin contact for mothers and their healthy newborn infants. *Cochrane Database of Systematic Reviews, 11,* CD003519.

Newton, M., Mosey, L. M., Egli, G. E., et al. (1961). Blood loss during and immediately after delivery. *Obstetrics and Gynaecology, 17,* 9–18.

Ng, P. S., Lai, C. Y., Sahota, D. S., & Yuen, P. M. (2007). A double-blind randomized controlled trial of oral misoprostol and intramuscular Syntometrine in the management of the third stage of labor. *Gynecologic and Obstetric Investigations, 63,* 55–60.

NICE (National Institute for Health and Care Excellence). (2017a). *Intrapartum care: Care for healthy women and babies, CG 190.* London: NICE.

NICE (National Institute for Health and Care Excellence). (2017b). *Quality Statement 6 Delayed cord clamping in intrapartum care: QS 105.* London: NICE. Available at: https://www.nice.org.uk/guidance/qs105/chapter/Quality-statement-6-Delayed-cord-clamping.

Oladapo, O. T., Okusanya, B. O., & Abalos, E. (2018). Intramuscular versus intravenous prophylactic oxytocin for the third stage of labour. *Cochrane Database of Systematic Reviews* (9), CD009332.

Patterson, D. (2005). The views and experiences of childbirth educators providing a breastfeeding intervention during pregnancy. In *Proceedings of 27th Congress of the International Confederation of Midwives on 'Midwifery: Pathways to Healthy Nations.'* Brisbane, Australia.

Patwardhan, M., Hernandez-Andrade, E., Ahn, H., et al. (2015). Dynamic changes in the myometrium during the third stage of labor, evaluated using two-dimensional ultrasound, in women with normal and abnormal third stage of labor and in women with obstetric complications. *Gynecologic and Obstetric Investigation*, 80, 26–37.

Prastertcharoensuk, W., Swadpanich, U., & Lumbiganon, P. (2000). Accuracy of the blood loss estimation in the third stage of labor. *International Journal Gynecological Obstetrics*, 71, 9–70.

Rabe, H., Diaz-Rossello, J. L., Duley, L., et al. (2012). Effect of timing of umbilical cord clamping and other strategies to influence placental transfusion at preterm birth on maternal and infant outcomes. *Cochrane Database of Systematic Reviews* (8), CD003248.

Saccone, G., Caissutti, C., Ciardulli, A., et al. (2018). Uterine massage as part of active management of the third stage of labour for preventing postpartum haemorrhage during vaginal delivery: A systematic review and meta-analysis of randomised trials. *British Journal of Obstetrics and Gynaecology*, 125(7), 778–781.

Shmueli, A., Benziv, R. G., & Hiersch, L. (2016). Episiotomy – risk factors and outcomes. *Journal of Maternal-Fetal and Neonatal Medicine*, 30(3), 251–256.

Singata, M., Tranmer, J., & Gyte, G. M. (2013). Restricting oral fluid and food intake during labour. *Cochrane Database of Systematic Reviews* (8), CD003930.

Soltan, M. H., Ibrahim, E. M., Tawfek, M., et al. (2012). Raised nitric oxide levels may cause atonic postpartum hemorrhage in women with anemia during pregnancy. *International Journal of Gynecology and Obstetrics*, 116, 143–147.

Soltani, H., Hutchon, D. R., & Poulose, T. A. (2010). Timing of prophylactic uterotonics for the third stage of labour after vaginal birth. *Cochrane Database of Systematic Reviews* (8), CD006173.

Soltani, H., Poulose, T. A., & Hutchon, D. R. (2011). Placental cord drainage after vaginal delivery as part of the management of the third stage of labour. *Cochrane Database of Systematic Reviews* (9), CD004665.

Sosa, C. G., Althabe, F., Belizan, J. M., et al. (2009). Risk factors for postpartum hemorrhage in vaginal deliveries in a Latin-American population. *Obstetrics and Gynecology*, 113, 1313–1319.

Torricelli, M., Vannuccini, S., Moncini, I., et al. (2015). Anterior placental location influences onset and progress of labor and postpartum outcome. *Placenta*, 36(4), 463–466.

Tunçalp, Ö., Hofmeyr, G. J., & Gülmezoglu, A. M. (2012). Prostaglandins for preventing postpartum haemorrhage. *Cochrane Database of Systematic Reviews* (8), CD000494.

van-Rheenen, P., & Brabin, B. J. (2004). Late umbilical cord clamping as an intervention for reducing iron deficiency anaemia in term infants in developing and industrialized countries: A systematic review. *Annals of Tropical Paediatrics*, 24, 3–16.

Van-Selm, M., Kanhai, H. H., & Keirse, M. J. (1995). Preventing the recurrence of atonic postpartum haemorrhage: A double-blind trial. *Acta Obstetrica et Gynecologica Scandinavica*, 74, 270–274.

Whitfield, M. F., & Salfield, S. A. (1980). Accidental administration of Syntometrine in adult dosage to the newborn. *Archives of Disease in Childhood*, 55, 68–70.

WHO (World Health Organization). (2012). *WHO recommendations for the prevention and treatment of postpartum haemorrhage*. Geneva: WHO.

WHO (World Health Organization). (2018a). *Maternal mortality. Fact sheet*. Geneva: WHO. Available at: http://www.who.int/news-room/fact-sheets/detail/maternal-mortality.

WHO (World Health Organization). (2018b). *Maternal mortality country profiles*. Geneva: WHO. Available at: http://www.who.int/gho/maternal_health/countries/en/#U.

Wiberg, N., Kallen, K., & Olofsson, P. (2008). Delayed umbilical cord clamping at birth has effects on arterial and venous blood gases and lactate concentrations. *BJOG: An International Journal of Obstetrics and Gynaecology*, 115, 697–703.

ANNOTATED FURTHER READING

Begley, C. M., Gyte, G. M., Devane, D., et al. (2019). Active versus expectant management for women in the third stage of labour. *Cochrane Database of Systematic Reviews* (2), CD007412.

This is an update of a Cochrane Review last published in 2015, albeit it is relatively small in terms of the number of studies and participants. Its aim was to examine different ways in which the placenta and membranes are born following the birth of the baby; e.g. expectant, active or mixed management, in order to establish the benefits and harms for all women of these methods, specifically those at low risk of severe bleeding. The authors provide advice for health professionals to discuss with women about the third stage of labour management so they can make an informed decision.

Mercer, J. S., & Erickson-Owens (2014). Is it time to rethink cord management when resuscitation is needed? *Journal of Midwifery and Women's Health, 59*(6), 635–644.

This is an interesting paper that challenges the reader to re-think about their practice of cord management at the birth and prior to the third stage of labour. It proposes that receiving an adequate blood volume from placental transfusion, at birth, is protective for the neonate, especially when distressed and requires resuscitation. Placental transfusion plays a major role in neonatal transition by preventing hypovolemia and providing better perfusion to all organs and the authors recommend delay in cord clamping.

USEFUL WEBSITES

MBRRACE-UK: Mothers and Babies: Reducing Risk through Audits and Confidential Enquiries across the UK: https://www.npeu.ox.ac.uk/mbrrace-uk

National Institute for Health and Care Excellence: https://www.nice.org.uk/

Prevention of Postpartum Hemorrhage Initiative: https://www.path.org/resources/prevention-of-post-partum-hemorrhage

Resuscitation Council UK (RCUK): https://www.re-sus.org.uk/#

Wait for White: Optimal Cord Clamping: https://www.facebook.com/optimalclamping/

World Health Organization: https://www.who.int/

22

Prolonged Pregnancy and Variations of Uterine Action

Karen Jackson

CHAPTER CONTENTS

This chapter examines the evidence relating to prolonged pregnancy, induction of labour, prolonged labour and precipitate labour. Any decision with regards to the management of a pregnancy that continues beyond term is based on discussion between the woman and obstetrician, but the midwife is in a unique position to help the woman make sense of such discussions, thereby enabling her to make an informed decision based on informed choice. When labour is induced, ceases or slows down, the midwife remains in a key position to ensure the woman is kept informed so that she is enabled to continue to exercise her ability to be autonomous in the plan of care of her own labour and birth and the subsequent execution of that plan. The role of the midwife in the care of the woman is discussed throughout.

THE CHAPTER AIMS TO

- explore the issues relating to prolonged pregnancy with reference to research and other evidence
- outline the indications for the induction of labour and examine the methods used to induce labour in contemporary practice
- explore non-medical options to induce labour
- describe the process where labour slows down or ceases or is prolonged and review the current evidence used to support the management and care in such cases

- explore midwifery approaches when labour progress slows or ceases
- describe the serious complication that is obstructed labour and discuss the importance of competent midwifery management and care of women during

the antenatal and intrapartum periods if such complications are to be avoided

- highlight the significant events in a precipitate labour.

PROLONGED PREGNANCY

Much of the confusion when exploring the research and other evidence on pregnancies that go beyond the expected date of birth (EDB) and, more specifically, beyond 42 weeks (294 days), lies in the terms used to describe such pregnancies, which include *post-term* pregnancy, *prolonged* pregnancy and *postdates* pregnancy. According to Galal et al. (2012) post-term pregnancy is defined as a pregnancy where the gestation exceeds 42 completed weeks (294 days). This definition is also used by others when referring to prolonged pregnancy (National Institute for Health and Care Excellence, NICE 2008; Simpson and Stanley 2011). Middleton et al. (2018) refer to pregnancies that go beyond 294 days as **both** *post-term* and *postdates*.

What is clear is that all these terms refer to a specific gestation of the pregnancy and **not** the fetus or neonate. For the purposes of this chapter, the term **prolonged pregnancy** will be used to describe a pregnancy *equal to or beyond 42 weeks*. **Postmaturity** on the other hand, refers to a description of the neonate with peeling of the epidermis, long nails, loose skin suggestive of recent weight loss, an alert face and there may be meconium staining of the umbilical cord and nails (Stavis 2017). The relationship between *'prolonged pregnancy'* and *'postmaturity'* is explored later.

If prolonged pregnancy is defined by weeks of gestation, whether this is based on a calculation of the EDB using Naegele's rule or by ultrasound scan no later than 16 weeks, is to consider women as a homogenous group and neglects, among other things, the racial variations with shorter gestational age in South Asian and Black women (Balchin et al. 2007). If the anxiety pertaining to prolonged pregnancy is possible adverse neonatal outcome, then perhaps consideration needs to be made as to how prolonged pregnancy is defined for these groups of women. Laursen et al. (2004) suggest the notion of prolonged pregnancy as *'a normal variation of human gestation'*. Indeed Jukic et al. (2013) found that giving an exact *'due date'* is not based on any sound scientific evidence. They suggest it may be

better to inform women that for first time mothers, half will have given birth by 40 weeks and 5 days' gestation and for women who have given birth before, half will have given birth by 40 weeks and 3 days. According to Hovi et al. (2006) only a small proportion of prolonged pregnancies culminate in a baby that is postmature.

INCIDENCE

According to NICE (2008), the frequency or incidence of prolonged pregnancy is between 5% and 10%. The wide variation is a reflection of the disparate definitions as highlighted above; the number of women where EDB is uncertain and different induction policies (Simpson and Stanley 2011). Based on a definition of equal to or more than (≥)42 weeks, a true incidence of prolonged pregnancy is difficult to assess because in many cases a woman's labour is induced before reaching that time for specific complications in the pregnancy, for maternal request or because the pregnancy has gone beyond the EDB. Over a decade ago, the Department of Health (DH 2006), affirmed that prolonged pregnancy was the most common indication given for induction of labour (IOL) in England, accounting for approximately 46% of inductions overall. However, the figures from the National Health Service (NHS Digital 2018) do not provide the same breakdown of statistics and only identify an overall induction rate for England of 32.6% in 2017–2018.

The use of an early ultrasound scan to date the pregnancy (see Chapter 13), whether or not there is uncertainty with the last menstrual period (LMP), is thought by many to reduce the number of pregnancies categorized as prolonged (Ragunath and McEwan 2007; NICE 2008; Simpson and Stanley 2011; Tun and Tuohy 2011; Oros et al. 2012). Both accurately defining prolonged pregnancy and the accurate dating of a pregnancy is important if the woman is to be advised appropriately regarding the possible risks and benefits when discussing the options of expectant management or IOL where pregnancy is prolonged in order to avoid unnecessary intervention in an otherwise *'low-risk'* pregnancy.

Possible Implications for Mother, Fetus and Baby

In exploring the research and other evidence, a number of studies suggest there is an increase in perinatal mortality and morbidity as the pregnancy goes beyond 41 weeks (Hermus et al. 2009; Simpson and Stanley 2011; Cheyne et al. 2012; Oros et al. 2012; Middleton et al. 2018). While many authors acknowledge that the *absolute risk is small* (NICE 2008; McCarthy and Kenny 2010; Simpson and Stanley 2011; Cheyne et al. 2012; Middleton et al. 2018), this information almost appears as an afterthought and not worthy of further discussion. If prolonged pregnancy is to be perceived as a *complication* the possible *risks* need to be viewed from the perspectives of the mother, fetus and neonate with regards to morbidity and mortality.

Simpson and Stanley (2011) suggest that if a pregnancy continues beyond 41 completed weeks, the risks for the mother are associated with a large for gestational age or macrosomic infant such as shoulder dystocia, genital tract trauma, operative birth and postpartum haemorrhage (PPH). In an otherwise low-risk pregnancy, the risks must be balanced with the risks of IOL, such as increased requirement for epidural anaesthesia, uterine hyperstimulation, operative birth, PPH and unsuccessful induction (Ragunath and McEwan 2007; Hermus et al. 2009; Bailit et al. 2010; McCarthy and Kenny 2010; Jowitt 2012; Oros et al. 2012; Middleton et al. 2018).

According to Simpson and Stanley (2011), the possible risks for the fetus and neonate in a prolonged pregnancy appear to be two-fold: placental dysfunction linked to oligohydramnios, restricted fetal growth, meconium aspiration, asphyxia and still birth; conversely the cases where growth continues resulting in a macrosomic infant at risk of bony injury, soft tissue trauma, hypoxia and cerebral haemorrhage. The work of Fox (1997) suggests that the changes in the placenta over the course of pregnancy are part of a process of maturation and an increase in functional efficiency as opposed to a decrease in functional efficiency. Given that few post-term neonates exhibit signs of postmaturity, possible changes in placental function might be more appropriately linked to pregnancies where the neonate displays such characteristics rather than in prolonged pregnancies *per se* (Stavis 2017).

Predisposing Factors

Factors that might predispose a woman to a prolonged pregnancy include:
- obesity
- nulliparity
- family history of prolonged pregnancy
- male fetus
- fetal anomaly such as anencephaly (Olesen et al. 2006; Biggar et al. 2010; Arrowsmith et al. 2011; Morken et al. 2011; Simpson and Stanley 2011).

Cardozo et al. (1986) suggest there might be three subgroups related to a prolonged pregnancy, which include:
- those whose dates are incorrect
- those with a normal but prolonged gestation where physiological maturity is achieved after 42 weeks
- those with correct dates and are functionally mature but who do not go into labour at term.

Biggar et al. (2010), examining whether the spontaneous onset of labour is immunologically mediated, found the risk of prolonged pregnancy is higher in first pregnancies, but subsequently reduces with each following pregnancy where the biological father is the same. If there is a different father, the risk of prolonged pregnancy is as if it were a first pregnancy. Morken et al. (2011) further discovered there was a familial factor in relation to the recurrence of prolonged pregnancy across generations, involving both the mother and the father. Laursen et al. (2004) demonstrate a lower perinatal mortality rate in prolonged pregnancies, where the mother has had a previous prolonged pregnancy, which would appear to support a possible genetic influence with a prolonged gestation as a normal variation on human gestation.

PLAN OF CARE FOR PROLONGED PREGNANCY: THE DEBATE AND CONTROVERSY

The concept of a *plan of care* for prolonged pregnancy implies more of a facilitative approach, where the healthcare professional works in partnership with the woman to determine the most appropriate way forward with the pregnancy in order to ensure the optimum outcome for both mother and baby. In a prolonged pregnancy, where there are any obstetric or medical complications, the priority should always follow the practice for the specific complication with the woman's consent. If the pregnancy is otherwise low risk, the plan of care can follow an expectant or active approach. The decision on which approach to take should be based on gaining a genuinely informed decision from the woman (and partner), ensuring they understand the possible benefits and risks of each approach (NICE 2008; Jowitt 2012; Nursing and Midwifery Council, NMC 2018).

If a woman chooses the *expectant* approach, the recommendations from NICE (2008) are increased antenatal surveillance, which includes cardiotocography (CTG) at least twice a week, and an ultrasound scan to estimate the maximum amniotic fluid pool depth. This is instead of a more complex approach to antenatal fetal surveillance, which according to NICE (2008) includes computerized CTG, amniotic fluid index and assessment of fetal breathing, tone and gross body movements.

The use of a cervical membrane sweep (CMS) at 41 weeks' gestation has been shown to increase the spontaneous onset of labour before 42 weeks in some nulliparous and parous women (Mitchell et al. 1977; de Miranda et al. 2006). The purpose of CMS is to attempt to initiate the onset of labour physiologically thus avoiding the intervention of IOL using prostaglandin, artificial rupture of membranes (ARM) and oxytocin. CMS is designed to separate the membranes from their cervical attachment by introducing the examining fingers into the cervical os and passing them circumferentially around the cervix. The process of detaching the membranes from the decidua results in an increase in the concentration of circulating prostaglandins that may contribute to the initiation of the onset of labour in some individuals (Mitchell et al. 1977). Massage of the cervix can be used when the cervical os remains closed and this process may also cause release of local prostaglandin. If, after an appropriate time, labour has not started spontaneously, the process can be repeated. However, Putnam et al. (2011) found no conclusive evidence that increasing the frequency of CMS reduces IOL at 41 weeks' gestation. The practice of CMS is not associated with any increase in maternal or neonatal infection although women report more vaginal blood loss and painful contractions in the 24-h period following the procedure. Simpson and Stanley (2011) state that to avoid IOL in one woman, CMS would need to performed for seven women and suggest the benefit is therefore small. However, when one compares this to the evidence from Stock et al. (2012), who state that 1040 women would need to be induced to avoid one perinatal death, while leading to seven additional admissions to the special care baby unit, the *'odds'* for CMS as a possible means to initiate labour seem extremely favourable.

Menticoglou and Hall (2002) argue *that ritual induction* at 41 weeks is based on flawed evidence and interferes with a normal physiological situation. Heimstad et al. (2007) compared IOL at 41 weeks' gestation with expectant management and found no difference between the two groups with regards to neonatal morbidity or mode of birth. A number of authors cite evidence that, where there is an active approach and IOL is undertaken beyond 41 weeks, there is a reduction in perinatal mortality (NICE 2008; Simpson and Stanley 2011; Tun and Tuohy 2011). However, as stated above, many authors acknowledge that the *absolute risk of perinatal death is* **small** (NICE 2008; McCarthy and Kenny 2010; Simpson and Stanley 2011; Cheyne et al. 2012; Middleton et al. 2018). Oros et al. (2012) found that IOL at 41 weeks led to an increase in the length of hospital stay for the mother and an increase in the caesarean section rate.

The debate on the management of prolonged pregnancy centres on the disparate evidence with regards to fetal risk and neonatal outcome in terms of perinatal mortality and morbidity, and implementing a policy of *'management'* rather than a *'plan of care'* is designed to reduce these risks. When looking at the evidence surrounding postdates ($40+^0$ weeks to $41+^6$ weeks) and prolonged pregnancy (42 weeks), what is clear is that *'nothing is clear'*! There is a plethora of evidence but much of it is contradictory and couched in emotive terms. Reference is consistently made to the *'risks of'* prolonged pregnancy or the *'risk of'* recurrence of prolonged pregnancy, which seems to imply that a poor outcome is inevitable. NICE (2008) refers to the *risks of* prolonged pregnancy against the harms and benefits of IOL to avoid prolonged pregnancy. The mechanisms leading to the onset of labour remain largely unknown and the possibility of a prolonged pregnancy being a variation on human gestation within normal parameters should be considered.

Like many authors, NICE (2008) seem to imply there are no benefits to a prolonged pregnancy, which questions how nature can have really got it so wrong. The emphasis appears to be that in human parturition, an EDB is calculated, to which subsequent care revolves around, perpetuating the ongoing debate and controversy. A number of women will readily accept, and may even request IOL once they go beyond their EDB and that decision must be respected, but the decision to decline induction of labour must also be respected.

The Midwife's Role

The woman and her partner must be given clear and unbiased information pertaining to the benefits and possible risks of any proposed plan of care to enable them to make an informed decision based on all available options. It is clear from the literature that this is not always the case, and the woman is being directed towards IOL by overemphasizing the risks of prolonged pregnancy, while downplaying the risks associated with IOL (Gatward et al. 2010; Cheyne et al. 2012; Stevens and Miller 2012). While the obstetrician will take the lead in such cases, the midwife has a key role in facilitating the woman's right to autonomy by ensuring she has been given clear and unbiased information; that she fully understands the options available to her; and in appropriate cases, acting as the woman's advocate (NMC 2018). Women are put in an unenviable situation at an extremely vulnerable time in their lives and they expect, quite rightly, that the experts will assist them to make sense of the choices available to them. The midwife has a duty of care to assist women at this time. It is, however, important to understand that whatever plan of care is put in place in any pregnancy, it is not always possible to avoid a perinatal death.

See Box 22.1 for a summary of the key points relating to prolonged pregnancy.

INDUCTION OF LABOUR

Labour is the process whereby the uterine muscle contracts and retracts leading to effacement and dilatation of the cervix, the birth of the baby, expulsion of the placenta and membranes and the control of bleeding (see Chapters 19–21). It is only one part of the passage in the childbirth experience but for the majority of women and their partners, it is the singular most important part and the care they receive will always be remembered.

'Induction of labour' (IOL) is an intervention to initiate the process of labour by artificial means and involves the use of prostaglandins, amniotomy (artificial rupture of membranes/ARM), intravenous oxytocin, or any combination of these (World Health Organization, WHO 2011). It is the term used when initiating this process in pregnancies from 24 weeks' gestation, which is the legal definition of fetal viability in the UK (House of Commons Select Committee 2007). Where labour is being induced, a full assessment must be made to ensure that any intervention planned will confer more benefit than risk for both mother and baby.

There has been a steady rise in IOL in recent years, with statistics showing an IOL rate of 32.6% (NHS Digital 2018). In the UK, it is an intervention that has become

---

BOX 22.1   Key Points in Planning the Care in a Prolonged Pregnancy

- Any intervention whether it is induction of labour or augmentation of labour should be **clinically indicated;** the intervention should be *more effective* than nature and has no side-effects that would otherwise outweigh its benefits.
- Accurate EDB determined by LMP and early ultrasound reduces the incidence of pregnancies being diagnosed as *prolonged.*
- The length of gestation in some racial groups must also be considered with regards to a definition of prolonged pregnancy in these groups of women to improve perinatal outcomes.
- A membrane sweep can be offered from 40 weeks of pregnancy as a means to initiate the onset of spontaneous labour.
- Where there is any complication in a pregnancy approaching or beyond term, the priority in the plan of care should follow the practice for the specific complication.
- Where the woman makes the choice for expectant management, she must be informed that any deviations highlighted in antenatal surveillance will necessitate a review of the plan of care and the options available to her.

---

routine practice in maternity units within the National Health Service (NHS). When comparing IOL to a spontaneous onset of labour, evidence affirms that women experience a more painful labour, increasing the requirement for epidural anaesthesia and an assisted mode of birth (NICE 2008; WHO 2011). While a Cochrane review confirmed earlier findings that IOL is not associated with an increase in caesarean sections (Middleton et al. 2018), a population-based cross-sectional analysis of 42,950 thousand births, found IOL in medically uncomplicated nulliparous women at term carried a more than doubling of risk of emergency caesarean sections compared with spontaneous labour (Davey and King 2016). The decision therefore to induce labour should only be made when it is clear that a vaginal birth is the most appropriate outcome in the pregnancy, at that moment in time, for that particular woman and her baby.

Indications for Induction of Labour

IOL is considered when the maternal or fetal condition suggests that a better outcome will be achieved by intervening

BOX 22.2   Indications for Induction of Labour

Maternal

- *Prolonged pregnancy:* one that exceeds 42 completed weeks or 294 days. The commonest reason for induction of labour due to the increased risk of perinatal mortality and morbidity when the pregnancy continues beyond term, although the absolute risk is small.
- *Hypertension, including pre-eclampsia:* the decision to induce labour and expedite birth is made in the best interests of the woman and her baby. The timing of induction is influenced by the severity of her symptoms.
- *Diabetes:* the type and severity of diabetes influences the decision to induce. The risk of fetal macrosomia is increased where diabetic control is poor. In women with pre-existing type 1 and type 2 diabetes, the risk of adverse perinatal outcome is significantly increased (NICE 2015). Where the fetus is within the parameters for normal growth for gestational age, IOL is offered after 38 weeks' gestation.
- *Pre-labour rupture of membranes:* the longer the interval between membrane rupture and birth of the baby, the higher the risk of infection to both mother and fetus. For the majority of women spontaneous labour will commence within 24 h of rupture of membranes. Women should be offered the choice of IOL after 24 h, or expectant management (NICE 2008).
- *Maternal request:* may be for psychological or social reasons. For some women there are compelling reasons for requesting IOL when there is no clinical indication. In such cases it is important the woman is quite clear about the implications of such a decision. IOL may be considered from 40 weeks (NICE 2008).

Fetal

- *Fetal death:* if there are no complications such as spontaneous rupture of the membranes (SRM), infection or bleeding, the choice of immediate IOL or expectant management should be offered. Where there are complications, IOL is recommended.
- *Fetal anomaly not compatible with life.*

BOX 22.3   Some Contraindications for Induction of Labour

- Placenta praevia
- Transverse/oblique lie or compound presentation
- HIV-positive women not receiving any antiretroviral therapy or women on any antiretroviral therapy with a viral load of ≥400 copies/mL (RCOG 2010; NICE 2011)
- Active genital herpes
- Cord presentation or cord prolapse when vaginal birth is not imminent
- Known cephalo–pelvic disproportion (CPD)
- Severe acute fetal compromise.

in the pregnancy than by allowing it to continue, physiologically. This most commonly applies to cases where there are deviations from the normal physiological processes of childbirth as a result of hypertension, diabetes, fetal growth restriction or macrosomia. A list of some of the indications for IOL can be seen in Box 22.2, although this should not be considered as a definitive list. The mother may also request to have labour induced, although NICE (2008) state this should only be agreed in exceptional circumstances. Ultimately, the grounds on which the decision is made to induce labour must be sound enough to support the outcome whatever that outcome might be. There is no guarantee IOL will result in a vaginal birth or positive outcome for mother and/or her baby.

The contraindications for IOL are situations that preclude a vaginal birth in the best interests of the mother and/or baby. These are listed in Box 22.3.

Methods of Induction

The cervix must maintain its integrity during pregnancy and then undergo remodelling prior to labour. For an induction to be successful, the cervix needs to have undergone the changes that will ensure the uterine contractions are effective in the progressive effacement and dilatation of the cervix, descent of the presenting part and the birth of the baby.

The cervix is considered to be *ripe* when it has undergone these changes. The Bishop score, devised in the 1960s (Bishop 1964), is the means by which the ripeness of the cervix is assessed using a scoring that examines four features of the cervix and the relationship of the presenting part to the ischial spines. Each of these five elements is scored between 0 and 3 on vaginal examination (VE). The scoring system has been modified and it is this version that is used in contemporary practice (Table 22.1). While a score of ≤6 is considered to be unfavourable, a score of ≥8 suggests a greater probability of a vaginal birth, similar to that when the onset of labour is spontaneous (NICE 2008). A ripe or favourable

TABLE 22.1 Modified Bishop's Pre-induction Pelvic Scoring System

Inducibility Features	0	1	2	3
Dilatation of the cervix (cm)	<1	1–2	2–4	>4
Consistency of the cervix	Firm	Firm	Med	Soft
Cervical canal length (cm)	>4	2–4	1–2	<1
Position of cervix	Posterior	Mid	Anterior	
Station of presenting part (cm above or below ischial spine)	−3	−2	−1/0	+1/+2

cervix is one that for the purpose of IOL is more compliant, offering less resistance as the contraction and retraction of the myometrium forces the presenting part down (NICE 2008).

A VE to assess the cervix and the likelihood of successful induction in this way is by nature a subjective examination and as such, there will be inter-observer variations. However, if the same individual undertakes the assessment each time, then inter-observer variation would not apply. This would also provide the woman with continuity of caregiver at an extremely vulnerable and anxious time and be in her best interests as well as the standard of care midwives should always aim to meet. Currently VE remains the most common method of cervical assessment for IOL.

Cervical Membrane Sweep

A cervical membrane sweep (CMS), is considered by NICE (2008) to be an addition to, rather than a method of IOL *per se*, with recommendations that it is offered to nulliparous women at the 40- and 41-week antenatal examination and to parous women at the 41-week review. It is commonly undertaken by a doctor or midwife experienced in the practice. However, the evidence that CMS reduces the need for further methods to induce labour remains inconclusive (Rogers 2010). Midwives need to ensure that women make an informed decision whether or not to go ahead with a CMS.

Some women may find the procedure uncomfortable or painful and they may experience vaginal spotting and abdominal cramps (McCarthy and Kenny 2010). Wong et al.'s (2002) study found that, while the procedure was safe in that it did not lead to pre-labour rupture of membranes, significant bleeding or maternal or neonatal infection, there was no reduction in the need for IOL but for some women, it caused significant discomfort. Boulvain et al. (2005) suggest the possible benefits in terms of a reduction in more formal induction methods need to be weighed against the discomfort of the VE and other adverse effects of bleeding and irregular contractions not leading to labour. The recommendation from NICE (2008) to offer CMS at 40/41 weeks is to avoid prolonged pregnancy and is ***not*** meant for high-risk cases. While the evidence on whether CMS leads to spontaneous labour is inconclusive, if the alternative is IOL for women whose only risk factor seems to be their EDB, it is perhaps an 'intervention' that is worthy of consideration.

Prostaglandin E$_2$

Prostaglandins are naturally occurring female hormones present in tissues throughout the body. Prostaglandin E$_2$ (PGE$_2$) and F$_2$ are known to be produced by tissues of the cervix, uterus, decidua and the fetal membranes and to act locally on these structures. *Dinoprostone* is the active ingredient in PGE$_2$ vaginal tablets, gel and pessaries (British National Formulary, BNF 2019). It replicates prostaglandin E$_2$ produced by the uterus in early labour to ripen the cervix and is seen as a more natural method than the use of oxytocin. PGE$_2$ placed high in the posterior fornix of the vagina, taking great care to avoid inserting it into the cervical canal (Fig. 22.1) is absorbed by the epithelium of the vagina and cervix leading to relaxation and dilatation of the muscle of the cervix and subsequent contraction of uterine muscle. According to Blackburn (2017), the use of a prostaglandin greatly increases the probability of birth occurring within 24 h, and prior to the use of oxytocin potentiates the effects of the oxytocic agent (BNF 2019).

There are a number of preparations of PGE$_2$, which have been found to be clinically equivalent; but not bio-equivalent. The recommendation from NICE (2008) is the use of gel, tablet or controlled release pessary. In a small study by Tomlinson et al. (2001), the women receiving the slow release pessary gave a higher satisfaction score with regards to their perception of labour. This preparation is marginally more expensive than the other forms, however, it is increasing in popularity across maternity units in the UK.

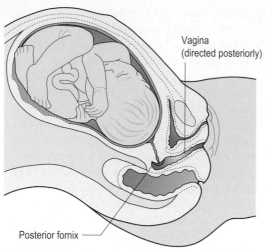

Vagina
(directed posteriorly)

Posterior fornix

Fig. 22.1 Insertion of prostaglandins. The posterior fornix of the vagina is used to insert prostaglandins for ripening or induction of labour. When undertaking a vaginal examination to assess the cervix, midwives should follow the direction of the vagina, which will be directed posteriorly if the woman is semi-recumbent. The uterus is anteverted and anteflexed, creating the posterior fornix. The cervix may appear 'difficult to reach', particularly when it is unfavourable (unripe).

Prior to the insertion of PGE$_2$, the midwife will carry out an abdominal examination to confirm the fetal lie, presentation, descent of the presenting part and assess fetal wellbeing, by use of electronic fetal monitoring (EFM). All findings are clearly recorded in the woman's maternity records and if there is any doubt or concern in the findings, the process must be stopped and the doctor informed (NMC 2018). Following insertion of PGE$_2$ the woman is advised to lie down for 30 min. When contractions begin, continuous EFM is used to assess fetal wellbeing. If the CTG is confirmed to be normal, i.e. all four features are considered to be reassuring (see Chapter 19), the CTG can be discontinued and intermittent auscultation used unless there are any other clear indications for the use of continuous EFM (NICE 2008).

The IOL process commonly takes place in a maternity unit, either on the antenatal ward or in the birthing/labour suite depending on the reason for the IOL. There is evidence to support starting the IOL process in the morning rather than the evening, citing increased maternal satisfaction with the process (Bakker et al. 2013). Prior to the administration of the PGE$_2$ the midwife must confirm there is a bed available on the birthing/labour suite in the event there is a need to transfer the woman as a *matter of urgency*. For the safety of the

woman and her baby, any decision to proceed with IOL must consider the current situation on the birthing/labour suite as the woman's response to the insertion of PGE$_2$ cannot be predicted. If there are any maternal or fetal risk factors in the pregnancy the IOL must always take place on the birthing/labour suite. In certain cases and under strict criteria, some women are able to return home for labour to establish following the administration of the PGE$_2$, to then return to the hospital for the later stages of labour and the birth (NICE 2014a).

Where the membranes are intact or ruptured, the recommended initial dose for all women, whether it is a first or subsequent pregnancy, is one dose of a 3 mg PGE$_2$ tablet or 2 mg gel, followed by reassessment in 6 h. If labour is not established at this point, a second dose of tablet or gel is inserted into the posterior fornix of the vagina with the woman's consent. **This equates to one cycle and is the maximum recommended** (NICE 2008). Alternatively, one pessary of 10 mg PGE$_2$ controlled-release pessary can be administered over 24 h, which also equates to one cycle. Side-effects of PGE$_2$ include nausea, vomiting and diarrhoea (BNF 2019).

If labour is not established after one cycle of treatment, the IOL is classed as unsuccessful. Following assessment that the woman and her baby remain in good health, discussion must take place between her and the doctor to determine further options:
- another attempt to induce labour *or*
- an elective caesarean section (NICE 2008).

Vaginal PGE$_2$ is currently the only recommended route for the use of prostaglandins for IOL. Misoprostol (PGE$_1$) is not licensed for use in the UK for IOL, except in cases of an intrauterine fetal death (IUFD). While it is thought to be more effective and less expensive than PGE$_2$ and oxytocin for the IOL, there remain questions about safety issues with regards to uterine hyperstimulation.

Risks Associated with Use of PGE$_2$. The use of PGE$_2$ can be unpredictable and may lead to uterine hyperstimulation, placental abruption, fetal hypoxia, pulmonary or amniotic fluid embolism (Kramer et al. 2006). The risk of uterine rupture is rare, occurring in between 0.3% and 7% of labours. However, with the rise in caesarean section rates in many middle- to high-income countries, it is inevitable that there will be increasingly more women with a uterine scar who in a subsequent pregnancy, may be faced with the decision to have their labour induced. While it is currently acceptable for PGE$_2$ to be administered to women with a scar in the *lower uterine segment* to induce labour, it is important for the midwife to understand the significance of a scarred uterus. In such a situation, the women should be fully informed of the increased risk of requiring an *emergency* caesarean section and increased risk of rupture of the uterus with vaginal PGE$_2$ induction.

Artificial Rupture of Membranes

There are two layers of membrane surrounding the fetus: the amnion is closest to the fetus, and the chorion is nearest to the decidua. ARM is a relatively simple process that can be used in an attempt to induce labour if the cervix is favourable and the presenting part is fixed in the pelvis. This method of induction is particularly useful where the woman does not want to use drugs such as PGE$_2$ or oxytocin, or where there is a risk of hyperstimulation if PGE$_2$ was to be used.

Prior to the procedure, an abdominal examination is carried out and if the lie is longitudinal, the presenting part is engaged and the fetal heart rate is within normal limits, a VE is done to assess the cervix, confirm the presentation and station and to exclude possible cord presentation or vasa praevia. If these findings are satisfactory, the bag of membranes lying in front of the presenting part (forewaters) is ruptured with the use of an amnihook or similar device to release the amniotic fluid. The fluid is assessed for colour and volume and following ARM, it may be possible to distinguish other features on the presenting part to identify the position of the fetus. After the procedure the woman is made comfortable, the fetal heart is auscultated and all findings are recorded in the maternity notes. The longer the interval between ARM and birth, the higher the risk of the woman developing chorioamnionitis as a result of an ascending infection from the genital tract leading to an increased risk of perinatal mortality (Bricker and Luckas 2012; Blackburn 2017). For this reason, if a decision has been made to induce labour for perceived risks it is common practice to start an oxytocin infusion within a few hours if labour has not been established following the ARM. In their review of two trials Bricker and Luckas (2012) found insufficient evidence to recommend amniotomy alone for IOL.

Changes to ripen the cervix are thought to be in response to prostaglandin produced by the amnion and cervix. In pregnancy, the chorion provides a barrier to the amnion and fetus from the vagina and cervix. Prostaglandin dehydrogenase (PGDH) is an enzyme produced by the chorion that breaks down prostaglandin. As a result of the actions of this enzyme the changes in the cervix do not take place and preterm labour is avoided (Smyth et al. 2013). Mitchell et al. (1977) found that VE in late pregnancy rapidly increases the concentration of circulating prostaglandins. This change occurs both in sweeping the membranes and with ARM. It is thought it is the disruption of the attachment of the membranes to the uterine wall that facilitates this change. In contrast, Van Meir et al. (1997) found that in labouring women, the part of the chorion that was in close contact with the cervical os released less PGDH allowing the prostaglandin from the amnion to come into contact with the cervix and facilitate ripening of the cervix. The theory is that if an ARM is performed too early the action of the amniotic prostaglandins on the cervix is lost.

Oxytocin

Oxytocin is synthesized in the hypothalamus and then transported to the posterior lobe of the pituitary gland from where it is episodically released to act on smooth muscle. The number of oxytocin receptors in the myometrium significantly increases by term, increasing uterine oxytocin sensitivity (Blackburn 2017).

In its synthetic form, oxytocin (Syntocinon) is a powerful uterotonic agent that may be used as part of the process for IOL following ARM. NICE (2008) do not recommend the use of oxytocin alone for IOL, or the use of ARM and oxytocin as a *'primary method'* of IOL, unless the use of vaginal PGE$_2$ is specifically contraindicated. There should be an interval of at least 6 h between the administration of prostaglandins and commencement of an oxytocin infusion. Oxytocin should be administered by slow intravenous infusion using an infusion pump or syringe driver with non-return valve. The infusion rate should follow the local protocol of the maternity unit and not exceed the maximum rate of 0.02 units oxytocin/min (BNF 2019). The dose is titrated against uterine activity, usually increasing the rate every 30 min with the aim of stimulating 3–4 contractions every 10 min, with each contraction lasting approximately 1 min, using the lowest possible dose. If contractions exceed this rate, or the contractions do not establish, the infusion must be stopped and the woman reviewed to determine the next step in the management of her labour.

When using an oxytocin infusion the fetal heart rate and uterine activity should be monitored using continuous EFM to ensure the fetus does not become compromised by the induced uterine contractions. There is a risk of hyperstimulation and hypertonic uterus leading to fetal compromise (Ragunath and McEwan 2007; McCarthy and Kenny 2010). In such cases, the infusion is decreased or discontinued and medical aid summoned. Even with the use of EFM the midwife still has an important role to play in assessing the woman's progress. The graphic representation on the CTG provides an indication of the frequency of the contractions but does not necessarily provide an accurate representation of the length and strength of the contractions, and for this reason it is important that the midwife continues to palpate the uterus to assess contractions for their length and strength. Whatever 'science' is being employed to assess maternal and fetal wellbeing, the midwife has a valuable opportunity to be with the woman and to use her 'art' to make a more holistic assessment of the woman and how she is responding to the process and what she wants and needs at this time.

Risks associated with use of intravenous oxytocin include:

- uterine hyperstimulation or hypertony
- fetal hypoxia and asphyxia
- uterine rupture
- fluid retention as a result of the antidiuretic effect of oxytocin
- postpartum haemorrhage
- amniotic fluid embolism (AFE).

In addition to the risks listed above, a recent study found that intravenous Syntocinon interferes with the physiology of lactation, affecting the initiation and maintenance of breastfeeding (Cadwell and Brimdyr 2017). This should be an important consideration before using Syntocinon as an intervention in labour.

The Midwife's Role when Caring for the Woman Undergoing Induction of Labour

The midwife's responsibilities regarding IOL include care during the antenatal and intrapartum period. Where a decision has been made to induce labour, it is important the midwife ensures the woman and her partner have been fully informed and understand the process and how it might be undertaken. There are a number of ways that labour can be induced and the manner the induction will take will depend on the individual circumstances of each woman. All information should be given in an objective manner to ensure the woman and her partner understand the reason for the induction, any possible consequences or risks of having/not having the procedure as well as any alternatives to IOL (NICE 2008). It is important for the woman and her partner to understand that induction may be delayed if the birthing/labour suite is busy, that it might take some time for contractions to be initiated, and a possibility that the induction process may be unsuccessful. While the assumption may be that this will already have been discussed with an obstetrician, it is incumbent upon the midwife to ensure the woman is always fully informed (NMC 2018). Time should be allowed for discussion with the midwife or obstetrician and it must be remembered that consent to a treatment can be withdrawn at any time and this decision by the woman must be respected (NMC 2018). The midwife or doctor should always record the discussions that take place and any requests made in the maternity notes.

During the induction process, all maternal and fetal observations should be recorded in the maternity notes. Until labour is established and the partogram is commenced, the midwife should record the observations in the antenatal section of the notes, ensuring that the detail is clear, concise and comprehensive (NMC 2018). The frequency and type of maternal and fetal monitoring will depend on the reason for and method of induction. The midwife is advised to follow the local maternity unit guidelines for IOL in each case, be conversant with the possible risks associated with each method of induction and be proficient and confident in recognizing and responding to any deviations from normal should they arise.

When the onset of labour is spontaneous, it is a more gradual process and as such, the woman has time to adjust to the changes in her body and is more able to cope with uterine contractions. When labour is induced, the sudden onset of strong painful contractions occurring every 3–4 min can be quite overwhelming and can result in an early request for pain relief. As well as this, the woman has to make a temporal shift from how she planned to birth her baby to what is now taking place. This can be extremely hard for the woman and her partner to come to terms with and may have a negative impact on this important time in their lives. Continuity of caregiver in labour is important as it enables the midwife to develop a trusting rapport with the woman and her partner as well more effectively assess progress and note any significant changes in body language and behaviour as labour advances (Laursen et al. 2009; Bohren et al. 2017). IOL can still be an affirmative, empowering experience and the midwife is in a key position to use their 'art' to enable the woman to have a positive birthing experience, whatever the outcome.

Non-Medical Approaches to Initiating Labour

For some women, avoidance of any surgical or pharmacological intervention in an otherwise low-risk pregnancy is extremely important and they might seek advice from the midwife on this matter. Non-medical approaches include the ingestion of castor oil, nipple stimulation, sexual intercourse, acupuncture and the use of homeopathic methods. While reviews by Kavanagh et al. (2008) and Smith and Crowther (2012) have found insufficient evidence to recommend some of these as a method to initiate labour, it is important for the midwife to develop a broad understanding of how they are thought to work and ensure that any advice given is in line with their sphere of practice (NMC 2018).

Stimulation of the breast either by massage or nipple stimulation has been found to be beneficial in women who had not gone into labour within 72 h and in reducing postpartum haemorrhage rates (Kavanagh et al. 2005). However, where the cervix is not ripe, stimulation of the breast has been found to be less effective. While stimulation of the nipple appears to cause the release of endogenous oxytocin, the effect of which initiates a uterine response, further studies are required before this method can be considered for use in high-risk groups.

SLOWER THAN EXPECTED PROGRESS AND PROLONGED LABOUR

The physiology of labour encompasses effective uterine contractions and cervical changes leading to progressive effacement and dilatation of the cervix, rotation of the fetus and descent of the presenting part, the birth of the baby, and expulsion of the placenta and membranes and the control of bleeding. The psychology of labour encompasses the need for a safe and stress-free environment, one in which the woman feels in control of events and has trust in those caring for her (Laursen et al. 2009) and is an equally important part of the process of labour (see Chapters 19–21).

For many women, the process of labour starts spontaneously and continues without the need to intercede.

For others the process may not adhere to medically ascribed time frames and the caregiver must assess whether this is a temporary slowing down in progress as the woman's mind and body adjusts to what is happening and is still to come, or whether it is the first signs of a delay in progress that may benefit from modifying the original plan of care.

There is no consistent view on what constitutes 'slow progress' of labour, but it appears to be an arbitrary assessment when progress does not follow the prescribed normal parameters (Bugg et al. 2013; Jackson 2017). Slow progress of labour appears to be a vague and ill-defined phenomenon, with no consensus on the diagnostic criteria for so-called 'dystocia' (Kjaergaard et al. 2009). Historically, there have been numerous terms used for slow progress of labour: *prolonged labour, labour dystocia, uterine inertia, failure to progress, delay in first/second stage of labour* and *dysfunctional labour* being just a few examples. What is striking is the explicit negativity of some of these terms, implying that women's bodies have not performed efficiently enough and have been defective in the childbearing process (Jackson 2017). Cluett et al. (2004) offer 'slower than expected labour' and Mobbs et al. (2018) simply suggests 'slow labour', which provide more positive and accurate terms in comparison to the typically unconstructive language often used in obstetrics. NICE (2014b) do not specify these terms but refer to a change in progress in the first or second stage of labour as 'suspected delay' or 'delay' depending on the findings.

When labour is prolonged, there is an increased risk of chorioamnionitis if there has been prolonged rupture of the membranes and an increased risk of postpartum haemorrhage as a result of an atonic uterus. Nonetheless, it must also be remembered the interventions used to correct a prolonged labour, such as amniotomy, oxytocin infusion and instrumental or operative birth, are not risk-free and therefore, any decision to intervene must take account of the full clinical picture and as importantly the wishes of the woman.

Delay in the Latent Phase of Labour

In the first stage of labour, the latent phase is the period when structural changes occur in the cervix and it becomes softer and shorter (from 3 cm to <0.5 cm); its position is more central in relation to the presenting part and there are often painful contractions (see Chapter 19). According to NICE (2014b), the cervix dilates up to 4 cm in the latent phase of labour. However, there is some debate that the *active/established* phase of labour should be defined from when cervical dilatation reaches 6 cm (American College of Obstetricians and Gynaecologists, ACOG 2014), thus extending the latent phase.

During the latent phase, the woman needs support and encouragement from those caring for her. The perceived result of painful contractions may be disappointing when hearing the cervix is 3 cm dilated after several hours. If progress in this phase of labour is considered to be slow, the emphasis is on conservative management rather than intervention (Tydeman and Rice 2016). The midwife must ensure the woman knows to eat and drink as she wishes to maintain her energy levels, which will help in bringing her a sense of normality and comfort. It is important for the woman to rest at this time, reassuring her that should she sleep, the contractions may **not** cease. Advice on how to relieve pain might include simple back massage, changes of position, a warm bath or some simple analgesia; all are an important part of midwifery care at this time. Any intervention such as an ARM during the latent phase can interfere with the action of amniotic prostaglandin on the cervix and as a result be counterproductive (Smyth et al. 2013).

Delay in the Active Phase of Labour: When Labour Slows or Ceases

NICE (2014b) refers to the *established* first stage of labour rather than the active phase, and defines this as the period when the uterine contractions are regular and painful and the cervix dilates progressively from 4 cm. Neal et al. (2010) suggest that the active phase begins between 3 and 5 cm when there are regular uterine contractions, whereas ACOG (2013) propose that a cervical dilatation of 6 cm marks active labour.

For nulliparous women, delay is suspected if their progress, in terms of cervical dilatation, is <2 cm in 4 h. For parous women it is the same, or there is considered to be a slowing in progress (NICE 2014b). This suggests the rate of cervical dilatation and duration of labour is measurable and such measurements can be applied to all nulliparous or multiparous women. It is, however, rather more complex and needs to take account of a wide range of variables in terms of maternal age, maternal size, fetal position, etc. Such factors may mean labour does not conform to a pre-determined rate of progression while still being physiological for that particular woman. Nonetheless, when caring for women in labour, midwives do need some parameters to work within in order to better understand what is considered acceptable in terms of progress (Neal et al. 2010). NICE (2014b) acknowledges the active phase of labour does not follow the trajectory that Friedman (1954) originally put forward and now suggest a rate of 0.5 cm/h. Although it is suggested that consideration should also be given to the rotation, descent and station of the presenting part, these observations do not appear to merit the same importance as cervical dilatation. For some women, good progress will be made in terms of rotation, descent and station of the presenting part, although such progress is not always reflected in a corresponding change in cervical dilatation. For low-risk, nulliparous women, with spontaneous onset of labour such expectations of active labour would appear to be overly stringent (Neal et al. 2010).

When delay is suspected, the midwife should discuss with the woman how the situation might be best managed from this point onwards, with appropriate consideration of all the facts, specific to their situation. Alleviating anxiety by ensuring there is continuous support in labour, changing maternal position, reducing pain using non-pharmacological means are some of the ways in which the midwife can help the woman at this time. Medical interventions to address the delay in progress, include ARM or an intravenous infusion of oxytocin, or a combination of both. The means to augment labour in this way has become common practice in the UK, with as many as 50% of nulliparous women receiving an oxytocin infusion in labour (Tydeman and Rice 2016). If these means are not successful, an instrumental or operative birth may be the only course of action depending on the stage of labour reached and the condition of the fetus. At the time of publication, the caesarean section rate in England was 29%, of which 13% were emergency caesarean sections and the proportion increasing with age accounting for 45% of births to women aged 40 years and over (NHS Digital 2018), many of which being for a diagnosis of *failure to progress*. Adopting less negative terminology is recommended to improve the woman's morale, such as *slower than expected labour* (Cluett et al. 2004), *slow labour* (Mobbs et al. 2018) or *prolonged labour*.

The partogram or partograph is a graphical representation of the maternal and fetal condition in established labour and the dilatation of the cervix against time. Information on a number of findings that are important in making an appropriate assessment of the ongoing progress of labour are usually recorded on a single sheet. NICE (2014b) recommends the use of a partogram once the woman is in established labour, despite the only evidence to support its use being studies from low-income countries. The findings from the review by Lavender et al. (2012) could not recommend the routine use of a partogram as part of the management of labour and suggested that its use should be determined at a local level. One of the most debated issues in the use of a partogram is the plotting of cervical dilatation on a graph, which has an *alert line* and an *action line*. The assumption is that the cervix dilates at a given rate in established labour, with the graph highlighting any perceived deviations from this pre-determined trajectory, suggesting progress in labour can be assessed based on cervical dilatation alone.

The Factors Influencing Slower than Expected Progress or Prolonged Labour

The influence of the '*3 Ps*': *the passages*, *the passenger* and *the powers*, on the process of labour, is considered to be a rather reductionist view of childbirth as there are so many other aspects that contribute to the rhythms of labour (Walsh 2012). Ineffective uterine contractions, malposition of the fetus leading to a relative or absolute CPD, malpresentation, emotional and psychological issues or any combination of these, may result in slower progress during the active phase or a cessation of cervical dilatation following a period of normal dilatation (Tydeman and Rice 2016). An understanding of the role of various mechanical, chemical and physiological/pathophysiological, emotional and psychological issues will help in determining why there is a delay in progress in the first or second stage of labour and what action might be taken.

In middle- to high-income countries, the majority of women will have grown up well-nourished and are fit and healthy, and thus *the passages* that the fetus must negotiate are unlikely to be seriously flawed, excluding possible trauma to the pelvis. Nonetheless, the impact of a full rectum, full bladder and fibroids cannot be ignored in causing a delay in the progress of labour. A malpresentation of *the passenger* such as shoulder, brow or face (mentoposterior) is one of the causes of slow progress or prolonged labour and this may occur as a result of a problem with the *passage* (see Chapter 23). A brow might revert to a face (mentoanterior) or vertex

presentation and the face in mentoposterior position may rotate to mentoanterior at the pelvic floor and if so a vaginal birth may be possible. The shoulder, brow or face (mentoposterior) cannot be born vaginally but a carefully executed abdominal and vaginal examination will exclude or confirm this so that the necessary action can be taken to prepare the woman for caesarean section.

When the fetus is adopting an attitude where the head is deflexed or slightly extended and the occiput is posterior the presenting diameters are larger and there will be a degree of asynclitism. This inevitably slows progress but does not necessarily mean progress is abnormal. This might be considered a relative CPD because with effective uterine contractions the fetus may adopt a more flexed attitude. On some occasions, more time is needed to do this safely. El Halta (1998) suggests that rupturing the membranes when the fetus is an occipitoposterior position may result in a sudden descent of the fetal head resulting in a deep transverse arrest whereby the occipitofrontal diameter (11.5 cm) is caught on the bispinous diameter of the outlet (10–11 cm).

Epidural anaesthesia has been found to slow the progress of labour in the first and second stage (Cheng et al. 2009), particularly so where there is an occipitoposterior position (see Chapter 23). The musculature of the pelvic floor plays an important part in assisting the rotation of the presenting part and epidural anaesthesia causes the pelvic floor to relax inhibiting rotation. It also has an impact on the stretching of the birth canal that normally triggers the neurohormonal reflex (*Ferguson's reflex*). In some cases, the head is simply (normally) large and any decision to intervene at this point with oxytocin may increase strength and frequency of uterine contractions in such a way as to unduly force this process with inevitable fetal heart rate changes prompting further intervention.

Although the uterus has prepared itself for the metabolic activity of labour, as labour continues the smooth muscle uses up its metabolic reserves and becomes tired. Any change to the strength, length or frequency of contractions (*the powers*) will affect progress and is indicative of inefficient uterine action. While some ketosis is considered normal in labour there remains a need for additional supplies of energy if the uterus is to continue contracting effectively and enable labour to progress without the need for medical intervention (Blackburn 2017). Women need to have adequate oral intake in order to cope with the very real demands that labour puts on their body.

Walsh (2012), Moberg (2015) and Simkin et al. (2017) highlight that interference with the progress of labour is not just down to mechanical or biophysical reasons as there is a complex interplay of hormones, particularly oxytocin, and how women labour. Midwives should be mindful of women who appear especially stressed and anxious that in turn can create psychological or emotional barriers to affecting a physiological labour. These may be attributed to the woman:

- feeling unsafe and vulnerable in their birthing environment
- being a survivor of previous sexual abuse
- having experienced a previous traumatic birth/post-traumatic stress.

Such influencing factors of a longer labour can be supported by simple strategies such as continuity of carer demonstrating compassionate and empathic care, a home like birthing environment and careful use of positive language (Simkin et al. 2017).

The Midwife's Role in Caring for a Woman in Prolonged Labour

A prolonged labour leads to increased levels of stress, anxiety, fear and fatigue, and increases the risk of infection, PPH and emergency caesarean section (Svärdby et al. 2006; Laursen et al. 2009). The importance of effective antenatal education in developing a plan of care for labour should not be underestimated. Advice on suitable food and drink to eat in the early stages of labour to maintain energy levels, positions and activities to encourage a forward rotation where there is an occipitoposterior position are just some of the ways that might help to assist the woman in the progress of labour.

When the woman and her partner come into a maternity unit/hospital to give birth, continuity of caregiver assists in creating a sense of trust between the woman, partner and the midwife but also allows for a more accurate assessment over time with non-interventionist ways in which progress can be maintained where appropriate. A change of position might help to facilitate more effective contractions or increase pelvic diameters when the fetal position is posterior. At this stage, it is also important to maintain hydration, to encourage voiding of urine and to suggest non-pharmacological ways to relieve pain. It is vital for midwives to respect the woman's autonomy (see Chapter 2) keeping her and

their partners informed of the progress in labour and the options available, which enables them to feel in control and to alleviate anxiety. Raised adrenalin levels as a result of fear, anxiety or pain can impact negatively on uterine activity and can slow progress in labour.

Accurate observations in labour are critical in assessing progress. Recognition and detection of variants in progress in labour with appropriate clinical response will improve the outcome of labour for both mother and baby (Neilson et al. 2003). An abdominal examination deftly undertaken can provide vital information about the labour with regard to the lie, presentation, position and descent of presenting part as well as the length, strength and frequency of contractions whereby any change in the pattern of the contractions can be identified. If the woman consents to VE the findings can be compared, to provide a more comprehensive picture of the progress of labour. On VE the midwife is assessing the presence and degree of moulding of the fetal skull, the presence and position of caput succedaneum in relation to the fetal skull sutures and fontanelles, and the dilatation of the cervix noting any thickening and its application to the presenting part. Noting changes in the colour of the liquor (once the membranes have ruptured) or in the fetal heart rate, will provide an indication of the health of the fetus in response to the progress of labour. Continuity of caregiver at this time reduces the likelihood of inter-observer variations while increasing the chance of spontaneous vaginal birth (Bohren et al. 2017).

When the decision to augment labour has been agreed by all parties, the woman and her partner will need additional support from the midwife, as the interventions necessary for this process may be very different from the birth they had previously imagined. Psychological as well as physical support is important at this time, as the control of the birth of their baby will appear to be in the hands of a third party which can lead to negative feelings of the childbirth experience (Nystedt et al. 2005, 2006).

The management of prolonged labour is a collaborative effort involving the woman and her partner, the midwife, obstetrician and anaesthetist. The normal pattern of observations and care in labour apply and any deviations from normal are reported to the obstetrician. When an ARM has been performed to augment labour an appropriate period of grace should be given for effective uterine contractions to resume before commencing an oxytocin infusion. The uterus responds with increased sensitivity to the oxytocin infused as the cervix dilates and it may be necessary to reduce the rate of the infusion as full dilatation is approached to avoid hyperstimulation of the uterus and the concomitant effects on mother and fetus. With the woman's consent, an assessment should be made 2–4 h after ARM or after commencing oxytocin to ascertain the likelihood of a successful vaginal birth. If there is persistent slow progress in the active phase despite optimal contractions (4–5 per 10 min, lasting >40 s), and the woman is well-hydrated and with an empty bladder, it is unlikely that continuing with an oxytocin infusion will lead to a vaginal birth.

The decision to augment labour in parous women or in women with prior caesarean section must be made by an experienced obstetrician because of the very real risk of hyperstimulation and uterine rupture.

Delay in the Second Stage of Labour

The second stage of labour can be divided into a passive (*pelvic*) phase and active (*perineal*) phase (see Chapter 20). Delay in this stage of labour may be due to malposition as the vertex does not descend and rotate; ineffective contractions due to a prolonged first stage; large fetus and large vertex; or absence of the desire to push with epidural analgesia. Assuming the woman is receiving active support and encouragement during the second stage, and has trust in those caring for her, some of these situations may be rectified with a change of position and further encouragement or the judicious use of an intravenous oxytocin infusion to avoid the need for an instrumental or operative birth.

According to NICE (2014b), birth would be expected to take place within 2 h for parous women and 3 h for nulliparous women when the cervix is fully dilated, but that a diagnosis of delay should take place after 1 h and 2 h, respectively, noting that there may be a suspicion of delay even before these timeframes. The variation in time limits should take into consideration the impact of epidural analgesia on the desire to push in the second stage. Birth should have occurred within 4 h, regardless of parity when an epidural is *in situ* (NICE 2014b). Walsh (2010) however, feels that this guidance is paradoxical, highlighting a *blatant double standard,* in that women are *'allowed'* less time when they are birthing physiologically.

The active phase when the mother is bearing down is the most critical time. When a diagnosis of delay in the second stage of labour has been made the case is referred to the obstetrician for review and assessment. The impact on both mother and fetus if the second stage exceeds a pre-determined time limit must be weighed against the risks of any interventions. Where there is any indication that the mother or the fetus is compromised the birth must be expedited as soon as possible but imposing an arbitrary time limit is felt by some to be unnecessary if both mother and fetus are doing well (Gilchrist et al. 2010; Tydeman and Rice 2016).

MIDWIFERY APPROACHES WHEN LABOUR PROGRESS SLOWS OR CEASES

Many midwives will recognize that women in straightforward physiological childbirth have individualized ebbs and flows throughout their labours. Indeed Walsh (2012) and many other midwives prefer to use *rhythms* in labour rather than stages of labour, as the latter are medically defined parameters. Downe (2006) refers to the *unique normality* of women's variations in the way they labour and the multifactorial influences on the experience of childbirth. It is therefore important that before any intervention occurs whether it is medicalized or not, is in response to a genuine problem rather than a physiological variation of normality. There are a number of approaches that can be utilized if women choose alternatives to traditional augmentation techniques (Tiran 2018).

There is some evidence that the following approaches including complementary therapies can be used for slow labour or labour that has ceased:

- water immersion: (Cluett et al. 2004; Zanetti-Dallenback et al. 2007; Thoni et al. 2010)
- continuous support in labour: (Bohren et al. 2017)
- massage: (Simkin and O'Hara 2002; Khodakarami et al. 2006; Field 2010)
- upright positions and mobilization: (Simkin and O'Hara 2002; Lawrence et al. 2013; Kumud et al. 2013)
- aromatherapy for reducing length of labour: (Luo et al. 2014)
- acupuncture and acupressure: (Skilnand et al. 2002; Kyeong et al. 2004).

It is important to note that some of the complementary therapies require an additional qualification or education and training for midwives or other practitioners (NMC 2018; Tiran 2018).

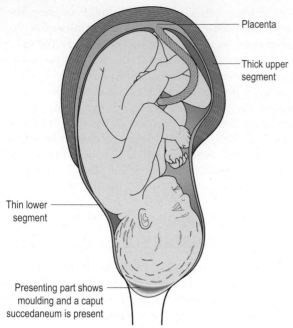

Placenta

Thick upper segment

Thin lower segment

Presenting part shows moulding and a caput succedaneum is present

Fig. 22.2 Obstructed labour. The uterus is moulded around the fetus; the thickened upper segment is obvious on abdominal palpation.

OBSTRUCTED LABOUR

While obstructed labour is not uncommon in low-income countries (Neilson et al. 2003), in the UK, it is only likely to be seen where a woman has laboured unattended at home for several hours and then seeks help at a hospital.

Obstructed labour occurs when, despite good uterine contractions, there appears to be no advancement of the presenting part. Possible causes of obstructed labour include:

- absolute CPD
- deep transverse arrest
- malpresentation
- lower segment fibroids
- fetal hydrocephaly
- multiple pregnancy with conjoined or locked twins.

If obstructed labour is not recognized, the woman's uterus will continue to contract to overcome the obstruction. She will become progressively more dehydrated, ketotic, pyrexial and tachycardic. The fetus will develop a bradycardia because of the relentless contractions. As the uterus continues to contract and retract the upper segment becomes progressively thicker, closely enveloping the fetus, and the lower segment becomes increasingly thinner. In nulliparous women the contractions may cease for a period before resuming again with increasing strength and frequency with little interval between contractions until the uterus assumes a state of tonic contraction. The difference between upper and lower segment may be seen as a ridge obliquely crossing the abdomen (*Bandl's ring*). The mother will be in severe and unrelenting pain. If VE is possible, the presenting part will be high with excessive moulding (Fig. 22.2). The uterus is in imminent danger of rupture and emergency measures must be taken if the situation has been allowed to get this far. Uterine rupture can lead to maternal mortality and the tonic contractions and uterine rupture cause the hypoxia, asphyxia and subsequent likely perinatal mortality (Neilson et al. 2003).

If the midwife attends a woman in this condition in the home setting, a paramedic ambulance should be called for immediate transfer to hospital. The birthing/labour suite should be informed, which, in turn, should contact the senior obstetrician, anaesthetist, neonatologist, theatre staff and special care baby unit. While waiting for the ambulance, the midwife should undertake venous cannulation, obtaining blood for urgent cross-match and site an intravenous infusion. The woman's GP can be called if close by, to provide additional help and support until the ambulance arrives. Observations of the woman and fetus, all actions taken and by whom, are recorded in the maternity notes as soon as possible (NMC 2018). If obstructed labour is diagnosed on admission to hospital an emergency caesarean section is performed.

During antenatal care, the midwife should highlight any predisposing maternal or fetal factors that could impact on the physiological progress of labour and appropriately refer to the obstetrician so that a full and frank discussion can take place and a decision made with the woman on the safest mode of birth. During labour, skilled observation and assessment of progress, particularly abdominal examination, will alert the midwife to any malpresentation or to the lack of advancement of the presenting part despite optimal uterine contractions. VE will confirm suspected malpresentation, and where the presentation is vertex, reveal increasing caput succedaneum or moulding. With a high presenting part, cervical dilatation will be extremely slow due to little if any application to the presenting part. The obstetrician is informed as soon as possible so that the birth can be expedited. Despite the very real threat to maternal and perinatal wellbeing these procedures should always only be undertaken with the woman's consent.

PRECIPITATE LABOUR

A precipitate labour is one where the fetus is born within 3 h of the commencement of contractions (NICE 2008). In some women, the uterus is over-efficient and much or all of the first stage is not recognized because contractions do not appear painful and the realization that the baby's head has been born may be the first indication that labour has actually started. In women with spontaneous onset of labour the incidence of precipitate labour is approximately 2%; such women being at greater risk of placental abruption (NICE 2008).

Other problems that may be associated with a precipitate labour include:

- soft tissue trauma of the maternal genital tract due to sudden stretching and distension as the baby is born
- fetal hypoxia as a result of the frequency and strength of the contractions
- intracranial haemorrhage from the sudden compression and decompression of the fetal skull as it passes through the birth canal with speed
- possible birth injury to the baby as the head and body emerge rapidly and fall to the floor.

It is likely that the birth would take place outside of where it was originally planned and thus the baby may be further compromised if it is not kept warm. The over-efficient uterus may relax after the birth of the baby, resulting in retained placenta and/or PPH. The psychological impact of such a rapid birth must not be underestimated, as not surprisingly some women will be in a state of shock after the event.

While precipitate labour will often recur in subsequent pregnancies there is no evidence to recommend IOL as a preventative measure. However, a woman who has experienced an *unattended* precipitate labour and birth may request IOL in order to ensure an attended birth in a safe environment (NICE 2008).

MAKING BIRTH A POSITIVE EXPERIENCE

For the woman who has a spontaneous onset of labour at term, has a single fetus in a cephalic presentation and who has no underlying medical disorders, labour should be a straightforward physiological event. The only intervention such a labour requires on the part of the midwife is to be there to meet the woman's needs and to offer continuous support and encouragement that enables the development of a trusting relationship.

The views of midwives and doctors on childbirth are often considered to be diametrically opposite, with midwives looking on childbirth as normal until proved otherwise and obstetricians viewing it as normal retrospectively (Walsh 2012). Whatever the perspective taken, the primary outcome must be the safety of the mother and baby. While a high-risk pregnancy and labour cannot be made low-risk it *can* still be a positive birthing experience for the woman and her partner. Childbearing is a time of major life transition and each woman and partner deserve to have a positive birth experience whether labour is spontaneous or induced and the birth is vaginal or by caesarean section. Interprofessional working together can only but help to contribute to that positive birth experience.

▮ REFLECTIVE ACTIVITY FOR SELF-ASSESSMENT

1. What are the risks and benefits of the various methods of induction of labour, including non-medical approaches?

2. Consider your place of work and reflect on women's autonomy and decision-making when they are offered induction of labour as an option. To what extent are women provided with all the information they need to make an informed decision? Are they given information regarding alternatives to induction of labour? How can you ensure that women in your maternity work place are enabled and empowered to make genuine informed decisions that are right for them?

3. List the evidence-based reasons for induction of labour and list the non-evidence-based reasons for induction of labour that you may have observed or been involved in during your clinical practice, How might you challenge the decisions that some doctors make to induce labour, which may be classed as inappropriate?

REFERENCES

ACOG (American College of Obstetricians and Gynaecologists). (2014). Obstetric Care Consensus No 1: Safe prevention of the primary cesarean section. *Obstetrics and Gynaecology, 123*(3), 693–711.

Arrowsmith, S., Wray, S., & Quenby, S. (2011). Maternal obesity and labour complications following induction of labour in prolonged pregnancy. *BJOG: An International Journal of Obstetrics and Gynaecology, 118*(5), 578–588.

Bailit, J. L., Gregory, K. D., Reddy, V. M., et al. (2010). Maternal and neonatal outcomes by labour onset type and gestational age. *American Journal of Obstetrics and Gynecology, 202*(3), 245.e1–245.e12.

Bakker, J., van der Goes, B., Pel, M., et al. (2013). Morning versus evening induction of labour for improving outcomes. *Cochrane Database of Systematic Reviews,* (2), CD007707.

Balchin, I., Whittaker, C., Patel, R., et al. (2007). Racial variation in the association between gestational age and perinatal mortality: Prospective study. *British Medical Journal, 334*(7598), 833.

Biggar, R. J., Poulsen, G., Melbye, M., et al. (2010). Spontaneous labor onset: Is it immunologically mediated? *American Journal of Obstetrics and Gynecology, 202*(3), 268.e1–268.e7.

Bishop, E. H. (1964). Pelvic scoring for elective induction. *Obstetrics and Gynecology, 24*(2), 266–268.

Blackburn, S. (2017). *Maternal, fetal, and neonatal physiology: A clinical perspective* (5th edn.). Philadelphia: Elsevier Saunders.

BNF (British National Formulary). (2019). *British National Formulary (BNF 78).* London: Pharmaceutical Press. Available at: https://bnf.nice.org.uk/.

Bohren, M. A., Hofmeyr, G. J., Sakala, C., et al. (2017). Continuous support for women during childbirth. *Cochrane Database of Systematic Reviews,* (7), CD003766.

Boulvain, M., Stan, C. M., & Irion, O. (2005). Membrane sweeping for induction of labour. *Cochrane Database of Systematic Reviews,* (1), CD000451.

Bricker, L., & Luckas, M. (2012). Amniotomy alone for induction of labour (Review). *Cochrane Database of Systematic Reviews,* (8), CD002862.

Bugg, G. J., Siddiqui, F., & Thornton, J. G. (2013). Oxytocin versus no treatment or delayed treatment for slow progress in the first stage of spontaneous labour. *Cochrane Database of Systematic Reviews,* (6), CD007123.

Cadwell, K., & Brimdyr, K. (2017). Intrapartum administration of synthetic oxytocin and downstream effects on breastfeeding: Elucidating physiologic pathways. *Annals of Nursing Research and Practice, 2*(3), 1024.

Cardozo, L., Fysh, J., & Pearce, J. M. (1986). Prolonged pregnancy: The management debate. *British Medical Journal, 293*(6554), 1059–1063.

Cheng, Y., Nicholson, J., Shaffer, B., et al. (2009). The second stage of labor and epidural use: A larger effect than previously stated. *American Journal of Obstetrics and Gynecology, 201*(6), S46.

Cheyne, H., Abhyankar, P., & Williams, B. (2012). Elective induction of labour: The problem of interpretation and communication of risks. *Midwifery, 28*(4), 412–415.

Cluett, E., Pickering, R., Getliffe, K., & Saunders, N. (2004). Randomised controlled trial of labouring in water compared with standard of augmentation for management of dystocia in first stage of labour. *British Medical Journal, 328*, 314–318.

de Miranda, E., van der Bom, J. G., Bonsel, G. J., et al. (2006). Membranse sweeping and prevention of post-term pregnancy in low-risk pregnancies: A randomised controlled trial. *BJOG: An International Journal of Obstetrics and Gynaecology, 113*(4A), 402–408.

Davey, M., & King, J. (2016). Caesarean section following induction of labour in uncomplicated first births- a population-based cross-sectional analysis of 42,950 births. *BMC Pregnancy and Childbirth, 16*, 92.

DH (Department of Health). (2006) NHS Maternity Statistics, England: 2004–2005. London: DH.

Downe, S. (2006). Engaging with the concept of unique normality in childbirth. *British Journal of Midwifery, 1*(6), 352–356.

El Halta, V. (1998). Preventing prolonged labor. *Midwifery Today. Summer,* 22–27.

Field, T. (2010). Pregnancy and labor massage therapy. *Expert Review of Obstetrics and Gynecology, 5*(2), 177–181.

Fox, H. (1997). Ageing of the placenta. *Archives of Diseases in Childhood, 77*(3), 171–175.

Friedman, E. (1954). The graphic analysis of labor. *American Journal of Obstetrics and Gynecology, 68*(6), 1568–1575.

Galal, M., Symonds, I., Murray, H., et al. (2012). Postterm pregnancy. *Facts Views and Vision in ObGyn, 4*(3), 175–187.

Gatward, H., Simpson, M., Woodhart, L., et al. (2010). Women's experiences of being induced for post-date pregnancy. *Women and Birth, 23*(1), 3–9.

Gilchrist L, Carrick-Sen D, Blott M, Loughney AD. (2010) Woman-centred second stage guidelines compared to time-limited guidelines: Evidence of benefit. *Archives of Disease in Childhood – Fetal and Neonatal Edition* 95:Fa8.

Heimstad, R., Skogvoll, E., Mattsson, L. A., et al. (2007). Induction of labour or serial antenatal fetal monitoring in post term pregnancy: A randomised controlled trial. *Obstetrics and Gynaecology, 109*(3), 609–617.

Hermus, M. A., Verhoeven, C. J., Mol, B. W., et al. (2009). Comparison of induction of labour and expectant management in postterm pregnancy: A matched cohort study. *Journal of Midwifery and Women's Health, 54*(5), 351–356.

House of Commons Select Committee on Science and Technology. (2007). *Twelfth report: Scientific developments relating to the abortion Act 1967. HC 1045–1*. London: The Stationery Office.

Hovi, M., Raatikainen, K., Heiskanen, N., et al. (2006). Obstetric outcome in post-term pregnancies: Time for reappraisal in clinical management. *Acta Obstetricia et Gynecologica Scandinavica, 85*(7), 805–809.

Jackson, K. (2017). When labour slows or stops. In K. B. Jackson, & H. Wightman (Eds.), *Normalising challenging or complex childbirth* (pp. 172–193). London: Open University Press.

Jukic, A. M., Baird, D. D., Weinberg, C. R., et al. (2013). Length of human pregnancy and contributors to its natural variation. *Human Reproduction, 28*(10), 2848–2855.

Jowitt, M. (2012). Should labour be induced for prolonged pregnancy? *Midwifery Matters, 134*, 7–13, Autumn.

Kavanagh, J., Kelly, A. J., & Thomas, J. (2005). Breast stimulation for cervical ripening and induction of labour (Review). *Cochrane Database of Systematic Reviews, (3)*, CD003392.

Kavanagh, J., Kelly, A. J., & Thomas, J. (2008). Sexual intercourse for cervical ripening and induction of labour (Review). *Cochrane Database of Systematic Reviews, (4)*, CD003093.

Kjaergaard, H., Olsen, J., Ottesen, B., & Dykes, A. K. (2009). Incidence and outcomes of dystocia in the active phase of labor in term nulliparous women with spontaneous labor onset. *Acta Obstetricia et Gynecologica, 88*, 402–407.

Khodakarami, N., Safarzadeh, A., & Fathizadeh, N. (2006). The effects of massage therapy on labour pain and pregnancy outcome. *European Journal of Pain, 10*(Suppl. S1), S214.

Kramer, M. S., Rouleau, J., Baskett, T. F., et al. (2006). Amniotic-fluid embolism and medical induction of labour: A retrospective, population-based cohort study. *Lancet, 368*, 1444–1448.

Kumud, A., Avinash, K., & Chopra, S. (2013). Effect of upright positions on the duration of first stage of labour among nulliparous mothers. *Nursing and Midwifery Research Journal, 9*(1), 10–20.

Kyeong Lee, M., Chang, S., & Kang, D. (2004). Effects of SP6 acupressure on labor pain and length of delivery time in women during labor. *Journal of Alternative and Complementary Medicine, 10*(6), 959–965.

Laursen, M., Bille, C., Olesen, A. W., et al. (2004). Genetic influence on prolonged gestation: A population-based Danish twin study. *American Journal of Obstetrics and Gynecology, 190*, 489–494.

Laursen, M., Johansen, C., & Hedegaar, M. (2009). Fear of childbirth and risk for birth complications in nulliparous women in Danish National Birth Cohort. *BJOG: An International Journal of Obstetrics and Gynaecology, 116*(10), 1350–1355.

Lavender, T., Hart, A., & Smyth, R. M. (2012). Effect of different partogram use on outcomes for women in spontaneous labour at term (Review). *Cochrane Database of Systematic Reviews, (8)*, CD005461.

Lawrence, A., Lewis, L., Hofmeyr, G. J., & Styles, C. (2013). Maternal positions and mobility during first stage labour. *Cochrane Database of Systematic Reviews, 10*, CD003934.

Luo, Z., Huang, L., Xia, H., & Zeng, Y. (2014). Aromatherapy for laboring women: Meta-analysis of randomized controlled trials. *Open Journal of Nursing, 4*, 163–168.

McCarthy, F. P., & Kenny, L. C. (2010). Induction of labour. *Obstetrics, Gynaecology and Reproductive Medicine, 21*(1), 1–6.

Menticoglou, S. M., & Hall, P. F. (2002). Routine induction of labour at 41 weeks' gestation: Nonsensus consensus. *BJOG: An International Journal of Obstetrics and Gynaecology, 109*(5), 485–491.

Middleton, P., Shepherd, E., & Crowther, C. A. (2018). Induction of labour for improving birth outcomes for women at or beyond term. *Cochrane Database of Systematic Reviews (5)*, CD004945.

Mitchell, M. D., Flint, A. P., Bibby, J., et al. (1977). Rapid increases in plasma prostaglandin concentrations after vaginal examination and amniotomy. *British Medical Journal, 2*(6096), 1183–1185.

Mobbs, N., Williams, C., & Weeks, A. (2018). Humanising birth: Does the language we use matter? *British Medical Journal Opinion*. Available at: https://blogs.bmj.com/bmj/2018/02/08/humanising-birth-does-the-language-we-use-matter/.

Moberg, K. (2015). How kindness, warmth, empathy and support promote the progress of labour: A physiological perspective. In S. Byrom, & S. Downe (Eds.), *The roar behind the silence* (pp. 86–93). London: Pinter and Martin.

Morken, N. H., Melve, K. K., & Skjaerven, R. (2011). Recurrence of prolonged and post-term gestational age across generations: Maternal and paternal contribution. *BJOG: An International Journal of Obstetrics and Gynaecology, 118*(13), 1630–1635.

NHS Digital. (2018). *NHS Maternity Statistics 2017–2018 Summary Report*. London: Health and Social Care Information Centre. Available at: https://files.digital.nhs.uk/C3/47466E/hosp-epis-stat-mat-summary-report%202017–18.pdf.

NICE (National Institute for Health and Care Excellence). (2008). *Inducing labour: CG70*. London: NICE. Available at: https://www.nice.org.uk/guidance/cg70/resources/inducing-labour-pdf-975621704389.

NICE (National Institute for Health and Care Excellence). (2011). *Caesarean section: CG132*. London: NICE. Available at: https://www.nice.org.uk/guidance/cg132/resources/caesarean-section-pdf-35109507009733.

NICE (National Institute for Health and Care Excellence). (2014a). *Inducing labour: QS60*. London: NICE. Available at: https://www.nice.org.uk/guidance/qs60/resources/inducing-labour-pdf-2098780923589.

NICE (National Institute for Health and Care Excellence). (2014b). *Intrapartum care for healthy women and babies: CG190*. London: NICE. Available at: https://www.nice.org.uk/guidance/cg190/resources/intrapartum-care-for-healthy-women-and-babies-pdf-35109866447557.

NICE (National Institute for Health and Care Excellence). (2015). *Diabetes in pregnancy: Management from pre-conception to the postnatal period: NG3*. London: NICE. Available at: https://www.nice.org.uk/guidance/ng3/resources/diabetes-in-pregnancy-management-from-pre-conception-to-the-postnatal-period-pdf-51038446021.

Neal, L., Lowe, N. K., Ahijevych, K., et al. (2010). 'Active labor' duration and dilation rates among low-risk, nulliparous women with spontaneous labor onset: A systematic review. *Journal of Midwifery and Women's Health*, 55(4), 308–318.

Neilson, J. P., Lavender, T., Quenby, S., et al. (2003). Obstructed labour. *British Medical Bulletin*, 67(1), 191–204.

NMC (Nursing and Midwifery Council). (2018). *The Code: Professional standards of practice and behaviour for nurses, midwives and nursing associates*. London: NMC.

Nystedt, A., Hogberg, U., & Lundman, B. (2005). The negative birth experience of prolonged labour: A case-referent study. *Journal of Clinical Nursing*, 14, 579–586.

Nystedt, A., Hogberg, U., & Lundman, B. (2006). Some Swedish women's experiences of prolonged labour. *Midwifery*, 22(1), 56–65.

Olesen, A. W., Westergaard, J. G., & Olsen, J. (2006). Prenatal risk indicators of a prolonged pregnancy. The Danish Birth Cohort 1998–2001. *Acta Obstetricia et Gynecologica Scandinavica*, 85(11), 1338–1341.

Oros, D., Bejarano, M. P., Cardiel, M. R., et al. (2012). Low-risk pregnancy at 41 weeks: When should we induce labor? *Journal of Maternal–Fetal and Neonatal Medicine*, 25(6), 728–731.

Putnam, K., Magann, E., Doherty, D., et al. (2011). Randomized clinical trial evaluating the frequency of membrane sweeping with an unfavourable cervix at 39 weeks. *International Journal of Women's Health*, 3, 287–294.

Ragunath, M., & McEwan, A. S. (2007). Induction of labour. *Obstetrics, Gynaecology and Reproductive Medicine*, 18(1), 1–6.

Rogers, H. (2010). Does a cervical membrane sweep in term healthy pregnancy reduce the length of gestation? *MIDIRS Midwifery Digest*, 20(3), 315–319.

RCOG (Royal College of Obstetricians and Gynaecologists). (2010). *Management of HIV in pregnancy. Green-top Guideline No 39*. London: RCOG. Available at: https://elearning.rcog.org.uk/sites/default/files/Sexually%20transmitted%20infections%20(including%20HIV)/RCOG_GT39_HIVPregnancy.pdf.

Simkin, P., & O'Hara, M. (2002). Non-pharmacologic relief of pain during labor: Systematic reviews of five methods. *American Journal of Obstetrics and Gynaecology*, 186(5 Suppl. Nature), S131–S159.

Simkin, P., Hanson, L., & Ancheta, R. (2017). *The labor progress handbook: Early interventions to prevent and treat dystocia* (4th ed.). Chichester: Wiley-Blackwell.

Simpson, P. D., & Stanley, K. P. (2011). Prolonged pregnancy. *Obstetrics, Gynaecology and Reproductive Medicine*, 21(9), 257–262.

Skilnand, E., Fossen, D., & Heiberg, E. (2002). Acupuncture in the management of pain in labour. *Acta Obstetricia et Gynecologica Scandinavica*, 81(10), 943–948.

Smith, C. A., & Crowther, C. A. (2012). Acupuncture for induction of labour (Review). *Cochrane Database of Systematic Reviews*, (7), CD002962.

Smyth, R., Alldred, S. K., & Markham, C. (2013). Amniotomy for shortening spontaneous labour (Protocol). *Cochrane Database of Systematic Reviews*, (1), CD006167.

Stavis, R. (2017). *Postmature (post term) infant. MSD Manual: Professional Version*. Available at: https://www.msdmanuals.com/en-gb/professional/pediatrics/perinatal-problems/postmature-postterm-infant.

Stevens, G., & Miller, Y. D. (2012). Overdue choices: How information and role in decision-making influence women's preferences for induction for prolonged pregnancy. *Birth*, 39(3), 248–257.

Stock, S. J., Ferguson, E., Duffy, A., et al. (2012). Outcomes of elective induction of labour compared with expectant management: Population based study. *British Medical Journal*, 344(e2838), 1–13.

Svärdby, K., Nordstrom, L., & Sellstrom, E. (2006). Primiparas with or without oxytocin augmentation: A prospective descriptive study. *Journal of Clinical Nursing*, 16, 179–184.

Tiran, D. (2018). *Complementary therapies in maternity care: An evidence based approach*. London: Singing Dragon.

Thoni, A., Mussner, K., & Ploner, F. (2010). Water birthing: Retrospective review of 2625 water births. Contamination of birth pool water and risk of microbial cross infection. *Minerva Ginecologica*, 62(3), 203–211.

Tomlinson, A. J., Archer, P. A., & Hobson, S. (2001). Induction of labour: A comparison of two methods with particular concern to patient acceptability. *Journal of Obstetrics and Gynaecology*, 21(3), 239–241.

Tun, M., & Tuohy, J. (2011). Rate of postdates induction using first-trimester ultrasound to determine estimated due date: Wellington Regional Hospital Audit. *Australian and New Zealand Journal of Obstetrics and Gynaecology*, 51(3), 216–219.

Tydeman, G., & Rice, A. (2016). Poor progress in labour. In D. M. Luesley, & M. Kilby (Eds.), *Obstetrics and Gynaecology. An evidence-based text for MRCOG* (3rd ed.). London: Arnold.

Van Meir, C. A., Ramirez, M. M., Matthews, et al. (1997). Chorionic prostaglandin metabolism is decreased in the lower uterine segment with term labour. *Placenta, 18*, 109–114.

Walsh, D. (2010). Labour rhythms. In D. Walsh, & S. Downe (Eds.), *Essential midwifery practice: Intrapartum care* (pp. 63–80). Chichester: Wiley-Blackwell.

Walsh, D. (2012). *Evidence and skills for normal labour and birth* (2nd ed.). London: Routledge.

WHO (World Health Organization). (2011). *WHO recommendations for induction of labour*. Geneva: WHO.

Wong, S. F., Hui, S. K., Choi, H., et al. (2002). Does sweeping of membranes beyond 40 weeks reduce the need for formal induction of labour? *BJOG: An International Journal of Obstetrics and Gynaecology, 109*(6), 632–636.

Zanetti-Dallenback, R., Tschudin, S., Zhong, X., et al. (2007). Maternal and neonatal infections and obstetrical outcome in water birth. *European Journal of Obstetrics and Gynecology and Reproductive Biology, 134*(2), 37–43.

ANNOTATED FURTHER READING

Jackson, K. (2017). When labour slows or stops. 2017. In K. B. Jackson, & H. Wightman (Eds.), *Normalising challenging or complex childbirth* (pp. 172–193). London: Open University Press.
This chapter explores midwifery approaches to labour which slows or stops. It aims to provide evidence-based alternative options that normalize and humanize labour in more challenging circumstances.

Jukic, A. M., Baird, D. D., Weinberg, C. R., et al. (2013). Length of human pregnancy and contributors to its natural variation. *Human Reproduction, 28*(10), 2848–2855.
Although the study appears underpowered in its small sample size, it provides useful information, highlighting that for a number of reasons, healthy human pregnancy varies considerably by as much as 37 days.

Mandruzzato, G., Alfirevic, Z., Chervenak, F., et al. (2010). Guidelines for the management of post-term pregnancy. *Journal of Perinatal Medicine, 38*(2), 111–119.
From an international perspective, this is a useful resource that addresses a number of salient issues relating to prolonged pregnancy. It highlights that there is no unequivocal evidence that prolonged pregnancy is a major risk per se.

Simkin, P., Hanson, L., & Ancheta, R. (2017). *The labor progress handbook: Early interventions to prevent and treat dystocia* (4th ed.). Chichester: Wiley-Blackwell.
This text is entirely devoted to the topic of labour 'dystocia'. It provides an excellent step by step guide with anecdotal and evidence based hints and tips for supporting women through labours that have slowed or ceased.

USEFUL WEBSITES

British National Formulary: https://bnf.nice.org.uk

Cochrane Library of Systematic Reviews: https://www.cochranelibrary.com/cdsr/table-of-contents

Health and Social Care Information Centre [HSCIC]: https://www.gov.uk/government/organisations/health-and-social-care-information-centre/about

National Health Service [NHS] Digital: https://digital.nhs.uk

National Institute for Health and Care [formerly Clinical] Excellence [NICE]: https://www.nice.org.uk

Royal College of Midwives [RCM]: https://www.rcm.org.uk

Royal College of Obstetricians and Gynaecologists [RCOG]: https://www.rcog.org.uk

World Health Organization [WHO]: https://www.who.int

23

Malpositions of the Occiput and Malpresentations

Terri Coates

CHAPTER CONTENTS

Malposition refers to any position other than occipitoanterior (OA) in a fetus with a vertex presentation. In a normal physiological labour, the fetal head presents with the occiput in the lateral position in the early stages of labour with anterior rotation as labour progresses. *Malpresentations* are all presentations of the fetus other than the vertex. Malpresentations that occur due to extension of the fetal head, causing brow or face to present, are usually diagnosed during active labour. Prompt and appropriate referral must be made. Both malpositions and malpresentations are associated with a difficult labour and an increased risk of operative intervention. The midwife must undertake regular clinical examinations to monitor the progress of labour to ensure fetal and maternal wellbeing. Effective open communication and record-keeping is crucial to provide safe care. The woman and her partner must be kept fully informed and supported throughout. Vaginal birth is possible in many cases, but intervention or operative birth become necessary when the malposition or malpresentation persist and labour slows down resulting in little or no progress.

THE CHAPTER AIMS TO

- examine the features of the malpresentations and malpositions
- recognize the predisposing factors
- outline possible causes of these positions and presentations

- describe the physical landmarks to aid recognition and diagnosis
- demonstrate sound knowledge of the mechanisms
- consider the outcomes for each position
- explore the midwife's management and the current uncertainties.

INTRODUCTION

Malpositions and malpresentations present the midwife with challenges of recognition and diagnosis both in the antenatal period and during labour. The midwife must ensure all examinations and discussions with the woman are documented and appropriate obstetric referral is made where a malpresentation or malposition has been found. The midwife should take time to discuss this with the woman to ensure they understand what may happen and the activities that may help (Munro and Jokinen 2012).

The presenting diameters do not fit well onto the cervix and therefore do not produce optimal stimulation for uterine contractions and labour. Labour with a fetus in a malposition or a malpresentation can be long, tedious and painful, requiring empathy, sustained encouragement and support for the woman and her partner. All the usual care in labour is provided by the midwife, paying attention to comfort and hydration (see Chapter 19). The woman should be encouraged to take an active part in decision-making and must be kept informed throughout.

In labour, women should be encouraged to adopt postures and positions they find comfortable and be encouraged to remain mobile. They should be supported to use coping methods to deal with their pattern of labour (Simkin 2010). The progress of labour may be slow, so midwives should take care to avoid the use of language that may demoralize the woman and her partner. Any sign of fetal or maternal distress or delay in labour must be referred promptly to an obstetrician (Sinha et al. 2018). Practices that are considered unhelpful include immobility and labouring on a bed, the setting of arbitrary time limits on the various stages of labour and the early use of epidural analgesia (Munro and Jokinen 2012).

OCCIPITOPOSTERIOR POSITIONS

Occipitoposterior (OP) positions are the most common type of malposition of the occiput and occur in approximately 10–30% of labours, but only in around 5% of births (Munro and Jokinen 2012; Le Ray et al. 2016). Women can be reassured that internal rotation to anterior positions can be expected in the majority of cases. A persistent OP position results from a failure of internal rotation or malrotation prior to birth (Gardberg et al. 1998; Peregrine et al. 2007). The vertex is presenting, but the occiput lies in the posterior rather than the anterior part of the pelvis. As a consequence, the fetal head is deflexed and larger diameters of the fetal skull present (Fig. 23.1).

Causes

The direct cause of the occipitoposterior position is often unknown, but it may be associated with an abnormally shaped pelvis. In an *android pelvis*, the *'forepelvis'* is narrow and the occiput tends to occupy the roomier *'hindpelvis'*. The oval shape of the *anthropoid pelvis*, with its narrow transverse diameter, favours a direct OP position.

Antenatal Diagnosis
Abdominal Examination

It is important to listen to the woman, as she may complain of backache and report feeling that her baby's bottom is very high up against her ribs. In addition, she may feel fetal movements across both sides of her abdomen.

On inspection. There is a saucer-shaped depression at or just below the umbilicus. This depression is created by the *'dip'* between the head and the lower limbs of the fetus. The outline created by the high, unengaged head can look like a full bladder (Fig. 23.2).

On palpation. While the breech is easily palpated at the fundus, the back is difficult to palpate, as it is well out to the maternal side, sometimes almost adjacent to the maternal spine. Limbs can be felt on both sides of the midline. The head is unusually high in an OP position, which is the most common cause of non-engagement in a primigravida at term. This is because the large presenting diameter, the occipitofrontal

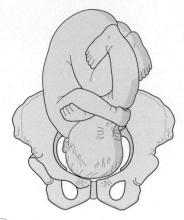

(A)   Right occipitoposterior position

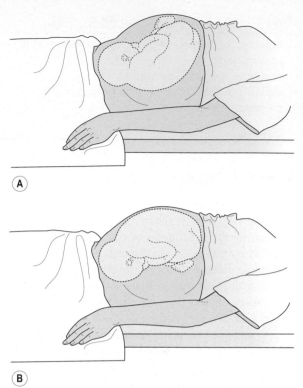

(A)

(B)

Fig. 23.2 Comparison of abdominal contour in (A) posterior and (B) anterior positions of the occiput.

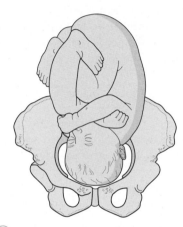

(B)   Left occipitoposterior position

Fig. 23.1 (A) Right occipitoposterior position. (B) Left occipitoposterior position.

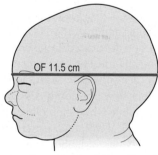

OF 11.5 cm

Fig. 23.3 Engaging diameter of a deflexed head: occipitofrontal (OF) 11.5 cm.

(11.5 cm), (Fig. 23.3) is unlikely to enter the pelvic brim until labour begins and flexion occurs (Fig. 23.4). The occiput and sinciput are on the same level. Flexion allows the engagement of the suboccipitofrontal diameter (10 cm).

The cause of the deflexion is a straightening of the fetal spine against the lumbar curve of the maternal spine. This makes the fetus straighten its neck and adopt a more erect attitude.

On auscultation. The fetal spine is not well flexed so the chest is thrust forward, therefore the fetal heart can be heard in the midline. However, the fetal heart may be heard more easily at the flank on the same side as the back.

Antenatal Preparation

There is no current evidence that suggests active changes of maternal posture will help to achieve an optimal fetal position before labour (Hunter et al. 2007; Munro and Jokinen 2012; Le Ray et al. 2016). Research has shown that the woman adopting a knee–chest position several times a day may achieve temporary rotation of the fetus to an anterior position but has only a short-term effect upon fetal presentation (Kariminia et al. 2004; Hunter et al. 2007). There is

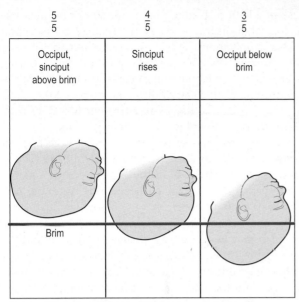

Fig. 23.4 Flexion with descent of the head.

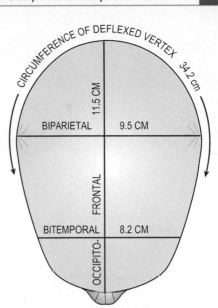

Fig. 23.5 Presenting dimensions of a deflexed head.

insufficient evidence to suggest that women should adopt the hands and knees posture, unless they find it comfortable (Simkin 2010; Munro and Jokinen 2012). Large research studies have concluded that hands and knees positioning in active labour does not facilitate rotation of the occiput to the anterior (Guittier et al. 2016) and lying on the side opposite that of the fetal back during labour does not facilitate fetal rotation (Le Ray et al. 2016). Both studies reported that women found these positions comfortable and concluded that positions adopted in labour should remain the women's choice.

For customary antenatal assessment of fetal position, Leopold's manoeuvres can be used during abdominal examination (see Chapter 11). These traditional methods of examination are only an assessment of the placement of the fetal spine and cannot estimate the direction of the fetal head. Peregrine et al. (2007) used ultrasound scans to confirm abdominal palpation and found that the fetal head is often aligned differently within the pelvis than the fetal spine within the uterus. In other words, the fetus may have turned its head to the right or left and the head may be anterior within the pelvis but the fetal back may palpate as lateral.

A review of current techniques used to diagnose fetal position such as Leopold's manoeuvres, the location of fetal heart sounds, vaginal examinations and presence of back pain are often unreliable (Simkin 2010). Failure to identify fetal position accurately can impact on the ability of the midwife to offer appropriate care. Consequently, it is considered that ultrasound is the most reliable way to accurately detect the fetal position (Munro and Jokinen 2012; Malvasi et al. 2016). More research studies are needed to examine the efficacy of midwifery skills in diagnosing fetal malpositions and non-technological approaches to improving the birth outcome for the woman and fetus.

Intrapartum Diagnosis

The large and irregularly-shaped presenting circumference (Fig. 23.5) does not fit well onto the cervix. This may hinder cervical ripening and predispose to a prolonged latent phase (Akmal and Paterson-Brown 2009). The contractions may also be in-coordinate. A high head predisposes to early spontaneous rupture of the membranes at an early stage of labour, which, together with an ill-fitting presenting part, may result in *cord prolapse* (see Chapter 25).

The woman may complain of continuous and severe backache, worsening with contractions. The absence of backache does not necessarily indicate an anteriorly positioned fetus. Descent of the head can be slow even with good contractions. The woman may have a strong desire to push early in labour because the occiput is pressing on the rectum.

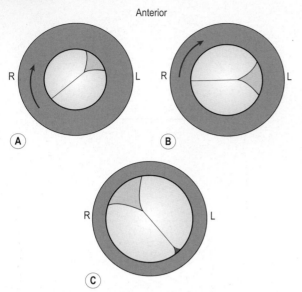

Anterior

Fig. 23.6 Vaginal touch pictures in a right occipitoposterior position. (A) Anterior fontanelle felt to left and anteriorly. Sagittal suture in the right oblique diameter of the pelvis. (B) Anterior fontanelle felt to left and laterally. Sagittal suture in the transverse diameter of the pelvis. (C) Following increased flexion, the posterior fontanelle is felt to the right and anteriorly. Sagittal suture in the left oblique diameter of the pelvis. The position is now right occipitoanterior.

Vaginal Examination

The findings (Fig. 23.6) will depend upon the degree of flexion of the head and degree of asynclitism (see Chapter 3). Locating the anterior fontanelle in the anterior part of the pelvis is diagnostic but this may be difficult if caput succedaneum is present. The direction of the sagittal suture and location of the posterior fontanelle will help to confirm the diagnosis. The position of the fetal head may be assessed using ultrasound where reason for the delay in labour requires accurate diagnosis (Malvasi et al. 2016).

Midwifery Care
First Stage of Labour

The woman may experience severe and unremitting backache, which is tiring and can be very demoralizing, especially if the progress of labour is slow. Continuous support from the midwife will help the woman and her partner to cope with the labour (Simkin 2010; Bohren et al. 2017) (see Chapter 19). The midwife can help by providing physical support such as massage and other comfort measures. Mobility should be encouraged with changes of posture and position and where possible, the

use of a bath or birthing pool and other non-pharmacological measures such as transcutaneous electrical nerve stimulation (TENS) or aromatherapy. There is no evidence that the *all-fours* position either during pregnancy or in labour will rotate a malpositioned baby (Kariminia et al. 2004; Munro and Jokinen 2012; Guittier et al. 2016; Le Ray et al. 2016) but it may provide comfort and help reduce persistent back pain.

The woman may experience a strong urge to push long before the cervix has become fully dilated. This is because of the pressure of the occiput on the rectum. However, if the woman pushes at this time, the cervix may become oedematous and this would further delay the onset of the second stage of labour. The urge to push may be eased by a change in position and the use of breathing techniques, inhalational analgesia or other methods to enhance relaxation. The woman's partner and the midwife can assist throughout labour with massage and physical support. The woman may choose a range of pain control methods (see Chapter 19) throughout her labour, depending on the level and intensity of pain she is experiencing at that time. The midwife must ensure that any delay in labour and fetal or maternal distress are promptly recognized and appropriate referrals made (Nursing and Midwifery Council, NMC 2018).

Second Stage of Labour

Full dilatation of the cervix may need to be confirmed by a vaginal examination because moulding and formation of a caput succedaneum may be in view while an anterior lip of cervix remains. The second stage of labour is usually characterized by significant anal dilatation some time before the head is visible. The midwife can encourage the woman to adopt upright positions that may help to shorten the length of the second stage and reduce the need for operative assistance (see Chapter 20). Squatting may increase the transverse diameter of the pelvic outlet which may improve the chance of a vaginal birth.

The length of the second stage of labour is usually increased when the occiput is posterior, and there is an increased likelihood of an operative birth (Le Ray et al. 2016; Sinha et al. 2018). In some cases where contractions are weak and ineffective, an oxytocin infusion may be administered to stimulate adequate contractions and achieve advancement/descent of the presenting part.

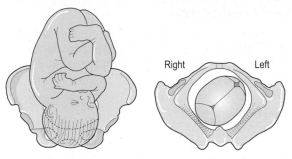

Fig. 23.7 Head descending with increased flexion. Sagittal suture in right oblique diameter of the pelvis.

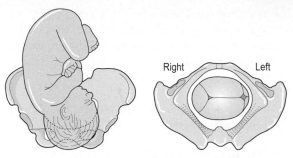

Fig. 23.8 Occiput and shoulders have rotated ⅛ of a circle forwards. Sagittal suture in transverse diameter of the pelvis.

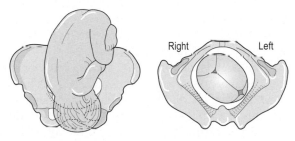

Fig. 23.9 Occiput and shoulders have rotated ⅜ of a circle forwards. Sagittal suture in the left oblique diameter of the pelvis. The position is right occipitoanterior.

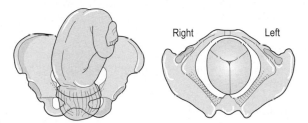

Fig. 23.10 Occiput has rotated ⅜ of a circle forwards. Note the twist in the neck. Sagittal suture in the anteroposterior diameter of the pelvis.

Fig. 23.7–23.10 Mechanism of labour in the right occipitoposterior position.

Manual Rotation

Manual rotation of the head from an occipitoposterior (OP) or occipitotransverse (OT) position to an anterior position has been shown to reduce the need for assisted birth and caesarean section by correcting the fetal malposition. This will facilitate the descent of the fetal head, to encourage a spontaneous vaginal birth (Shaffer et al. 2011, Tempest et al. 2017).

There are two techniques for undertaking manual rotation either by an obstetrician or an experienced and trained midwife. Both techniques require informed consent from the woman and adequate analgesia. The woman's bladder must be empty, and the cervix should be fully dilated. Either, constant pressure is exerted with the tips of the fingers against the lambdoidal suture to rotate the fetal head into the occiput anterior position, or the whole hand is introduced into the birth canal and fingers and thumb positioned under the lateral posterior parietal bone and the anterior parietal bone (Phipps et al. 2014); the head is then rotated to the anterior position. Using either method, the rotation may take two or three contractions to complete and then should be held for two contractions while the woman bears down to

reduce the risk of the rotation reverting (Phipps et al. 2014; Shaffer et al. 2011). If a midwife is practising in a setting where operative birth is not readily available, such as in a birthing centre, this timely intervention may reduce maternal and neonatal morbidity and mortality (Shaffer et al. 2011; Tempest et al. 2017).

Malpositions and malpresentations are generally associated with a higher incidence of interventions in labour, complications and instrumental birth (Guittier et al. 2016; Sinha et al. 2018). Immediate and subsequent postnatal care of the woman and her baby following an instrumental birth are discussed in Chapters 24 and 35.

Mechanism of Right Occipitoposterior Position (Long Rotation)

See Figs 23.7–23.10.
- The lie is longitudinal.
- The attitude of the head is deflexed.
- The presentation is vertex.
- The position is right occipitoposterior.
- The denominator is the occiput.
- The presenting part is the middle or anterior area of the left parietal bone.

- The occipitofrontal diameter, 11.5 cm, lies in the right oblique diameter of the pelvic brim. The occiput points to the right sacroiliac joint and the sinciput to the left iliopectineal eminence.

Flexion

Descent takes place with increasing flexion. The occiput becomes the leading part.

Internal Rotation of the Head

The occiput reaches the pelvic floor first and rotates forwards ⅜ of a circle along the right side of the pelvis to lie under the symphysis pubis. The shoulders follow, turning ⅔ of a circle from the left to the right oblique diameter.

Crowning

The occiput escapes under the symphysis pubis and the head is crowned.

Extension

The sinciput, face and chin sweep the perineum and the head is born by a movement of extension.

Restitution

The occiput turns ⅛ of a circle to the right and the head realigns itself with the shoulders.

Internal Rotation of the Shoulders

The shoulders enter the pelvis in the right oblique diameter; the anterior shoulder reaches the pelvic floor first and rotates forwards ⅛ of a circle to lie under the symphysis pubis.

External Rotation of the Head

At the same time the occiput turns a further ⅛ of a circle to the right.

Lateral Flexion

The anterior shoulder escapes under the symphysis pubis, the posterior shoulder sweeps the perineum and the body is born by a movement of lateral flexion.

Possible Course and Outcomes of Labour
Long Internal Rotation

This is the commonest outcome. With good uterine contractions producing flexion and descent of the head, the occiput will rotate forward ⅜ of a circle, as described above.

Short Internal Rotation

The term *persistent occipitoposterior position* (Figs 23.11, 23.12) indicates that the occiput fails to rotate forwards. Instead, the sinciput reaches the pelvic floor first and rotates forwards. As a result, the occiput moves into the hollow of the sacrum. The baby is born facing the pubic bone (*face to pubis*).

Cause. Failure of flexion: the head descends without increased flexion and the sinciput becomes the leading part. It reaches the pelvic floor first and rotates forwards to lie under the symphysis pubis.

Diagnosis. In the first stage of labour: signs are those of any posterior position of the occiput, namely a deflexed head and a fetal heart heard in the flank or in the midline. Descent is slow.

In the second stage of labour: delay is common. On vaginal examination the anterior fontanelle is felt behind the symphysis pubis, but a large caput succedaneum may mask this. If the pinna of the ear is felt pointing towards the woman's sacrum, this indicates a posterior position. Ultrasound may be useful to confirm the current fetal position (Malvasi et al. 2016).

The long occipitofrontal diameter causes considerable dilatation of the anus and gaping of the vagina, while the fetal head is barely visible, and the broad biparietal diameter distends the perineum and may cause excessive bulging. As the head advances, the anterior fontanelle can be felt just behind the symphysis pubis. Consequently, the fetus is born facing the pubis. Characteristic upward moulding is present with the caput succedaneum on the anterior part of the parietal bone (Fig. 23.13).

The Birth

The sinciput will first emerge from under the symphysis pubis as far as the root of the nose and the midwife maintains flexion by restraining it from escaping further than the glabella, allowing the occiput to sweep the perineum and be born. The face should then come down from under the symphysis pubis, with maternal effort carefully guided by the midwife (Figs 23.14–23.17). Perineal trauma is common and the midwife should watch for signs of rupture in the centre of the perineum (*button-hole* tear). An episiotomy may be required, owing to the larger presenting diameters.

Undiagnosed Face to Pubis

If the signs are not recognized at an earlier stage, the midwife may first be aware that the occiput is posterior

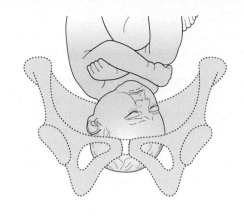

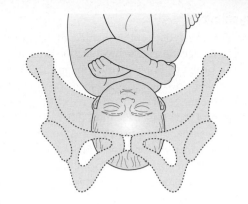

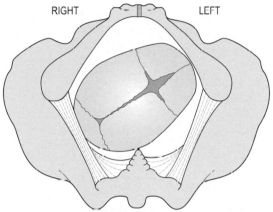

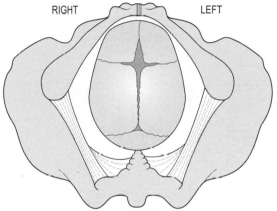

Fig. 23.11 Persistent occipitoposterior position before rotation of the occiput: position is right occipitoposterior.

Fig. 23.12 Persistent occipitoposterior position after short rotation: position direct occipitoposterior.

when the hairless forehead is seen escaping beneath the pubic arch. Any accidental extension of the fetal head should be corrected by flexion towards the symphysis pubis.

Deep Transverse Arrest

The head descends with some increase in flexion. The occiput reaches the pelvic floor and begins to rotate forwards. Flexion is not maintained and the occipitofrontal diameter becomes caught at the narrow bispinous diameter of the outlet. Arrest may be due to weak contractions, a straight sacrum or a narrowed pelvic outlet.

The sagittal suture is found in the transverse diameter of the pelvis and both fontanelles are palpable. Neither sinciput nor occiput leads. The head is deep in the pelvic cavity at the level of the ischial spines although the

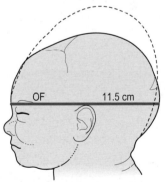

Fig. 23.13 Upward moulding (dotted line) following persistent occipitoposterior position. OF, occipitofrontal.

caput may be lower still. There is no advance and obstetric assistance will be required. Manual rotation may be attempted first, and then vaginal birth may follow with the woman's effort.

Management

The woman must be kept informed of progress and participate in decisions. Pushing at this time may not resolve the problem but the midwife and the woman's partner can help by encouraging *sigh out slowly* (SOS) breathing. A change of position may help to overcome the urge to bear down (see Chapter 20).

Where assistance is required for a safe birth the woman's informed consent is required. Procedures should be undertaken under appropriate local, regional or more rarely general anaesthesia (see Chapter 24). The considerations are the woman's choice, her condition and that of her unborn baby. The baby's head will be brought into an anterior position and the birth completed using forceps or vacuum extraction (see Chapter 24).

Conversion to Face or Brow Presentation

When the head is deflexed at the onset of labour, extension occasionally occurs instead of flexion. If extension is complete, then a *face presentation* results, but if incomplete, the head is arrested at the brim with the brow presenting. This is a rare complication of posterior positions and is more commonly found in multigravidae.

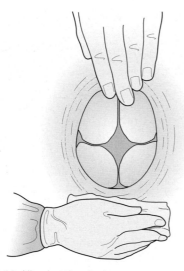

Fig. 23.14 Allowing the sinciput to escape as far as the glabella.

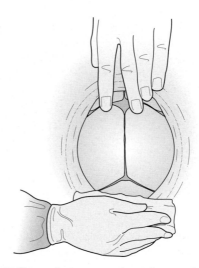

Fig. 23.15 The occiput sweeps the perineum, sinciput held back to maintain flexion.

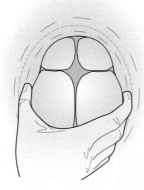

Fig. 23.16 Grasping the head to bring the face down from under the symphysis pubis.

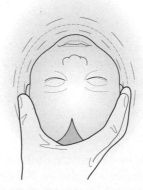

Fig. 23.17 Extension of the head.

Figs. 23.14–23.17 Birth of head in a persistent occipitoposterior position.

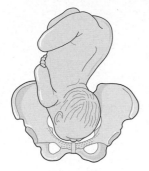

Fig. 23.18 Right mentoposterior.

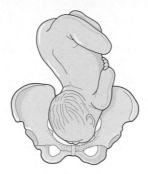

Fig. 23.19 Left mentoposterior.

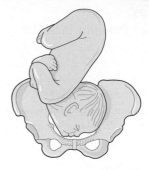

Fig. 23.20 Right mentolateral.

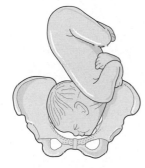

Fig. 23.21 Left mentolateral.

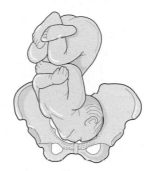

Fig. 23.22 Right mentoanterior.

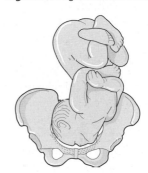

Fig. 23.23 Left mentoanterior.

Figs. 23.18–23.23 Six positions of face presentation.

Complications

Apart from prolonged labour with its attendant risks to the woman and fetus and the increased likelihood of instrumental birth, there are a number of complications that may occur which the midwife should consider.

Obstructed Labour

This may occur when the head is deflexed or partially extended and becomes impacted in the pelvis (see Chapter 22).

Maternal Trauma

A forceps birth will result in perineal bruising and trauma. Birth of a baby in the persistent occipitoposterior position, particularly if previously undiagnosed, may cause a third- or fourth-degree tear (Melamed et al. 2013).

Neonatal Trauma

The unfavourable upward moulding of the fetal skull, found in an occipitoposterior position, can cause intracranial haemorrhage, as a result of the falx cerebri being pulled away from the tentorium cerebelli. The larger presenting diameters also predispose to a greater degree of compression. Cerebral haemorrhage (see Chapter 35) may also result from chronic hypoxia, which may accompany prolonged labour.

Neonatal trauma occurring following birth from an occipitoposterior position has also been associated with forceps or ventouse births.

FACE PRESENTATION

When the attitude of the head is one of complete extension, the occiput of the fetus will be in contact with its spine and the face will present. The incidence is about ≤1:500 (Bhal et al. 1998; Akmal and Paterson-Brown 2009) and the majority develop during labour from vertex presentations with the occiput posterior; this is termed *secondary face presentation*. Less commonly, the face presents before labour; this is termed *primary face presentation*. There are six positions in a face presentation; the denominator is the *mentum* and the presenting diameters are the *submentobregmatic* (9.5 cm) and the *bitemporal* (8.2 cm) (Figs 23.18–23.23).

Causes
Anterior Obliquity of the Uterus

The uterus of a multigravida with slack abdominal muscles and a pendulous abdomen will lean forward and alter the direction of the uterine axis. This causes the fetal buttocks to lean forwards and the force of the contractions to be directed in a line towards the mentum rather than the occiput, resulting in extension of the head.

Contracted Pelvis

In the flat pelvis, the head enters in the transverse diameter of the brim and the parietal eminences may be held up in the obstetrical conjugate causing the head to become extended such that a face presentation develops. Alternatively, if the head is in the posterior position with the vertex presenting, and remains deflexed, the parietal eminences may be caught in the sacrocotyloid dimension of the maternal pelvis so that the occiput cannot descend, and the head becomes extended resulting in a face presentation. This is more likely in the presence of an android pelvis, in which the sacrocotyloid dimension is reduced.

Hydramnios (Polyhydramnios)

If the vertex is presenting and the membranes rupture spontaneously, the resulting rush of an excess of amniotic fluid may cause the head to extend as it sinks into the lower uterine segment.

Congenital Malformation

Anencephaly can be a fetal cause of a face presentation. In a cephalic presentation, because the vertex is absent the face is thrust forward and presents. More rarely, a tumour of the fetal neck may cause extension of the head.

Antenatal Diagnosis

Antenatal diagnosis is rare, since in most cases, a face presentation develops during labour. A cephalic presentation in a known anencephalic fetus may be presumed to be a face presentation.

Intrapartum Diagnosis
Abdominal Palpation

Face presentation may not be detected, especially if the mentum is anterior. The occiput feels prominent, with a groove between the head and back, but it may be mistaken for the sinciput. The limbs may be palpated on the side opposite to the occiput and the fetal heart is best

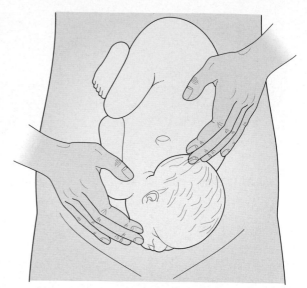

Fig. 23.24 Abdominal palpation of the head in a face presentation. Position right mentoposterior.

heard through the fetal chest on the same side as the limbs. In a mentoposterior position the fetal heart is difficult to hear because the fetal chest is in contact with the maternal spine (Fig. 23.24).

Vaginal Examination

The presenting part is high, soft and irregular. When the cervix is sufficiently dilated, the orbital ridges, eyes, nose and mouth may be felt. However, confusion between the mouth and anus could arise. The mouth may be open, and the hard gums are diagnostic with the possibility of the fetus sucking the examining finger. As labour progresses the face becomes oedematous, making it more difficult to distinguish from a breech presentation. To determine the position, the mentum must be located. If it is posterior, the midwife should decide whether it is lower than the sinciput, and if it can advance, it will rotate forwards. In a *left* mentoanterior position, the orbital ridges will be in the *left* oblique diameter of the pelvis (Fig. 23.25A). Care must be taken not to injure or infect the eyes with the examining finger; alternatively, ultrasound may be used to assess progress.

Mechanism of a Left Mentoanterior Position

- The lie is longitudinal.
- The attitude is one of extension of the fetal head and neck.
- The presentation is the face (Fig. 23.26).

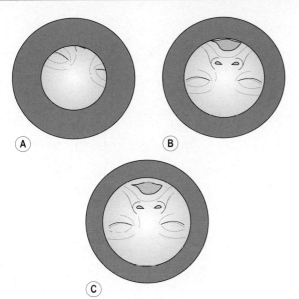

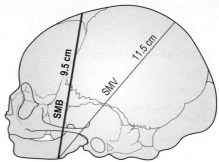

Fig. 23.26 Diameters involved in the birth of a face presentation. Engaging diameter, submentobregmatic (SMB) 9.5 cm. The submentovertical (SMV) diameter, 11.5 cm, sweeps the perineum.

Fig. 23.25 Vaginal touch pictures of left mentoanterior position. (A) The mentum is felt to left and anteriorly. Orbital ridges in left oblique diameter of the pelvis. (B) Following increased extension of the head, the mouth can be felt. (C) The face has rotated ⅛ of a circle forwards. Orbital ridges in transverse diameter of the pelvis. Position direct mentoanterior.

- The position is left mentoanterior.
- The denominator is the mentum.
- The presenting part is the left malar bone.

Extension

Descent takes place with increasing extension. The mentum becomes the leading part.

Internal Rotation of the Head

This occurs when the chin reaches the pelvic floor and rotates forwards ⅛ of a circle. The chin escapes under the symphysis pubis (Fig. 23.27A).

Flexion

This takes place and the sinciput, vertex and occiput sweep the perineum; the head is born (Fig. 23.27B).

Restitution

This occurs when the chin turns ⅛ of a circle to the woman's left side.

Internal Rotation of the Shoulders

The shoulders enter the pelvis in the left oblique diameter of the maternal pelvis and the anterior shoulder

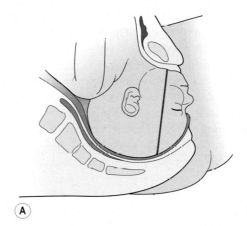

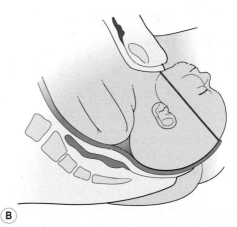

Fig. 23.27 Birth of the head in the mentoanterior position. (A) The chin escapes under the symphysis pubis. Submentobregmatic diameter at outlet. (B) The head is born by a movement of flexion.

reaches the pelvic floor first, rotating forwards ⅛ of a circle along the right side of the pelvis.

External Rotation of the Head

This occurs simultaneously. The chin moves a further ⅛ of a circle to the left.

Lateral Flexion

The anterior shoulder escapes under the symphysis pubis, the posterior shoulder sweeps the perineum and the baby's body is born by a movement of lateral flexion.

Possible Course and Outcomes of Labour
Prolonged Labour

Labour is often prolonged because the face is an ill-fitting presenting part and does not therefore stimulate effective uterine contractions. The woman should be kept informed of her progress and any proposed intervention throughout labour. In addition, the facial bones do not mould and, in order to enable the mentum to reach the pelvic floor and rotate forwards, the shoulders must enter the pelvic cavity at the same time as the head. The fetal axis pressure is directed to the mentum and the head is extended almost at right-angles to the spine, increasing the diameters to be accommodated in the pelvis.

Mentoanterior Positions

With good uterine contractions, descent and rotation of the head occur (Fig. 23.27) and labour progresses to a spontaneous birth as described above.

Mentoposterior Positions

If the head is completely extended, so that the mentum reaches the pelvic floor first, and the contractions are effective, the mentum will rotate forwards and the position becomes anterior.

Persistent Mentoposterior Position

In this case, the head is incompletely extended and the sinciput reaches the pelvic floor first and rotates forwards ⅛ of a circle, which brings the mentum into the hollow of the sacrum (Fig. 23.28). There is no further mechanism. The face becomes impacted because, in order to descend further, both head and chest would have to be accommodated in the pelvis. Whatever emerges anteriorly from the vagina must pivot around the subpubic arch. When the mentum is posterior this is impossible because the head can extend no further.

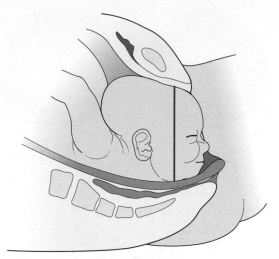

Fig. 23.28 Persistent mentoposterior position.

Reversal of Face Presentation

A face presentation in a persistent mentoposterior position may, in some cases, be manipulated to an occipitoanterior position using bimanual pressure (Neuman et al. 1994; Gimovsky and Hennigan 1995). This method was developed to reduce the likelihood of an operative birth for those women who refused caesarean section. Using a tocolytic drug, such as terbutaline, to relax the uterus, the fetal head is disengaged using upward transvaginal pressure. The fetal head is then flexed with bimanual pressure under ultrasound guidance to achieve an occipitoanterior position.

Management of Labour
First Stage of Labour

Upon diagnosis of a face presentation, the midwife should inform the obstetrician of this deviation from the normal. Routine observations of maternal and fetal conditions are made as in a normal physiological labour (see Chapter 19). A fetal scalp electrode must *not* be applied, and care should be taken not to infect or injure the eyes during vaginal examinations.

Immediately following rupture of the membranes, a vaginal examination should be performed to exclude cord prolapse, which is more likely because the face is an ill-fitting presenting part. Progress and descent of the fetal head should be assessed by ultrasound (Malvasi et al. 2016) or abdominal palpation, and careful vaginal examination to determine cervical dilatation and descent of the head.

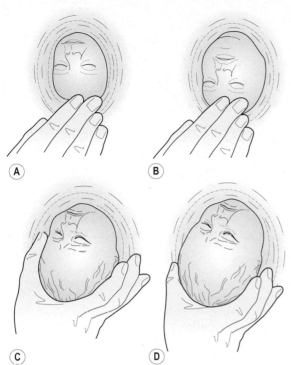

Fig. 23.29 Birth of face presentation. (A) The sinciput is held back to increase extension until the chin is born. (B) The chin is born. (C) Flexing the head to bring the occiput over the perineum. (D) Flexion is completed; the head is born.

In mentoposterior positions the midwife should note whether the mentum is lower than the sinciput, since rotation and descent depend on this. If the head remains high in spite of good contractions, caesarean section is likely. The woman may be prescribed an H2 blocker such as oral ranitidine, 150 mg every 6 h throughout labour if it is considered that an anaesthetic may be necessary.

Birth of the Head

When the face appears at the vulva, extension must be maintained by holding back the sinciput and permitting the mentum to escape under the symphysis pubis before the occiput is allowed to sweep the perineum. In this way, the submentovertical diameter (11.5 cm) instead of the mentovertical diameter (13.5 cm) distends the vaginal orifice. Because the perineum is also distended by the biparietal diameter (9.5 cm), an elective episiotomy may be performed to avoid extensive perineal lacerations (Fig. 23.29).

If the head does not descend in the second stage of labour, the obstetrician should be informed. In a mentoanterior position it may be possible for the obstetrician

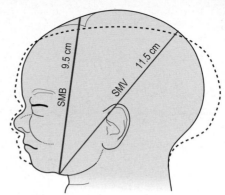

Fig. 23.30 Moulding in a face presentation (dotted line). SMB, submentobregmatic; SMV, submentovertical.

to assist the baby's birth with forceps when rotation is incomplete. If the position remains mentoposterior, the head has become impacted, or there is any suspicion of disproportion, a caesarean section will be necessary.

Complications
Obstructed Labour

Because the face, unlike the vertex, does not mould, a minor degree of pelvic contraction may result in obstructed labour (see Chapter 22). In a persistent mentoposterior position the face becomes impacted and caesarean section is necessary.

Cord Prolapse

A prolapsed cord is more common when the membranes rupture because the face is an ill-fitting presenting part. The midwife should always perform a vaginal examination when the membranes rupture to rule out cord prolapse (see Chapter 25).

Facial Bruising

The baby's face is always bruised and swollen at birth, with oedematous eyelids and lips. The head is elongated (Fig. 23.30) and the baby will initially lie with the head extended. The midwife should warn the parents in advance of the baby's *bruised* appearance, reassuring them that this is only temporary as the oedema will disappear within 1 or 2 days, with the contusion usually resolving within a week. Trauma during labour may cause tracheal and laryngeal oedema immediately after the birth, which can result in neonatal respiratory distress. In addition, fetal anomalies or tumours, such as fetal goitres that may have contributed to fetal

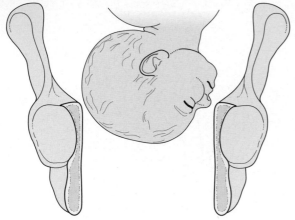

Fig. 23.31 Brow presentation.

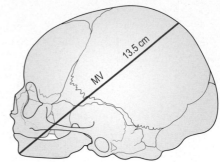

Fig. 23.32 Brow presentation. The mentovertical (MV) diameter, 13.5 cm, lies at the pelvic brim.

malpresentation, may make intubation difficult. As a result, a clinician with expertise in neonatal resuscitation should be present at the birth.

Cerebral Haemorrhage

The lack of moulding of the facial bones can lead to intracranial haemorrhage caused by excessive compression of the fetal skull or by rearward compression, in the typical moulding of the fetal skull found in this presentation (Fig. 23.30).

Maternal Trauma

Extensive perineal lacerations may occur at birth owing to the large submentovertical and biparietal diameters distending the vagina and perineum. There is an increased incidence of operative birth by either forceps or by caesarean section, both of which increase maternal morbidity.

BROW PRESENTATION

In the brow presentation, the fetal head is partially extended with the frontal bone, which is bounded by the anterior fontanelle and the orbital ridges, lying at the pelvic brim (Fig. 23.31). The presenting diameter of 13.5 cm is the mentovertical (Fig. 23.32), which exceeds all diameters in an average-sized gynaecoid pelvis. This presentation is rare, with an incidence of approximately 1 in 1000 births (Bhal et al. 1998).

Causes

These are the same as for a secondary face presentation (see above); during the process of extension from a

vertex presentation to a face presentation, the brow will present temporarily and in a few cases, this will persist.

Diagnosis

Brow presentation is *not* usually detected before the onset of labour.

Abdominal Palpation

The head is high, appears unduly large and does not descend into the pelvis despite good uterine contractions.

Vaginal Examination

The presenting part is high and may be difficult to reach. The anterior fontanelle may be felt on one side of the maternal pelvis and the orbital ridges, and possibly the root of the nose, at the other. A large caput succedaneum may mask these landmarks if the woman has been in labour for some hours (Fig. 23.33).

Management

The obstetrician must be informed immediately this presentation is suspected. This is because vaginal birth is extremely rare and obstructed labour usually results. It is possible that a woman with a large pelvis and a small baby may give birth vaginally. When the brow reaches the pelvic floor the maxilla rotates forwards and the head is born by a mechanism somewhat similar to that of a persistent occipitoposterior position. However, the midwife should never expect such a favourable outcome. The woman should be warned about the possible course of labour and that a vaginal birth is unlikely.

If there is no evidence of fetal compromise, the obstetrician may suggest that labour continues for a short while in case further extension of the head converts the

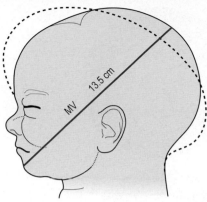

Fig. 23.33 Moulding in a brow presentation (dotted line). MV, mentovertical.

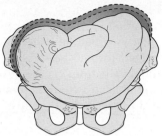

Fig. 23.34 Shoulder presentation, dorsoanterior.

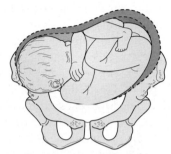

Fig. 23.35 Shoulder presentation, dorsoposterior.

brow presentation to a face presentation. Occasionally, spontaneous flexion may occur, resulting in a vertex presentation. If the head fails to descend and the brow presentation persists, a caesarean section is performed, with the woman's consent.

Complications

These are the same as in a face presentation, except that obstructed labour requiring caesarean section is the *probable* rather than a *possible* outcome.

SHOULDER PRESENTATION

When the fetus lies with its long axis across the long axis of the uterus (transverse lie) the shoulder is most likely to present. Occasionally, the lie is oblique but this does not persist as the uterine contractions during labour make it longitudinal or transverse.

Shoulder presentation occurs in approximately 1:300 pregnancies near term. Only 17% of these cases remain as a transverse lie at the onset of labour, of which the majority are multigravidae (Gimovsky and Hennigan 1995; Akmal and Paterson-Brown 2009). The head lies on one side of the abdomen, with the breech at a slightly higher level on the other. The fetal back may be anterior or posterior (Figs 23.34, 23.35).

Causes
Maternal

Before term, transverse or oblique lie may be transitory, related to the woman's position or displacement of the presenting part by an overextended bladder prior to ultrasound examination. Other causes are also described.

Lax abdominal and uterine muscles. This is the most common cause and is found in multigravidae, particularly those of high parity.

Uterine malformation. A bicornuate or subseptate uterus may result in a transverse lie, and in more rare of cases a cervical or low uterine fibroid may be a cause.

Contracted pelvis. Rarely, this may prevent the head from entering the pelvic brim.

Fetal

Pre-term pregnancy. The amount of amniotic fluid in relation to the fetus is greater, allowing the fetus more mobility than at term.

Multiple pregnancy. There is a possibility of hydramnios but the presence of more than one fetus reduces the room for manoeuvre when amounts of amniotic fluid are within normal limits. It is the second twin that more commonly adopts a transverse lie after the birth of the first baby.

Hydramnios. The distended uterus is globular in shape and the fetus can move freely in the excessive amniotic fluid volume.

Macerated fetus. Lack of muscle tone causes the fetus to slump down into the lower pole of the uterus.

Placenta praevia. This may prevent the fetal head from entering the pelvic brim.

Antenatal Diagnosis
Abdominal Palpation
The uterus appears broad and the fundal height is less than expected for the period of gestation. On pelvic and fundal palpation, neither head nor breech is felt. The mobile head is found on one side of the abdomen and the breech at a slightly higher level on the other.

Antenatal Management
A cause for the shoulder presentation must be sought before deciding on a course of management and requires a medical referral. Ultrasound examination can detect placenta praevia or uterine malformations, while X-ray pelvimetry will demonstrate a contracted pelvis (see Chapter 3). Any of these causes requires elective caesarean section. Once such causes have been excluded, external cephalic version (ECV) may be attempted. If this fails, or if the lie is transverse again at the next antenatal visit, the woman is admitted to hospital while further investigations into the cause are made. The woman frequently remains in hospital until labour commences because of the risk of cord prolapse if the membranes rupture.

Intrapartum Diagnosis
The findings are as above but when the membranes have ruptured the irregular outline of the uterus is more marked. If the uterus is contracting strongly and becomes moulded around the fetus, palpation is very difficult. The pelvis is no longer empty as the shoulder is wedged into the brim.

Vaginal Examination
In early labour, the presenting part may not be felt. The membranes usually rupture early because of the ill-fitting presenting part, with a high risk of cord prolapse. If the labour has been in progress for some time, the shoulder may be felt as a soft irregular mass. It is sometimes possible to palpate the ribs, with their characteristic grid-iron pattern being diagnostic (Fig. 23.36). When the shoulder enters the pelvic brim an arm may prolapse, which should be differentiated from a leg, i.e. the hand is not at right-angles to the arm, the fingers are longer than the toes and of unequal length, and the thumb can be opposed. No *os calcis* can be felt and the palm is shorter than the

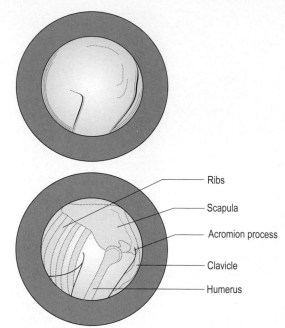

Fig. 23.36 Vaginal touch picture of shoulder presentation.

sole. If the arm is flexed, an elbow feels sharper than a knee.

Possible Outcome
Whenever the midwife detects a transverse lie, she must obtain medical assistance. There is no mechanism for the birth of a shoulder presentation.

If a transverse lie is detected in early labour while the membranes are still intact, the obstetrician doctor may attempt an ECV. If this is successful, the doctor may then undertake a controlled rupture of the membranes. (This may be considered before labour in some cases; Hutton et al. 2015; Hofmeyr et al. 2015). If the membranes have already ruptured spontaneously, a vaginal examination must be performed immediately to detect possible cord prolapse.

If a shoulder presentation persists in labour, the birth of the baby must be by caesarean section to avoid obstructed labour and subsequent uterine rupture (see Chapter 25).

Immediate caesarean section must be performed:
- when ECV is unsuccessful
- when the membranes are already ruptured
- if the cord prolapses
- when labour has already been in progress for some hours.

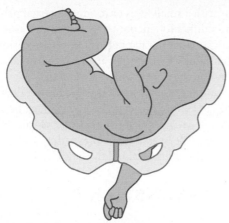

Fig. 23.37 Shoulder presentation with prolapse of the arm. (With permission from S MacDonald, G Johnson (Eds). (2017) Mayes Midwifery. Edinburgh: Elsevier.)

Complications
Prolapsed cord
This may occur when the membranes rupture (see Chapter 25).

Prolapsed Arm
This may occur when the membranes have ruptured and the shoulder has become impacted. Birth should be by immediate caesarean section (Fig. 23.37).

Neglected Shoulder Presentation
With adequate supervision both antenatally and during labour, this should never occur.

The fetal shoulder becomes impacted, having been forced down and wedged into the maternal pelvic brim. The membranes have ruptured spontaneously and if the arm has prolapsed it becomes blue and oedematous. The uterus goes into a state of tonic contraction, the overstretched lower segment is tender to touch and the fetal heartbeat may be absent. All the maternal signs of obstructed labour are present (see Chapter 22) and the outcome, if not treated in time, is a ruptured uterus and a stillbirth.

Management
An immediate caesarean section is performed regardless of whether the fetus is alive or dead, as attempts at manipulative procedures or destructive operations can be dangerous for the woman and may result in uterine rupture.

UNSTABLE LIE
The lie is defined as *unstable* when after 36 weeks' gestation, instead of remaining longitudinal, it varies from one examination to another between longitudinal and oblique or transverse.

Causes
Any condition in late pregnancy that increases the mobility of the fetus or prevents the fetal head from entering the pelvic brim may cause this.

Maternal Causes
These include:
- lax uterine muscles in multigravidae
- contracted pelvis.

Fetal Causes
These include:
- hydramnios
- placenta praevia.

Management
Antenatal
Where a transverse lie has been identified, the woman should be advised to admit herself to the hospital maternity unit as soon as labour commences. In some cases, it may be advisable for her to be admitted to hospital to avoid unsupervised onset of labour. The midwife should explain the risks associated with the possibility of rupture of membranes and cord prolapse. With consent, ultrasonography is used to assess the volume of liquor and exclude placenta praevia or fetal pathology. Attempts should be made to correct the malpresentation by ECV and if unsuccessful, caesarean section is considered.

Intrapartum
Obstetricians may recommend induction of labour after 38 weeks' gestation, when the lie is unstable. Having first ensured that the lie is longitudinal, a controlled rupture of the membranes is performed so that the fetal head enters the pelvis and an intravenous infusion of oxytocin is commenced to stimulate contractions.

The midwife should ensure that the woman has an empty rectum and bladder before the procedure, as a loaded rectum or full bladder can prevent the presenting part from entering the pelvis. The abdomen should be palpated at frequent intervals to ensure that the lie **remains** longitudinal and to assess the descent of the fetal head. If labour commences with the lie other than longitudinal, the complications are the same as for a transverse lie.

COMPOUND PRESENTATION

When a hand, or occasionally a foot, lies alongside the head, the presentation is said to be *compound*. This tends to occur with a small fetus or roomy maternal pelvis and seldom is difficulty encountered except in cases where it is associated with a flat pelvis. On rare occasions, the head, hand and foot are felt in the vagina – a serious situation that may occur with a dead fetus.

If a compound presentation is diagnosed during the first stage of labour, obstetric assistance must be sought. If diagnosis occurs during the second stage of labour and the midwife sees a hand presenting alongside the vertex, she should try to hold the hand back.

REFLECTIVE ACTIVITY FOR SELF-ASSESSMENT

1. In what circumstances would you suspect the fetus was presenting in an occipitoposterior position?
2. Using a doll and pelvis or mannequin, practise the mechanisms of a right occipitoposterior position as a long internal rotation and then as a short internal rotation. What are the signs that the fetus is likely to be born face to pubis?
3. How would you diagnose a face presentation in labour, abdominally and vaginally?
4. What may be the complication of an unstable lie and what advice would you give to a woman where the lie of the fetus varies from one examination to the other in late pregnancy?
5. What trauma could the woman and baby sustain as a result of a malposition of the occiput or a malpresentation and how could you as a midwife, attempt to prevent them from occurring or reduce the extent?

REFERENCES

Akmal, S., & Paterson-Brown, S. (2009). Malpositions and malpresentations of the foetal head. *Obstetrics and Gynecology and Reproductive Medicine, 199*, 240–246.

Bhal, P. S., Davies, N. J., & Chung, T. (1998). A population study of face and brow presentation. *Journal of Obstetrics and Gynecology, 18*(3), 231–235.

Bohren, M. A., Hofmeyr, G. J., Sakala, C., et al. (2017). Continuous support for women during childbirth. *Cochrane Database of Systematic Reviews*, (7), CD003766.

Gardberg, M., Laakkonen, E., & Salevaara, M. (1998). Intra-partum sonography and persistent occiput posterior position: A study of 408 deliveries. *Obstetrics and Gynecology, 91*(5), 1746–1749.

Gimovsky, M., & Hennigan, C. (1995). Abnormal fetal presentations. *Current Opinion in Obstetrics and Gynecology, 7*(6), 482–485.

Guittier, M. J., Othenin-Girard, V., de Gasquet, B., et al. (2016). Maternal positioning to correct occiput posterior fetal position during the first stage of labour: A randomised controlled trial. *British Journal of Obstetrics and Gynaecology, 123*(13), 2199–2207.

Hunter, S., Hofmeyr, G. J., & Kulier, R. (2007). Hands and knees posture in late pregnancy or labour for fetal malposition (lateral or posterior). *Cochrane Database of Systematic Reviews*, (4), CD001063.

Hofmeyr, G. J., Kulier, R., & West, H. M. (2015). External cephalic version for breech presentation at term. *Cochrane Database of Systematic Reviews*, (4), CD000083.

Hutton, E. K., Hofmeyr, G. J., & Dowswell, T. (2015). External cephalic version for breech presentation before term. *Cochrane Database of Systematic Reviews*, (7), CD000084.

Kariminia, A., Chamberlain, M. E., & Keogh, J. (2004). Randomised controlled trial of effect of hands and knees posturing on incidence of occiput posterior position at birth. *British Medical Journal, 328*(7438), 490–493.

Le Ray, C., Lepleux, F., De La Calle, A., et al. (2016). Lateral asymmetric decubitus position for the rotation of occipito-posterior positions: Multicenter randomized controlled trial EVADELA. *American Journal of Obstetrics and Gynecology, 215*(511), e1–e7.

Malvasi, A., Giacci, F., Gustapane, S., et al. (2016). Intrapartum sonographic signs: New diagnostic tools in malposition and malrotation. *Journal of Maternal-Fetal and Neonatal Medicine, 29*(15), 2408–2413.

Melamed, N., Gavish, O., & Eisner, M. (2013). Third- and fourth-degree perineal tears – incidence and risk factors. *Journal of Maternal–Fetal and Neonatal Medicine, 26*(7), 660–664.

Munro, J., & Jokinen, M. (2012). *RCM evidence-based guidelines for midwifery-led care in labour. Persistent lateral and posterior fetal positions at the onset of labour*. London: Royal College of Midwives Trust.

Neuman, M., Beller, U., & Lavie, O. (1994). Intrapartum bimanual tocolytic-assisted reversal of face presentation: Preliminary report. *Obstetrics and Gynecology, 84*(10), 146–148.

NMC (Nursing and Midwifery Council). (2018). *The Code: Professional standards of practice and behaviour for nurses, midwives and nursing associates.* London: NMC.

Peregrine, E., O'Brian, P., & Jauniaux, E. (2007). Impact on delivery outcome of ultrasonographic fetal head position prior to induction of labor. *Obstetrics and Gynecology, 109*(3), 618–625.

Phipps, H., de Vries, B., Hyett, J., et al. (2014). Prophylactic manual rotation for fetal malposition to reduce operative delivery (Protocol). *Cochrane Database of Systematic Reviews, 12*, CD009298.

Shaffer, B. L., Cheng, Y. W., Vargas, J. E., & Caughey, A. B. (2011). Manual rotation to reduce caesarean delivery in occiput posterior or transverse position. *Journal of Maternal–Fetal and Neonatal Medicine, 24*(1), 65–72.

Simkin, P. (2010). The fetal occiput position: State of the science and a new perspective. *Birth, 37*(1), 61–71.

Sinha, S., Talaulikar, V. S., & Arulkumaran, S. (2018). Malpositions and malpresentations of the fetal head. *Obstetrics, Gynaecology and Reproductive Medicine, 28*(3), 83–91.

Tempest, N., McGuinness, N., Lane, S., & Hapangama, D. K. (2017). Neonatal and maternal outcomes of successful manual rotation to correct malposition of the fetal head; A retrospective and prospective observational study. *PloS One, 12*(5), e0176861.

ANNOTATED FURTHER READING

Chapman, K. (2000). Aetiology and management of the secondary brow. *Journal of Obstetrics and Gynaecology, 20*(1), 39–44.

Six cases of vaginal birth from a brow presentation over a career of 39 years are recorded in this article. Most midwives will never see a brow presentation birth vaginally; this is a fascinating record from a long career.

Malvasi, A., Barbera, A., Di Vagno, G., et al. (2015). Asynclitism: A literature review of an often forgotten clinical condition. *Journal of Maternal–Fetal and Neonatal Medicine, 28*(16), 1890–1894.

Marked asynclitism is often associated with malpositions and malpresentations. Accurate assessment of asynclitism may help with diagnosis of the position of the fetal head.

Malvasi, A., Giacci, F., Gustapane, S., et al. (2016). Intrapartum sonographic signs: New diagnostic tools in malposition and malrotation. *Journal of Maternal–Fetal and Neonatal Medicine, 29*(15), 2408–2413.

Transvaginal digital examinations are subjective. If a malposition or malpresentation is suspected upon digital examination, ultrasound can be used to improve the accuracy in determining the position of the head. This review suggests the use of ultrasound to determine the head position.

Reichman, O., Gdansky, E., Latinsky, B., et al. (2008). Digital rotation from occipito-posterior to occipito-anterior decreases the need for caesarean section. *European Journal of Obstetrics and Gynecology and Reproductive Biology, 136*, 25–28.

The results of a prospective study suggest that digital rotation should be considered when managing the labour with a fetus in the occipitoposterior position. This paper affirms that such a manoeuvre has a high success rate, in experienced hands, reducing the need for vacuum extraction and caesarean section and so shortens the duration of hospital stay. Furthermore, the authors claim the intervention has the potential to reduce maternal and neonatal morbidity and mortality.

Shaffer, B. L., Cheng, Y. W., Vargas, J. E., & Caughey, A. B. (2011). Manual rotation to reduce caesarean delivery in occiput posterior or transverse position. *Journal of Maternal–Fetal and Neonatal Medicine, 24*(1), 65–72.

This paper examines manual rotation of the fetal head from occipitotransverse to occipitoposterior positions and its association with a reduction of caesarean sections and adverse maternal outcomes and no adverse neonatal outcomes when compared with expectant management. If a midwife is practising in a setting where operative birth is not readily available, this intervention may reduce maternal and neonatal morbidity and mortality.

USEFUL WEBSITES

Association of Radical Midwives: https://www.midwifery.org.uk/

Nursing and Midwifery Council: https://www.nmc.org.uk/

Royal College of Midwives: https://www.rcm.org.uk/

Royal College of Obstetricians and Gynaecologists: https://www.rcog.org.uk/

Spinning babies: https://spinningbabies.com/

24

Operative Births

Richard Hayman, Maureen D. Raynor

CHAPTER CONTENTS

This chapter describes the methods of operative birth that may be used when the mother is unable to give birth without medical or surgical assistance. The role of the midwife in these procedures will be explored, as will the principles of 'keeping the normal, normal'.

THE CHAPTER AIMS TO

- identify the areas of midwifery care that relate to the preparation for an assisted vaginal birth (ventouse/forceps) or birth by caesarean section (CS)
- describe the role of the midwife in relation to the issues of informed consent and the management of complications following assisted birth
- consider the various techniques used for assisted vaginal birth (ventouse/forceps) and birth by CS, plus the skills required by the midwife to improve the experience for both the mother and her partner
- discuss the changing role of the midwife in relation to operative births.

ASSISTING A VAGINAL BIRTH

Globally assisted vaginal birth is a frequently and widely practised intervention in the provision of care to women during childbirth. In the UK for example, there were 626,203 births in NHS hospitals in England during 2017–2018, reflecting a slight decline by 1.6% compared with 2016–2017. Moreover, the proportion of births with a spontaneous onset of labour has decreased from 68.6% in 2007–2008 to 52.2% in 2017–2018. Conversely, births where labour was induced has increased from 20.4% in 2007–2008 to 32.6% in 2017–2018. Of those births reported, 77,511 (12.4%) were assisted by ventouse or forceps with the latter being the more ubiquitous instrument used during 2017–2018 (NHS Digital 2018). That said, the incidence of instrumental intervention varies widely both between and within countries, and may be performed as infrequently as 1.5% or as often as 28%. Such differences may be linked to the alternative management strategies employed during labour in different units (Merriam et al. 2017). Various techniques have been championed to help lower the rates of operative births. These are summarized in Box 24.1.

It should be noted, however, that other interventions, such as epidural analgesia, have been observed to be associated with an increased risk of instrumental vaginal birth and have been suggested to be linked to an increased risk of birth by caesarean section (CS) (Anim-Somuah et al. 2018). However, such 'disadvantages' must be balanced against the higher rates of maternal satisfaction that this form of analgesia provides. It is up to the woman to make an informed choice as to which of the benefits and risks are most important, not up to the attending medical staff to make didactic

decisions on her behalf. Indeed, while it has been commented (Johanson and Menon 2010) that, in general, maternal outcomes would be improved by lowering instrumental birth rates, no evidence to support such a statement has ever been forthcoming, as it is not easy to see what the alternatives are for a woman who, despite her own best efforts, has not been able to secure a 'normal birth'.

INDICATIONS FOR VENTOUSE OR FORCEPS

The indications for assisted vaginal birth may be simply categorized into fetal and maternal. However, the reasons cited for intervention are frequently imprecise as multiple factors often interact.

Fetal

- Malposition of the fetal head (occipitolateral and occipitoposterior), see Chapter 23. Such positions occur more frequently in the presence of regional anaesthesia, as alterations in the tone of the pelvic floor may impede the spontaneous rotation to the optimal occipitoanterior position during the decent of the presenting part (vertex of the fetal head).
- Fetal 'distress' is a commonly cited indication for instrumental intervention; however, *presumed fetal compromise* is a more comprehensive term (unless a fetal blood sample has been obtained showing hypoxia and acidosis, in which case *fetal hypoxia* should be used) (National Institute for Health and Care Excellence, NICE 2014).
- Elective instrumental intervention for infants of reduced weight. In infants weighing <1.5 kg, birth with forceps does not confer an advantage over spontaneous birth and may increase the incidence of intracranial haemorrhage. Ventouse carries the same risks, but in addition, should be avoided in infants of <34+[6] weeks' gestation.
- Assisted vaginal breech birth. Forceps can be applied to the after-coming head to control the birth of the vertex, a situation where the ventouse is contraindicated.

Maternal

- The commonest maternal indications are those of maternal distress, exhaustion or prolongation of the second stage of labour. This has been suggested as

---

BOX 24.1 Useful Techniques to Help Lower the Operative Birth Rate

- One-to-one care in labour (Hodnett et al. 2013)
- Active management of the second stage with Syntocinon (O'Driscoll et al. 1993; Brown et al. 2013)
- Upright birth posture/mobilization (NICE 2014; Gupta et al. 2017)
- Delaying the onset of the active second stage by 1–2 h in women with regional analgesia/anaesthesia (NICE 2014)
- Fetal blood sampling rather than expediting birth when fetal heart rate abnormalities occur (NICE 2014).

>2 h in a primigravida (3 h if an epidural is *in situ*), or >1 h in a multipara (2 h if an epidural is *in situ*) (NICE 2014).

- Medically significant conditions such as: aortic valve disease with significant outflow obstruction; myasthenia gravis; significant antepartum haemorrhage due to placental abruption or vasa praevia; severe hypertensive disease; and previous CS (to minimize the risk of scar rupture).

CONTRAINDICATIONS TO AN INSTRUMENTAL VAGINAL BIRTH

Absolute

- The fetal head is ≥⅕ palpable abdominally
- The position as determined by a vaginal examination (occipitoanterior/posterior or lateral) of the fetal head is unknown
- Before full dilatation of the cervix (although a possible exception occurs with the ventouse birth of a second twin)
- When the operator is inexperienced in instrumental vaginal birth
- In addition, the ventouse *should not* be used:
  - in gestations of <34+⁶ weeks because of the increased risk of intracranial haemorrhage in the fetus
  - with the fetus presenting by the face
  - if there is a significant degree of caput that may either preclude correct placement of the cup or, more sinisterly, indicate a substantial degree of cephalopelvic disproportion (CPD).

Relative Contraindications (for Forceps or Ventouse)

- Fetal bleeding disorders (e.g. alloimmune thrombocytopaenia) or a predisposition to fractures (e.g. osteogenesis imperfecta) are relative contraindications specifically to an operative birth with the ventouse. However, the comparative risks of a birth by a difficult second stage caesarean section must also be considered and a discussion undertaken antenatally about the most appropriate plan for birth (it may be wiser to recommend that such women have an elective CS).
- There is minimal risk of fetal haemorrhage if the vacuum extractor is employed following fetal blood sampling or application of a scalp electrode.

PREREQUISITES FOR ANY OPERATIVE VAGINAL BIRTH

- Rupture of the membranes must be confirmed.
- The cervix must be fully dilated.
- Cephalic presentation with identification of the position (occipitoanterior/posterior or lateral).
- Adequate pelvis as ascertained by clinical pelvimetry.
- The fetal head must be <⅕ palpable per abdomen, with the presenting part at or below the ischial spines.
- Adequate analgesia/anaesthesia.
- Empty bladder/no obstruction below the fetal head (contracted pelvis/ovarian cyst).
- A knowledgeable and experienced operator with adequate preparation to proceed with an alternative approach if necessary.
- An adequately informed woman (with signed consent form detailing appropriate risks/benefits/complications as the situation demands).

BIRTH BY VENTOUSE

The ventouse is essentially a suction cup (made from plastic or metal) that is connected (via tubing) to a vacuum source. Following the placement of the cup onto the fetal head, traction can be applied to assist the birth.

There is no definitive guide as to which instrument to use on which occasion. However, the ventouse cup may not be successful at securing birth and therefore obstetric forceps should be chosen if there is:

- suspected fetal macrosomia
- excessive caput or moulding
- poor maternal effort due to exhaustion (which may be compounded by epidural analgesia and poor sensation)
- gestation <34 completed weeks.

Types of Ventouse

Until recently, the most commonly used ventouse in use in the UK was that of the 'soft' or silicone cup design (Fig. 24.1A). While these cups have the undoubted advantages of being extremely malleable (reducing maternal trauma by being more easy to correctly place within the vagina) and having a reduced incidence of fetal scalp trauma when compared with other cup designs, soft cups have a poorer success rate than metal cups in achieving a vaginal birth (Royal College of Obstetricians and Gynaecologists, RCOG 2011).

Metal cup ventouse designs are of the Bird or Malmström types, which have a centrally placed traction chain with a laterally located vacuum conduit. They come in diameters of 4, 5 and 6 cm.

Both the standard soft and metal cup designs require the generation of an operating vacuum from an external source – and as such, these pieces of equipment require two operators for their successful use (one to control the placement of the ventouse and assist the birth, the other (most commonly the attending midwife) to control the degree of vacuum that is generated.

More recent advances in design have removed the need for the external suction generators by incorporating the vacuum mechanism into 'handheld' pumps (e.g. Kiwi OmniCup) as illustrated in Fig. 24.1B. Such devices are

safe and may be useful for rotational births because they are low profile and are easily manoeuvred into the correct position. However, they have a significantly higher failure rate than the conventional metal cup ventouse, with cup detachments occurring more frequently (Turkmen 2014).

The Use of the Ventouse

The ventouse is more frequently employed by obstetricians than the obstetric forceps due to its apparent ease of use and comparative safety. However, repeated meta-analyses have demonstrated that the ventouse is less likely to achieve a successful vaginal birth than forceps, although both types of instruments are associated with a lowering of the overall CS rate (Johanson and Menon 2010). While the ventouse is associated with an increased risk of neonatal complications

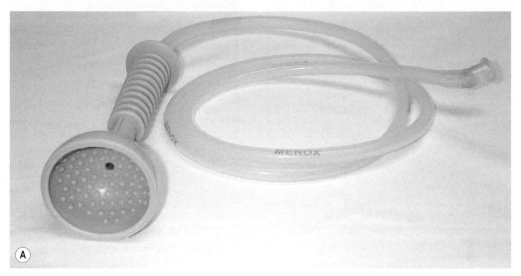

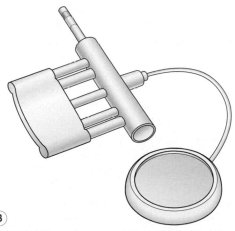

Fig. 24.1 (A) The soft cup ventouse. (B) The Kiwi OmniCup.

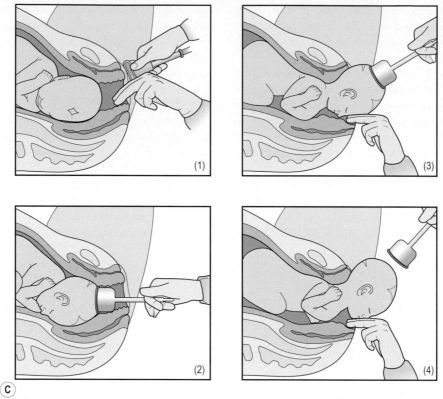

Fig. 24.1, cont'd. (C) An assisted vertex delivery employing a ventouse. The cup should be positioned over the flexion point to ensure optimal technique for the assisted vaginal birth.

such as cephalohaematoma (see Chapter 35), other facial (nerve palsies) and significant cranial injuries (fractures) are more common with forceps.

Procedure

- The rationale for the birth is discussed with the woman and her partner. The procedure is explained and consent obtained (written consent should be obtained if time allows).
- The woman's legs should be placed into the lithotomy position.
- While inhalational analgesia may be sufficient (Entonox – N_2O), more commonly a pudendal nerve block with perineal infiltration may be administered, or an epidural, if already *in situ*, may be topped up.
- Once adequate analgesia is assured, the maternal bladder is emptied.
- The fetal heart rate (FHR) must be continuously monitored (with a cardiotocograph – CTG).
- For the successful use of the ventouse, it is essential to determine the flexion point, which is located, in

an average term infant, along the sagittal suture 3 cm anterior to the posterior fontanelle (and thus 6 cm posterior to the anterior fontanelle). The centre of the cup should be placed directly over this, as failure to adequately position the cup can lead to a progressive deflexion of the fetal head during traction.

The *operating vacuum pressure* for nearly all ventouse is between 0.6 and 0.8 kg/cm² (60–80 kPa/500–800 cm H_2O). No evidence exists that a stepwise reduction in pressure improves the rate of successful birth when compared with a linear reduction. Using the latter technique with a silastic cup, a caput succedaneum (see Chapter 35) is formed instantly, and with the metal cup or OmniCup, an adequate chignon is produced in <2 min. It is important to note that a cup of 5 cm diameter is suitable for nearly all births, even with larger babies.

When the vacuum is achieved, traction must be applied to coincide with a contraction and thus maternal expulsive efforts. Without both of these contributing factors, birth with a ventouse will fail. Traction is provided along a track defined by the curve of Carus (see Chapter 3); initially in a downwards and backwards direction, then in a forward and upward manner. Once the fetal head has crowned, the vacuum is released, the cup removed and with further maternal efforts the baby will be born. In addition to the relative ease of use and low risk of complications, it is undoubtedly this sense of contribution to the birth that makes the ventouse a more satisfactory birthing experience for the mother and her partner, than an operative birth with obstetric forceps.

Precautions in Use

With the ventouse, the operator should allow ≤2 episodes of breaking the suction in any vacuum-assisted birth, and the maximum time from application to birth should ideally be ≤15 min. If there is no evidence of descent with the first pull, the woman should be reassessed to ascertain the reason for failure-to-progress. In addition, care should be taken to ensure that no vaginal skin is trapped in the edges of the cup as this can result in complex degrees of perineal trauma (see Chapter 17) that can be extremely difficult to repair in a satisfactory fashion.

The Midwife Ventouse Practitioner

Some midwives feel that women will be better served by a midwife ventouse practitioner rather than an obstetrician and embrace such innovations (Tinsley 2010). However, others might see it as exceeding the limits of normal midwifery practice. The fact is that midwifery care is changing and developing, specifically with the advancement of care within stand-alone midwife-led units.

While the idea of reducing the psychological trauma to a woman during a birth by limiting the number of carers in attendance at this crucial and critical time is to be commended, it would be foolhardy to assume that the midwife ventouse practitioner would be the primary carer for every pregnant women on every occasion that required an assisted vaginal birth. As such, it is likely that a midwife previously unknown to the labouring woman would be asked to assist at the moment when help is required, an event that would therefore be no less 'traumatic' for a woman or her partner than asking an obstetrician to attend. All accoucheurs, including midwife ventouse practitioners, must be well educated and trained before carrying out a ventouse birth – although it is highly unlikely that the more complex surgical skills required of a birth by forceps or CS would be mastered in

addition. It should be remembered that as a ventouse will fail in up to 20% of cases, even in the most skilled hands, having no ability to change instruments or resort to birth by CS will place those midwives who work as ventouse practitioners in isolation in a most unenviable position.

BIRTH BY FORCEPS

Characteristics of the Obstetric Forceps

All obstetric forceps are composed of two separate blades (determined as right and left by reference to their insertion around the fetal head within the maternal vagina), two shanks (shafts) of varying length and two handles. Forceps are often described as non-rotational or rotational. Non-rotational forceps are 'held' together by either an English (non-sliding) lock on the shank or, in the case of rotational forceps, by a sliding lock on the shank. The blades have a cephalic curve to accommodate the form of the baby's head and are fenestrated (and not solid) to minimize the trauma to the baby's head during both placement and birth. They also have a pelvic curve to reduce the risks of trauma to the maternal tissues during the birth process.

When the blades are correctly positioned around the fetal skull, the handles will be neatly aligned in the hands of the doctor who applies them and will be noted to 'lock with ease'. Forceps that do not lock are most commonly incorrectly placed.

Classification of Obstetric Forceps

Forceps operations fall into two categories: mid- and low-cavity. Mid-cavity forceps are used when the leading part of the fetal head has reached below the level of the ischial spines; low-cavity forceps are used when the head has descended to the level of the pelvic floor. High-cavity forceps (with the leading part of the fetal head above the level of the ischial spines) are now considered unsafe and a CS will be the preferred method of birth in nearly all cases.

Types of Obstetric Forceps
Wrigley's forceps

These are designed for use in outlet lift-out when the head is on the perineum or to assist the birth of the fetal head at caesarean section. They have a short shank, fenestrated blades with both pelvic and cephalic curves, and an English lock (Fig. 24.2).

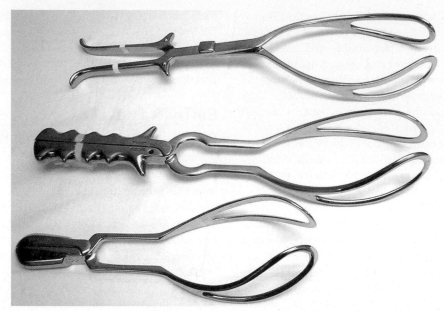

Fig. 24.2 Types of forceps. From top: Kielland's, Neville–Barnes/Simpson's and Wrigley's. Note the difference in cephalic curve. The rotational forceps (Kielland's) have a long shaft and little pelvic curve. Wrigley's forceps have a shorter shank.

Neville–Barnes or Simpson's forceps

These are generally used for a low- or mid-cavity forceps birth when the sagittal suture is in the anteroposterior diameter of the cavity of the pelvis. While they have cephalic and pelvic curves to the fenestrated blades, the handles are longer and heavier (Fig. 24.2) than those of the Wrigley's. Anderson's and Haig–Ferguson's forceps are also similar in shape and size.

Kielland's forceps

These were originally designed to deliver the fetal head at a station at, or above, the pelvic brim. They are now more commonly used for the rotation and extraction of a baby whose head is in the deep transverse or occipitoposterior malpositions. By comparison to the non-rotational forceps, the Kielland's forceps blades have fenestrated blades with a much-reduced pelvic curve (in order to allow for the safe rotation of the fetus), longer shanks (to enable rotation within the mid-cavity of the pelvis) and a sliding lock to allow for correction of any degree of asynclitism of the fetal head. These forceps (Fig. 24.2) should be used only by an obstetrician skilled in their application and use, and indeed in many units their use has been abandoned.

Procedure

In addition to the key points outlined for ventouse above, i.e. rationale, consent, urinary bladder catheterization, FHR monitoring and position of the woman's legs, specific issues need consideration:

- Consideration should be given as to the location of the birth – in the birthing room (lift-out or low-cavity – non-rotational deliveries) or in the obstetric theatre (all other forceps births).
- Unlike the ventouse, inhalational analgesia or a pudendal nerve block with perineal infiltration is unlikely to be sufficient for a forceps birth. In the majority of instances an epidural, if already *in situ*, may be topped up, or a spinal anaesthetic should be administered. These are mandatory before consideration is given to using Kielland's forceps.
- The forceps should be held discretely in front of the woman (to visualize how they will be inserted *per vaginum*) and placed around the fetal head. The left blade is inserted before the right blade, with the accoucheur's hand protecting the vaginal wall from direct trauma.
- The forceps blades come to lie parallel to the axis of the fetal head, and between the fetal head and the pelvic wall. The operator then articulates and locks

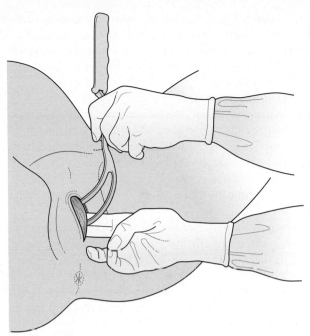

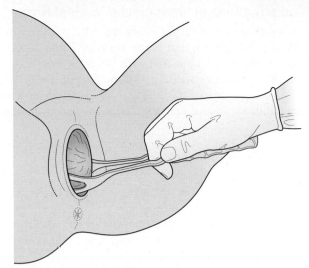

Fig. 24.5 Traction of the head is downwards until this point; when the head is low, the direction of pull is outward, towards the operator.

Fig. 24.3 Left blade being inserted. The fingers of the right hand guard the vaginal tissue.

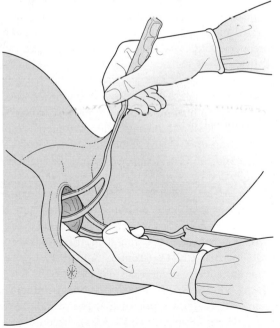

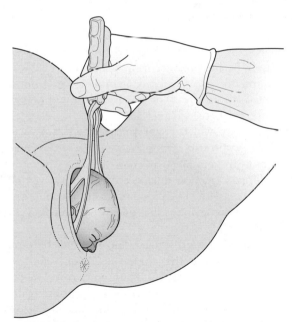

Fig. 24.6 As the head crowns it is guided upwards.

Fig. 24.4 Right blade being inserted.

the blades, checking their application before applying traction. The blades **must** be repositioned or the procedure abandoned if the application is incorrect.

- Traction should be applied in concert with uterine contractions and maternal expulsive efforts.
- As with the ventouse, the axis of traction changes during the birth and is guided along the curve of Carus, the blades being directed to the vertical as the head crowns (Figs 24.3–24.6).

Complications of Instrumental Vaginal Birth

Although forceps are less likely than the ventouse to fail to achieve a vaginal birth, they are significantly more likely to be associated with third- or fourth-degree tears (with or without the concurrent use of an episiotomy), vaginal trauma, use of general anaesthesia, flatal, faecal and urinary continence (see Chapter 17).

Maternal complications

Complications may include:
- trauma or soft tissue damage – occurring to the cervix, vagina or perineum
- dysuria or urinary retention, which may result from bruising or oedema to the tissues around the urethra
- perineal discomfort
- haemorrhage (both from tissue trauma and also uterine atony – the risk of which is always increased following an assisted vaginal birth).

Neonatal complications

Complications may include:
- marks on the baby's face and bruising (commonly caused by the pressure from the forceps blades and around the caput succedaneum/chignon from the ventouse – nearly all of which resolve within 48–72 h after birth; see Chapter 35)
- facial palsy, which may result from pressure from a blade compressing a facial nerve (a transient problem in most instances)
- prolonged traction during a birth with a ventouse will increase the likelihood of scalp abrasions, cephalohaematoma or subaponeurotic bleeding (see Chapter 35).

Some authors suggest that failure rates of <1% should be achieved using the correct technique and with well-maintained equipment. Many authors feel that this is an unrealistic target. Failure of the ventouse realistically arises in up to 20% of cases and indeed Johanson and Menon (2010) achieved vaginal birth with the first instrument in only 86% of assisted births.

The following as factors will often be found to have contributed to failure:

With the ventouse.
- Failure to select the correct cup type – inappropriate use of the silastic cup – especially in the presence of deflexion of the fetal head, excess caput, 'dense' epidural block or fetal macrosomia (true CPD)
- Failure of the equipment to provide adequate traction as a consequence of a leakage of the vacuum
- Incorrect cup placement – too anterior or lateral, with or without inclusion of maternal soft tissues within the cup.

With any instrument
- Inadequate initial case assessment – high head, misdiagnosis of the position and attitude of the head
- Traction along the wrong plane (often too anteriorly and not along the curve of Carus)
- Poor maternal effort with inadequate use of Syntocinon to maximize the contribution from coordinated uterine activity.

Whatever the outcome, the midwife in attendance is vital to the success of any manoeuvres undertaken, encouraging the mother to be an active participant in her birth, supporting the mother and her partner through what may be perceived to be a 'deviation from normal' and importantly, to support the clinician undertaking the assisted birth.

CAESAREAN SECTION

Caesarean section is an operative procedure, which is carried out under anaesthesia (regional or general), whereby the fetus, placenta and membranes are delivered through an incision made in the abdominal wall and uterus.

Globally the latest data from 150 countries, reveals that 18.6% of all births occur by CS, ranging from 6% to 27.2% in the least and most developed regions, respectively (Betrán et al. 2016). Table 24.1 shows that Latin America and the Caribbean region has the highest CS rates, followed by North America with the lowest rates being in Africa. However, regardless of the country the CS rate is increasing. Betrán et al. (2016) state that data from 121 countries in terms of the trend analysis, showed that between 1990 and 2014, the global average CS rate increased 12.4% (from 6.7% to 19.1%), with an average annual rate of increase of 4.4%.

In the UK, the RCOG (2001) National Sentinel Caesarean Section Audit reported that the overall CS rate was 21.5% (in England and Wales), accounting for approximately 120,000 births per year. While the CS rates for maternity units ranged from 10% to 65%, 10% of women had CS before labour (range between maternity units 4% to 59%), and 12% of women who went into labour had a CS (range between maternity units 2% to

TABLE 24.1 Caesarean Section (CS) Rate by World Region

Region and ranking in terms of CS rate	CS rate (%)
1. Latin America and the Caribbean	40.5
2. Northern America	32.3
3. Oceania	31.1
4. Europe	25
5. Asia	19.2
6. Africa	7.3

Adapted from Betrán et al 2016. The Increasing Trend in Caesarean Section Rates: Global, Regional and National Estimates: 1990 2014.

22%). Older mothers also impact the CS rate. NHS Digital (2018) data shows that the proportion of births by CS increase with age group and accounts for 45% of births to those women aged ≥40.

It is believed that some of the differences in CS rates observed may be explained by differences in the demographic and clinical characteristics of the population, such as maternal age, ethnicity, previous CS, breech presentation, prematurity and induction of labour; resources play a major role in less developed countries. However, the exact reasons for these differences remain unclear (Bragg et al. 2010).

Although there has been an increase in CS rates over the past 20 years, the four major clinical determinants of the CS rate have not changed. Common primary indications reported for women having a primary CS were: failure to progress in labour (25%), presumed fetal compromise (28%) and breech presentation (14%). The most common indications for women having a repeat CS were: previous CS (44%); maternal request as reported by clinicians (12%); failure to progress (10%); presumed fetal compromise (9%); and breech presentation (3%).

Currently in the UK, slightly more than one in seven women experience complications during labour that provide an indication for CS. These problems can be life-threatening for the mother and/or baby (e.g. eclampsia, abruptio placenta) and, in approximately 40% of such cases, a CS provides the safest route for birth. In all cases, the principal aims must be to ensure that those women and babies who need birth by CS are so delivered, and that those who do not are saved from an unnecessary intervention.

In 1985, concern regarding the increasing frequency of caesarean section led the World Health Organization (WHO) to hold a Consensus Conference (Stephenson 1992). This conference concluded that there were no 'health benefits' above a CS rate of 10–15%. The Scandinavian countries managed to hold CS rates at this level during the 1990s, with outcomes comparable to or better than those of countries with higher CS rates. However, this is no longer the case and CS rates in these countries have now increased towards those in the other developed nations.

Although many factors have been associated with an increase in the CS rate, not all have been to the detriment of the mother or baby. Interestingly, while the CS rate has risen over the two preceding decades, the instrumental vaginal birth rate has remained relatively constant.

Clarifying the Indications for Caesarean Section

NICE (2011) recommends that the urgency of CS should be documented using the following standardized scheme in order to aid clear communication between healthcare professionals about the urgency of a CS:

1. Immediate threat to the life of the woman or fetus
2. Maternal or fetal compromise which is not immediately life-threatening
3. No maternal or fetal compromise but an early birth is indicated
4. Birth timed to suit woman or staff.

The need for birth by a category 1 ('crash') CS is fortunately a rare event, as it can be a psychologically traumatic event for the woman and her partner. It is also extremely stressful for the clinical staff in attendance. Resources may have to be obtained from other areas of clinical care to facilitate such a birth and care standards risk being compromised in the rush to secure a 'safe' outcome. Care should therefore be exercised before making this decision, and *in utero* fetal resuscitation (fluids and tocolytics) may give enough time for a more considered and careful approach.

Indications why elective caesarean section would be the strongly recommended mode of birth:

- past obstetric history
- previous classical caesarean section
- complex pelvic floor or anal sphincter repair where woman is still symptomatic/experiencing morbidity

- previous severe shoulder dystocia with significant neonatal injury
- current pregnancy events:
  - significant fetal disease likely to lead to poor tolerance of labour
  - monoamniotic twins or higher-order multiple pregnancy
  - placenta praevia
  - obstructing pelvic mass
  - active primary herpes at onset of labour
- intrapartum events:
  - presumed fetal compromise in the first stage
  - maternal disease for which delay in the birth process may compromise the safety of the mother
  - absolute cephalopelvic disproportion (brow presentations, etc., see Chapter 23).

These lists are not comprehensive and factors or other indicators may coexist to influence the decision-making process.

The Operative Procedure

- The rationale for the intervention is discussed with the woman and her partner. The procedure is explained and consent obtained (written consent must be obtained in all cases other than a category 1 or 'crash section'). For elective procedures, consent may be taken in a dedicated preoperative assessment (the decision having been previously discussed and agreed in the antenatal clinic by a senior clinician in consultation with the woman and her partner).
- A preoperative assessment includes: weight and observations of blood pressure, pulse and temperature. The woman is gowned, make-up, the presence of any nail varnish and jewellery removed (rings/earrings taped).
- The woman is visited by the anaesthetist and the operating department practitioner preoperatively, and assessed. An anaesthetic chart will be commenced.
- Results of any blood tests that have been requested are obtained (full blood count, group and save and cross-match, if required).
- The woman will have fasted and have taken the prescribed antacid therapy.
- Many women prefer to have urinary catheterization in the theatre once the regional or general anaesthetic has been administered. However, some women will prefer to have this procedure undertaken in the

privacy of their room before entering the operating theatre.
- As the woman will need to lie flat, it is essential that a wedge or cushion is used, or the table is tilted, to direct the gravid uterus away from the inferior vena cava. The risks of supine hypotension syndrome will thus be reduced.
- The regional or general anaesthetics will be administered.
- The WHO (2008) surgical safety checklist has been widely accepted globally, contributing to reduce postoperative mortality and morbidity. For this reason, a surgical 'time out' on every woman entering the operating theatre prior to the preparation of the skin should be employed. In competent hands, this takes a matter of seconds dramatically improving safety, while not delaying the birth to any perceptible degree.
- The skin is prepared in accordance with local and national guidelines. Currently, it remains unclear what kind of skin preparation might be the most efficacious in the prevention of post-CS surgical wound infection (Hadiati et al. 2012; WHO 2015).
- Intravenous antibiotics should be administered as surgical prophylaxis before the skin is incised. This reduces the risk of maternal infection more than prophylactic antibiotics given after skin incision, and no effect on the baby has been demonstrated.

The anatomical layers that need to be breached in order to reach the fetus are: skin, subcutaneous fat, rectus sheath, muscle (rectus abdominis), abdominal peritoneum, pelvic peritoneum and uterine muscle.

A transverse lower abdominal incision (bikini-line incision) is usually performed with the skin and subcutaneous tissues incised using a transverse curvilinear incision at a level of two fingerbreadths above the symphysis pubis. The subcutaneous tissues are subsequently separated by blunt dissection and the rectus sheath incised transversely for 2 cm either side of the midline. This incision is then extended with scissors or blunt dissection before the facial sheath is separated from the underlying muscle. The recti are separated from each other, the peritoneum incised and the abdominal cavity entered.

The fold of the peritoneum over the anterior aspect of the lower uterine segment and above the bladder is incised and the bladder mobilized and reflected down. The uterus is incised transversely taking care not to cause surgical trauma to the fetus (a significant risk in the presence of low levels of amniotic fluid). The surgeon, with help from the surgical assistant (who must apply fundal pressure), will then secure the safe birth of the baby.

The main reason for preferring the lower uterine segment technique is the reduced incidence of dehiscence of the uterine scar in any subsequent pregnancy and/or birth when compared to a classical or vertical incision (which may be the only surgical approach that is suitable in situations such as anterior wall placenta praevia, in extreme prematurity (where no lower uterine segment may be formed) or in the presence of dense adhesions from previous surgery.

Oxytocics (a bolus of 5 IU of Syntocinon administered intravenously) should be given by the anaesthetist after birth of the baby and clamping of the umbilical cord. When the baby and placenta have been delivered, the uterus is closed in two layers and the rectus sheath and skin sutured. Most surgeons use a braided polyglactin suture (Vicryl) for all layers. The wound is then dressed and the vagina swabbed to remove any clots. This also allows a final intraoperative assessment of any ongoing bleeding from within the uterus.

In the UK, the triennial report from MBRRACE for 2014–2016 and 2015–2017 on maternal morbidity and mortality identified thromboembolic disorder as the leading cause of maternal deaths (Knight et al. 2018; Knight et al. 2019). Therefore, women having a CS should be offered thromboprophylaxis because they are at increased risk of venous thromboembolism. The choice of method of prophylaxis (e.g. graduated stockings, hydration, early mobilization, low-molecular-weight heparin) should take into account risk of thromboembolic disease, although in most cases it is simplest, and safest, to administer low molecular weight heparin to all women until they are fully mobile. Those with an increased risk (e.g. maternal obesity or concurrent maternal morbidity) should have a more formal assessment of risk and an individualized care plan put in place.

Early skin-to-skin contact between the woman and her baby should be encouraged and facilitated as it improves maternal perceptions of the infant, mothering skills, maternal behaviour, breastfeeding outcomes and reduces infant crying (see Chapter 27). In addition, women who have had a CS should be offered additional support to help them to start breastfeeding as soon as possible after the birth of their baby. This is because women who have had a caesarean section are less likely to start breastfeeding in the first few hours after the birth, but, when breastfeeding is established, they are as likely to continue as women who have had a vaginal birth.

Women's Request for Caesarean Section

The reasons behind the 'demands' for birth by CS are complex (Nama and Wilcock 2011). Despite the focus of attention in the media, evidence suggests that very few women actually request CS in the absence of medical indications and the 'too posh to push cohort' are in an extreme minority (Weaver and Magill-Cuerden 2013; Hutcherson and Ayers 2017). However, the accounts of women who have had difficult experiences of childbirth describe 'knowing something was wrong but believe that they were not listened to' are all too familiar (Karlström et al. 2009). Such women frequently publicize their problems via Facebook or other social media networks, fuelling the idea of 'them against us', and the joys of any future pregnancy risk being overwhelmed by the focus for a birth by CS whatever the rationale behind their beliefs.

Psychological Support and the Role of the Midwife

Choice is an important element in understanding this sequence. Women expect to be actively involved in their care and all staff involved must ensure that recent, valid and relevant information is provided in a comprehensible manner. This will help women to decide what is best for them, in relation to their own specific circumstances. The midwife, as an informed, confident and competent practitioner, will have a pivotal role in this process and be able to provide women with clear and unbiased information concerning the choices available (Feeley et al. 2019; WHO 2012). This will often relieve the stress of the situation and help women make a competent decision, supporting them in the midst of any misgivings.

One-to-one care from a support person during labour can influence the rate of birth by CS, as a continual, supportive presence in labour is undoubtedly of considerable benefit, both to the woman and to her family (Tracy et al. 2013; Hodnett et al. 2013). It is important that midwives recognize the positive impact on outcomes of their continuous presence during established labour (NICE 2014; Hodnett et al. 2013). Caseload midwifery is a tried and tested means of achieving continuity of care with carer, which culminates in positive outcomes for both mother and neonate (Tracy et al. 2013; NHS England 2017).

Psychological support mechanisms may also help these women to overcome their fears and, as such, it may be appropriate to develop links with trained counsellors to enable women to explore their anxieties and reach a more informed and rational decision prior to electing to undergo major abdominal surgery (see Chapter 18). However, NICE (2011) recommends for women requesting a CS that if, after discussion and offer of support (including perinatal mental health support for women with anxiety about childbirth, see Chapter 25), a vaginal birth is still not an acceptable option, a planned caesarean section should be offered.

Vaginal Birth after Caesarean Section

Ziadeh and Sunna (1995) reported that the widespread adoption of a policy whereby 80% of women with a prior CS should have a vaginal birth after caesarean section (VBAC) would potentially eliminate up to one-third of births by CS. In contemporary practice, this is still the target towards which those providing care to women in pregnancy strive.

When advising about the mode of birth after a previous CS, it is important to consider the maternal preferences and priorities, the risks and benefits of repeat CS and the risks and benefits of planned VBAC, including the risk of unplanned (i.e. emergency) CS (RCOG 2015). A woman's sense of control in the decision-making process is vital to her overall satisfaction and emotional adjustment postpartum (Alderdice et al. 2019).

NICE (2011) recommends that women who have had up to and including four caesarean sections should be informed that the risks of fever, bladder injuries and surgical injuries do not vary with the planned mode of birth and that the risk of uterine rupture, although higher for planned vaginal birth, is rare. However it is a 'brave' clinician who would choose to recommend vaginal birth as a safe option in those women who have had two previous CS.

It is also important to remember that pregnant women with both a previous CS and a previous vaginal birth should be informed that they have an increased likelihood of achieving a vaginal birth than women who have had a previous CS but no previous vaginal birth.

Pare et al. (2005) argued that the concerns around the safety of VBAC ignored the potential downstream consequences of a strategy whereby multiple elective repeat caesarean sections are considered to be the safer option. These include an increased length of stay in hospital and increased risks of placenta praevia and accreta in future pregnancies. They confirmed that for women who desire two or more additional children, the risks of multiple caesarean sections outweigh the risks of a VBAC attempt.

Criteria for a successful VBAC:
- Adequate supervision must be available, including continuous electronic fetal monitoring with cardiotography (CTG).
- All the facilities for assisted birth should be readily available.
- Progress of the labour is sufficient, observed both in the descent of the presenting part and by the dilatation of the cervix.
- The woman and her partner should be fully informed about the risks and benefits.

Postoperative Care

After birth by CS, women should receive enhanced recovery care, i.e. be observed on a one-to-one basis by a properly trained member of staff until they have regained airway control, have observed cardiorespiratory stability and are able to communicate effectively. Enhanced recovery (see Chapter 26) is an evidence-based approach that helps women recover more speedily post-CS and includes the enter perioperative period. In essence, the key aims of this approach are to ensure:
- women are in the optimal health preoperatively CS
- women receive effective care intraoperatively
- women receive optimum care postoperatively.

After recovery from anaesthesia, observations (respiratory rate, heart rate, blood pressure, pain and sedation) should be recorded every 15 min in the immediate recovery period (for the first 30 min) and thereafter every half-hour for 2 h, and hourly thereafter provided that the observations are stable or satisfactory. Such vital signs or physiological parameters should be recorded using a 'track and trigger' system such as the Modified Obstetrics Early Warning Score (MOEWS) chart (see Chapter 26). If these observations are not stable, more frequent observations and medical review are recommended. In addition, the wound and lochia must be inspected every 30 min to detect any ongoing blood loss. If the mother intends to breastfeed, skin-to-skin contact with mother and baby can be facilitated as soon as possible in the operating theatre. This will assist with early breastfeeding, a process that can usually be achieved with minimal disturbance to the undertaking of these routine observations.

For women who have had intrathecal opioids, there should be a minimum hourly observation of respiratory rate, sedation and pain scores for at least 12 h if diamorphine has been administered and for 24 h in the case of morphine. For women who have had epidural opioids or patient-controlled analgesia (PCA) with opioids, there should be routine hourly monitoring of respiratory rate, sedation and pain scores throughout treatment and for at least 2 h after discontinuation of treatment.

Postoperative analgesia

Postoperative analgesia should be given on a regular basis and may be given in a variety of ways:

- Ongoing epidural anaesthesia/analgesia. Women should have diamorphine (3 mg) or fentanyl (100 µg) administered into the epidural space for intra- and postoperative analgesia, as it reduces the need for supplemental analgesia after a caesarean section. Intravenous or intramuscular administration of diamorphine (2.5–5 mg) is a suitable alternative. However, intramuscular or intravenous analgesia should never be given in conjunction with epidural opioids for at least the first 4 h after administration of the epidural dose because of the cumulative effects and risks of respiratory depression.
- PCA using opioid analgesics may be offered after caesarean section as an alternative pain relief regimen.
- Antiemetics (e.g. cyclizine; prochlorperazine) are usually prescribed when opioids are required.
- Analgesia, such as diclofenac (oral or rectal) or paracetamol (oral, intravenous or rectal) are the mainstays of postoperative analgesia.
- Oral drugs (e.g. dihydrocodeine, codydramol, ibuprofen or paracetamol).
- Providing there are no contraindications (history of kidney disease, sensitivity to nonsteroidal anti-inflammatory drugs [NSAIDs], peptic ulcer, severe brittle asthma), NSAIDs should be offered post-caesarean section as an adjunct to other analgesics, as they reduce the need for the administration of opioids.

Care following regional block

Following birth under epidural or spinal anaesthesia, the woman may sit up as soon as she wishes, provided her blood pressure is not low. All observations must be recorded as described above.

Women who are recovering well after CS and who do not have complications can eat and drink when they feel hungry or thirsty, at which point the intravenous fluid infusion can be discontinued.

The baby should remain with the mother unless there is a medical reason for care being provided elsewhere (e.g. on a special care or neonatal intensive care unit) and indeed they should be transferred to the postnatal ward together once it is safe to do so. Such care is undoubtedly of benefit to a woman's psychological health and long-term wellbeing.

Care in the postnatal ward

Once care is transferred to the postnatal ward, the blood pressure, temperature, respirations and pulse must be checked every 4 h and recorded as previously mentioned using a MOEWS chart (Knight et al. 2018). In addition, the wound and lochia should be inspected at the same time. Removal of the urinary bladder catheter should be carried out once a woman is mobile after a regional anaesthetic and not sooner than 12 h after the last epidural 'top-up' dose. Healthcare professionals caring for women who have had a CS and who have urinary symptoms should consider the possible diagnosis of: urinary tract infection, stress incontinence (which occurs in about 4% of women after CS) or urinary tract injury (which occurs in about 1 per 1000 women after birth by CS) (NICE 2011).

The mother should be encouraged to move her legs and to perform leg and breathing exercises, however routine respiratory physiotherapy does not need to be offered to women after a caesarean section under general or regional anaesthesia, as it does not improve respiratory outcomes such as coughing, phlegm, body temperature, chest palpation and auscultatory changes.

The woman should be helped to get out of bed as soon as possible following a CS, and should also be encouraged to become fully mobile. Prophylactic low-molecular-weight heparin and antiembolic or thromboembolic deterrent ('TED') stockings should be prescribed (Knight et al. 2019). However, the first dose of low-molecular-weight heparin should be delayed until 4 h after the intrathecal injection or removal of the epidural catheter.

Women who have had a general anaesthetic for CS may feel very tired and drowsy for some hours. A woman

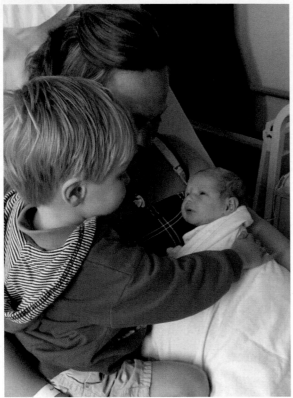

Fig. 24.7 Mother and family post-birth.

may complain of a feeling of detachment and unreality and may feel that she does not relate well to the baby. The woman who is concerned should be reassured and be given the opportunity to talk freely.

The mother must be encouraged to rest as much as possible and tactful advice may need to be given to her visitors. If the mother becomes too tired, help is needed with care for the baby. This should, preferably, take place at the mother's bedside and should include support with breastfeeding. Early parent(s)-baby interactions and family relationships should be fostered (Fig. 24.7) with little disruption in the way of hospital routines, custom and practice.

NICE (2011) guidelines state that caesarean section wound care should include: removing the dressing 24 hours after the birth; assessing the wound for signs of infection (such as increasing pain, redness or discharge) separation or dehiscence; encouraging the woman to wear loose comfortable clothes and cotton underwear; gently cleaning and drying the wound daily if needed; and planning the removal of sutures or clips if required.

Some women may have a lingering feeling of failure or disappointment at having had an emergency CS and may value the opportunity to talk this over with the mid-wife or other clinicians involved in her care. Indeed it is considered to be good practice for the obstetrician who undertook the CS to review the woman postpartum, not only in order to discuss the problems that necessitated the surgical intervention, but also to counsel about the options for any future pregnancy.

Healthcare professionals caring for women who have heavy and/or irregular vaginal bleeding following CS should be aware that this is more likely to be due to endometritis than retained products of conception. As a consequence, should this complication be suspected, first-line treatment with broad spectrum antibiotics should be implemented rather than referral for ultrasound assessment. However, if there are any concerns about the completeness of the placental tissue or membranes, referral for senior review at an early stage should be the preferred course of action.

While the length of hospital stay is likely to be longer after a caesarean section (an average of 3–4 days) than after a vaginal birth (average 1–2 days), women who are recovering well, are apyrexial and do not have complications following CS should be offered early transfer home (after 24 h) from hospital and follow-up at home, as this is not associated with more infant or maternal readmissions compared with later transfer (NICE 2011).

Analgesia/Anaesthesia
Pudendal block

This is the procedure where local anaesthetic is infiltrated into the tissue around the pudendal nerve within the pelvis (Fig. 24.8). The pudendal nerve emerges from the spine at the level of the S2–S4 vertebrae and 'descends' into the pelvis crossing behind the ischial spine as it does so. The pudendal nerve supplies the levator ani muscles, the deep and superficial perineal muscles and the sensory nerves (pain/stretch and temperature) of the lower vagina and perineum. A pudendal needle (a specifically designed needle incorporating a sheath guard) is employed with up to 20 mL of local anaesthetic, usually 1% lidocaine (lignocaine), being injected into the region around and below the ischial spine. As both motor and sensory nerves are affected with this technique it may be used to provide analgesia

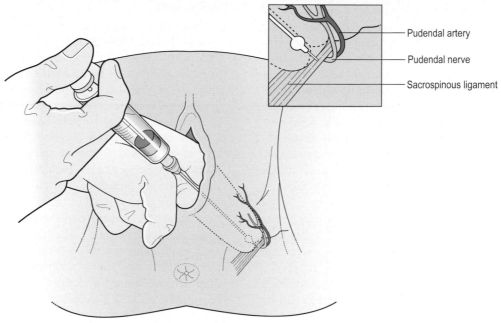

Pudendal artery

Pudendal nerve

Sacrospinous ligament

Fig. 24.8 Locating the pudendal nerve.

for the lower vagina and perineum, and is therefore used during forceps and ventouse instrumental births.

Perineal infiltration

See Chapter 17 for infiltration and repair of episiotomy, as well as third- and fourth-degree perineal trauma.

Regional anaesthesia

The two most commonly employed regional anaesthetic techniques are those of epidural and intrathecal (spinal) anaesthetic.

The epidural space is the space located within the bony spinal canal just outside the dura mater. In contact with the inner surface of the dura is another membrane called the 'arachnoid mater'. The cerebrospinal fluid (CSF) is contained between the arachnoid mater and the 'pia mater', another membrane that lies directly in contact with the spinal cord. In adults, the spinal cord terminates at the level of the lower border of the L2 vertebra below which lies a bundle of nerves known as the cauda equina ('horse's tail').

Insertion of an epidural needle involves threading a needle between the spinal vertebrae, through the ligaments and into the epidural potential space taking great care not to puncture the dura mater immediately below, which contains the CSF.

Techniques

Procedures involving injection of any substance into the epidural space require the operator to be technically proficient in order to avoid complications.

The subject is most commonly placed in the seated or lateral positions. Intravenous access is mandatory. Following a standard aseptic technique protocol, the level of the spine at which the catheter/spinal needle is to be placed is identified.

Epidural. The iliac crest is a commonly used anatomical landmark for lumbar epidural injections, as this level roughly corresponds with the fourth lumbar vertebra, which is usually below the termination of the spinal cord. Following the infiltration of local anaesthetic, a Tuohy needle is usually inserted in the midline, between the spinous processes, passing below the vertebral lamina until reaching the ligamentum flavum and the epidural space. A slight clicking sensation may be felt by the operator as the tip of the needle breaches the ligamentum flavum and enters the epidural space.

A syringe containing saline is attached to the Tuohy needle – most practitioners using the loss of resistance to pressure to identify that the needle is correctly placed.

A catheter is then threaded through the needle (typically 3–5 cm into the epidural space), the needle withdrawn and the catheter secured to the skin with adhesive tape or dressings to prevent it becoming dislodged. The catheter is a fine plastic tube, through which anaesthetic drugs may be injected into the epidural space. Many epidural catheters have three or more orifices along the shaft at the distal tip (far end) of the catheter to allow rapid and even dispersal of the injected agents more widely around the catheter and reduce the incidence of catheter blockage.

A person receiving an epidural for pain relief may receive local anaesthetic (most commonly levobupivacaine), with or without an opioid (most commonly fentanyl). These are injected in relatively small doses, compared with when they are injected intravenously or intramuscularly.

For a short procedure, the anaesthetist may introduce a single dose of medication (the 'bolus' technique), although the effects of this will eventually wear off. Thereafter, the anaesthetist or midwife may repeat the bolus provided the catheter remains undisturbed. For a prolonged effect, a continuous infusion of drugs may be employed. However, there is evidence that patient-controlled epidural analgesia (PCEA), whereby the administration of the boluses is controlled by the patient (up to a predetermined maximum dose) provides better analgesia than a continuous infusion technique, although the total doses received by the individual are often identical (Kwok et al. 2014).

Typically, the effects of the epidural block are noted below a specific level on the body – a block at or below the T10 sensory level is ideal for women in labour or during birth. Nonetheless, giving very large volumes into the epidural space may spread the block higher.

The epidural catheter is usually removed prior to transfer to the postnatal ward.

Spinal anaesthesia. Intrathecal (spinal) anaesthesia is a technique whereby a local anaesthetic drug is injected into the cerebrospinal fluid through a fine (24–26 gauge) spinal needle. The technique has some similarity to epidural anaesthesia. However, important differences include the following:

- Intrathecal anaesthesia requires a lower dose of drug and has a faster onset than epidural anaesthesia.
- The block achieved with spinal anaesthesia is typically described as being more dense.
- A spinal anaesthetic block typically lasts for 2 h, however it cannot be topped up, as no catheter is inserted.
- Intrathecal injections are performed below the second lumbar vertebral body to avoid damaging the spinal cord.

Complications

According to the Association of Anaesthetists of Great Britain and Ireland (AAGBI 2002):

- Failure to achieve analgesia or anaesthesia occurs in about 5% of cases, while another 15% experience only partial analgesia or anaesthesia. If analgesia is inadequate, another epidural may be attempted.
- The following factors are associated with failure to achieve epidural analgesia/anaesthesia: obesity, history of a previous failure of epidural anaesthesia, history of substance abuse (with opiates), advanced labour (cervical dilatation of >7 cm at insertion) and previous history of spinal surgery.
- Accidental dural puncture with headache (common, about 1 in 100 insertions). The epidural space in the adult lumbar spine is only 3–5 mm deep. It is therefore comparatively easy to accidentally puncture the dura (and arachnoid) with the needle, causing cerebrospinal fluid (CSF) to leak out into the epidural space. This may, in turn, cause a post-dural puncture headache (PDPH). This can be severe and last several days, and in some rare cases, weeks or months. It is caused by a reduction in CSF pressure and is characterized by postural exacerbation when the subject raises his/her head above the lying position. If severe, it may be successfully treated with an epidural blood patch, however most cases resolve spontaneously with time.
- Bloody tap (about 1 in 30–50). It is easy to injure an epidural vein with the needle. In people who have normal blood clotting, it is extremely rare for significant complications to develop. However, people who have a coagulopathy may be at increased risk.
- Catheter misplaced into the subarachnoid space (rare, less than 1 in 1000). If the catheter is accidentally misplaced into the subarachnoid space (e.g. after an unrecognized accidental dural puncture), normally cerebrospinal fluid can be freely aspirated from the catheter (which would usually prompt the anaesthetist to withdraw the catheter and resite it elsewhere). If, however, this is not recognized, large doses of anaesthetic may be delivered directly into the cerebrospinal fluid. This may result in a high block, or, more rarely, a total spinal, where anaesthetic is delivered directly to the brain stem, causing unconsciousness and sometimes seizures.
- Neurological injury lasting less than 1 year (rare, about 1 in 6700).

- Death (very rare, less than 1 in 100,000).
- Epidural haematoma formation (very rare, about 1 in 168,000)
- Neurological injury lasting longer than 1 year (extremely rare, about 1 in 240,000).
- Paraplegia (extremely rare, 1 in 250,000).

General anaesthesia

Despite the increasing use of regional anaesthesia, general anaesthesia is required in up to 5% of women requiring anaesthesia during birth. General anaesthesia can usually be more rapidly administered than a regional block, and is therefore of value when speed is important (such as when the fetus is in serious jeopardy). Women are pre-oxygenated (they are given oxygen to breathe for several minutes) prior to the 'rapid sequence' induction of anaesthesia with the intravenous administration of anaesthetic (e.g. thiopentone or propofol) followed by a muscle relaxant (e.g. suxamethonium) and cricoid pressure is applied (essential to reduce the risks of aspiration of stomach contents). Maternal unconsciousness ensues within seconds and orotracheal intubation is secured with a cuffed tube. There are minimal side-effects and relatively little negative fetal consequence at the time of birth provided meticulous practices are in place.

Anaesthesia is sustained by inhalational anaesthetic means (commonly enflurane or sevoflurane) with an opioid administered intravenously after clamping the cord.

Difficult or failed intubation. This condition is more likely to occur in pregnant women, particularly with those who have pregnancy-induced hypertension or who are obese. Access to the larynx may be obstructed or difficult to view in these women and therefore anticipation of the disorder is the key to its management. Should difficulties be anticipated, anaesthetists should carry out the intubation using a well-lubricated stylet or bougie to aid the endotracheal intubation.

The management of a failed intubation is primarily to maintain adequate oxygenation via assisted ventilation of the woman until the effects of suxamethonium and thiopentone have worn off and the woman has regained consciousness. This is done through the continued application of cricoid pressure and ventilation via a face mask.

It is therefore imperative that surgery is not commenced until the anaesthetist has secured the airway and confirmed that the woman is adequately ventilated.

Complications. Although surgical and anaesthetic techniques have improved, women are still more liable to suffer from complications and to have increased morbidity following caesarean section under general anaesthetic when compared to regional blockade.

Mendelson's syndrome. This condition was described by Mendelson in 1946 (see Levy 2006). It is a chemical pneumonitis caused by the reflux of gastric contents into the maternal lungs during a general anaesthetic. The acidic gastric contents damage the alveoli, impairing gaseous exchange. It may become impossible to oxygenate the woman and death may result. The predisposing factors are: the pressure from the gravid uterus when the woman is lying down, and the effect of the progesterone relaxing smooth muscle and the cardiac sphincter of the stomach. Analgesics administered during labour (e.g. pethidine) can cause significant delay in gastric emptying and will thereby exacerbate these risks.

Prevention of Mendelson's syndrome

Antacid therapy. Prophylactic treatment should be administered to all women in whom a caesarean is planned or anticipated. A usual regimen is for women having an elective operation to be given a single dose of oral omperazole 40 mg 12 hours preoperatively. If a general anaesthetic is anticipated, 30 mL of sodium citrate should be orally administered immediately before induction.

Cricoid pressure. This is a technique whereby pressure is exerted on the cartilaginous ring below the larynx, the cricoid, to occlude the oesophagus and prevent reflux (Fig. 24.9). This is the most important measure in preventing pulmonary aspiration. Cricoid pressure is administered during the induction of a general anaesthetic (most commonly by an operating department practitioner) and is maintained until the tracheal tube is confirmed as being correctly positioned and the seal of the cuff inflated.

Currently in the UK, the rate of maternal deaths directly attributed to anaesthesia has decreased significantly in the last 40 years from double figures in 1976–1978 to well below 1:100,000 maternities in the triennium 2015–2017 (Knight et al. 2019).

Research and the Incidence of Caesarean Section: Tackling High and Rising Caesarean Section Rates

Low CS rates are associated with low levels of intervention and high levels of psychological support. It is difficult to decipher whether caesarean section rates have

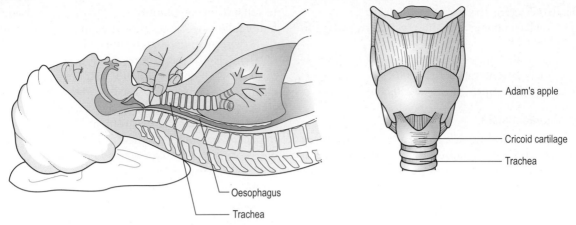

Adam's apple

Cricoid cartilage

Trachea

Oesophagus

Trachea

Fig. 24.9 Cricoid pressure showing occlusion of the oesophagus by pressure applied to the cricoid cartilage.

BOX 24.2 Clinical Interventions Proven to Reduce the Rates of Birth by CS

- External cephalic version (ECV) after 36 weeks for fetuses in a breech presentation
- Continuous support in labour
- Induction of labour for pregnancies beyond 41 weeks
- Use of a partogram with a 4-hour action line in labour
- Fetal blood sampling before caesarean section for abnormal cardiotocograph in labour
- Support for women who choose vaginal birth after caesarean section.

From NICE (National Institute for Health and Clinical Excellence). (2011) Caesarean section. CG 132. London: NICE.

been affected by interventions, such as proactive management of labour – that is, artificial rupture of membranes and use of oxytocin – or whether other factors have influenced these.

NICE (2011) guidelines recommend that the clinical interventions proven to reduce the rates of birth by CS include all the key points highlighted in Box 24.2.

While there is no accepted optimal rate for CS in the UK, some units manage to keep their CS rate below 25%. If reductions in the rate are to be achieved, efforts should focus on where there is the most potential for reduction: reducing primary CS, particularly in first-time mothers, and increasing rates of VBAC.

To provide more meaningful information to women when they are choosing their mode of birth, NICE (2011) has recommended that there is a pressing need to document the medium- to long-term outcomes in women and their babies after a planned CS or a planned vaginal birth. They note that it should be possible to gather data using standardized questions (traditional paper-based questionnaires, face-to-face interviews and internet-based questionnaires) about maternal septic morbidities and emotional wellbeing up to 1 year after a planned CS in a population of women who have consented for follow-up.

NICE (2011) also comment that it would be important to collect high-quality data on infant morbidities after a planned CS compared with a planned vaginal birth. A long-term morbidity evaluation (between 5 and 10 years after the CS) could use similar methodology to assess additional symptoms related to urinary and gastrointestinal function.

REFLECTIVE ACTIVITY FOR SELF-ASSESSMENT

1. What are the maternal and fetal indications for an assisted vaginal birth?
2. In the perioperative period how can enhanced recovery boost maternal outcomes?
3. What is the role of the midwife when caring for women whose mode of birth is an operative one, i.e. assisted vaginal birth (forceps or ventouse) or caesarean section?

REFERENCES

AAGBI (Association of Anaesthetists of Great Britain and Ireland). (2002). *Immediate: Post anaesthetic recovery*. London: AAGBI.

Alderdice, F., Henderson, J., Opondo, C., et al. (2019). Psychosocial factors that mediate the association between mode of birth and maternal postnatal adjustment: Findings from a population-based survey. *BMC Women's Health, 19*(1), 42.

Anim-Somuah, M., Smyth, R. M., Cyna, A. M., & Cuthbert, A. (2018). Epidural versus non-epidural or no analgesia for pain management in labour. *Cochrane Database of Systematic Reviews*, (5), CD000331.

Betrán, A. P., Torloni, M. R., Zhang, J. J., Gülmezoglu, A. M., & WHO Working Group on Caesarean Section (2016). WHO statement on caesarean section rates. *British Journal of Obstetrics and Gynaecology, 123*(5), 667–670.

Bragg, F., Cromwell, D. A., Edozien, L. C., et al. (2010). Variation in rates of caesarean section among English NHS trusts after accounting for maternal and clinical risk: Cross sectional study. *British Medical Journal, 341*, c5065 (correction c65749).

Brown, H. C., Paranjothy, S., Dowswell, T., et al. (2013). Package of care for active management in labour for reducing caesarean section rates in low–risk women. *Cochrane Database of Systematic Reviews*, (9), CD004907.

Feeley, C., Thomson, G., & Downe, S. (2019). Caring for women making unconventional birth choices: A meta-ethnography exploring the views, attitudes, and experiences of midwives. *Midwifery, 72*, 50–59.

Gupta, J. K., Sood, A., Hofmeyr, G., et al. (2017). Position in the second stage of labour for women without epidural anaesthesia. *Cochrane Database of Systematic Reviews*, (5), CD002006.

Hadiati, D. R., Hakimi, M., & Nurdiati, D. S. (2012). Skin preparation for preventing infection following caesarean section. *Cochrane Database of Systematic Reviews*, (9), CD007462.

Hodnett, E. D., Gates, S., Hofmeyr, G. J., et al. (2013). Continuous support for women during childbirth. *Cochrane Database of Systematic Reviews*, (7), CD003766.

Hutcherson, A., & Ayers, S. (2017). Maternal expectations and satisfaction with caesarean section. In G. Capogna (Ed.), *Anesthesia for cesarean section*. Cham: Springer.

Johanson, R. B., & Menon, V. (2010). Vacuum extraction versus forceps for assisted vaginal delivery. *Cochrane Database of Systematic Reviews, 11*, CD000224.

Karlström, A., Engström-Olofsson, R., Nysted, A., et al. (2009). Swedish caregivers' attitudes towards caesarean section on maternal request. *Women and Birth, 22*, 57–63.

Knight, M., Bunch, K., Tuffnell, D., et al. (Eds.). (2018). *MBRRACE-UK. Saving Lives, improving mothers' care – Lessons learned to inform maternity care from the UK and Ireland Confidential Enquiries into maternal deaths and morbidity 2014–2016*. Oxford: National Perinatal Epidemiology Unit, University of Oxford.

Knight, M., Bunch, K., Tuffnell, D., et al. (Eds.). (2019). On behalf of MBRRACE-UK. *Saving Lives, Improving Mothers' Care - Lessons learned to inform maternity care from the UK and Ireland Confidential Enquiries into Maternal Deaths and Morbidity 2015-17*. Oxford: National Perinatal Epidemiology Unit, University of Oxford.

Kwok, S., Wang, H., & Leong Sng, B. (2014). Post-caesarean analgesia. *Trends in Anaesthesia and Critical Care, 4*(6), 189–194.

Levy, D. M. (2006). Pre-operative fasting – 60 years on from Mendelson. *Continuing Education in Anaesthesia, Critical Care & Pain, 6*(6), 215–218.

Merriam, A. A., Ananth, C. V., Wright, J. D., et al. (2017). Trends in operative vaginal delivery, 2005–13: A population-based study. *British Journal of Obstetrics and Gynaecology, 124*, 1365–1372.

Nama, V., & Wilcock, F. (2011). Caesarean section on maternal request: Is justification necessary? *The Obstetrician and Gynaecologist, 13*, 263–269.

NHS Digital. (2018) *NHS Maternity Statistics, England 2017–8*. Available at: https://digital.nhs.uk/data-and-information/publications/statistical/nhs-maternity-statistics/2017-18#summary.

NHS England. (2017). *Implementing better births: Continuity of carer*. Available at: https://www.england.nhs.uk/publication/local-maternity-systems-resource-pack.

NICE (National Institute for Health and Care Excellence). (2014). *Intrapartum care. Care of healthy women and their babies during childbirth: CG 190*. London: NICE.

NICE (National Institute for Health and Clinical Excellence). (2011). *Caesarean section CG 0132*. London: NICE.

O'Driscoll, K., Meagher, D., & Boylan, P. (1993). *Active management of labour* (3rd ed.). London: Mosby.

Pare, E., Quiñones, J., & Macones, G. (2005). Vaginal birth after caesarean section versus elective repeat caesarean section: Assessment of maternal downstream health outcomes. *BJOG: An International Journal of Obstetrics and Gynaecology, 113*, 75–85.

RCOG (Royal College of Obstetricians and Gynaecologists). (2001). *Clinical Effectiveness support Unit. The national Sentinel caesarean section audit report*. London: RCOG.

RCOG (Royal College of Obstetricians and Gynaecologists). (2011). *Operative vaginal delivery. Green-top Guideline No 26*. London: RCOG.

RCOG (Royal College of Obstetricians and Gynaecologists). (2015). *Birth after previous caesarean birth. Green-top Guideline No 45*. London: RCOG.

Stephenson, P. A. (1992). *International differences in the use of obstetrical interventions.* Copenhagen: World Health Organization. WHO EUR/ICP of MCH, 112.

Tinsley, V. (2010). Midwives undertaking ventouse births. In J. E. Marshall, & M. D. Raynor (Eds.), *Advancing skills in midwifery practice* (pp. 67–75). Edinburgh: Churchill Livingstone.

Tracy, S. K., Hartz, D. L., Tracy, M. B., et al. (2013). Caseload midwifery care versus standard maternity care for women of any risk: M@NGO, a randomised controlled trial. *Lancet, 382*(9906), 1723–1732.

Turkmen, S. (2014). Maternal and neonatal outcomes in vacuum–assisted delivery with the Kiwi OmniCup and Malmström metal cup. *Journal of Obstetrics and Gynaecology Research, 41*(2), 207–213.

Weaver, J., & Magill-Cuerden, J. (2013). 'Too posh to push': The rise and rise of a catchphrase. *Birth, 40*(4), 264–271.

WHO (World Health Organization). (2008). *Surgical safety checklist.* Available at: https://www.who.int/patientsafety/safesurgery/ss_checklist/en/.

WHO (World Health Organization). (2012). *Respectful maternity care: The universal rights of childbearing women.* Washington: White Ribbon Alliance.

WHO (World Health Organization). (2015). *WHO recommendation on choice of an antiseptic agent and its method of application for skin preparation prior to caesarean section.* The WHO Reproductive Health Library. Geneva: World Health Organization.

Ziadeh, S. M., & Sunna, E. I. (1995). Decreased cesarean birth rates and improved perinatal outcome: A seven year study. *Birth, 22*(3), 144–147.

ANNOTATED FURTHER READING

Draper, E. S., Gallimore, I. D., Kurinczuk, J. J., & on behalf of the MBRRACE-UK Collaboration., et al. (2018). *MBRRACE-UK perinatal mortality Surveillance report, UK perinatal deaths for births from January to December 2016. The infant mortality and morbidity studies.* Leicester: Department of Health Sciences, University of Leicester.

Luesley, D. M., & Kilby, M. D. (Eds.). (2016). *Obstetrics and gynaecology: An evidence-based text for MRCOG* (3rd ed.) London: Hodder/Arnold.
This book, written by obstetricians approaching their Part 2 MRCOG examination, is a useful handbook for students of midwifery and midwives alike. The perspective is evidence-based and very woman-centred. Sections D and E focus on the first and second stages of labour, their complications and management. It contains useful references at the end of each chapter.

National Patient Safety National Patient Safety Agency Surgical Safety Checklist for Maternity. Available at: https://improvement.nhs.uk/resources/learning-from-patient-safety-incidents/.
A useful modification of the checklist from the WHO (2008) specific to the maternity context as the majority of women having a CS are awake at the occasion of 'time out'.

Simms, R., & Hayman, R. (2011). Instrumental vaginal delivery. *Obstetrics, Gynaecology and Reproductive Medicine, 21*(1), 7–14.
A general reference that informs some sections of this chapter.

USEFUL WEBSITES

Mothers and Babies: Reducing Risk Through Audits and Confidential Enquiries Across the UK: www.mbrrace.ox.ac.uk

National Confidential Enquiry into Patient Outcome and Death: www.ncepod.org.uk

National Institute for Health and Care Excellence: www.nice.org.uk

NHS UK: https://www.nhs.uk/conditions/enhanced-recovery/

National Patient Safety Agency: www.npsa.nhs.uk

Royal College of Midwives: www.rcm.org.uk

Royal College of Obstetricians and Gynaecologists: www.rcog.org.uk

Scottish Intercollegiate Guideline Network: www.sign.ac.uk

White Ribbon Alliance: https://www.whiteribbonalliance.org/resources

World Health Organization: www.who.net

25

Maternity Emergencies

Terri Coates, Kerry Green

CHAPTER CONTENTS

The emergency situations covered in this chapter are rare, but the communication and actions of the midwife are fundamental to the wellbeing of the woman, her baby and also her partner and family. Early detection of severe illness in childbearing women remains a challenge to all healthcare professionals involved in their care. Awareness of local emergency procedures and knowledge of correct use of any supportive equipment are essential, and midwives in all practice settings must maintain skills that enable them to act appropriately in an emergency. The use of multiprofessional workshops to rehearse simulated situations can ensure that all members of the care team know exactly what is required when needed. Midwives need also to engage in reviews of practice to ensure that policies and protocols are regularly reviewed to incorporate best practice and current evidence.

THE CHAPTER AIMS TO

- highlight the importance of effective communication between members of the multiprofessional team in critical clinical situations
- heighten awareness of sudden changes in maternal condition
- identify symptoms suggestive of serious illness
- explore the possible causes of midwifery and obstetric emergencies and the subsequent action to be taken

- discuss the rare obstetric conditions of uterine rupture, acute inversion of the uterus and vasa praevia
- discuss amniotic fluid embolism and the prompt action required to preserve the woman's life
- review the treatment of hypovolemic shock and maternal sepsis in midwifery practice.

INTRODUCTION

The immediate management of the emergencies discussed in this chapter is dependent on the prompt action of the midwife. Recognition of the problem and the instigation of emergency measures will determine the outcome for the mother or the fetus. The midwife should remain calm and aim to keep the woman and her partner fully informed in order to obtain her consent and cooperation for procedures that may be needed.

It is recognized that pregnancy and labour are normal physiological events, however regular routine observations of vital signs must be an integral part of midwifery care. There is potential for pregnant women and those who have recently given birth to be at risk of physiological deterioration that is not always predicted or recognized (Knight et al. 2019 on behalf of MBRRACE-UK, Mothers and Babies: Reducing Risk through Audits and Confidential Enquiries across the UK). Abnormalities in maternal vital signs often precede deterioration in maternal condition. To improve recognition of women who are unwell before they become critically ill, the modified early obstetric warning score (MEOWS) chart should be used (Knight et al. 2019).

All midwifery and medical staff must be updated on signs and symptoms of critical illness in respect of midwifery, obstetric and non-obstetric causes. The national maternity review (NHS England 2016) highlights the importance of multiprofessional education and training of emergency situations to enhance safety in maternity care. Emergency skills training should facilitate the opportunity to practise and maintain skills in the management of maternity emergencies. Effective communication between the multiprofessional team is essential to ensure the optimum outcome for the childbearing woman who becomes ill and her baby (Knight et al. 2019).

COMMUNICATION

Health services are often criticized for poor communication among their staff, especially when the outcome is unexpected. Effective communication involves the sharing of accurate and precise information (NHS Improvement 2018). The SBAR: *Situation, Background, Assessment* and *Recommendations* tool is a framework that midwives can use during clinical conversations that require immediate focus and action.

Use of the SBAR Tool

The tool (see Chapter 26) consists of standardized prompt questions about the condition of an individual in four stages:

- **S**ituation
- **B**ackground
- **A**ssessment
- **R**ecommendation.

These prompts can assist the midwife to assertively and effectively share concise and focused information about a woman's condition, reducing repetition. The SBAR tool can be used in *all* clinical conversations: face-to-face, by telephone or through collaborative multiprofessional team meetings. In each of the following maternity emergencies, the use of the SBAR tool should be paramount in facilitating appropriate action that is always in the best interest of the woman and her baby.

VASA PRAEVIA

The term *'vasa praevia'* is used when a fetal blood vessel lies over the cervical os, in front of the presenting part. This occurs when fetal vessels from a velamentous insertion of the cord or to a succenturiate lobe (see Chapter 6) cross the area of the internal os to the placenta. The fetal life is at risk due to the possibility of the rupture of a fetal vessel leading to haemorrhage of fetal blood, which will present as maternal vaginal bleeding. Blood loss of even small quantities can have serious implications for the fetus owing to the relatively small blood volume of the fetus (O'Connor et al. 2016). Where vasa praevia is identified in the third trimester, recommended management includes birth by caesarean section before the membranes rupture (Juaniaux et al. 2018).

Diagnosis

Vasa praevia may be diagnosed antenatally using ultrasound scan. Sometimes vasa praevia will be palpated on vaginal examination when the membranes are still intact. If vasa praevia is suspected, the vaginal examination should be discontinued and the obstetrician informed. Fresh vaginal bleeding, particularly if it commences at the same time as the membranes rupture may be due to ruptured vasa praevia. Fetal distress disproportionate to blood loss may be suggestive of vasa praevia.

Management

The midwife should seek urgent medical assistance and the situation calmly explained to the mother and her birth partner. The maternal vital signs should be monitored and the abdomen palpated to assess uterine tone. The blood loss should be estimated and the fetal heart rate monitored via a cardiotocograph (CTG). The birth should not be delayed if the fetal condition is deteriorating and emergency caesarean section may be indicated to expedite the birth (Juaniaux et al. 2018). There is high fetal mortality associated with this emergency and a paediatrician should be present for the birth. If the baby is born in poor condition, resuscitation, urgent haemoglobin estimation and a blood transfusion with O-negative blood may be necessary.

PRESENTATION AND PROLAPSE OF THE UMBILICAL CORD

Predisposing Factors

These are the same for both presentation and prolapse of the cord (see Box 25.1 for definitions). Any situation where the presenting part is neither well applied to the

---

BOX 25.1 Definitions

Cord Presentation
This occurs when the umbilical cord lies in front of the presenting part, with the fetal membranes still intact.

Cord Prolapse
The cord lies in front of the presenting part and the fetal membranes are ruptured (see Fig. 25.3).

Occult Cord Prolapse
This is said to occur when the cord lies alongside, but not in front of, the presenting part.

---

cervix nor well down in the pelvis may result in a loop of cord slipping down in front of the presenting part. Such situations (Lin 2006; Holbrook and Phelan 2013; Royal College of Obstetricians and Gynaecologists, RCOG 2014) include:

- high or ill-fitting presenting part
- high parity
- prematurity
- malpresentation
- multiple pregnancy
- polyhydramnios.

High head

If the membranes rupture spontaneously when the fetal head is high, a loop of cord is able to pass between the uterine wall and the fetus resulting in its lying in front of the presenting part. As the presenting part descends, the cord becomes trapped and occluded. If the presenting part is high or unengaged in the pelvis the midwife should avoid artificial rupture of the membranes where possible.

Multiparity

The presenting part may not be engaged when the membranes rupture and malpresentation is more common.

Prematurity

The smaller size of the fetus in relation to the pelvis and the uterus allows the cord to prolapse. Babies of very low birth weight (<1500 g) are particularly vulnerable (Lin 2006; Holbrook and Phelan 2013).

Malpresentation

Cord prolapse is associated with breech presentation, especially a *complete* or footling breech. This relates to the ill-fitting nature of the presenting parts and also the proximity of the umbilicus to the buttocks. In this situation, the degree of compression may be less than with a cephalic presentation, but there is still a danger of asphyxia.

Shoulder and compound presentation and transverse lie (see Chapter 23) carry a high risk of prolapse of the cord, occurring with spontaneous rupture of the membranes.

Multiple pregnancy

Malpresentation, particularly of the second twin, is more common in multiple pregnancy with the consequences of possible cord prolapse.

Polyhydramnios

The cord is liable to be swept down in a gush of liquor if the membranes rupture spontaneously. Controlled release of liquor during artificial rupture of the membranes is sometimes performed to try to prevent this.

Cord Presentation

This is diagnosed on vaginal examination when the cord is felt behind intact membranes. It may be associated with aberrations found during fetal heart monitoring such as decelerations, which occur if the cord becomes compressed.

Cord presentation management

Under no circumstances should the membranes be ruptured. The midwife should discontinue the vaginal examination in order to reduce the risk of rupturing the membranes. Medical aid should be summoned. To assess fetal wellbeing, continuous electronic fetal monitoring should be commenced, or the fetal heart should be auscultated as frequently as possible. The woman should be assisted into a position that will reduce the likelihood of cord compression (Figs 25.1, 25.2). Unless birth is imminent, caesarean section is the most likely outcome.

Cord Prolapse
Diagnosis

Whenever there are factors present that predispose to cord prolapse (Fig. 25.3), a vaginal examination should be performed immediately on spontaneous rupture of the membranes.

Bradycardia and variable or prolonged decelerations of the fetal heart are associated with cord compression,

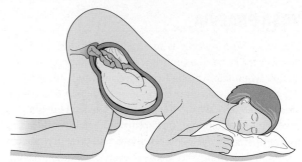

Fig. 25.1 Knee–chest position. Pressure on the umbilical cord is relieved as the fetus gravitates towards the fundus.

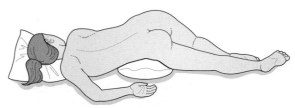

Fig. 25.2 Exaggerated Sims' position. Pillows or wedges are used to elevate the woman's buttocks to relieve pressure on the umbilical cord.

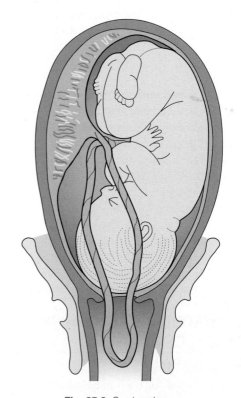

Fig. 25.3 Cord prolapse.

which may be caused by cord prolapse. The diagnosis of cord prolapse is made when the cord is felt below or beside the presenting part on vaginal examination. The cord may be felt in the vagina or in the cervical os or a loop of cord may be visible at the vulva.

Immediate action

Where the diagnosis of cord prolapse is made, the time should be noted, and the midwife must call for urgent assistance. The midwife should explain to the woman and her birth partner her findings and any emergency measures that may be needed. If an oxytocin infusion is in progress this should be discontinued. Handling the cord should be avoided as this may cause vasospasm (RCOG 2014). If the cord lies outside of the vagina it should be gently replaced back into the vagina with a dry pad (Winter et al. 2017), however this must be undertaken with care to avoid vasospasm. Administering oxygen to the woman by face mask at 4 L/min may improve fetal oxygenation.

Relieving pressure on the cord

The midwife may need to keep her fingers in the vagina and hold the presenting part of the umbilical cord, especially during a contraction, as shown in Fig. 25.4. The woman can be supported to change position and further reduce pressure on the cord. If the woman raises her pelvis and buttocks or adopts the knee–chest position, the fetus will be encouraged to gravitate towards the diaphragm (Fig. 25.1). The foot of the bed may also be raised (*Trendelenburg* position) to relieve compression on the cord. Alternatively, the woman can be helped to lie on her left side, with a wedge or pillow elevating her hips (*exaggerated Sims'* position) (Fig. 25.2).

There is some evidence to suggest that bladder filling may also be an effective technique for managing cord prolapse (Houghton 2006; Bord et al. 2011). This may be useful if there is an anticipated delay in transfer to theatre or if cord prolapse occurs in the community (Winter et al. 2017). A self-retaining 16G Foley catheter is used to instill approximately 500–700 mL of sterile saline into the bladder (Fig. 25.5). The full bladder can relieve compression of the cord by elevating the presenting part about 2 cm above the ischial spines until birth by caesarean section. The bladder should be drained before the caesarean section commences.

Birth must be expedited without delay to reduce the mortality and morbidity associated with this emergency.

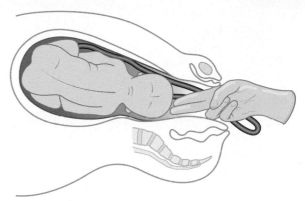

Fig. 25.4 Displacement of the presenting part away from the pelvic inlet. (With permission from S MacDonald, G Johnson (Eds). (2017) Mayes Midwifery. Edinburgh: Elsevier.)

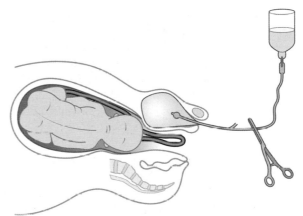

Fig. 25.5 Filling the bladder. (With permission from S MacDonald, G Johnson (Eds). (2017) Mayes Midwifery. Edinburgh: Elsevier.)

Caesarean section is the treatment of choice in those instances where the fetus is still alive and vaginal birth is not imminent. If a cord prolapse is diagnosed in the second stage of labour, with a multigravida, the midwife may perform an episiotomy to expedite the birth. Where the presentation is cephalic, assisted birth may be achieved through ventouse or forceps (see Chapter 24).

If a cord prolapse occurs in the *community setting*, emergency transfer to a consultant-led maternity unit is essential. The midwife should carry out the same procedures to relieve the compression on the cord. Senior obstetric and anaesthetic staff should be informed and be prepared to perform an emergency caesarean section. An experienced paediatrician should be available to resuscitate the baby, should it be born alive.

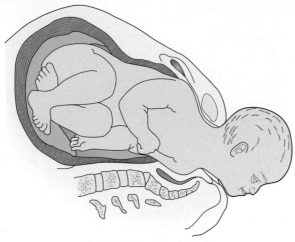

Fig. 25.6 Shoulder dystocia.

SHOULDER DYSTOCIA

The term *'shoulder dystocia'* describes failure of the shoulders to traverse the pelvis spontaneously requiring additional manoeuvres after the birth of the head (RCOG 2012a). However, a universally accepted definition of shoulder dystocia has yet to be produced (RCOG 2012a).

The anterior shoulder becomes trapped behind, or, on the symphysis pubis, while the posterior shoulder may be in the hollow of the sacrum or high above the sacral promontory (Fig. 25.6). This is, therefore, a **bony** dystocia, and traction at this point will further impact the anterior shoulder, impeding attempts to assist the baby's birth.

Incidence

Shoulder dystocia is not a common emergency: the incidence is reported as varying between 0.58% and 0.7% in collected data (RCOG 2012a).

Risk Factors

Although it would be useful to identify those women at risk from a birth complicated by shoulder dystocia, most risk factors can give only a high index of suspicion. Antenatal risk factors include diabetes, post-term pregnancy, high parity, maternal age over 35 and maternal obesity (weight >90 kg). It is recommended that shoulder dystocia is discussed with all pregnant women and a record of the conversation is made in the woman's notes (Michelotti et al. 2018).

Fetal macrosomia (birth weight >4000 g) has been associated with an increased risk of shoulder dystocia. The incidence increases as birth weight increases, although many cases of shoulder dystocia occur with infants of normal weight. Ultrasound scanning for prediction of macrosomia to prevent shoulder dystocia still has a poor record of success though it is anticipated that ultrasound detection of macrosomia can be improved (Siggelkow et al. 2011). If a large baby is suspected, then this fact must be communicated clearly to the team caring for the woman in labour (RCOG 2012a).

Maternal diabetes and gestational diabetes have been identified as important risk factors (Athukorala et al. 2007). In diabetic women, a previous birth complicated by shoulder dystocia increases the risk of recurrence to 9.8%; this compares with a risk of recurrence of 0.58% in the general population (Ouzounian et al. 2012). The National Institute for Health and Care Excellence (NICE 2015) guidelines for pregnancy and diabetes are described in Chapter 15.

In labour, risk factors that have been consistently linked with shoulder dystocia include oxytocin augmentation, prolonged labour, prolonged second stage of labour and operative births (Keller et al. 1991; Bahar 1996; Gupta et al. 2010). For a clinically suspected large baby, the multiprofessional team must be alert for the possibility of shoulder dystocia (RCOG 2012a).

Warning Signs and Diagnosis

The birth may have been uncomplicated initially, but the head may have advanced slowly, with the chin having difficulty in sweeping over the perineum. Once the head is born, it may look as if it is trying to return into the vagina (the *turtle sign*). Shoulder dystocia is diagnosed when manoeuvres such as gentle downward axial traction on the head, that may normally be undertaken by the midwife, fail to complete the birth (RCOG 2012a). The woman should be discouraged from pushing and any further traction must be avoided.

Management and Manoeuvres

Upon diagnosing shoulder dystocia, the midwife must summon help immediately: the midwife coordinator, an experienced obstetrician, an anaesthetist and a person proficient in neonatal resuscitation. Stating the problem early to the team has been associated with improvements in outcomes in shoulder dystocia (RCOG 2012a).

Shoulder dystocia is a frightening experience for the woman, for her partner and for the midwife. The midwife should remain calm and explain as much as possible to the woman with the aim to obtain her full cooperation should any manoeuvres be required to complete the birth.

The purpose of all these manoeuvres is to *disimpact* the shoulders and move them into a wider pelvic diameter and complete the birth using only routine traction. The principle of using the simplest of manoeuvres first should be applied. The midwife will need to make an accurate and detailed record of the time help was summoned and those who attended, the type of manoeuvre(s) used and the time taken, the amount of force used and the outcome of each manoeuvre attempted (Nursing and Midwifery Council, NMC 2018). It is also important to record which of the fetal shoulders was anterior.

The skills required to relive shoulder dystocia should primarily be concerned with comprehension, learning and regular opportunities to practice and use clinical judgement, e.g. mandatory multi-disciplinary '*skills and drills*' training. The HELPERR mnemonic approach to the management of shoulder dystocia (American Academy for Family Physicians 2004) is considered limited and unhelpful, with a study reporting a poor correlation between healthcare professionals' knowledge of manoeuvres and their eponyms (Jan et al. 2014).

Non-invasive Procedures

Change in maternal position

Any change in the maternal position may be useful to help release the fetal shoulders as shoulder dystocia is a bony, mechanical obstruction. However, certain manoeuvres have proved useful and are described below. It is anticipated that following the use of one or more of these manoeuvres, the birth is likely to proceed.

The McRoberts manoeuvre

This manoeuvre involves assisting the woman to lie completely flat (pillows removed) with her buttocks off the bed with hyperflexion of her hips to bring her knees up to her chest as far as possible (Fig. 25.7). This manoeuvre will rotate the angle of the symphysis pubis superiorly and use the weight of the woman's legs to create gentle pressure on her abdomen, releasing the impaction of the anterior shoulder (Gonik et al. 1983, 1989). The McRoberts manoeuvre is associated with the lowest level of morbidity and requires the least force to assist the birth (Bahar 1996; RCOG 2012a).

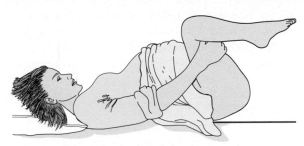

Fig. 25.7 The McRoberts manoeuvre.

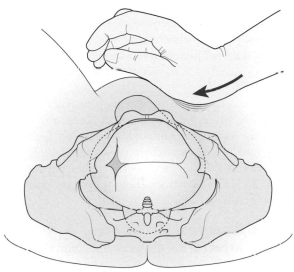

Fig. 25.8 Correct application of suprapubic pressure for shoulder dystocia. (After Pauerstein C (Ed.) (1987) Clinical obstetrics. New York. Churchill Livingstone, with permission.)

Suprapubic pressure

Pressure should be exerted on the side of the fetal back and towards the fetal chest. This manoeuvre may help to adduct the shoulders and push the anterior shoulder away from the symphysis pubis into the larger oblique or transverse diameter (Fig. 25.8). Suprapubic pressure can be employed together with the McRoberts manoeuvre to improve success rates (RCOG 2012a).

All-fours position

The all-fours position (or *Gaskin manoeuvre*) is achieved by assisting the woman onto her hands and knees. The act of the woman turning may be the most useful aspect of this manoeuvre (Bruner et al. 1998). In shoulder dystocia, the impaction is at the pelvic inlet and the force of gravity will keep the fetus against the anterior aspect of the mother's uterus and pelvis. However, this manoeuvre may be especially helpful if the posterior shoulder is impacted behind the sacral promontory as this position optimizes space available in the sacral curve and may allow the posterior arm/shoulder to be born first. Manipulative manoeuvres can be performed while the woman is on all fours but clear verbal communication is needed as eye contact is difficult.

Where non-invasive procedures have not been successful, direct manipulation of the fetus must be attempted, requiring the midwife to insert a whole hand into the vagina. The McRoberts position as detailed above can be used, or the woman could be placed in the lithotomy position with her buttocks well over the end of the bed so that there is no restriction on the sacrum.

Episiotomy

The problem facing the midwife is an obstruction at the pelvic inlet, which is a bony dystocia, not an obstruction caused by soft tissue. Although episiotomy (see Chapters 17 and 20) will not help to release the shoulders *per se*, the midwife should consider the need to perform one to gain access to the fetus without tearing the perineum and vaginal walls.

Internal Rotational Manoeuvres

Posterior aspect of the posterior shoulder: the Rubin manoeuvre

The midwife inserts a whole hand into the vagina and identifies the most accessible or lowest shoulder, which is usually the posterior shoulder and pushes that shoulder in the direction of the fetal chest. This process adducts the shoulders and allows rotation away from the symphysis pubis. This manoeuvre reduces the 12 cm bisacromial diameter to effect the birth (Fig. 25.9).

Anterior aspect of the posterior shoulder: the Woods manoeuvre

The midwife inserts a whole hand into the vagina and identifies the fetal chest. Then, by exerting pressure on to the posterior fetal shoulder, rotation is achieved. Although this manoeuvre does abduct the shoulders, it will rotate the shoulders into a more favourable diameter and enable the midwife to complete the birth (Fig. 25.10).

If rotation in one direction does not disimpact the shoulders then the midwife should be prepared to try a 180° rotation in the opposite direction.

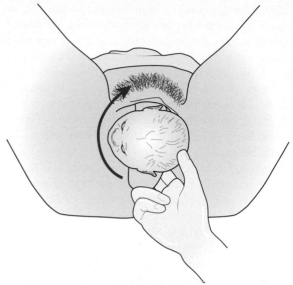

Fig. 25.9 The posterior aspect of the posterior shoulder manoeuvre (The Rubin manoeuvre).

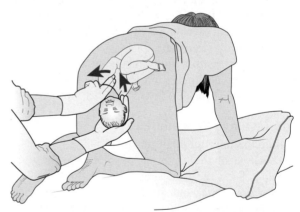

Fig. 25.10 The anterior aspect of the posterior shoulder manoeuvre (The Woods manoeuvre). (After Sweet BR, Tiran D. (1996) Mayes' Midwifery. London: Baillière Tindall, with permission.)

Birth of the posterior arm

The midwife has to insert a hand into the vagina, making use of the space created by the hollow of the sacrum, as shown in Fig. 25.11A,B. Then two fingers grasp the wrist of the posterior arm (Fig. 25.11C), to flex the elbow and sweep the forearm over the chest for the hand to be born, as shown in Fig. 25.11D (O'Leary 2009). If the rest of the birth is not then accomplished, the birth of the second arm is assisted following rotation of the shoulder using either the Woods or Rubin

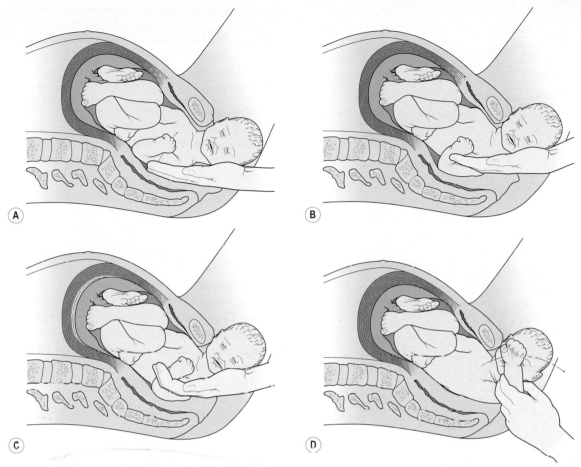

Fig. 25.11 Birth of the posterior arm. (A) Location of the posterior arm. (B) Directing the arm into the hollow of the sacrum. (C) Grasping and splinting the wrist and forearm. (D) Sweeping the arm over the chest and delivering the hand.

manoeuvre or by reversing the Løvset manoeuvre (see Chapter 20).

Zavanelli manoeuvre

If the manoeuvres described above have been unsuccessful, the obstetrician may consider the *Zavanelli manoeuvre* (Sandberg 1985, 1999) as a last option for the birth of a live baby. The Zavanelli manoeuvre requires the reversal of the mechanisms of birth so far achieved and reinsertion of the fetal head into the vagina. The birth is then completed by caesarean section.

Method: The head is returned to its pre-restitution position (Fig. 25.12A). Pressure is then exerted onto the occiput and the head is returned to the vagina (Fig.

25.12B). Prompt birth of the baby by caesarean section is then required.

Symphysiotomy

Symphysiotomy is the surgical separation of the symphysis pubis and is used to enlarge the pelvis to enable the birth. It is usually performed in cases of cephalo-pelvic disproportion (CPD) and is used more routinely in low-income countries. There are a few recorded cases where symphysiotomy has been used successfully to relieve shoulder dystocia (Wykes et al. 2003; Wilson et al. 2016), but the procedure has usually been associated with a high level of maternal morbidity. The rarity of reported cases makes it difficult to assess the technique for the relief of shoulder dystocia.

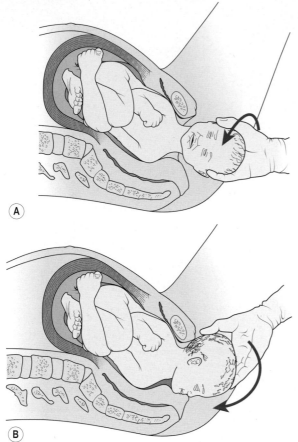

Fig. 25.12 The Zavanelli manoeuvre. (A) Head being returned to direct anteroposterior (pre-restitution) position. (B) Head being returned to the vagina. (After Sandberg EC. (1985) The Zavanelli maneuver: a potentially revolutionary method for the resolution of shoulder dystocia. American Journal of Obstetrics and Gynecology 152: 479–487, with permission.)

Outcomes Following Shoulder Dystocia
Maternal

Approximately two-thirds of women will have a blood loss of >1000 mL from injury associated with the birth (O'Leary 2009). Maternal death from uterine rupture has been reported following the use of fundal pressure and from haemorrhage during and following the birth (O'Leary 2009).

Fetal

Shoulder dystocia remains a cause of intrapartum fetal death, as Draper et al. (2017) highlight in the MBRRACE-UK Perinatal Confidential Enquiry, reporting on six perinatal deaths (four stillbirths and two neonatal deaths) that occurred during the timeframe of the audit. Neonatal asphyxia may occur following shoulder dystocia in 5.7–9.7% of cases and the attending paediatrician must be experienced in neonatal resuscitation (RCOG 2012a).

Fetal damage may occur even with excellent management using appropriate obstetric manoeuvres. Following shoulder dystocia, examination of the newborn should be carried out by a senior neonatal clinician (RCOG 2012a).

Brachial plexus injury is commonly associated with shoulder dystocia especially when more than one manoeuvre has been required, complicating from 2.3% to up to 16% of such births (Gurewitsch et al. 2006; Sandmire and DeMott 2009; RCOG 2012a). Damage to cervical nerve roots 5 and 6 may result in an Erb's palsy (see Chapter 35).

The midwife must ensure that simulation training and practice drills are attended annually to maintain skills (RCOG 2012a). Record-keeping following shoulder dystocia, as shown in Box 25.2, should include identification of the anterior shoulder and the direction of the fetal head (RCOG 2012a; NMC 2018).

RUPTURE OF THE UTERUS

Rupture of the uterus is one of the most serious complications in midwifery and obstetrics. It is often fatal for the fetus and may also contribute to the death of the mother, being a significant problem worldwide. Rupture of the uterus is defined as being *complete* or *incomplete*:

- *Complete rupture* involves a tear in the wall of the uterus with or without expulsion of the fetus.
- *Incomplete rupture* involves tearing of the uterine wall but not the perimetrium.

Dehiscence of an existing uterine scar may also occur. This involves rupture of the uterine wall but the fetal membranes remain intact. The fetus is retained within the uterus and is not expelled into the peritoneal cavity (Nahum 2018). Familiarity with the potential risk factors and signs and symptoms for uterine rupture may aid the midwife's recognition and management of this rare emergency.

Risk Factors

A scarred uterus is a recognized risk factor for uterine rupture (Al-Zirqi et al. 2017; Fitzpatrick et al. 2012). Caesarean section is a common cause of a scarred uterus. A vaginal birth following caesarean section is associated with a 0.5% risk of uterine rupture (RCOG 2015). However, a short interval since a previous caesarean section and previous classical (longitudinal) incision are associated with an increase in the risk of uterine rupture. Labour and/or augmentation of labour with oxytocin and prostaglandins in scarred uteri are risk factors for uterine rupture (Al-Zirqi et al. 2017) and is associated with a two- to three-fold increase in the risk of uterine rupture (RCOG 2015).

Cases of spontaneous rupture of an unscarred uterus in primigravidae are reported in the literature (Roberts and Trew 1991; Uccella et al. 2011) but are rare in high-income countries (Hofmeyr et al. 2005). Misuse of oxytocin and prostaglandins in an unscarred uterus is also associated with uterine rupture (Knight et al. 2014).

In addition, uterine rupture can be precipitated in the following circumstances:

- high parity
- obstructed labour; the uterus ruptures owing to excessive thinning of the lower segment *(Bandl's ring)*
- extension of severe cervical laceration upwards into the lower uterine segment as a result of trauma during an assisted birth
- trauma to the abdomen, as a result of a blast injury or an accident (Michiels et al. 2007).

Signs of Intrapartum Rupture of the Uterus

Clinical signs of uterine rupture can be inconsistent and may depend on the site and extent of the rupture

> **BOX 25.3 Key Signs of Rupture of the Uterus**
>
> - Abnormalities of the fetal heart rate and pattern
> - Abdominal pain or pain over previous caesarean section scar
> - Vaginal bleeding
> - Maternal tachycardia
> - Slow progress in labour

(Nahum 2018). Classic signs of uterine rupture are outlined in Box 25.3. However, the most commonly reported marker for uterine rupture is fetal heart rate abnormalities and bradycardia (Guiliano et al. 2014; Fitzpatrick et al. 2012).

Complete rupture of the uterus may be accompanied by sudden collapse of the woman, who complains of severe abdominal pain. The maternal pulse rate increases and, simultaneously, alterations of the fetal heart may occur, including the presence of variable decelerations (Landon 2010). There may be evidence of fresh vaginal bleeding. The uterine contractions may cease and the contour of the abdomen changes. The fetus becomes palpable in the abdomen as the presenting part regresses. The degree and speed of the woman's collapse and shock depend on the extent of the rupture and the blood loss.

Incomplete rupture may have an insidious onset found only after the birth or during a caesarean section. This type is more commonly associated with previous caesarean section. Blood loss associated with dehiscence, or incomplete rupture, can be scanty, as the rupture occurs along the fibrous scar tissue, which is avascular (Landon 2010).

Whenever shock during the third stage of labour is more severe than the type of birth or blood loss would indicate, or the woman fails to respond to the treatment given, the possibility of incomplete rupture should be considered. Incomplete rupture may also manifest as abdominal pain and/or postpartum haemorrhage following vaginal birth.

Management

All maternity units should have a protocol for dealing with uterine rupture. An immediate caesarean section is performed in the hope of procuring a live baby. Following the birth of the baby and placenta, the extent of the rupture can be assessed. Choice between the options to perform a hysterectomy or to repair the rupture depends on the extent of the trauma and the woman's condition. Further clinical assessment will include evaluation of the need for blood replacement and management of any shock.

The woman will be unprepared for such events that have occurred and therefore may be totally opposed to hysterectomy. It is worth noting however, that there are few reports of successful pregnancy following repair of uterine rupture.

AMNIOTIC FLUID EMBOLISM

Amniotic fluid embolism (AFE) is a rare, unpredictable and unpreventable obstetric emergency. The total incidence of AFE in the UK is reported to be 0.26 per 100,000 maternities, of which there were 6 deaths in the triennium 2015–2017 (Knight et al. 2019). Amniotic fluid embolism continues to be a direct cause of maternal death and although it is no longer considered universally fatal due to improvements in identification of AFE and resuscitation, it is associated with significant morbidity for both the mother and baby (Tuffnell and Slemeck 2017).

Amniotic fluid embolism is thought to occur when amniotic fluid enters the maternal circulation via the uterus or placental site leading rapidly to maternal collapse. The body responds to AFE in two phases. The initial phase is one of pulmonary vasospasm causing hypoxia, hypotension, pulmonary oedema and cardiovascular collapse. The second phase sees the development of left ventricular failure, with coagulopathy and potentially uncontrollable haemorrhage.

Amniotic fluid embolism should be considered as a possible diagnosis in the event of maternal collapse in pregnancy, labour, or following birth where there is no other obvious cause (Tuffnell and Slemeck 2017).

Predisposing Factors

Amniotic fluid embolism can occur at any gestation. Chance entry of amniotic fluid into the circulation under pressure may occur through the uterine sinuses of the placental bed. The barrier between the maternal circulation and the amniotic sac may be breached during periods of raised intra-amniotic pressure, such as termination of pregnancy or during placental abruption. Procedures such as artificial rupture of the membranes (ARM) and insertion of an intrauterine catheter, have

---

BOX 25.4 Key Signs and Symptoms of Amniotic Fluid Embolism

- Respiratory
  - Cyanosis
  - Dyspnoea
  - Respiratory arrest
- Cardiovascular
  - Tachycardia
  - Hypotension
  - Pale clammy skin/shivering
  - Cardiac arrest
- Haematological
  - Haemorrhage from placental site
  - Coagulation disorders, DIC
- Neurological
  - Restlessness, panic
  - Convulsions
- Fetal compromise

---

been associated with AFE. Amniotic fluid embolism can also occur during an intrauterine manipulation, such as internal podalic version or during a caesarean section.

Clinical Signs and Symptoms

Premonitory signs and symptoms (restlessness, abnormal behaviour, respiratory distress and cyanosis) may occur before collapse (Tuffnell and Slemeck 2017). There is maternal hypotension and uterine hypertonus. The latter will induce fetal compromise and is in response to uterine hypoxia. Cardiopulmonary arrest follows quickly and only minutes may elapse before cardiac arrest. Coagulopathy develops following the initial collapse (Liao and Luo 2016). The key signs and symptoms are summarized in Box 25.4.

Emergency Action

Any one of the symptoms highlighted in Box 25.4, is indicative of an acute emergency. As the woman is likely to be in a state of collapse, effective resuscitation must be started immediately. An emergency team should be called as the midwife will require immediate assistance in caring for the woman. In both community and hospital settings the midwife should commence basic life support while awaiting arrival of emergency services or the multidisciplinary team (see Chapter 26). Early involvement of the multidisciplinary team that includes a haematologist, is important in the management of this emergency (Tuffnell and Slemeck 2017). A perimortem caesarean section may also be required if cardiac arrest has occurred (see Chapter 26). Specific management for the condition is life support with high levels of oxygen and early intubation. Correction of coagulopathy should also form part of the management.

Complications of Amniotic Fluid Embolism

Disseminated intravascular coagulation (DIC) is likely to occur within 30 min of the initial collapse. In some cases, the woman bleeds heavily prior to developing amniotic fluid embolism, which contributes to the severity of her condition. It has also been reported that the amniotic fluid has the ability to suppress the myometrium, resulting in uterine atony. Acute kidney injury is a complication of the excessive blood loss and the prolonged hypovolaemic hypotension. Prompt transfer to a critical care unit for specialized care improves the outcome in AFE (Tuffnell and Slemeck 2017).

Midwifery support and advice should be continued for the family. When the woman has recovered sufficiently, an opportunity to talk about the emergency should be provided with the midwifery and obstetric team, particularly in addressing perinatal mental health (Futura et al. 2014).

Effect of Amniotic Fluid Embolism on the Fetus

Perinatal mortality and morbidity are high where amniotic fluid embolism occurs before the birth of the baby. Delay in the time from initial maternal collapse to the baby's birth needs to be minimal if fetal compromise or death is to be avoided. However, maternal resuscitation may, at that time, be a priority. Box 25.5 summarizes the key points relating to amniotic fluid embolism.

To date, there has been no comprehensive study of the epidemiology and management of amniotic fluid

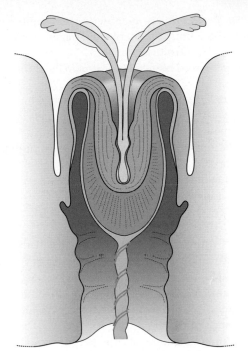

Fig. 25.13 Second-degree inversion of the uterus.

embolism in order to inform earlier diagnosis, which may lead to better outcomes. However, a database of voluntary notifications has been established through the UK Obstetric Surveillance System (UKOSS) to collect information on suspected or proven amniotic fluid embolism, whether fatal or not.

ACUTE INVERSION OF THE UTERUS

This is a rare but potentially life-threatening complication of the third stage of labour. It occurs in approximately 1 in 20,000 births (Witteveen et al. 2013). Midwives' awareness of the precipitating factors enables them to take preventive measures to avoid this emergency.

Classification of Inversion

Inversion can be classified according to severity as follows:
- *first-degree*: the fundus reaches the internal os
- *second-degree*: the body or corpus of the uterus is inverted to the internal os (Fig. 25.13)
- *third-degree*: the fundus protrudes to or beyond the introitus and is visible

- *fourth-degree*: this is *total* uterine and vaginal inversion where both the uterus and vagina are inverted beyond the introitus.

Inversion is also classified according to the timing of the event:

- *acute inversion*: occurs within the first 24 h
- *subacute inversion*: occurs after the first 24 h, and within 4 weeks
- *chronic inversion*: occurs after 4 weeks and is rare (Bhalia et al. 2009).

It is the first of these, *acute inversion,* that the remainder of this section considers.

Causes

Causes of acute inversion are associated with uterine atony and cervical dilatation (Witteveen et al. 2013), and include:

- mismanagement in the third stage of labour, involving excessive cord traction to manage the birth of the placenta
- combining fundal pressure and cord traction to expel the placenta
- use of fundal pressure to expel the placenta while the uterus is atonic
- pathologically adherent placenta
- spontaneous occurrence, of unknown cause
- primiparity
- fetal macrosomia
- short umbilical cord
- sudden emptying of a distended uterus.

  Careful management of the third stage of labour is needed to prevent uterine inversion. In active management of the third stage of labour, palpation of the fundus is essential to confirm that contraction has taken place, prior to undertaking controlled cord traction (see Chapter 21).

Warning Signs and Diagnosis

The major sign of acute inversion of the uterus is profound shock and usually haemorrhage. The blood loss is within a range of 800–1800 mL. Inversion of the uterus will cause the woman severe abdominal pain. On palpation of the uterus, the midwife may feel an indentation of the fundus. Where there is a major degree of inversion the uterus may not be palpable abdominally but may be felt upon vaginal examination or, in a severe case, the uterus may be seen at the vulva.

  The pain is thought to be caused by the stretching of the peritoneal nerves and the ovaries being pulled as the fundus inverts. Bleeding may or may not be present, depending on the degree of placental adherence to the uterine wall. The cause of the symptoms may not be readily apparent and diagnosis may be missed if inversion is incomplete.

Management
Immediate action

A swift response is needed to reduce the risks to the woman. Throughout the events the woman and her partner should be kept informed of what is happening. Assessment of vital signs, including level of consciousness is of the utmost importance.

1. Urgent medical help is summoned and emergency ambulance transfer to hospital is expedited if the woman is at home/in the community setting.
2. Vital signs, including level of consciousness is assessed and high flow oxygen administered (depending on setting).
3. The midwife in attendance should immediately attempt to replace the uterus. If replacement is delayed, the uterus can become oedematous and replacement will become increasingly difficult. Replacement may be achieved by pushing the fundus with the palm of the hand, along the direction of the vagina, towards the posterior fornix. The uterus is then lifted towards the umbilicus and returned to position with a steady pressure known as *Johnson's manoeuvre.* If replacement cannot be achieved immediately, the foot of the bed can be raised to reduce traction on the uterine ligaments and ovaries (Witteveen et al. 2013).
4. An intravenous cannula should be inserted, and blood taken for: full blood count, clotting studies and cross-matching prior to commencing an infusion.
5. Analgesia such as morphine may be administered to the woman.
6. If the placenta is still attached, it should be left *in situ* as attempts to remove it at this stage may result in uncontrollable haemorrhage.
7. Once the uterus is repositioned, the midwife or obstetrician should keep their hand *in situ* until a firm contraction is palpated. Oxytocics should be given to maintain the contraction (Witteveen et al. 2013; Winter et al. 2017).

Medical management

The hydrostatic method of replacement involves the instillation of several litres of warm saline infused through a giving set into the vagina. The pressure of the fluid builds up in the vagina and restores the uterus to the normal position, while the midwife or obstetrician seals off the introitus by hand or using a soft ventouse cup.

If the inverted uterus cannot be replaced manually, a cervical constriction ring may have developed. Drugs can be given to relax the constriction and facilitate the return of the uterus to its normal position however this may exacerbate a postpartum haemorrhage once the uterus is replaced as the drugs relax the uterus (Winter et al. 2017). Surgical correction via a laparotomy may be required to correct the inversion. Full support and explanation of the emergency should be offered to the woman in the postnatal period (Witteveen et al. 2013).

SHOCK

Shock is a complex syndrome involving a reduction in blood flow to the tissues that may result in irreversible organ damage and progressive collapse of the circulatory system (Mulryan 2011; Chandraharan and Arulkumaran 2013). If left untreated it will result in death. Shock can be acute but prompt treatment results in recovery, with little detrimental effect on the woman. However, failure to initiate effective treatment, or inadequate treatment, can result in a chronic condition ending in multisystem organ failure, which may be fatal (NICE 2019a).

Shock can be classified as follows:
- *hypovolaemic*: the result of a reduction in intravascular volume such as in severe haemorrhage during childbirth
- *septic or toxic*: occurs with a severe generalized infection
- *cardiogenic*: impaired ability of the heart to pump blood; in midwifery it may be apparent following a pulmonary embolism or in women with cardiac defects
- *neurogenic*: results from an insult to the nervous system as in uterine inversion
- *anaphylactic*: may occur as the result of a severe allergy or drug reaction.

This section deals with the principles of *hypovolaemic shock* and *maternal sepsis/septic shock*, either of which may develop as a consequence of childbirth.

Hypovolaemic Shock

This is caused by any loss of circulating fluid volume as in haemorrhage, but may also occur when there is severe vomiting. The body reacts to the loss of circulating fluid in stages as described below.

Initial stage

The reduction in fluid or blood decreases the venous return to the heart. The ventricles of the heart are inadequately filled, causing a reduction in stroke volume and cardiac output. As cardiac output and venous return fall, the blood pressure is reduced. The fall in blood pressure decreases the supply of oxygen to the tissues and cell function is affected.

Compensatory stage

The fall in cardiac output produces a response from the sympathetic nervous system through the activation of receptors in the aorta and carotid arteries. Blood is redistributed to the vital organs. Vessels in the gastrointestinal tract, kidneys, skin and lungs constrict. This response is seen by the skin becoming pale and cool. Peristalsis slows down, urinary output is reduced and exchange of gas in the lungs is impaired as blood flow diminishes. The heart rate increases in an attempt to improve cardiac output and blood pressure. The pupils of the eyes dilate. The sweat glands are stimulated and the skin becomes moist and clammy. Adrenaline (epinephrine) is released from the adrenal medulla and aldosterone from the adrenal cortex. Antidiuretic hormone (ADH) is secreted from the posterior lobe of the pituitary. Their combined effect is to cause vasoconstriction, increased cardiac output and a decrease in urinary output. Venous return to the heart will increase but, unless the fluid loss is replaced, this will not be sustained.

Progressive stage

This stage leads to multisystem organ failure. Compensatory mechanisms begin to fail, with vital organs lacking adequate perfusion. Volume depletion causes a further fall in blood pressure and cardiac output. The coronary arteries suffer lack of blood supply and peripheral circulation is poor, with weak or absent pulses.

Final, irreversible stage of shock

Multisystem organ failure and cell destruction are irreparable and death ensues.

Effect of Shock on Organs and Systems

The human body is able to compensate for loss of up to 10% of blood volume, principally by vasoconstriction.

When that loss reaches 20–25%, however, the compensatory mechanisms begin to decline and fail. In pregnancy, the plasma volume increases, as does the red cell mass. The increase is not proportionate, but allows a healthy pregnant woman to sustain significant blood loss at birth as the plasma volume is reduced with little disturbance to normal haemodynamics. In cases where the increase in plasma volume is reduced or there has been an antepartum haemorrhage, the woman is more susceptible to experience a pathological effect on the body and its systems following a much lower blood loss during childbirth. Individual organs are affected as below.

Brain

The level of consciousness deteriorates as cerebral blood flow is compromised. The woman will become increasingly unresponsive to verbal stimuli and there is a gradual reduction in the response elicited from painful stimulation.

Lungs

Gas exchange is impaired as the physiological dead space increases within the lungs. Levels of carbon dioxide rise and arterial oxygen levels fall. Ischaemia within the lungs alters the production of surfactant and, as a result of this, the alveoli collapse. Oedema in the lungs, due to increased permeability, exacerbates the existing problem of diffusion of oxygen. Atelectasis, oedema and reduced compliance impair ventilation and gaseous exchange, leading ultimately to respiratory failure. This is known as *adult respiratory distress syndrome* (ARDS).

Kidneys

The renal tubules become ischaemic owing to the reduction in blood supply. As the kidneys fail, urine output falls to <20 mL/h. The body does not excrete waste products such as urea and creatinine, so levels of these in the blood rise.

Gastrointestinal tract

The gut becomes ischaemic and its ability to function as a barrier against infection wanes. Gram-negative bacteria are able to enter the circulation.

Liver

Drug and hormone metabolism ceases, as does the conjugation of bilirubin. Unconjugated bilirubin builds up and jaundice develops. Protection from infection is further reduced as the liver fails to act as a filter. Metabolism of waste products does not occur, so there is a build-up of lactic acid and ammonia in the blood. Death of hepatic cells releases liver enzymes into the circulation.

Management

Urgent resuscitation is needed to prevent the woman's condition deteriorating and causing irreversible damage (Chandraharan and Arulkumaran 2013). Women who decline blood products must have their wishes respected and a treatment plan in case of haemorrhage should be discussed with them before labour (Winter et al. 2017).

The priorities are to:

1. *Call for help*: shock is a progressive condition and delay in correcting hypovolaemia can lead ultimately to maternal death.
2. *Maintain the airway*: if the woman is severely collapsed, she should be turned on to her side and 40% oxygen administered at a rate of 4–6 L/min. If she is unconscious, an airway should be inserted.
3. *Replace fluids*: two wide-bore intravenous cannulae should be inserted to enable fluids and drugs to be administered swiftly. Blood should be taken for cross-matching prior to commencing intravenous fluids. A systematic review of the evidence found that colloids were not associated with any difference in survival and were more expensive than crystalloids (Perel et al. 2013). Crystalloids are, however, associated with loss of fluid to the tissues, and therefore to maintain the intravascular volume colloids may be considered after 2 L of crystalloid have been infused. Where possible, all intravenous fluids should be warmed using a fluid warmer (Nolan and Pullinger 2014). Packed red cells and fresh frozen plasma are infused when the condition of the woman is stable and these are available.
4. *Arrest haemorrhage*: the source of the bleeding needs to be identified and stopped. Any underlying condition should be managed promptly and appropriately.
5. *Warmth*: it is important to keep the woman warm, but not over warmed or warmed too quickly, as this will cause peripheral vasodilatation and result in hypotension.

Assessment of Clinical Condition

An interprofessional team approach to management should be adopted to ensure that the correct level of expertise is available. A clear protocol for the management of shock should be used, with the midwife fully aware of key personnel required. Once the woman's immediate condition is stable, the midwife should continue to assess and record the woman's condition or liaise with staff on the critical care unit if the woman has been transferred there for subsequent care (Chandraharan and Arulkumaran 2013).

Hypovolaemic shock in pregnancy will reduce placental perfusion and oxygenation to the fetus, resulting in fetal distress and possibly death. Where maternal shock is caused by antepartum factors, the midwife should determine whether the fetal heart is present, but as swift and aggressive treatment may be required to *save the woman's life*, this should always be *the first priority*.

Detailed MEOWS observation charts including fluid balance should be accurately maintained. The extent of the woman's condition may require her to be transferred to a critical care unit.

Observations and clinical signs of deterioration in hypovolaemic shock

1. Assess the level of consciousness in association with the *Glasgow Coma Score* (GCS). This is a reliable, objective tool for measuring coma, using eye opening, motor response and verbal response. A total of 15 points can be achieved, and a measure of <12 is cause for concern. Any signs of restlessness or confusion should be noted (Dougherty and Lister 2011).
2. Assess the respiratory status using respiratory rate, depth and pattern, pulse oximetry and blood gases. Humidified oxygen should be used if oxygen therapy is to be administered for any length of time.
3. Monitor the blood pressure continuously, or at least every 30 min, with note taken of any fall in blood pressure.
4. Monitor the cardiac rhythm continuously.
5. Measure the urine output hourly, using an indwelling catheter and urometer.
6. Assess the skin colour of the woman, including the core and peripheral temperature hourly.
7. If a central venous pressure (CVP) line has been sited, haemodynamic measures of the pressure in

---

BOX 25.6   Key Points for Managing Hypovolaemic Shock

- Call for help
- Identify the source of bleeding and control temporarily if able
- Gain venous access using two wide-bore cannulae
- Rapidly infuse intravenous fluid to correct loss
- Assess for coagulopathy and correct
- Manage the underlying condition

---

the right atrium are taken to monitor the infusion rate and quantities. The fluid balance should be maintained and recorded accurately.
8. Observe for further bleeding, including the lochia, or any oozing from a wound or puncture site.
9. Undertake venepuncture for haemoglobin and haematocrit estimation to assess the degree of blood loss.
10. The woman is likely to be nursed flat in the acute stages of shock. Clinical assessment will also include a review and recording of pressure areas, with positional changes made as necessary to prevent deterioration. A lateral tilt should be maintained to prevent aortocaval compression if a gravid uterus is likely to compress the major vessels.

Box 25.6 summarizes the key points relating to the management of hypovolaemic shock.

Central Venous Pressure

It is unlikely that a midwife will experience central venous pressure (CVP) being measured outside of an intensive care unit (Fig. 25.14). CVP is the pressure in the right atrium or superior vena cava and is an indicator of the volume of blood returning to the heart, reflecting the competence of the heart as a pump and the peripheral vascular resistance. Normal CVP values will change with gestation and can vary between +5 and +10 cm H_2O. Values within this range indicate that the vascular space is well filled and red cell transfusion would not be necessary. However, in the presence of acute peripheral circulatory failure, which accompanies severe shock, the monitoring of CVP aids assessment of blood loss with a negative value indicating the necessity for fluid replacement. An isolated CVP recording is of little clinical value. Trends in CVP results are more useful clinically and are interpreted in conjunction with fluid balance and peripheral perfusion.

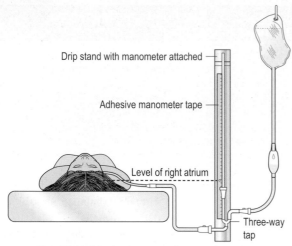

Fig. 25.14 Monitoring central venous pressure.

It is extremely dangerous to base an intravenous regimen on guesswork, as hypervolaemia or hypovolaemia, cardiac and renal failure may result.

Maternal Sepsis

Maternal sepsis (septic shock) is a life-threatening condition where there is an abnormal host response to infection resulting in damage to the body's organs and tissues (Bonet, et al. 2017). This may occur in pregnancy, following birth or in the postnatal period. Septic shock is a continuum of sepsis, where there is persistent hypotension requiring vasopressors to maintain blood pressure and serum lactate level >2 mmol/L (Singer et al. 2016; NICE 2019b). In the UK and Ireland, between 2015 and 2017, a total of 20 women died of sepsis. Of these, 10 died from genital tract/urinary tract sepsis; one woman died from influenza; and a further nine women died from pneumonia/other causes (Knight et al. 2019).Women and their families should be made aware of the importance of disclosing significant symptoms to enable earlier interventions in treatment of any underlying infection.

Certain organisms produce toxins that cause fluid to be lost from the circulation into the tissues. One of the commonest forms of sepsis causing death in childbearing in the UK is that caused by Lancefield group A beta-haemolytic *Streptococcus pyrogenes* (RCOG 2012b). This is a Gram-positive organism, responding to intravenous antibiotics, specifically those that are penicillin-based. Gram-negative organisms such as *Escherichia coli*, *Proteus* or *Pseudomonas pyocyaneus* are common pathogens in the female genital tract. The

placental site and perineal wounds are the main points of entry for an infection associated with pregnancy and childbirth. This may occur following prolonged rupture of fetal membranes, birth trauma, septic abortion or in the presence of retained placental tissue.

Clinical signs

Sepsis is often insidious in onset but requires prompt recognition and immediate medical referral. It is paramount that the midwife observes maternal vital signs in the event of caring for a woman who reports feeling unwell in addition to assessing her clinical condition. The woman may present with tachypnoea, tachycardia, pyrexia or extremely low temperature, or rigors. However, a temperature recording may appear normal if the woman has taken paracetamol as this will reduce pyrexia. The woman may seem confused or anxious, exhibiting a change in her mental state. Abdominal pain and gastrointestinal symptoms are common in pelvic sepsis. Other symptoms, including hypotension, develop in septic shock as the condition progresses. Haemorrhage may be apparent, which could be a direct result of events due to childbearing however, it occurs in septic shock due to disseminated intravascular coagulation (DIC) (see Chapter 14). In hospital, all observations should be recorded on a MEOWS chart to determine any further deterioration in the woman's condition and prompt any subsequent action.

Management

The principles of the management of maternal sepsis are early recognition and rapid treatment (NICE 2019b). If sepsis is suspected in the community setting, immediate transfer to hospital is required so that the multidisciplinary team can effect treatment at an early stage. There are actions which should be undertaken as quickly as possible, within the first hour where sepsis is suspected:

1. Administer high flow oxygen and monitor oxygen saturation aiming to achieve oxygenation within the range of 94–98%. Oxygen delivery is compromised secondary to hypotension, interstitial oedema and abnormal capillary blood flow (Daniels and Nutbeam 2017).
2. An infection screen should be undertaken to identify the aetiology and source of infection. This should include: blood cultures, high vaginal swab, throat swab and midstream specimen of urine.

3. Measure serum lactate as this marker can become raised when, as a result of tissue hypoperfusion, oxygen delivery does not meet oxygen demand (Daniels and Nutbeam 2017). The following blood tests should also be undertaken: FBC, clotting screen, C-reactive protein, renal and liver tests (NICE 2019b).

4. Rigorous treatment with intravenous broad spectrum antibiotics is essential to halt the illness.

5. Further deterioration in the woman's condition can be prevented by restoring circulatory volume. Replacement of fluid volume will restore perfusion of the vital organs. NICE (2019b) recommend an initial infusion of 500 mL of crystalloid over <15 min. Fluid replacement requirements should be discussed with the anaesthetist and obstetrician if the lactate level is normal, the woman is normotensive, or has pre-eclampsia (UK Sepsis Trust 2018).

6. Fluid balance is essential as fluid overload may lead to fatal pulmonary or cerebral oedema. The midwife must maintain careful monitoring and clear, accurate documentation of the woman's condition at all times during the acute and recovery stages of maternal shock (NMC 2018).

In all situations where the woman requires to be transferred to a critical care unit, relatives should be kept informed of her progress. The midwife may be the person with whom the relatives have formed a relationship and therefore is relied upon to give them information on the woman's condition and progress.

DRUG TOXICITY/OVERDOSE

Drug toxicity and illicit drug overdose should be considered as a cause in all cases of maternal collapse in any type of setting. The principles of observation and resuscitation already discussed in this chapter (and Chapter 26) apply to such a scenario. Common sources of drug toxicity in midwifery and obstetric practice are local anaesthetic agents injected intravenously by accident and magnesium sulphate given in the presence of renal impairment (RCOG 2011).

REFLECTIVE ACTIVITY FOR SELF-ASSESSMENT

1. What would lead you to suspect a childbearing woman was developing sepsis? Utilizing the SBAR tool, plan how you would effectively communicate your observations to the obstetrician and members of the multiprofessional team?

2. You are attending a multigravida in labour at home and, on vaginal examination, following spontaneous rupture of membranes, you discover the umbilical cord has prolapsed. What would be your plan of action in order to optimize the birth outcome for both the mother and baby?

3. With a doll and pelvis and assistance from one of your peers or a midwife practice supervisor/mentor, demonstrate the various manoeuvres that may assist in releasing the shoulders when there is an apparent delay in the emergence of the baby's body following birth of the head. What could be the possible outcomes for the mother and baby following shoulder dystocia?

4. As a practising midwife, what are your responsibilities and duty of care to a woman, her baby (depending on the birth outcome) and family, following a midwifery or obstetric emergency?

REFERENCES

Al-Zirqi, I., Daltveit, A. K., Forsen, L., et al. (2017). Risk factors for complete uterine rupture. *American Journal of Obstetrics and Gynecology, 216,* 165 e1–7.

American Academy for Family Physicians. (2004). *Advanced Life Support in Obstetrics (ALSO): Shoulder Dystocia.* Kansas: AAFP.

Athukorala, C., Crowther, C., Wilson, K., et al. (2007). Women with gestational diabetes mellitus in the ACHOIS trial: Risk factors for shoulder dystocia. *Australian and New Zealand Journal of Obstetrics and Gynaecology, 47,* 37–41.

Bahar, A. M. (1996). Risk factors and fetal outcome in cases of shoulder dystocia compared with normal deliveries of a similar birthweight. *British Journal of Obstetrics and Gynaecology, 103,* 868–872.

Bhalia, R., Wuntakal, R., Odejinmi, F., et al. (2009). Acute inversion of the uterus. *The Obstetrician and Gynaecologist, 11*(1), 13–18.

Bonet, M., Noguiera Pileggi, V., Rijken, M. J., et al. (2017). Towards a consensus definition of maternal sepsis: Results of a systematic review and expert consultation. *Reproductive Health, 14*(67), 1–13.

Bord, I., Gemer, O., Anteby, E. Y., et al. (2011). The value of bladder filling in addition to manual elevation of presenting fetal part in cases of cord prolapse. *Archives of Gynecology and Obstetrics*, *283*(5), 989–991.

Bruner, J. P., Drummond, S. B., Meenan, A. L., et al. (1998). All-fours maneuver for reducing shoulder dystocia during labor. *Journal of Reproductive Medicine*, *43*(5), 439–443.

Chandraharan, E., & Arulkumaran, S. (Eds.). (2013). *Obstetric and intrapartum emergencies: A practical guide to management*. Cambridge: Cambridge University Press.

Daniels R, Nutbeam T (Eds). On behalf of the United Kingdom (UK) Sepsis Trust. (2017) *The sepsis manual 2017–2018* (4th ed.). Birmingham: UK Sepsis Trust. Available at: https://sepsistrust.org/wp-content/uploads/2018/06/Sepsis_Manual_2017_web_download.pdf.

Dougherty, L., & Lister, S. (Eds.). (2011). *The Royal Marsden Hospital manual of clinical nursing procedures* (8th ed.) Oxford: Blackwell Science.

Draper, E. S., KurinczukJ. J., Kenyon, S., (Eds); on behalf of MBRRACE-UK Collaboration. MBRRACE-UK. (2017). *Perinatal Confidential Enquiry: term, singleton, intraprtum stillbirth and intrapartum-related neonatal death. Leicester: The Infant Mortality and Morbidity Studies*. Department of Health Sciences, University of Leicester. Available at: www.npeu.ox.ac.uk/downfiles/mbrrace-uk/reports/MBRRACE-UK%20In20Confidential%20Enquiry%20Report%20-%20final%20version.pdf.

Fitzpatrick, K. E., Kurinczuk, J. J., Alfirevic, Z., et al. (2012). Uterine rupture by intended mode of delivery in the UK: A national case-control study. *PLoS Med*, *9*(3), e1001184.

Futura, M., Sandall, J., & Bick, D. (2014). Women's perceptions and experiences of severe maternal morbidity: A Synthesis of qualitative studies using a meta-ethnographic approach. *Midwifery*, *30*, 158–169.

Gonik, B., Stringer, C. A., & Held, B. (1983). An alternate maneuver for management of shoulder dystocia. *American Journal of Obstetrics and Gynecology*, *145*, 882–883.

Gonik, B., Allen, R., & Sorab, J. (1989). Objective evaluation of the shoulder dystocia phenomenon: Effect of maternal pelvic orientation on force reduction. *Obstetrics and Gynecology*, *74*(1), 44–48.

Guiliano, M., Closset, E., Thereby, D., et al. (2014). Signs, symptoms and complications of complete and partial uterine ruptures during pregnancy and delivery. *European Journal of Obstetrics, Gynecology and Reproductive Biology*, *179*, 130–134.

Gupta, M., Hockley, C., Quigley, M. A., et al. (2010). Antenatal and intrapartum prediction of shoulder dystocia. *European Journal of Obstetrics and Gynecology and Reproductive Biology*, *151*(2), 134–139.

Gurewitsch, G. T., Johnson, E., Hamzehzadeh, S., et al. (2006). Risk factors for brachial plexus injury with and without shoulder dystocia. *American Journal of Obstetrics and Gynecology*, *2*(194), 486–492.

Hofmeyr, G. J., Say, L., & Gülmezoglu, A. M. (2005). World Health Organization (WHO) systematic review of maternal mortality and morbidity: The prevalence of uterine rupture. *British Journal Obstetrics and Gynaecology*, *112*(9), 1221–1228.

Holbrook, B. D., & Phelan, S. T. (2013). Umbilical cord prolapse. *Obstetrics and Gynecology Clinics of North America*, *40*(1), 1–14.

Houghton, G. (2006). Bladder filling: an effective technique for managing cord prolapse. *British Journal of Midwifery*, *14*(2), 88–89.

Jan, H., Guimicheva, B., Gosh, S., et al. (2014). Evaluation of healthcare professionals' understanding of eponymous maneuvers and mnemonics in emergency obstetric care. *International Journal of Gynaecology and Obstetrics*, *125*(3), 228–231.

Juaniaux, E., Alfirevic, Z., Bhide, A. G., et al. On behalf of the Royal College of Obstetricians and Gynecologists, et al. (2018). *Vasa praevia: Diagnosis and management. Green-top Guideline No 27b*. London: RCOG. Available at: https://obgyn.onlinelibrary.wiley.com/doi/epdf/10.1111/1471-0528.15307.

Keller, J. D., Lopez, J. A., Dooley, S. L., et al. (1991). Shoulder dystocia and birth trauma in gestational diabetes: A five year experience. *American Journal of Obstetrics and Gynecology*, *165*, 928–930.

Knight, S., Kenyon, P., Brocklehurst , (Eds.). (2014). On behalf of MBRRACE-UK. *Saving Lives, Improving Mothers' Care - Lessons learned to inform maternity care from the UK and Ireland Confidential Enquiries into Maternal Deaths and Morbidity 2015–2017*. Oxford: National Perinatal Epidemiology Unit , University of Oxford.

Knight, M., Bunch, K., Tuffnell, D. , et al. , (Eds.). (2019). On behalf of MBRRACE-UK. *Saving Lives, Improving Mothers' Care - Lessons learned to inform maternity care from the UK and Ireland confidential enquiries into maternal deaths and morbidity 2015–2017*. Oxford: National Perinatal Epidemiology Unit , University of Oxford. Available at: Available at: www.npeu. ox.ac.uk/downloads/files/mbrrace-uk/reports/MBRRACE-UK-%20Maternal%20Report%202018%20-%20Web%20Version.pdf.

Landon, M. B. (2010). Predicting uterine rupture in women undergoing trial of labor after prior cesarean delivery. *Seminars in Perinatology*, *34*(4), 267–271.

Liao, C. Y., & Luo, F. J. (2016). Amniotic fluid embolism with isolated coagulopathy: A report of two cases. *Journal of Clinical Diagnostic Research*, *10*(10) 0D03–5.

Lin, M. G. (2006). Umbilical cord prolapse. *Obstetrical and Gynecological Survey*, *61*(4), 269–277.

Michelotti, F., Flatley, C., & Kumar, S. (2018). Impact of shoulder dystocia, stratified by type of manoeuvre, on severe neonatal outcome and maternal morbidity. *Australian and New Zealand Journal of Obstetrics and Gynaecology, 58,* 298–305.

Michiels, I., De Valck, C., De Loor, J., et al. (2007). Spontaneous uterine rupture during pregnancy, related to a horse fall 8 weeks earlier. *Acta Obstetrica et Gynecologica Scandinavica, 86*(3), 380–381.

Mulryan, C. (2011). *Acute illness management.* London: Sage.

Nahum, G. (2018). Uterine rupture in pregnancy. *Medscape.* Available at: https://reference.medscape.com/article/275854-overview.

NHS England. (2016). *The National Maternity Review. Better Births. Improving outcomes in maternity services in England: A five year forward view for maternity care.* London: NHS England. Available at: https://www.england.nhs.uk/wp-content/uploads/2016/02/national-maternity-review-report.pdf.

NHS Improvement. (2018). *Spoken communication and patient safety in the NHS.* Available at: https://improvement.nhs.uk/documents/3345/Much_more_than_words_summary_v2.pdf.

NICE (National Institute for Health and Care Excellence). (2015). *Diabetes in pregnancy. Management from pre-conception to the postnatal period: NG3.* London: NICE. Available at: https://www.nice.org.uk/guidance/ng3/resources/diabetes-in-pregnancy-management-from-preconception-to-the-postnatal-period-pdf-51038446021.

NICE (National Institute for Health and Care Excellence). (2019a). *Acutely ill adults in hospital: Recognizing and responding to deterioration. Clinical Guideline 50.* London: NICE. Available at: https://www.nice.org.uk/guidance/cg50/resources/acutely-ill-adults-in-hospital-recognising-and-responding-to-deterioration-pdf-975500772037.

NICE (National Institute for Health and Care Excellence). (2019b). *Sepsis: Recognition, diagnosis and early management. Clinical Guideline 51.* London: NICE. Available at: https://www.nice.org.uk/guidance/ng51/resources/sepsis-recognition-diagnosis-and-early-management-pdf-1837508256709.

Nolan, J., & Pullinger, R. (2014). Hypovolemic shock. *British Medical Journal, 348,* g1139.

NMC (Nursing and Midwifery Council). (2018). *The Code: Standards of practice and behaviour for nurses, midwives and nursing associates.* London: NMC. Available at: https://www.nmc.org.uk/globalassets/sitedocuments/nmc-publications/nmc-code.pdf.

O'Connor M, Nair M, Kurinczuk JJ, Knight M. (2016) *UKOSS (UK Obstetric Surveillance System) Annual Report 2016.* Oxford: National Perinatal Epidemiology Unit. Available at: https://www.npeu.ox.ac.uk/downloads/files/ukoss/annual-reports/UKOSS%20Annual%20Report%202016.pdf.

O'Leary, J. A. (2009). *Shoulder dystocia and birth injury: prevention and treatment* (3rd ed.). Totowa: Humana Press.

Ouzounian, J. G., Gherman, R. B., Chauhan, S., et al. (2012). Recurrent shoulder dystocia: Analysis of incidence and risk factors. *American Journal of Perinatology, 29*(7), 515–518.

Perel, P., Roberts, I., & Ker, K. (2013). Colloids versus crystalloids for fluid resuscitation in critically ill patients. *Cochrane Database of Systematic Reviews* (2), CD000567.

Roberts, L., & Trew, G. (1991). Uterine rupture in a primigravida. *Journal of Obstetrics and Gynaecology, 11*(4), 261–262.

RCOG (Royal College of Obstetricians and Gynaecologists). (2011). *Maternal collapse in pregnancy and the puerperium. Green-top Guideline No 56.* London: RCOG. Available at: https://www.rcog.org.uk/globalassets/documents/guidelines/gtg_56.pdf.

RCOG (Royal College of Obstetricians and Gynaecologists). (2012a). *Shoulder dystocia. Green-top Guideline No 42* (2nd ed.). London: RCOG. Available at: https://www.rcog.org.uk/globalassets/documents/guidelines/gtg_42.pdf.

RCOG (Royal College of Obstetricians and Gynaecologists). (2012b). *Bacterial sepsis in pregnancy: Green-top Guideline No 64a.* London: RCOG. Available at: https://www.rcog.org.uk/globalassets/documents/guidelines/gtg 64a.pdf.

RCOG (Royal College of Obstetricians and Gynaecologists). (2014). *Umbilical cord prolapse. Green-top Guideline No 50.* London: RCOG. Available at: https://www.rcog.org.uk/globalassets/documents/guidelines/gtg-50-umbilicalcord-prolapse-2014.pdf.

RCOG (Royal College of Obstetricians and Gynaecologists). (2015). *Birth after previous caesarean birth. Green top Guideline No 45.* London: RCOG. Available at: https://www.rcog.org.uk/globalassets/documents/guidelines/gtg_45.pdf.

Sandberg, E. C. (1985). The Zavanelli maneuver: a potentially revolutionary method for the resolution of shoulder dystocia. *American Journal of Obstetrics and Gynecology, 152,* 479–487.

Sandberg, E. C. (1999). The Zavanelli maneuver: 12 years of recorded experience. *Obstetrics and Gynecology, 93*(2), 312–317.

Sandmire, H. F., & DeMott, R. K. (2009). Controversies surrounding the causes of brachial plexus injury. *International Journal of Gynecology and Obstetrics, 104*(1), 9–13.

Siggelkow, W., Schmidt, M., Skala, C., et al. (2011). A new algorithm for improving fetal weight estimation from ultrasound data at term. *Archives of Gynecology and Obstetrics, 283*(3), 469–474.

Singer, M., Deutschman, C. S., Seymour, C. W., et al. (2016). The Third International Consensus Definitions for Sepsis and Septic Shock (Sepsis-3). *Journal of the American Medical Association, 315*(8), 801–810.

Tuffnell, D., & Slemeck, E. (2017). Amniotic fluid embolism. *Obstetrics, Gynaecology and Reproductive Medicine, 27*(3), 86–90.

Uccella, S., Cromi, A., Boganim, G., et al. (2011). Spontaneous prelabor uterine rupture in a primigravida: a case report and review of the literature. *American Journal of Obstetrics and Gynecology, 205*(5), e6–8.

UK Sepsis Trust. (2018). *The sepsis manual 2017–2018* (4th ed.). Birmingham: United Kingdom Sepsis Trust. Available at: https://sepsistrust.org/wp-content/uploads/2018/06/Sepsis_Manual_2017_web_download.pdf.

Wilson, A., Truchanowicz, E. G., Elmoghazy, D., et al. (2016). Symphysiotomy for obstructed labour: A systematic review and meta-analysis. *British Journal of Obstetrics and Gynaecology, 123*, 1453–1461.

Winter, C., Crofts, J., Draycott, T., et al. (2017). *Practical obstetric multi-professional training PROMPT* (3rd ed.). Cambridge: Cambridge University Press.

Witteveen, T., van Stralen, G., Zwart, J., et al. (2013). Puerperal uterine inversion in the Netherlands: A nationwide cohort study. *Acta Obstetricia et Gynecologica Scandinavica, 92*(3), 334–337.

Wykes, C. B., Johnston, T. A., Paterson-Brown, S., et al. (2003). Symphysiotomy: A lifesaving procedure. *British Journal of Obstetrics and Gynaecology, 110*(2), 19–21.

ANNOTATED FURTHER READING

National Institute for Health and Care Excellence. (2019). *Acutely ill adults in hospital: recognizing and responding to deterioration: Clinical Guideline 50.* London: NICE.

This guideline details how patients in hospital should be monitored to identify those whose health may suddenly become worse and the care they should receive. It aims to reduce the risk of patients needing to stay longer in hospital, not recovering fully or dying. It was updated in April 2019 to include the national early warning score (NEWS2), endorsed by NHS England.

National Institute for Health and Care Excellence. (2019). *Sepsis: recognition, diagnosis and early management. Clinical Guideline 51.* London: NICE.

This guideline covers the recognition, diagnosis and early management of sepsis for all populations and was updated in April 2019 to include the national early warning score (NEWS2), endorsed by NHS England.

Raynor, M. D., Marshall, J. E., & Jackson, K. (2012). *Midwifery practice: critical illness, complications and emergencies case book.* Maidenhead: Open University Press.

This text provides a case study approach to several critical conditions and emergencies that can prove a challenge to all healthcare professionals working in midwifery practice, with particular importance being placed on multiprofessional team working. Each case explores and explains the pathology, pharmacology and care principles and uses test questions and answers to assist learning.

Royal College of Obstetricians and Gynaecologists. (2011). *Maternal collapse in pregnancy and the puerperium. Greentop Guideline No 56.* London: RCOG.

This guideline provides details of the different causes of maternal collapse, the identification of women at increased risk and the management of maternal collapse within both hospital and community settings, and includes all gestations and the postpartum period. The resuscitation team and equipment and training requirements are also provided.

Winter, C., Crofts, J., Draycott, T., et al. (Eds.). (2017). *PROMPT PRactical Obstetric Multi-Professional Training Course Manual* (3rd ed.) London: RCOG Press.

The PROMPT (Practical Obstetric Multi-Professional Training) course covers the management of a range of obstetric emergency situations. There has been increasing evidence that PROMPT training is having significant impact on outcomes in the UK, and internationally. In 2016, PROMPT was recognized in the NHS England: National Maternity Review. The PROMPT training package consists of interactive lectures, drills and workshops, providing hands-on experience of practical skills and team-working in simulated obstetric emergency situations. This 3rd edition has been updated in line with recent evidence and national and international guidelines to reflect the latest research and current clinical practice. There are new modules, algorithms, implementation tools, scenarios and videos.

Wylie, L., & Bryce, H. (2016). *The midwives' guide to key medical conditions. Pregnancy and childbirth* (2nd ed.). London: Elsevier.

This text is designed to help practitioners manage pregnancy and childbirth in women with systemic disease, recognize the early onset of disease-related pregnancy complications, and determine when it may be necessary to refer patients to another member of the healthcare team.

USEFUL WEBSITES

Erb's Palsy Group: https://www.erbspalsygroup.co.uk/

Mothers and Babies: Reducing Risk through Audits and Confidential Enquiries across the UK (MBRRACE-UK): https://www.npeu.ox.ac.uk/mbrrace-uk

National Institute for Health and Care Excellence: https://www.nicc.org.uk/

NHS Improvement: https://improvement.nhs.uk/

Resuscitation Council UK: https://www.resus.org.uk/#

Royal College of Obstetricians and Gynaecologists: https://www.rcog.org.uk/

The UK Sepsis Trust: https://sepsistrust.org/

United Kingdom Obstetric Surveillance System (UKOSS): https://www.npeu.ox.ac.uk/ukoss

26

Recognition of the Acutely Unwell Woman: Maternal Collapse and Resuscitation

Lindsey Ryan

CHAPTER CONTENTS

Maternal collapse is a rare but life-threatening event with wide-ranging causes. The outcomes for the mother and also for her fetus depend on prompt recognition and effective resuscitation involving the whole of the multidisciplinary team (MDT). Midwives and student midwives are at the frontline of caregiving, so while maternal collapse is infrequent, there is a high probability that they will be involved in care-giving to the acutely unwell woman. This chapter will highlight the repertoire of skills and tools needed by midwives in order to recognize and manage acute illness as part of the multidisciplinary team providing maternity care for women (RCOG 2011).

THE CHAPTER AIMS TO

- define maternal collapse/acute illness
- explore the MBRRACE-UK report as an example of good practice to provide context of maternal morbidity/mortality
- identify how to recognize acute illness through using the A–E approach to assessment plus the 'track and trigger' changing physiology tool such as MEWS (Maternity Early Warning Score)
- highlight how to effectively escalate concerns for the deteriorating woman through use of the communication tool SBAR (Situation Background Assessment Recommendation)
- provide an overview of the Resuscitation Council-UK (RCUK) Guidelines 'Adult Basic Life Support' and use of an automated external defibrillator (AED)
- outline the physiological changes in the pregnant woman that impede resuscitation

INTRODUCTION

Maternal collapse is defined as a sudden event involving the cardiorespiratory systems and/or brain, resulting in a reduced or absent conscious level (and potentially death), at any stage in pregnancy and up to 6 weeks after birth (RCOG 2011). Many women now present in pregnancy with complex comorbidities. Therefore critical care skills are now key in contemporary midwifery practice to recognize early those women at risk of developing morbidity as a result of pregnancy and childbirth. Globally, this is a major issue and in the UK for example, the recent triennial report on Maternal Morbidity and Mortality for 2015–2017 by Knight et al. (2019) on behalf of MBRRACE, identified that 9.2 women per 100,000 died during pregnancy or up to 6 weeks after childbirth or the end of pregnancy. This Confidential Enquiry into Maternal Deaths (CEMD) is in its 67th year of providing triennial reports highlighting the lessons learnt around maternal collapse in the UK. MBRRACE currently produce a yearly report; investigating the causes, management of maternal deaths and making recommendations to care providers and policy-makers. Globally, this is one example of good practice, where a national audit contributes to decision-making at local level. Nonetheless, while it can be acknowledged that since its conception a dramatic decline in maternal morbidity and mortality has been demonstrated, women within maternity services in the UK still continue to experience suboptimal care that contributes to poor outcome in some cases (Royal College of Anaesthetist, RCOA 2011; Knight et al. 2018). The United Nations (UN 2015) Sustainable Development Programme recognized the need to improve quality of living standards, reduce extreme poverty and tackle climate change through the production of 17 global goals and collaborative international working. Raising the standards of sanitation, eliminating hunger and improving nutrition are closely interrelated with reducing maternal morbidity and mortality on a global perspective (see Chapter 1). The focussed aim of the UN (2015) is to reduce the global maternal mortality rates to less than 70 by 2030. In order to help achieve this, skilled care is required from educated and highly trained midwives. Indeed the *Lancet* (2014: 1) executive summary on the midwifery series states:

> *Midwifery is a vital solution to the challenges of providing high-quality maternal and newborn care for all women and newborn infants, in all countries.*

Globally, according to statistics from the World Health Organization (WHO 2015) there is a steady decline in maternal mortality rates. They state that the approximate global lifetime risk of a maternal death fell markedly from 1 in 73 to 1 in 180. In the UK, the overall fall in maternal mortality is mainly due to a decrease in the number of deaths from direct causes – these are the conditions resulting from the pregnant state (e.g. haemorrhage, amniotic fluid embolism and thromboembolism). Mortality due to indirect causes (e.g. medical conditions such as cardiac disease or mental illness worsened by pregnancy) has been prominently reported in successive triennial reports on maternal morbidity and mortality in the UK since 2000. The most recent UK data (Knight et al. 2019) demonstrates the rate of maternal mortality was higher among older women, those living in the most deprived areas and among women from particular ethnic minority groups; specifically black, Asian or mixed ethnic groups. Sepsis remained a major cause of concern and in the triennium 2009–12 re-emerging as one of the leading causes of maternal death (Knight et al. 2014). This triggered enhanced recognition and management pathways within the UK National Health Service (NHS) hospital Trusts; in conjunction within ongoing work on a national level (www.sepsistrust.org). This chapter will revisit some of these conditions in more detail. These changes are set against the backdrop of demographic changes in the pregnant population; for example increased levels of obesity, pre-existing health problems, older women, sedentary behaviours and different expectations, including increased demand for elective caesarean sections. Data also suggest iatrogenic causes of major obstetric haemorrhage from abnormally invasive placenta and excessive use of uterotonic agents (see Chapter 21) (Knight et al. 2018). Box 26.1 highlights some key messages from MBRRACE-UK (Knight et al. 2018).

RECOGNIZING ACUTE ILLNESS

MBRRACE-UK (Knight et al. 2019) highlights that some women died in the UK despite receiving excellent care, due to the severity of their conditions. However, there is evidence that suboptimal care contributes to the death of a significant number of women. Examples include failure to recognize impending acute illness early in order to escalate care and mobilize early management (e.g. fluid replacement, antibiotics and oxygen therapy) to help stabilize ill women. The presence of human factors in high pressure

---

BOX 26 1   Key Messages from MBRRACE

- Do not presume normality – prove it using a MEWS chart.
- Challenge assumptions – both your own and others to avoid the normalization of symptoms as always pregnancy related.
- Share your concerns within the team – involve senior staff (Midwives, Obstetricians and Anaesthetists) use SBAR for effective communication.
- Wherever possible attend multiprofessional training, and student midwives should be rostered to attend 'skills and drills' within the multidisciplinary team prior to registration as midwives.

Adapted from Knight M, Bunch K, Tuffnell D, Jayakody H, et al. (Eds). On Behalf of MBRRACE-UK (2018) Saving Lives, Improving Mothers' Care – Lessons Learned to Inform Maternity Care from the UK and Ireland Confidential Enquiries into Maternal Deaths and Morbidity 2014–2016. Oxford: NPEU.

situations such as health care all too often contribute to failure of the team and poor outcomes. Doing 'too little too late' or 'too much too soon' are both themes highlighted in the case studies within MBRRACE-UK (Knight et al. 2019). Using a standardized tool for tracking changes in physiology, such as a MEWS or MOEWS (Modified Obstetric Early Warning Score) chart, helps identify changes in physiology that require review and possible action, often before other clinical symptoms become apparent. A physiological *track and trigger* system should be used to monitor all antepartum and postpartum admissions and be employed in conjunction with the partogram in labour. The tool will have a graded response strategy for women identified as being at risk of clinical deterioration; initially suggesting repeating of observations within a more frequent time frame, progressing to senior review and clinical interventions. To develop competency, student midwives should practise completion of the tool and escalation to the team as per local guidelines. Fig. 26.1 is an example of a MEWS/MOEWS chart.

The physiology of shock is covered in detail in Chapter 25, discussing how failure of the cardiovascular system to deliver oxygen to the tissues may cause irreversible organ damage. Shock is initially reversible however, when detected early using the 'track and trigger' system described above. It is worth noting that pregnancy equips women with the physiological buffers to compensate in the event of shock. Due to the increase in circulating blood volume, compared with a non-pregnant woman, a pregnant woman could lose up to 1200–1500 mL of blood (35% of blood volume) before showing signs of shock. The MEWS chart clearly indicates the subtle changes that serve as warning signs in physiology, namely, tachypnoea (raised respiratory rate) and tachycardia (raised heart rate). If detected and treated early with 'resuscitation measures', while also addressing the cause of the shock, the effects are reversed, with little detrimental effect on the woman (Chandraharan and Arulkumaran 2013). There could be a significant delay in the development of further symptoms and signs of hypovolaemia in a pregnant woman such as hypotension (low blood pressure), pallor, reduced urine output or altered levels of consciousness, due to this buffer zone. It is important to note however, that the first physiological parameter to be noticeably altered is the woman's respiratory rate. Other features such as tachycardia and hypotension are late signs. Therefore, significant changes in respiration should act as a red flag to arrest any further deterioration in the woman's condition that could have a catastrophic effect. Given this, an early warning score system modified for the maternity context should be used in the care of all women presenting to acute care services who are pregnant or within 42 days of having given birth (RCOA 2018a). Fig. 26.2 highlights the chain of survival identified by the Resuscitation Council UK (RCUK 2010a).

THE ABCDE APPROACH TO MANAGING CRITICAL ILLNESS

A further expanded understanding of the physiological status in an acutely unwell woman can be obtained through undertaking an A–E assessment approach. Similar to the MEWS, it is systematic and addresses all aspects of the woman's clinical status. It differs from a MEWS chart however, as it prescribes necessary interventions to address the abnormal features detected, prior to moving onto the next level of assessment. It is included within Resuscitation Council UK (RCUK 2010b) guidance as essential action in the management of the acutely unwell woman, as the key to preventing maternal collapse/arrest (see Table 26.1). This A–E assessment tool is historically favoured by medical staff, although now common place in resuscitation 'skills and drills' teaching (RCUK 2010b) for midwives and other members of the MDT delivering maternity care. It also references the non-technical skills employed in health care; listening to the woman, subconsciously assessing level of consciousness, assessing any changes in skin

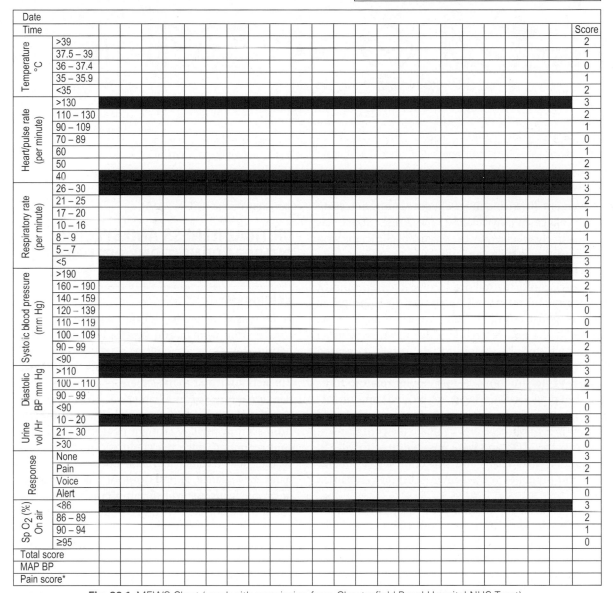

Fig. 26.1 MEWS Chart (used with permission from Chesterfield Royal Hospital NHS Trust).

colour and allowing the midwife to use her intuition or 'gut feeling'. Women who are critically unwell will relate when they can, both verbally through expressions of an 'impending sense of doom' and through changes in their physiology. The underlying principles of RCUK (2010b) are outlined in Box 26.2.

SBAR COMMUNICATION TOOL

SBAR is a simple to use, structured format for communication between the multidisciplinary team, which allows for the effective transfer of information. Following its introduction into healthcare settings within the

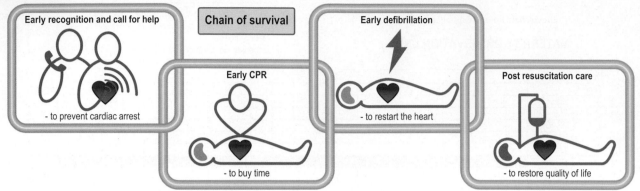

Fig. 26.2 Chain of survival. (Reproduced with permission from RCUK (Resuscitation Council UK). (2010a) Adult basic life support and automated external defibrillation. Available at: www.resus.org.uk.)

UK, it has led to improvements in patient safety (NHS Improvement 2018) and more effective communication (Royal College of Physicians (RCP 2018). SBAR has been positively received by the variety of clinicians who have adopted it for sharing and focussing information. The deteriorating woman is an excellent example of when concise information needs to be shared promptly, intelligently and assertively to trigger the appropriate level of response required. Communication is two way; both the giving and receiving of detail, which is often over-complicated by inappropriate detail, confused message and uncertain sense of importance. In high pressure, acute situations, teams cannot rely on 'hinting and hoping' that messages are received and understood. Those working within maternity services should take the time to observe and evaluate the communication across the MDT and were possible, practice SBAR, utilizing SBAR notepads and stickers where available. The salient points to the acronym SBAR are explained below.

Situation: state who you are, your location/the clinical area you are calling from and why you are calling.

Background: provide pertinent background to the woman's history.

Assessment: emphasize the parts of your assessment of the woman that concern you the most/what interventions have you already done.

Recommendation: state clearly what you need from the recipient of the communication/timeframe for attending to review.

Table 26.1 outlines the ABCDE approach to resuscitation (RCUK 2010b) and Table 26.2 provides an algorithm to perform basic life support to an adult using a step-by-step approach (RCUK 2015).

CRITICAL ILLNESS AND SPECIFIC CLINICAL CONDITIONS PERTINENT TO PREGNANCY, LABOUR AND BIRTH

Eclampsia

Hypertensive disorders during pregnancy carry severe risks for the woman and developing fetus; the fulmination of eclampsia should be considered acute critical illness, hence why it is covered briefly in this chapter. The aetiology and management of hypertensive disorders are addressed in Chapter 15. The rate of eclampsia related deaths are falling globally, with the greatest drop seen in the UK (Knight et al. 2019). The significant reduction since the commencement of reporting to the most recent triennia is due to increased antenatal surveillance, appreciation of risk factors and use of prophylactic Aspirin. Eclampsia is the neurological condition associated with pre-eclampsia that becomes apparent with the woman experiencing tonic-clonic convulsions. While most seizures are self-limiting, urgent medical assistance from the midwife and other members of the MDT is required to protect the airway and stabilize the woman. She is at increased risk of aspiration and hypoxia associated with loss of airway in the post-ictal phase, when reduced levels of consciousness require urgent assessment and intervention. Tonic-clonic seizures present challenges to the normal airway manoeuvres of head-tilt-chin-lift (Fig. 26.3) and rolling the woman onto her left side may be more practical in first-line management of the situation until help

TABLE 26.1 ABCDE Approach to Resuscitation (Resuscitation Council UK 2010b)

	Assessment – Look/Listen and Feel	Management
On Approach	Is it safe for you to approach? Wear personal protective equipment where indicated. How does the woman look? Ask 'how are you?' This quick assessment highlights those who are unconscious and most at risk.	If there are concerns regarding colour and response of – formalize assessment as per the BLS sequence below. Call for help at any point during the assessment
Airway	• Look for signs of obstruction • Can they speak? • Evidence of cyanosis? • Abnormal sounds or movements suggestive of obstruction?	• Call for help immediately when you suspect airway obstruction – immediate threat to life • Airway opening manoeuvres (head-tilt/chin-lift), airways suction, insertion of an oropharyngeal or nasopharyngeal airway (Fig. 26.3) • Provide high-concentration oxygen using a mask with oxygen reservoir
Breathing	• Count the respiratory rate – 12–20 is normal • Oxygen saturations? • Noisy breathing? • Use of accessory muscles? • Both sides of the chest moving equally? • Depth of respiration?	• Critically ill women need supplementary oxygen • If the woman's depth or rate of breathing is judged to be inadequate or absent, use bag-mask or pocket-mask ventilation to improve oxygenation and ventilation, while calling immediately for expert help
Circulation	• What is the woman's colour like? Pale/flushed/grey/ashen/clammy? • What is her peripheral temperature like to the touch? • Formally take and record the temperature • Pulse (radial and carotid)? Count the beat and feel the strength/volume • Peripheral refill time (compress nailbed with hand held at level of the heart for 5 s, hard enough until it blanches. Colour should return in <2 s) • Blood pressure? • Urine output?	• Insert ×2 large, wide-bore IV cannulae and take bloods for routine haematological, biochemical, coagulation and microbiological investigations and cross-matching, before infusing intravenous fluid. • In signs of cardiovascular shock, infuse 500 mL crystalloid IV – preferably through a warming device • Arrest haemorrhage where possible • Keep the woman warm – be aware of wet sheets, clothes, exposure to draft and environmental temperature • Reassess BP and HR every 5 min and aim for woman's normal rate

Continued

TABLE 26.1 ABCDE Approach to Resuscitation (Resuscitation Council UK 2010b)—cont'd

	Assessment – Look/Listen and Feel	Management
Disability	Common causes of unconsciousness include profound hypoxia, hypercapnia, cerebral hypoperfusion (low BP) or the recent administration of sedatives or analgesic drugs. • Review and treat the ABCs: exclude or treat hypoxia and hypotension • Check the medication/prescription chart • Examine the pupils of the eyes (size, equality and reaction to light) • Make a rapid initial assessment of the woman's conscious level using the AVPU method: Alert; responds to Vocal stimuli; responds to Painful stimuli; or Unresponsive to all stimuli • Measure the blood glucose to exclude hypoglycaemia	• Re-visit airway if any concerns with level of consciousness • Further drugs may be required – call for senior help (if haven't already done so) • Treat blood sugar accordingly – IV preparations where level of consciousness/airway is threatened • Care for the unconscious woman in the lateral position if her airway is not protected
Exposure	To examine the woman properly, full exposure of the body may be necessary. Respect her dignity and minimize heat loss.	Remember EVERYTHING else: • Take a full clinical history from the woman, any relatives or friends and other staff. Assess thoroughly the full clinical picture • Review the woman's notes and charts: MEWS trends/drugs prescribed • Review the results of laboratory or radiological investigations • Consider definitive treatment of the underlying condition
	Record the woman's response to any interventions started throughout the A–E approach to resuscitation and repeat full assessment. Remember to document all actions/care interventions and individuals involved in the care/decision-making from the MDT. Also communicate and provide thorough handover of care using SBAR or RSVP.	

Adapted from RCUK (Resuscitation Council UK). (2015) Adult Basic Life Support and Automated External Defibrillation. Available at: www.resus.org.uk.

BOX 26.2 The ABCDE Approach – Underlying Principles

The approach to all deteriorating or critically ill women/ or patients is the same. The underlying principles are:

1. Use the **A**irway, **B**reathing, **C**irculation, **D**isability, **E**xposure (ABCDE) approach to assess and treat the woman.
2. Do a complete initial assessment and reassess regularly.
3. Treat life-threatening problems before moving to the next part of the assessment.
4. Assess the effects of treatment.
5. Recognize when extra help is needed. Call for appropriate help early.
6. Use all members of the team. This enables interventions (e.g. assessment, attaching monitors, intravenous access) to be undertaken simultaneously.
7. Communicate effectively – use the **S**ituation, **B**ackground, **A**ssessment, **R**ecommendation (SBAR) or **R**eason, **S**tory, **V**ital signs, **P**lan (RSVP) approach.
8. The aim of the initial treatment is to keep the woman alive, and achieve some clinical improvement. This will buy time for further treatment and making a diagnosis.

Remember it can take a few minutes for treatments to work, so use clinical judgement and skilled decision-making and wait a short while before reassessing the woman after an intervention. Assess the whole clinical scenario.

Adapted from RUCK (Resuscitation Council UK). (2010b) The ABCDE Approach – Underlying Principles. Available at: www.resus.org.uk.

---

arrives. The midwife will still have a key role to play within the MDT in the ABCDE of resuscitation, airway management, fetal monitoring, ongoing assessment of maternal wellbeing via measurement of physiological parameters/vital signs following the administration of anticonvulsant and antihypertensive medication using the skills already discussed.

Pulmonary Embolism

At the time of writing this chapter the most recent MBRRACE-UK report highlighted that thrombosis and thromboembolism continue to be the leading cause of direct deaths occurring within 42 days of the end of pregnancy (Knight et al. 2019). This might suggest that although risk assessment and prophylactic treatment with low-molecular-weight heparin is routine in current practice, the risk of a venous thromboembolism (VTE) event is compounded by maternal obesity, medical comorbidity, more prevalent acute illness such as sepsis and also increased surgical interventions. The skills of history-taking and challenging assumptions when recognizing and managing acute illness are paramount, as clinical symptoms of pulmonary embolism (PE) can be easily confused for features of cardiac symptoms and pneumonia. Chapter 15 discusses thromboembolic disease alongside the other comorbidities outlined above in more depth; Boxes 26.3 and 26.4 cover the key messages about VTE and cardiac disease.

Anaphylaxis

Anaphylaxis is a severe, life-threatening generalized or systemic hypersensitivity reaction, resulting in respiratory, skin and circulatory changes and possibly collapse (RCUK 2016). Significant changes to circulating volume distribution are displayed through rapid hypotension and tachycardia. Upper airway occlusion can occur, caused by swelling in the mouth and throat and causing ventilation failure. Allergic triggers include a variety of drugs (intravenous, intramuscular, oral or topical preparations), latex, food and animal allergens. Swift recognition and call for help is required to manage the life-threatening airway and/or breathing and/or circulation problems. Exposure to a known allergen for the woman supports the diagnosis, but many cases occur with no previous history being reported (RCOG 2011). Midwives should have heightened awareness to possible anaphylaxis in administering Anti-D, and vaccination programmes in the community setting. Best practice would be to undertake such intervention in the acute setting where access to the medical team and resources to manage anaphylaxis are available. Fig. 26.4 provides an example of an algorithm that might be in place to help towards the first-line management of cardiac arrest from anaphylaxis in hospital from a multidisciplinary perspective.

Anaesthetic Emergencies

Care of the pregnant woman is provided by teams made up of midwives, obstetricians and anaesthetists, not individuals working in isolation (Bogod et al. 2018; RCOA 2018a). The role of the anaesthetist in providing anaesthesia and regional analgesia during labour and birth is achieved through effective team work within the MDT. Anaesthetists are pivotal members of the team in the recognition and management of the acutely unwell

TABLE 26.2   Technical Details on How to Perform Adult Basic Life Support

Sequence	Technical Description
Safety	Make sure you, the woman and any bystanders are safe
Response	**Check the woman for a response** • Gently shake her shoulders and ask loudly: 'Are you all right?' If she responds, leave her in the position in which you find her, provided there is no further danger; try to find out what is wrong with her and get help if needed; reassess her regularly. **See final section of the flowchart for how to achieve the recovery position.**
Airway	**Open the airway** • Turn the woman onto her back initially for assessment • Place your hand on her forehead and gently tilt her head back; with your fingertips under the point of the chin, lift the chin to open the airway (Fig. 26.3)
Breathing	**Look, listen and feel for normal breathing for no more than 10 seconds** In the first few minutes after cardiac arrest, the individual may be barely breathing, or taking infrequent, slow and noisy gasps. Do not confuse this with normal breathing. If you have any doubt whether breathing is normal, act as if it is they are not breathing normally and prepare to start CPR.
Call for Help	Call a time critical ambulance in accordance with local and national guidance. Call for an 'adult arrest team'/'medical emergency team' within the hospital. You will also need an 'obstetric/maternity emergency team'. • Ask a helper to call if possible, otherwise call them yourself • Stay with the woman when making the call if possible • Pre-hospital when working alone, activate the speaker function on the phone (if this facility is available) to aid communication with the ambulance service • Make sure you are familiar with the terms used locally to call the various teams
Send for an AED	**Send someone to get an Automated External Defibrillator (AED), if available/adult resuscitation trolley/grab bag.** If you are on your own, do not leave the woman, start CPR
Address need to tilt	**Where others are available to help, manual displacement of the gravid uterus is more effective at increasing cardiac return during CPR. If this is not possible, rolls of towels under the right hip can be used.** • To move the woman's pregnant abdomen, push or pull towards the woman's left hand side and hold in place (see Figs 26.5, 26.7, 26.8). Release only to allow for AED

Continued

Circulation	**Start chest compressions.** • Stand/kneel by the side of the woman depending on her position • Place the heel of one hand in the centre of her chest (which is the lower half of the breastbone (sternum) • Place the heel of your other hand on top of the first hand (Fig. 26.6) • Interlock the fingers of your hands and ensure that pressure is not applied over the woman's ribs (Fig. 26.6) • Keep your arms straight • Do not apply any pressure over the upper abdomen or the bottom end of the bony sternum (breastbone) • Position your shoulders vertically above the woman's chest and press down on the sternum to a depth of 5–6 cm • After each compression, release all the pressure on the chest without losing contact between your hands and the sternum • Repeat at a rate of 100–120 minutes
Rescue breaths	**After 30 compressions, open the airway again using head-tilt and chin-lift (Fig. 26.3) and give *two* rescue breaths.** • If in the hospital setting, the relevant kit is available and if you are trained to do so, use a pocket-mask or bag-valve-mask to deliver ventilation breaths. • If performing mouth-to-mouth resuscitation – pinch the soft part of the nose closed, using the index finger and thumb of your hand on the forehead. • Allow the mouth to open, but maintain chin-lift. • Take a normal breath and place your lips around the woman's mouth, making sure that you have a good seal. • Blow steadily into the mouth, while watching for the chest to rise, taking about 1 second as in normal breathing; this is an effective rescue breath. • Maintaining head-tilt and chin-lift, take your mouth away from the woman and watch for her chest to fall as air comes out. • Take another normal breath and blow into the woman's mouth once more to achieve a total of two effective rescue breaths. Do not interrupt compressions by more than 10 seconds to deliver two breaths. Then return your hands without delay to the correct position on the sternum and give a further 30 chest compressions. **Continue with chest compressions and rescue breaths in a ratio of 30:2.** If you are untrained or unable to do rescue breaths, give chest compression only CPR (i.e. continuous compressions at a rate of at least 100–120/min).
If an AED arrives	**Switch on the AED.** Attach the electrode pads on the woman's bare chest. • If more than one rescuer is present, CPR should be continued while electrode pads are being attached to the chest. • Follow the spoken/visual directions. • Ensure that nobody is touching the woman while the AED is analysing the rhythm. **If a shock is indicated, deliver shock.** • Ensure that nobody is touching the woman. • Push shock button as directed (fully automatic AEDs will deliver the shock automatically). • Immediately restart CPR at a ratio of 30:2 with left tilt/manual displacement of gravid uterus. • Continue as directed by the voice/visual prompts. **If no shock is indicated, continue CPR.** • Immediately resume CPR. • Continue as directed by the voice/visual prompts.

TABLE 26.2   Technical Details on How to Perform Adult Basic Life Support—cont'd

Sequence	Technical Description
Continue CPR	**Do not interrupt resuscitation until:** • A health professional tells you to stop. • You become exhausted. • The woman is definitely waking up, moving, opening eyes and breathing normally – it is rare for CPR alone to restart the heart. Unless you are certain the person has recovered, continue CPR.
Recovery position	**If you are certain the woman is breathing normally but is still unresponsive, place in the recovery position.** • Remove the woman's glasses/spectacles, if worn. • Kneel/stand beside the woman and make sure that both her legs are straight. • Place the arm nearest to you out at right angles to her body, elbow bent with the hand palm-up. • Bring the far arm across the chest, and hold the back of the hand against the woman's cheek nearest to you. • With your other hand, grasp the far leg just above the knee and pull it up, keeping the foot on the ground. • Keeping the woman's hand pressed against her cheek, pull on the far leg to roll her towards you but onto her side. • Adjust the upper leg so that both the hip and knee are bent at right angles. • Tilt the head back to make sure that the airway remains open. • If necessary, adjust the hand under the cheek to keep the head tilted and facing downwards to allow secretions/liquid material such as mucous, vomitus, etc. to drain from the mouth. • Check breathing regularly. **Be prepared to restart CPR immediately if the woman deteriorates or stops breathing normally.**

Adapted from RCUK (Resuscitation Council UK). (2015) Adult Basic Life Support and Automated External Defibrillation. Available at: www.resus.org.uk.

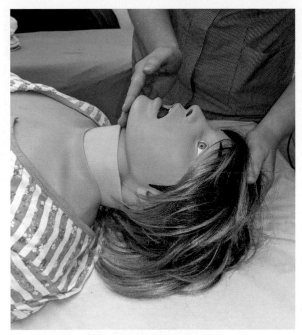

Fig. 26.3 Head-tilt-chin-lift.

BOX 26.3 Key Messages on Pulmonary Embolism

- PE can occur in the antenatal, intrapartum and post-natal period
- Difficult and laboured breathing
- Chest pain and discomfort
- Haemoptysis
- Low-grade pyrexia
- Acuteness of symptoms is seen with larger a embolism – severe central chest pain due to ischaemia
- Tachycardia and hypotension
- Syncope and altered level of consciousness due to hypoxia.

Adapted from Knight M, Bunch K, Tuffnell D, Jayakody H, et al. (Eds). On Behalf of MBRRACE-UK (2018) Saving Lives, Improving Mothers' Care – Lessons Learned to Inform Maternity Care from the UK and Ireland Confidential Enquiries into Maternal Deaths and Morbidity 2014–2016. Oxford: NPEU.

BOX 26.4 Key Messages on Cardiac Disease

- Cardiac disease can affect women of all ages.
- Women with known heart disease are high risk and need early access to specialist and obstetric care.
- Persistent breathlessness when lying flat is not normal in pregnancy and may suggest cardiac problems.
- Be aware of severe band-like chest pain/squeezing/pressure symptoms that radiate to the arm or back – they may be cardiac in nature.

Adapted from Knight M, Bunch K, Tuffnell D, Jayakody H, et al. (Eds). On Behalf of MBRRACE-UK (2018) Saving Lives, Improving Mothers' Care – Lessons Learned to Inform Maternity Care from the UK and Ireland Confidential Enquiries into Maternal Deaths and Morbidity 2014–2016. Oxford: NPEU

woman. However, it is often the midwife delivering care in the room with the woman, who is frontline in detecting complications of epidural and spinal analgesia. These complications can be life-threatening and are possible causes of acute deterioration and maternal collapse. Critical care skills are vital in the early recognition of the woman who is showing signs of deterioration (RCOA 2018b). Local anaesthetic toxicity occurs with an excessive dose of local anaesthetic drugs or they are inadvertently administered intravenously. Early recognition and swift reporting of local anaesthetic toxicity during regional anaesthesia is vital (Box 26.5).

Total (Complete) Spinal Block

Total/high spinal block is an uncommon but significant complication of neuraxial anaesthesia and it occurs when inadvertently a high dose of local anaesthetic is administered into the subarachnoid space within the spinal column. The level of sensory block goes well above the intended level and causes block of the sympathetic nerves that supply the heart and respiratory muscles; potentially causing respiratory and cardiac arrest. Box 26.6 summarizes the clinical features of this critical life-threatening event.

Sepsis

Globally, sepsis remains a cause of acute critical illness that can result in maternal mortality if not recognized and treated promptly and effectively. The latest estimates as reported by the WHO (2019) indicate that sepsis is the underlying cause of 11% of maternal direct deaths, although the true burden of maternal infection and its sequelae is not well known. This has necessitated the WHO (2019) to launch the Global Maternal Sepsis Study (GLOSS) and awareness campaign that was implemented in 53 countries by the end of 2017. They

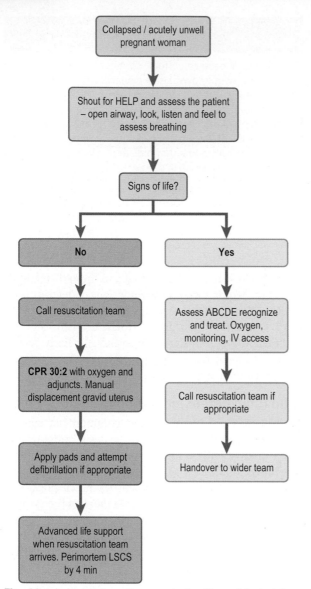

Fig. 26.4 In-hospital cardiac arrest algorithm. Adapted from RCUK (Resuscitation Council UK). (2010c). In-house cardiac arrest algorithm. Available at: www.resus.org.uk.

have provided a website about the study, the findings of which will help to empower healthcare professionals in the prevention, early recognition and treatment of sepsis in women and their babies: https://srhr.org/sepsis/. Further information about the WHO GLOSS study can also be accessed at: www.npeu.ox.ac.uk/ukoss/current-surveillance/who-gloss-global-maternal-sepsis-study.

Box 26.7 summarizes the key points relating to sepsis.

> **BOX 26.5** **Recognition and Management of Local Anaesthetic Toxicity: Epidural or Spinal**
>
> | | |
> |---|---|
> | Recognition | • Sudden alteration in mental status/confusion |
> | | • Severe cardiovascular changes/collapse (bradycardia) |
> | | • LA toxicity may occur sometime after an initial injection |
> | Immediate management | • Stop injecting the LA/epidural infusion |
> | | • Call for help |
> | | • Follow the ABCDE approach |
> | Treatment | • Start CPR if in cardiac arrest |
> | | • Start intravenous lipid emulsion – usually used for intravenous nutrition, also serves to mop up the toxic local anaesthetic drugs in the blood |
> | | • The woman will need to transfer to Critical Care for organ support |

WHAT ARE THE PHYSIOLOGICAL AND ANATOMICAL CHANGES IN PREGNANCY THAT AFFECT RESUSCITATION?

Airway

The increased weight in pregnancy can cause challenges in maintaining an airway on the unconscious pregnant woman; hence early intubation during cardiopulmonary resuscitation (CPR) is necessary. Anaesthetists with specialist training in obstetrics are well rehearsed in difficult airway management. An early call for appropriate assistance from obstetric and medical teams, as detailed in Table 26.2, ensure those with these skills are there to assist midwives.

Aspiration

Successful securing of the airway helps reduce the risk of regurgitation and aspiration of stomach contents into the lungs. Pregnant women are at increased risk of this due to progesterone relaxing the smooth muscle in the oesophagus, delayed gastric emptying and raised intra-abdominal pressure on the stomach due to the

---

BOX 26.6 Clinical Manifestations and Management of Complete Spinal Block

Recognition: **A**irway, **B**reathing and **C**ardiovascular	• Loss of consciousness* • Hypotension* • Bradycardia* • Respiratory compromise* • Apnoea* • Reduced oxygen saturation • Difficulty speaking/coughing • Cardiac arrest (asystole) (*most common symptoms)
Neurological	• Nausea and anxiety* • Arm/hand abnormal, unpleasant sensations when touched or paralysis* • High sensory level BLOCK • Cranial nerve involvement (*most common symptoms)
Management	• Verbal reassurance – woman will experience an 'impending sense of doom' • Immediate call for help and follow algorithm for basic life support/resuscitation if woman collapses and until medical help arrives • The anaesthetist will provide organs support and if necessary general anaesthesia to support her breathing until the local anaesthetic wears off • The woman will need to be transferred to the critical care unit for treatment and organ support as indicated

---

BOX 26.7 Key Messages on Sepsis

• 'Think Sepsis' – early recognition and management makes a difference to the outcome.
• Use the A–E assessment tool to identify physiological concerns and address these with the early interventions ('Sepsis Six' care bundle).
• Clinical red flags are: pyrexia, hypothermia, tachycardia, tachypnoea, hypoxia, hypotension, oliguria and reduced consciousness.

Adapted from NICE (National Institute for Health and Care Excellence). (2016) Sepsis: recognition, diagnosis and early management: CG 51. Available at: www.nice.org.uk.

weight of the gravid uterus. (See Chapter 10 for physiological changes and adaptation during pregnancy in the gastrointestinal system.)

Breathing

As highlighted in Chapter 10, pregnancy causes a variety of physiological changes that accelerate the development of hypoxia and make effective pulmonary ventilation more difficult during CPR. Changes in lung function, diaphragmatic splinting and increased oxygen consumption, make the pregnant woman become hypoxic easily upon cessation of breathing in primary apnoea or in respiratory arrest.

Circulation

Aortocaval (inferior vena cava and aorta) compression by the gravid uterus from 20 weeks' gestation reduces venous return to the woman's heart. This in turn then reduces her cardiac output by 30–40%, which causes supine hypotension. This can be experienced by the conscious woman through lying too flat, however is alleviated through rolling onto her left side and thus allowing the weight of the gravid uterus to fall away approximately 15 degrees from the major blood vessels, returning her circulation. During reduced consciousness, clinicians must achieve this function for the woman, or resuscitation will be severely impeded and chances of successful outcomes reduced. Left lateral tilt can be achieved by wedging the woman's right hip using multiple blankets or pillows (Fig. 26.5) or through manually displacing the gravid uterus (Figs 26.7, 26.8).

The first of these techniques then presents challenges to achieving effective chest compressions as the woman's body is no longer flat. The second technique is easy to achieve in the unconscious woman due to lack of tone and is effective, however it requires another member of the team to perform this continuously. This would need to be released for defibrillation. Effective chest compressions are physically demanding and require the adequate depth and rate described in Table 26.2. The

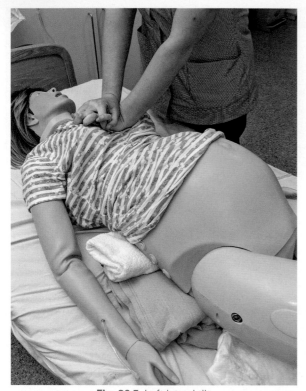

Fig. 26.5 Left-lateral tilt.

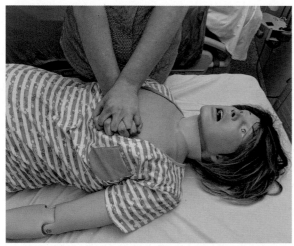

Fig. 26.6 Hand placement for chest compressions.

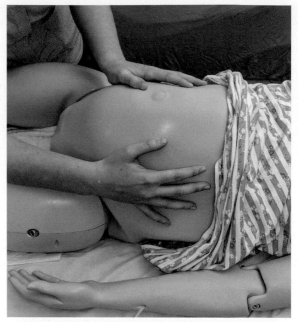

Fig. 26.7 Manual displacement of the gravid uterus.

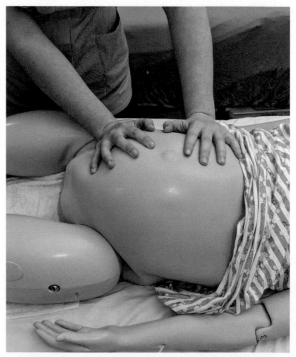

Fig. 26.8 Alternative hand placement for manual displacement of the gravid uterus.

mechanical changes to the woman, in particular her thoracic upper-body further add to this challenge and stressful situation. The increased cardiac output in pregnancy means that large volumes of blood can be lost very rapidly, especially from the uterus during haemorrhage, which by term is receiving 10% of the woman's cardiac output. Otherwise healthy women will tolerate blood loss remarkably well, and can lose up to 35% of their circulation before becoming symptomatic (hypotension). The key to preventing arrest however, is the early recognition and treatment of the early warning signs (tachypnoea, tachycardia) as outlined earlier in the A–E assessment (Table 26.1). Haemorrhage is tolerated less well in pre-existing physiological conditions of anaemia and dehydration. Sudden changes to maternal circulation through blood loss is further complicated in cases of pre-eclampsia and sepsis, where their circulation may already be haemodynamically unstable and impaired, depending on the severity of the condition. Heightened awareness to subtle hypovolemia, often due to concealed blood loss can be easily missed when hypertension or hypotension are already present.

Perimortem Caesarean

Perimortem caesarean section (CS) is the surgical intervention to expedite the birth of the fetus and placenta during CPR, performed primarily in the interests of maternal, not fetal, survival. In women ≥20 weeks' gestation, if there is no response to correctly performed CPR within 4 min of maternal collapse or if resuscitation is continued beyond this, birth via CS should be undertaken to aid effective maternal resuscitation. It should be achieved within 5 min of the collapse and undertaken at the point of collapse regardless of clinical setting. Birth of the fetus and placenta removes the cardiac impairment through mechanical and haematological adaptations described above. Emergence of the fetus to the waiting Neonatal Emergency Team improves the chances of survival, but is not the reason *per se* for the perimortem CS. Associated with this decision would be the outcome of a child with potentially severely damaged brain function (hypoxic ischemic encephalopathy), however the needs of the mother must come first (RCOG 2011).

Human Factors

The majority of errors made in clinical practice are caused by humans making mistakes. Midwives working within high pressured situations are required to recognize complex, sometimes infrequently seen clinical scenarios while challenged by shift patterns and cultural factors that influence behaviours and decision-making. National audits in the UK such as MBRRACE (2016) and the 'Each Baby Counts' report (RCOG 2017) highlight the impact *human factors* have over caregiving and functioning of the MDT within both everyday situations such as electronic monitoring fetal cardiotocography (CTG) interpretation and emergencies such as maternal collapse. Human factors will always be present and continue to have a potentially detrimental impact on midwives and doctors, unless the MDT starts to focus training also on the non-technical skills. Multiprofessional rehearsal of critical scenarios must include the practical skills of airway management, chest compression, etc., alongside effective communication and leadership. Many of the lessons learned in relation to human error have historically come from other high pressured industries including aviation and the military, with the development of a 'human factors framework' within health care being a more recent discipline. Understanding human factors and raising awareness within the team is crucial, as is the exploration following a critical incident to unpick their impact and to learn lessons, to avoid any repetition. To truly learn lessons, midwives must draw parallels across health care to mitigate and minimize future potential through implementing human-factors tools and thinking during everyday practice. Using a framework, such as Dupont's 1993 (see Nzelu et al. 2018) 'Dirty Dozen' (Table 26.3) to reflect on clinical experiences and heighten self-awareness on how being human impacts on caregiving, is a useful exercise in reducing error potential. Acceptance that as humans we will always continue to make mistakes is vital, exploration of ways to mitigate as a team is pivotal.

Enhanced Maternity Care

Enhanced maternity care (EMC) put simply, is the care of an unwell childbearing woman who can be treated and cared for by an MDT within the maternity unit (RCOA 2018b). It is seen as a new standard of care beyond normal maternity care for women with medical or surgical problems during pregnancy or the postpartum period, but without the severity of illness that requires full critical care support. Through EMC training, the focus on early recognition and response to deterioration and closer working between maternity and critical care teams to optimize care. After childbirth, admission to

TABLE 26.3 Dupont's 'Dirty Dozen' in CTG Misinterpretation

What's Happening in Practice?	The Human Factors	How to Mitigate Misinterpretation
Ineffective communication/not being heard/misleading communication.	Lack of communication	Using a structured communication tool such as SBAR (Situation, Background, Assessment, Recommendations)
Over-confident clinicians, relying on pattern recognition and not seeking out alternative explanations/diagnosis.	Complacency	Think outside the box. Challenge assumptions.
Incomplete handover/poor history-taking/not listening to the woman.	Lack of knowledge	Effective training as a team/live multidisciplinary 'skills drills'.
The complexity of maternity care, and the multitude of variables that require attention at the same time (MEWS, fetal monitoring, supporting the woman, etc.) Possibly further complicated by caring for more than one woman at a time.	Distraction	Stop moments with the team to help determine priorities and focus the team. Maintain situational awareness/helicopter view over full clinical picture.
Feeling unsure of what's happening/unsure of the plan. Not knowing the team's strengths and weaknesses.	Lack of teamwork	MDT handovers including introductions. Team training that includes student midwives. Recognition of everyone in the team. Leadership within emergencies. Team debriefs following critical incidents to identify key learning points – what was done well and what the team could do better if anything.
Tiredness and inability to perform tasks. Making errors.	Fatigue	Use checklists (WHO theatre sign in/out, 'fresh eyes' for CTGs, etc.) and simplified guideline algorithms in practice. Take your break and support others to take theirs. Acknowledge the fatigue associated with nightshifts in particular.
Searching for equipment in an emergency, not having necessary equipment easily to hand in emergency situations.	Lack of resources	Develop standardized kit boxes to deal with emergencies. Respect for resources – individual responsibilities for replacing stock, managing broken equipment.
Feelings of being overwhelmed and not in control.	Pressure	Prioritize, delegate and ask for help when you need it.
Noticing significant factors in practice but feeling unable to speak up within the team. Sharing information and not being listened to.	Lack of assertiveness	Break down hierarchy and the chain of command. Open channels of communication to all members of the team. Promote a culture that is safe to work within.
Subconscious response to pressure and demands that have a physical feeling over us; can drain our energy levels and reduce our ability to concentrate.	Stress	Conscious awareness of stress levels. Promote wellbeing within the team. Make the most of days off.
When our alertness diminishes, or we are distracted by the complexity and fail to see the whole clinical picture. Not noticing recording of maternal pulse instead of fetal; failing to associate deteriorating patient to concealed haemorrhage, etc.	Lack of awareness	Maintain situational awareness through MDT stop moments/safety huddles. Work as a team to overcome task fixation (focussing on one object or factor to the detriment of everything else).
Working to a set of unwritten rules or beliefs, which can detract from safety standards (e.g. 'second-stage CTG').	Norms	Challenge assumptions within the team and yourself.

Adapted from Nzelu O, Chandraharan E, Pereira S. (2018). Human Factors: The Dirty Dozen in CTG misinterpretation. Glob J Reprod Med, 6(2): 555683. DOI: 10.19080/GJORM.2018.06.555683

a critical care unit should not automatically mean the separation of a mother from her baby. If the baby is well, then critical care units should do all they can to facilitate contact between the mother and her baby. EMC will commonly be delivered by midwives; however, in large centres, there may be scope for critical care nurses to provide EMC competencies in tandem with midwives. Critical care outreach teams are critical care-trained nurses who support ward teams across the hospital, who are caring for acutely ill 'inpatients', outside of the critical care environment. In recent years, governing medical and midwifery bodies have recommended broad-based training and this approach is of particular relevance to the multispecialty area of the maternity unit. Recognition of the need for broader understanding and depth of knowledge into medical conditions such as cardiac disease for midwives is clear (see Case Study 26.1: Vanessa's story).

CASE STUDY 26.1   Vanessa's Story of Surviving a Critical Illness

I became unwell in my third pregnancy with a chest infection when I was 31 weeks and initially I was treated by my GP ... until I was at home cooking tea for my other children and experienced a horrible sharp pain every time I took a breath. I was 32 weeks and 3 days pregnant when I presented at the ED [Emergency Department]. They gave me strong painkillers which eased my pain and then a series of tests to find the causes. A chest X-ray revealed I had pneumonia in both lungs and part of one of my lungs was collapsed. I can remember the doctors telling me I had sepsis and as I work as support staff in the hospital I knew what this was. They admitted me and I was transferred to the HDU [High Dependency Unit]. This was now late into the night, my mother had come to look after our children so my husband, Paul came to join me. They carried out further tests on HDU to rule out that I didn't have a blood clot on my lung and I remember being visited by an obstetrician and midwife, who checked that my baby was well, with a scan and monitoring. I felt reassured by my baby's movements, and to be honest I didn't realize just how unwell I was at this point.

The following morning my blood pressure became unstable and very low for me and the doctors on HDU explained they wanted to put a central line into my neck so they could give me medicines and monitor me closely. I can recall I was on the CTG at the same time and just as they finished his heartbeat dropped and didn't recover. Suddenly there was lots more staff in the room and they asked my consent to take me to theatre to perform an emergency caesarean. Because of my anti-blood clot drugs it had to be under a general anaesthetic. My husband wasn't with me at this time; he was at home with the kids. Within minutes of my baby's heart rate slowing down, they ran me down the corridor, straight to theatre. It was like an out of body experience. I knew it was me, but felt like it was all happening to someone else. I understood the need, staff were explaining everything they could to me, but it was still immensely scary. I have a strong memory

of everyone in the theatre talking over me; there must have been at least 15 people. Our baby Connor was born at 10.27 and gave a healthy cry apparently. He was well grown and obviously healthy, but because he was only 32 weeks and my sepsis, he went straight to the Neonatal Unit. Paul arrived during my operation to be told of the quick decision to deliver our baby and the need for me to be put to sleep. A midwife went and spoke with him and tried to reassure him.

They decided to keep me asleep and intubated to rest my lungs and allow me to recover. I woke up on ITU the following day – very disorientated, confused and unable to understand the timeline of what had happened to me. My last memory of being in the busy and noisy theatre was a blur. It felt like I had lost 24 hours of my life. Paul was there when I woke up, sitting in the chair next to my bed – I tried to get out of bed, but he stopped me, explaining the surgery and the need to lie still. Once again, many people rushed into my room and removed my breathing tube. It was then that Paul told me that our baby had been transferred to another unit for neonatal care.

As I became more awake I saw the messages on my phone and social media from our friends and family who had been told of Connor's arrival. It just didn't seem real. The conversations with the nurses and midwives felt surreal. It was my husband who helped me piece the pieces back together. Paul had wanted to be the person that helped me do this; we talked through the events, like it was someone else's bad experience. I can remember being very worried for Paul, he was being so strong for us both and perhaps I was still not appreciating that I was the poorly one.

The care from the midwives included helping express breastmilk for my baby – I questioned her whether he would be able to have the breastmilk given all the drugs they had given me. She didn't know and left me while she went to find out. I prepared myself for the news that it would probably need to be thrown away. Pumping with wires, tubes and drips was hard work and felt so unnatural and so different to my first

Continued

CASE STUDY 26.1   Vanessa's Story of Surviving a Critical Illness—cont'd

two breastfeeding experiences. Being separated from Connor was agony. Lots of our friends and family were also coming to terms with what had happened to us. On day 3 they transferred me back to the care of the midwives on the labour suite – but still without my baby. When they wheeled me into the room there was an empty cot beside the bed. This was the first time that I cried. Over the next 2 days, I remained in the observations bay, getting limited rest or sleep as other women and their babies came in to share the room with me. The littlest of tasks, such as getting up to the toilet on my own, were just exhausting. I was moved into my own room, still on the labour suite on day 5. My Connor returned to the same hospital as me on the Wednesday. My window overlooked the ambulance bay and I heard his ambulance and transfer team arrive – I literally ran out to meet him! I was offered a wheelchair but didn't need it, my baby was on his way to meet me at last. I hugged the neonatal transfer team, so grateful to them for bringing him to me. I recognized him as my baby instantly thanks to the endless photos Paul had taken of him. Our first cuddle happened within minutes of him arriving on the neonatal unit. It was the first time Paul had seen him out of the incubator also. He was placed skin to skin on my chest – it felt amazing! I didn't want to put him back in that incubator.

My first shower on day 6 was the first time I brushed my hair and saw myself in the mirror since my birth experience – I was bruised all over; my neck, my arms, my hands. I lost over 2 stone in weight, in 6 days. I looked so different. That first shower had been so significant to me, to start to wash the trauma away and begin processing what I had been through. Sadly, my expressing had stopped producing milk, despite lots of trying and support from neonatal nurses, I guess my body was just too un-

well. I had had no emotional preparation for what the surgery involved, the pain, the discomfort or the recovery.

I was discharged home the next day, deemed well enough to physically manage with the daily visits to see Connor, and being a mum to my other two at the same time. I was exhausted. I couldn't walk up my own stairs and I slept on the sofa the first night of being home. Relieved but still in shock. It took months to recover physically – I had to be readmitted twice postnatally as I was too ill to stay at home. More antibiotics through a drip and drugs for chest pain associated with the infection. I didn't start eating and drinking properly until about a month later. I was just too tired and too weak to think about food. The cough persisted for months.

Emotional recovery took much longer and the following year, both Paul and I experienced lots of highs and lows. I was obviously grateful to have survived and have our beautiful son, but I was now battling new anxieties about everything. When Connor was about 6 months old I realized I was suffering with postnatal depression, which I was able to share with Paul. Together we shared our emotional memories. At Connor's 1st birthday party, Paul was really withdrawn, choosing to not join in, too upset from everything he had been through and watched happen to me. He experienced flashbacks and went to the GP support. We are both so grateful for all the love and support our family showed us in those difficult first few weeks and continue to do so. With their help we are moving on and enjoying family life again. Connor is thriving and the perfect addition to our family.

With thanks to Vanessa and Paul – parents to Connor

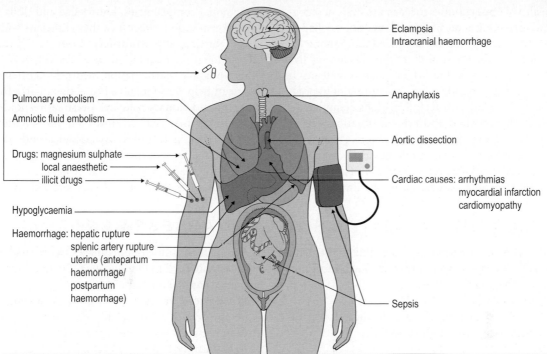

Fig. 26.9 Causes of maternal collapse. (Reproduced with permission from RCOG (Royal College of Obstetricians and Gynaecologists). (2011) Maternal collapse in pregnancy and the puerperium. Green-top Guideline No 56. London: RCOG.)

	Reversible cause	Cause in pregnancy
4 Hs	Hypovolaemia	Bleeding (may be concealed) (obstetric/other) or relative hypovolaemia of dense spinal block; septic or neurogenic shock
	Hypoxia	Pregnant patients can become hypoxic more quickly
		Cardiac events: peripartum cardiomyopathy, myocardial infarction, aortic dissection, large-vessel aneurysms
	Hypo/hyperkalaemia and other electrolyte disturbances	No more likely
	Hypothermia	No more likely
4 Ts	Thromboembolism	Amniotic fluid embolus, pulmonary embolus, air embolus, myocardial infarction
	Toxicity	Local anaesthetic, magnesium, other
	Tension pneumothorax	Following trauma/suicide attempt
	Tamponade (cardiac)	Following trauma/suicide attempt
Eclampsia and pre-eclampsia		Includes intracranial haemorrhage

SUMMARY

Of the women aged 16–50 admitted to UK Intensive Care Units (ICU), 1 in 10 are obstetric-related cases (RCOA 2011). In addition, there are likely to be significant numbers of critically ill perinatal women who are cared for within the maternity unit given the complexities of modern-day practice and changes in demographics globally. This affords midwives to strengthen their knowledge and skills of critical care and provide student midwives with a wealth of opportunities to learn the skills in recognizing and managing acute illness and maternal collapse; such opportunities should be facilitated and embraced. Participation in education and training including live 'skills drills', as part of the wider maternity team is encouraged as they provide a 'safe' environment to practise the technical and non-technical skills required for managing high pressured and critical situation. Delivering effective teamwork in acute situations requires all members of the MDT to communicate clearly, using the tools described in this chapter, to aid prompt and appropriate treatment, while also accepting the limitations of

professional competencies, knowledge and skills as well as demonstrating respect for other clinicians within the team (Nursing and Midwifery Council, NMC 2018; International Confederation of Midwives, ICM 2018). Where possible, participation in timely debriefing as a team can help those involved to contextualize the incident, the individual's role and personal response to it. Exposure to maternal collapse and resuscitation may serve to be traumatic unless psychological and emotional needs are met within the individual through reflecting, sharing and learning from such critical incidents. Fig. 26.9 summarizes the causes of maternal collapse.

▌ REFLECTIVE ACTIVITY FOR SELF-ASSESSMENT

1. Recall a clinical situation of acute illness you have had involvement in – what was your role in recognizing and managing the situation?
   a. Which 'tools' have you used?
   b. Where did your intuition fit into these tools and the physiology they highlighted?

2. Following training opportunities to rehearse resuscitation, how did *human factors* influence your performance and the outcome?
3. Having read Vanessa's story above that captures her perspective of a critical illness – what elements of caregiving, if any, could have made her experience different?

REFERENCES

Bogod, D., Plaat, F., Mushambi, M., et al. (2018). Guidelines for the Provision of Anaesthesia Services for an Obstetric Population. Available at: www.rcoa.ac.uk/document-store/guidelines-the-provision-of-anaesthesia-services-obstetric-population-2018.

Chandraharan, E., & Arulkumaran, S. (2013). *Obstetric and intrapartum emergencies A practical guide to management.* Cambridge: Cambridge University Press.

ICM (International Confederation of Midwives). (2018). Essential competencies for midwifery practice 2018. UPDATE. Available at: www.internationalmidwives.org/assets/files/general-files/2018/10/icm-competencies--english-document_final_oct-2018.pdf.

Knight M, Kenyon S, Brocklehurst P, et al. (eds.). On behalf of MBRRACEUK. (2014). *Saving Lives, Improving Mothers' Care – Lessons learned to inform future maternity care from the UK and Ireland Confidential Enquiries into Maternal Deaths and Morbidity 2009–2012.* Oxford: NPEU, Oxford.

Knight, M., Bunch, K., Tuffnell, D., et al. (Eds.). On Behalf of MBRRACE-UK. (2018). *Saving lives, improving mothers' care – lessons learned to inform maternity care from the UK and Ireland Confidential enquiries into maternal deaths and morbidity 2014–2016.* Oxford: NPEU.

Knight, M., K., Bunch, K., Tuffnell, D., et al. (Eds.). On Behalf of MBRRACE-UK . (2019). *Saving Lives, Improving Mothers' Care – Lessons Learned to inform maternity care from the UK and Ireland Confidential Enquiries into Maternal Deaths and Morbidity 2015–17.* Oxford: NPEU.

Lancet. (2014). Midwifery: An executive summary for The Lancet's series. Available at: www.thelancet.com/pb/assets/raw/Lancet/stories/series/midwifery/midwifery_exec_summ.pdf.

MBRRACE-UK. (2016). *Saving lives, improving mothers' care 2016 – lay summary.* Oxford: NPEU.

MBRRACE-UK. (2019). *Saving lives, improving mothers' care 2019 – lay report.* Oxford: NPEU.

NHS Improvement. (2018) ACT Academy. Online Library of Quality, Service Improvement and Redesign Tools: SBAR Communication tool – Situation, Background, Assessment, Recommendation. (This Safety Guideline is Endorsed by the Australian and New Zealand College of Anaesthetists, ANZCA). Available at: https://improvement.nhs.uk/documents/2162/sbar-communication-tool.pdf.

NICE (National Institute for Health and Care Excellence). (2016). Sepsis: Recognition, Diagnosis and Early Management: CG 51. Available at: www.nice.org.uk.

NMC Nursing and Midwifery Council. (2018). *The Code: professional standards of practice and behaviour for nurses, midwives and nursing associates.* London: NMC. Available at: www.resus.org.uk.

Nzelu, O., Chandraharan, E., & Pereira, S. (2018). Human FACTORS: The Dirty Dozen in CTG misinterpretation. *Global Journal of Reproductive Medicine, 6*(2), 555683.

RCUK (Resuscitation Council UK). (2010a). Adult basic life support and automated external defibrillation. Available at: www.resus.org.uk.

RCUK (Resuscitation Council UK). (2010b). The ABCDE approach – underlying principles. Available at: www.resus.org.uk.

RCUK (Resuscitation Council UK). (2010c). In-house cardiac arrest algorithm. Available at: www.resus.org.uk.

RCUK (Resuscitation Council UK). (2015). Adult basic life support and automated external defibrillation. Available at: www.resus.org.uk.

RCUK (Resuscitation Council UK). (2016). Emergency treatment of anaphylactic reactions. Available at: www.resus.org.uk.

RCOA (Royal College of Anaesthetists) and the Maternal Critical Care Working Group. (2011). *Providing equity of critical and maternity care for the critically ill pregnant or recently pregnant woman*. London: RCOA.

RCOA (Royal College of Anaesthetists). (2018a). *Guidelines for the Provision of Anaesthetic Services (GPAS) 2018.* Available at: www.rcoa.ac.uk/gpas2018.

RCOA (Royal College of Anaesthetists). (2018b). *Maternity Critical Care/Enhanced Maternal Care Standards Development Working Group: Care of the critically ill woman in childbirth; enhanced maternal care.* London: RCOA.

RCOG (Royal College of Obstetricians and Gynaecologists). (2011). *Maternal collapse in pregnancy and the puerperium. Green-top Guideline No 56.* London: RCOG.

RCOG (Royal College of Obstetricians and Gynaecologists). (2017). *Each Baby Counts: 2015 Full Report.* London: RCOG.

RCP (Royal College of Physicians). (2018). Never too busy to learn – how the modern team can learn together in the busy workplace. Available at: www.rcplondon.ac.uk.

UN (United Nations). (2015). Sustainable Development Goals. United Nations. Available at: www.un.org.

WHO (World Health Organization). (2015). *Trends in maternal mortality: 1990 to 2015: Estimates by WHO, UNICEF, UNFPA, World Bank Group and the United Nations Population Division.* Geneva: WHO. WHO/RHR/15.23.

WHO (World Health Organization). (2019). Global Maternal Sepsis Study (GLOSS) and Awareness Campaign. Available at: www.who.int/reproductivehealth/projects/Project-brief-GLOSS.pdf.

ANNOTATED FURTHER READING

Department of Health and Social Care. (2016). Improving the safety of maternity care in the NHS. Available at: www.gov.uk/government/news/improving-the-safety-of-maternity-care-in-the-nhs.
Outlines an overview of how safety can be improved in the contemporary maternity service in the UK.

Hinton, L., Locock, L., & Knight, M. (2015). Maternal critical care: what can we learn from patient experience? A qualitative study. *BMJ Open, 5*, e006676.
Details some interesting insights into women's experience of being on the receiving end of critical care.

Nzelu, O., Chandraharan, E., & Pereira, S. (2018). Human Factors: The Dirty Dozen in CTG misinterpretation. *Global Journal of Reproductive Medicine, 6*(2), 555683.
Provides a good working example on how the Dupont (1993) checklist can be applied to the context of electronic fetal heart monitoring.

Renfrew, M., McFadden, A., Bastos, M. H., et al. (2014). Midwifery and quality care: findings from a new evidence-informed framework for maternal and newborn care. *Lancet, 384*(9948), 1129–1145.
This paper along with the other three papers in the Lancet series on midwifery, examines the central contribution by midwives to the survival and wellbeing of childbearing women and newborn infants globally. The framework is a useful tool for all midwives around the world, as the researchers reported that when midwives were educated, trained effectively that resources were used more efficiently and maternal and neonatal outcomes improved.

The UK Sepsis Trust. (2017). The sepsis manual. Available at: www.sepsistrust.org.
A useful manual with detailed information about sepsis.

USEFUL WEBSITES

MBRRACE-UK: Mothers and Babies: Reducing Risk through Audits and Confidential Enquiries across the UK: www.npeu.ox.ac.uk/mbrrace-uk

Resuscitation Council (UK): Information for professionals: www.resus.org.uk/information-for-professionals

Royal College of Anaesthetists: www.rcoa.ac.uk

Royal College of Midwives: www.rcm.org.uk

Royal College of Obstetricians and Gynaecologists: www.rcog.org.uk/en/guidelines-research-services/audit-quality-improvement/each-baby-counts/implementation/improving-human-factors/video-briefing

TED: Time Escalation Decision: "The Little Voice Inside": http://voiceinside.co.uk

UK Sepsis Trust: www.sepsistrust.org

World Health Organization: www.who.int

VIDEO RESOURCE

https://youtu.be/YiJBG8jDvnE
This link provides access via YouTube of the 2nd World Sepsis Congress held in 2018 by the Global Sepsis Alliance. Details of the full Congress proceedings and keynote speakers' talks can be viewed.
www.youtube.com/watch?v=Zx4vezE5iHM
Features a short video from Professor Mary Renfrew about the four research papers in the Lancet series on midwifery.

Puerperium

27

Optimal Infant Feeding

Helen McIntyre, Jayne E. Marshall

CHAPTER CONTENTS

Women decide to feed their baby within a psychosocial context, which is not always supportive of breastfeeding as the expected norm. Midwives have a key role informing and facilitating mothers to breastfeed successfully. It is strongly in the interest of the individual mother and community that women who choose to breastfeed are enabled to do so for as long as they choose. The reasons women give for discontinuation are consistent over time and internationally; they think they do not have enough milk, breastfeeding is painful and they have problems getting the baby to feed. Preventing these distressing problems requires a multifaceted approach that starts with an enabling attitude and effective, practical and evidence-based training of all those who facilitate and support breastfeeding mothers, especially in the first week of their baby's life. For those mothers who cannot, or choose not to breastfeed, the midwife has an equally important role in ensuring that the baby is fed safely and appropriately (Brown 2016; Dixley 2014; McAndrew et al. 2012; DiGiroloma et al. 2008; Schmied et al. 2011).

THE CHAPTER AIMS TO

- explain the structure and function of the female breast
- describe the properties and components of breastmilk and some comparison with formula milk
- outline the recommendations and requirements of the Baby Friendly Hospital Initiative and the *International Code of Marketing of Breast-milk Substitutes*

- emphasize the role of the midwife in ensuring breastfeeding success for both mother and baby
- discuss the role of breastmilk expression and human milk banking
- describe some causes of difficulty with breastfeeding
- discuss the use of formula feeding and the various products available.

INTRODUCTION

Breastfeeding for the first 6 months of life and extending up to 3 years (World Health Organization, WHO 2018) is the ideal start for babies. Breastfeeding improves the physical and mental health of the infant and mother as well as infant cognitive development in high and low-income countries. It is the single most important preventative approach for saving children's lives, as highlighted in the agenda for Sustainable Development by the United Nations (UN) General Assembly and subsequent Sustainable Development Goals (SDGs) (UN 2015; Renfrew and Hall 2008). Furthermore, the benefits of breastfeeding are seen in all countries. Victora et al. (2016) found that increasing breastfeeding rates around the world to near universal levels could prevent 823,000 annual deaths in children under 5 years and 20,000 annual maternal deaths from breast cancer.

Low breastfeeding rates in the UK, which in 2018–19 were 47.3% at 6 weeks (Public Health England, PHE 2019) compared with 71% in Norway, have led to a progressive increase in the incidence of illness that has a significant cost to the National Health Service (NHS).

The problems that deter women from breastfeeding can mostly be prevented (Renfrew and Hall 2008). This requires a multifaceted approach (Brown 2016; Dixley 2014) with implementation of the UNICEF-UK Baby Friendly Initiative at its core.

THE BREAST AND BREASTMILK

Anatomy and Physiology of the Breast

The breasts are bilateral compound secretory glands, positioned between the 2nd and 6th rib of the thorax, extending laterally from the sternum to the axilla and lying anterior to the pectoralis major muscle. Each breast is composed of varying proportions of fat and glandular tissue separated by connective tissue, into lobes. Each lobe is subdivided into lobules consisting of alveoli and ducts (Fig. 27.1).

The intimate connection between fat and glandular tissue within the breast (Nickell and Skelton 2005), make the proportions difficult to calculate non-invasively. However, analysis of 21 non-lactating breasts (surgically removed for carcinoma *in situ*) (Vandeweyer and Hertens 2002) revealed that the percentage weight of fat per breast varied from 3.6% to 37.6%. Mammographic studies of non-lactating breasts have reported breast glandularity decreasing with age (Jamal et al. 2004).

Investigations on 25 sections of central breast tissue removed during breast reduction operations performed on women with an average body mass index (BMI) of 28, found a mean of 61% fat (Cruz-Korchin et al. 2002). On average, the women's central breast area contained only 7% glandular tissue and 29% connective tissue. Nickell and Skelton (2005) observed larger breasts contain relatively more fat in 136 patients with an average BMI of 32, undergoing breast reduction surgery. Furthermore, fat cells negatively impact prolactin activity on acini cells (Hale and Hartmann 2007) and more crucially, Geddes (2008) noted a *2:1 ratio of glandular to fat tissue in lactating breasts* when using ultrasound scanning.

Research on the volumes of 20 complete duct systems (*lobes*) in an autopsied breast, found considerable variation in the proportion of breast tissue serviced by each duct. The largest lobe released 23% of breast volume, 50% of the breast was supplied by three ducts and 75% by the largest six. Conversely, eight small duct systems together accounted for only 1.6% of breast volume (Going and Moffat 2004).

Ultrasound investigations of the *lactating* breasts of 21 subjects (Ramsay et al. 2005) identified on average nine milk ducts per breast (range being 4–18), fewer than previously believed but commensurate with the investigations conducted by Love and Barsky (2004). Taneri et al. (2006) examined 226 mastectomy specimens and found the mean number of ducts in the nipple duct bundle was 17.5. This is significantly higher than the number reported to open on the nipple surface. Taneri et al. (2006) reflected that this discrepancy could be due to duct branching within the nipple or the presence of some ducts that do not reach the nipple surface.

The complexity of breast tissue has implications for women undergoing breast surgery and their subsequent ability to successfully breastfeed requiring honest pre-operative counselling. The *alveoli* contain milk-producing *acini cells*, surrounded by myoepithelial cells, which contract and propel the milk out (Fig. 27.2). Some 65% of glandular tissue is within a 30 mm radius of the nipple (Geddes 2008), perfect for a baby's mouth to close over, reducing transportation time and wastage in the ducts. Small lactiferous ducts, carrying milk from the alveoli, unite to form larger ducts. Several large ducts (lactiferous tubules) conveying milk from one or more lobes emerge on the surface of the nipple. Myoepithelial cells are also oriented longitudinally along the ducts and, under the influence of oxytocin, these smooth muscle cells contract and the tubule becomes shorter and wider in a similar action to peristalsis (Woolridge 1986; Ramsay et al. 2004). The tubule distends during active milk flow, while the myoepithelial cells are maintained in a state of contraction by circulating oxytocin for about 2–3 min. The fuller the breast when let-down occurs, the greater the degree of ductal distension. The

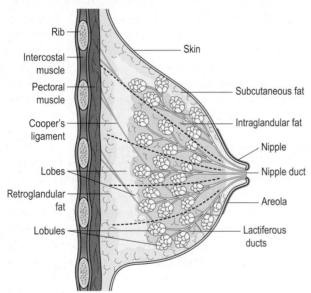

Fig. 27.1 Anatomy of the breast. (Reproduced with permission of Liz Ellis.)

Labels: Rib, Intercostal muscle, Pectoral muscle, Cooper's ligament, Lobes, Retroglandular fat, Lobules, Skin, Subcutaneous fat, Intraglandular fat, Nipple, Nipple duct, Areola, Lactiferous ducts

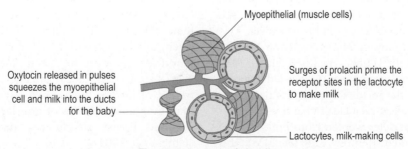

Myoepithelial (muscle cells)

Oxytocin released in pulses squeezes the myoepithelial cell and milk into the ducts for the baby

Surges of prolactin prime the receptor sites in the lactocyte to make milk

Lactocytes, milk-making cells

Fig. 27.2 A bunch of alveoli.

lactiferous ducts are able to dilate from a resting 1.0–1.4 mm by 58%, therefore also acting as a storage repository for breastmilk (Ramsay et al. 2004).

The human *nipple*, which follows the mammalian line, is covered with epithelium and contains cylindrically arranged smooth muscle and elastic fibres. When this contracts and the nipple becomes erect, a tight sphincter is formed (Cross 1977) to prevent unwanted loss of milk from the mammary gland when it is not being suckled.

Surrounding the nipple is an area of pigmented skin called the *areola*, which increases in size from a primary to secondary areola in pregnancy and darkens under the influence of melanin. The areola protects the area from friction, acts as a marker for the infant to attach to the breast and contains Montgomery's glands. These glands produce a sebum-like substance, which lubricates the nipple during pregnancy and throughout breastfeeding. Breasts, nipples and areolae vary considerably in size between women but bear no reflection on their ability to effectively lactate.

The breast is supplied with blood from the internal and external mammary arteries and branches of the intercostal arteries. The corresponding veins are arranged in a circular fashion around the nipple. Increased venous access in pregnancy supplies essential nutrients for glandular and ductal growth, often seen as *'blue lines'* on the surface of the breasts. Lymph drains freely from the two breasts into lymph nodes in the axillae and the mediastinum.

During pregnancy, progesterone induces alveolar/glandular growth and oestrogen, ductal growth. Other hormones (such as growth hormone, prolactin, epidermal growth factor, fibroblast growth factor, human placental lactogen, parathyroid hormone-related protein and insulin-like growth factor) are involved, governing a complex sequence of events that prepares the breast for lactation (Neville et al. 2002). The rise in prolactin can stimulate the secretion of colostrum from around 16 weeks of pregnancy.

Lactogenesis

Once the alveolar epithelial cells have developed into acini cells/lactocytes, around mid-pregnancy (**Lactogenesis I**), they are able to produce small quantities of secretion: colostrum. Although some women may produce as much as 30 mL/day in late pregnancy (Cox et al. 1999), the production of milk is held in abeyance until after 30–40 h following the birth, when levels of placental hormones have fallen sufficiently to allow the already high

levels of prolactin to initiate milk production (**Lactogenesis II**). Continued production of prolactin is caused by milk removal as the baby feeds at the breast, with concentrations highest during night feeds and following a feed. Prolactin is involved in the suppression of ovulation, and some women may remain anovular until lactation ceases, known as lactation amenorrhea, although for others the effect is not so prolonged (Labbok 2016; Guillebaud and MacGregor 2017) (see Chapter 28).

Maternal nutritional intake and nutritional status are known to affect birth outcome, and the fetus *in utero*. The mother's diet before and during pregnancy may also *programme* the fetus, affecting health in adult life (Hall Moran 2012), but the effects of maternal nutrition on the development of the mammary gland in pregnancy are less well known. Evidence from rats (Kim and Park 2004) suggests that undernutrition may actually enhance cell growth and milk production. Torgersen et al. (2010) found no differences in the risk of cessation of exclusive breastfeeding in mothers with and without eating disorders. Over-nutrition (*obesity*), however, has been shown to adversely affect Lactogenesis II (Rasmussen 2007).

If breastfeeding (or expressing) is delayed for a few days, lactation can still be initiated as prolactin levels remain high, even in the absence of breast use, for at least the first week (Kochenour 1980). However, the establishment of lactation is more secure if breastfeeding or expressing begins as soon after birth as possible.

Endocrine release of prolactin from the anterior pituitary gland during and following a feed is important in opening and stimulating the acini receptor sites to initiate lactation. As lactation progresses, the prolactin response to suckling diminishes and milk removal becomes the driving force behind milk production. This is due to a whey protein secreted in the milk that inhibits the synthesis of milk (Prentice et al. 1989; Daly 1993; Wilde et al. 1995).

The protein collects in the breast as the milk accumulates, exerting a negative feedback control on the continued production of milk. Removal of this autocrine inhibitory factor (sometimes referred to as *Feedback Inhibitor of Lactation: FIL*) by milk removal, allows milk production to accelerate as shown in Fig. 27.3.

This mechanism acts locally within the breast, enabling each breast to function independently. For this reason, milk production slows as the baby is gradually weaned from the breast or increased again if the baby is put back to the breast more often, perhaps because of illness.

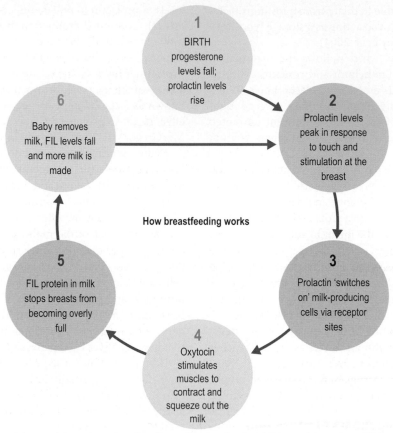

Fig. 27.3 Physiology of lactation showing how the feedback inhibitor of lactation (FIL) works. (From S Macdonald, G Johnson (Eds) Mayes Midwifery (15th ed.). London: Elsevier).

Milk is synthesized continuously into the alveolar lumen, where it is stored until milk removal from the breast is initiated. Only when stored oxytocin is released from the posterior pituitary gland prior to and during a breastfeed, will the myoepithelial cells contract, making milk available to the suckling baby. Milk release is also under neuroendocrine control. Tactile stimulation of the breast, thoughts of their baby, a picture, smell or sound of their baby stimulate oxytocin release, causing contraction of the myoepithelial cells. This process is known as the *let-down* or *milk-ejection* reflex and makes the milk available to the baby. Oxytocin release occurs in discrete pulses throughout the feed and may trigger bursts of active feeding or a flood of milk.

This initial unconditioned reflex becomes positively or negatively conditioned over time. In one small study, psychological stress (mental arithmetic or noise) was found to reduce the frequency of the oxytocin pulses but did not affect the amplitude of the pulse. In addition, there was no effect on either prolactin levels or the amount of milk the baby received (Ueda et al. 1994).

Milk Production and the Mother

Human lactation does not follow non-primate dairy models (Woolridge 1995) and adequate milk production is largely independent of the mother's nutritional status and BMI (Prentice et al. 1994).

Dietary surveys in moderate- to high-income countries have consistently found calorie intake to be less than the recommended amount (Whitehead et al. 1981; Butte et al. 1984). Controlled trials conducted in low-income countries have demonstrated that giving extra food to mothers, even those who were poorly nourished, did not increase the rate of growth of their babies (Prentice et al. 1980, 1983). It has been suggested that metabolic efficiency is enhanced in lactating women, enabling them to conserve energy and subsidize the cost of their milk production (Illingworth et al. 1986). However, the lactational performance of the human female is compromised when undernutrition reaches famine or near-famine conditions. Milk production appears to drive appetite, rather than the reverse. Hunger effectively regulates the calorie intake of a breastfeeding mother, therefore eating a balanced diet to satisfy appetite is sufficient. Similarly, if healthy breastfeeding women wish to undertake strenuous exercise from 6–8 weeks after birth, or to lose weight (500–1000 g/week), they can be assured that neither the quality nor the quantity of their milk will be affected (Dewey et al. 1994; Dusdieker et al. 1994). However, a high BMI can negatively affect the baby's feeding cues, glucose management and the mother's lactation (Hale and Hartmann 2007). Exclusive breastfeeding combined with a low fat diet and exercise will result in more effective weight loss than diet and exercise alone (Hammer et al. 1996; Dewey 1998).

Milk production is similarly unaffected by fluctuations in the woman's fluid intake. It has been repeatedly demonstrated that neither a significant decrease (Dearlove and Dearlove 1981) nor a significant increase (Morse et al. 1992) in maternal fluid intake has any effect on milk production or the baby's weight.

Properties and Components of Breastmilk

Human milk has nutritional, digestive, immune, microbiome and epigenetic properties unique to each mother-baby pairing, unlike formula milk, which only has generic nutritional components, predominantly derived from cow's milk: a summary of which is shown in Table 27.1.

Human milk varies in its composition:

- with the time of day (e.g. fat content is lowest in the morning and highest in the afternoon)
- with the stage of lactation (e.g. the fat and protein content of colostrum is higher than in mature milk)
- with the gestational age of the baby
- in response to maternal nutrition (e.g. although the total amount of fat is not influenced by diet, the type of fat that appears in the milk will be influenced by what the mother eats)
- because of individual variations.

The most dramatic change in the composition of milk occurs during the course of a feed. At the beginning of a feed, the baby receives a high volume of relatively low fat, high protein and lactose milk: the foremilk. As the feed progresses, the volume of milk decreases but the proportion of fat in the milk increases, by as much as five times the initial value: the hindmilk (Jackson et al. 1987). The baby's ability to obtain this fat-rich milk is not determined by the length of time they spend suckling at the breast, but by the quality of the attachment to the breast. The baby needs to be well attached so that the tongue can be used to maximum effect, massaging the milk from the breast and maintaining a vacuum rather than relying solely on the mother's milk ejection reflex. A poorly attached baby may have difficulty in obtaining enough fat to meet their calorific needs, resorting to very frequent feeds making the mother's breast sore. A well-attached baby can obtain all they require in a very short time.

Provided the baby is well attached, the length of the feed is thus determined by the **rate of milk transfer** from mother to baby. If milk transfer occurs at a high rate, feeds will be relatively short; if it occurs slowly, feeds will be longer (Woolridge et al. 1982). Milk transfer seems to be more efficient with feeds being shorter in a second lactation than in a first (Ingram et al. 2001).

Fats and fatty acids

For the human baby, with its unique and rapidly growing brain, fat, not protein, in human milk has particular significance. Some 98% of the lipid in human milk is in the form of triglycerides. Of particular importance are the long chain polyunsaturated fats (LC-PUFAs), because of their role in brain growth and myelination (Fernstrom 1999). Two of them, arachidonic acid (AA) and docosahexanoic acid (DHA) appear to play an important role in the development of the retina and visual cortex of the newborn. AA is required for development of the brain, nervous system and vascular tissue. Despite formula manufacturers attempting to incorporate these in new products, DHA levels in the brains of breastfed babies is high compared with those who are formula fed, therefore the stereo-specific addition in plant form appears ineffective.

High quantities of linoleic acid and linolenic acid are found in breastmilk. These long chain fatty acids are required for prostaglandin synthesis maturing the intestinal cells. They aid digestion, add to the anti-infective properties of breastmilk and are precursors to AA and DHA.

Fat also provides babies with >50% of their calorific requirements (Picciano 2001). Fat is digested and rapidly absorbed due to lingual and gastric lipases and because

TABLE 27.1 **Summary and Comparisons of the Components of Human Breastmilk and Formula Milk**

Nutrient	Human Milk	Formula Milk	Comment
Fats and fatty acids	• Rich in brain-building omega 3s, namely DHA and AA • Automatically adjusts to infant's needs • Levels decline as baby gets older • Rich in cholesterol • Nearly completely absorbed • Contains fat-digesting enzyme, lipase	• No DHA • Does not adjust to infant's needs • No cholesterol • Not completely absorbed • No lipase	Fat is the most important nutrient in breastmilk. The absence of cholesterol and DHA (vital nutrients for growing brains and bodies), may predispose a child to adult heart and central nervous system diseases. Waste and unabsorbed fat accounts for unpleasant smelling stools in formula-fed babies
Carbohydrates	• Rich in lactose • Rich in oligosaccharides, which promote intestinal health	• No lactose in some formulae • Deficient in oligosaccharides	Lactose is considered an important carbohydrate for brain development
Protein	• Soft, easily-digestible whey • More completely absorbed; higher in the milk of mothers who give birth to preterm infants • Lactoferrin for intestinal health • Lysozyme, an antimicrobial rich in brain and body building protein components • Rich in growth factors • Contains sleep-inducing proteins	• Harder to digest non-human whey and casein curds • Not completely absorbed, more waste, harder on kidneys • No or only a trace of lactoferrin • No lysozyme • Deficient or low in some brain- and body-building proteins • Deficient in growth factors • Does not contain as many sleep-inducing proteins	Human infants are **not** allergic to human milk protein
Vitamins and minerals	• Better absorbed, especially iron, zinc and calcium • 50–75% iron is absorbed • Contains more selenium (an antioxidant)	• Not absorbed as well • 5–10% iron is absorbed • Contains less selenium (an antioxidant)	A greater percentage of vitamins and minerals in breastmilk are absorbed, i.e. enjoy a higher bioavailability. To compensate, more vitamins and minerals are added to formulae, which makes it harder for the baby to digest

TABLE 27.1 Summary and Comparisons of the Components of Human Breastmilk and Formula Milk—cont'd

Nutrient	Human Milk	Formula Milk	Comment
Anti-infective factors	• Rich in living white blood cells (leucocytes): millions per feed • Rich in immunoglobulins M, A, D, G, E • Contains lactoferrin and bifidus factor	• No live white blood cells – or any other cells • Dead food has less immunological benefit • Few immunoglobulins (bovine)	When the mother is exposed to an infection, antibodies are made in response that are transferred to the baby via her breastmilk
Enzymes and hormones	• Rich in digestive enzymes, such as lipase and amylase • Rich in many hormones, e.g. thyroid, prolactin, oxytocin • Epidermal growth factor and insulin growth factor increases maturity of baby's digestive system and reduces susceptibility to infection • Varies with mother's diet	• Processing destroys digestive enzymes • Processing destroys (bovine) hormones • Always tastes the same	Digestive enzymes promote intestinal health. Hormones contribute to the overall biochemical balance and wellbeing of the baby. By taking on the flavour of the mother's diet, breastmilk shapes the tastes of the child to family foods

the uniquely human milk enzyme bile-salt-stimulated *lipase*, activates once it reaches the baby's intestine. Pancreatic lipase is not plentiful in the newborn, so a baby who is not fed human milk is less able to digest fat.

Cholesterol, a risk factor for coronary heart disease (CHD) in adults, occurs in human milk at higher levels than are currently present in infant formulae (Kamelska et al. 2012). These high levels play an important role in brain growth and development (Scholtz et al. 2013), but paradoxically lower the blood cholesterol concentration in later life (Owen et al. 2008).

Carbohydrate

The main carbohydrate component of human milk is *lactose*: a disaccharide, providing the baby with about 40% of its calorific requirements. Lactose is converted into *galactose* and glucose by the action of the enzyme *lactase* for rapid breakdown and absorption requiring frequent breastfeeding. This ensures a regular energy supply to the rapidly growing brain. Lactose accelerates gut transit time of meconium through the intestine, enhances the absorption of calcium and promotes the growth of *lactobacillus bifidus* ('friendly bacteria'), which increases intestinal acidity, thus reducing the growth of

pathogenic organisms in the baby. Lactase in the intestinal brush borders from 24 weeks' gestation supports the active breakdown of lactose.

Oligosaccharides prevent the binding of Gram-negative bacteria to the intestinal brush border by offering another binding site acting as a probiotic.

Protein

Colostrum contains *pancreatic secretory trypsin inhibitor* (PSTI) in a seven-fold concentration compared with mature milk, protecting the gastrointestinal tract from damage and apoptosis (Marchbank et al. 2009). Human milk contains less protein than any other mammalian milk, which accounts in part for its more transparent appearance. Human milk is whey-dominant, mainly *α-lactalbumin*, which forms soft, flocculent curds when acidified in the stomach and has the capacity with oleic acid to induce cell death in tumour cells, but not healthy cells (**HAMLET** = **H**uman **A**lpha-lactalbumin **M**ade **LE**thal to **T**umour cells). The proportion of whey to casein protein changes in breastmilk in synchrony with infant development: 90:10 in early lactation, 60:40 in mature lactation and 50:50 in late lactation; a variation not possible in formula milk.

Allergies occur less frequently in breastfed babies than in those fed with formula milk for two main reasons:

1. The infant's intestinal mucosa is permeable to proteins before the age of 6–9 months, which in a human milk-fed baby is protected by the acidity in the intestine, IgA and lactose which supports a rapid gut transit time.
2. Proteins in cow's milk can act as allergens. In particular, *bovine β-lactoglobulin,* which has no human milk protein counterpart, is capable of producing antigenic responses in atopic infants (Brostoff and Gamlin 2008).

Occasionally, a baby may react adversely to substances in their mother's milk that come from her diet. However, this is very rare and can usually be resolved by the mother identifying and avoiding the foods that cause the adverse reaction and can then continue to breastfeed. Another bovine whey protein, *bovine serum albumin,* has been implicated as the trigger for the development of insulin-dependent diabetes mellitus (Paronen et al. 2000; Horta et al. 2015). Human insulin released in breastmilk supports gut maturation and serum glucose balance in the infant.

High concentrations of *taurine* are found in human milk, which is required for the conjugation of bile salts and fat absorption in the first week of life. It is also essential for the myelination of the nervous system.

Vitamins

All the vitamins required for good nutrition and health are supplied in breastmilk without overload, and although the actual amounts vary from mother to mother, none of the normal variations poses any risk to the infant (Hopkinson 2007). Larger proportions are present in formula milk, however their bioavailability is unclear and the concentrations vary depending on the longevity of the remaining shelf-life.

Fat-soluble vitamins: A, D, E and K

Vitamin A. Vitamin A is present in human milk *as retinol, retinyl esters* and *beta carotene.* Colostrum contains twice the amount present in mature human milk, giving colostrum its yellow colour and supporting developing eye acuity in the infant. Bile-salt-stimulated lipase (present in human milk) assists the hydrolysation of the retinyl esters and may account for the rarity of vitamin A deficiency in breastfed babies in high-income countries (Leaf 2007).

Vitamin D. Vitamin D plays an essential role in the metabolism of calcium and phosphorus in the body, preventing osteomalacia in adults and rickets in children. It is not strictly a vitamin, but a hormone triggered by ultraviolet light. Naturally occurring dietary sources of vitamin D are fish liver oils, butter, eggs and cheese with some foods such as margarine being fortified with Vitamin D. Vitamin D is the name given to two fat-soluble compounds: *calciferol* (vitamin D_2) and *cholecalciferol* (vitamin D_3). The latter is generated through exposure to sufficient ultraviolet light (≤30 min of summer sunlight a day) on human skin.

For light-skinned babies, *safe* exposure to sunlight for short periods will help to keep vitamin D requirements within the lower limits of the normal range. However, latitude and strength of the sunlight is important. Those living in regions where exposure to the sun is low have always been at risk for vitamin D deficiency as Moan et al. (2008) found in Scandinavia, where photo-conversion of 7-dehydrocholesterol occurred only between March and October, with a maximum in June and July. In the UK, researchers in Aberdeen discovered that sunlight exposure in summer and spring provided 80% of the baby's total annual intake of vitamin D (Macdonald et al. 2011). Social mobility, cultural considerations and concerns over skin cancer from sunlight have increased the risk of vitamin D deficiency by reducing the skin's exposure to sunlight. In the UK, this is of particular concern in women and infants of Asian and Afro-Caribbean ethnic origin (National Institute for Health and Care Excellence, NICE 2017). It is therefore a recommendation that *everyone* in the UK should take Vitamin D supplementation (Scientific Advisory Committee on Nutrition, SACN 2016).

Maternal vitamin D deficiency during pregnancy has been implicated as a risk factor for diabetes, ischaemic heart disease and tuberculosis. In addition to the previously known paediatric problems of hypocalcaemic convulsions, dental enamel hypoplasia, infantile rickets and congenital cataracts in early life, vitamin D deficiency has been shown to affect neonatal head and linear growth and may adversely affect the developing fetal brain (Shaw and Pal 2002).

NICE (2017) recommend women take vitamin D supplements of 10 µg/day during pregnancy and while breastfeeding, as the concentration of vitamin D in human milk is low. As a precaution, breastfed babies from birth up to 1 year of age should also be given a supplement of 8.5–10 µg/day (340–400 IU) of vitamin D per day (NICE 2016, 2017; SACN 2018).

Babies who are formula fed do not require vitamin D if they are having 500 mL/day of infant formula or more, as infant formula already has added vitamin D, unless the baby is considered to be at risk (NICE 2016, 2017; SACN 2018).

Vitamin E. Although vitamin E is present in human milk, its role is uncertain. It appears to prevent the oxidization of polyunsaturated fatty acids and may prevent certain types of anaemia to which preterm infants are susceptible.

Vitamin K. Vitamin K is the generic name for a group of structurally similar, fat-soluble vitamins. The two naturally occurring forms of this vitamin are vitamin K1 (*phytonadione*) found in green leafy vegetables, and K2 (*menaquinone*), which is synthesized by gut flora. By 2 weeks of age, the breastfed baby's gut flora should be synthesizing adequate amounts of vitamin K2.

Vitamin K is essential for the synthesis of blood-clotting factors II, VII, IX and X. It is present in human milk and absorbed efficiently. Because it is fat-soluble, it is present in greater concentrations in colostrum and in the high-fat *hindmilk* (Kries et al. 1987). The increased volume of milk as lactation progresses means that the baby obtains twice as much vitamin K from mature milk (3 days onwards) than from colostrum (Canfield et al. 1991).

Vitamin K deficiency bleeding (VKDB), formerly called '*haemorrhagic disease of the newborn*' (HDN), is a coagulation disturbance in newborns due to vitamin K deficiency. The incidence of classic VKDB, occurring between 1 and 7 days of life, ranges from 0.25 to 1.7 cases per 100 births (see Chapter 37). However, those instances where VKDB occurs in the first 24 h of life are largely confined to the babies of mothers who were taking medications such as isoniazid, rifampicin, anti-coagulants and anticonvulsant agents in pregnancy. Late VKDB occurs between 2 weeks and 6 months of life with an incidence of 4.4 to 7.2 per 100,000 and occurs predominantly in exclusively breastfed babies as vitamin K is added to infant formula milks, but may also occur in any baby who is unable to absorb the fat-soluble vitamin K (see Chapter 35).

There has been much debate over which babies are more susceptible to developing VKDB, and if supplements should be given after birth and how these should be given. As VKDB is a potentially fatal condition, prophylactic administration of vitamin K is recommended for *all* babies and is routinely administered to all preterm and ill babies as part of their treatment regime (Blackburn 2018). NICE (2015) recommend that vitamin K_1 1 mg given intramuscularly after birth to all healthy term babies is the most effective prophylaxis for prevention of early onset VKDB. Some vitamin K_1 remains within the muscle and acts as a slow release depot, providing prophylaxis for classic and probably also for late VKDB (Hey 2003).

For healthy term babies whose parents decline a single intramuscular injection of vitamin K_1, an oral prophylaxis regimen is recommended (NICE 2015), although there is not a consensus on the most effective oral regime. If vitamin K_1 is administered orally, multiple doses are required in the first week of life and if the baby is breastfed, a further dosing regime is required until at least 12 weeks of age, if not longer. Medical advice should be sought if the baby vomits within 1 h of oral administration or is too unwell to take the preparation orally.

Water-soluble vitamins: B complex and C. Unless the mother's diet is seriously deficient, breastmilk will contain adequate levels of the water-soluble vitamins, B and C. Since they are generally widely distributed in foods (vitamin C is found in most fruit and vegetables), a diet significantly deficient in one vitamin will be deficient in others as well. Thus, an improved diet will be more beneficial than artificial supplements. Water-soluble vitamins are actively transported across the placenta throughout pregnancy.

Vitamin B complex. Vitamin B complex consists of eight water-soluble vitamins: *thiamine* (B1), *riboflavin* (B2), *niacin* (B3), *pantothenic acid* (B5), *pyridoxine* (B6), *biotin* (B7), *folic acid* (B9) and *cyanocobalamin* (B12). All play an important role in metabolism in the body and stabilizing the nervous system.

Vitamin C. Vitamin C (*L-ascorbic acid*) is an antioxidant that helps protect cells from free radical damage. It is necessary to form collagen, and thus plays a role in growth and repair of bone, skin and connective tissue. It also assists the body to absorb iron. With some vitamins, e.g. vitamin C and thiamine, a plateau may be reached where increased maternal intake has no further impact on breastmilk.

Minerals and trace elements

Iron. Healthy term babies are usually born with high fetal haemoglobin levels (16–22 g/dL), which decreases rapidly after birth, albeit if delayed cord clamping of between 1–3 min following birth has been practised at birth, the incidence of neonatal anaemia is reduced (WHO 2013). The iron recovered from haemoglobin breakdown is reutilized. Babies also have ample iron stores that are sufficient for at least 4–6 months. Although the amounts of iron are less in human milk, 70% is absorbed compared with 10% of that found in formula milks (Saarinen and Siimes 1979). The difference is due to a complex series of interactions taking place within the gut. The extra iron from formula milk in the babies gut has also been implicated in the growth of Gram-negative bacteria (Jaeggi et al. 2015). Babies receiving fresh cow's milk or formula may become anaemic because the cow's milk protein, especially if unmodified, can irritate the lining of the stomach and intestine, leading to loss of blood into the stools (Ziegler 2011).

Zinc. A deficiency of this essential trace mineral may result in the baby's failure to thrive and development of typical skin lesions. Breastfed babies maintain high plasma zinc values compared with formula-fed babies, even when the concentration of zinc is three times that of human milk (Khaghani et al. 2010), as zinc is actively transported from the maternal circulation to the mammary gland (Krebs 1999). Preterm babies may need zinc supplements.

Calcium. Calcium is more efficiently absorbed from human milk than from breastmilk substitutes because of the higher calcium: phosphorus ratio of human milk. Formula milks based on cow's milk inevitably have higher phosphorus content than human milk.

Other minerals. Human milk has significantly lower levels of calcium, phosphorus, sodium and potassium than formula milk. Copper, cobalt and selenium, however, are present at higher levels. The higher bioavailability of these minerals and trace elements ensures that the baby's needs are met while also imposing a lower solute load on the neonatal kidney than do breastmilk substitutes.

Anti-infective factors

Leucocytes. During the first 10 days following birth, there are more white cells/mL in breastmilk than in blood. The nonspecific macrophages and neutrophils are among the most common leucocytes in human milk protecting the infant through their phagocytic activity on harmful bacteria.

Immunoglobulins. Five types of immunoglobulin proteins have been identified in human milk: IgM, IgA, IgD, IgG and IgE (**MADGE**).

Immunoglobulin A (IgA). This is the most important of the immunoglobulins, which appears to be synthesized and stored in the breast. Although some IgA is absorbed by the baby, the majority is not. Instead, it coats the intestinal epithelium and protects the mucosal surfaces against entry of pathogenic bacteria and enteroviruses. It affords protection against: *Escherichia coli* (*E. coli*), *salmonellae*, *shigellae*, *streptococci*, *staphylococci*, *pneumococci*, *poliovirus* and the *rotaviruses*.

The mother's body also monitors and responds to pathogens in her infant's environment when they remain together via **GALT** (*gut-associated lymphoid tissue*); **BALT** (*bronchus-associated lymphoid tissue*); and **MALT** (*mucosa-associated lymphoid tissue*) or the entero-mammary, broncho-mammary or muco-mammary circulation. Pathogens that enter the mother's gastrointestinal or respiratory tract stimulate pre-committed lymphocytes in the Peyer's patches of the small intestine or in the bronchial submucosa. The activated Beta cells migrate via the blood to the mammary (and salivary) glands, where they become transformed into plasma cells that start secreting large quantities of the appropriate neutralizing antibody into the milk.

Immunoglobulin G (IgG). IgG transfers across the placenta and through breastmilk, therefore passive immunity will be maintained while the baby is being breastfed by its mother. Maintaining contact between mother and baby further enhances the specificity of antibody development by the mother.

Immunoglobulin E (IgE). This immunoglobulin is raised in the presence of an allergic reaction but is also found in small quantities in breastmilk for a longer period than in cow's milk (Sultana 2015). The implication of this is unclear.

Immunoglobulin M (IgM). This immunoglobulin is especially large and is one that the baby develops for itself via immunizations. It is known that a breastfed baby is able to increase the responsiveness to the immunization, based on the frequency and length of breastfeeding compared with a formula-feeding baby (Saso and Kampmann 2017).

Immunoglobulin D (IgD). IgD acts to combat disease without causing inflammation (Sultana 2015).

Lysozyme. Lysozyme destroys bacteria by disrupting their cell walls. The concentration of lysozyme increases with prolonged lactation (Montagne et al. 2001).

Lactoferrin. Lactoferrin is a protein that binds to enteric iron for absorption by the baby, thus preventing potentially pathogenic *E. coli* from obtaining the iron they need for survival. There are seven times the levels of lactoferrin in colostrum than in mature milk and it can be found in many externally facing surfaces such as mucosal, respiratory and gut. It has antiviral activity against human immunodeficiency virus (HIV), cytomegalovirus (CMV) and herpes simplex virus (HSV), by interfering with virus absorption or penetration (Liu and Newburg 2013).

Bifidus factor. Bifidus factor in human milk promotes the growth of Gram-positive bacilli ('friendly bacteria') in the gut flora, particularly *Lactobacillus bifidus*, which discourages the multiplication of Gram-negative pathogens. Babies fed on cow's-milk-based formulae, however, have more potentially pathogenic bacilli present in the flora of their gut. If a breastfed baby is given one supplementary formula feed, they will produce *a formula feeding microbiome* within 24 h, which can take between 2 and 4 weeks to be reversed once the baby is exclusively breastfed again; consequently compromising the baby in the short and long term (Walker 2016).

Hormones and growth factors. Epidermal growth factor and insulin-like growth factor stimulate the baby's digestive tract to mature more quickly and strengthen the barrier properties of the gastrointestinal epithelium. Once the initially leaky membrane lining of the gut matures, it is less likely to allow the passage of large molecules, and becomes less vulnerable to microorganisms. The earlier the first breastfeed takes place after birth the greater the reduction in gut permeability.

THE BABY FRIENDLY INITIATIVE

As an international child rights organization, UNICEF has always had the interests of children at its heart in everything it does, based on the United Nations (UN) Convention on the Rights of the Child (UNCRC). Whenever decisions are made about children throughout the world, they must always be based on what is best for the child and not what is convenient for national governments, organizations or individual adults. As a consequence, the overarching principle of the WHO/UNICEF UK Baby Friendly Initiative (BFI) is based on the UNCRC such that every standard must have the best interests of babies at its core (UNICEF-UK 1990; UN 2016).

The WHO/UNICEF UK Baby Friendly Hospital Initiative (BFHI) is a globally recognized programme that

---

BOX 27.1 International Ten Steps to Successful Breastfeeding

1. Have a written breastfeeding policy that is routinely communicated to all healthcare staff.
2. Train all healthcare staff in the skills necessary to implement this policy.
3. Inform all pregnant women about the benefits and management of breastfeeding.
4. Help mothers initiate breastfeeding soon after birth.
5. Show mothers how to breastfeed and how to maintain lactation even if they should be separated from their infants.
6. Give newborn infants no food or drink other than breastmilk, unless *medically* indicated.
7. Practice rooming in: allow mothers and infants to remain together 24 hours a day.
8. Encourage breastfeeding on demand.
9. Give no artificial teats or dummies to breastfeeding infants.
10. Foster the establishment of breastfeeding support groups and refer mothers to them on discharge from hospital or clinic.

WHO/UNICEF (1989). Joint statement – protecting, promoting and supporting breastfeeding: the role of maternity services. Geneva: WHO.

---

forms a key part of the *WHO Global Strategy on Infant and Young Child Feeding* (WHO/UNICEF 2003). It was launched worldwide in 1991 (and in the UK in 1994) following the adoption of the *Innocenti Declaration on the Protection, Promotion and Support of Breastfeeding* in 1990, to encourage healthcare organizations to promote practices supportive of breastfeeding. At that time, the initiation and continuation rates of breastfeeding were low and this initiative provided the evidence to support women to breastfeed their babies. This meant educating healthcare professionals on BFHI principles as well as implementing evidenced-based infant feeding practices that were underpinned by the minimum standards.

The World Health Organization: Ten Steps to Successful Breastfeeding

The BFHI was focused around the 10 steps to successful breastfeeding (Box 27.1), with which all organizations who wish to achieve Baby Friendly status must comply (WHO/UNICEF 1989). This has subsequently been extended to community-based facilities, neonatal units and university education programmes for midwifery and health visiting (specialist community public health nursing, SCPHN), all of which can be BFI-accredited in their own right. In addition, all accredited Baby Friendly facilities must fully implement the *International Code of Marketing of Breast-milk Substitutes* (WHO 1981). By 2019, 64% of all UK maternity services and 68% of health visiting services were fully accredited as Baby Friendly organizations, with 91% of all maternity services and 89% health visiting services being at some stage of the accreditation process (UNICEF-UK 2019a). Similarly, 43% of midwifery education programmes and 17% of SCPHN programmes have achieved BFI accreditation for universities, with 74% of midwifery programmes and 20% of SCPHN programmes being at some stage of the process (UNICEF-UK 2019a).

In the UK, BFI has become recognized as the minimum standard by government and policy-makers across the four countries, such that all maternity care providers should implement an externally evaluated, structured programme encouraging breastfeeding. Consequently, areas of good practice have now become common practice in many maternity care settings, e.g. skin-to-skin contact, rooming in (Waldenström and Swensen 1991), exclusive breastfeeding, etc. The introduction of breastfeeding guardians/champions in strategic positions of organizations have supported greater implementation and sustainability of the standards and with the development of an All Party Parliamentary Group on Infant Feeding and a new focus on corporate social responsibility to increase breastfeeding acceptability, it is anticipated that breastfeeding rates will continue to improve in subsequent years.

The last *Infant Feeding Survey* in the UK was conducted a decade ago, in 2010 by McAndrew et al. (2012), and revealed an increase in breastfeeding initiation at birth from 76% in 2005 to 81% in the subsequent 5 years. Exclusive breastfeeding however, had fallen to 24% by 6 weeks in England compared with 17% in Wales and 13% in Northern Ireland in the same period. Despite there being a rise from 25% to 34% of any breastfeeding at 6 months, exclusive breastfeeding (as recommended by the WHO) remained at 1%. A later survey conducted in Scotland revealed a marked improvement in breastfeeding rates, notably the increase in breastfeeding at 6 months from 32% in 2010 to 43% by 2017. These results highlight the positive impact of national infant feeding strategy that incorporates 100% maternity and

community services in Scotland achieving BFHI accreditation (NHS Scotland 2018).

Further evidence has emerged over the past couple of decades, with an increasing understanding of how mothers can effectively be supported to recognize and respond to their baby's cues and form a close and lasting relationship. Such evidence focuses on early brain development, emotional attachment and positive parenting interactions and highlights the importance of early care practices and a broader approach to the BFI resulting in better outcomes for all children (Del Bono and Rabe 2012). UNICEF-UK implemented new enhanced Baby Friendly standards in 2012, based on a universal multifaceted approach (Box 27.2) involving maternity, neonatal, health visiting and children's centres services, with the overall aim of enabling every mother to get breastfeeding off to a good start and build a close and loving relationship with her baby (UNICEF-UK 2017).

Exclusive Breastfeeding for the First 6 Months of Life

Human milk is species-specific. In 2003, the *Global Strategy for Infant and Young Child Feeding* called for all mothers to have access to skilled support to initiate and sustain exclusive breastfeeding for 6 months and ensure the timely introduction of adequate and safe complementary foods with continued breastfeeding up to 3 years and beyond (WHO 2003, 2018; UNICEF-UK/DH 2015a). Breastmilk is perfectly balanced to meet the nutritional demands of the newborn baby and is the ***only food*** required until 6 months of age. In order for mothers to establish and sustain exclusive breastfeeding for 6 months, WHO and UNICEF recommend the following practices:

- initiation of breastfeeding within the first hour of life
- exclusive breastfeeding – that is the infant only receives breastmilk without any additional food or drink, not even water
- reciprocal breastfeeding – that is as often as the baby or mother requires, day and night
- no use of bottles, teats or pacifiers.

In 2006, WHO published findings from a global multisited study, which plotted the growth pattern of exclusively breastfed babies. This has revolutionized the expectation of growth velocity from the previous growth charts that were based on Caucasian, American formula-fed babies (WHO 1978). The plateau of growth at around 4–6 months, which had been a concern, was

BOX 27.2   The UNICEF-UK Enhanced Baby Friendly Standards 2012

Building a Firm Foundation

1. Have written policies and guidelines to support the standards.
2. Plan an education programme that will allow staff to implement the standards according to their role.
3. Have processes for implementing, auditing and evaluating the standards.
4. Ensure that there is no promotion of breastmilk substitutes, bottles, teats or dummies in any part of the facility or by any of the staff.

↓

An Educated Workforce

Educate staff to implement the standards according to their role and the service provided.

↓

Parent's Experiences of Maternity Services	**Parent's Experiences of Health Visiting/Public Health Nursing Services**
1. Support pregnant women to recognize the importance of breastfeeding and early relationships for the health and wellbeing of their baby.	1. Support pregnant women to recognize the importance of breastfeeding and early relationships for the health and wellbeing of their baby.
2. Support all mothers and babies to initiate a close relationship and feeding soon after birth.	2. Enable mothers to continue breastfeeding for as long as they wish.
3. Enable mothers to get breastfeeding off to a good start.	3. Support mothers to make informed decisions regarding the introduction of food or fluids other than breastmilk.
4. Support mothers to make informed decisions regarding the introduction of food or fluids other than breastmilk.	4. Support parents to have a close and loving relationship with their baby.
5. Support parents to have a close and loving relationship with their baby.	

Parent's Experiences of Neonatal Services	**Parent's Experiences of Children's Centres**
1. Support parents to have a close and loving relationship with their baby.	1. Support pregnant women to recognize the importance of early relationships for the health and wellbeing of their baby.
2. Enable babies to receive breastmilk and to breastfeed when possible.	2. Protect and support breastfeeding in all areas of the service.
3. Value parents as partners in care.	3. Support parents to have a close and loving relationship with their baby.

↓

Building on Good Practice

Embed all the standards to support excellent practice for mothers, babies and their families.

---

proven to be consistent with normal infant growth of *breastfeeding* babies. The recent introduction of the UK–WHO growth chart produced by the Royal College of Paediatrics and Child Health (RCPCH 2013: updated), combines WHO growth standards with UK preterm and term birth data and is used for all babies and children from 2 weeks to 4 years of age. This chart depicts a more representative healthy pattern of growth that is desirable for **all** children, whether breastfed or formula-fed (see Chapter 34).

In addition to the UNICEF-UK Baby Friendly Hospital Initiative (BFHI) standards being revised in 2012 (UNICEF-UK 2017) to reflect current knowledge and ensure they were fit for purpose, the *Ten steps to successful breastfeeding* (first introduced in 1989) were also updated in 2018 (WHO/UNICEF 2018) as shown in Fig. 27.4. These are both compliant with the *International Code of Marketing of Breast-milk Substitutes* (WHO 1981) and relevant World Health Assembly resolutions.

The following sections aim to place the *Ten Steps to Successful Breastfeeding* (WHO/UNICEF 1989, 2018) in context to assist the reader in understanding the relevance to their practice as midwives/healthcare professionals.

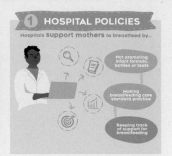
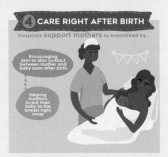
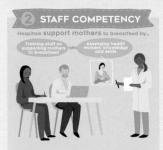
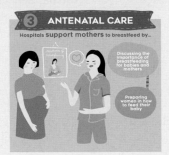
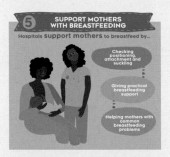
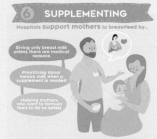
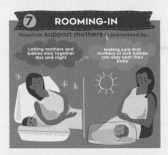
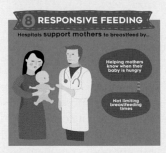
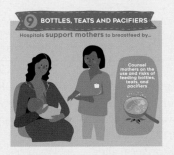
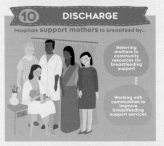
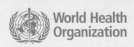
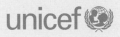

Fig. 27.4 The WHO/UNICEF Ten Steps to Successful Breastfeeding Poster. (Available at: www.who.int/nutrition/bfhi/bfhi-poster-A2.pdf)

BOX 27.3 The *International Code of Marketing of Breast-milk Substitutes*

Recommendations Include

- No advertising or promotion in hospitals, shops or to the general public (this includes posters, pens, calendars, EDB calculators and advertisements in mother-and-baby books).
- Not giving free samples of breastmilk substitutes to mothers.
- No free gifts relating to products within the scope of the Code to be given to mothers (including discount coupons or special offers).
- No financial or material gifts to health workers for the purpose of promoting products, nor free or subsidized supplies to hospitals or maternity wards.
- Information provided by manufacturers to health workers should include only scientific and factual material, and not create or imply a belief that formula feeding is equivalent or superior to breastfeeding.
- Health workers should encourage and protect breastfeeding.

World Health Organization. (1981) *International Code of Marketing of Breast-milk Substitutes.* Geneva: WHO. Available at: https://apps.who.int/iris/bitstream/handle/10665/40382/9241541601.pdf;jsessionid=C49C790D718A64FA8801A01D5B004337?sequence=1.

Midwives and the *International Code of Marketing of Breast-milk Substitutes* (BFI Step 1)

In 1981, the combined forces of WHO and UNICEF produced the *International Code of Marketing of Breast-milk Substitutes* (WHO 1981), which was adopted at the 34th World Health Assembly. The Code has major implications for the work of midwives as all staff need to be aware of and adhere to it, avoiding using documentation that promotes the use of breastmilk substitutes. Healthcare staff should always provide impartial information about breastmilk substitutes to parents as needed (NICE 2014). Although it is a voluntary Code in most countries, some countries now have the Code enshrined in law.

The Code as shown in Box 27.3, does not prevent mothers from feeding their babies with infant formula, but strengthens safe, adequate nutrition for babies and maintains, promotes and protects the supremacy of breastfeeding and breastmilk feeding (WHO 2007).

All maternity staff should be conversant with the infant feeding policies and practices within their employing organizations, which must be compliant with contemporary evidence and the *International Code of Marketing of Breast-milk Substitutes* in order to meet the requirements of UNICEF Baby Friendly status. The BFI standards require regular auditing from a quantitative and qualitative perspective, as the manner of support is just as important as the support mechanisms.

Facilitating Breastfeeding (BFI Step 2)

To be accredited as Baby Friendly, an organization, be it a maternity/neonatal service or an education provider, there should be a clearly defined infant feeding policy/education strategy that supports the UNICEF-UK BFI standards. All healthcare professionals who work in the maternity setting within hospital and community settings should be educated and trained to develop their knowledge, skills and professional values to facilitate optimal infant feeding based on the BFHI standards (Fallon et al. 2019; NICE 2014, 2015; UNICEF-UK 2016, 2017). A training programme for new staff and annual infant feeding updates provide the basis for sustaining an effective Baby Friendly service.

The BFI education standards (UNICEF-UK 2014) comprise five themes and 14 learning outcomes based on the BFI standards that must be incorporated into the curricula and successfully achieved by students at the point of registration as a midwife or SCPHN. This includes: the fundamental knowledge of the anatomy of the breast and physiology of lactation; the practical skills required to support mothers in feeding their babies; communication skills development; and an understanding of the psychosocial and political factors affecting successful breastfeeding. As a result, newly qualified midwives and SCPHNs are equipped with the essential knowledge and skills they need to support breastfeeding and relationship building effectively, which further supports sustaining an effective Baby Friendly service.

In 2019, UNICEF-UK introduced new infant feeding learning outcomes for healthcare students and trainees who are involved in the care of new babies, their mothers and families, namely medical, children's nursing, dietetic and pharmacy students as well as maternity support workers and nursery nurses (UNICEF-UK 2019b). The purpose of these learning outcomes is to provide a stimulus for universities to consider the inclusion of infant feeding content within a wider range of healthcare professional curricula and training programmes to help aid understanding and further improve practice and the subsequent health of babies and mothers. While these learning outcomes are an extension of the UNICEF-BFI university accredited programme for midwifery and SCPHN, there are no plans to provide full assessment and accreditation for these courses at the time of publication.

Infant Feeding Choices (BFI Step 3)

The subject of infant feeding should be part of an ongoing conversation that the woman has with her midwife as her pregnancy progresses. Providing information to women/family about the benefits of breastmilk and the breastfeeding process during the antenatal period has been shown to increase the initiation of breastfeeding by 10% (McAndrew et al. 2012).

During the antenatal period, time should be taken for the woman to get to know her baby by naming the 'bump' and sharing the baby's development with their family as well as discussing the management of early breastfeeding. The woman should be aware that:

- breastfeeding is a learned skill
- it should not hurt
- she does not need to be taught the major practical details of feeding until after the baby is born.

The midwife's responsibility to the woman is to ensure that her choice is fully informed, rather than to persuade her to breastfeed. This cannot be achieved if the midwife withholds information from her, based on BFI Standards and the *International Code of Marketing of Breast-milk Substitutes* (WHO 1981). The nutritional and immunological consequences of not breastfeeding are seen in population studies, and concerned with relative risks. It is not possible to narrow the risk down to the individual. Nevertheless, all pregnant women should be made aware that, compared with a fully breastfed baby, a baby fed on formula milk from birth is:

- five times more likely to be hospitalized with gastroenteritis (within the first 3 months of life)
- five times more likely to suffer from urine infections (within the first 6 months of life)
- twice as likely to suffer from chest infections (within the first 7 years of life)
- twice as likely to suffer from ear infections (within the 1st year of life)
- twice as likely to develop atopic disease where there is a family history

- up to 20 times more likely to develop necrotizing enterocolitis if born prematurely.

Additionally, the pregnant woman should know that she may increase her own risk of postnatal depression, premenopausal breast cancer, ovarian cancer and osteoporosis if she does not breastfeed (WHO 2018).

Although the greatest benefits are gained through exclusive breastfeeding up to 6 months and continued to 3 years (WHO 2018), the length of time a woman breastfeeds her baby should always be applauded. The many benefits of skin-to-skin care of the mother and baby at birth and beyond that may also include key family members, need to be stressed with all mothers irrespective of feeding intention. Skin-to-skin care stabilizes the baby's physiological parameters such as heart-rate, respiratory rate, metabolic rate, temperature and immunology (UNICEF-UK 2017). In addition, psychological adaptation to embedded neuronal pathways of the brain's limbic system in the mother and baby enhances their attachment/'bonding' (Cooijmans et al. 2017).

Observing a baby being breastfed can strongly influence the decision to breastfeed either positively or negatively, depending on the context (Brown 2016). This is of particular relevance for women for whom theoretical knowledge may have less influence than embodied knowledge (Dykes 2006). Peer group support can influence both initiation and continuation of breastfeeding (Pollard 2017) and introducing pregnant women to other mothers who are breastfeeding young babies may also be helpful. This is now facilitated in many 'Baby Cafés' throughout the UK.

Breasts and nipples are altered by pregnancy and sebum secretion obviates the need for cream to lubricate the nipple (see Chapter 10). Women who have inverted and non-protractile (flat) nipples often find that they improve spontaneously during pregnancy. The previous antenatal preparation of breasts and nipples (e.g. the wearing of Woolwich shells and Hoffman's exercises), have not been proven to be efficacious but may still perpetuate.

Initiating the First Feed (BFI Step 4)

The midwife's role in facilitating the initiation of the first few feeds is to:

- keep the mother and baby together (unless resuscitative measures are required for either the baby or mother) and ensure that feeding cues are understood
- ensure that the baby is adequately fed at the breast

- support the mother in developing the necessary practical skills and confidence to feed her baby by her chosen feeding method.

While babies are instinctively equipped to want to seek a feed, feeding is a learned and socially acquired skill for mothers (Brown 2016; Dixley 2014). Therefore all new mothers, but particularly those who have never experienced or witnessed breastfeeding before, require encouragement and reassurance (*emotional support*), advice and guidance on the fundamentals of effective attachment so that feeding is pain free (*practical support*), and factual information about breastfeeding (*informational support*) in small, manageable quantities. Some mothers will need more help and support than others, however, providing this from the start is good investment in the long term such that any remedial intervention is less likely to be required.

Many mothers who have already had babies may require as much support with breastfeeding as first-time mothers due to:

- previous unsuccessful breastfeeding
- breastfeeding may have previously gone well by chance rather than knowledge
- the new baby may behave very differently, or have different needs, from the mother's previous baby/babies
- the mother may have recently fed (or still be feeding) a toddler and has forgotten quite how much help a new baby requires to breastfeed
- their previous baby may have been born at a time when the underpinning information that was contemporary at that time, is now considered to be outdated.

A mother who chooses to formula feed her baby will also need sensitive and appropriate guidance on positioning and attachment to facilitate effective bottle-feeding using the same principles in a *classical* breastfeeding position. The *laid back* approach is not suitable when formula-feeding babies.

Observational studies have identified nine steps to the initiation of the first feed that enable babies to have uninterrupted skin-to-skin contact with their mother/parent (Widström et al. 2011; Brimdyr et al. 2017), as shown in Box 27.4.

The rest periods which are interspersed, are particularly important, as this is when the baby assimilates the information gathered from the reconnaissance it has undertaken. Further, if the nine steps are interrupted,

---

BOX 27.4 Nine Steps to Initiating the First Feed

During the first hour after birth, the baby goes through the following innate and instinctive stages. Observing the natural and instinctive behaviour during this time helps to eliminate possible iatrogenic effects from the test period.

1. The birth cry is a distinct and specific cry as the baby's lungs expand for the first time.
2. Relaxation is a time immediately after the birth cry ends, when the baby becomes still and has no visible movements.
3. Awakening begins as the baby opens their eyes for the first time, blinks, has small mouth movements and limited hand and shoulder motions.
4. Activity involves larger body movements, including whole arm motions, specific finger movements, shoulder motion, head lifting and stable open eyes.
5. Rest could happen at any point during the first hour, interspersed between stages or as a transition between stages.
6. Crawling involves the baby moving purposely toward the breast and nipple. It could be accomplished through sliding, leaping, bobbing or pushing (Fig. 27.5).
7. Familiarization is a stage at the mother's nipple where the baby licks, tastes, touches and moves around the nipple and areola area.
8. Suckling involves the baby self-attaching to the nipple and initiating breastfeeding.
9. Sleeping is an involuntary activity of the baby around 1.5–2 hours after birth.

Widström AM, Lilja G, Aaltomaa-Michalias P, et al. (2011) Newborn behaviour to locate the breast when skin-to-skin: a possible method for enabling early self-regulation. ACTA Paediatrica: Nurturing the Child 100(1): 79–85.

---

the baby has to recommence at the first step, therefore delaying its first breastfeed. Enabling this process has been demonstrated to approximately double maternal self-efficacy with breastfeeding (Aghdas et al. 2014). The length of skin-to-skin (Fig. 27.5) is also directly related to breastfeeding exclusivity on discharge from maternity care. A baby having more than 1 h of skin-to-skin is more than three times as likely to be breastfeeding exclusively on discharge from maternity care (Bramson et al. 2010).

The early work by (Widström et al. 1987; Righard and Alade 1990) demonstrated that separation had a greater effect on poor and delayed attachment to the breast

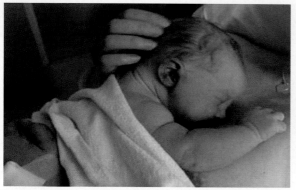

Fig. 27.5 Skin-to-skin post-birth in readiness for the first feed.

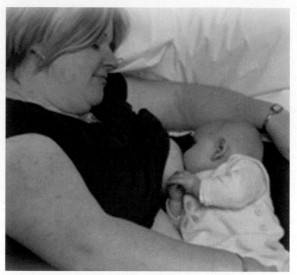

Fig. 27.6 Mother lying on her side.

than opiates. However, the impact of opiates cannot be ignored, as there are delays in feeding due to sleepiness leading to potential weight loss (Dewey et al. 2003). Fentanyl used in regional anaesthesia during labour doubles the difficulty in breastfeeding at day 1 and increases the chance of discontinuation of breastfeeding at 6 weeks from 2% to 17% (Beilin et al. 2005).

The impact of iatrogenic oxytocin during induction or augmentation of labour and the active management of the third stage of labour have demonstrated a negative effect on the breastfeeding competence of the baby and lactation efficacy in the mother (Cadwell and Brimdyr 2017).

Should a mother choose to formula-feed, the importance of skin-to-skin contact remains and should be facilitated. This may encourage the mother to give a first breastfeed, which should be praised and a future decision on feeding method be assessed at each feed.

Subsequent Feeds (BFI Steps 5, 7, 8, 10)

As part of the completion of the first feed, the cues that the baby exhibits for the next and subsequent feeds require reinforcing with the mother and family. These include:

- rapid eye movement
- stirring from sleep
- yawning
- rooting
- licking of lips
- sucking fingers
- making small noises and
- ultimately crying.

However, it is worth noting that crying is a sign the baby is distressed, which increases their adrenaline and

combined with the mother's subsequent delay in oxytocin release, is likely to create difficulty with feeding.

When facilitating a breastfeed, the midwife should use a *non-touch/hands-off* technique at all times unless the mother requests and gives consent to do otherwise (Spencer 2013; Weimers et al. 2006). This requires empathic communication and clear instructions (McIntyre 2013). Empowering women's self-efficacy enables successful breastfeeding continuation and good future problem-solving by the mother (DiGiroloma et al. 2008; Schmied et al. 2011).

There are presently two styles of supporting breastfeeding: the **classical** and **laid back** (Coulson 2012, 2019) approach. The principles in terms of attachment of the baby to the breast still apply, although the position of the baby to mother is different.

EFFECTIVE POSITIONING

Positioning of the Mother

A comfortable and sustainable position is a prerequisite of effective breastfeeding. A woman who has recently given birth, especially one new to breastfeeding, may need some help with this. Where the perineum is very painful of following a caesarean section, the mother may be more comfortable *lying on her side,* as shown in Fig. 27.6 or in the *'laid back'* positioning in the first few days after birth. It is likely that the mother will need assistance in placing the baby at the breast in a lying position.

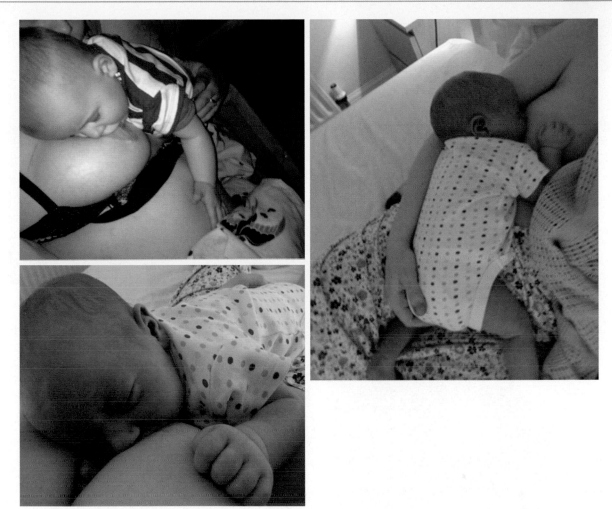

Fig. 27.7 Note the different alignment of the baby's body in relation to the mother in the 'laid back' breast-feeding position.

Alternatively, the *laid back* approach could have the mother lying on her back with the baby lying transversely or obliquely across the mother's abdomen as shown in Fig. 27.7. This approach requires the mother to sit in a chair that has a deep backward sloping seat, providing good support, and with her legs outstretched.

Alternatively, the mother may prefer to sit up to feed her baby (*'classical'* position) as in Fig. 27.8, with her back upright at a right-angle to her lap and her feet supported.

Positioning of the Baby

Whether using a classical or laid back approach the baby's body should be turned towards the mother's body (Fig. 27.9), so that the baby is coming up to her breast at the same angle as her breast is coming down to the baby.

The more the mother's breast points down, the more the baby needs to be on their back (Fig. 27.10) taking account of the *angle of the dangle*. The mantra *tummy to tummy* is not always helpful and should be discouraged, as the mother may be supporting the baby across her own body with her forearm (Fig. 27.11) or in an under-arm hold (Fig. 27.8). The baby's head and body need to be in line without a twisted neck. In a laid back position, the baby requires three points of contact to feel secure, therefore the feet, hands and body need to be stabilized.

If the baby's nose is opposite the mother's nipple, being brought to the breast with the neck slightly

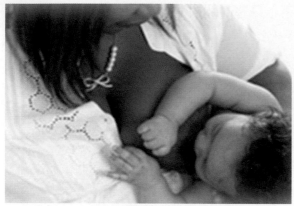

Fig. 27.8 The classical breastfeeding position. Mother feeding sitting up using an underarm hold.

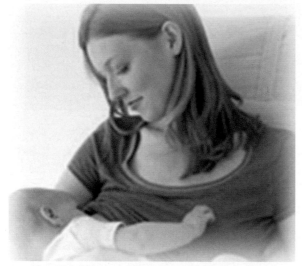

Fig. 27.9 Baby turned towards the mother's body.

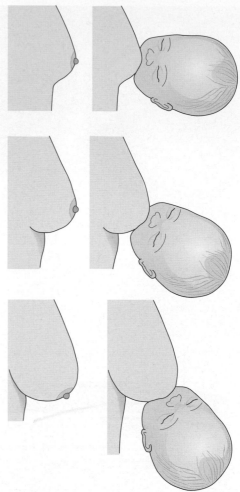

Fig. 27.10 Baby's body in relation to the mother's body, depending on the angle of the breast.

extended, the baby's mouth will be in the correct relationship to the nipple enabling easier swallowing (Fig. 27.12). The CHINS acronym is one way of remembering the principles, as shown in Box 27.5.

Attaching the Baby to the Breast

The baby should be supported across the shoulders, so that slight extension of the neck can be maintained with the head free to move as required by the baby.

Healthy term babies are equipped with a number of primitive reflexes that enable them to obtain the nourishment they require. At birth, all reflexes are of brainstem origin, with minimal cortical control. As the baby matures, higher, cortical pathways develop and

the reflexes disappear sequentially: rooting at about 4 months of age and tongue protrusion by about 6 months of age (Bagnall 2005).

If the newborn baby's mouth is moved gently against the mother's nipple, the baby will open the mouth wide. As the baby drops their lower jaw and darts the tongue down and forward, they should be moved quickly to the breast as shown in Fig. 27.13. The intention of the mother should be to aim the baby's bottom lip as far away from the base of the nipple as is possible, with the chin touching the breast. This allows the baby to draw breast tissue as well as the nipple into the mouth with the tongue, therefore leaving minimal areolar visible above the baby's top lip (Fig. 27.14) (Woolridge 1986; Monaci and Woolridge 2011).

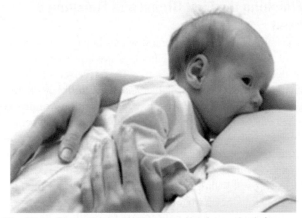

Fig. 27.11 The baby's head is supported by the mother's forearm.

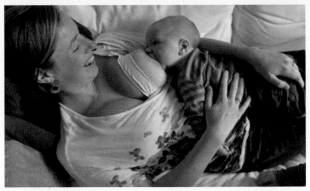

Fig. 27.13 A wide gape: the baby takes in a generous amount of the areola.

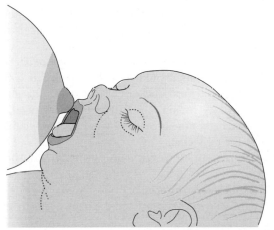

Fig. 27.12 The baby's mouth is opposite the nipple, the neck slightly extended.

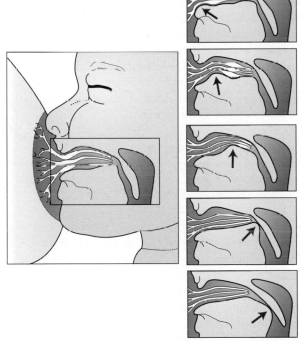

Fig. 27.14 The baby has formed a 'teat' from the breast and the nipple, which causes the nipple to extend back as far as the junction of the hard and soft palates. The lactiferous ducts are within the baby's mouth. A generous portion of areola is covered by the bottom lip. (Reproduced from Woolridge MW. (1986) The 'anatomy' of sucking. Midwifery 2: 164–71, with permission.)

BOX 27.5 Principles of Positioning the Baby at the Breast (UNICEF-UK)

- **C**lose
- **H**ead free to tilt
- **I**n line
- **N**ose to nipple
- **S**ustainability

The nipple should extend almost as far as the junction of the hard and soft palate. Contact with the hard palate triggers the sucking reflex. The baby's lower jaw moves up and down, following the action of the tongue. Although the mother may be startled by the physical sensation, she should not experience pain. If the baby is well attached, minimal suction is required to hold the breast within the oral cavity due to the buccal fat pads, large tongue to mouth ratio and strong *orbicularis aurous* muscles around the lips. The tongue can then apply rhythmical cycles of compression and relaxation so that milk is removed from the ducts. This view of the main mechanism a baby uses to remove milk from the breast was challenged (Geddes et al. 2008), but confirmed by further ultrasound studies (Monaci and Woolridge 2011). Although the tongue is used from time to time to generate increased suction pressure aiding milk removal, this is superimposed on the peristaltic action and does not occur in isolation (Monaci and Woolridge 2011). Milk transfers when breastfeeding occurs through the pulsatile effects of oxytocin, the creation of a vacuum and peristaltic action of the tongue to control the volume of each bolus swallowed. The baby may also spontaneously 'knead' the breast with their hands. The baby feeds from the breast, therefore the mother should guide her baby towards her breast without distorting its shape. The shape of the nipple should be the same before and following a feed.

FEEDING BEHAVIOUR

A breastfeeding baby typically performs one of three activities (Monaci and Woolridge 2011):
1. Rests
2. Stimulates the mother's nipple, without swallowing milk (*non-nutritive sucking/simply sucking*)
3. Sucks and swallows milk (*nutritive sucking including flutter sucking/swallowing*).

After an initial burst of nipple stimulation (short frequent sucking, two sucks per second), the baby begins swallowing – slow, deep, one suck per second (*nutritive*) sucking or 1–2 sucks per swallow – and feeds vigorously with few pauses. As the feed progresses, pausing occurs more frequently and lasts longer. Pausing is an integral part of all human's feeding rhythm and should not be interrupted. The midwife should simply encourage the mother to allow the baby to pace the feed. The change in the pattern generally relates to milk flow. *Flutter sucking* occurs at the end of the feed and appears like a '*jaw judder*', enabling the thicker fat rich milk to be transferred.

Finishing the First Breast and Finishing a Feed

The baby will release the breast when they have had sufficient milk from it. Their ability to know this may be controlled either by the calories they have received or by the change in the volume available. The baby should be offered the second breast after they have had the opportunity to expel any wind, which they will take according to appetite.

The baby should not be deliberately removed from the breast before they release it spontaneously, unless the mother is experiencing pain, in which case the baby should be re-attached, if still willing to feed. Taking the baby off the first breast before they have finished may cause three problems:
1. The baby will have volumes of foremilk and lactose, which can induce colic
2. The baby is deprived of the high calorie hindmilk that is slower to digest
3. If adequate milk removal has not taken place, milk stasis may occur, ultimately leading to the mother developing mastitis or experiencing reduced milk production, or both.

Provided that the baby starts each feed on alternate sides, both breasts should be used equally. If a baby does not release the breast or will not settle after a feed, the most likely reason is that they have not been correctly attached to the breast and was therefore unable to remove the milk efficiently.

Other reasons for babies withdrawing from the breast are:
• incorrect attachment
• the milk flow is very fast and the baby needs to let go and pause
• the baby has swallowed air with the generous flow of milk that occurs at the beginning of a feed and requires an opportunity to expel wind.

There is no justification for imposing either one breast per feed or alternatively both breasts per feed as a feeding regimen.

Timing and Frequency of Feeds

A healthy term *unmedicated* baby knows how often and for how long they need to be fed. This is known as **responsive feeding,** superseding the terms *reciprocal, baby-led and demand feeding* (UNICEF-UK 2016). This enables the mother to choose to feed her baby to fit her lifestyle and physiology as well as the baby to request attention from their mother as required. The individual mother–baby pair therefore develops their own unique pattern of feeding and nurture. Providing the baby is thriving and the mother is happy, there is no need to change it. Unmedicated mothers and babies may breast-feed up to 12 feeds in 24 h.

Mothers of medicated labours and births will need guidance to not leave their babies to sleep for prolonged periods (i.e. over 6 h) and ensure feeding cues are acted upon promptly. It is not unusual in the first day or so for the baby to feed infrequently, and have 6–8 h gaps between effective feeds, each of which may be quite long.

Volume of the Feed

Well-grown term babies are born with good glycogen reserves, high levels of antidiuretic hormone (ADH) and a stomach volume of 5–7 mL on day 1 and 22–38 mL by day 3. Consequently, babies do not need large volumes of milk or colostrum before they become available physiologically. In the first 24 h, the baby takes an average of 2 mL/kg per feed and by the second 24 h, this has increased to 4 mL/kg per feed (Santoro et al. 2010; Walker 2016). No precise information is available on the actual volume of breastmilk an individual baby requires in order to grow satisfactorily.

Weight loss and weight gain

Most newborn babies lose some weight during their first week of life. There is a general expectation that the baby will regain their birth weight by 10–14 days, however acceptable weight loss is disputed. Conventionally, 10% is often cited as the upper limit of normal, but there is little evidence to support a figure as high as this.

Monitoring milk transfer

A noticeable change in the baby's sucking/swallowing pattern is the most consistent sign of milk transfer. Soft but audible swallows may also be heard at the beginning of the feed. Most mothers are aware that their breast feels softer after the baby has fed well. A well-fed baby will release the breast spontaneously, appear satisfied and content.

Over the first 4 days of life, the breastfed baby should defecate twice every 24 h, with stools changing from the initial black meconium stool to the bright yellow, sweet smelling stool that is typical of a baby fed on breastmilk, by day 3. A stool that is still changing at 96 hours of life could indicate that further attention needs to be paid to the way the mother is feeding her baby. A formula-fed baby's stools would change at the same rate but would be pale yellow in colour and smell sour by day 3. Urine output should increase from one or more wet nappies per

day in the first day to about 6–8 by the end of the first week (i.e. the number of days born + 1 day). The urine is described as straw in colour. Pink staining in the urine/nappy is indicative of urates and is usually rectified by increasing the frequency of feeds.

An assessment of milk transfer should be made at each postnatal contact. This should ideally be done daily for the first week, to reduce the risk of babies losing an unacceptable amount of weight. An assessment tool, suitable for use by face-to-face or telephone contact, has been developed by UNICEF-UK (2018) for this purpose. Furthermore, introducing the mother to local infant feeding groups/networks is an essential part of community support to enhance successful lactation.

Difficulty with attachment is the commonest reason for babies failing to obtain enough milk and mothers developing painful nipples/breasts. If attachment is difficult, because the baby is sleepy, the breast tissue is inelastic or the mother and baby are separated due to illness, the mother should be encouraged to hand expression to establish lactation. If ineffective milk transfer continues, a full assessment of the baby and mother are required and active breastmilk expression either manually or mechanically should be facilitated.

Expressing Breastmilk

Although all women who choose to breastfeed their babies should know how to hand express milk, *routine* expression of the breasts should not be part of the normal management of lactation. This applies to mothers who have given birth by caesarean section, are diabetic or obese, despite these women being known to have delayed lactation (NICE 2014, 2015; Forster et al. 2017). It is essential that no limitation is placed on either feed *frequency* or *duration*, and the baby is attached effectively, for the volume of milk produced to be in accordance with the requirements of the baby. This should prevent the occurrence of problems such as breast engorgement requiring removal of milk by hand/pump.

Expression *is* appropriate in the following situations, if:

- there is concern about the interval between feeds in the early perinatal period (expressed colostrum should always be given in preference to formula milk to healthy term babies)
- there are difficulties in attaching the baby to the breast
- the baby is separated from the mother, due to prematurity or illness

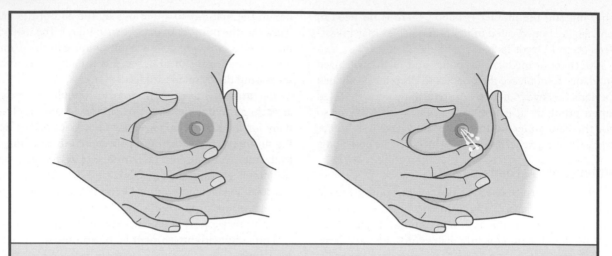

1. Wash hands and have a wide-necked sterile container ready.

2. Begin by gently massaging the breast.

3. Cup the breast with the thumb and finger in a 'C' shape about 2–3 cm back from the base of the nipple.

4. Gently squeeze, bringing the fingers and thumb together in a rhythmic action (if no milk appears after a few minutes, move the fingers a fraction forward or back to find the right spot.

5. Continue until no more milk drops appear (avoid sliding the fingers as this can cause damage to the breast).

6. Milk can be collected in a sterile cup or bottle (or drawn up into a syringe for colostrum).

7. When flow from one breast slows down, swap to the other side and repeat.

8. Breastmilk can be stored for up to 5 days in a fridge at 4° C or 6 months in a freezer.

Fig. 27.15 Hand expression.

- there is concern about the baby's rate of growth, or the mother's milk supply (expressing to top-up with the mother's own milk may be necessary in the short term, while the cause of the problem is resolved)
- the mother needs to be separated from her baby for periods (occasionally or regularly), as the baby gets older.

Prior to any breast expressing, the mother should be provided with a warm, private and non-interrupted space and have her chosen equipment for expressing. She will need to encourage the release of oxytocin, which can be achieved in a variety of ways: breast massage, having a photograph of the baby, a '*comforter*' smelling of the baby, having the baby close by or in skin-to-skin contact.

Manual expression of milk

Manual expression is flexible and can be undertaken easily anywhere and should be taught to all mothers, as it is often an easy solution to start with. It is usually the most efficient method of obtaining colostrum. Some mothers will find hand expressing superior to any breast pump (Fig. 27.15).

Expressing with a breast pump

If it is possible and practical, the mother should be able to experiment with a variety of breast pumps to discover what will suit her best, as not all pumps suit every woman.

Manually-operated pumps. Manually operated pumps are cheap to buy but most are not efficient enough to allow initiation of full lactation. However, they can be useful when expressing is required once lactation is established. It is helpful for midwives to explain to mothers that these pumps function most efficiently if the vacuum phase is considerably longer than the release phase.

Electrically-controlled pumps. Some electrically-controlled pumps provide a regular vacuum and

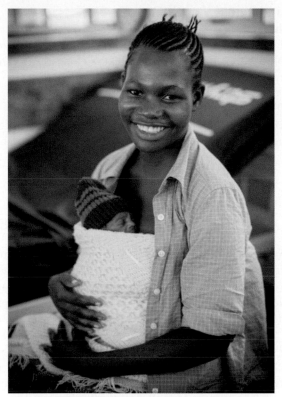

Fig. 27.16 Kangaroo mother care.

release cycle, with variability in the strength of the suction and others also vary the frequency of the cycle. The cup/funnel size should always be a good fit for the mother's breast. *Double pumping* is possible with most models, and this has repeatedly been shown to be of benefit, either reducing the time for which the mother needs to use the pump at each session to obtain the available milk or increasing the volume of milk obtained for term babies and preterm babies (Wambach and Riordan 2016).

How much and how often?

Mothers of preterm babies are encouraged to begin expressing milk by a pump as soon as possible after birth *at least* 8 times in 24 h, including once overnight to successfully sustain lactation at adequate levels compared with those who delay expressing or express less frequently (UNICEF 2017). Breast massage and *kangaroo mother care* (Fig. 27.16): holding the baby in skin-to-skin contact between the mother's breasts for prolonged periods of time have also been positively associated with enhanced milk production (Wambach and Riordan 2016).

No time limit should be set for the length of each expressing session. The mother should be guided by the *milk flow*, not the clock. Expressing should continue until milk flow slows, followed by a short break, and each breast should be expressed twice, either separately (*sequential pumping*) or together (*double pumping*). Switching encourages another surge of oxytocin. When milk flow slows for the second time, the session should end. Frequent expressing sessions are more likely to have the desired effect than lengthy, infrequent sessions.

Inadequate milk volume, followed by declining production, is a common problem for mothers who are expressing their milk for their preterm baby. In order to *prevent* this from happening, the midwife should discuss with the mother, the value of early initiation of expressing, the appropriate use and correct size of equipment and the importance of the frequency of expression, rather than trying to rescue failing lactation pharmacologically. It may also be helpful to show the mother how to express *hands free*, using an expressing brassiere to hold the breast shields securely in place (Fig. 27.17)

Storage of breastmilk

NICE (2014, 2015) advises that expressed milk can be stored for up to:

- 6 hours at room temperature
- 5 days in the main part of a fridge, at 4°C or lower
- 2 weeks in the freezer compartment of a refrigerator
- 6 months in a domestic freezer, at −18°C or lower.

CARE OF THE BREASTS

Daily washing is all that is necessary for breast hygiene. Brassieres may be worn in order to provide comfortable support and are useful if the breasts leak and breast pads (or breast shells) are used.

Breast Problems
Sore and damaged nipples

The cause is almost always trauma from the baby's mouth and tongue, which results from incorrect attachment of the baby to the breast. Correcting this will provide immediate relief from pain and allow rapid healing to take place. Epithelial growth factor, contained in fresh human milk and saliva, may aid this process.

Resting the nipple enables healing to take place but makes the continuation of lactation much more complicated because it is necessary to express the milk

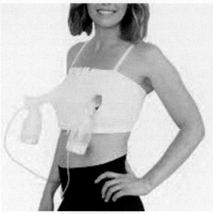

Fig. 27.17 Hands free expressing brassiere.

and to use some other means of feeding it to the baby (hand expression being less painful). Nipple shields should be used with caution, and never before the mother has begun to lactate, as the baby is unlikely to extract colostrum via a shield. They may make feeding less painful, but their use does not enable the mother to learn how to feed her baby correctly, and their longer-term use may result in reduced milk transfer from mother to baby. This in turn may result in mastitis in the mother as a consequence of reduced milk removal, slow weight gain or prolonged feeds in the baby due to reduced milk transfer, or both. If mothers choose to use them, they should be advised to seek help with learning to attach the baby comfortably without a nipple shield as soon as practicable (McKechnie and Eglash 2010).

Other causes of soreness

Infection with *Candida albicans* (thrush) can occur, although it is not common during the first week following the baby's birth. Sudden development of pain after a period of trouble-free feeding is suggestive of thrush. The nipple and areola are inflamed and shiny, and pain typically persists throughout the feed. The baby may show signs of oral or anal thrush. Both mother and baby should receive concurrent fungicidal treatment, such as miconazole, and it may take several days for the pain in the nipple to disappear.

Dermatitis

Sensitivity may develop to topical applications such as creams, ointments or sprays, including those used to treat thrush.

Anatomical Variations
Short nipples

Short nipples should not cause problems as the baby is able to receive stimulation to suckle so long as sufficient breast tissue is taken in by the baby.

Long nipples

Long nipples can lead to poor feeding because although the baby would be stimulated to suckle, they are unable to draw sufficient breast tissue into their mouth, due to the length of the nipple.

Abnormally large nipples

If the baby is small, their mouth may not be able to get beyond the nipple and onto the breast. Lactation can be initiated through expressing, by hand or by pump, provided the nipple fits into the breast shield. As the baby grows and the breast and nipple become more protractile, breastfeeding should become possible. Supporting the weight of the breast may be required.

Inverted and flat nipples

If the nipple is deeply inverted it may be necessary to initiate lactation by expressing and delay attempting to attach the baby to the breast until lactation is established, the breasts have become soft and the breast tissue more elastic. Many inverted nipples become everted with breastfeeding or nipple rolling which stimulates the erectile tissue in the nipple.

DIFFICULTIES WITH BREASTFEEDING
Engorgement

This condition occurs around the 3rd or 4th day following the baby's birth and venous engorgement. The breasts become hard, often oedematous, painful and sometimes appear flushed. The mother may be pyrexial. Engorgement is usually an indication that the baby is not keeping pace with the stage of lactation. Engorgement may occur if feeds are delayed or restricted or if the baby is unable to feed efficiently because they are not correctly attached to the breast.

Management should be aimed at enabling the baby to feed well (Box 27.6). In severe cases, the only solution will be the gentle use of a pump. This will reduce the tension in the breast and *will not* cause excessive milk production. The mother's fluid intake should not be restricted, as this has no effect on milk production.

BOX 27.6 Challenges of Attaching Babies to the Breast

Inelastic breast tissue, overfull or engorged breasts or deeply inverted nipples may present the baby with more of a challenge.

- If the breast is engorged, pushing away the oedema by gently manipulating the tissue that lies under the areola may be all that is required.
- Hand expression, or the use of a breast pump, may relieve fullness to the point where the baby can draw in the inner tissue to create the necessary teat from the breast.
- If attachment is still difficult, the mother should be asked to lie on her side with the short edge of a pillow under her ribs to raise the breast off the bed. The midwife may need to assist the baby in attaching.
- Using the *'laid back'* approach may enable the baby to self-attach. *Re-birthing* may also be an option to relax both mother and baby.
- If the baby is still unable to attach to the breast, the mother should be shown how to hand express and how to give her colostrum to her baby.
- It may also be necessary to show the mother how to use a breast pump (hand or electric). However, in the first 24–48 h, colostrum is usually best expressed by hand.

  When attachment is difficult, the priorities should be to ensure that the baby is adequately fed on their mother's milk, and to work on making the breast tissue more elastic (both of which can be facilitated by hand or electrical expressing). Attaching the baby to the breast directly can come later.

Deep Breast Pain

In most cases, deep breast pain responds to improvement in breastfeeding technique and is likely to be due to raised intraductal pressure caused by inefficient milk removal. Although it may occur during the feed, it typically occurs afterwards. This distinguishes it from the sensation of the *let-down reflex*, which some mothers experience as a fleeting pain before and during feeds. Very rarely, deep breast pain may be the result of ductal thrush infection.

Mastitis

In the majority of cases, mastitis, an inflammation of the breast, is the result of milk stasis, not infection, although infection may follow (NICE 2018). Typically, one or more adjacent lobes of breast tissue are inflamed through milk being forced into the connective tissue of the breast, and appear as wedge-shaped areas of redness and swelling. If milk is forced back into the bloodstream, the woman's pulse and temperature may rise and in some cases flu-like symptoms, including shivering attacks or rigors, may occur. The presence or absence of systemic symptoms does not help to distinguish infectious from noninfectious mastitis (WHO 2000; NICE 2018).

Noninfective (acute intramammary) mastitis

Noninfective (acute intramammary) mastitis results from milk stasis and may occur during the early days of breastfeeding as the result of unresolved engorgement or at any time due to poor feeding technique when milk from one or more segments of the breast is not being efficiently drained by the baby. It occurs much more frequently in the breast that is opposite the mother's dominant side for holding her baby (Inch and Fisher 1995). Pressure from fingers or clothing has been blamed for causing the condition, without any supporting evidence. It is essential that breastfeeding from the affected breast continues, otherwise milk stasis will increase further, providing ideal conditions for pathogenic bacteria to replicate. An infective condition could then arise, leading to abscess formation if left untreated.

Where supervision is available from the midwife, 12–24 h could elapse to ascertain whether the mastitis can be resolved by helping the mother to improve her feeding technique and encouraging her to allow the baby to complete the first breast initially. If supervision is not available or if there is no improvement during the 24-h period, antibiotics such as cephalexin, flucloxacillin or erythromycin should be given as prescribed (WHO 2000). However, Arroyo et al. (2010) demonstrated positive outcomes taking oral breastmilk lactobacilli.

Infective mastitis

The main cause of superficial breast infection is damage to the epithelium, allowing bacteria to enter the underlying tissues. The damage usually results from incorrect attachment of the baby to the breast, which has caused trauma to the nipple. The mother therefore requires urgent assistance to improve her feeding technique, as well as a 10–14 day course of appropriate antibiotics. Multiplication of bacteria may be enhanced by the use of breast pads or shells. In spite of antibiotic therapy, abscess formation may occur. Infection may also enter the breast via the milk ducts if milk stasis remains unresolved (WHO 2000).

Breast Abscess

A fluctuant swelling develops in a previously inflamed area: namely a *breast abscess*. Pus may be discharged from the nipple. Simple needle aspiration may be effective, or incision and drainage may be necessary (NICE 2018). It may not be possible for the baby to feed from the affected breast for a few days, however milk removal should continue by expression with breastfeeding recommencing as soon as practicable as this would reduce the chances of further abscess formation (WHO 2000). A sinus that drains milk may form, but it is likely to heal in time.

Blocked Ducts

Lumpy areas in the breast are not uncommon, due to distended glandular tissue. If such lumps become very firm and tender and sometimes flushed, they are often described as *blocked ducts*. This description carries with it the image of a physical obstruction within the lumen of the duct. However, this is very rarely the cause of the symptoms. It is much more likely that milk removal has been uneven due to suboptimal attachment and that secreted milk is trying to occupy more space than is actually available, causing the alveoli to distend. Milk may subsequently be forced out into the connective tissue of the breast where it causes inflammation. The inflammatory process narrows the lumen of the duct by exerting pressure on it from the outside as the tissue swells, resulting in *mastitis* or *incipient mastitis*. Consequently, the solution is to improve milk removal by effective attachment, or breastmilk expression, and to treat the accompanying pain and inflammation. Massage, often advocated to clear the imagined blockage, may make matters worse, as all it does is force more milk into the surrounding tissue.

White Spots/Epithelial Overgrowth

Very occasionally, a ductal opening in the tip of the nipple may become obstructed by epithelial overgrowth. A white blister is evident on the surface of the nipple, effectively causing a physical obstruction closing off the exit points from one or more milk-producing sections of the breast. This may sometimes be resolved by the baby feeding and massaging the breast simultaneously. Alternatively, after the baby has fed and the skin is softened, the blister may be removed with a clean fingernail or a rough flannel. True blockages of this sort tend to recur, but once the woman understands how to deal with them, the progression to mastitis can be avoided.

FEEDING DIFFICULTIES DUE TO THE BABY

Colic in the Breastfed Baby

Fig. 27.18 diagrammatically represents the causes and effects of secondary lactose intolerance – or *'colic'* – in the breastfed baby.

Although not all abdominal discomfort is due to poor attachment, symptoms of *colic* in a breastfed baby, such as abdominal discomfort, excessive flatus/wind, explosive stools, light green stools, may often be explained in terms of the foremilk/hindmilk mixture that the baby receives during the course of the feed/day.

If the baby is ***not*** well attached, they may not be able to access the fat-rich milk as the feed volume diminishes. Since it is the fat that provides most of the calories and, along with the slowing gastric emptying time, the poorly attached baby will feel hungry again sooner than they would be if they had been well attached. Only a change in attachment will break this cycle.

Over 24 h, the baby will have consumed a much greater volume of milk than they would have done if they had been better attached. *Since the concentration of lactose in milk is fairly constant*, the baby will have also received much more lactose than otherwise. This excess lactose in the gut may transitorily exceed the amount of the enzyme lactase that the baby's intestinal brush border is able to generate. The baby thus exhibits the signs of lactose intolerance/lactase deficiency. The accumulated undigested lactose creates an osmotic gradient that draws water into the bowel; added to which the bacteria in the baby's gut are provided with more substrate than usual, which they eagerly attack as an energy source producing large quantities of gas in the process (mostly carbon dioxide and methane). Distension of the gut by both fluid and gas produces pain (cramping) and looser stools. These are often green in colour due to the presence of bile that has not been reabsorbed. Depending on the extent of the lactase deficiency and the quantity of lactose ingested, symptoms can range from mild abdominal discomfort to severe dehydrating diarrhoea.

'Over the counter' *simethicone* and *lactase*, can be purchased, however there are no good quality trials demonstrating their effectiveness in alleviating the abdominal discomfort in breastfed babies. The simpler, safer solution is to improve attachment.

If a poorly attached baby can consume sufficient milk in each 24-h period to get the calories they require, they will grow, but they may have to feed very frequently to achieve this. Frequent feeds may in turn increase the mother's milk

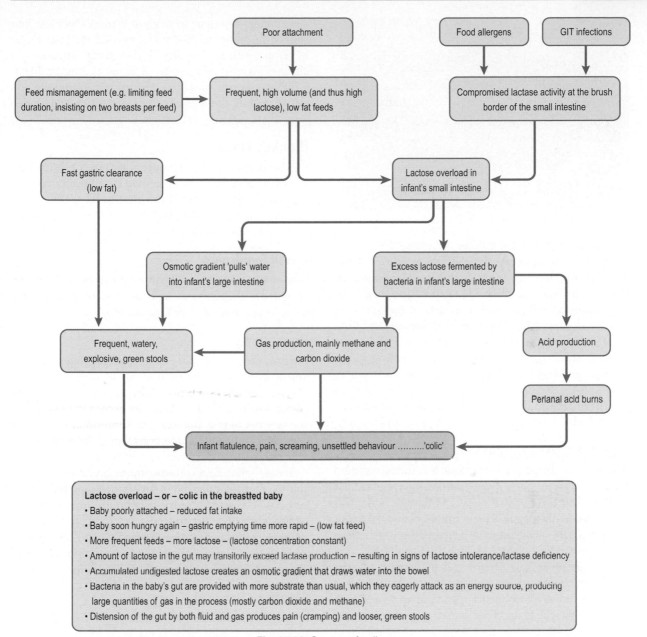

Fig. 27.18 Causes of colic.

supply, giving rise to the frustrating scenario of a mother with an abundant supply, yet a baby who is feeding *'round the clock'*. If the baby simply cannot hold enough milk, the situation above will be compounded by a baby who is not growing well according to their growth charts.

Cleft Lip

Provided that the palate is intact, the presence of a cleft in the lip should not interfere with breastfeeding because the vacuum that is necessary to enable the baby to attach to the breast is created between the tongue and the hard palate, not the breast and the lips (see Chapters 32 and 36).

Cleft Palate

The cleft in the roof of the baby's mouth prevents a vacuum or stimulation to suckle effectively from the breast and *milk is likely to exude from the nose*. There is no

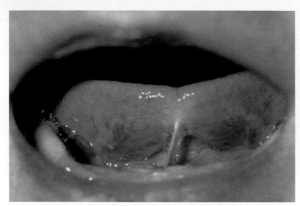

Fig. 27.19 Tongue-tie (ankyloglossia).

reason why the mother should be discouraged from putting the baby to the breast, for comfort, pleasure or food, provided that they are aware of the above and appreciate that it is likely that they will need to give their baby their expressed milk as well. A variety of measures are available to support feeding in infants thus affected until surgery can take place (around 6 months of age). Success with breastfeeding rather than breastmilk feeding will be reliant on good support (Cleft Lip and Palate Association, CLAPA 2015). Expressed breastmilk is still the best form of nutrition if the mother is able to maintain volumes and give to the baby using bespoke feeding teats and bottles.

Tongue Tie (Ankyloglossia)

If the baby cannot extend their tongue over their lower gum they are unlikely to be able to draw the breast deeply into their mouth to feed effectively (Brookes and Bowley 2014). This may be due to the tongue being short or because the frenulum, which is the membrane attaching the tongue to the floor of the mouth, is too tight or inflexible (see Chapter 32).

A significant tongue-tie can give the tongue a heart-shaped appearance, which is detrimental to breastfeeding and also considered to impact speech development (Fig. 27.19). The tongue is anchored preventing it from curling around the nipple and pushing it to the roof of the mouth to establish an adequate latch. As a result, the baby is unable in most instances to maintain an adequate latch, which prevents effective milk transfer and causes trauma to the nipple due to its misplacement and subsequent friction on the hard palate. In those cases where feeding is affected, a frenulotomy, recommended by NICE (2005), is offered which involves dividing the frenulum linguae and freeing the tongue.

Increasingly it is argued that more emphasis should be placed on tongue function rather than simply its appearance, as tongue movement is more complex than simply the ability to protrude it beyond the gum ridge. Many practitioners maintain that when attention to attachment does not resolve a breastfeeding problem, a full assessment should be carried out, observing any impairment of activities that require a functional tongue (Hazelbaker 2010).

Blocked Nose

Babies normally breathe through their noses. Obstruction causes great difficulty with feeding because they have to interrupt the process in order to breathe. Blockages caused by mucus may be relieved with a twist of damp cotton wool, or by instilling drops of normal saline before a feed.

Down Syndrome

Babies who have Down syndrome can be successfully breastfed, although extra help and encouragement may be necessary initially (see Chapter 36).

Prematurity

Preterm infants who have developed sucking and swallowing reflexes occurring around 28 weeks' gestation may successfully breastfeed, which is less tiring than taking a feed by bottle. However, if the reflexes are not strongly developed, the baby may tire before the feed is complete and complementary feeding by nasogastric tube may be necessary.

Babies who are too immature to breastfeed may be able to cup-feed, as an alternative to being tube-fed (Pollard 2017). Less mature babies who are unable to suck or swallow will be dependent on receiving nutrition via artificial methods such as tube-feeding and intravenous alimentation. The mother should be strongly advised and supported to provide expressed breastmilk for her infant.

Illness or Surgery

In general, babies recover quickly following illness or surgery, but if they have never been to the breast, or if feeding has been interrupted for a long period, the mother will require skilled help from the midwife to initiate or re-establish feeding.

COMPLEXITY AND BREASTFEEDING

Breastfeeding may have to be suspended temporarily following the administration of certain drugs, e.g. chloramphenicol, or following diagnostic techniques using radiopharmaceuticals. Most regions have drug centres and hospital pharmacy information services where advice may be sought about the safety of drugs for lactating women (see: https://www.breastfeedingnetwork.org.uk-drugs-factsheets). Temporary use of donor milk should be considered.

Carcinoma

If the mother has carcinoma, the cytotoxic treatment she receives will make it impossible to breastfeed without causing harm to the baby. However, if she wishes to, she could express and discard her milk for the duration of the treatment and resume breastfeeding later. If she has had a mastectomy, she may feed successfully from the other breast. The mother may also be able to breastfeed following a lumpectomy for carcinoma, but it is advisable to seek advice from her surgeon. Breastfeeding is known to protect against breast cancer in a dose-related manner (Gonzalez-Jimenez et al. 2013). Donor breastmilk should be offered as an alternative to formula milk.

Breast Surgery

Neither breast reduction nor augmentation is an inevitable contraindication to breastfeeding, but much depends on the techniques used. Where possible, advice should be sought from the surgeon. If the nipple has been displaced, the duct system may not be patent. If surgery is proposed for a woman who wishes to breastfeed in the future, it may be possible that the surgery can be altered to preserve the ductal system. The only method of assessing if the breast will function effectively is to support and encourage the baby to attach and feed at the breast.

Breast Injury

Injuries caused by scalding to the chest in childhood may cause such severe scarring that breastfeeding is impossible. Burns or other accidents may also cause serious damage.

One Breast Only

It is perfectly possible to feed a baby effectively using just one breast. If the mother has only one functioning breast, she should be reassured that each breast works independently of the other. If the baby is offered only one breast, that breast will make enough milk to feed the baby. There are documented cases of women feeding two babies with just one breast (Nicolls 1997).

Human Immunodeficiency Virus (HIV) Infection

Human immunodeficiency virus (HIV) may be transmitted in breastmilk. The current WHO recommendations on HIV and infant feeding stated that mothers living with HIV should breastfeed for at least 12 months and may continue breastfeeding for up to 24 months or longer (similar to the general population) while being fully supported for Antiretroviral Therapy (ART) adherence (WHO/UNICEF/UNAIDS 2016). This reflects the fact that there are areas in the world where the risks from formula feeding are higher than the risks to the infant from HIV transmission through breastmilk (Fawzy et al. 2011; Kafulafala et al. 2010). However guidance in the UK (British HIV Association, BHIVA 2019) remains that mothers known to be HIV-positive and regardless of ART, should be advised to exclusively formula-feed from birth. The differences in guidance make advising HIV-positive mothers and promoting breastfeeding problematic for midwives and healthcare professionals (see Chapter 15).

Cessation of Lactation
Suppression of lactation

If a mother chooses not to breastfeed, or if she has a late miscarriage or stillbirth, lactation will still commence. The woman may experience discomfort for a day or two, but if not stimulated, the breasts will naturally cease to produce milk. Very rarely, severe discomfort with engorgement occurs. Expressing small amounts of milk once or twice can afford great relief without interfering with the rapid regression of the condition. The mother will be more comfortable if her breasts are supported, but it is doubtful if binding the breasts contributes anything towards suppression (Swift and Janke 2003).

There is no basis on which to advise the mother to restrict her fluid intake or to seek a prescription for a diuretic, which will be equally ineffective as these measures merely add to the woman's discomfort by making her thirsty. Pharmacological suppression of lactation with dopamine receptor agonists such as bromocriptine and cabergoline is effective but is not recommended for routine use.

Discontinuation of breastfeeding

Discontinuing lactation abruptly once breastfeeding has become established may cause serious problems for the mother, leading to engorgement, mastitis or even a breast abscess. The mother should be encouraged to mimic normal weaning by expressing her breasts, reducing the frequency over several days or possibly weeks. The gradual reduction in the volume of milk removed from the breasts results in a corresponding diminution in the production of milk. Eventually, the woman should be encouraged to express only if she feels uncomfortable. Pharmacological suppression using cabergoline may be considered following the death of a baby.

Returning to work

If the breastfeeding mother returns to work, her baby will require feeding in her absence. If the mother wishes her baby to continue taking breastmilk, she will need to express her milk in advance. However, should the mother find it difficult to express her milk at work, her baby could receive a formula-feed (or *solid* food, if over 6 months), while she is away, but continue breastfeeding at all other times. *Pregnancy and maternity* is one of nine features known in law as a *protected characteristic* that is covered by the Equality Act (2010) and which should be applied in the workplace. This means that when a mother returns to work, the employer should provide an appropriate safe space, fridge and running water as a minimum for the mother to breastfeed or express breastmilk and store it somewhere cool to take home (Advisory Conciliation and Arbitration Service, ACAS 2017).

Weaning from the breast

When the mother or the baby decides to stop breastfeeding, feeds should be tailed off gradually. Breastfeeds may be omitted, one at a time, and spaced further apart. Adding supplementary foods should not begin until about 6 months of age (UNICEF-UK/DH 2015a). If the mother uses solid food to give the baby *tasters* and the experience of different textures before weaning, should be given *after* the breastfeed as the breastmilk is still providing the baby's nutritional requirements at this stage. Solid foods given to the baby before the breastfeed (weaning) will result in them taking less milk from the breast and less milk being produced. Allowing the baby to lead the process of weaning (Rapley 2012) may make the transition much easier. The different flavours experienced through breastmilk also supports an easier transition to tolerating solids.

Complementary and Supplementary Feeds (BFI Steps 6, 9)

Complementary feeds or *top-ups* are feeds given to the baby *after* a breastfeed. Complementary feeds of breastmilk substitutes (formula milk) should be given as a *last resort*, not

---

BOX 27.7 'Sleepy' Babies

*Provided that the baby is otherwise well, which will be determined by examining the baby from time to time, there is no evidence that long intervals between feeds have any adverse effect. As few as **three feeds** in the first 24 hours of life is within the normal range.*

Be wary of the mother and baby who have been exposed to opiates and/or iatrogenic oxytocin.

- The baby should remain close to the mother and/or skin-to-skin contact to enable an immediate response to her baby's feeding cues (UNICEF-UK 2017).
- The baby should be roused at intervals, possibly by changing the nappy, and being offered the breast.
- The mother should be shown how to hand express some colostrum, and how to give this to the baby.
- It is *unnecessary* to measure the baby's blood glucose levels (see Chapter 37).

---

as an alternative to helping the mother with breastfeeding or expressing milk. Exposure to non-human milk proteins has been implicated in the development of type 1 diabetes, eczema and wheeze/asthma (Renfrew et al. 2012). Even a single exposure can sensitize susceptible infants.

In the last *Infant Feeding Survey* in the UK, McAndrew et al. (2012) found that 31% of babies born in UK hospitals received breastmilk substitutes while in hospital. The mothers of these babies were three times more likely to have given up breastfeeding by the time their baby was a week old, in comparison with mothers whose babies received only breastmilk.

About 10% of newborns are at risk of hypoglycaemia (see Chapter 37), and may require a higher calorific intake in the immediate neonatal period than their mothers can provide. Where possible this should be the mother's expressed colostrum or human milk obtained from a human milk bank.

Babies who are well but sleepy (Box 27.7), jaundiced (see Chapter 37), unsettled (Box 27.8), or have difficulty attaching to the breast (Box 27.6), should be given their mother's own expressed milk if necessary, in addition to being offered the breast.

If complementary feeds are clinically indicated and the mother cannot express sufficiently, donor milk from a human milk bank could be used. Donors are serologically tested, as for blood donations.

If the baby is very young, additional feeds should be given by oral syringe, spoon or cup, rather than by bottle. An oral syringe (or dropper) will reduce wastage and

BOX 27.8 'Unsettled' Babies

An unsettled baby of any age who is crying again soon after they have been fed may not have been well attached or have colic.

- A full observation of a feed is necessary, to guide the mother.
- If the attachment is good, then the baby may be reacting to being removed from the closeness of the mother's body. If the mother needs to sleep, suggest that she feeds lying down and help her if necessary. However, it is imperative that the baby's safety is maintained should the feed take place in the bed. *Laid back positioning* may also be considered.
- The mother might try to express some colostrum/milk to give to the baby if she is concerned that the baby has not received all that they can from the breast.
- Some babies will appear unsettled even if they have fed well at the breast. The baby may be uncomfortable. The act of changing the nappy may help; so may wrapping the baby comfortably but securely and providing rhythmic motion, such as walking or holding the baby over the shoulder or over the forearm, both of which will enable any wind to be released and to settle the baby.
- Always facilitate confidence in the mother, by explaining appropriate coping strategies that she can learn and use.
- If *you* give the baby formula or a pacifier to settle them, that is what the mother will do when she goes home, therefore **neither** of these are recommended
- *Do not offer* to remove the baby. Separating mother and baby, particularly at night reduces breastfeeding success.
- If the mother *asks* you to, and you agree to take the baby away to settle, return the baby to her when they wake again to be fed.

BOX 27.9 Donated Breastmilk

If you are offering a mother donated human milk for her baby for any reason, she might find the information below helpful in deciding whether to accept it.

- All human milk donors meet the same criteria as blood donors; they are in a low risk group and give consent to an HIV blood test.
- All human milk donors sign a form to have their blood tested.
- Almost all donors are currently feeding their own baby while donating.
- No donated milk is used for any baby until the results of the donor's blood test have been received.
- All donated milk is collected in sterilized bottles, kept in the fridge and frozen within 24 hours of expression.
- When it arrives, still frozen, at the milk bank, the donated milk is thawed, a small sample taken for bacteriological screening and the rest is pasteurized.
- After pasteurization, another small sample is taken (for post-pasteurization bacteriological screening) and the rest is refrozen in a holding freezer.
- Only when the results of both samples have been received is the milk transferred to the freezer from which it can be used for preterm and term babies.
- Donors are not paid for the milk they donate: it is freely given!

the use of a cup would allow the baby to remain more in control of their intake. If the difficulty persists, for example with attachment, the mother may find it quicker and more efficient to give her expressed milk to the baby by bottle. There is no evidence that the baby will subsequently refuse the breast in these circumstances (Flint et al. 2016).

Supplementary feeds are feeds given **in place** of a breastfeed. There is no justification for their use except in exceptional circumstances, such as severe illness or unconsciousness. This is because each breastfeed that is missed by the baby interferes with the establishment of lactation and affects the mother's confidence in being able to successfully breastfeed her baby.

Human Milk Banking

Research has demonstrated the effectiveness of pasteurization as a means of destroying HIV (Eglin and Wilkinson 1987) and the importance of human milk in preventing necrotizing enterocolitis (NEC) (Chauchan et al. 2008). This resulted in the formation of the UK Association for Milk Banking (UKAMB) in 1998 and re-establishing human milk banks.

Banked human milk is used predominantly for preterm and ill babies. Occasionally, if there is sufficient, it is used for term babies whose mothers are temporarily unable to meet their babies' needs with their own expressed milk or due to illness and treatment regimes. Mothers who are offered donated milk for their babies must have sufficient information about the collection and screening of human milk to enable them to make an informed choice whether or not to accept it (Box 27.9).

FEEDING WITH FORMULA MILK

Most breastmilk substitutes (infant formulae) are modified cow's milk. The minimum and maximum permitted levels of named ingredients, and named prohibited ingredients in all cow's milk-based (and soya infant) formulae have to meet set legislation as defined by the *Infant Formula and Follow-on Formula Regulations* (Her Majesty's Government 2007). However, considerable variations in composition exist within the legally permitted ranges.

The two main components are *skimmed milk*, which is a by-product of butter manufacture, and *whey*, which is a by-product of cheese manufacture. Breastmilk substitutes may contain fats from any source, animal or vegetable, except from sesame and cotton, provided that they do not contain >8% trans isomers of fatty acids. The fat source may not always be apparent from reading the label: for example *oleo* is beef fat and would be unacceptable to Hindus and vegetarians, and *oils of vegetable origin* may have come from marine algae. Formula milks may also contain soya protein, maltodextrin, dried glucose syrup and gelatinized and precooked starch.

Types of Formula Milk

There are two main types of formula milk: *whey-dominant and casein-dominant.* Only *whey-dominant milks* (first milks) should be used for the first year of life. There is a comprehensive and quarterly updated report: '*Infant Milks in the UK*' produced by an independent charity, *First Steps Nutrition Trust* (see Useful Websites, below) that health professionals can access for contemporary information and advice.

Whey-dominant formulae

In these, a small amount of skimmed milk is combined with demineralized whey. The ratio of proteins in the formulae approximates to the ratio of whey to casein found in mature human milk (60:40). These feeds are more easily digested, emulating the feeding patterns of breastfed babies than the casein-dominant formulae, which slow gastric emptying times. Only whey-based formula milk should be given to a baby up to 12 months of age.

Casein-dominant formulae

These formulae are advertised for *hungrier* babies, and are **not** recommended for **all babies.** While the macronutrient proportions (fat, carbohydrate, protein, etc.) are the same as in whey-dominant formulae, more of the protein is in the form of casein (20:80). The higher casein content causes large, relatively indigestible curds to form in the baby's stomach, intending to make them *feel full* for longer. However, there is no evidence that babies settle better or sleep longer if given these milks.

Milks for babies intolerant of standard formulae

Predicting which babies will be prone to allergies is an inexact science. It is estimated that the likelihood of a baby being predisposed to allergy is about 20–35% if one parent is affected, 40–60% if both parents are affected and 50–70% if both parents have the same allergy (Brostoff and Gamlin 2008).

Hydrolysate formula. Hydrolysate formula (prescription-only) is made of cow's milk, cornstarch and other foods, treated with digestive enzymes so that the milk proteins are partially broken down. It has been thought in the past that these alternatives carry less risk of allergy than standard formulae.

Some of these hydrolysates are intended to *treat* an existing allergy, and others are designed for *preventative* use in babies who are at high risk of developing cow's milk protein allergy and who are not breastfeeding (Brostoff and Gamlin 2008). Not only are these substances considerably more expensive than either standard or soya-based formula, NICE (2014) guidance now maintains that there is *insufficient evidence that infant formula based on partially or extensively hydrolysed cow's milk protein helps prevent allergies* (Boyle et al. 2016).

Whey hydrolysates. These formulae are made from the whey of cow's milk (rather than from whole milk) and have been thought to be potentially more useful for highly allergenic babies.

Amino-acid-based formula, or elemental formula. Amino-acid-based formulae, or elemental formulae has a completely synthetic protein base, providing essential and non-essential amino acids, together with fat, maltodextrin, vitamins, minerals and trace elements. However, this type of formula milk is very expensive.

Soya-based formula. Soya-based formula was developed as a response to the emergence of cow's milk protein intolerance in babies fed on formula milk. However, there is evidence that soya-based formula's high phytoestrogen content can pose a risk to the long-term reproductive health of infants (Adgent et al. 2018).

Consequently, soya-based formula milk should be used only in exceptional circumstances to ensure adequate nutrition, for example with babies of vegan parents who are not breastfeeding or babies who are unable to tolerate alternatives, such as amino-acid formulae (Crawley and Westland 2019).

Many babies who are intolerant of cow's milk are also intolerant of soya. Early soya formula feeding runs the risk of inducing soya protein intolerance in the child and soya protein is much harder to avoid in the weaning diet than dairy products.

Goat's milk formula. Goat's milk formula was approved by the European Food Standards Agency (EFSA) in 2012 and introduced in the UK as a further source of infant nutrition in 2013. To date its benefit over bovine milk based formula is not known.

Choosing a Breastmilk Substitute

Although not always enforced, it is an offence under UK law to sell any infant formula as being suitable from birth unless it meets the *Infant Formula and Follow-on Formula Regulations* (Her Majesty's Government 2007). Despite claims made by formula manufacturers, there is no obvious scientific basis on which to recommend one brand over another. Only *follow-on* milk advertising is permitted.

It is not necessary for the mother to stick to one brand, and if she finds that one formula milk does not suit her baby she can try an alternative brand. This has been made easier by the availability of ready-to-feed sachets or cartons, with which mothers can experiment without having to buy large quantities of formula milk. Babies with underlying metabolic disorders, such as galactosaemia or phenylketonuria, however, require the appropriate, ***prescribed*** breastmilk substitute.

As formula milks are highly processed, factory-produced products, there inevitably can arise inadvertent errors, such as too much or too little of an ingredient, accidental contamination, incorrect labelling and 'foreign bodies'. It is therefore imperative that mothers are advised to inspect the contents of the tin or packet before use and if it looks or smells strange, return it to the vendor.

Preparation of an Artificial Feed

The introduction of ready-to-feed formula in hospital may save staff time, but it reduces women's confidence in safely preparing a formula milk feed if that is their chosen

---

BOX 27.10 Principles of Reconstituting Formula Milk Powder

1. Wash your hands and work on a clean surface.
2. Boil the kettle with fresh tap water.
3. Leave to cool for a maximum of 20 minutes.
4. Use a clean, sterile bottle and teat.
5. Pour cooled water into the sterile bottle and measure water volume required at eye level.
6. Add required number of level scoops using the manufacturer's scoop from the tin/package.
7. Screw the teat, cap and lid in place then shake to mix.
8. Test the temperature of the reconstituted milk on the inside of your forearm.
9. Feed to your baby in a responsive manner.
10. Discard any remaining milk after 2 hours.

---

feeding method (Khan and McIntyre 2016). It is good practice that all mothers intending to formula-feed their baby are given the information they need to do so in a way that reduces the risk to the baby (UNICEF-UK 2017).

All powdered formula feed available in the UK is now reconstituted using one flat scoopful (from that specific powder) to 1 fluid ounce/28 mL of *cooled* boiled water (Box 27.10). Clear instructions about the volumes of powder and water are also printed on the container. Many of the major UK manufacturers of formula milk now produce ready-to-feed cartons, reducing the risk of over- or under-concentration, but precluding universal use through higher cost. The heat treatment also renders ready-to-feed formulae sterile. Powdered milk stored in tins or packets in contrast are not and contain latent *Enterobacter sakazakii* (*Cronobacter* species), *E. coli* and *Salmonella*, which multiply on reconstitution.

In response to growing concerns about bacterial contaminants in these powders, the WHO produced guidelines on the safe preparation, storage and handling of powdered infant formula (WHO 2007), and the Food Standards Agency (FSA) and Department of Health subsequently changed their recommendations in relation to reconstitution. Each feed should be prepared **just before** it is required using fresh water that has boiled **only once** (as repeated boiling concentrates the mineral salts) and cooled for approximately 20 min to 70°C, adding the powder, allowing the milk to cool and giving the feed straight away. Any remaining milk should be discarded by 2 h (UNICEF-UK/DH 2015b). The use of automated milk reconstitution machines is not advised as the boiled water is cooled with cold water that has been standing in the tank and pipes of the machine.

The water supply

It is essential that the water used to reconstitute powdered milk is free from bacterial contamination and any harmful chemicals. It is generally assumed in the UK that boiled tap water will meet these criteria, but from time to time, this is shown not to be the case. If bottled water is used, a still, non-mineralized variety suitable for babies must be chosen and it should be boiled as usual. Softened water is usually unsuitable.

Feeding equipment

Bottle teats. Concern over the nitrosamine content of rubber teats and dummies as well as plastic feeding bottles containing Bisphenol A (BPA), have prohibited their use in the European Union (EU) since 2011. In the UK, this has also been embedded in specific Regulations pertaining to Consumer Protection Law (Her Majesty's Government 1995; European Food Safety Authority, EFSA 2011). As the surface of all types of teats and bottles can become damaged with repeated use, it is therefore recommended that mothers should always check their equipment regularly and discard them if in any doubt of their integrity and ultimately the safety of their babies.

No bottle teat is like a breast as they do not lengthen like the human nipple to aid feeding. Although there are a range of teats available, no type of teat has any advantage over another. The mother should feel free to experiment, and use the type of teat that seems to suit her baby. It may be easier for the baby to use a simple soft long teat than industry-labelled orthodontic teats.

The size of the hole in the teat causes much anxiety to mothers. It is probably a good idea to have several teats with holes of different sizes so that the mother can experiment as necessary. *To test the hole size, turn the bottle upside down and the milk should drip at a rate of about one drop per second.*

Feeding bottles. Feeding bottles will have relatively smooth interiors. Crevices and grooves in a bottle make cleaning difficult. Patterned or decorated bottles make it less easy to see whether the bottle is clean. Although not widely available, there are glass feeding bottles that parents may purchase should they be concerned about the safety of plastic bottles. Furthermore, the parents may also be conscious of the environmental disadvantages of using plastic products to spur them into selecting an alternative feeding bottle.

Sterilization of feeding equipment

Effective cleaning of all feeding equipment used should be demonstrated to the mother and methods of sterilization discussed using the following principles:
- The most important prerequisite is that all equipment is thoroughly washed in hot, soapy water and well rinsed before proceeding further.
- If ***boiling*** is to be used, full immersion with no air bubbles, is essential and the contents must be boiled for 10 minutes.
- If ***cold sterilization*** using a hypochlorite solution is the method of choice, the utensils must be fully immersed in the solution, with no air bubbles for the recommended time. The manufacturer's advice must be followed when rinsing items removed from the solution. If the item is to be rinsed, previously boiled water should be used and not water directly from the tap.
- ***Steam and microwave sterilization*** are also possible, but the mother should check that her equipment can withstand such methods. Once the batch of equipment has been sterilized and the lid removed, self-contained sterile bottles need to be created as they will all become de-sterilized.

Feeding the Baby with the Bottle

The importance of formula feeding in a responsive and reciprocal manner needs to be highlighted to the parents. The mother should try to simulate breastfeeding conditions for the baby by holding the baby close, maintaining eye-to-eye contact and allowing the baby to determine their intake (e.g. 5–10 mL at the first feed in line with the infant's stomach volume). The baby should be held in a semi-recumbent position with their shoulders supported in a comfortable, neutral position. The baby must never be left unattended while feeding from a bottle and mothers should be warned about the dangers of *bottle propping with or without any accompanying devices.*

The innate skills a baby has for breastfeeding should also be used when feeding from a bottle. The baby's lips should be touched to elicit the mouth to open wide and the teat should follow the line of the baby's tongue, so that the baby uses the teat effectively. The bottle should be held horizontal to the ground, tilted just enough to ensure the baby is taking milk, not air, through the teat (UNICEF-UK/First Steps Nutrition Trust 2019). Recent findings using opaque weighted feeding bottles have demonstrated increased attention of feeding cues and self-regulation of volumes taken by the baby (Ventura and Hernandez 2019).

When *correctly* prepared, modern formula milks should not cause hypernatraemia. There is therefore no need to give the baby extra water. The stools and vomit of a baby fed on formula milk have an unpleasant sour smell. Unlike a breastfed baby, the formula-fed baby may become constipated.

THE HEALTHY START INITIATIVE

In 2006, the *Healthy Start Initiative* replaced the UK Welfare Food Scheme that had existed for 80 years, providing tokens to disadvantaged and low-income families that were exchanged for liquid milk or breastmilk substitutes. The Healthy Start Initiative Scheme has broadened the nutritional base of the former Welfare Food Scheme to allow fruit and vegetables as well as milk or breast-milk substitutes to be obtained through the exchange of fixed value vouchers at a range of food and supermarket outlets. Those eligible to receive the vouchers are listed below.

Women who are at least 10 weeks pregnant or have a child under 4 years of age **and** receive:
- Income Support
- Income-based Jobseeker's Allowance
- Income-related Employment and Support Allowance *or*
- Child Tax Credit with an annual family income of ≤£16,190 per tax year)
- Pension Credit
- Universal Credit with no earned income or total earned income of £408 or less per month for the family.
- All pregnant women under the age of 18, whether or not they are receiving benefits or tax credit.

Those eligible for vouchers are also entitled to free vitamin supplements for themselves, and for their babies *from birth* until their 4th birthday.

REFLECTIVE ACTIVITY FOR SELF-ASSESSMENT

1. During the antenatal period, what information would you give to all pregnant women to inform their choice in infant feeding to support their mothering skills? What is the evidence to support your discussion?
2. List the components of breastmilk and formula feed. How do they affect infant growth and development?
3. How can the midwife encourage the engagement of fathers/partners in supporting infant feeding practices?
4. How does the *International Code of Marketing of Breast-milk Substitutes* affect the manner in which health professionals work?

REFERENCES

ACAS (Advisory Conciliation and Arbitration Service). (2017). *Pregnancy and maternity discrimination: key points for the workplace*. London: ACAS.

Adgent, M. A., Umbach, D. M., Zemel, B. S., et al. (2018). A longitudinal study of estrogen-responsive tissues and hormone concentrations in infants fed soy formula. *Journal of Clinical Endocrinology and Metabolism, 103*(5), 1899–1909.

Aghdas, K., Talak, K., & Sepideh, B. (2014). Effect of immediate and continuous mother-infant skin-to-skin, contact on breastfeeding self-efficacy of primiparous women: a randomized control trial. *Women and Birth, 27*, 37–40.

Arroyo, R., Martín, V., Maldonado, A., et al. (2010). Treatment of infectious mastitis during lactation: antibiotics versus oral administration of lactobacilli isolated from breast milk. *Clinical Infectious Diseases, 50*(12), 1551–1558.

Bagnall, A. (2005). Feeding development. In E. Jones, & C. King (Eds.), *Feeding and nutrition in the pre-term infant* (p. 141). Edinburgh: Elsevier/Churchill Livingstone.

Beilin, Y., Bodian, C. A., Weiser, J., et al. (2005). Effect of labor epidural analgesia with and without fentanyl on infant breast-feeding: a prospective, randomized, double-blind study. *Anesthesiology, 103*, 1211–1217.

Blackburn, S. T. (2018). Haematologic and Hemostatic systems, *Maternal, Fetal, & Neonatal Physiology: A Clinical Perspective* (5th ed.). Ch. 8. Philadelphia: Saunders/Elsevier. .

Boyle, R. J., Ierodiakonou, D., Khan, T., et al. (2016). Hydrolysed formula and risk of allergic or autoimmune disease; systematic review and metanalysis. *British Medical Journal, 352*, i974.

Bramson, L., Lee, J. W., Moore, E., et al. (2010). Effect of early skin-to-skin mother–infant contact during the first 3 hours following birth on exclusive breastfeeding during the maternity hospital stay. *Journal of Human Lactation, 26*(2), 130–137.

Brimdyr, K., Cadwell, K., Stevens, J., & Takahashi, Y. (2017). An implementation algorithm to improve skin-to-skin practice in the first hour after birth. *Maternal and Child Nutrition, 14*(2), 1–15.

BHIVA (British HIV Association). (2019). *BHIVA guidelines for the management of HIV in pregnancy and postpartum 2018* (2019 interim update). Available at: www.bhiva.org/pregnancy-guidelines.

Brookes, A., & Bowley, D. M. (2014). Tongue tie: The evidence for frenotomy. *Early Human Development, 90*(11), 765–768.

Brostoff, J., & Gamlin, L. (2008). *The complete guide to allergy and food intolerance*. London: Bloomsbury.

Brown, A. (2016). *Breastfeeding uncovered: who really decides how we feed our babies?* London: Pinter and Martin.

Butte, N. F., Garza, C., Stuff, J. E., et al. (1984). Effect of maternal diet and body composition on lactational performance. *American Journal of Clinical Nutrition, 39*, 296–306.

Cadwell, K., & Brimdyr, K. (2017). Intrapartum administration of synthetic oxytocin and downstream effects on breastfeeding: elucidating physiologic pathways. *Annals of Nursing Research and Practice, 2*(3), 1024–1032.

Canfield, L. M., Hopkinson, J. M., Lima, A. F., et al. (1991). Vitamin K in colostrum and mature human milk over the lactation period – a cross-sectional study. *American Journal of Clinical Nutrition, 53*(3), 730–735.

Chauchan, M., Henderson, G., & Quigley, M. (2008). Formula milk versus donor breast milk for feeding preterm or low birth weight infants. *Archives of Disease in Childhood. Fetal and Neonatal Edition, 93*, 162–166.

CLAPA (Cleft Lip and Palate Association). (2015). *Help with feeding*. London: CLAPA. Available at: www.clapa.com/wp-content/uploads/2015/12/Help-with-Feeding.pdf.

Cooijmans, K., Beijers, R., Rovers, A., & de Weerth, C. (2017). Effectiveness of skin-to-skin contact versus care-as-usual in mothers and their full-term infants: study protocol for a parallel-group randomized controlled trial. *BMC Pediatrics, 17*(1), 54.

Coulson, S. (2012). *An introduction to biological nurturing: new angles on breastfeeding*. London: Pinter and Martin.

Coulson, S. (2019). *Biological nurturing – breastfeeding instinctively*. London: Pinter and Martin.

Cox, D. B., Kent, J. C., Casey, T. M., et al. (1999). Breast growth and the urinary excretion of lactose during human pregnancy and early lactation: endocrine relationships. *Experimental Physiology, 84*(2), 421–434.

Crawley, H., & Westland, S. (2019). *Infant milks in the UK: a practical guide for health professionals*. London: First Steps Nutrition.

Cross, B. A. (1977). Comparative physiology of milk removal. *Symposium of the Zoological Society (London), 41*, 193–210.

Cruz-Korchin, N., Korchin, L., Gonzalez-Keelan, C., et al. (2002). Macromastia: how much of it is fat? *Plastic Reconstruction Surgery, 109*(1), 64–68.

Daly, S. (1993). The short term synthesis and infant regulated removal of milk in lactating women. *Experimental Physiology, 78*, 209–220.

Dearlove, J. C., & Dearlove, B. M. (1981). Prolactin, fluid balance and lactation. *British Journal of Obstetrics and Gynecology, 123*, 845–846.

Del Bono, E., & Rabe, B. (2012). *Breastfeeding and child cognitive outcomes: Evidence from a hospital-based breastfeeding support policy: Working Paper Series 2012–29*. Essex: University of Essex, Institute for Social and Economic Research.

Dewey, K. G. (1998). Effects of maternal caloric restriction and exercise during lactation. *Journal of Nutrition, 128*(2 Suppl), 386S–3899S.

Dewey, K. G., Lovelady, C. A., Nommsen-Rivers, L. A., et al. (1994). A randomized study of the effects of aerobic exercise by lactating women on breast-milk volume and composition. *New England Journal of Medicine, 330*(7), 449–453.

Dewey, K. G., Nommsen-Rivers, L. A., Heinig, M. J., & Cohen, R. J. (2003). Risk factors for suboptimal infant breastfeeding behavior, delayed onset of lactation, and excess neonatal weight loss. *Pediatrics, 112*(3 Pt 1), 607–619.

DiGiroloma, A. M., Gummer-Strawn, L. M., & Fein, S. B. (2008). Effect of maternity-care practices on breastfeeding. *Pediatrics, 122*(Suppl. 2), S43–S49.

Dixley, A. (2014). *Breast intentions: How women sabotage breastfeeding for themselves and others*. London: Pinter and Martin.

Dusdieker, L. B., Hemingway, D. L., & Stumbo, P. J. (1994). Is milk production impaired by dieting during lactation? *American Journal of Clinical Nutrition, 59*, 833–840.

Dykes, F. (2006). The education of health practitioners supporting breastfeeding women: time for critical reflection. *Maternal and Child Nutrition, 2*, 204–216.

Eglin, R. P., & Wilkinson, A. R. (1987). HIV infection and pasteurization of breast milk. *Lancet, 1*(8541), 1093.

EFSA (European Food Safety Authority). (2011). Commission Directive 2011/8/EU of 28 January 2011; amending Directive 2002/72/EC as regards the restriction of use of Bisphenol A in plastic infant feeding bottles. *Official Journal of the European Union*. Available at: https://eur-lex.europa.eu/legal-content/EN/TXT/PDF/?uri=CELEX:32011L0008&from=EN.

The Equality Act. (2010) London: TSO.

Fallon, V. M., Harrold, J. A., & Chisholm, A. (2019). The impact of the UK Baby Friendly Initiative on maternal and infant health outcomes: a mixed-methods systematic review. *Maternal and Child Nutrition*, 15(3), 12778–12800.

Fawzy, A., Arpadi, S., Kankasa, C., et al. (2011). Early weaning increases diarrhoea morbidity and mortality among uninfected children born to HIV-infected mothers in Zambia. *Journal of Infectious Diseases*, 203, 1222–1230.

Fernstrom, J. D. (1999). Effects of dietary polyunsaturated fatty acids on neuronal function. *Lipids*, 34(2), 161–169.

Flint, A., New, K., & Davies, M. W. (2016). Cup feeding versus other forms of supplemental enteral feeding for newborn infants unable to fully breastfeed. *Cochrane Database of Systematic Reviews*, (8), CD005092.

Forster, D. A., Moorhead, A. M., Jacobs, S. E., et al. (2017). Advising women with diabetes in pregnancy to express breastmilk in late pregnancy (Diabetes and Antenatal Milk Expressing [DAME]): a multicentre, unblinded, randomised controlled trial. *Lancet*, 389(10085), 2204–2213.

Geddes, D. T., Kent, J. C., Mitoulas, L. R., & Hartmann, P. E. (2008). Tongue movement and intra-oral vacuum in breastfeeding infants. *Early Human Development*, 84(7), 471–477.

Geddes, L. (2008). Breastmilk provides menu of different flavours. *New Scientist*, 199(2666), 14.

Going, J. J., & Moffat, D. F. (2004). Escaping from Flatland: clinical and biological aspects of human mammary duct anatomy in three dimensions. *Journal of Pathology*, 203(1), 538–544.

Gonzalez-Jimenez, E., Garcia, P., Aguilar, J., et al. (2013). Breastfeeding and the prevention of breast cancer: a retrospective review of clinical histories. *Journal of Clinical Nursing*, 23, 2397–2403.

Guillebaud, J., & MacGregor, A. (2017). *Contraception: your questions answered* (7th ed.). Edinburgh: Churchill Livingstone.

Hale, T. V., & Hartmann, P. F. (2007). *Hale and Hartmann's textbook of human lactation*. Amarillo TX: Hale.

Hall Moran, V. (2012). Nutrition in pregnant and breastfeeding adolescents: a biopsychosocial perspective. In V. Hall Moran (Ed.), *Maternal and infant nutrition and nurture: controversies and challenges* (2nd ed.) (pp. 45–88). London: Quay Books.

Hammer, R. L., Babcock, G., & Fisher, A. G. (1996). Low-fat diet and exercise in obese lactating women. *Breast-feeding Review*, 4(1), 29–34.

Hazelbaker, A. K. (2010). *Tongue-tie: morphogenesis, impact, assessment and treatment*. Ohio: Aidan and Eva Press.

Her Majesty's Government. (1995). *Statutory Instrument 1995: No 1012: Consumer Protection: The N-nitrosamines and N-nitrosatable substances in elastomer or rubber teats and dummies (Safety) Regulations 1995*. London: The Stationery Office. Available at: www.legislation.gov.uk/uksi/1995/1012/made/data.pdf.

Her Majesty's Government. (2007). *Statutory Instrument: 2007: No 3521: Food [England] Infant Formula and Follow-on Formula [England] Regulations (first introduced 1995; updated 2007)*. London: The Stationery Office. Available at www.legislation.gov.uk/uksi/2007/3521/pdfs/uksi_20073521_en.pdf.

Hey, E. (2003). Vitamin K – what, why and when. *Archives of Disease in Childhood Fetal and Neonatal edition*, 88(2), F80–F83.

Hopkinson, J. (2007). Nutrition in lactation. In T. V. Hale, & P. F. Hartmann (Eds.), *Hale and Hartman's textbook of human lactation* (pp. 379–381). Amarillo, TX: Hale.

Horta, B., De Mola, C., & Victora, C. (2015). Long–term consequences of breastfeeding on cholesterol, obesity, systolic blood pressure and type 2 diabetes: a systematic review and meta-analysis. *Acta Paediatrica*, 104(S467), 30–37.

Illingworth, P. J., Jong, R. T., Howie, P. W., et al. (1986). Diminution in energy expenditure during lactation. *British Medical Journal*, 292, 437–441.

Inch, S., & Fisher, C. (1995). Mastitis in lactating women. *The Practitioner*, 239, 472–476.

Ingram, J., Woolridge, M., & Greenwood, R. (2001). Breast-feeding: it is worth trying with the second baby. *Lancet*, 358(9286), 986–987.

Jackson, D. A., Woolridge, M. W., Imong, S. M., et al. (1987). The automatic sampling shield: a device for sampling suckled breast milk. *Early Human Development*, 15(5), 295–306.

Jamal, N., Ng, K. H., McLean, D., et al. (2004). Mammographic breast glandularity in Malaysian women: data derived from radiography. *American Journal of Roentgenology*, 182(3), 713–717.

Jaeggi, T., Kortman, G. A. M., Moretti, D., et al. (2015). Iron fortification adversely affects the gut microbiome, increases pathogen abundance and induces intestinal inflammation in Kenyan infants. *Gut*, 64(5), 731–742.

Kafulafala, G., Hoover, D., Taha, T., et al. (2010). Frequency of gastroenteritis and gastroenteritis-associated mortality with early weaning in HIV-1-uninfected children born to HIV-infected women in Malawi. *Journal of Acquired Immune Deficiency Syndrome*, 53, 6–13.

Khan, K., & McIntyre, H. (2016). A literature review of hospital postnatal care. *MIDIRS Midwifery Digest*, 26(3), 345–352.

Kamelska, A. M., Pietrzak-Fiećko, R., & Bryl, K. (2012). Variation of the cholesterol content in breast milk during 10 days collection at early stages of lactation. *Acta Biochimica Polonica*, 59(2), 243–247.

Khaghani, S., Ezzatpanah, H., Mazhari, N., et al. (2010). Zinc and copper concentrations in human milk and infant formulas. *Iranian Journal of Pediatrics*, 20(1), 53–57.

Kim, H. H., & Park, C. S. (2004). A compensatory nutrition regimen during gestation stimulates mammary development and lactation potential in rats. *Journal of Nutrition, 134*(4), 756–761.

Kochenour, N. K. (1980). Lactation suppression. *Clinical Obstetrics and Gynecology, 23*, 1052–1059.

Krebs, N. F. (1999). Zinc transfer to the breastfed infant. *Journal of Mammary Gland Biology and Neoplasia, 4*(3), 259–268.

Kries, R. V., Shearer, M., McCarthy, P. T., et al. (1987). Vitamin K1 content of maternal milk: influence of the stage of lactation, lipid composition, and vitamin K1 supplements given to the mother. *Pediatric Research, 22*(5), 513–517.

Labbok, M. (2016). *The lactational amenorrhoea method (LAM) for postnatal contraception.* Melbourne, Australian Breastfeeding Association. Available at: www.breastfeeding.asn.au/bfinfo/lactational-amenorrhea-method-lam-postpartum-contraception.

Leaf, A. A. (2007). Vitamins for babies and young children: RCPCH Standing Committee on Nutrition. *Archives of Disease in Childhood, 92*(2), 160–164.

Liu, B., & Newburg, D. S. (2013). Human milk glycoproteins protect infants against human pathogens. *Breastfeeding Medicine, 8*(4), 354–362.

Love, S. M., & Barsky, S. H. (2004). Anatomy of the nipple and breast ducts revisited. *Cancer, 101*(9), 1947–1957.

Macdonald, H. M., Mavroeidi, A., Fraser, W. D., et al. (2011). Sunlight and dietary contributions to the seasonal vitamin D status of cohorts of healthy postmenopausal women living at northerly latitudes: a major cause for concern? *Osteoporosis International, 22*(9), 2461–2472.

Marchbank, T., Weaver, G., Nilsen-Hamilton, M., & Playford, R. J. (2009). Pancreatic secretory trypsin inhibitor is a major motogenic and protective factor in human breast milk. *American Journal of Physiology-Gastrointestinal and Liver Physiology, 296*(4), G697–G703.

McAndrew, F., Thompson, J., Fellows, L., et al. (2012). *Infant Feeding Survey 2010.* A survey carried out on behalf of Health and Social Care Information Centre by IFF Research in partnership with Professor Mary Renfrew, Professor of Mother and Infant Health, College of Medicine, Dentistry and Nursing, University of Dundee. Available at: https://sp.ukdataservice.ac.uk/doc/7281/mrdoc/pdf/7281_ifs-uk-2010_report.pdf.

McKechnie, A. C., & Eglash, A. (2010). Nipple shields: a review of the literature. *Breastfeeding Medicine, 5*(6), 309–314.

McIntyre, H. (2013). Factors influencing student midwives' competence and confidence when incorporating UNICEF Baby Friendly Initiative Education Standards in clinical practice. Unpublished DHSci Thesis, University of Nottingham. Available at: http://eprints.nottingham.ac.uk/27802.

Moan, J., Porojnicu, A. C., Dahlback, A., & Setlow, R. B. (2008). Addressing the health benefits and risks, involving vitamin D or skin cancer, of increased sun exposure. *Proceedings of the National Academy of Science, 105*(2), 668–673.

Monaci, G., & Woolridge, M. (2011). Ultrasound video analysis for understanding infant breastfeeding. *Proceedings of the 18th Institut d'Economia Ecològica i Ecologia Política International (IEEEP) International Conference on Image Processing (ICIP)* (pp.1765–1768). Brussels, Belguim.

Montagne, P., Cuillière, M. L., Molé, C., et al. (2001). Changes in lactoferrin and lysozyme levels in human milk during the first twelve weeks of lactation. *Advances in Experimental and Medical Biology, 501*, 241–247.

Morse, J. M., Ewing, G., Gamble, D., et al. (1992). The effect of maternal fluid intake on breast milk supply: a pilot study. *Canadian Journal of Public Health, 83*(3), 213–216.

Neville, M. C., McFadden, T. B., & Forsyth, I. (2002). Hormonal regulation of mammary differentiation and milk secretion. *Journal of Mammary Gland Biology and Neoplasia, 7*(1), 49–66.

NHS Scotland. (2018). *Maternal and Infant Nutrition Survey, Scottish Government.* Available at: www.gov.scot/publications/scottish-maternal-infant-nutrition-survey-2017/pages/1/.

NICE (National Institute for Health and Care Excellence). (2005). *Division of ankyloglossia (tongue tie) for breastfeeding IPG 149.* London: NICE. Available at: https://www.nice.org.uk/guidance/ipg149/resources/division-of-ankyloglossia-tonguetie-for-breastfeeding-pdf-1899863228061637.

NICE (National Institute for Health and Care Excellence). (2014). *Maternal and Child Nutrition PH11.* London: NICE. Available at: https://www.nice.org.uk/guidance/ph11/resources/maternal-and-child-nutrition-pdf-1996171502533.

NICE (National Institute for Health and Care Excellence). (2015). *Postnatal care up to 8 weeks after birth CG37.* London: NICE. Available at: https://www.nice.org.uk/guidance/cg37/resources/postnatal-care-up-to-8-weeks-after-birth-pdf-975391596997.

NICE (National Institute for Health and Care Excellence). (2016). *Vitamin D deficiency in children (CKS).* London: NICE. Available at: https://cks.nice.org.uk/vitamin-d-deficiency-in-children#!scenario:1.

NICE (National Institute for Health and Care Excellence). (2017). *Vitamin D supplement use in specific population groups PH56.* London: NICE. Available at: https://www.nice.org.uk/guidance/ph56/resources/vitamin-d-supplement-use-in-specific-population-groups-pdf-1996421765317.

NICE (National Institute for Health and Care Excellence). (2018). *Mastitis and breast abscess: Management of mastitis and breast abscess in lactating women*. London: NICE. Available at: https://cks.nice.org.uk/mastitis-and-breast-abscess#!scenario.

Nickell, W. B., & Skelton, J. (2005). Breast fat and fallacies: more than 100 years of anatomical fantasy. *Journal of Human Lactation, 21*(2), 126–130.

Nicolls, H. (1997). Two on to one will go. *Midwifery Matters, 73*, 6–7.

Owen, C. G., Whincup, P. H., Kaye, S. J., et al. (2008). Does initial breastfeeding lead to lower blood cholesterol in adult life? A quantitative review of the evidence. *American Journal of Clinical Nutrition, 88*, 305–314.

Paronen, J., Knip, M., Savilahti, E., et al. (2000). Effect of cow's milk exposure and maternal type 1 diabetes on cellular and humeral immunization to dietary insulin in infants at genetic risk for type 1 diabetes. Finnish Trial to Reduce IDDM in the Genetically at Risk Study Group. *Diabetes, 49*(10), 1657–1665.

Picciano, M. F. (2001). Nutrient composition of human milk. *Pediatric Clinics of North America, 48*(1), 53–67.

Pollard, M. (2017). *Evidence-based care for breastfeeding mothers: A resource for midwives and allied healthcare professionals* (2nd ed.). London: Routledge.

Prentice, A. M., Addey, C. V., & Wilde, C. J. (1989). Evidence for local feedback control of human milk secretion. *Biochemical Society Transactions, 17*(122), 489–492.

Prentice, A. M., Roberts, S. B., & Whitehead, R. G. (1980). Dietary supplementation of Gambian nursing mothers and lactational performance. *Lancet ii*, 886–888.

Prentice, A. M., Lunn, P. G., Watkinson, M. M., & Whitehead, R. G. (1983). Dietary supplementation of lactating Gambian women II. Effect on maternal health, nutritional status and biochemistry. *Human Nutrition and Clinical Nutrition, 37*(1), 65–74.

Prentice, A. M., Goldberg, G. R., & Prentice, A. (1994). Body mass index and lactational performance. *European Journal of Clinical Nutrition, 48*(Suppl. 3), S78–S89.

PHE (Public Health England). (2019). *Official Statistics: breastfeeding prevalence at 6–8 weeks after birth: Experiential Statistics Quarter 4 2018/19 Statistical Commentary*. London: PHE. Available at: https://assets.publishing.service.gov.uk/government/uploads/system/uploads/attachment_data/file/818429/2018-19_Q4_-_FINAL_Breastfeeding_Statistical_Commentary.pdf.

Ramsay, D. T., Kent, J. C., Owens, R. A., & Hartmann, P. E. (2004). Ultrasound imaging of milk ejection in the breast of lactating women. *Pediatrics, 113*, 361–367.

Ramsay, D. T., Kent, J. C., Hartmann, R. A., & Hartmann, P. E. (2005). Anatomy of the lactating human breast redefined with ultrasound imaging. *Journal of Anatomy, 206*(6), 525–534.

Rapley, G. (2012). Baby-led weaning. In V. Hall Moran (Ed.), *Maternal and infant nutrition and nurture: controversies and challenges* (2nd ed.) (pp. 261–284). London: Quay Books.

Rasmussen, K. M. (2007). Maternal obesity and the outcome of breastfeeding. In T. W. Hale, & P. E. Hartmann (Eds.), *Hale and Hartmann's textbook on human lactation* (pp. 387–402). Amarillo, TX: Hale.

Renfrew, M. J., & Hall, D. (2008). Enabling women to breast feed. Editorial. *British Medical Journal, 337*, a1570.

Renfrew, M. J., Pokhrel, S., Quigley, M., et al. (2012). *Preventing disease and saving resources: the potential contribution of increasing breastfeeding rates in the UK*. London: UNICEF-UK.

Righard, L., & Alade, M. O. (1990). Effect of delivery room routines on success of first breast-feed. *Lancet, 336*, 1105–1107.

RCPCH (Royal College of Paediatrics and Child Health). (2013). *UK-WHO Growth Charts 0–4 years* (2nd ed.). Available at: www.rcpch.ac.uk/resources/uk-who-growth-charts-0-4-years.

Saarinen, U. M., & Siimes, M. A. (1979). Iron absorption from breast milk, cow's milk and iron supplemented formula: an opportunistic use of changes in total body iron determined by hemoglobin, ferritin and body weight in 132 infants. *Pediatric Research, 13*, 143–147.

Santoro, W., Jr., Martinez, F. E., Ricco, R. G., & Jorge, S. M. (2010). Colostrum ingested during the first day of life by exclusively breastfed healthy newborn infants. *Journal of Pediatrics, 156*(1), 29–32.

Saso, A., & Kampmann, B. (2017). Vaccine responses in newborns. *Seminars in Immunopathology, 39*(6), 627–664.

Schmied, V., Beake, S., Sheehan, A., et al. (2011). Women's perception and experiences of breastfeeding support: a metasynthesis. *Birth Issues in Perinatal Care, 38*(10), 49–60.

Scholtz, S. A., Gottipati, B. S., Gajewski, B. J., et al. (2013). Dietary sialic acid and cholesterol influence cortical composition in developing rats. *Journal of Nutrition, 143*(2), 132–135.

SACN (Scientific Advisory Committee on Nutrition). (2016). *Vitamin D and Health*. London: Public Health England. Available at: https://assets.publishing.service.gov.uk/government/uploads/system/uploads/attachment_data/file/537616/SACN_Vitamin_D_and_Health_report.pdf.

SACN (Scientific Advisory Committee on Nutrition). (2018). *Feeding in the First year of Life*. London: Public Health England. Available at: https://assets.publishing.service.gov.uk/government/uploads/system/uploads/attachment_data/file/725530/SACN_report_on_Feeding_in_the_First_Year_of_Life.pdf.

Shaw, N. J., & Pal, B. R. (2002). Vitamin D deficiency in UK Asian families: activating a new concern. *Archives of Disease in Childhood, 86*, 147–149.

Spencer, R. L. (2013). *Women's experiences of breastfeeding: An interpretive phenomenological study.* Unpublished DHSci Thesis, University of Nottingham. Available at: http://e-prints.nottingham.ac.uk/27881.

Sultana, R. R. (2015). Comparison of Immunoglobulin levels in human milk. *KAAV International Journal of Science, Engineering and Technology, 2*(1), 25–46.

Swift, K., Janke, J. (2003). Breast binding ... is it all that it's wrapped up to be? *Journal of Obstetrics, Gynecology and Neonatal Nursing, 32*(3), 332–339.

Taneri, F., Kurukahvecioglu, O., Akyurek, N., et al. (2006). Micro-anatomy of milk ducts in the nipple. *European Surgery Research, 38*(6), 545–549.

Torgersen, T., Ystrom, E., Haugen, M., et al. (2010). Breastfeeding practice in mothers with eating disorders. *Maternal Child Nutrition, 6*(3), 243–252.

Ueda, T., Yokoyama, Y., Irahara, M., & Aono, T. (1994). Influence of psychological stress on suckling-induced pulsatile oxytocin release. *Obstetrics and Gynecology, 84,* 259–262.

UNICEF-UK. (1990). *UN Convention on the Rights of the Child.* (Enforced in the UK: 15th January 1992). Available at: https://downloads.unicef.org.uk/wp-content/uploads/2010/05/UNCRC_united_nations_convention_on_the_rights_of_the_child.pdf?_ga=2.104793024.1304908563.1564320273–51810980.1528748516.

UNICEF-UK. (2014). *Implementing the UNICEF-UK Baby Friendly standards in universities: learning outcomes and topic areas.* Available at: www.unicef.org.uk/babyfriendly/wp-content/uploads/sites/2/2010/11/University_learning_outcomes.pdf.

UNICEF-UK. (2016). *Responsive feeding: supporting close and loving relationships.* Available at: www.unicef.org.uk/babyfriendly/wp-content/uploads/sites/2/2017/12/Responsive-Feeding-Infosheet-Unicef-UK-Baby-Friendly-Initiative.pdf.

UNICEF-UK. (2017). *Guide to the Baby Friendly Initiative standards* (2nd ed.). Available at: www.unicef.org.uk/babyfriendly/wp-content/uploads/sites/2/2014/02/Guide-to-the-Unicef-UK-Baby-Friendly-Initiative-Standards.pdf.

UNICEF-UK. (2018). *Breastfeeding assessment tool: how you and your midwife can recognize that your baby is feeding well.* Available at: www.unicef.org.uk/babyfriendly/wp-content/uploads/sites/2/2018/07/breastfeeding_assessment_tool_mat.pdf.

UNICEF-UK. (2019a). *Accreditation statistics and awards.* Available at: www.unicef.org.uk/babyfriendly/about/accreditation-statistics-and-awards-table.

UNICEF-UK. (2019b). *Learning outcomes: medical, dietetic, pharmacy students and more.* Available at: www.unicef.org.uk/babyfriendly/accreditation/universities/learning-outcomes.

UNICEF-UK/DH. (2015a). *Your baby's first solid foods: your pregnancy and baby guide.* Available at: www.unicef.org.uk/babyfriendly/wp-content/uploads/sites/2/2008/02/Start4Life-Introducing-Solid-Foods-2015.pdf.

UNICEF-UK/DH. (2015b). *A guide to bottle feeding: how to prepare infant formula and sterile feeding equipment to minimise the risks to your baby.* London: PHE. Available at: www.unicef.org.uk/babyfriendly/wp-content/uploads/sites/2/2008/02/start4life_guide_to_bottle_-feeding.pdf.

UNICEF-UK/First Steps Nutrition Trust. (2019). *Responsive bottle feeding.* Available at: www.unicef.org.uk/babyfriendly/wp-content/uploads/sites/2/2019/04/Infant-formula-and-responsive-bottle-feeding.pdf.

UN (United Nations). (2015). *Transforming our world: The 2030 Agenda for Sustainable Development (A/RES/70/1).* New York: UN.

UN (United Nations). (2016). Human Rights Office of the High Commissioner (UN) Joint statement of the UN Special Rapporteurs on the Right to Food, Right to Health. The Working Group on Discrimination against Women in law and in practice and the Committee on the Rights of the Child in support of increased efforts to promote, support and protect breastfeeding. *States should do more to support and protect breastfeeding, and end inappropriate marketing of breast-milk.* Available at: www.humanitarianresponse.info/sites/www.humanitarianresponse.info/files/documents/files/joint_statement_breastfeeding_final-web_1.pdf.

Vandeweyer, E., & Hertens, D. (2002). Quantification of glands and fat in breast tissue: an experimental determination. *Annals of Anatomy, 184*(2), 181–184.

Ventura, A. K., & Hernandez, A. (2019). Effects of opaque weighted bottles on maternal sensitivity and infant intake. *Maternal and child nutrition, 15*(2), e12737.

Victora, C. G., Bahl, R., Barros, A. J., et al. (2016). Breastfeeding in the 21st century: epidemiology, mechanisms, and lifelong effect. *Lancet Breastfeeding Series, 387*(10017), 475–490.

Waldenström, U., & Swensen, Å. (1991). Rooming-in at night in the postpartum ward. *Midwifery, 7,* 82–89.

Walker, M. (2016). *Breastfeeding management for the clinician: using the evidence* (4th ed.). Burlington, MA: Jones and Bartlett Learning.

Wambach, K., & Riordan, J. (2016). *Breastfeeding and human lactation* (5th ed.). Burlington, MA: Jones and Bartlett Learning.

Weimers, L., Svensson, K., Dumas, L., et al. (2006). Hands-on approach during breastfeeding support in a neonatal intensive care unit: a qualitative study of Swedish mother's experiences. *International Breastfeeding Journal, 1,* 20.

Whitehead, R. G., Paul, A. A., Black, A. E., & Wiles, S. J. (1981). Recommended dietary amounts of energy for pregnancy or lactation in the UK. In B. Torun, V. R. Young, & W. M. Rang (Eds.), *Protein energy requirements of developing countries: evaluation of new data* (pp. 259–265). Tokyo: United Nations University.

Widström, A. M., Ransjo-Arvidson, A. B., Christensson, K., et al. (1987). Gastric suction in healthy newborn infants. *Acta Paediatrica: Nurturing the Child, 76*(4), 566–572.

Widström, A. M., Lilja, G., Aaltomaa–Michalias, P., et al. (2011). Newborn behaviour to locate the breast when skin–to–skin: a possible method for enabling early self–regulation. *ACTA Paediatrica: Nurturing the Child, 100*(1), 79–85.

Wilde, C. J., Addey, C. V., Boddy, L. M., & Peaker, M. (1995). Autocrine regulation of milk secretion by a protein in milk. *Biochemical Journal, 305,* 51–58.

Woolridge, M. W. (1986). The 'anatomy' of sucking. *Midwifery, 2,* 164–171.

Woolridge, M. W. (1995). Breast-feeding: physiology into practice. In D. P. Davis (Ed.), *Nutrition in child health* (pp. 13–31). London: Royal College of Physicians.

Woolridge, M. W., Baum, J. D., & Drewett, R. F. (1982). Individual patterns of milk intake during breast-feeding. *Early Human Development, 7,* 265–272.

WHO (World Health Organization). (1978). *A growth chart for international use in maternal and child health care: guidelines for primary health care personnel.* Geneva: WHO.

WHO (World Health Organization). (1981). *International Code of Marketing of Breast-milk Substitutes.* Geneva: WHO. Available at: https://apps.who.int/iris/bitstream/handle/10665/40382/9241541601.pdf;jsessionid=C-49C790D718A64FA8801A01D5B00433/?sequence=1.

WHO (World Health Organization). (1989). *Evidence for the ten steps to successful breastfeeding.* Geneva: WHO.

WHO (World Health Organization). (2000). *Mastitis: causes and management* (WHO/RCH/CAH/00.13). Geneva: Department of Child and Adolescent Health and Development, WHO.

WHO (World Health Organization). (2003). *Global strategy for infant and young child feeding.* Geneva: WHO.

WHO (World Health Organization). (2007). *Guidelines for the safe preparation, storage and handling of powdered infant formula.* Geneva: WHO.

WHO (World Health Organization). (2013). *Delayed clamping of the umbilical cord to reduce infant anaemia.* Available at: https://apps.who.int/iris/bitstream/handle/10665/120074/WHO_RHR_14.19_eng.pdf;sequence=1.

WHO (World Health Organization). (2018). *WHO highlights the importance of safeguarding breastfeeding for children up to 3 years of age.* Available at: www.unicef.org.uk/baby-friendly/who-highlights-importance-of-safeguarding-breastfeeding-for-children-up-to-three-years-of-age.

WHO/UNICEF. (1989). *Joint statement – protecting, promoting and supporting breastfeeding: the role of maternity services.* Geneva: WHO.

WHO/UNICEF. (2003). *Global strategy on infant and young child feeding.* Geneva: WHO.

WHO/UNICEF. (2018). *Ten steps to successful breastfeeding.* Geneva: WHO. Available at: www.who.int/nutrition/bf-hi/ten-steps/en.

WHO/UNICEF/UNAIDS. (2016). *Guideline updates on HIV and infant feeding. The duration of breastfeeding and support from health services to improve feeding practices among mothers living with HIV.* Geneva: WHO/UNICEF.

Ziegler, E. E. (2011). Consumption of cow's milk as a cause of iron deficiency in infants and toddlers. *Nutritional Review, 69*(Suppl. 1), S37–S42.

ANNOTATED FURTHER READING

Brown, A. (2016). *Breastfeeding uncovered: who really decides how we feed our babies?* London: Pinter and Martin.
This text examines why breastfeeding, a biologically normal behaviour, can appear so challenging in reality. The author reveals how complex social and cultural messages work against new mothers, damaging the normal physiology of breastfeeding and making it seem unmanageable. In so doing, the focus is removed from the mother to society as a whole, urging it to rethink its attitude towards breastfeeding and mothering and instead being more supportive and encouraging in protecting mothers to feed their babies.

Hale, T., & Hartmann, P. (2007). *Hale and Hartmann's textbook of human lactation.* Amarillo, TX: Hale.
This multi-author textbook written by experts in their fields, provides a comprehensive resource on all aspects of human lactation and infant feeding. It is comprised of six sections that cover: anatomy and biochemistry, immunobiology, management of the infant, management of the mother, maternal and infant nutrition and medications, to effectively guide the reader in understanding the theory and its application to practice.

Hall Moran, V. (Ed.). (2012). *Maternal and infant nutrition and nurture: controversies and challenges* (2nd ed.) London: Quay Books.
This multi-author book uses a socio-biological perspective to examine the complex interaction between political, socio-cultural and biological factors in food and health in relation to maternal and infant nutrition.

Hall Moran, V., & Lowe, N. M. (Eds.). (2016). *Nutrition and the developing brain.* London: CRC Press.
This text reviews the evidence from animal and human research and considers the impact of the biospecificity of

breastmilk on brain function and cognitive development, something which cannot be replicated with formula substitutes. Exploration of issues such as single versus multiple limiting nutrients, critical periods of deficiency, and the impact of the child–parent relationship on the architecture of the developing brain are also key features.

Palmer, G. (2009). *The politics of breast-feeding. When breasts are bad for business* (3rd ed.). London: Pinter and Martin.

This book offers a profound exploration of the global and personal costs of artificial feeding in terms of infant mortality and morbidity and how breast feeding can be perceived as being 'bad for business'. While the book presents the authority about the evidence for breastfeeding, it discusses the social and commercial forces that prevent this vital function of early life and parenting from being the norm. It therefore challenges the reader to examine their own values and attitudes in supporting infant feeding practices and the impact this can have on global health and wellbeing.

Pollard, M. (2017). *Evidence-based care for breastfeeding mothers: A resource for midwives and allied healthcare professionals* (2nd ed.). London: Routledge.

This book provides a thorough but accessible rationale and explanation of support available to postnatal women with infant feeding. It is based on the UNICEF-UK BFI University Learning Outcomes and includes key fact boxes, clinical scenarios and activities to help the readers assimilate the contents in order to promote and support breastfeeding mothers.

UNICEF: A short video 'How to hand express' is Available at: www.unicef.org.uk/babyfriendly/baby-friendly-resources/breastfeeding-resources/hand-expression-

World Health Organization. (1981). *International Code of Marketing of Breast-milk Substitutes.* Geneva: WHO. Available at: www.who.int/nutrition/publications/code_english.pdf.

This Code was adopted by a resolution (WHA34.22) of the World Health Assembly in 1981, creating a set of core principles to ensure adequate nutrition for infants across the world by protecting and promoting breastfeeding and by ensuring the proper use of breastmilk substitutes, when necessary, on the basis of adequate information and through appropriate marketing and distribution.

World Health Organization. (1989). *Protecting, promoting and supporting breast-feeding: the special role of maternity services. A Joint WHO/UNICEF Statement.* Geneva: WHO.

This is a useful historical reference source that first sets out the 10 steps for successful breastfeeding, which subsequently formed the basis of the global Baby Friendly Hospital Initiative, making recommendations concerning the structure and function of maternity/healthcare services.

USEFUL WEBSITES

Association of Breastfeeding Mothers: https://abm.me.uk/

Baby Feeding Law Group: www.bflg-uk.org/

Baby Milk Action: www.babymilkaction.org/

Breastfeeding Network: www.breastfeedingnetwork.org.uk/

British HIV Association (BHIVA): www.bhiva.org/

Cleft Lip And Palate Association (CLAPA): www.clapa.com/

European Food Safety Authority: www.efsa.europa.eu/

First Steps Nutrition: www.firststepsnutrition.org/

Healthy Start Initiative: www.healthystart.nhs.uk/

La Leche League: www.laleche.org.uk/

Royal College of Paediatrics and Child Health: www.rcpch.ac.uk/

UNICEF UK Baby Friendly Initiative: www.unicef.org.uk/babyfriendly/

World Health Organization: www.who.int/

28

Physiology and Care During the Puerperium

Mary Steen, Karen Jackson, Angela Brown

CHAPTER CONTENTS

There is current evidence that postnatal care is often under-valued and under-resourced, even though it is an important and challenging time for a mother who has recently given birth, her partner and the family. Current postnatal care in the UK can involve several healthcare practitioners. Midwives are the lead health professionals, with support from maternity support workers (MSWs), general practitioners (GPs), health visitors, specialist community public health nurses (SCPHNs) and other practitioners, depending on the mother's individual needs and circumstances. Both public and non-government services can work together to support the mother, father, baby and other family members to cope and adjust following the birth of a new baby. This approach to postnatal care differs from that offered to women in most other high-income countries where the provision for regular contact with midwives as the main healthcare professional responsible for postnatal care is less well defined. Potential postnatal morbidity and in some cases mortality for the mother is discussed in Chapter 29. (Dixon and Schmied 2019; Care Quality Commission, CQC 2019; National Institute for Health and Care Excellence, NICE 2014, 2015; Nursing and Midwifery Council, NMC 2018, 2019).

THE CHAPTER AIMS TO

- review the historical background of postnatal care
- explore the role of the midwife in the assessment and care of women's postnatal health and wellbeing
- review the current evidence for women's general health and wellbeing after childbirth
- discuss contemporary challenges for the provision of maternity care during the postnatal period
- explore fertility awareness and methods of contraception following the birth of a baby
- consider women's and their partners views and experiences of postnatal care.

THE POSTNATAL PERIOD

Following the birth of a baby, placenta and membranes, the newly birthed mother enters a period of physical and emotional/psychological recuperation (Steen 2017; Baddock 2019). Skin-to-skin contact is recommended immediately following birth and during the postnatal period, as there is clear evidence of benefit to the mother and father (Moore et al. 2012; NICE 2014). The *puerperium* starts immediately after birth of the placenta and membranes and continues for approximately 6–8 weeks. In many cultures around the world, 40 days for recuperation is a time-honoured practice (Waugh 2011; Steen 2017). A general expectation is that by 6–8 weeks after birth, a woman's body will have recovered sufficiently from the effects of pregnancy and the process of parturition. However, there has now been recognition that the return to a non-pregnant state of health and wellbeing can take much longer (Bick et al. 2011; World Health Organization, WHO 2013). Some women continue to experience health issues and complications related to childbirth that extend well beyond the 6-week period defined as the early puerperium (WHO 2013) (see Chapter 29). In some cases, healing and recovery can take up to a year following birth Wray and Bick 2012; Steen 2017; Dahlen and Priddis 2019).

Today, the focus is for a midwife to work in partnership with a woman and other care providers to deliver a seamless service and care (NMC 2019). In the UK, the transformation of maternity services is ongoing, following the recommendations of the *National Maternity Review: Better Births* (NHS England 2016). It has been highlighted that women need more opportunities to make choices about their maternity care and receive continuity of care throughout the childbirth continuum (NHS England 2016). Improved postnatal care, including extending the period of postnatal care and introducing community hubs are being implemented in some areas of the UK and evaluation of the impact and women's satisfaction will be reported upon in 2020.

It is envisaged that offering more flexibility to the provision of postnatal care will make a positive impact on the health and wellbeing of women, babies and their families. In addition, the availability of a maternity support worker (MSW) or doula can help some mothers adjust and support midwives to provide individualized postnatal care (Royal College of Midwives, RCM 2016; Bohren et al. 2017).

The quality of postnatal care provided to women and families in the first days and weeks after birth can have a huge impact and affect mothers' and families'
experiences of the transition to parenthood. However, in the present climate, when there is an ever-increasing birth rate, a shortage of midwives and ongoing financial constraints, postnatal care remains a challenging task for maternity service providers.

HISTORICAL BACKGROUND

Postnatal care in the UK has been an integral part of the midwife's role since the beginning of the last century following the introduction of the Midwives Act in 1902. This was instigated by the high maternal mortality rates: the majority of maternal deaths at this time resulting from puerperal infection. However, the more recent leading causes of direct maternal deaths are related to heart disease and incidences of thrombosis, thromboembolism and haemorrhage have been recorded (Knight et al. 2019). However, mental health conditions have been identified as a risk factor for direct maternal deaths and as a consequence, suicide has become a major concern (Knight et al. 2019).

Over time, maternal mortality and morbidity rates have influenced the provision of postnatal care. This led to routine observations, such as temperature, pulse, respirations, blood pressure, breast examination, uterine involution and observation of lochia, being introduced as well as a set pattern of postnatal visits.

Midwives were expected to visit women and their babies twice a day for the first 3 days following birth at home and then daily until day 10, commonly referred to as the 'lying in period' (Leap and Hunter 1993). Further legislation extended the regulatory maximum duration of postnatal care from 10 to 14 days in 1936, and then this was increased to 28 days in 1962. This approach to postnatal care was considered appropriate to meet the needs of women at that time. However, a considerable decline in maternal mortality rates began in the 1930s and has continued up to the present day. A traditional pattern and content of postnatal care continued until the 1980s, during which time there had been a shift of the place of birth from the home to the hospital.

In 1986, *selective visiting* in the postnatal period was introduced by the former Professional Statutory Regulatory Body (PSRB), the United Kingdom Central Council (UKCC) For Nursing, Midwifery and Health Visiting, rather than the midwife visiting on specified days (UKCC 1986). This was essentially to meet the service demands of women returning home much sooner after having given birth. A postal survey undertaken in England in 1991 reported that most maternity services had changed from the daily home visits up to the 10th postnatal day to selective home visits, but there was wide variation in patterns of selective visiting (Garcia et al. 1994). This was probably as a result of there being little guidance as to how to plan and implement this change, including there being no evaluation with regard to the implications this would have for the women. A House of Commons Health Committee report (Winterton 1992) highlighted that postnatal care was neglected, with a distinct lack of research in this area. This was followed by the establishment of the Expert Maternity Committee, whose remit was to examine policy and make recommendations for the maternity services in England and Wales. Their report *Changing Childbirth* (Department of Health, DH 1993) recommended that the maternity services should offer women more choice, greater continuity of care and more involvement and control in the planning of their care, which should be midwifery-led. The *Maternity Matters* report (DH 2007) further affirmed these recommendations.

In the present day, a partnership approach, where the woman is encouraged to explore how she is feeling physically and emotionally and to seek the advice and support of the midwife, is advocated (Steen 2017; NMC 2019). The importance of all newly birthed mothers having access to postnatal care that will meet their individual needs is underpinned by the NMC (2019) Standards of Proficiency for midwives and by the national quality standard defining core care, and what should be provided for the mother and baby in the days and weeks following birth (NICE 2015, 2017).

FRAMEWORK AND REGULATION FOR POSTNATAL CARE

The initial framework for hospital postnatal care in the early 20th century involved a regimented approach with the newly birthed mother being viewed as a patient; a period of prescribed bed rest, compliance with hospital regimens such as vulval swabbing, binding of legs and separation from her baby were thus routine procedures. Renfrew (2010) describes how mothers in the late 1970s and early 1980s remained in postnatal wards for a week or more after birth and their babies kept in nurseries with their feeds timed and measured, regardless of whether they were being breastfed or formula-fed. In the 1990s, the provision of postnatal care was reviewed with regard to its content, purpose or effectiveness (Marsh and Sargent 1991; Garcia and Marchant 1993; Twaddle et al. 1993); this led to research investigating and challenging

regimented and ritual patterns of postnatal care (Shaw et al. 2006; Wray 2006; Goodwin et al. 2018). Length of postnatal stay in hospital has since significantly decreased with a movement towards de-medicalization of childbirth (Gibbon and Steen 2012; Goodwin et al. 2018).

It is now acceptable practice for healthy mothers and babies to return home a few hours after the birth and by the 3rd day, the majority of women will have returned home to be cared for by a community midwife. Early transfer home enables the newly birthed mother to recuperate in her own familiar surroundings with the support of her family and friends. In addition, the introduction of digital resources provided via *NHS Choices* and the availability of maternity mobile Apps that will provide important user-friendly information relating to postnatal care to be recommended by the NHS, are evolving (NHS England 2018).

MIDWIVES AND POSTNATAL CARE

It is vitally important that midwives have the knowledge and skills to determine when to be proactive and undertake specific observations when there are indications to do so. Therefore, the midwife needs to be able to acknowledge and recognize what are the expected physiological outcomes following birth. Furthermore, being able to identify signs of what is not normal and when to instigate care that will necessitate investigation, tests and the support of other health professionals, is essential. It is the midwives' responsibility to ensure they remain proficient and able to undertake any further necessary education and training if required to provide extended care (NMC 2018, 2019) (Box 28.1).

Public Health Care

It has long been recognized that poverty and being socially disadvantaged in society leads to increased risk of poor health and wellbeing (Hart 1971; Acheson 1998). In England, at the beginning of the 21st century, the Department of Health acknowledged that the key in providing healthy babies a healthy start in life was **healthy mothers** (DH 2004). This essential message prevails and it is important that mothers and their family members receive information and advice about healthy lifestyles; indeed the NHS Long Term Plan policy in the UK highlights new emphasis on targeting smoking, alcohol and the mental health of both new mothers and fathers (NHS England 2019a). Midwives have a vital role to address public health targets and are ideally placed to promote healthy lifestyles to the mother, her partner and extended family during the postnatal period. However, midwives cannot address public

---

BOX 28.1   The Standards for Proficiency for Midwives (NMC 2019)

The standards of proficiency specify the knowledge, understanding and skills that midwives must demonstrate at the point of qualification when caring for women across the maternity journey, newborn infants, partners and families across all care settings. They reflect what the public can expect *ALL* midwives to know and be able to do, in order to deliver safe, effective, respectful, kind, compassionate, person-centred midwifery care.

The standards of proficiency are grouped under six Domains that are interrelated and build on each other:

- **Domain 1**: *Being an accountable, autonomous, professional midwife:*

Midwives are fully accountable as the lead professional for the care and support of childbearing women and newborn infants. Respecting human rights, they work in partnership with women, enabling their views, preferences, and decisions, and helping to strengthen their capabilities. They promote safe and effective care, drawing on the best available evidence at all times They communicate effectively and with kindness and compassion.

- **Domain 2:** *Safe and effective midwifery care: promoting and providing continuity of care and carer:*

Midwives promote continuity of care, and work across the continuum from pre-pregnancy, labour and birth, postpartum and the early weeks of the newborn infant's life. They work in the woman's home, hospitals, the community, midwifery-led units and all other environments where women require care by midwives. The midwife is responsible for creating an environment that is safe, respectful, kind, nurturing and empowering, ensuring that the woman's experience of care during her whole maternity journey is seamless.

- **Domain 3:** *Universal care for all women and newborn infants:*

Midwives work in partnership with women to care for and support all childbearing women, newborn infants and their families. They make an important contribution to population health, promoting psychological and physical health and wellbeing. Midwives optimise normal physiological processes, and support safe psychological, social, cultural and spiritual situations, working to promote positive outcomes and to anticipate and prevent complications.

- **Domain 4:** *Additional care for women and newborn infants with complications:*

Midwives are ideally placed to recognize any changes that may lead to complications. The midwife is responsible for immediate emergency response and first-line management and in ensuring timely collaboration with and referral to interdisciplinary and multiagency colleagues. The midwife has specific responsibility for continuity and coordination of care, providing ongoing midwifery care as part of the interdisciplinary team, and acting as an advocate for women and newborn infants to ensure that they are always the focus of care.

- **Domain 5:** *Promoting excellence: the midwife as colleague, scholar and leader:*

Midwives make a critically important contribution to the quality and safety of maternity care, avoiding harm and promoting positive outcomes and experiences. They play a leading role in enabling effective team working, promoting continuous improvement. Midwives recognize their own strengths as well as the strength of others. They take responsibility for engaging in continuing professional development and know how they can support and supervise others, including students and colleagues. They recognize that their careers may develop in practice, education, research, management, leadership and policy settings.

- **Domain 6:** *The midwife as skilled practitioner:*

Midwives are skilled, autonomous practitioners who apply knowledge safely and effectively, to optimize outcomes for all women and newborn infants. They combine clinical knowledge, understanding, skills and interpersonal and cultural competence, to provide quality care that is tailored to individual circumstances. They assess, plan, provide and evaluate care in partnership with women, referring to and collaborating with other health and social care professionals as needed. They continue to enhance their midwifery practice for the benefit of women, newborn infants, partners and families.

Nursing and Midwifery Council. (2019) Standards of proficiency for midwives. London: NMC. Available at: https://www.nmc.org.uk/globalassets/sitedocuments/standards/standards-of-proficiency-for-midwives.pdf.

---

health issues alone and working collaboratively with other health and social care professionals and local communities, including the signposting to other essential services, needs to be more effective. Models of care to give more intense care and support to disadvantaged groups have been developed, such as Sure Start Children's Centres (a statutory requirement under the Apprenticeships, Skills, Children and Learning Act, Section 198; Her Majesty's Government 2009; Department for Education, DE 2013). These centres were originally set up to provide accessible community-based services including family healthcare and parenting skills delivered by midwives and health visitors with support from other professionals that would enable families with children and young people up to the age of

19 to improve their health and wellbeing (Bate and Foster 2017).Targets were linked to public health issues such as smoking cessation, breastfeeding rates, particularly aimed at reaching disadvantaged groups.

Positive benefits for mothers and their families who lived within the designated postcode for Children's Centre services have been reported (Tanner et al. 2012). A sustained continued commitment from local authorities to provide ongoing funding and services to meet local needs to benefit mothers and their families is not without its challenges affecting the functioning of some Children's Centres (Bate and Foster 2017). However, the introduction of community hubs and additional funding for early adaptors for the implementation of the 'Better Births' initiative (NHS England 2016, 2017) is expected to provide some assistance in meeting local needs.

The Provision of and Need for Postnatal Care

It is essential that compassionate midwifery care and support to newly birthed mothers is woman-focused and family-orientated. As underpinned by the common conduct and standards of behaviour set out in The Code (NMC 2018) and Standards of Proficiency for Midwives (NMC 2019), good communication explaining what is considered to be normal physical, emotional/psychological, occurrences during the postnatal period will reassure a mother that she is experiencing a normal physiological process. **Building a trusting and caring relationship** will give a mother the confidence to ask questions when she has concerns or is anxious about her health and wellbeing.

A survey undertaken on behalf of the National Childbirth Trust (NCT) (Bhavani and Newburn 2010) involving 1260 first-time mothers reported that mothers felt that midwives were always or mostly kind and understanding (80%) and treated them with respect (83%). There were still gaps in the provision and satisfaction with regards to postnatal care reported. Only 4% of mothers reported being involved in the development of a postnatal care plan to meet their individual needs as recommended by NICE (2014, 2015). Mothers who had undergone either an operative or surgical procedure to aid their birth were reported to be the least satisfied with their postnatal care. Similar issues have been highlighted by a more recent survey of women's views undertaken by the Care Quality Commission (CQC 2019). Although, these surveys do not represent the whole of the UK maternal population, these do give some insight into women's views and knowledge of where improvements in postnatal care provision should be targeted.

A social model of compassionate care that encompasses the continued observation and monitoring of the health and wellbeing of the mother, father and their baby from the birth and into the postnatal period in the full range of settings, will support both parents to adjust to their new parenting role. Guidance and reassurance is an important aspect of midwifery care. Working in partnership with the parents will assist them to develop confidence in their parenting abilities and caring for their baby. There is growing evidence that when fathers are included, this is beneficial to both the mother's and the baby's health and wellbeing (Steen et al. 2012; Lee et al. 2018; Yuan et al. 2018). Fathers can play an important role in breastfeeding support (Daniele et al. 2018; Dennis et al. 2018) and skin-to-skin contact (SSC) has been found to have a positive impact on babies, on fathers and on family relationships (Shorey et al. 2016).Therefore, it is vital that fathers are included in discussions and pathways of care. Yet, there is also evidence that many fathers feel excluded, unsure and fearful (RCM 2011; Steen et al. 2012). Subsequently, an international collaboration of educators and researchers was set up to gather data and summarize studies that investigate and explore the engagement of fathers and family in maternity care, producing a useful online resource (www.familyincluded.com)

In the UK, it is still usual for a midwife to 'attend' a woman on a regular basis for the first few days following birth, regardless of whether the mother is in hospital or at home. During the course of contact visits, midwifery practice has been to undertake a routine physical examination to assess the new mother's recovery from the birth (Wray and Bick 2012; NMC 2019; Baddock 2019). From an international perspective, this practice is unusual. It is only relatively recently that postnatal home visits, and postnatal support programmes have been initiated in America, Canada and Australia (Boulvain et al. 2004; Peterson et al. 2005; Vernon 2007) and that women in these countries have a recognized need for and their satisfaction with maternity services to be considered (Dixon and Schmied 2019).

A common reference to postnatal services being the 'Cinderella' or the 'Poor cousin' of maternity services has led to repeated reports from women, of poor support, disappointment in the services and in some cases, evidence of negligence as a result of substandard care (Redshaw and Heikkila 2010; Warwick 2017; Dahlen and Priddis, 2019).

The birth of a baby does not attract the same level of funding as the needs of those with long-term conditions or terminal diseases and postnatal care remains fragmented, is seldom individualized and is often inflexible in some areas. However, there has been an increasing awareness that there are important aspects around promoting good health and wellbeing of the newly birthed mother and baby, as this can have implications for the nation's healthcare costs (NICE 2014, 2015; NHS England 2018). It is important that at each postnatal contact the midwife should provide the mother with information and advice (NICE 2014) to enable them to:

- assess their baby's general condition
- identify signs and symptoms of common health problems
- contact a healthcare professional or emergency service if required.

Postnatal Contact, Visits and Support

In the UK, the midwife is the main provider of postnatal care for the majority of women, which can take place in a range of settings such as the woman's/a relative's home or in postnatal clinics/community hubs. Expectations of mothers about the purpose of home visits by the midwife may vary according to their cultural backgrounds and individual needs. Some faiths hold important ceremonies for the newborn baby and a home visit from a midwife will need to be mutually arranged to fit around these. Newly birthed mothers who have experienced motherhood before may feel that they need minimal support from a midwife and this can also be mutually arranged. In contrast, a first-time mother or a mother who has had complications will more likely require further support and additional contact.

If financially able, a woman may choose to employ a *doula* to provide valuable physical, emotional and social support and help her during her transition to motherhood. Employing a doula is common practice in Norway and is increasingly becoming more popular in the UK.

The concept of postnatal care is one that aims to assist the mother, her baby and family towards attaining an optimum health and wellbeing status. Where the visit from the midwife can be seen as supportive and helpful to the mother and her family, this purpose is more likely to be achieved. There is however, limited research that has explored the experiences of women from different ethnic backgrounds although an earlier study demonstrated marked inequalities in both the provision of services as well as the actual direct contact with caregivers (Hirst and Hewison 2002). When midwifery postnatal care is extended, there is greater opportunity for midwives to continue midwifery support where this might be appropriate (NHS England 2018).

In many areas of maternity care, maternity support workers (MSWs) are employed to undertake certain aspects of care that have been previously the role of the midwife. This can involve undertaking postnatal visits and providing breastfeeding support. While it is expected the MSW is educated and trained for such activities, there is no nationally agreed role and concern has been expressed regarding this lack of clarity that could affect the safety and professional accountability of midwives if they delegate the MSW inappropriate tasks (Hussain and Marshall 2011; Lindsay 2014; RCM 2016). As the role suggests, the MSW is to *support* the midwife and should therefore **not** be employed as a substitute for the midwife. *When care is undertaken by the MSW, the midwife is always the lead accountable professional.*

It is usual that a health visitor (Specialist Community Public Health Nurse, SCPHN) will attend the mother during the postnatal period, having already made contact during pregnancy. There should always be clear communication between the midwife and health visitor should these visits commence before the midwife discharges the mother and baby from maternity care to ensure the care and advice is consistent. The particular role of the health visitor is focused on reducing inequalities in health and promoting health working in partnership with members of the multiprofessional team and community agencies. The health visitor maintains contact with the family until the child reaches school age. Family nurse practitioners (FNPs) can also offer further support in some deprived areas.

PHYSIOLOGICAL CHANGES AND OBSERVATIONS

The postnatal period is often termed the *fourth stage of labour* and it has three distinct but continuous phases (Romano et al. 2010) as shown in Table 28.1.

Regardless of place of birth, the midwife is primarily concerned with the observation of the health of the newly birthed mother and her baby. As such, it has been common practice to have an overall framework upon which to base the assessment of the mother's state of health and for the observations contained within the examination to link with pre-stated categories in the postnatal midwifery records. This formalized approach to the postnatal review might be an appropriate tool to use if there is concern about a woman who is feeling unwell and there is a need for a comprehensive picture of the woman's state of health and wellbeing (see Chapters 15 and 29). Where this is not the case, such an approach might be less useful from the viewpoint of the needs of a healthy woman who has recently given birth (Redshaw and Heikkila 2010; Steen 2017). The concern focuses on whether in the time taken to complete

TABLE 28.1	**The Three Phases of the Postnatal Period**	
The initial phase: *acute period*	The first 6–12 h	• a time of rapid change • potential for immediate crises such as postpartum haemorrhage, uterine inversion, amniotic fluid embolism and eclampsia
The second phase: *subacute postpartum period*	Lasting 2–6 weeks	• changes are less rapid • body undergoes major changes in terms of haemodynamics, genitourinary recovery, metabolism and emotional status
The third phase: *delayed postpartum period*	Can last up to 6 months	• changes are extremely gradual • pathology is rare

a 'holistic top to toe' examination as a thorough review of someone who is generally well, the midwife might ignore or give less attention to what the mother really wants to talk about (Steen 2017). However, Wray (2011) highlights that women wish to be physically checked over as a means of receiving contact and feedback from the midwife about their bodies and recovery separate from that of their baby.

The skill of the midwife's care is to achieve a balance when deciding which observations are appropriate so that they do not fail to detect potential aspects of morbidity. The following section of this chapter identifies areas of physiology that are likely either to cause women the most anxiety or to have the greatest outcome with regard to morbidity. These descriptions relate to observations undertaken for women who have had vaginal births and uncomplicated pregnancies.

Returning to the Non-Pregnant Status

During the puerperium, all body systems of the mother gradually adjust from the pregnant state back to the pre-pregnant state. Mothers go through a transitional period and the period of physiological adjustment and recovery following birth is closely related to her overall health status. The intricate relationships between physiological, emotional/psychological and cultural and sociological factors are all encompassed in the scope of caring for the postnatal woman and her newborn (Steen 2017; Baddock 2019).

Vital Signs: General Health and Wellbeing

The following information is based on the premise that the midwife is exploring the health of the postnatal woman from a viewpoint of confirming normality. *Common sense*, although a concept that is very difficult to define, is probably a well-understood paradigm and taking such an approach is an important part of midwifery care with regard to addressing the issues that are visible before seeking out the less obvious. In this instance, an overall assessment of the woman's physical appearance prior to continuing any further investigation for her or her baby, will add considerably to the care that will subsequently be undertaken.

Observations of temperature, pulse and respiration

During the first 6 h, postnatal care observations to record vital signs of temperature, pulse and respiration (TPR) will need to be taken and these should be within a normal range before a woman returns home if she has opted for an early transfer. A Modified Early Obstetric Warning Score (MEOWS) is utilized in some maternity units (Gibbon and Steen 2012; Knight et al. 2019). If the woman has had a home birth, the midwife must not leave the new mother's home until she is satisfied that her vital signs are stable (Gibbon and Steen 2012).

It is not necessary to undertake observations of temperature routinely for women who appear to be physically well and who do not complain of any symptoms that could be associated with an infection. However, where the woman complains of feeling unwell with flu-like symptoms, or there are signs of possible infection or an association with a potential environment for infection, the midwife should undertake and record the mother's temperature. This will enhance the amount of clinical information available where further decisions about potential morbidity may need to be made.

Making a note of the pulse rate is probably one of the least invasive and most cost-effective observations a midwife can undertake. If undertaken when seated alongside or at the same level as the woman, it can create positive feelings of care, while also obtaining valuable clinical information. While assessing the pulse rate for a full minute, the midwife can also observe a number of related signs of wellbeing: *the respiratory rate, the overall body temperature, any untoward body odour, skin condition* and the *woman's overall colour and complexion*, as well as listening to what the woman is saying.

Blood pressure

Following the birth of the baby, a baseline recording of the woman's blood pressure (BP) will be made within 6 h of the birth (NICE 2014). In the absence of any previous history of morbidity associated with hypertension, it is usual for the blood pressure to return to a normal range within 24 h following the birth. Routinely undertaking observations of blood pressure without a clinical reason is therefore not required once a baseline recording has been taken.

Circulation

The body has to reabsorb a quantity of excess fluid following the birth and for the majority of women, this results in passing large quantities of urine, particularly in the first day, as diuresis is increased (Cunningham et al. 2005; Steen 2013). Women may also experience oedema of their ankles and feet, which may be greater than that experienced in pregnancy. These are variations of normal physiological processes and should resolve within the puerperal timescale as the woman's activity levels also increase. Advice should be related to taking reasonable exercise, avoiding standing for long periods and elevating the feet and legs when sitting where possible. Swollen ankles should be bilateral and not accompanied by pain; the midwife should particularly observe if this is present in one calf only, which could indicate pathology associated with a deep vein thrombosis (Steen 2017).

Skin and nutrition

Women who have experienced urticaria of pregnancy or cholestasis of the liver should achieve relief following the birth of the baby. The pace of life once the baby is born can lead to women having a reduced fluid intake or eating a different diet than they had formerly (Steen 2017). This in turn might affect their skin and overall physiological state. Women should be encouraged to maintain a balanced fluid intake and a diet that has a greater proportion of fresh food in it (Steen et al. 2017; Othman et al. 2018). This will improve gastrointestinal activity, the absorption of iron and minerals and reduce the potential for constipation and feelings of fatigue.

Breast care

It is essential that midwives offer support and advice on common breast and breastfeeding problems. With a woman's permission, a midwife should examine the woman's breasts for any physical problems such as engorgement, cracked or bleeding nipples, mastitis, or signs of thrush. Engorgement on the 3rd to 4th postnatal day is a common problem for most mothers, regardless of whether they have chosen to breastfeed or formula-feed their babies. It is important that mothers are made aware of this in the antenatal period, so it does not come as a complete surprise to the woman. If breastfeeding and the breasts become engorged, the midwife should advise the mother to feed on demand, perform breast massage from under her axilla and towards the nipple, to hand express the milk, take analgesia as required and to wear a well-fitting bra. (Chapter 27 discusses optimal infant feeding and Chapter 29 explores complications in the puerperium.)

The uterus

Once the baby is born, oxytocin is secreted from the posterior lobe of the pituitary gland to act upon the uterine muscle and assist separation of the placenta. Following the birth of the placenta and membranes, the uterine cavity collapses inwards; the now opposed walls of the uterus compress the newly exposed placental site and effectively seal the exposed ends of the major blood vessels. The muscle layers of the myometrium act as *living ligatures* that compress the large sinuses of the blood vessels exposed by placental separation. These occlude the exposed ends of the large blood vessels and contribute further to reducing blood loss. In addition, vasoconstriction in the overall blood supply to the uterus results in the tissues receiving a reduced blood supply; therefore, deoxygenation and a state of ischaemia arise. Through the process of autolysis, autodigestion of the ischaemic muscle fibres occurs by proteolytic enzymes, resulting in an overall reduction in their size. There is phagocytic action of polymorphs and macrophages in the blood and lymphatic systems upon the waste products of autolysis, which are then excreted via the renal system in the urine. Coagulation takes place through platelet aggregation and the release of thromboplastin and fibrin (Cunningham et al. 2005; Stables and Rankin 2017). What remains of the inner surface of the uterine lining apart from the placental site, regenerates rapidly to produce a covering of epithelium. Partial coverage occurs within 7–10 days after the birth and total coverage is complete by 2–3 weeks after the birth of the baby (Cunningham et al. 2005; Stables and Rankin 2017).

Once the placenta has separated, the circulating levels of oestrogen, progesterone, human chorionic gonadotrophin (HCG) and human placental lactogen (HPL) are reduced. This leads to further physiological changes in muscle and connective tissues, as well as having a major influence on the secretion of prolactin from the anterior lobe of the pituitary gland.

Abdominal palpation (*anthropometry*) of the uterus is usually performed soon after placental expulsion to

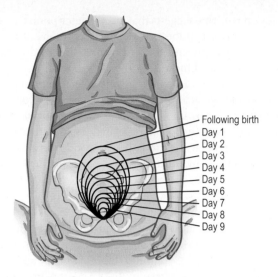

Following birth
Day 1
Day 2
Day 3
Day 4
Day 5
Day 6
Day 7
Day 8
Day 9

Fig. 28.1 The daily progress of the involution process.

ensure that the physiological processes are beginning to take place (see Chapter 21). On abdominal palpation, the fundus of the uterus should be located centrally, its position being at the same level or slightly below the umbilicus, and should be in a state of contraction, feeling firm under the palpating hand. The woman may experience some uterine or abdominal discomfort, especially where uterotonic drugs have been administered to augment the physiological process (Steen 2017).

Uterine involution. The *process of involution* is essential for midwives to understand in order to assess and monitor the physiological process of the return of the uterus to its non-pregnant state (Fig. 28.1). Involution involves the gradual return and reduction in size of the uterus to a pelvic organ until it is no longer palpable above the symphysis pubis (Stables and Rankin 2017). This process is usually assessed by measuring the symphysio-fundal height (S-FH). This is the distance from the top of the uterine fundus to the symphysis pubis and is commonly assessed by abdominal palpation (Bick et al. 2009). NICE (2014) has concluded that there is insufficient evidence to recommend the routine measurement of fundal height and how often this should take place as the process of involution is highly variable between individual women. Therefore, involution of the uterus should be placed into context alongside the colour, amount and duration of the woman's vaginal fluid loss and her general state of health at that time. Uterine involution in combination with other observations such as a raised or lowered temperature abdominal tenderness and offensive lochia can be helpful to detect

maternal morbidity, such as sepsis (Royal College of Obstetricians and Gynaecologists, RCOG 2012). (See also Chapter 25.)

Assessment of postpartum uterine involution. There are several aspects to the abdominal palpation of the postpartum uterus that contribute to the observation as a whole. The first is to identify height and location of the fundus (the upper parameter of the uterus). Assessment should then be made of the condition of the uterus with regard to uterine muscle contraction and finally whether palpation of the uterus causes the woman any pain. When all these dimensions are combined, this provides an overall assessment of the state of the uterus and the progress of uterine involution can be described. Findings from such an assessment should clearly record the *position of the uterus* in relation to the umbilicus or the symphysis pubis, *the state of uterine contraction* and the *presence of any pain during palpation*. A suggested approach to how this is undertaken in clinical practice can be found in Box 28.2.

BOX 28.2 Suggested Approach to Undertaking Postnatal Assessment of Uterine Involution

- Discuss the need for uterine assessment with the woman and obtain her agreement to proceed. She should have emptied her bladder within the previous 30 min.
- Ensure privacy and an environment where the woman can lie down on her back with her head supported. Locate a covering to put over her lower body.
- Ensure your hands are clean and warm and assist the woman to expose her abdomen as necessary; the assessment **should not** be undertaken through the woman's clothing.
- Place the lower edge of your hand at the umbilical area and gently palpate inwards towards the spine until the uterine fundus is located.
- The fundus is palpated to assess its location and the degree of uterine contraction, noting any pain or tenderness.
- Once the assessment is complete, assist the woman to sit up and dress as necessary.
- Ask the woman about the colour and amount of her vaginal loss and whether she has passed any clots or if she has any concerns about the loss.
- Following the assessment, inform the woman of what you have found and of any further action that may be required.
- Record all the details of the assessment in the woman's maternity records.

Afterpains. 'Afterpains' are caused by involutionary contractions and usually last for 2–3 days after the birth of the baby. These cramping types of pains are more commonly associated with multiparity and breastfeeding. The production of the oxytocin in relation to the let-down response that initiates the contraction in the uterus, results in the woman experiencing pain. Women have described the pain as equal to the severity of moderate labour pains, with some requiring analgesia (Marchant et al. 2002; Jangsten et al. 2011). A systematic review concluded that nonsteroidal anti-inflammatory drugs (NSAIDs) were better than placebos at relieving afterpains and NSAIDs were better than paracetamol, but there were insufficient data to make conclusions regarding the effectiveness of opioids at relieving afterpains (Deussen et al. 2011).

It is helpful to explain the cause of afterpains to women and that they might experience a heavier loss at this time, even to the extent of passing clots. Pain in the uterus that is constant or present on abdominal palpation is unlikely to be associated with afterpains and further enquiry should be made about this. Women might also confuse afterpains with flatus pain, especially after an operative birth or where they are constipated. Identifying and treating the cause is likely to relieve the symptoms or raise concern about a more complex condition that requires further investigation.

Postpartum vaginal blood loss. Blood products constitute the major part of the vaginal loss immediately after the birth of the baby and expulsion of the placenta and membranes. As involution progresses, the vaginal loss reflects this and changes from a predominantly fresh blood loss to one that contains stale blood products, lanugo, vernix casseosa and other debris from the redundant products of the conception. This loss varies from woman to woman, being a lighter or darker colour, but for any woman the shade and density tends to be consistent (Marchant et al. 2002).

Lochia is a Latin word traditionally used to describe the vaginal loss following the birth (Cunningham et al. 2005). Medical and midwifery textbooks have described three phases of lochia and have given the duration over which these phases persist. Research has explored the relevance of these descriptions for women and raised questions about the use of these descriptions in clinical practice. Marchant et al. (2002) reported that not all women are aware they will have a vaginal blood loss after the birth and that this loss can range widely in terms of the colour, amount and duration in the first 12 weeks following the

baby's birth. This suggests that overall descriptions of normality ascribed to the traditional descriptions of lochia are outdated and unhelpful to women and midwives in accurately describing a clinical observation.

Most women can clearly identify the colour and consistency of vaginal loss if asked and will be able to describe any changes. It is important for a midwife to ask direct questions about the woman's vaginal loss: whether this is more or less, lighter or darker than previously and whether the woman has any concerns. It is of particular importance to record any clots passed and when these occurred. Clots can be associated with future episodes of excessive or prolonged postpartum bleeding (see Chapter 29).

Assessment that attempts to quantify the amount of loss or the size of clot is problematic. However, the use of descriptions that are common to both woman and midwife can improve accuracy in these assessments, such as asking the mother how often she has to change her maternity pad and describing her blood loss in her own words.

Continence after birth

The majority of women will revert back to their non-pregnant status during the puerperium without any major urinary or bowel problems. Any minor changes to women's urinary and bowel habits should resolve within the first few days of giving birth. Women suffering from perineal injury may need extra reassurance that having their bowels open may be uncomfortable but will not disrupt and dislodge any stitches in the perineal region (see Chapter 17). A systematic review has reported that there is sufficient evidence to suggest that pelvic floor exercise training during pregnancy and after birth can prevent and treat urinary incontinence (Mørkved and Bø 2013). NICE (2014) recommends that pelvic floor muscle exercises should be taught as first line treatment for urinary incontinence.

It is important that women are given opportunities to discuss any urinary or bowel problems at each visit as these are often considered taboo subjects. Some women may find such subject matter as embarrassing and will not seek help and advice, while others may put up with urinary and bowel problems believing that it is an accepted outcome following childbirth. Therefore, it is essential that a midwife builds a trusting, caring relationship to encourage every woman to disclose any urinary or bowel problems.

Usually, urinary and bowel symptoms resolve within the first 2 weeks following birth but some problems do persist. If a woman continues to notice a change to her pre-pregnant urinary and bowel pattern by the end of the puerperal period, they should be advised to have this reviewed (Steen 2013). Initially, conservative management is advocated and then if the symptoms are persistent, a referral to a specialist may be required (Gerrard and ten Hove 2013) (see Chapter 29).

Perineal trauma

Perineal and vaginal injury during childbirth continues to affect the majority of women (East et al. 2012a; Steen and Diaz 2018). Morbidity associated with perineal injury and repair is a major health problem for women throughout the world. It is well reported that perineal trauma can have long-term social, psychological and physical health consequences for women with the associated pain and discomfort disrupting breastfeeding, family life and sexual relationships (Priddis et al. 2014; Webb et al. 2014).

It is important that midwives are educated and trained to recognize the extent of perineal and vaginal trauma, and, have gained the confidence and clinical skills to suture competently, as failure to do so can contribute to negative consequences for women in both the short and long term (Steen 2010; Webb et al. 2014; RCOG 2015; Steen and Diaz 2018). In addition, it is important to consider how to alleviate the associated pain and discomfort attributed to perineal injuries following birth. Up-to-date knowledge and an understanding of the negative consequences for women will assist midwives in advising women on how to alleviate perineal pain, prevent further trauma and promote healing (see Chapter 17).

Perineal pain. Regardless of whether the birth resulted in actual perineal trauma, women are likely to feel swollen and bruised around the vaginal and perineal tissues for the first few days after a vaginal birth. Women who have undergone any degree of actual perineal injury will experience pain for several days until healing takes place (East et al. 2012a; Steen and Diaz 2018). It is essential that women are offered adequate pain relief initially following birth and then for them to be advised on how to alleviate the inflammation associated with perineal injuries and any pain felt during the postnatal period. In the first few days after the birth all women should be asked if they have any pain or discomfort in the perineal area, regardless of whether there is a record of actual perineal trauma (Steen and Diaz 2018; NICE 2014).

Where women appear to have no discomfort or anxieties about their perineum, it is **not essential** for the midwife to examine this area specifically and arguably, it is an intrusion on the woman's privacy to do so. The basic principles of morbidity or infection (Cunningham et al. 2005) indicate that it is unusual for morbidity to occur without inflammation and pain, although these factors are also integral to the healing process (Steen 2007a). Although the perineal area might be causing the woman some discomfort from the original trauma, where this is unchanged or absent, a pathological condition should **not** be developing. There may be occasions, however, where the midwife might consider that the woman is declining this observation because of embarrassment or anxiety. In such cases, the midwife should use her skills of communication to explore whether there is a clinical need for this observation to be undertaken and, if so, to advise the woman accordingly. Examining the perineal area is undertaken to assess healing after birth. Standardized scales to assist the midwife in this assessment are not readily available and formal evaluation appears to be an ongoing neglected area of women's health care (Steen and Diaz 2018). Fortunately, for the majority of women, the perineal wound gradually becomes less painful and initial healing should occur by 10–14 days after the birth (Steen 2007a; Steen and Diaz 2018).

Alleviating perineal pain and discomfort. Evidence suggests that a combination of systemic and localized treatments may be necessary to achieve adequate pain relief, which will meet individual women's needs (Steen and Roberts 2011; Steen and Diaz 2018).

There is some evidence that oral analgesia, bathing, diclofenac suppositories, lignocaine gel and localized cooling treatment can alleviate perineal pain. No adverse effects on healing have been reported when localized cooling is applied (East et al. 2012b; Francisco et al. 2018).

The treatments that appear to achieve pain relief are summarized in Box 28.3.

Tiredness and fatigue

Most women will complain of tiredness and fatigue during the first few weeks following birth (Woolhouse et al. 2014) and lack of sleep at the end of pregnancy, giving birth and establishing feeding can take its toll on the new mother. It is therefore, vitally important that a newly birthed mother is advised to consciously make time to rest and sleep during the postnatal period, taking the opportunity to have a 'nap' during the day when her baby is sleeping and not to feel guilty about doing

> **BOX 28.3 Summary of Methods to Alleviate Postnatal Perineal Pain and Discomfort**
>
> - **Oral analgesia:** self-administered, effective for mild to severe pain, e.g. paracetamol
> - **Bathing**
> - **Diclofenac suppositories:** effective in the first 24–48 h, provides some relief
> - **Lignocaine gel:** effective in the first 48 h
> - **Localized cooling:** crushed ice or gel pads.

this. A midwife may need to reassure a mother that household chores can wait, as it takes time to adjust to caring for a newborn. Tiredness and fatigue can have an adverse effect on a mother's health and wellbeing status. Being tired and fatigued will inevitably have a negative effect on a woman's ability to care for her baby (Troy and Dalgas-Pelish 2003; Steen 2017). Tiredness and fatigue can lead to maternal exhaustion and has been associated with maternal depression (Taylor and Johnson 2010) (see Chapter 30).

Midwives can play a vital role in supporting a woman to have realistic expectations about life after birth and advising her to nurture herself and on the importance of finding time to rest and recuperate as maternal anxiety has been found to be associated with tiredness and fatigue (Taylor and Johnson 2013).

EXPECTATIONS OF HEALTH

It is reasonable for women to expect to regain their body shape for themselves once the baby is born (Steen 2007b; Steen 2017). However, this is not the immediate outcome for many women and, once again, individual women will have their own expectations about the nature and speed at which they would like this recovery to occur. The role of the midwife at this point is to assist the woman to identify actual symptoms of disorder from the gradual process of reorder and advise what action the woman can do for herself in the way of progressive recovery. Advice for new mothers in recovering from the birth is limited and often superficial; also women may feel they should know what to do, or have unrealistic expectations of motherhood and their ability to cope with these new experiences. This is one area where taking the time to talk about, what might seem to the midwife a range of peripheral or even superficial,

issues that might be worrying the otherwise healthy new mother could be of benefit during a visit, rather than the range of routine clinical observations (Redshaw et al. 2013; Steen 2017).

Balancing diet and exercise with rest and relaxation

It is vitally important that women are well nourished during the postnatal period to aid their recovery (Dixon and Schmied 2019). Some mothers can be susceptible to what is known as *maternal nutritional depletion* that can be caused by a lack of micronutrients, frequent pregnancies, lactating and overexertion (Merchant 2015). Therefore, the midwife must be alert and enquire about a woman's diet and eating habits. In addition, there is substantial evidence that suggests exercising during the postnatal period also has many positive effects in combination with eating a healthy diet (Berk 2004; Steen 2007b). Women who exercise regularly are more likely to recover more quickly after the birth, particularly when combined with healthy eating (Amorim Adelegove and Linne 2013).

Exploring a woman's level of activity will encourage a discussion in relation to appropriate exercise and, by association, nutritional intake and rest or relaxation and sleep. Furthermore, undertaking regular pelvic floor exercises is of benefit to women's long-term health (Mørkved and Bø 2013).

Future Health, Future Fertility

Advice on managing fertility is within the sphere of practice of the midwife and it is an important aspect of postpartum care. Midwives need to be aware of a range of different needs with regard to women's sexuality and should be able to offer sensitive and appropriate advice on contraception where this is needed.

FERTILITY AWARENESS (NATURAL FAMILY PLANNING)

The study of fertility awareness, previously (and sometimes still) referred to as *natural family planning*, is a fascinating observation of the way in which the female body works to produce the optimum conditions for conception. According to UK Medical Eligibility Criteria for Contraceptive Use (Faculty of Sexual and Reproductive Healthcare Clinical Effectiveness Unit, FSRH 2016), natural family planning includes all the methods of contraception based on the identification of the fertile time in the menstrual cycle. The effectiveness of these methods depends on accurately identifying the fertile time and modifying sexual behaviour. If used according to teaching and instruction and depending on the method used, natural family planning can be up to 99% effective (Family Planning Association, FPA 2014). To avoid pregnancy, the couple can either abstain from sexual intercourse or use a barrier method of contraception during the fertile time. Natural methods are attractive to couples who do not wish to use hormonal or mechanical methods of contraception. The midwife can provide the appropriate FPA leaflet, signpost the couple to the local contraception clinic or find local information on fertility awareness and available education from the website: www.fertilityuk.org.

The method can also be used as a guide to women wishing to become pregnant, by concentrating sexual intercourse on the days they are most fertile. The fertile time lasts around 8–9 days of each menstrual cycle. The oocyte survives for up to 24 h, however the FPA (2014) suggests that a second oocyte could, occasionally, be released within 24 h of the first. In addition, FPA (2014) state that as a sperm can live inside a female body for up to 7 days, this means that should sexual intercourse occur 7 days before ovulation, a pregnancy could result.

Fertility Awareness Methods

Physiological signs of fertility are:

- cervical secretions (Billings or ovulation method)
- basal body (waking) temperature
- cervical palpation
- calendar calculation.

Cervical secretions

Following menstruation, the vagina will become dry. As oestrogen levels rise, the fluid and nutrient content of the secretions increases to facilitate sperm motility, consequently, a sticky white, creamy or opaque secretion is noticed. As ovulation approaches, the secretions become wetter, more transparent and slippery with the appearance of raw egg white and are capable of considerable stretching between the finger and thumb. The last day of the transparent slippery secretions is called the *peak day*, which coincides closely with ovulation (FSRH 2015). Following ovulation, the hormone *progesterone* causes the secretions to thicken forming a plug of mucus in the cervical canal, acting as a barrier to sperm. The secretions will then appear sticky and dry until the next menstrual period.

When practising this method of contraception, the cervical secretions are observed daily. The fertile time starts when secretions are first noticed following menstruation and ends on the third morning after the peak day. If the secretions are used as a single indicator of fertility, the presence of seminal fluid can make observation difficult. Changes in secretions will be affected by seminal fluid, menstrual blood, spermicidal products, vaginal infections and some medications (Guillebaud and MacGregor 2017).

Postnatal considerations. In the first 6 months following childbirth, the majority of women who are fully breastfeeding will be able to rely on the *lactational amenorrhoea method* (LAM) for contraception. Women who wish to continue using natural methods of contraception should begin observing cervical secretions for the last 2 weeks before the LAM criteria will no longer apply (i.e. 5 months and 2 weeks following birth), in order to establish their basic infertile pattern.

Basal body temperature

A woman can calculate her ovulation by recording her temperature immediately on waking each day. Should the woman have arisen during the night, she must take at least 3 h rest before recording her temperature. After ovulation, the hormone progesterone produced by the corpus luteum causes the temperature to rise by about 0.2°C. The temperature remains at this higher level until the next menstrual period. The infertile phase of the menstrual cycle will begin on the 3rd day after the temperature rise has been observed. Temperature can be affected by a number of factors such as infection and certain medications, therefore care needs to be taken when interpreting temperature charts (FPA 2014).

Postnatal considerations. A mother with the demands of a new baby may find difficulty in recording her temperature at the same time every day. Consequently, many women prefer to rely on examining cervical secretions, or combine noting secretions with cervical changes at this time.

Cervical palpation

Changes in the cervix throughout the menstrual cycle can be detected by daily palpation of the cervix by the woman or her partner. After menstruation, the cervix is low, easy to reach, feels firm and dry and the os is closed. As ovulation approaches, the cervix shortens, softens, sits higher in the vagina and the os dilates slightly under the influence of oestrogen.

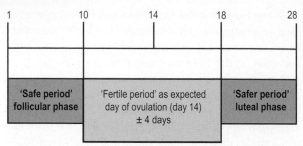

Fig. 28.2 Natural family planning: the fertility awareness (rhythm) method of contraception in a 28-day menstrual cycle.

Postnatal considerations. Hormonal changes in pregnancy take around 12 weeks to settle following the birth of a baby. The cervix will not revert completely to its pre-pregnant state as the os will remain slightly dilated even in the infertile time.

Calendar calculation

The calendar method (Fig. 28.2) is based on observation of the woman's past menstrual cycles. When commencing to use this method, the specialist practitioner and the woman should examine the previous 12 menstrual cycles (FSRH 2015). The shortest and longest cycles over the previous 12 months are used to identify the likely fertile time. The *first fertile day* is calculated by subtracting 20 days from the end of the shortest menstrual cycle. In a 28-day cycle, this would be day 8. The *last fertile day* is calculated by subtracting 10 days from the end of the longest menstrual cycle. In a 28-day cycle, this would be day 18. Cycle length is constantly reassessed and appropriate calculations made. Guillebaud and MacGregor (2017) indicate that the calendar method is not sufficiently reliable to be recommended as a single indicator of fertility, but is useful when combined with other indicators of fertility. Ovulation usually takes place 14 days before the 1st day of the next menstrual period. Therefore a woman who has a 28-day cycle would ovulate on approximately day 14 of her cycle and a woman who has a 30-day cycle would ovulate on approximately day 16 of her cycle.

Postnatal considerations. Calendar calculations must be re-calculated once normal menstruation has recommenced.

Symptothermal method

This is a combination of temperature charting, observing cervical secretions and calendar calculation, with the option of observing cervical palpation in order to identify the most fertile time. Some include in this method, the observation of *ovulation pain* or *Mittelschmerz* and cyclic changes such as breast tenderness but these do not correlate closely with physiological ovulation. Use of more than one indicator increases the accuracy in identification of the **fertile time**. When combining indicators, a couple should avoid sexual intercourse from the first fertile day by calculation, or the first change in the cervix until the 3rd day of elevated temperature, provided all elevated temperatures occur *after* the peak day.

Fertility monitoring device

These handheld computerized devices monitor luteinizing hormone (LH) and oestrone-3-gluronide (a metabolite of oestradiol) through testing the urine. The most well known in the UK is the *'Persona'* monitoring device, which is about 94% effective and will detect from the urine test when a woman is fertile, indicating this through a series of lights. A green light indicates the infertile phase and a red light indicates the fertile phase, when barrier methods **must** be used should sexual intercourse be contemplated. A yellow light indicates that the database requires more information and a further urine test is required.

Postnatal considerations. The fertility monitor is *not* recommended as a method of contraception during lactation. The manufacturers of the *Persona* recommend that a woman has had **two** normal menstruations with cycle lengths from 23 to 35 days before using the monitor at the beginning of the third period (Guillebaud and MacGregor 2017).

Lactational amenorrhoea method

It is thought that the action of the infant suckling at the breast causes neural inputs to the hypothalamus. This results in the inhibition of gonadotrophin release from the anterior pituitary gland, leading to suppression of ovarian activity. The delay in return of postnatal fertility in lactating mothers varies greatly as it depends on patterns of breastfeeding, which are influenced by local culture and socioeconomic status. The time taken for the return of ovulation is directly related to sucking frequency and duration. The maintenance of night-feeds and the introduction of supplementary feeds also affects the return of ovulation.

The LAM is a very effective method of contraception when used according to the Bellagio consensus

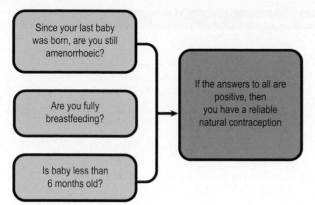

Fig. 28.3 Natural contraception: lactational amenorrhoea method (LAM).

statement (Guillebaud and MacGregor 2017). Research data concludes that there is over 98% protection against pregnancy during the first 6 months following birth if a woman is still amenorrhoeic and fully or almost fully breastfeeding her baby (FPA 2014). In order to confirm that LAM remains effective as a contraceptive method, the woman should be asked if three questions (as indicated in Fig. 28.3) still apply. It has been postulated that mothers who work outside the home can still be considered to be nearly fully breastfeeding, provided they stimulate their breasts by expressing breastmilk several times a day. However, the FSRH (2017) states that expression of milk may reduce the efficacy of using LAM as a contraceptive.

LAM is not recommended for use after 6 months following birth, because of the increased likelihood of ovulation. Studies throughout the world have been conducted on the effectiveness of LAM as a contraceptive, confirming a rate of over 98% protection against pregnancy (Labbok 2016), suggesting it is a viable option for some postnatal breastfeeding mothers.

Overview of Postnatal Contraceptive Methods

An overview of contraceptive methods available to women in the postnatal period is illustrated in Table 28.2.

In addition to the methods shown in Table 28.2, women, who are **not** breastfeeding their babies can use the combined oral contraceptive pill, the contraceptive patch *Evra*, or the vaginal ring *NuvaRing* from day 21 following birth (see Table 28.3). For women who **are** breastfeeding, as these methods may reduce milk production, it is therefore advised that combined contraceptive

methods are *not used* until 6 weeks after giving birth. Other non-oestrogen containing contraceptive methods are recommended, if required up to this 6-week period.

RECORD-KEEPING AND DOCUMENTATION

A midwife has to provide high standards of practice and care at all times (NMC 2019). Clear and accurate records of any observations and discussions that have taken place during the postnatal period are a key tool in safeguarding the health and wellbeing of the mother and her baby. In the Code, the NMC (2018) clearly states that a midwife (and nurse) must keep clear and accurate records (Box 28.4).

Evidence and Best Practice

Every midwife is responsible for ensuring their knowledge is contemporary and their practice is always based on the best available evidence (NMC 2018, 2019). As a consequence, the midwife should gain a considerable amount of information during each contact with the mother and baby. The wide range for normality and the individuality within this can make it difficult for the midwife to decide whether an observation is related to morbidity. It is more likely to be the relationship between several observations that raises cause for concern. Where these observations appear to be more related to variations from the usual physiological processes, the midwife has a responsibility to make appropriate and timely referral to a medical practitioner, such as the GP, or other appropriate healthcare professional (NMC 2018, 2019).

TRANSITION TO PARENTHOOD

The transition to parenthood involves major adjustments within a family and some mothers will welcome and actively seek help and support from a midwife during the postnatal period, but others, for a range of reasons, may not. Women from different cultural backgrounds may have traditions that conflict with the current organization of postnatal care (Ockleford et al. 2004; Steen 2017), or consider that they already have sufficient skills and experience. Not being able to understand or speak English may also prevent a woman from seeking help and support.

Although a visit to the home might have been planned, there will also be times when women are not

TABLE 28.2   Contraceptive Options for Postnatal Women

Contraceptive	When to Use/Fit postnatally	Additional Notes
Barrier methods: (*condom, Femidom*)	As soon as required	If used correctly can be very effective and in addition offers some protection against sexually transmitted infections (STIs). Some vaginal lubrication may be required. Sometimes used with spermicides (although there is no evidence that they are effective against pregnancy or STIs). With perfect use, male condoms are 98% effective, but can be much lower with typical use. With perfect use, the female condom is 95% effective, but can be much lower with typical use.
Diaphragms and caps	6 weeks	They do not interfere with lactation but the device should be refitted postnatally when the uterus has resumed a non-pregnant size. Usually used with spermicides.
Intrauterine contraceptive devices (*IUCDs*)	From 4 weeks (28 days), but can be fitted 48 h after birth	These devices last for 5–10 years depending on the type used, but may cause the menstrual period to be longer, heavier or more painful in some women. If inserted on day 28, additional contraception is required from day 21 until the IUCD is fitted. IUCDs are 99% effective.
The IUS system (*MIRENA* or *Jaydess*)	From 4 weeks (28 days), but can be fitted 48 h after birth	Mirena is licensed for 5 years. Jaydess is a smaller IUS and is licensed for 3 years. Some women experience irregular bleeding but after 3 months, this will normally settle. The menstrual period usually becomes much lighter and shorter; amenorrhoea can also occur. Additional contraception should be used from day 21 until the IUS is fitted. The IUS is over 99% effective.
Implant, e.g. *Nexplanon*	3 weeks (21 days)	Implants are effective for 3 years but cause irregular bleeding in most women during the first year. Nexplanon is over 99% effective.
Contraceptive injection, e.g. *Depo-Provera, Sayana Press*	6 weeks (42 days) if breastfeeding; 3 weeks (21 days) if not breastfeeding	Injections can be given sooner than 6 weeks but can then give rise to heavy irregular bleeding. They are effective for up to 13 weeks. Appointments for injections may be every 12 weeks. Fertility may not return for several months after stopping the injection. Some young women using Depo-Provera long term, may be at risk of osteoporosis. Depo-Provera and Sayana Press are over 99% effective.
Progesterone only pill (*POP/ mini-pill*)	3 weeks (21 days)	The POP/mini-pill has been known to increase milk volume, but it has to be taken at the same time every day. If the pill is commenced on day 21, efficacy is immediate, if taken after day 21 additional contraception should be used. If a pill is taken >3 h late (over 12 h if Cerazette or equivalent), extra precautions must be taken. Some of the hormone may pass into the breastmilk but there is no evidence of adverse effects on the infant. If taken correctly, the POP is 99% effective.

TABLE 28.2	**Contraceptive Options for Postnatal Women—cont'd**	
Contraceptive	**When to Use/Fit postnatally**	**Additional Notes**
Natural family planning methods	As soon as required	May be appropriate for some women on cultural or religious grounds, but extended periods of abstinence may be required as it is more difficult to interpret signs of fertility during breastfeeding.
Lactational amenorrhoea method (*LAM*)	Immediately following birth	LAM is over 98% effective provided that the Bellagio criteria are adhered to, i.e. the baby is fully or almost fully breastfeeding, the baby is <6 months old and the woman is amenorrhoeic. Some researchers recommend regular feeding throughout the day and night for LAM to be most effective.
Vasectomy	Not advisable shortly after birth	Vasectomy is almost 100% effective, but it is considered to be irreversible and some minor side-effects can be experienced.
Female sterilization	Not advisable shortly after birth	Female sterilization is almost 100% effective. This procedure can involve mother–infant separation and anaesthesia can pass into breastmilk causing sedation to the infant. Side-effects of surgery must be considered. General anaesthesia is normally used. The woman needs to be counselled prior to the operation. Consider alternative reversible contraception.
Emergency contraception (*Levonelle, ellaOne, emergency IUCD*)	From 3 weeks (21 days) for Levonelle and ellaOne. From 4 weeks (28 days) for the IUCD	Used following unprotected sexual intercourse or contraceptive failure. Three methods available: progestogen only emergency contraception (Levonelle), ellaOne, any time after day 21, and insertion of IUCD recommended after 28 days due to risk of perforation and expulsion. Levonelle can be used by breastfeeding and non-breastfeeding women. The earlier Levonelle is taken the more effective it is, e.g. if taken within 24 h, it is 95% effective. Can usually be taken up to 72 h following unprotected sexual intercourse (UPSI). **ellaOne is more likely to be used for non–breastfeeding women.** If ellaOne is taken while breastfeeding, breastfeeding must be avoided for a week. Breastmilk must be expressed and discarded for 1 week following administration. ellaOne is thought to be slightly more effective than Levonelle. It can usually be taken up to 120 h following UPSI. **The IUCD can be inserted 5 days (120 h) after unprotected sex or within 5 days of the earliest time an ovum could have been released.** It is almost 100% effective.

at home when the midwife visits. It is important to keep in mind individual circumstances and whether these might have any bearing on a no-access visit. Parents who have a physical disability such as hearing loss or poor mobility may take time to answer a door bell. It is, therefore, important to make arrangements for contact to be made by alternative means, e.g. a visual alarm or telephone to alert the woman of the visit beforehand. An online resource that provides an insight into parents' lived experiences is the Disability, Pregnancy and Parenthood website (listed in Useful websites, below). The midwife can assist parents who have an intellectual

disability to find and access local services available in their community to meet their specific individual needs (Llewellyn and Hindmarsh 2015). The introduction of postnatal clinics/drop-in centres in parts of the UK for maternity services to meet local needs, offers some degree of flexibility around postnatal follow-up care (Gibbon and Steen 2012).

A meta-synthesis has reported that fathers must feel well supported, included and prepared for parenthood themselves, in order to support their partner effectively in achieving a positive parenthood experience (Steen et al. 2012). However, providing antenatal education for

TABLE 28.3   Hormonal Contraception

Contraceptive	When to Use/ Fit Postnatally	Summary
Combined oral contraceptive pill (COC)	3 weeks (21 days)	• Highly effective if taken correctly. • There are a whole range of COCs (i.e. containing oestrogen and progestogen), e.g. Microgynon, Marvelon. • The woman may have a preference if she has taken a COC before which suited her. • If started on day 21, efficacy starts immediately. • If commenced after day 21 post-birth, additional methods, i.e. barrier methods should be used. • If taken correctly, the COC is 99% effective.
Contraceptive patch *Evra*	3 weeks (21 days)	• Recently developed, containing oestrogen and progestogen, this patch is applied to the skin and changed every 7 days. • After 3 weeks, there is a patch-free week where a withdrawal bleed will occur. • The patch-free week should not be extended as contraceptive cover will be lost. • If used correctly, this method of contraception is over 99% effective.
Contraceptive ring *NuvaRing*	3 weeks (21 days)	• Relatively newly developed vaginal ring containing oestrogen and progesterone. • The ring is inserted into the vagina for 3 weeks, removed for 7 days (ring-free week), then a new ring is inserted no more than 7 days later. • If used correctly, this method of contraception is over 99% effective.

BOX 28.4   The Midwife's Record-Keeping

Keep clear and accurate records relevant to your practice. This applies to the records that are relevant to your scope of practice. It includes but is not limited to patient records.

To achieve this you must:

1. Complete records at the time or as soon as possible after an event, recording if the notes are written some time after the event.
2. Identify any risks or problems that have arisen and the steps taken to deal with them, so that colleagues who use the records have all the information they need.
3. Complete records accurately and without any falsification, taking immediate and appropriate action if you become aware that someone has not kept to these requirements.
4. Attribute any entries you make in any paper or electronic records to yourself, making sure they are clearly written, dated and timed, and do not include unnecessary abbreviations, jargon or speculation.
5. Take all steps to make sure that records are kept securely.
6. Collect, treat and store all data and research findings appropriately.

Adapted from the Nursing and Midwifery Council. (2018) The Code: Professional standards of practice and behaviour for nurses, midwives and nursing associates. London: NMC. Available at: www.nmc.org.uk/globalassets/sitedocuments/nmc-publications/nmc-code.pdf.

birth and parenting for all, particularly those parents who are most in need, remains a challenge for maternity services providers as well as midwives to facilitate (see Chapter 9).

Becoming a parent is often a stressful event and can contribute to relationship difficulties and attachments within the family and studies have reported that parents would have benefited from education and being aware of some early warning of challenges they may face as new parents (Deave and Johnson 2008; Steen et al. 2011). The midwife has an important role in supporting both parents during the transition to parenthood as there are clear health and wellbeing benefits for the mother and baby. In addition, the midwife may have an important role with regard to referral and support for women who are in abusive relationships (Steen and Keeling 2012; Steen 2017).

Where there are concerns about the safety or protection of the newborn baby, advice from the local social services and children's centres/community hubs can offer a range of services to assist disadvantaged groups and local communities during the transition to parenthood (see Chapter 2). Family nurse practitioners (FNPs) can also offer further support in some deprived areas. In addition, there is good evidence that new parents benefit from the support that their families, friends and other parents can offer.

THE 6–8 WEEK POSTNATAL EXAMINATION

The role of the GP in postnatal care is usually limited to undertaking the 6–8 week examination that ultimately discharges the women from maternity care. However, the NHS England Standard General Medical Services Contract defines the duration of GP contact as ending on the 14th day after the birth (NHS England 2019b). Bick et al. (2015) highlights that there is evidence the routine 6–8 week postnatal examination does not always meet the needs of women, and recommendations have been made that the content, timing and care provider are reviewed. Furthermore, a wide range of persistent morbidity, including backache, urinary and faecal incontinence, depression, perineal pain and dyspareunia, tend to not be reported to, or identified by, midwives or GPs within postnatal care, causing delay in the woman's recovery from childbirth.

The 6–8 week postnatal examination should be thorough, holistic and include a review of the woman's physical, social and emotional wellbeing and can be undertaken by a healthcare professional with the required proficiency, taking into consideration any screening and medical history (NICE 2014). This would indicate there is the potential for midwives to take on the responsibility for discharging healthy women who have experienced a physiological birth on completion of their maternity care at 6–8 weeks. This would warrant the midwife undertaking additional education and training, such as cervical cytology screening and prescribing contraception (NMC 2018).

The continued surveillance of the new mother and baby by the midwife for up to 6–8 weeks can only but help in improving breastfeeding rates beyond the first few days following birth, as well as being more alert to the early signs of the mother developing a perinatal mental health disorder. Such practice would also support the recommendations of 'Better Births' (NHS England 2016) in facilitating continuity of care and subsequently improve the childbirth experiences of women and their families, albeit not without its challenges to implement throughout the entire maternity services.

REFLECTIVE ACTIVITY FOR SELF-ASSESSMENT

1. What are the processes involved in the involution of the uterus?

    How would you assess that these processes are taking place physiologically following a vaginal birth?

2. Consider the postnatal visiting practice in your locality.

    How does it compare with national guidelines?

3. How are women and their partners prepared and supported in their transition to parenthood by the midwife, other healthcare professionals and voluntary and independent services within the local community of your practice?

    How can this be enhanced?

4. Explain the features/essential criteria of the lactational amenorrhoea method (LAM) to be an effective contraceptive to women following childbirth.

    What advice and support would you give to a couple who choose to use LAM as a medium-term contraceptive?

REFERENCES

Acheson, D. (1998). *Independent inquiry into inequalities in health*. London: HMSO.

Amorim Adelegove, A. R., & Linne, Y. M. (2013). Diet or exercise, or both, for weight reduction in women after childbirth. *Cochrane Database of Systematic Reviews* (7), CD005627.

Baddock, S. (2019). Overview of physiological changes during the postnatal period. In S. Pairman, S. K. Tracy, H. G. Dahlen, & L. Dixon (Eds.), *Midwifery: Preparation for practice Book 2* (4th ed.) (pp. 589–599). Chatswood, NSW: Elsevier.

Bate, A., & Foster, D. (2017). *Sure Start (England). Commons Briefing Paper 7257*. London: House of Commons Library. Available at: https://researchbriefings.files.parliament.uk/documents/CBP-7257/CBP-7257.pdf.

Berk, B. (2004). Recommending exercise during and after pregnancy: what the evidence says. *International Journal of Childbirth Education*, 19(2), 18–22.

Bhavani, V., & Newburn, M. (2010). *Left to your own devices: The postnatal care experiences of 1260 first-time mothers*. London: NCT. Available at: www.nct.org.uk/sites/default/files/related_documents/PostnatalCareSurveyReport5.pdf.

Bick, D., MacArthur, C., & Winter, H. (2009). *Postnatal care: Evidence and guidelines for management* (2nd ed.). Edinburgh: Churchill Livingstone.

Bick, D., Rose, V., Weavers, A., et al. (2011). Improving inpatient postnatal services: midwives views and perspectives of engagement in a quality improvement initiative. *BMC Health Services Research, 11*(1), 293.

Bick, D., MacArthur, C., Knight, M., et al. (2015). Post-pregnancy care: Missed opportunities in the reproductive years. In S. Davies (Ed.), *Annual Report of the Chief Medical Officer 2014. The Health of the 51%: Women.* (pp. 95–107). London: DH. A vailable at: https://assets.publishing.service.gov.uk/government/uploads/system/uploads/attachment_data/file/595439/CMO_annual_report_2014.pdf.

Bohren, M. A., Hofmeyr, G. L., Sakala, C., et al. (2017). Continuous support for women during childbirth. *Cochrane Database of Systematic Reviews* (7), CD003766.

Boulvain, M., Perneger, T. V., Othenin-Girard, V., et al. (2004). Home-based versus hospital-based postnatal care: A randomised trial. *BJOG: An International Journal of Obstetrics and Gynaecology, 111*(8), 807–813.

CQC (Care Quality Commission). (2019). 2018 Survey of women's experiences of maternity care: Statistical release. *NHS patient survey programme.* Available at: www.cqc.org.uk/sites/default/files/20190424_mat18_statisticalrelease.pdf.

Cunningham, F. G., Leveno, K. J., Bloom, S., et al. (2005). *Williams Obstetrics* (22nd ed.). New York: McGraw-Hill Medical, 121–150. 695–710.

Dahlen, H., & Priddis, H. (2019). Perineal care and repair. In S. Pairman, S. K. Tracy, H. G. Dahlen, & L. Dixon (Eds.), *Midwifery: Preparation for practice, Book 2* (4th edn.) (pp. 567–633). Chatswood, NSW: Elsevier.

Daniele, M. A., Ganaba, R., Sarrassat, S., et al. (2018). Involving male partners in maternity care in Burkina Faso: A randomized controlled trial. *Bulletin of the World Health Organisation, 96*(7), 450–461.

Deave, T., & Johnson, D. (2008). The transition to parenthood: What does it mean for fathers? *Journal of Advanced Nursing, 63*(6), 626–633.

Dennis, C. L., Brennenstuhl, S., & Abbass-Dick, J. (2018). Measuring parental breastfeeding self-efficacy: A psychometric evaluation on the Breastfeeding Self-Efficacy Scale-Short Form among fathers. *Midwifery, 64*, 17–22.

Deussen, A. R., Ashwood, P., & Martis, R. (2011). Analgesia for relief of pain due to uterine cramping/involution after birth. *Cochrane Database of Systematic Reviews* (5), CD004908.

DfE (Department for Education). (2013). *Sure Start Children's Centres statutory guidance for local authorities, local health services and Jobcentre Plus.* London: DfE. Available at: https://assets.publishing.service.gov.uk/government/uploads/system/uploads/attachment_data/file/678913/childrens_centre_stat_guidance_april-2013.pdf.

DH (Department of Health). (1993). *Changing childbirth: The Report of the Expert Maternity Group.* London: The Stationery Office.

DH (Department of Health). Department for Education and Skills. (2004) *National Service Framework for children, young people and maternity services core standards: Change for children – every child matters.* London: DH Publications. Available at: https://assets.publishing.service.gov.uk/government/uploads/system/uploads/attachment_data/file/199952/National_Service_Framework_for_Children_Young_People_and_Maternity_Services_-_Core_Standards.pdf.

DH (Department of Health). (2007). *Maternity matters: choice, access and continuity of care in a safe service.* London: DH Publications. Available at: http://familieslink.co.uk/download/july07/Maternity%20matters.pdf.

Dixon, L., & Schmied, V. (2019). Support women becoming mothers. In S. Pairman, S. K. Tracy, H. G. Dahlen, & L. Dixon (Eds.), *Midwifery: Preparation for practice Book 2* (4th ed.) (pp. 600–633). Chatswood, NSW: Elsevier.

East, C. E., Sherburn, M., Nagle, C., et al. (2012a). Perineal pain following childbirth: Prevalence, effects on postnatal recovery and analgesia usage. *Midwifery, 28*(1), 93–97.

East, C. E., Begg, L., Henshall, N. E., et al. (2012b). Local cooling for relieving pain from perineal trauma sustained during childbirth. *Cochrane Database of Systematic Reviews* (5), CD006304.

FSRH. (Faculty of Sexual and Reproductive Healthcare Clinical Effectiveness Unit). (2015). *Fertility awareness methods.* London: FSRH/RCOG.

FSRH. (Faculty of Sexual and Reproductive Healthcare Clinical Effectiveness Unit). (2016). *UK medical eligibility criteria for contraceptive use.* London: FSRH/RCOG (updated 2017).

FSRH. (Faculty of Sexual and Reproductive Healthcare Clinical Effectiveness Unit). (2017). *Contraception after pregnancy.* London: FSRH/RCOG.

FPA (Family Planning Association). (2014). *Your guide to natural family planning: Helping you choose the best method of contraception that is best for you.* London: FPA. Available at: www.fpa.org.uk/sites/default/files/natural-family-planning-your-guide.pdf.

Francisco, A. A., de Oliveira, S. M. J. V., Steen, M., et al. (2018). Ice pack induced perineal analgesia after spontaneous vaginal birth: A randomised controlled trial. *Women and Birth, 31*(5), e334–e340.

Garcia, J., & Marchant, S. (1993). Back to normal? Postpartum health and illness. In *Research and the midwife conference proceedings 1992* (pp. 2–9). Manchester: University of Manchester.

Garcia, J., Renfrew, M., & Marchant, S. (1994). Postnatal home visiting by midwives. *Midwifery, 19*(10), 40–43.

Gibbon, K., & Steen, M. (2012). Postnatal care. Caring for women during a homebirth. In M. Steen (Ed.), *Supporting* women to give birth at home: *A practical guide for midwives* (pp. 148–154). Abingdon: Routledge.

Goodwin, L., Taylor, B., Kokab, F., & Kenyon, S. (2018). Postnatal care in the context of decreasing length of stay in hospital after birth: The perspectives of community midwives. *Midwifery, 60*, 36–40.

Guillebaud, J., & MacGregor, A. (2017). *Contraception: Your questions answered* (7th ed.). Edinburgh: Churchill Livingstone.

Hart, J. T. (1971). The inverse care law. *Lancet, 297*, 405–412.

Hirst, J., & Hewison, J. (2002). Hospital postnatal care: Obtaining the views of Pakistani indigenous 'white' women. *Clinical Effectiveness in Nursing, 6*(1), 10–18.

Her Majesty's Government. (2009). *Apprenticeships, Skills, Children and Learning Act 2009 c.22. s.198 Arrangements for children's centres*. London: The Stationery Office. Available at: www.legislation.gov.uk/ukpga/2009/22/pdfs/ukpga_20090022_en.pdf.

Hussain, C. J., & Marshall, J. E. (2011). The effect of the developing role of the maternity support worker on the professional accountability of the midwife. *Midwifery, 27*, 336–341.

Jangsten, E., Bergh, I., Mattsson, L., et al. (2011). Afterpains: a comparison between active and expectant management of the third stage of labor. *Birth, 38*(4), 294–301.

Knight M, Bunch K, Tuffnell D, et al. (Eds) on behalf of MBRRACE-UK. (2019). *Saving Lives, Improving Mothers' Care – Lessons learned to inform maternity care from the UK and Ireland Confidential Enquiries into Maternal Deaths and Morbidity 2015–2017*. Oxford: National Perinatal Epidemiology Unit, University of Oxford.

Labbok, M. (2016). *The lactational amenorrhoea method (LAM) for postnatal contraception*. Melbourne: Australian Breastfeeding Association. Available at: www.breastfeeding.asn.au/bfinfo/lactational-amenorrhea-method-lam-postpartum-contraception.

Leap, N., & Hunter, B. (1993). *The midwife's tale. An oral history from handywoman to professional midwife*. London: Scarlet Press.

Lee, S. J., Sanchez, D. T., Grogan-Kaylor, A., et al. (2018). Father early engagement behaviors and infant low birth weight. *Maternal and Child Health Journal, 22*(10), 1407–1417.

Lindsay, P. (2014). Maternity support workers and safety in maternity care in England. *Practising Midwife, 17*, 20–23.

Llewellyn, G., & Hindmarsh, G. (2015). Parents with intellectual disability in a population context. *Current Developmental Disorders Report, 2*(2), 119–126.

Marchant, S., Alexander, J., & Garcia, J. (2002). Postnatal vaginal bleeding problems and general practice. *Midwifery, 18*(1), 21–24.

Marsh, J., & Sargent, E. (1991). Factors affecting the duration of postnatal visits. *Midwifery, 7*, 177–182.

Merchant, K. (2015). *Maternal nutritional depletion*. Washington: Policy Research Institute.

Moore, E. R., Anderson, G. C., Bergman, N., et al. (2012). Early skin-to-skin contact for mothers and their healthy newborn infants. *Cochrane Database of Systematic Reviews* (5), CD003519.

Mørkved, S., & Bø, K. (2013). Effect of pelvic floor muscle training during pregnancy and after childbirth on prevention and treatment of urinary incontinence: A systematic review. *British Journal of Sports Medicine, 48*(4), 299–310.

NHS England. (2016). *The National Maternity Review. Better Births. Improving outcomes in maternity services in England: a five year forward view for maternity care*. London: NHS England. Available at: www.england.nhs.uk/wp-content/uploads/2016/02/national-maternity-review-report.pdf.

NHS England. (2017). *Implementing better births. A resource pack for local maternity systems*. London: NHS England. Available at: www.england.nhs.uk/wp-content/uploads/2017/03/nhs-guidance-maternity-services-v1.pdf.

NHS England. (2018). *Maternity Transformation Programme. Update*. Board paper PB.24.05.2018/04. Available at: www.england.nhs.uk/wp-content/uploads/2018/05/04-pb-24-05-2018-maternity-transformation-programme.pdf.

NHS England. (2019a). *Long term plan*. London: NHS England. Available at: www.longtermplan.nhs.uk/wp-content/uploads/2019/01/nhs-long-term-plan-june-2019.pdf.

NHS England. (2019b). *NHS England Standard General Medical Services Contract 2018/2019*. London: NHS England. Available at: www.england.nhs.uk/wp-content/uploads/2019/04/general-medical-services-contract-19-20.pdf.

NICE (National Institute for Health and Care Excellence). (2014). *Postnatal care up to 8 weeks after birth: CG 37*. London: NICE. Available at: www.nice.org.uk/guidance/cg37/resources/postnatal-care-up-to-8-weeks-after-birth-pdf-975391596997.

NICE (National Institute for Health and Care Excellence). (2015). *Postnatal care: QS 37*. London: NICE. Available at: www.nice.org.uk/guidance/qs37/resources/postnatal-care-pdf-2098611282373.

NICE (National Institute for Health and Care Excellence). (2017). *Intrapartum care for healthy women and babies: CG 190*. London: NICE. Available at: www.nice.org.uk/guidance/cg190/resources/intrapartum-care-for-healthy-women-and-babies-pdf-35109866447557.

NMC (Nursing and Midwifery Council). (2018). *The Code: Professional Standards of Practice and Behaviour for Nurses, Midwives and Nursing Associates*. London: NMC. Available at: www.nmc.org.uk/globalassets/sitedocuments/nmc-publications/nmc-code.pdf.

NMC (Nursing and Midwifery Council). (2019). *Standards of Proficiency for Midwives*. London: NMC. Available at: https://www.nmc.org.uk/globalassets/sitedocuments/standards/standards-of-proficiency-for-midwives.pdf.

Ockleford, E. M., Berryman, J. C., & Hsu, R. (2004). Postnatal care: What new mothers say. *British Journal of Midwifery*, 12(3), 166–171.

Othman, S. M. E., Steen, M. P., Jayasekara, R., & Fleet, J. A. (2018). A healthy eating education program for midwives to investigate and explore their knowledge, understanding, and confidence to support pregnant women to eat healthily: Protocol for a mixed-methods study. *JMIR Research Protocols*, 7(5), e143.

Peterson, W. E., Charles, C., DiCenso, A., et al. (2005). The Newcastle satisfaction with nursing scales: A valid measure of maternal satisfaction with inpatient postpartum nursing care. *Journal of Advanced Nursing*, 52(6), 672–681.

Priddis, H., Schmied, V., & Dahlen, H. (2014). Women's experiences following severe perineal trauma: A qualitative study. *BMC Women's Health*, 14, 32.

Romano, M., Cacciatore, A., Giordano, R., & La Rosa, B. (2010). Postpartum period: Three distinct but continuous phases. *Journal of Prenatal Medicine*, 4(2), 22–25.

RCM (Royal College of Midwives). (2011). *Reaching out: Involving fathers in maternity care*. London: RCM. Available at: www.drfogarty.co.uk/FathersGuide.pdf.

RCM (Royal College of Midwives). (2016). *The roles and responsibilities of the maternity support workers*. London: RCM. Available at: www.rcm.org.uk/media/2338/role-responsibilities-maternity-support-workers.pdf.

RCOG (Royal College of Obstetricians and Gynaecologists). (2012). *Bacterial sepsis in pregnancy: Green-top Guideline No 64b*. London: RCOG. Available at: www.rcog.org.uk/globalassets/documents/guidelines/gtg_64a.pdf.

RCOG (Royal College of Obstetricians and Gynaecologists). (2015). *The management of third- and fourth-degree perineal tears. Green-top Guideline No 29*. London: RCOG. Available at: www.rcog.org.uk/globalassets/documents/guidelines/gtg-29.pdf.

Gerrard, J., & ten Hove, R. (2013). *Chartered Society of Physiotherapists and Royal College of Midwives Joint statement on pelvic floor muscle exercises: Improving health outcomes for women following pregnancy and birth*. London: CSP/RCM. Available at: www.csp.org.uk/system/files/csp_rcm_pelvicfloorstatement_2013.pdf.

Redshaw, M., & Heikkila, K. (2010). *Delivered with care: A national survey of women's experience of maternity care 2010*. Oxford: National Perinatal Epidemiology, University of Oxford.

Redshaw, M., Hennegan, J., & Kruske, S. (2013). Holding the baby: Early mother-infant contact after childbirth and outcomes. *Midwifery*, 30(5), e177–e187.

Renfrew, M. J. (2010). Making a difference for women, babies and families. *Evidence-based Midwifery*, 8(2), 40–46.

Shaw, E., Levitt, C., Wong, S., et al. (2006). Systematic review of the literature on postpartum care: Effectiveness of postpartum support to improve maternal parenting, mental health, quality of life and physical health. *Birth*, 33(30), 210–220.

Shorey, S., He, H. G., & Morelius, E. (2016). Skin to skin contact by fathers and the impact on infant and paternal outcomes: An integrative review. *Midwifery*, 40, 207–217.

Stables, D., & Rankin, J. (2017). The puerperium: The mother. In J. Rankin (Ed.), *Physiology in childbearing with anatomy and related biosciences* (4th ed.) (pp. 587–595). Edinburgh: Elsevier.

Steen, M. (2007a). Perineal tears and episiotomy: How do wounds heal? *British Journal of Midwifery*, 15(5), 273–280.

Steen, M. (2007b). Wellbeing and beyond. *Midwives*, 10(3), 116–119.

Steen, M. (2010). Care and consequences of perineal trauma. *British Journal of Midwifery*, 18(6), 358–362.

Steen, M. (2013). Continence in women following childbirth. *Nursing Standard*, 28(1), 47–55.

Steen, M. (2017). Maternal morbidity following childbirth. In S. MacDonald, & G. Johnson (Eds.), *Mayes' Midwifery* (15th ed.) (pp. 1079–1090). Edinburgh: Elsevier.

Steen, M., & Roberts, T. (2011). The consequences of pregnancy and birth for the pelvic floor. *British Journal of Midwifery*, 19(11), 692–698.

Steen, M., & Keeling, J. (2012). STOP! Silent screams. *Practising Midwife*, 15(2), 28–30.

Steen, M., & Diaz, M. (2018). Perineal trauma: A women's health and wellbeing issue. *British Journal of Midwifery*, 26(9), 574–584.

Steen, M., Downe, S., Bamford, N., et al. (2012). 'Not-patient' and 'not-visitor': A metasynthesis of fathers' encounters with pregnancy, birth and maternity care. *Midwifery*, 28(4), 362–371.

Steen, M., Downe, S., & Graham-Kevan, N. (2011). Development of antenatal education to raise awareness of the risk of relationship conflict. *Evidence Based Midwifery*, 8(2), 53–57.

Steen, M., Mottershead, R., Idriss, J., et al. (2017). Diet and eating habits of expectant parents and families in Ras Al Khaimah, Emirates: An exploratory study. *Evidence Based Midwifery*, 15(2), 46–53.

Tanner, E., Agur, M., Hussey, D., et al. (2012). *Evaluation of Children's Centres in England (ECCE): Strand 1: First Survey of Children's Centres in the Most Deprived Areas (Research Report DFE-RR230)*. London: DfE.

Taylor, J., & Johnson, M. (2010). How women manage fatigue after childbirth. *Midwifery*, 26(3), 367–375.

Taylor, J., & Johnson, M. (2013). The role of anxiety and other factors in predicting postnatal fatigue: From birth to 6 months. *Midwifery*, 29(5), 526–534.

Troy, N. A., & Dalgas-Pelish, P. (2003). The effectiveness of a self care intervention for the management of postpartum fatigue. *Applied Nursing Research*, 16(1), 38–45.

Twaddle, S., Liao, X. H., & Fyvie, H. (1993). An evaluation of postnatal care individualised to the needs of the woman. *Midwifery*, 9(3), 154–160.

UKCC. (United Kingdom Central Council). (1986). *United Kingdom Central Council for Nursing, Midwifery and*

Health Visiting. A Midwife's Code of Practice. London: UKCC.

Vernon, D. (Ed.). (2007). *With women: Midwives' experiences: From shift work to continuity of care.* Canberra: Australian College of Midwives.

Warwick. (2017). *Postnatal services are the Cinderella of maternity services say midwives.* RCM Press Release, 4th May 2017. Available at www.rcm.org.uk/media-releases/2017/may/postnatal-services-are-the-cinderella-of-maternity-services-say-midwives.

Waugh, L. J. (2011). Beliefs associated with Mexican immigrant families' practice of la cuarentena during postpartum recovery. *Journal of Obstetric, Gynecologic and Neonatal Nursing, 40*(6), 732–741.

Webb, S., Sherburn, M., & Ismail, K. M. (2014). Managing perineal trauma after childbirth. *British Medical Journal, 349*, g6829, 27–31.

Winterton, N. (1992). *House of Commons Health Committee Second report: Maternity Services, 1.* London: Her Majesty's Stationery Office.

Woolhouse, H., Gartland, D., Perlen, S., et al. (2014). Physical health after childbirth and maternal depression in the first 12 months postpartum: Results of an Australian nulliparous pregnancy cohort study. *Midwifery, 30*(3), 378–384.

Wray, J. (2006). Seeking to explore what matters to women about postnatal care. *British Journal of Midwifery, 14*, 246–254.

Wray, J. (2011). *Bouncing back? An ethnographic study exploring the context of care and recovery after birth through the experiences and voices of mothers.* Unpublished PhD Thesis, Salford, University of Salford.

Wray, J., & Bick, D. (2012). Is there a future for universal midwifery postnatal care in the UK? *MIDIRS Midwifery Digest, 22*(4), 495–498.

WHO (World Health Organization). (2013). *Postnatal care of the mother and newborn.* Geneva: WHO. Available at: https://apps.who.int/iris/bitstream/handle/10665/97603/9789241506649_eng.pdf.

Yuan, L., Gu, Z., Peng, H., & Zhao, L. (2018). A paternal-fetal attachment pilot intervention on mental health for pregnant mothers. *NeuroQuantology, 16*(1), 71–76.

ANNOTATED FURTHER READING

Baston, H., & Hall, J. (2017). *Midwifery essentials: Postnatal.* Edinburgh: Elsevier.

The second edition includes the latest, national and international guidelines and embraces the principles of 'Better Births' in the context of postnatal care. It provides a user-friendly source of information to reflect the latest evidence-base for current postnatal practice. There is focus on the importance of communication and contemporary women-centred care with useful scenarios to encourage debate and reflection among learners.

Guillebaud, J., & MacGregor, A. (2017). *Contraception: Your questions answered* (7th ed.). Edinburgh: Churchill Livingstone.

The latest edition of this book is extremely comprehensive and up-to-date, covering all available contraceptive methods not just available in the UK but worldwide. It is in a question and answer style regarding each particular contraceptive method and provides the best available evidence to guide and support clinical practice.

National Institute for Health and Care Excellence. (2014). *Postnatal care up to 8 weeks after birth: CG 37.* London: NICE. Available at: www.nice.org.uk/guidance/cg37/resources/postnatal-care-up-to-8-weeks-after-birth-pdf-975391596997.

This guideline was originally published in 2006 and was updated in 2014. It covers the routine postnatal care that women and their babies should receive for 6–8 weeks after the birth. Details of the advice on breastfeeding and the management of common and serious health problems in women and their babies after the birth are also included.

USEFUL WEBSITES

Best Beginnings: Out of the blue: www.bestbeginnings.org.uk/out-of-the-blue

Brook (Sexual health and wellbeing for the under 25s): www.brook.org.uk

Care Quality Commission: https://cqc.org.uk

Cry-sis: www.cry-sis.org.uk

Department for Education: www.gov.uk/government/organisations/department-for-education

Department of Health: www.gov.uk/government/organisations/department-of-health-and-social-care

Disability, Pregnancy and Parenthood: www.disabledparent.org.uk

Doula UK: https://doula.org.uk

Family Planning Association: www.fpa.org.uk

Faculty of Sexual and Reproductive Health Care: www.fsrh.org/home

Family Included Initiative: https://familyincluded.com

Fertility UK: www.fertilityuk.org

Maternity Action: https://maternityaction.org.uk

Mumsnet: www.mumsnet.com

National Childbirth Trust: www.nct.org.uk

National Health Service (NHS) Digital: https://digital.nhs.uk

National Health Service (NHS) England: www.england.nhs.uk

National Institute for Health and Care [formerly Clinical] Excellence (NICE): www.nice.org.uk

Nursing and Midwifery Council: www.nmc.org.uk

World Health Organization (WHO): www.who.int

29

Physical Health Issues and Complications in the Postnatal Period

Angela Brown, Mary Steen

CHAPTER CONTENTS

This chapter reviews the care of women who either entered the postpartum period having experienced obstetric or medical complications, including those who did not undergo a vaginal birth, or whose postpartum recovery, regardless of the mode of birth, did not follow a normal pattern. It includes the care for women with signs and symptoms of life-threatening conditions and those with obvious risks for increased postpartum physical morbidity. (The effects of morbidity related to psychological trauma are covered in Chapter 30.)

THE CHAPTER AIMS TO

- discuss the role of midwifery care in the detection and management of life-threatening conditions and postpartum morbidity
- review best practice in the management of complications associated with trauma and pathology arising from pregnancy and childbirth

- review the role of the midwife (and family) where postpartum health is complicated by an instrumental or operative birth.

THE NEED FOR WOMAN-FOCUSED AND FAMILY-CENTRED POSTPARTUM CARE

A woman-focused approach to care in the postpartum period alongside individualized care planning developed with the woman and her family will assist her physical and psychological recovery (National Institute for Health and Care Excellence, NICE 2014a; 2015, Royal College of Obstetricians and Gynaecologists, RCOG 2016). Midwives must focus on the needs of women as individuals rather than fitting women into a routine care package (NICE 2015; RCOG 2016; NHS England 2016). The midwife needs to be familiar with the woman's background and antenatal and labour history, irrespective of the care setting (NICE 2015; NHS England 2016) when assessing whether or not the woman's progress is following the expected postpartum recovery pattern (Care Quality Commission, CQC 2018; Schmied and Bick 2014).

All women should be offered appropriate and timely information with regard to their own health and well-being (and their babies) including recognition of, and responding to, concerns (NICE 2015; Bick et al. 2011; World Health Organization, WHO 2013). Postnatal care should be considered from a viewpoint of confirming 'normality' (Steen 2017). Where there has been obstetric or medical complications, the woman will be assessed and reviewed within the context of the immediate and ongoing care by the midwife of the woman's health over the postnatal period. The role of the midwife in these cases is first, to identify whether a potentially life-threatening condition exists and, if so, to refer the woman for appropriate emergency investigations and care (NICE 2014b, 2015; Knight et al. 2018; Nursing and Midwifery Council, NMC 2018a). Where the birth involves obstetric or medical complications, a woman's postpartum care is likely to differ from those women whose pregnancy and labour are considered straightforward. Some women may perceive that their birth experience was traumatic, despite no obvious traumatic events noted by the obstetric or midwifery staff (Reed et al. 2017; NHS England 2016).

POTENTIALLY LIFE-THREATENING CONDITIONS AND MORBIDITY AFTER THE BIRTH

Despite the apparent advances in medication and practice, women still die postpartum. The discovery of penicillin, the provision of blood transfusions and the introduction of ergometrine were major contributions to saving women's lives over the 20th century (Loudon 1992), and maternal death after childbirth where there has been no preceding antenatal complication is now a rare occurrence in the UK (Knight et al. 2019) and in other developed countries (Alkema et al. 2015). Between 2015 and 2017, two-thirds of all maternal deaths in the UK were to women who had pre-existing physical or mental health problems (Knight et al. 2019). Thrombosis or thromboembolism and haemorrhage were major causes of direct maternal deaths in the UK. Maternal suicide is the second largest cause of direct maternal deaths in the UK (during and to 42 days postpartum) and it remains a leading cause of direct deaths occurring during pregnancy or up to a year after the end of pregnancy from 2015 to 2017 (Knight et al. 2019). Indirect maternal mortality has reduced by 23% since 2010–2012, mostly attributed to fewer deaths from influenza and sepsis, and cardiac disease remains the most common cause of indirect death (Knight et al. 2018).

Being aware of this information is vital for all those involved in giving postnatal care as good quality care can contribute to the prevention as well as the detection and management of potentially fatal outcomes (Wray and Bick 2012; Knight et al. 2019).

Postnatal care is not always meeting the needs of women. Health challenges can manifest in the days and weeks following the birth of a baby (Yonemoto et al. 2017). Midwifery care in this postnatal period is important, to address any developing issues and to prevent health issues from becoming long-term problems (Yonemoto et al. 2017).

The midwife provides midwifery care in partnership with the woman to meet her individual needs and according to NICE (2014a, 2015) all women should receive essential 'core' routine care in the first 6–8 weeks after birth. In the postnatal period, the midwife aims to support the woman and her family transition to parenthood by monitoring her recovery after the birth and to offer her appropriate information and advice.

Women with complex and multiple health issues need additional care following their transfer home from hospital after birth (Knight et al. 2019). They should have a senior medical review prior to discharge with a clear, documented care plan for their postnatal care (Knight et al. 2019). The care plan should include the timing and booking of all follow-up appointments (Knight et al. 2019).

At a woman's first postnatal contact, she should be advised of the signs and symptoms of potentially life-threatening conditions that could arise in the days and weeks following birth (NICE 2014b, 2015; NHS England 2016). These include signs of postpartum haemorrhage (PPH), infection, pre-eclampsia and eclampsia plus thromboembolism (NICE 2014b, 2015).

IMMEDIATE MATERNAL COMPLICATIONS FOLLOWING THE BIRTH OF THE BABY

Immediate (primary) PPH is a potentially life-threatening event that occurs at the point of or within 24 h of expulsion of the placenta and membranes and presents as a sudden and excessive vaginal blood loss (see Chapter 21). Secondary PPH is defined as any significant bleeding from the genital tract (from any route – vaginal or abdominal) from 24 h post-birth and for up to 6 weeks' postpartum (Dossou et al. 2015). The most common causes of secondary PPH are retained products of conception, subinvolution of the placental bed and/or infection (Belfort 2018; Mavrides et al. 2016). Unlike primary PPH, which includes a defined volume of blood loss (>500 mL) as part of its definition, there is no volume of blood specified for a secondary PPH and management differs according to apparent clinical need and suspected cause (Belfort 2018; Mavrides et al. 2016).

Regardless of the timing of any haemorrhage, it is most frequently the placental site that is the source. Alternatively, a cervical or deep vaginal wall tear or trauma to the perineum might be the cause in women who have recently given birth. Retained placental fragments or other products of conception are likely to inhibit the process of involution, or reopen the placental wound. The diagnosis is likely to be determined more by the woman's condition and pattern of events (Belfort 2018; Mavrides et al. 2016).

Maternal Collapse Within 24 Hours of the Birth Without Overt Bleeding

Where no signs of haemorrhage are apparent, other causes need to be considered (see Chapter 15). Management of all these conditions requires ensuring the woman is in a safe environment until effective treatment can be administered by the most appropriate health professionals, and meanwhile maintaining the woman's airway, basic circulatory support as needed and providing oxygen (see Chapter 26). It is important to remember that, regardless of the apparent state of collapse, the woman may still be able to hear and so verbally reassuring the woman (and her partner or relatives if present) is an important aspect of the immediate emergency and ongoing care.

POSTPARTUM COMPLICATIONS

Identifying Deviations from the Normal

Following the birth of their baby, women should be offered information and reassurance on the normal pattern of postpartum recovery. This helps the women to understand that many of the symptoms they are experiencing are normal healing from birth and then can recognize deviations from normal. Women should be given the appropriate knowledge around expected recovery and the signs and symptoms that should be reported to their midwife. Coupled with careful questioning during postnatal visits, the midwife can determine deviations from normal and offer appropriate counselling and referral.

The postpartum visit enables a review of the woman's physical and psychological health. The midwife will need to collate and evaluate the information to develop a plan of management with the woman. Women will probably give information about events or symptoms that are the most worrying or most painful to them at that time and the midwife determines with careful questioning, the significance of the symptoms. The midwife must establish whether there are any other signs of possible morbidity and determine whether these might indicate the need for referral. Fig. 29.1 suggests a model for linking together key observations that suggest potential risk of, or actual, morbidity.

The central point, as with any personal contact, is the midwife's initial review of the woman's appearance and psychological state. This is underpinned by an assessment of the woman's vital signs, where any general state of illness is evident, including signs of infection. The accumulation of a number of clinical signs will assist the midwife in making decisions about the presence or potential for morbidity. Where there is a rise in temperature above 38°C it is usual for this to be considered a deviation from normal and of clinical significance. If puerperal infection is suspected, the woman must be referred back to the obstetric services as soon as possible (Knight et al. 2019). Adherence to local infection control policies and awareness of the signs and symptoms of sepsis in postnatal women is important for all practitioners caring for women.

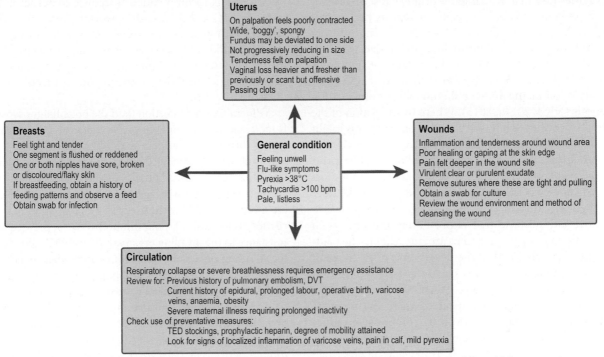

Uterus
On palpation feels poorly contracted
Wide, 'boggy', spongy
Fundus may be deviated to one side
Not progressively reducing in size
Tenderness felt on palpation
Vaginal loss heavier and fresher than
previously or scant but offensive
Passing clots

Breasts
Feel tight and tender
One segment is flushed or reddened
One or both nipples have sore, broken
or discoloured/flaky skin
If breastfeeding, obtain a history of
feeding patterns and observe a feed
Obtain swab for infection

General condition
Feeling unwell
Flu-like symptoms
Pyrexia >38°C
Tachycardia >100 bpm
Pale, listless

Wounds
Inflammation and tenderness around wound area
Poor healing or gaping at the skin edge
Pain felt deeper in the wound site
Virulent clear or purulent exudate
Remove sutures where these are tight and pulling
Obtain a swab for culture
Review the wound environment and method of
cleansing the wound

Circulation
Respiratory collapse or severe breathlessness requires emergency assistance
Review for: Previous history of pulmonary embolism, DVT
             Current history of epidural, prolonged labour, operative birth, varicose
             veins, anaemia, obesity
             Severe maternal illness requiring prolonged inactivity
Check use of preventative measures:
             TED stockings, prophylactic heparin, degree of mobility attained
             Look for signs of localized inflammation of varicose veins, pain in calf, mild pyrexia

Fig. 29.1 The relationship between deviation from normal physiology and potential morbidity.

The pulse rate and respirations are also significant observations when accumulating clinical evidence. Although there may be no evidence of vaginal haemorrhage, for example, a weak and rapid pulse rate (>100 bpm) in conjunction with a woman who is in a state of collapse with signs of shock and a low blood pressure (systolic <90 mmHg) may indicate the formation of a haematoma, where there is an excessive leakage of blood from damaged blood vessels into the surrounding tissues. A rapid pulse rate in an otherwise well woman might suggest that she is anaemic but could also indicate increased thyroid or other dysfunctional hormonal activity. A good understanding of each individual woman's history is important in order to link clinical findings to potential morbidity in the postnatal period.

The midwife needs to be alert to any possible relationship between the observations overall and their potential cause with regard to common illnesses, e.g. that the woman has a common cold, and that the morbidity is associated with or affected by having recently given birth. Where the midwife is in conversation with the woman as part of the postpartum assessment, if she receives information that suggests the woman has signs deviating from what is expected to be normal, it is important that a range of clinical observations are undertaken to refute or confirm this, followed by timely and appropriate referral.

Midwives develop skills and processes from their experience to accumulate evidence from their observations and conversations about the overall wellbeing of the woman and her baby (NICE 2014a, 2015). However, this process is mainly covert and difficult to adapt in any formal way to help less experienced midwives or even explain the course of action to the women themselves (Marchant 2006). To clarify the actions necessary, when NICE guidelines were published and updated, a quick guide was also produced providing a table of the action required for possible signs/symptoms of complications and common health problems in women (NICE 2014a, 2015).

The Uterus and Vaginal Loss Following a Vaginal Birth

It is expected that the midwife will undertake assessment of uterine involution and position at intervals throughout the period of midwifery care (see Chapter 28). It is recommended that this should always be undertaken when: the woman is feeling generally unwell; has abdominal pain and tenderness; in the presence of fever;

a vaginal loss that is markedly brighter red or heavier than previously; is passing clots; or reports her vaginal loss to be offensive (NICE 2014a, 2015). The midwife should assess for any abnormalities in the size, tone and position of the uterus that could explain the symptoms (NICE 2014a, 2015; WHO 2013). If no uterine abnormality is found, the midwife should look for other explanations (NICE 2014a, 2015). Where the palpation of the uterus identifies that it is deviated to one side, this might be as a result of a full bladder. Where the midwife has ensured that the woman had emptied her bladder prior to the palpation, the presence of urinary retention must be considered. Catheterization of the woman's bladder in these circumstances is indicated for two reasons: to remove any obstacle that is preventing the process of involution taking place; and to provide relief to the bladder itself (Steen 2013). If the deviation is not as a result of a full bladder, further investigations need to be undertaken to determine the cause (Steen 2013).

Morbidity might be suspected where the woman's uterus fails to follow the expected progressive reduction in size, feels wide or 'boggy' on palpation and is less well-contracted than expected. This might be described as *subinvolution* of the uterus, which can indicate postpartum infection, or the presence of retained products of the placenta or membranes, or both (Aiken et al. 2012). If this is suspected, the midwife should review the woman's birth records to review placental details recorded at the time.

Treatment is by antibiotics, oxytocic medications that act on the uterine muscle, hormonal preparations or evacuation of the uterus (ERPC), usually under a spinal or general anaesthetic. Consultation and referral to obstetric services is important for appropriate follow-up.

Sepsis and Vulnerability to Infection
Potential Causes and Prevention
Infection is the invasion of tissues by pathogenic microorganisms; the degree to which this results in ill-health relates to their virulence and number. Sepsis is defined as the presence of infection with systemic manifestations; severe sepsis is defined as sepsis with organ dysfunction or tissue hypoperfusion (Dellinger et al. 2013). Severe sepsis with associated multiorgan dysfunction has a high mortality (20–40%); this rises to approximately 60% if septicaemic shock develops (RCOG 2012). Administration of intravenous broad-spectrum antibiotics within 1 h of suspicion of severe sepsis is indicated and prompt antibiotic treatment for genital tract sepsis is recommended to reduce maternal mortality (RCOG 2012). Midwives working in community settings with postpartum women must refer suspected cases back to health services for urgent care. Sepsis is a medical emergency and the midwife may have a role in determining clinical deterioration and ensuring immediate medical care.

Vulnerability for infection (and the potential for sepsis) is increased where conditions exist that enable the organism to thrive and reproduce and where there is access to and from entry points in the body. Organisms are transferred between sources and a potential host by hands, air currents and fomites (i.e. agents such as bed linen). Hosts are more vulnerable when they are in a condition of susceptibility because of poor immunity or a pre-existing resistance to the invading organism. The body responds to the invading organisms by forming antibodies, which in turn produce inflammation initiating other physiological changes such as pain and an increase in body temperature.

Acquisition of an infective organism can be **endogenous**, where the organisms are already present in or on the body, e.g. *Streptococcus faecalis* (Lancefield group B); *Clostridium perfringens (formerly known as C. welchii)* (both present in the vagina); or *Escherichia coli* (present in the bowel), or organisms in a dormant state are reactivated, e.g. tuberculosis bacteria. Other routes are **exogenous**, where the organisms are transferred from other people (or animal) body surfaces or the environment. Other transfer mechanisms include *droplets* – inhalations of respiratory pathogens on liquid particles (e.g. β-haemolytic *Streptococcus* and *Chlamydia trachomatis*), *cross-infection* and *nosocomial* (hospital-acquired) transfer from an infected person or place to an uninfected one (e.g. *Staphylococcus aureus*).

The bacteria responsible for the majority of puerperal infection arise from the Streptococcal or Staphylococcal species, with community acquired GAS (group A β-haemolytic streptococci) (RCOG 2012). The *Streptococcus* bacterium has a chain-like formation and may be haemolytic or non-haemolytic, and aerobic or anaerobic; the most common species associated with puerperal sepsis is the β-haemolytic *S. pyogenes* (Lancefield group A), although other strains of the streptococcal bacteria have also been identified as the source of serious morbidity (Muller et al. 2006). The *Staphylococcus* bacterium has a grape-like structure, of which the most important species is *S. aureus* or *pyogenes*. Staphylococci are the most frequent cause of wound infections; where these bacteria are coagulase-positive they form clots on the plasma, which can lead to more widely spread systemic morbidity.

There is additional concern about their resistance to antibiotics and subsequent management to control spread of the infection. The most common site of sepsis for postnatal women is the genital tract and in particular, the uterus, resulting in endometritis (RCOG 2012). Regardless of the location of care, postpartum women and healthcare professionals should be aware of how infection can be acquired and should pay particular attention to effective hand-washing techniques. They should adhere to the accepted practice for aseptic technique such as local infection control policies when in contact with wound care, including the use of gloves for this, and where there is direct contact with areas in the body where bacteria of potential morbidity are prevalent. Avoiding the spread of infection is especially necessary when the woman or her family or close contacts have a sore throat or upper respiratory tract infection (RCOG 2012). Educating women and their family about the basic principles of good hand hygiene is a key public health role of the midwife in staving off infection (Wound Healing Institute Australia 2019). Midwives must be aware of the signs and symptoms of sepsis, as prompt referral and treatment is required to prevent maternal deaths. See Box 29.1 for the signs and symptoms of sepsis.

The Uterus and Vaginal Loss Following Operative Birth

A lower segment caesarean section (CS) will have involved cutting of the major abdominal muscles and trauma to other soft tissues (see Chapter 24). Palpation of the abdomen is therefore likely to be very painful for the woman in the first few days after surgery. The woman who has undergone a CS will have a very different level of physical activity from the woman who has had a vaginal birth. It may be some hours after the operation until the woman feels able to sit up or move about. Blood and debris will have been slowly released from the uterus during this time and, when the woman begins to move, this will be expelled through the vagina and may appear as a substantial fresh-looking red loss. Following this initial loss, it is usual for the amount of vaginal loss to lessen and for further fresh loss to be minimal. All this can be observed without actually palpating the uterus. For women who have undergone an operative birth, once 3 or 4 days have elapsed, abdominal palpation to assess uterine involution can be undertaken by the midwife where this appears to be clinically necessary. By this

> ### BOX 29.1 Signs and Symptoms of Sepsis
>
> - Fever
> - Shivering
> - Hypothermia
> - Tachycardia
> - Tachypnoea
> - Altered mental status
> - Significant oedema
> - Hyperglycaemia in the absence of diabetes
> - Hypotension
> - Oliguria
> - Ileus
> - Raised inflammatory blood ranges
> - Thrombocytopenia
> - Hyperbilirubinemia
> - Hyperlactatemia
> - Decreased capillary refill or mottling
> - Abdominal pain
> - Offensive vaginal loss.

From Dellinger R, Levy M, Rhodes A, et al. (2013) Surviving Sepsis Campaign: international guidelines for management of severe sepsis and septic shock. Intensive Care Medicine 39(2): 165–228.

time, the uterus or area around the uterus should not be overly painful on palpation.

Where clinically indicated, e.g. where the vaginal bleeding is heavier than expected, the uterine fundus can be gently palpated. If the uterus is not well contracted then medical intervention is needed. Uterine stimulants (uterotonics) are usually prescribed in the form of an intravenous infusion of oxytocin or an intramuscular injection of oxytocin/ergometrine, if not contraindicated (see Chapter 21). If the bleeding continues where such treatment has been commenced, further investigations might include obtaining a venous blood sample for clotting factors, or the woman might need to return to theatre for further exploration of the uterine cavity. Midwives should be aware that in women who have had a CS and who have heavy and/or irregular vaginal bleeding, it is more likely to be from endometritis than retained products of conception (NICE 2011).

Ultrasound scans are now commonly used in the postpartum period to facilitate early detection of postpartum uterine complications (Paliulyte et al. 2017). Ultrasound scans are frequently used for excluding retained placental tissue and assist clinicians with more accurate identification of women who require surgical intervention (Üçyiğit and Johns 2016).

Wound Complications

Perineal Complications

All postnatal women should be asked at every visit about any concerns that they may have on the healing of perineal injury (NICE 2015). It is important that the midwife has an understanding of the effect of trauma as a physiological process and the normal pattern for wound healing (Steen 2007; Steen and Diaz 2018). Knowledge and an understanding of the physiological process and the nutrients that are necessary to promote healing will assist a midwife to recognize when there is a delay in healing and also enable the midwife to advise a woman on her dietary requirements (Fig. 29.2 and Table 29.1).

Perineal pain is a result of perineal injury and is surgically or naturally induced as a result of the birth. Women complain of varying degrees of severity of perineal pain. Perineal injury that requires suturing predisposes women to an increased risk of severe perineal pain (see Chapter 17). This might be as a result of the analgesia no longer being effective, the presence

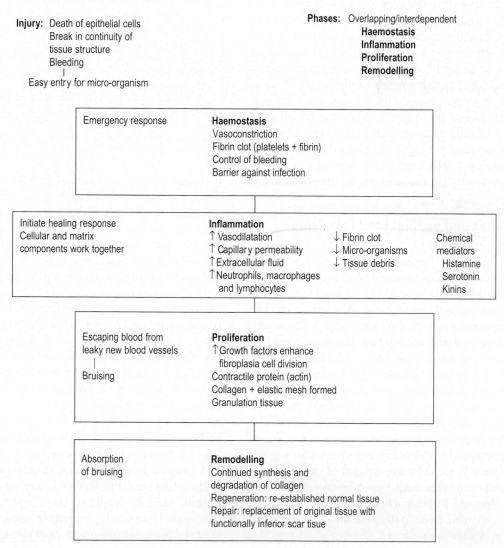

Injury: Death of epithelial cells
Break in continuity of
tissue structure
Bleeding
|
Easy entry for micro-organism

Phases: Overlapping/interdependent
Haemostasis
Inflammation
Proliferation
Remodelling

Emergency response — **Haemostasis**
Vasoconstriction
Fibrin clot (platelets + fibrin)
Control of bleeding
Barrier against infection

Initiate healing response
Cellular and matrix
components work together — **Inflammation**
↑ Vasodilatation
↑ Capillary permeability
↑ Extracellular fluid
↑ Neutrophils, macrophages
and lymphocytes
↓ Fibrin clot
↓ Micro-organisms
↓ Tissue debris
Chemical
mediators
Histamine
Serotonin
Kinins

Escaping blood from
leaky new blood vessels
|
Bruising — **Proliferation**
↑ Growth factors enhance
fibroplasia cell division
Contractile protein (actin)
Collagen + elastic mesh formed
Granulation tissue

Absorption
of bruising — **Remodelling**
Continued synthesis and
degradation of collagen
Regeneration: re-established normal tissue
Repair: replacement of original tissue with
functionally inferior scar tissue

Fig. 29.2 The phases of wound healing. (Reproduced with permission from Steen M. (2007) Perineal tears and episiotomy: how do wounds heal? British Journal of Midwifery Perineal Care Supplement 15(5):273–80.)

TABLE 29.1 Nutrients and their Contribution to Healing

Nutrient	Contribution
Carbohydrates	Energy for leucocyte, macrophage and fibroblast function
Proteins	Immune response, phagocytosis, angiogenesis, fibroblast proliferation, collagen synthesis, wound maturation
Fats	Provision of energy, formation of new cells
Vitamins	
Vitamin A	Collagen synthesis and cross-linking, tensile strength
Vitamin B (complex)	Immune response, collagen cross-linking, tensile strength
Vitamin C	Collagen synthesis tensile strength, neutrophil function, macrophage migration, immune response
Vitamin E	Reduce tissue damage from free radical formation
Minerals	
Copper	Collagen synthesis, leucocyte formation
Iron	Collagen synthesis, oxygen delivery
Zinc	Increases cell proliferation, epithelialization, collagen strength

Adapted from Dellinger R, Levy M, Rhodes A, et al. (2013). Surviving Sepsis Campaign: International guidelines for management of severe sepsis and septic shock. Intensive Care Medicine, 39(2), 165–228.

of inflammation in the surrounding tissues or, more seriously, the formation of a haematoma. A haematoma usually develops deep in the perineal fascia tissues and may not be easily visible if the perineal tissues are already inflamed. Inadequate perineal repair or a traumatic vaginal birth can increase the risk of a haematoma. The blood contained within a haematoma can exceed 1000 mL and may significantly affect the overall state of the woman, who can present with signs of acute hypovolemic shock. Treatment is by evacuation of the haematoma and resuturing of the perineal wound, usually under a general anaesthetic and management of the associated morbidity from the blood loss.

Perineal pain that is severe and is not caused by a haematoma might arise as a result of inflammation causing the stitches to feel excessively tight. Local application of cold packs can bring relief as they reduce the immediate oedema and continue to provide relief over the first few days following the birth (Steen et al. 2006; Steen and Diaz 2018; Steen 2017). The length of cooling effects lasts up to 2 h post-application (de Souza et al. 2016; Francisco et al. 2018; Steen and Diaz 2018). Other methods for reduction of perineal pain include oral analgesia, bathing, diclofenac (oral and suppositories) and lignocaine gel (Steen and Diaz 2018; Steen 2017). It is recommended that a combination of systemic and localized treatments will be needed to meet women's analgesic needs (Steen and Diaz 2018; Steen 2017).

Factors that are associated with poor healing include poor diet, obesity, pre-existing medical disorders and negative social conditions such as poor housing, increased stress and smoking (Steen 2007). Where pain in the perineal area occurs at a later stage, or re-occurs, this might be associated with an infection. The skin edges are likely to have a moist, puffy and dull appearance; there may also be an offensive odour and evidence of pus in the wound. A swab should be obtained for microorganism culture and referral made to a GP. Antibiotics might be commenced immediately when there is specific information about any infective agent. The midwife should pay attention to the woman's whole clinical picture as sepsis can progress quickly and a woman can become extremely unwell in a short period of time (see Chapter 26). If any concerns are present, it is better to request a second opinion early rather than later. Where the perineal tissues appear to be infected, it is important to discuss with the woman about cleaning the area and making an attempt to reduce constant moisture and heat. Women might be advised about using cotton underwear, avoiding tights and trousers and frequently changing sanitary pads. They should also be advised to avoid using perfumed bath additives, perfumed soap or talcum powder.

If the perineal area fails to heal, or continues to cause pain, a referral should be made for a medical review. There is currently insufficient evidence to either recommend or refute resuturing to manage perineal wound breakdown after birth (Dudley et al. 2013). There is evidence to suggest that a substantial proportion of women continue to experience long-term perineal complications following birth and often do not report these to healthcare professionals (Steen and Diaz 2018). Therefore, it is important to advise women to seek help and encourage them to discuss any concerns with their GP. Most women should be pain-free and be able to resume sexual intercourse within a few weeks after the birth; this will vary in individual women. Some women may still experience discomfort, depending on the severity of trauma and the healing process. Dyspareunia (painful sexual intercourse) can be related to severe perineal trauma/obstetric anal sphincter injury (see Geeta's story in Chapter 17) and this can impact the woman's relationship with her partner (Fodstad et al. 2016; Steen and Diaz 2018). Women should be asked about the resumption of sexual intercourse from approximately 2 weeks post-birth, at each contact (NICE 2014a, 2015). Some women experience anxiety about the resumption of sexual activity and this should be explored with each woman when she expresses concern (NICE 2015). Women with perineal trauma who experience dyspareunia should be offered review of her perineum (NICE 2015). Midwives can recommend a water-based lubricant gel to reduce discomfort during intercourse (NICE 2014b, 2015).

Caesarean Section Wound Complications

It is now common practice for women undergoing an operative birth to have prophylactic antibiotics at the time of the surgery (NICE 2011). This has been demonstrated to significantly reduce the incidence of subsequent wound infection and endometritis. It is recommended that the wound dressing is removed at approximately 24 h post-birth (Berghella 2018; NICE 2011). Advice needs to be offered to the woman about care of her wound and adequate drying when taking a bath or shower, or for more obese women, where abdominal skin folds are present and are likely to create an environment that is constantly warm and moist. For these women, a dry dressing over the suture line might be appropriate.

Wound infections generally occur between 4 and 7 days after the caesarean. Midwives should be aware of risk factors that include: obesity, chorioamnionitis, blood transfusion, anticoagulation therapy, alcohol or drug misuse, second stage caesarean birth and subcutaneous haematoma (Berghella 2018). Infections that develop within the first 24–48 h are usually attributed to group A or B β-hemolytic *Streptococcus* (Berghella 2018). Women will experience high temperatures and wound cellulitis. Infections that develop later are usually attributed to *Staphylococcus epidermidis* or

aureus, *Escherichia coli*, *Proteus mirabilis*, or cervico-vaginal flora (Berghella 2018). A wound that is hot, tender and inflamed and is accompanied by a pyrexia is highly suggestive of an infection. Where this is observed, a swab should be obtained for microorganism culture and medical advice should be sought. Haematomas and abscesses can also form underneath the wound and women may identify increased pain around the wound where these are present. Rarely, a wound may need to be probed to reduce the pressure and allow infected material to drain, reducing the likelihood of the formation of an abscess. With shorter hospital stays for women post-surgery, these problems increasingly occur after the woman has left hospital, so asking the woman about her pain in the postnatal period and visually inspecting the wound is important.

Circulation

A total of 34 women died from venous thromboembolism in the UK and Ireland between 2015 and 2017, during pregnancy or up to 6 weeks after pregnancy (Knight et al. 2019). Midwives and GPs need to be alert to identify high-risk women and the possibility of thromboembolism in puerperal women with unilateral calf pain, redness or swelling and shortness of breath or chest pain (NICE 2014, 2015).

Women who have a previous history of pulmonary embolism, deep vein thrombosis (DVT), are obese or who have varicose veins, have a higher risk of postpartum morbidity. Postpartum care of women who have pre-existing or pregnancy-related medical complications relies on prophylactic precautions and should be undertaken for women who undergo surgery and have these pre-existing factors. Thromboembolic D (TED) stockings should be provided during, or as soon as possible after, the birth and prophylactic heparin prescribed until women attain normal mobility. All women who undergo an epidural anaesthetic, are anaemic or have a prolonged labour or an operative birth are slightly more at risk of developing complications linked to blood clots. Women with pre-existing medical issues are at higher risk because of their overall health status and environment of care postpartum. For example, women who undergo a CS as a result of maternal illness are more likely to spend longer in bed, thereby reducing their mobility and increasing their risk of morbidity.

Clinical signs that women might report include the following (from the most common to the most serious):

- Circulatory problems related to varicose veins, usually localized inflammation or tenderness around the varicose vein, sometimes accompanied by a mild pyrexia. This is *superficial thrombophlebitis*, which is usually resolved by applying support to the affected area and administering anti-inflammatory drugs, where these are not in conflict with other medication being taken or with breastfeeding.
- Some degree of *oedema* of the lower legs and ankles and feet can be viewed as being within normal limits where it is not accompanied by calf pain (especially unilaterally), pyrexia or a raised blood pressure.
- Unilateral oedema of an ankle or calf accompanied by stiffness or pain; increased unilateral calf diameter might indicate a *DVT* that has the potential to cause a pulmonary embolism (Kearon and Bauer 2018). Urgent medical referral must be made to confirm the diagnosis and commence anticoagulant or other appropriate therapy.
- The most serious outcome is the development of a *pulmonary embolism*. The first sign might be the sudden onset of breathlessness, which may not be associated with any obvious clinical sign of a blood clot. Women with this condition are likely to become seriously ill and could suffer a respiratory collapse with very little prior warning.

Hypertension

Women who have had previous episodes of hypertension in pregnancy may continue to be hypertensive for up to 12 weeks postpartum (August 2018). There is still a risk that women who have clinical signs of pregnancy-induced hypertension can develop eclampsia in the hours and days following the birth, although this is a relatively rare outcome in the normal population (August 2018; Bigelow et al. 2014).

In addition, some women can develop pre-eclampsia or HELLP syndrome that presents as postpartum hypertension where there has been no previous history of raised blood pressure or proteinuria (August 2018; Bigelow et al. 2014). Late, new onset postnatal pre-eclampsia can manifest from approximately 48 hours until 6 weeks (Bigelow et al. 2014). Blood pressure monitoring in the postnatal period should be as per hospital protocols and then as per clinically indicated following discharge. Medical advice should determine optimal systolic and diastolic levels, with instructions for treatment with antihypertensive medication if the blood pressure exceeds these levels. As women can develop postnatal pre-eclampsia without having antenatal symptoms as the symptoms can be fairly nonspecific, such as a headache or epigastric pain or vomiting, the woman may delay or fail to contact a healthcare professional for advice. Where they do seek advice, the healthcare professional may not be alert to the possibility of the development of postpartum eclampsia (Chames et al. 2002). If a postpartum woman presents with symptoms associated with pre-eclampsia, the midwife should be alert to this possibility and undertake observations of the blood pressure and urine and obtain medical advice (Bigelow et al. 2014).

For women with essential hypertension, the management of their overall medical condition will be reviewed postpartum by their usual caregivers.

Headache

This is a common ailment in the general population; concern in relation to postpartum morbidity should therefore centre around the history of the severity, duration and frequency of the headaches, the medication being taken to alleviate them and how effective this is. As this is also associated with hypertension, a recording of the blood pressure should be undertaken to exclude this as a primary factor. In taking the history, if an epidural analgesic was administered, medical advice should be sought. Headaches from a dural tap typically arise once the woman has become mobile after the birth and they are at their most severe when standing, lessening when the woman lies down. They are often accompanied by neck stiffness, vomiting and visual disturbances. These headaches are very debilitating and are best managed by stopping the leakage of cerebral spinal fluid by the insertion of 10–20 mL of blood into the epidural space; this should resolve the clinical symptoms. Where women have returned home after the birth, they would need to return to the hospital to have this procedure.

Headaches might also be precursors of psychological distress and it is important that other issues related to birth are explored, taking the time and opportunity to do this in a sensitive manner. Factors that might be overlooked include dehydration, sleep loss and a greater than usual stressful environment (see Chapter 30). However, the midwife should take time to discuss the woman's feelings and offer advice or reassurance about these where possible.

Backache

Many women experience pain or discomfort from backache in pregnancy as a result of separation or diastasis of the abdominal muscles (rectus abdominis diastasis, RAD). Where backache is causing pain that affects the woman's activities of daily living, referral can be made to local physiotherapy services. Pelvic girdle pain has a significant impact on women's daily life and ongoing complaints after pregnancy need referral to further services to prevent the psychological sequelae that can develop as a result of the impact on the women's mobility (Mackenzie et al. 2018).

Urinary Complications

Urinary complications can have short- and long-term social, psychological and physical health consequences and women often do not receive adequate follow-up in the 12 months following birth (Brown et al. 2015). Urinary symptoms can persist for up to 4 years post-birth (Gartland et al. 2016), which can have a major impact on a woman's life. About one-third of all postnatal women will experience urinary incontinence (Woodley et al. 2017). Some women who have had a complicated birth (including prolonged second stage) may be susceptible to the risk of urinary infections, which may lead to cystitis and in some severe cases, pyelonephritis (Mulder et al. 2014). Where a woman has undergone an epidural or spinal anaesthetic, this can have an effect on the neurological sensors that control urine release and flow, which may cause acute retention. The main complication of any form of urine retention is that the uterus might be prevented from effective contraction, which leads to increased vaginal blood loss. There is also increased potential for the woman to contract a urine infection with possible kidney involvement and long-term effects on bladder function.

In addition, women who have sustained pelvic floor damage during birth may suffer from continence problems in the short and long term. Stress and urge incontinence of urine, uterovaginal prolapse (cystocele and rectocele) and dyspareunia are all associated with pelvic floor damage (Handa 2018; McDonald et al. 2015). Very rarely, urinary incontinence might be the result of a urethral fistula following complications from the labour or birth.

Midwives are in a prime position to safeguard bladder management and promote normal bladder functioning (Lamb and Sanders 2016). A midwife will need to be alert to any urinary concerns a woman may have, as sometimes these can be missed. Being alert to the risks and being able to recognize ongoing urinary problems is an essential component of care (Steen 2013; Lamb and Sanders 2016). Abdominal tenderness in association with other urinary symptoms, for example a poor output, dysuria or offensive urine and a raised temperature or general flu-like symptoms, might indicate a urinary tract infection (UTI). Midwives can perform a urine dipstick test and if the urine tests positive for both leucocytes and nitrites, a mid-stream urine specimen should be sent for culture and analysis of antibiotic sensitivities (NICE 2013). Antibiotic treatment should be recommended, and the woman should consult her doctor.

Women might feel embarrassed about having urinary problems and midwives may need to consider appropriate ways of encouraging women to talk about any symptoms so that they can inform them about their future management (Steen 2013). Specific enquiry about these issues should be made when women attend for their 6–8-week postnatal examination; further investigations should be made for women who are encountering these problems. Keeping a bladder diary can be a useful aid. NICE (2013) have suggested that women should complete a bladder diary for 3 consecutive days to allow for variation in day-to-day activities to be captured.

It is essential that midwives have knowledge and an understanding of the risks and symptoms of urinary problems and are able to ask sensitive questions to identify women at risk, as failure to do so can lead to poor psychological health. These women will need additional social and psychological support (Steen 2013).

Bowel Complications

Bowel complications following birth can have short- and long-term social, psychological and physical health consequences for women (Brown et al. 2015). The incidence of anal incontinence post-birth is typically under-reported, which makes it difficult to determine the true prevalence of the complication (Frasson and Dodi 2016). Careful questioning in a trusting relationship may encourage a woman to share her concerns if she experiences symptomology. All of the associated symptoms require medical follow-up and investigation (Frasson and Dodi 2016). Faecal incontinence is associated with primiparity, instrumental birth, prolonged second stage, shoulder dystocia and severe perineal injury, secondary to acute structural or neurological injury (Shin et al. 2015).

Constipation and haemorrhoids are a frequent post-natal complication for many women. It is estimated that about 40% of women will suffer from constipation following birth (Shin et al. 2015). Haemorrhoids are also frequently experienced by women during pregnancy and in the postnatal period (Åhlund et al. 2018). Estimations for prevalence of postnatal haemorrhoids range from 10% to 40% (Åhlund et al. 2018). Symptoms include flatus, incontinence, itching, burning, passive leakage, painful swelling at the anus, urge and faecal incontinence (Åhlund et al. 2018). The prevalence of bowel complications may be higher than reported, as many women may suffer in silence and may be too embarrassed to ask for help (Steen 2013).

A midwife needs to be alert to any bowel symptoms and should ask a woman sensitively about her bowel habits. Being alert to the risks and being able to recognize ongoing bowel complications is an essential component of midwifery care. Enquiring about the pattern and frequency of bowel movements and comparing this to the woman's previous experience is likely to assist a midwife in identifying whether or not there is an issue. Factors such as dietary intake, a degree of dehydration during labour and concern about further pain from any perineal trauma can contribute to bowel problems. A diet that includes soft fibre and increased fluids can be recommended to alleviate constipation. A Cochrane review found that there is insufficient evidence on the safety and effectiveness of laxatives (including lactulose) during the early postpartum period to make recommendations about their use to prevent constipation (Turawa et al. 2015). However, some women may require additional measures to relieve their constipation and may wish to try an aperient. Women need advice that any disruption to their normal bowel pattern should resolve within days of the birth, taking into consideration the recovery required by the presence of perineal trauma. They should also be reassured about the effect of a bowel movement on the area that has been sutured, as many women may be unnecessarily anxious about the possibility of tearing their perineal stitches. Where women have prolonged difficulty with constipation, anal fissures can result (Steen 2013). These are painful and difficult to resolve and therefore advice about bowel management is important in avoiding this situation. Women who have haemorrhoids should also be given advice on following a diet high in fibre and fluids, preferably water and the use of appropriate aperients to soften the stools as well as topical applications to reduce the oedema and pain.

It is also of concern where women might experience loss of bowel control and whether this is faecal incontinence. It is important to determine the nature of the incontinence and distinguish it from an episode of diarrhoea. It might be helpful to ask whether the woman has taken any laxatives in the previous 24 h and to explore what food was eaten. Where the problems do not seem to be associated with other factors, the woman should first be advised to see her GP.

The role of the midwife is to encourage women to talk about these concerns by being proactive in asking about any bowel changes. Where women identify any change to their pre-pregnant bowel pattern by the end of the puerperal period, they should be advised to have this reviewed further, whether it is constipation or loss of bowel control (Steen 2013).

Postpartum Anaemia

Postpartum iron deficiency is a common occurrence caused by bleeding or inadequate intake or uptake. Symptoms include tiredness, shortness of breath and dizziness (Markova et al. 2015). Postpartum anaemia is defined as Hb <100 g/L (Pavord et al. 2012). While severe anaemia (haemoglobin <70 g/dL) is rare in resource-rich countries, it is a serious problem for many women in resource-poor countries. The impact, however, of the events of the labour and birth may leave many women looking pale and tired for a day or so afterwards. Symptomatic women can have a diagnosis of postpartum anaemia confirmed with a blood test; treatment should be aimed at reducing any symptoms (Markova et al. 2015). Women who have had an estimated blood loss >500 mL, untreated anaemia antenatally or postpartum symptoms of anaemia, should have their Hb checked within 48 h of birth (Pavord et al. 2012). Oral iron supplements should be recommended for mild cases of iron deficiency anaemia and intravenous iron supplementation for moderate to severe cases. Ferric carboxymaltose is the first choice for intravenous iron therapy. For women undergoing an iron infusion, midwives should be alert to avoid extravasation due to the risk of permanent skin discolouration (Breymann et al. 2017). Less commonly now, blood transfusions may also be recommended for treatment of postpartum anaemia but the risk and benefits of a transfusion should be carefully considered by the woman and her doctor. Blood transfusions have demonstrated a temporary improvement in fatigue but the risks of transfusion must be balanced

(Markova et al. 2015). The degree to which the haemoglobin level has fallen should determine the appropriate management and this is particularly important in the presence of pre-existing haemoglobinopathies, sickle cell and thalassaemia.

Serum ferritin levels measure the amount of stored iron, however, ferritin levels can be raised if infection or inflammation is present, even if iron stores are low. Levels below 15 µg/L are diagnostic of established iron deficiency (Pavord et al. 2012). Serum ferritin should be checked prior to starting iron in women who have a known haemoglobinopathy (Pavord et al. 2012). In iron depletion anaemia, the amount of stored iron is reduced but the functional or transport levels of iron remain unaffected. Elemental iron 100–200 mg daily is recommended (Pavord et al. 2012). Alternatively, iron suspensions may be better tolerated and oral iron should be continued for 3 months after the iron deficiency is corrected to replenish the woman's stores of iron. Ascorbic acid may be recommended to enhance iron absorption. Tannins in tea and coffee can also interfere with iron absorption (Breymann et al. 2017).

Where the woman has returned home soon after the birth, her postpartum haemoglobin values might not have been undertaken where there was no history of anaemia prior to labour and the blood loss at birth was not assessed as excessive. If there is no clinical information to hand, the midwife needs to rely on the woman's clinical symptoms; if these include lethargy, tachycardia and breathlessness, as well as a clinical picture of pale mucous membranes, the midwife should organize a blood test.

Breast Complications

Regardless of whether women are breastfeeding, they may experience tightening and enlargement of their breasts towards the 3rd or 4th day, as hormonal influences encourage the breasts to produce milk (see Chapter 27). For women who are breastfeeding, the general advice is to feed their baby and avoid excessive handling of the breasts. Simple analgesics may be required to reduce discomfort. For women who are not breastfeeding, the advice is to ensure that the breasts are well supported but that this is not too constrictive and, again, that taking regular analgesia for 24–48 h should reduce the discomfort. Heat and cold applied to the breasts via a shower or a soaking in the bath, acupuncture, cabbage leaves and proteolytic enzymes may temporarily relieve

acute discomfort, a recent Cochrane review found that there was insufficient evidence to recommend widespread implementation (Mangesi and Zakarija-Grkovic 2016). A randomized controlled trial (RCT) in 2017 demonstrated a reduction in pain and hardness caused from breast engorgement for women using cold cabbage leaves (Wong et al. 2017).

MIDWIFERY CARE AFTER AN OPERATIVE BIRTH

In the immediate period after an operative birth, the attendant will be closely monitoring recovery from the anaesthetic used for CS (see Chapter 24). Regular observation of vaginal loss, leakage onto wound dressings and fluid loss in any drain system should also be undertaken.

Once the woman has fully recovered from the operation she should be transferred to a ward environment. Midwifery care involves the overall framework of core care (see Chapter 28). Appropriate care is to assess the needs of the individual woman and to formalize this within a documented postnatal care plan, so that she and caregivers have a clear framework by which to promote recovery (NICE 2014, 2015).

Women who have undergone an operative birth will require assistance with a number of activities they would otherwise have done themselves. During their hospital stay, they will need help to maintain their personal hygiene, to get out of bed and mobilize and to start to care for their baby. The rate at which each woman will be able to regain control over these areas of activity is highly individual. It is strongly suggested that caregivers should not expect all women to have reached a certain level of recovery in line with their 'postnatal day'.

It is now common for women to have a much shorter period in hospital after birth; some women might return home between 24 and 72 h after a major operation, with very minimal support (Wray and Bick 2012; Steen 2017). Practical advice about the management of their recovery and self-care at home is also within the remit of midwifery postpartum care. For example; the midwife might suggest that the woman identifies the ways in which she could reduce the need to go upstairs. Alongside this, women can be encouraged to go out with their baby when someone is available to help with all the baby transportation equipment; this will encourage venous return and cardiac output at a level that is beneficial rather than exhausting.

The benefits of mobility after surgery are well known and although women may be supplied with thromboembolic stockings prior to the operation and be prescribed an anticoagulant regimen such as heparin, women need to be encouraged to mobilize as soon as practicable after the operation to reduce the risk of circulatory problems. Women need an explanation that mobility is of benefit soon after the birth, but it is also an important part of care to recognize when the woman has reached her limit with regard to physical activity and may need to rest (Wray 2011; Steen 2017). Women should be encouraged to use analgesia as required in order to encourage mobilization. Good information about self-care and recovery is important to every woman and the midwife has a key role to play in this process. Each woman is unique, so her recovery from surgery alongside her adaptation to motherhood needs to be considered and tailored to meet her individual needs (Wray 2011; Steen 2017).

EMOTIONAL WELLBEING

Psychological Deviation from Normal

Psychological distress and psychiatric illness in relation to childbirth are covered in depth in Chapter 30. Birth is a significant life effect that can lead to trauma for some women. Birth trauma can have a major impact on a woman's life, her relationships with her family and new baby and her long-term health and wellbeing (Bastos et al. 2015). Postnatal support from healthcare providers is important to women who have experienced trauma (Priddis et al. 2018).

Midwives can find it easier to determine a woman's needs if they have a pre-existing relationship with the woman (Dahlberg et al. 2016). Women also value the trusting relationship with a known midwife (Dahlberg et al. 2016). This prior knowledge can mean that the midwife might detect or be concerned about a change in the woman's behaviour that has not been noticed by her family. Any initial concerns of the woman or the family should be explored by the midwife making use of open questions and listening skills during the postnatal contact either in the home or in the hospital setting (NICE 2015; Bick et al. 2011). Midwives should ask women about their emotional wellbeing, social supports and strategies for managing at every postnatal visit (Steen and Green 2016; RCOG 2016). Behavioural changes may be very subtle, but, however small, they might be of importance in the woman's overall psychological state;

it is the balance between the woman's physical condition and her psychological state that might influence an eventual decision to refer for further expert advice. Midwives should also be aware that women from culturally and linguistically diverse cultures (CALD) are at an increased risk of psychiatric disorders in the postnatal period (Steen 2017).

Postnatal fatigue is an extremely common occurrence thought to effect as many as 64% of new mothers (Badr and Zauszniewski 2017). Although the woman and her partner are likely to have an expectation of reduced sleep once the baby is born, the actual experience of this can have varied effects on individual women (Steen 2017; Wray 2012). The cause of the lack of sleep or tiredness is important – is the insomnia a result of anxiety about the future? This might include fears about the possibility of a cot death, a lack of confidence in coping as a mother, financial or relationship worries. The opportunity to sleep might be reduced because the feeding is not yet established or the baby is not in a settled environment and so the woman is constantly disturbed when she tries to sleep. Seeking to unravel the issues can help the midwife and the woman to determine the underlying cause and whether simple interventions could improve the situation. As a result of this enquiry, women who come into the category where chronic fatigue or anxiety prevents them from sleeping when the opportunity arises, may benefit from interagency referral and support. The midwife is in a prime position to determine the cause of the fatigue and facilitate referral as needed. This includes the identification of physiological reasons for the woman's fatigue. The midwife is an important member of the primary healthcare team and should practice within an interagency context (see Chapter 30). Enabling women to plan and set realistic goals as part of their own recovery from childbirth is ongoing and extends beyond the 6–8 weeks (Bick et al. 2011; Wray 2012).

WOMAN/MIDWIFE RELATIONSHIP

The essence of the contact between the woman and the midwife after the birth is to strive to maintain a therapeutic relationship – one of support and advice that builds on the relationship formed, ideally, antenatally. Within the current provision of care, it is not always possible to achieve the objective of continuity of carer postnatally, and some women will have postnatal home visits from several different midwives, possibly previously unknown to them. Indeed, other healthcare workers such as maternity support workers (MSWs) or nursing associates (NMC 2018b) may form part of the postnatal care-giving process under the supervision of midwives.

Once the woman has given birth and returned to her home environment, there may be aspects of the birth that she does not understand or that cause her distress. Where appropriate, a midwife undertaking postnatal care in the woman's home might be able to help the woman review and reflect on the birth by talking about it and listening to her concerns. Where necessary, the midwife can facilitate referral to the key people involved, in order that the woman can discuss the birth or see the records of the birth and clarify any outstanding issues (NICE 2014, 2015; Morrow et al. 2013). Other forms of support, for instance specific counselling for those with traumatic emotional experiences, might also be appropriate under professional guidance (NICE 2014a) (see Chapter 30).

REFLECTIVE ACTIVITY FOR SELF-ASSESSMENT

The postnatal time is one where the midwife needs to facilitate family bonding and be alert for any deviations in the woman's clinical state.

1. Describe at least three ways the midwife can achieve the above while ensuring these measures are woman-centred, family-centred and will support the midwife to gather the appropriate information.

2. Identify the ways that sepsis can present in the postnatal period for women and the role of the midwife in identification and prevention of more serious complications from developing.

3. Discuss how a documented care plan can facilitate optimal postnatal care for a woman.

REFERENCES

Åhlund, S., Rådestad, I., Zwedberg, S., et al. (2018). Haemorrhoids – A neglected problem faced by women after birth. *Sexual & Reproductive Healthcare, 18*, 30–36.

Aiken, C., Mehasseb, M., & Prentice, A. (2012). Secondary postpartum haemorrhage. *Fetal and Maternal Medicine Review, 23*(1), 1–14.

Alkema, L., Chou, D., Hogan, D., et al. (2015). Global, regional, and national levels and trends in maternal mortality between 1990 and 2015, with scenario-based projections to 2030: A systematic analysis by the UN Maternal Mortality Estimation Inter-Agency Group; United Nations Maternal Mortality Estimation Inter-Agency Group collaborators and technical advisory group. *Lancet, 387*(10017), 462–474.

August, P. (2018). Management of hypertension in pregnant and postpartum women. In C. Lockwood, & G. Bakris (Eds.), *UptoDate* Available at: www.uptodate.com.

Badr, H. A., & Zauszniewski, J. A. (2017). Meta-analysis of the predictive factors of postpartum fatigue. *Applied Nursing Research, 36*, 122–127.

Bastos, M. H., Furuta, M., Small, R., et al. (2015). Debriefing interventions for the prevention of psychological trauma in women following childbirth. *Cochrane Database of Systematic Reviews* (4), CD007194.

Belfort, M. (2018). Secondary (late) postpartum haemorrhage. In L. Simpson, & D. Levine (Eds.), *UptoDate*. Available at: www.uptodate.com.

Berghella, V. (2018). Cesarean delivery: Postoperative issues. In C. Lockwood (Ed.), *UptoDate*. Available at: www.uptodate.com.

Bick, D. E., Rose, V., Weavers, A., et al. (2011). Improving inpatient postnatal services: Midwives' views and perspectives of engagement in a quality improvement initiative. *BMC Health Services Research, 11*, 293.

Bigelow, A., Pereira, G., Warmsley, A., et al. (2014). Risk factors for new-onset late postpartum preeclampsia in women without a history of preeclampsia. *Obstetric Anesthesia Digest, 35*(2), 84.

Breymann, C., Honegger, C., Hösli, I., & Surbek, D. (2017). Diagnosis and treatment of iron-deficiency anaemia in pregnancy and postpartum. *Archives of Gynecology and Obstetrics, 296*(6), 1229–1234.

Brown, S., Gartland, D., Perlen, S., et al. (2015). Consultation about urinary and faecal incontinence in the year after childbirth: A cohort study. *BJOG: An International Journal of Obstetrics and Gynaecology, 122*(7), 954–962.

Chames, M., Livingston, J., Ivester, T., et al. (2002). Late postpartum eclampsia: A preventable disease? *American Journal of Obstetrics and Gynecology, 186*(6), 1174–1177.

CQC (Care Quality Commission). (2018). *NHS 2017 Survey of Women's Experiences of Maternity Care Quality Commission*. London: CQC. Available at: www.cqc.org.uk.

Dahlberg, U., Haugan, G., & Aune, I. (2016). Women's experiences of home visits by midwives in the early postnatal period. *Midwifery, 39*, 57–62.

Dellinger, R., Levy, M., Rhodes, A., et al. (2013). Surviving Sepsis Campaign: International guidelines for management of severe sepsis and septic shock. *Intensive Care Medicine, 39*(2), 165–228.

de Souza Bosco Paiva, C., Junqueira Vasconcellos de Oliveira, S., Amorim Francisco, A., et al. (2016). Length of perineal pain relief after ice pack application: A quasi-experimental study. *Women and Birth, 29*(2), 117–122.

Dossou, M., Debost-Legrand, A., Déchelotte, P., et al. (2015). Severe secondary postpartum hemorrhage: A historical cohort. *Birth, 42*(2), 149–155.

Dudley, L., Kettle, C., & Ismail, K. (2013). Secondary suturing compared to non–suturing for broken down perineal wounds following childbirth. *Cochrane Database of Systematic Reviews* (9), CD008977.

Fodstad, K., Staff, A. C., & Laine, K. (2016). Sexual activity and dyspareunia the first year postpartum in relation to degree of perineal trauma. *International Urogynecology Journal, 27*(10), 1513–1523.

Francisco, A., de Oliveira, S., Steen, M., et al. (2018). Ice pack induced perineal analgesia after spontaneous vaginal birth: A randomized controlled trial. *Women and Birth, 31*(5), e334–e340.

Frasson, A., & Dodi, G. (2016). Fecal incontinence after childbirth: Diagnostic and clinical aspects. In D. Riva, & G. Minini (Eds.), *Childbirth-related pelvic floor dysfunction*. Cham: Springer.

Gartland, D., MacArthur, C., Woolhouse, H., et al. (2016). Frequency, severity and risk factors for urinary and faecal incontinence at 4 years postpartum: A prospective cohort. *BJOG: An International Journal of Obstetrics & Gynaecology, 123*(7), 1203–1211.

Handa, V. (2018). Effect of pregnancy and childbirth on urinary incontinence and pelvic organ prolapse. In L. Brubaker (Ed.), *UptoDate*. Available at: www.uptodate.com.

Kearon, C., & Bauer, K. A. (2018). Clinical presentation and diagnosis of the non-pregnant adult with suspected deep vein thrombosis of the lower extremity. In L. Leung, & J. Mandel (Eds.), *UptoDate*. Available at: www.uptodate.com.

Knight, M., Bunch, K., Tuffnell, D., et al. (Eds.). (2018). On behalf of MBRRACE-UK. *Saving Lives, Improving Mothers' Care – Lessons Learned to Inform Maternity Care from the UK and Ireland Confidential Enquiries into Maternal Deaths and Morbidity 2014–16*. Oxford: National Perinatal Epidemiology Unit, University of Oxford.

Knight, M., Bunch, K., Tuffnell, D., et al. (Eds.). (2019). On behalf of MBRRACE-UK. *Saving Lives, Improving Mothers' Care – Lessons learned to inform maternity care from the UK and Ireland Confidential Enquiries into Maternal Deaths and Morbidity 2015–17*. Oxford: National Perinatal Epidemiology Unit, University of Oxford.

Lamb, K., & Sanders, R. (2016). Bladder care in the context of motherhood: Ensuring holistic midwifery practice. *British Journal of Midwifery, 24*(6), 415–421.

Loudon, I. (1992). The transformation of maternal mortality. *British Medical Journal, 305*, 1557–1560.

Mackenzie, J., Murray, E., & Lusher, J. (2018). Women's experiences of pregnancy related pelvic girdle pain: A systematic review. *Midwifery, 1*(56), 102–111.

Mangesi, L., & Zakarija-Grkovic, I. (2016). Treatments for breast engorgement during lactation. *Cochrane Database of Systematic Reviews* (6), CD006946.

Marchant, S. (2006). The postnatal care journey – are we nearly there yet? *MIDIRS Midwifery Digest, 16*(3), 295 304.

Markova, V., Norgaard, A., Jørgensen, K. J., & Langhoff-Roos, J. (2015). Treatment for women with postpartum iron deficiency anaemia. *Cochrane Database of Systematic Reviews* (8), CD010861.

Mavrides, E., Allard, S., Chandraharan, E., & on behalf of the Royal College of Obstetricians and Gynaecologists., et al. (2016). Prevention and management of postpartum haemorrhage. *An International Journal of Obstetrics and Gynaecology, 124*(5), e106 e149.

McDonald, E. A., Gartland, D., Small, R., & Brown, S. J. (2015). Dyspareunia and childbirth: A prospective cohort study. *BJOG: An International Journal of Obstetrics & Gynaecology, 122*(5), 672–679.

Morrow, J., McLachlan, H., Forster, D., et al. (2013). Redesigning postnatal care: Exploring the views and experiences of midwives. *Midwifery, 29*(2), 159–166.

Mulder, F. E., Hakvoort, R. A., Schoffelmeer, M. A., et al. (2014). Postpartum urinary retention: A systematic review of adverse effects and management. *International Urogynecology Journal, 25*(12), 1605–1612.

Muller, A. E., Oostvogel, P. M., Steegers, E. A., & Dörr, P. J. (2006). Morbidity related to maternal group B streptococcal infections. *Acta Obstetrica et Gynecologica Scandinavica, 85*(9), 1027–1037.

NHS England. (2016). *National Maternity Review, Better Births: Improving outcomes of maternity services in England – A five year forward view for maternity care*. Available at: www.england.nhs.uk/publication/better-births-improving-outcomes-of-maternity-services-in-england-a-five-year-forward-view-for-maternity-care.

NICE (National Institute for Health and Care Excellence). (2011). *Caesarean section. Clinical Guideline 132*. London: NICE.

NICE (National Institute for Health and Care Excellence). (2013). *Urinary incontinence in women: Management. Clinical Guideline 171*. London: NICE.

NICE (National Institute for Health and Care Excellence). (2014a). *Antenatal and postnatal mental health: Clinical management and service guidance: CG 192*. London: NICE.

NICE (National Institute for Health and Care Excellence). (2014b). *Intrapartum care for healthy women and babies. Clinical Guideline 190*. London: NICE.

NICE (National Institute for Health and Care Excellence). (2015). *Postnatal care up to 8 weeks after birth. Clinical Guideline 37*. London: NICE.

NMC (Nursing and Midwifery Council). (2018a). *Standards for competence for Registered midwives*. London: NMC. Available at: www.nmc.org.uk.

NMC (Nursing and Midwifery Council). (2018b). *The Code: Professional standards of practice and behaviour for nurses, midwives and nursing associates*. Available at: www.nmc.org.uk/standards/code.

Paliulyte, V., Drasutiene, G., Ramasauskaite, D., et al. (2017). Physiological uterine involution in primiparous and multiparous women: Ultrasound study. *Obstetrics and Gynecology International*, *2017*, 6739345.

Pavord, S., Myers, B., Robinson, S., & on behalf of the British committee for Standards in Haematology., et al. (2012). UK guidelines on the management of iron deficiency in pregnancy. *British Journal of Haematology*, *156*, 588–600.

Priddis, H. S., Keedle, H., & Dahlen, H. (2018). The perfect storm of trauma: The experiences of women who have experienced birth trauma and subsequently accessed residential parenting services in Australia. *Women and Birth*, *31*(1), 17–24.

RCOG (Royal College of Obstetricians and Gynaecologists). (2012). *Bacterial sepsis in pregnancy. Green-top Guideline No 64a April*. London: RCOG.

RCOG (Royal College of Obstetricians and Gynaecologists). (2016). *Providing quality care for women – A framework for maternity service standards*. London: RCOG.

Reed, R., Sharman, R., & Inglis, C. (2017). Women's descriptions of childbirth trauma relating to care provider actions and interactions. *BMC Pregnancy and Childbirth*, *17*, 21.

Schmied, V., & Bick, D. (2014). Postnatal care – Current issues and future challenges. *Midwifery*, *30*(6), 571–574.

Shin, G. H., Toto, E. L., & Schey, R. (2015). Pregnancy and postpartum bowel changes: Constipation and fecal incontinence. *American Journal of Gastroenterology*, *10*(4), 521.

Steen, M. (2007). Perineal tears and episiotomy: How do wounds heal? *British Journal of Midwifery Perineal Care Supplement*, *15*(5), 273–280.

Steen, M. (2013). Continence in women following childbirth. *Nursing Standard*, *28*(1), 47–55.

Steen, M. (2017). Maternal morbidity following childbirth. In S. MacDonald, & G. Johnson (Eds.), *Mayes' Midwifery* (15th edn.) (pp. 1079–1090). London: Elsevier.

Steen, M., & Diaz, M. (2018). Perineal trauma: A women's health and wellbeing issue. *British Journal of Midwifery*, *26*(9), 574–584.

Steen, M., & Green, B. (2016). Mental health during pregnancy and early parenthood. In M. Steen, & Michael Thomas (Eds.), *Mental health across the lifespan: A handbook*. New York: Taylor and Francis.

Steen, M., Briggs, M., & King, D. (2006). Alleviating postnatal perineal trauma: To cool or not to cool? *British Journal of Midwifery*, *14*(5), 304–308.

Turawa, E. B., Musekiwa, A., & Rohwer, A. C. (2015). Interventions for preventing postpartum constipation. *Cochrane Database of Systematic Reviews* (9), CD011625.

Üçyiğit, A., & Johns, J. (2016). The postpartum ultrasound scan. *Ultrasound*, *24*(3), 163–169.

WHO (World Health Organization). (2013). *Recommendations on postnatal care of the mother and newborn*. Geneva: WHO. Available at: www.who.int.

Wong, B. B., Chan, Y. H., Leow, M. Q., et al. (2017). Application of cabbage leaves compared to gel packs for mothers with breast engorgement: Randomised controlled trial. *International Journal of Nursing Studies*, *76*, 92–99.

Woodley, S. J., Boyle, R., Cody, J. D., et al. (2017). Pelvic floor muscle training for prevention and treatment of urinary and faecal incontinence in antenatal and postnatal women. *Cochrane Database of Systematic Reviews* (12), CD007471.

Wound Healing Institute Australia. (2019). *Wound innovations, perineal care module*. Available at: www.woundinnovations.com.au/product/perineal-care-module.

Wray J. (2011) Bouncing back? An ethnographic study exploring the context of care and recovery after birth through the experiences and voices of mothers. Unpublished PhD thesis, University of Salford.

Wray, J. (2012). Impact of place upon celebration of birth – experiences of new mothers on a postnatal ward. *MIDIRS Midwifery Digest*, *23*(3), 357–361.

Wray, J., & Bick, D. (2012). Is there a future for universal midwifery postnatal care in the UK? *MIDIRS Midwifery Digest*, *22*(44), 495–498.

Yonemoto, N., Dowswell, T., Nagai, S., & Mori, R. (2017). Schedules for home visits in the early postpartum period. *Cochrane Database Systematic Reviews* (8), CD009326.

ANNOTATED FURTHER READING

National Maternity Review. Better Births. Improving outcomes of maternity services in England. A five year forward view for maternity care. Available at: www.england.nhs.uk/publication/better-births-improving-outcomes-of-maternity-services-in-england-a-five-year-forward-view-for-maternity-care/

The National Maternity Review explores the requirements for planning, design and safe implementation of maternity care. More specifically, it explores how women and families can get the care that they want and how staff can be supported to provide the care.

NICE Postnatal Care Quality Standard, 16 July 2013. Available at: nice.org.uk/guidance/qs37

The Postnatal Quality Standard outlines routine postnatal care for women and babies. It is inclusive of feeding support, recognizing when deviations from normal occur, safe sleeping and outlines high quality care and areas that need improvement.

Redshaw, M., & Henderson, J. (2015). *Safely delivered: A national survey of women's experience of maternity care 2014.* Available at: www.npeu.ox.ac.uk/downloads/files/reports/Safely%20delivered%20NMS%202014.pdf.

Ten thousand women giving birth in England were surveyed in a 2-week period in 2006 and 2010. The survey response rate was 47%. Key findings from the survey are reported that provide a snapshot of maternity care in 2014.

Surviving Sepsis Campaign. Available at: www.survivingsepsis.org/Guidelines/Pages/default.aspx

The Surviving Sepsis Campaign is a joint collaboration of the Society of Critical Care Medicine and the European Society of Intensive Care Medicine committed to reducing mortality and morbidity from sepsis and septic shock worldwide. Up-to-date recommendations can be found through the site.

The Royal College of Midwives. (2014). *Postnatal care planning (Postnatal Pressure Points – a series).* Available at: https://uat.rcm.org.uk/media/2358/pressure-points-postnatal-care-planning.pdf.

This report focuses on postnatal care planning and demonstrates how the situation could be improved through the funding of more midwives.

USEFUL WEBSITES

MBRRACE-UK Mothers and Babies: Reducing Risk through Audits and Confidential Enquiries across the UK: www.npeu.ox.ac.uk/mbrrace-uk

National Childbirth Trust: www.nct.org.uk/parenting/you-after-birth

National Institute for Health and Care [formerly Clinical] Excellence: www.nice.org.uk

NICE Quality Standard for postnatal care: www.nice.org.uk/guidance/qs37

Open University. Postnatal Care HEAT module – Lab space, Open University: www.open.edu/openlearncreate/mod/oucontent/view.php?id=339

Royal College of Midwives (RCM): www.rcm.org.uk/search/node/postnatal?f%5B0%5D=field_topic%3A41

World Health Organization: www.who.int/maternal_child_adolescent/topics/newborn/postnatal_care/en/

30

Perinatal Mental Health

Maureen D. Raynor, Amy Mason, Mark Williams,
Pete Wallroth, Gill Skene, Sherry Whibley

CHAPTER CONTENTS

In psychological terms, pregnancy, childbirth and the puerperium are major life events or life crises. Having children is associated with an immense increase in individual life changes that may lead to anxiety and chronic stressors, for example a new baby may result in a change of housing and brings increased financial demands. Pregnant women in employment will inevitably take maternity leave and may return to work in a different capacity or even on a part-time basis. A new baby may cause disruption to the family unit. Roles and responsibilities alter with changes to the dynamics of family relationships. Having a child may place strains on relationships and there is a higher rate of relationship discord and breakdown around this time. Many women find coping with the physiological adaptation to pregnancy, the plethora of antenatal screening tests and advice, issues around choice, control and communication emotionally draining. Therefore, while many women and their partners experience pregnancy and childbirth as a joyous, exciting and life-affirming event, the transition to parenthood is an emotionally charged time, bringing common anxieties, a certain degree of loss and periods of self-doubt. This can culminate in pregnancy and postpartum being a fragile time of physical, psychological and social upheavals. Like other stressful life events, childbirth can be associated with depression and anxiety. However, it is also known to be associated with an increased risk of serious psychiatric illness. Pregnancy provides a wealth of opportunities for promoting emotional health while predicting and preventing mental illness. It is important for midwives to be able to identify emotional changes and adjustment reactions as a woman transitions to motherhood, and distinguish them from the early warning signs of emotional distress or indeed, mental illness.

THIS CHAPTER IS FORMED OF TWO DISTINCT BUT INTERRELATED PARTS

Part A of the chapter aims to:

- explore the psychological context of pregnancy, childbirth and the puerperium by examining the full range of human emotions that may affect women as they adjust to change and make the transition to motherhood
- emphasize that awareness of the multiplicity of psychosocial factors and what constitutes emotions and behaviours are key components in enhancing understanding of perinatal mental health.

Part B of the chapter aims to:

- identify the range of perinatal mental illness (PMI) or psychiatric conditions that pre-exist or co-exist with pregnancy as well as those conditions presenting within the puerperium
- highlight key recommendations from national and international reports that act as the key drivers for change in the prevention, early recognition and management of PMI.

PART A: PREGNANCY, CHILDBIRTH, PUERPERIUM: THE PSYCHOLOGICAL CONTEXT

STRESS/ANXIETY

Although pregnancy and the transition to motherhood are normal life events, they are periods of heightened vulnerability for the onset of anxiety and depression in a woman's life. Stress and anxiety are the psychopathology of humans' existence and a part of normal human emotion. A degree of stress during pregnancy is both essential and normal for the psychological adjustment of pregnant women. The 'worry work' that women encounter assists in their psychological adaptation to the emotional demands and changes of pregnancy. Conversely, elevated levels of stress hormones and unnecessary anxiety will stretch coping reserves, and could prove disabling. Stress is the body's psychophysical response to any type of demand or threat, whether good or bad. Anxiety on the other hand is a state of angst, worry or unease,

often triggered by an element of perceived threat or an event where there is an uncertain outcome, such as a written examination or when important decisions have to be made. The brain plays a key role in how an individual responds and processes the perception of a threat. This is realized via a neurohormonal response by both the neocortex and limbic system. The 'fight or flight' reflex is produced when there is a threat to the self. Anxiety and fear causes the individual to become stressed, releasing stress response hormones, namely catecholamines (adrenaline/noradrenaline) and cortisol. A host of psycho-physical symptoms can manifest, such as:

- hyper-alertness
- tension
- sense of unease
- restlessness
- insomnia
- fear and forgetfulness.

Gastrointestinal upset and marked changes in the cardiovascular system may also be experienced, e.g. dry mouth and nausea, sweating, palpitations, tachycardia, shortness of breath and dizziness. Stress and anxiety therefore have a cognitive, somatic, emotional, physiological and behavioural component.

Anxiety disorders, on the other hand, are a group of mental illness that cause such marked distress that they disrupt normal function, overwhelm or impair the individual's ability to lead a normal life. Examples of anxiety disorders such as obsessional–compulsive and phobic anxiety states are discussed in more detail in Part B of the chapter.

A number of studies have raised the profile of elevated levels of stress hormones during the antenatal period, having the potential to lead to deleterious effects on the fetus (Dunkel Schetter and Tanner 2012; Glover et al. 2010; O'Donnell et al. 2009; Talge et al. 2007; Teixeira et al. 2009). Persistent antenatal anxiety may act as a possible precursor to maternal mental illness postpartum, however this is still an emerging field. The mechanism by which raised levels of stress hormones may affect fetal development is not yet fully understood. However, Biaggi et al. (2015) and Glover and Barlow (2014) highlight the importance of identifying women at risk antenatally and having strategies in place to help guide midwifery practice plus alleviate stress and anxiety for pregnant women. In the UK, this view resonates with the National Institute for Health and Care Excellence's (NICE 2014a) clinical guidelines on antenatal and postnatal mental health.

It can be concluded that there are many factors in women's lives that can impact on their happiness (Fig. 30.1) and affect their emotional health and wellbeing. Understanding the root cause and expression of anxiety, stress and mental distress in women is complex, as the social circumstances in which women live and into which children are born play a major role in their health and wellbeing. Midwives have a pivotal role to play in directing women and their partner to antenatal education programme (see Chapter 9) and where appropriate, counselling such as in the case of an overwhelming fear of pregnancy/childbirth known as *tocophobia* (see Chapter 18). Such strategies can be empowering in terms of behaviour control, development of self-efficacy and promotion of self-confidence coupled with a sense of satisfaction and positive feelings towards parenthood.

TRANSITION TO PARENTHOOD

Postnatally, parents may find coping with the demands of a new baby, e.g. infant feeding, financial constraints, the whole process of lifestyle adjustments and role changes a real strain. For new mothers, this will involve diverse emotional responses ranging from joy and elation to sadness and utter exhaustion. Fatigue, pain and discomfort commonly result once the elation that follows the safe arrival of the baby wears off. Disturbed sleep is inevitable with a new baby. Mothers who are trying to establish breastfeeding, older women, women who are recovering from a caesarean section or those who have had a long and difficult labour/birth, twins or higher multiples, may feel wretched and constantly weary for months following childbirth. Soreness and pain being experienced from perineal trauma will affect libido, so too will feelings of exhaustion, despair and unhappiness that may be associated with the round-the-clock demands of caring for a new baby or higher multiples. Little wonder then that women may be left feeling bereft and quite miserable after giving birth.

ROLE CHANGE/ROLE CONFLICT

Having a baby, and particularly the transition to parenthood that accompanies the first child, leads to a significant shift in a couple's relationship; social networks are disrupted, especially those of the mother, and the quality and quantity of social support such networks can and do provide. There is a strong possibility that old relationships, particularly with those who are childless or single, may be weakened, leading to a sense of social isolation. However, some relationships are strengthened or even replaced gradually by new contacts established with other parents. The dynamics of relationships with family members are also altered during this process of transition and change. The relationship with the woman's/man's parents for example alters as their daughter/son becomes a mother/father and their parents develop new roles as grandparents. The competing demands on time of caring for a new baby may lead to role conflict and confusion for parents. Mothers may find that there is little time for them to pursue other activities, which can diminish any opportunity for contact with and support from others. Partners, especially young fathers, can also experience a sense of isolation as the dynamic within the couple's relation alters, becoming more baby-centred (Doss et al. 2009; Werner-Bierwisch et al. 2018). Postnatal care is therefore essential to women's emotional wellbeing and should be a continuation of the care given during pregnancy (Royal College of Midwives, RCM 2012). Its contribution plays a significant part in the positive adjustment to parenthood, as it

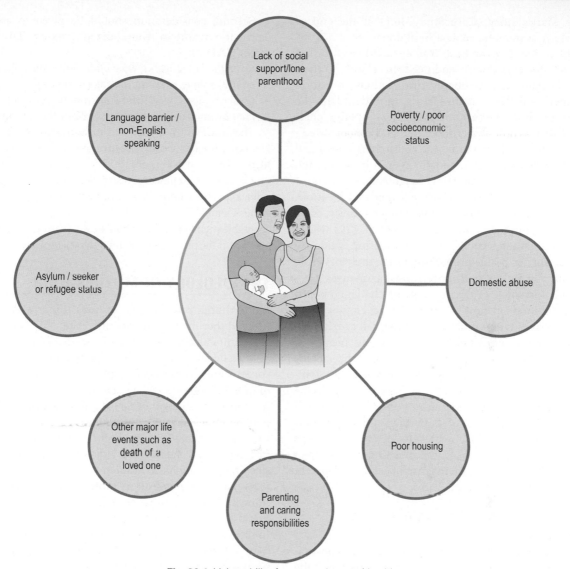

Fig. 30.1 Vulnerability factors and mental health.

assists in the acquisition of confident and well-informed parenting skills (Barlow et al. 2011; Baldwin et al. 2018; Mihelic et al. 2018).

Fatherhood

Like motherhood, men's transition to fatherhood is guided by the sociocultural context in which they live and work and by the personal characteristics that interplay with the quality of the relationship with their partner. A detailed analysis by Genesoni and Tallandini (2009) revealed that pregnancy experienced by their partner was found to be the most demanding period in terms of psychological reorganization of the self for men.

Labour and birth were reported to be the most intensely emotional moments with the postnatal period being mostly influenced by environmental factors and being viewed as the most challenging during the transition and adjustment to fatherhood. Not surprisingly, many new fathers adjusting to the demands and disruption to routine that a new baby brings may struggle to reconcile their personal and work-related needs with those of their new families (Kaźmierczak and Karasiewicz 2018; Philpott et al. 2017).

It is postulated that approximately 10% of new fathers experience mental health problems, including depression and anxiety (Singley and Edwards 2015)

– see Mark's story (Case Study 30.1) at the end of Part A. A systematic review by Baldwin et al. (2018) sought to identify the best available evidence on first time fathers' experiences and needs in relation to their mental health and wellbeing during their transition to fatherhood. Three main factors were identified: the formation of the fatherhood identity, competing challenges of the new fatherhood role and negative feelings and fears relating to it. The researchers concluded that the role restrictions and changes in lifestyle often resulted in fathers reporting heightened feelings of stress, for which denial or escape activities, e.g. smoking, working longer hours or listening to music, were used as coping techniques. Baldwin et al. (2018) also found that fathers wanted more information, guidance and support to better prepare them for their new role as a father as well as partner relationship changes. Crespi and Ruspini (2015) state that the challenge posed by parenthood on how to balance paid employment, leisure activities and other interests as well as relationships brings responsibilities, anxieties and pleasures. The issues outlined are real childrearing concerns for both men and women in contemporary society. Strikingly fatherhood in modernity requires men to be simultaneously provider, guide, household help and nurturer. The difficulties of these roles, and the tensions they sometimes produce is a test to men's relationships with their female partners, the meaning and place of work in their lives and their sense of self as competent adults (Crespi and Ruspini 2015).

Routine Screening for Mental Health/Wellbeing

In the UK, NICE (2014a) guidance on ante- and postnatal mental health provides clarity on routine screening for PMI during a pregnant woman's first contact with primary care or her antenatal 'booking' visit, which is repeated early postpartum. The (Whooley) questions posed are to aid with the early identification of common mental health problems such as anxiety and depression, as part of a general discussion about a woman's mental health and emotional wellbeing:

Whooley Questions

- *During the past month, have you often been bothered by feeling down, depressed or hopeless?*
- *During the past month, have you often been bothered by having little interest or pleasure in doing things?*

Second, consideration should be given to anxiety using the two-item **Generalized Anxiety Disorder scale (GAD-2)**:

- *Over the last 2 weeks, how often have you been bothered by feeling nervous, anxious or on edge?*
- *Over the last 2 weeks, how often have you been bothered by not being able to stop or control worrying?*

The NICE (2014a) key recommendation is that if a woman responds positively to either of the depression identification questions or is at risk of developing a mental illness, or there is clinical concern, the midwife should consider, as part of a thorough assessment, referring the woman to her General Practitioner (GP) or escalate the referral to a suitable member of the mental health team such as a psychiatrist if the problem is deemed to be serious.

THE IDEOLOGY OF MOTHERHOOD

Motherhood, it is thought, ensures that a woman has fulfilled her biological destiny, confirms a woman's femininity and raises her status in society, but without financial gain. Instead of feeling elated by motherhood, some women experience displeasure, harbour feelings of unhappiness and feel dismayed or even disappointed in their role as new mothers (Grabowska 2017). Many may be afraid to speak out about their feelings in case they are judged a 'bad' mother. Painful emotions may be internalized, magnifying difficulties with coping and sleeping, leading many women to suffer in silence. Distress may then manifest as mothers rage against their impossible situation. Some women may even grieve for the loss of their former lifestyle, career or status. Feminist ideology contends that healthcare professionals have defined women's postnatal experience through proposing that well-adjusted, 'normal' and therefore 'good' mothers are those who are happy and fulfilled, but those who are unfulfilled, anxious or distressed are 'ill' and may be perceived as 'bad' mothers (Nicholson 2010). This may lead to feelings of isolation, inadequacy and confusion. The ideology of motherhood is therefore an assumption and a paradox with inherent dichotomies as the woman strives to be 'super mum, super wife, super everything' (Choi et al. 2005). Midwives have a pivotal role to play in assisting women and their partners to prepare for the physical, social, emotional and psychological demands of pregnancy, labour, the puerperium and, perhaps more importantly, their transition to parenthood (Barlow et al. 2011; Department of Health and Social Care, DHSC 2011; RCM 2012).

SOCIAL SUPPORT

Social support refers to empathy relations, emotional support, intelligence support and economic or financial support. During periods of stress, supportive and holistic care from midwives will not only assist in promoting emotional wellbeing of women, but will also help to ameliorate threatened psychological morbidity in the postnatal period (East et al. 2019; NICE 2016). Women who are socially isolated or who have poor socioeconomic circumstances are particularly vulnerable to mental health problems and need additional help and support. This includes women from minority ethnic groups who do not speak English, and often have problems accessing health care (Knight et al. 2018). The psychosocial benefits of midwifery care well beyond the historical boundaries of the traditionally defined postnatal period should not be underestimated (World Health Organization, WHO 2014). That said, the restructuring of postnatal care means the majority of women who birth in a hospital setting are transferred home within hours or the first day following birth (Jones et al. 2016; Bowden et al. 2019). Consequently, there is now a social expectation that midwives will respond more flexibly and responsively to women's emotional needs on an individual basis (NHS England 2016; NICE 2006). This calls for skilled multidisciplinary and multiagency collaboration as well as effective teamwork, taking into account the diversity within teams, for example the invaluable contribution of the maternity support worker in maternity care. Social support is further explored in Part B.

EMOTIONAL CHANGES DURING PREGNANCY, LABOUR AND THE PUERPERIUM

Pregnancy

Since many decisions have to be made, it is perfectly normal for women to have periods of self-doubt and crises of confidence. Box 30.1 outlines the many and varied emotions women may experience during the different trimesters of pregnancy. The reality for many women will encompass fluctuations between ambivalence to positive and negative emotions.

Labour

During labour, midwives must facilitate choice to help women maintain control. Factors that induce stress should be prevented, or at least minimized, as the

---

> **BOX 30.1 Common Emotional Changes that Might be Experienced during Pregnancy**
>
> **First trimester**
> - pleasure, excitement, elation
> - dismay, disappointment
> - ambivalence, emotional lability (e.g. episodes of weepiness exacerbated by physiological events such as nausea, vomiting and tiredness)
> - increased femininity
>
> **Second trimester**
> - a feeling of wellbeing, especially as the physiological effects of tiredness, nausea and vomiting start to abate
> - a sense of increased attachment to the fetus; the impact of ultrasound scanning generating images for the prospective parents may intensify the experience
> - stress and anxiety about antenatal screening and diagnostic tests
> - increased demand for knowledge and information as preparations are now on the way for the birth
> - feelings of the need for increasing detachment from work commitments
>
> **Third trimester**
> - loss of or increased libido
> - altered body image
> - psychological effects from physiological discomforts such as backache and heartburn
> - anxiety about labour (e.g. pain)
> - anxiety about fetal abnormality, which may disturb sleep or cause nightmares
> - increased vulnerability to major life events such as financial status, moving house or lack of a supportive partner.

woman's long-term emotional health may be severely compromised by an adverse birth experience (Care Quality Commission, CQC 2018). Choice and control are important psychological concepts to mental health and wellbeing. Evidence suggests that having choice in pregnancy and childbirth, and a sense of being in control, lead to a more satisfying birth experience (Cook and Loomis 2012). The publication of *Better Births* (NHS England 2016) signals a real philosophical shift in maternity care in terms of the guaranteed choices for women.

Ongoing research to determine the relationship between women's perception of control during childbirth and postnatal outcomes is needed in order to measure factors such as postnatal depression, positive parenting relationships and self-esteem. Common emotional responses during labour are detailed in Box 30.2.

BOX 30.2 **Emotional Changes during Labour**

- Ranging from great excitement and anticipation, to utter dread
- Fear of the unknown
- Fear of technology, intervention and hospitalization
- Tension, fear and anxiety about pain and the ability to exercise control during labour
- Concerns about the wellbeing of the baby and ability of the partner to cope
- Fear of death: hospitals may be construed as places of illness, death and dying; the magnitude of such feelings may intensify if the woman experiences life-threatening complications or even an emergency caesarean section
- The process of birth thrusts a lot of private data into the realms of the public, so there could be a fear of lack of privacy or utter embarrassment.

BOX 30.3 **Common Emotional Changes during the Puerperium**

- Immediately following birth, the woman might experience relief. The woman might convey a cool detachment from events, especially if labour was protracted, complicated and difficult
- Contradictory and conflicting feelings ranging from satisfaction, joy and elation to exhaustion, helplessness, discontentment and disappointment as the early weeks seem to be dominated by the novelty and unpredictability of the new baby
- A feeling of closeness to partner or baby; equally the woman may feel disinterested in the baby
- Early skin-to-skin contact and breastfeeding will help to nurture the early stages of relationship building between mother and baby
- Being very attentive towards the baby; equally the woman may show disinterest in the baby
- Fear of the unknown and sudden realization of overwhelming responsibility
- Exhaustion and increased emotionality
- Pain (e.g. perineal, in nipples)
- Increased vulnerability, indecisiveness (e.g. in feeding), loss of libido, disturbed sleep and anxiety.

The Puerperium

The puerperium is hailed as the 'fourth trimester' – an emotionally complex transitional phase. By definition, it is the period from birth to 6–8 weeks postpartum, when the woman is readjusting physiologically, socially and psychologically to motherhood. Emotional responses may be just as intense and powerful for experienced as well as for new mothers. The major psychological changes are therefore emotional. The woman's mood appears to be a barometer, reflecting the baby's needs of feeding, sleeping and crying patterns. New mothers tend to be easily upset and oversensitive. A sense of proportion is easily lost, as women may feel overwhelmed and agitated by minor mishaps. The woman might start to regain a sense of proportion and 'normality' between 6 and 12 weeks. Exhaustion is also a major factor of women's emotional state (Giallo et al. 2015). Perhaps the most important factor in regaining any semblance of normality is the mother's ability to sleep throughout the night. A woman's sexual urges, emotional stability and intellectual acuity may take months, if not longer, to return. Some of the more common emotional changes in the puerperium are summarized in Box 30.3.

POSTNATAL 'BLUES'

Childbirth is an emotionally intense experience. Mood changes in the early days postpartum are particularly common. The postnatal 'blues' is a transitory state, experienced by 50–80% of women depending on parity

(Harris et al. 1994). Many women experience this well-known phenomenon depicted as a mild mood disruption that occurs within the early postpartum period O'Keane et al. 2011; Miller et al. 2017). It has been identified as an antecedent to depression following childbirth (Cooper and Murray 1997; Beck 2001). The onset typically occurs between day 3 and 5 postpartum, but may last up to 1 week or more, though rarely persisting longer than 48 h. The main features are mild and may include:

- a state whereby the woman experiences labile emotions (e.g. tearfulness, despair, irritability to euphoria and laughter)
- a state whereby the woman feels overwhelmed by the sudden realization of the relentless responsibility of the baby's 24-h dependency and vulnerability.

The actual aetiology is unclear but hormonal influences (e.g. changes in oestrogen, progesterone and prolactin levels) seem to be implicated as the period of increased emotionality appears to coincide with the production of milk in the breasts. This state of heightened emotionality is self-limiting and will resolve spontaneously, assisted by support from loved ones. The midwife should be vigilant during this time, as persistent features could be indicative of depressive illness.

DISTRESS OR DEPRESSION?

Repeated contact with women during pregnancy and the puerperium afford a wealth of opportunity to explore feelings, experience and emotions, and for midwives to provide clear explanations to women about the differences between distress – a normal reaction to major life events – and depressive illness. However, midwives should be mindful of over-reliance on the medical model to describe women's moods, as such an approach may serve to pathologize or medicalize normal emotional changes (Nicholson 2010).

Emotional Distress Associated with Traumatic Birth Events

Understanding the root cause and expression of mental distress associated with pregnancy and childbirth is complex. It is important to recognize the interrelationship between traumatic life events and women's mental health. Vulnerability factors such as a history of childhood domestic abuse, sexual abuse or a morbid fear of childbirth can negate a woman's experience of childbirth. What is intended to be one of the happiest days in a woman's life can quickly turn into anguish and distress. Furthermore, environmental factors may lead to a sense of loss of control, for example effects of intense pain, use of technological interventions, insensitive and disrespectful care or an emergency caesarean section (CS) may prove very distressing and frightening. There is increasing recognition that childbirth can be a cause of post-traumatic stress disorder (PTSD) (Furuta et al. 2012). *PTSD*, a term most commonly associated with individuals who have suffered the onslaught of war, has emerged in the literature around maternity care. PTSD is defined as a clinical syndrome typified by re-experiencing, avoidance, negative cognition and mood plus hyperarousal symptoms, which persist for more than 1 month after exposure to a traumatic event (Regier et al. 2013; Cook et al. 2018; de Graaff et al. 2018) (see Case Studies 30.1–30.3).

Regier et al. (2013) states that PTSD is categorized as a trauma and stress-related disorder in the *Diagnostic and Statistical Manual* (DSM)-5, when a person has been exposed directly or indirectly to, or have witnessed death, threatened death, actual or threatened serious injury or sexual violence. Such a traumatizing experience should have led to a myriad of symptomatology highlighted above before the diagnosis of PTSD can be made. Obstetric PTSD occurs when women feared they or their baby were in danger of dying. Not surprisingly it is commonest after emergency

> ### BOX 30.4 Reported Symptoms of Obstetric PTSD
>
> - Features of obstetric PTSD – applies where symptoms are present for >1 month (Beck 2009)
> - Intrusive thoughts or images resulting in nightmares, panic attacks or 'flashbacks' about the birth
> - Detachment from loved ones and difficulty with mother–baby relationship (attachment)
> - Avoidance, especially of issues relating to pregnancy/birth
> - Hypervigilance/increased arousal – having a sense of imminent disaster
> - Sleep disturbances
> - Irritability or angry outbursts
> - Anxiety/depression
> - Other features are not dissimilar to those previously discussed in the text relating to stress and anxiety.

CS or obstetric emergencies, particularly involving intensive care. It is estimated 6% of emergency CS are followed by obstetric PTSD (Beck 2009). Box 30.4 highlights some of the reported symptoms of obstetric PTSD.

Unlike mild to moderate depression in the postpartum period, which seems to have its roots in the biophysical and psychosocial domains, obstetric distress after childbirth appears to be directly linked to the stress, fear and trauma of birth, yet its prevalence is not well recognized. de Graaff et al. (2018) claim there is still no research on primary prevention of traumatic childbirth and the research that exists on secondary prevention remains equivocal and insufficient. Psychological interventions such as 'debriefing' have been suggested to manage immediate symptomatology but there is no reliable evidence that it is a useful intervention in reducing psychological morbidity. Moreover, clinical guidelines from NICE (2014a) have stated that following a traumatic birth, women should not routinely be offered 'single-session formal debriefing focused on the birth'. Instead midwives and other healthcare professionals should support women who wish to talk about their experience and draw on the love and support of family and friends. Neither should midwives overlook the impact of birth on the partner.

Association between Domestic Violence/Abuse and Depressive Illness

The definition of domestic violence and abuse is: any incident or pattern of incidents of controlling, coercive or threatening behaviour, violence or abuse between those aged 16 or over who are or have been intimate partners or family members regardless of gender or sexuality. This can encompass but is not limited to the following types of abuse: psychological, physical, sexual, financial and emotional (Strickland and Allen 2018).

There is an association between domestic abuse/violence and perinatal mental illness, with a significant predisposition to depression in the postpartum period (Howard et al. 2013; Ferrar et al. 2016; Zhanga et al. 2019). Violence against women, particularly intimate partner violence and sexual abuse/violence, is not a new phenomenon, nor are its consequences to women's physical, mental and reproductive health. It is therefore a major public health problem and a violation of women's human rights (WHO 2017). Global estimates published by WHO (2017) indicate that about 1 in 3 (35%) of women worldwide have experienced either physical and/or sexual intimate partner violence or non-partner sexual violence in their lifetime. Most of this violence is intimate partner violence. Worldwide, almost one-third (30%) of women who have been in a relationship report that they have experienced some form of physical and/or sexual violence by their intimate partner in their lifetime. Furthermore globally, as many as 38% of murders of women are committed by a male intimate partner (WHO 2017). These crimes include domestic abuse, rape, sexual offences, stalking, harassment, so-called 'honour-based' violence, including forced marriage, female genital mutilation, child abuse, human trafficking focusing on sexual exploitation, prostitution, pornography and obscenity (Strickland and Allen 2018).

In the UK, a recent report by the National Rural Crime Network (NRCN 2019) identified that there is under-reporting of domestic abuse in rural areas and highlighted the barriers to reporting, how to improve reporting and improve services to survivors of domestic abuse. This is the culmination of results from an 18-month intensive research study that analysed the evidence after speaking in-depth to survivors of abuse, assessing local support services and examining the approach adopted by the police. Knight et al. (2019) conveyed that all the women who were murdered in the triennial period of 2014–16 were killed by a partner or former partner. In a number of instances, there was no written evidence women had been asked about domestic abuse, or they had only ever been seen in the presence of their partner and thus had no opportunity to report abuse. In the triennium 2015–2017, Knight et al. (2019) reported that 6% of the women who died during or

up to a year after pregnancy in the UK were at severe and multiple disadvantage. The main factors linked to multiple disadvantage were a mental health diagnosis, substance use and domestic abuse. Knight et al. (2019) stressed that healthcare professionals need to be alert to the symptoms or signs of domestic abuse, and women should be given the opportunity to disclose domestic abuse in an environment in which they feel secure.

Antenatal Screening for Domestic Abuse/Violence

Although O'Doherty et al. (2015) concluded in their Cochrane Review that, while screening increases identification and that there is insufficient evidence to justify screening in healthcare settings, antenatal care provides midwives and other healthcare professionals a window of opportunity for identifying women who experience intimate partner violence. Not only is it often the only point of contact for women within a healthcare setting, but also provision of health services and support through the duration of a pregnancy, and the possibility for follow-up, make antenatal care a suitable setting for addressing issues of abuse (NICE 2014b; WHO 2017). The NICE (2008) antenatal care guidelines recommendation is for healthcare professionals to be alert to the symptoms or signs of domestic violence. Sensitive enquiry will ensure that women are given the opportunity to disclose domestic violence in an environment in which they feel secure (see Chapters 11 and 18).

CONCLUSION

A plethora of significant social and health policies and clinical guidelines have resulted in wider consideration being given to the social and psychological context of pregnancy and the puerperium. The transition to parenthood can be challenging for both mothers and fathers. Their experience will be influenced by their sociocultural background, as well as the interplay of a myriad of other factors. Midwives need to have knowledge and understanding of how they influence care provision, and develop a toolkit of skills and information on how they can best support women and their partner to make positive adjustment to their parenting role. Box 30.5 provides a summary of key points.

CASE STUDY 30.1   Mark's Story – Depression and ADHD

Never in a million years would I have said that I would end up with depression, let alone in the postnatal period. I was so uneducated back in 2004, when my life changed forever.

It started from the labour ward when I had my first and only panic attack to date when the doctors came rushing in and telling me that my wife, Michelle had to have an emergency C- Section straight away … and thinking my wife and baby where going to die.

When my son was born I didn't get that overwhelming feeling of love that I was expecting, I was just glad they were both alive.

Michelle, the lady I love, went on to have severe postnatal depression and the care teams came to be involved after 2 weeks. I didn't have a clue about postnatal depression and was now thinking maybe it was down to me. It made me wonder if I was going to be a good dad. My life totally changed and within months, things got much worse. I had to give up my job. With no money coming in and a new mortgage to pay, I felt so isolated looking after them. I had to do things I had never done before and started to drink to cope with my racing thoughts.

I was now starting to feel depressed myself but didn't know if it was just low mood. I kept telling myself it would be better tomorrow but it never was at all during this time.

My mother-in-law came to live with us and my personality totally changed within the first few months after my son was born. At one point I got so angry and punched the sofa. As a result I broke my hand. I started fights and just wanted someone to take away the pain inside me. Four to five months after my son was born I began to have suicidal thoughts.

The one great thing that came from staying home was the bond I developed with my son. But I couldn't tell Michelle how I was truly feeling as I didn't want it to affect her recovery.

Michelle's illness after 18 months had subsided. However I was now struggling. I would come home after not really going to work, saying I was 'fine'. I changed jobs more and more with my drinking slowly getting worse.

I struggled but everything settled down until another trauma happened 5 years later in 2011.

I had a full mental breakdown in a car one day outside work.

I was put on medication and learned about positive coping skills with counselling. I was under community mental health teams and after a few years was diagnosed with ADHD at 40. So many men have undiagnosed mental health disorders such as a history of anxiety depression and emotional trauma before becoming a parent, like mums.

See. www.reachingoutpmh.co.uk/daddy-blues-by-mark-williams

CASE STUDY 30.2   Gill's Story – PTSD

I thought parenthood would change me emotionally but had imagined those changes would be (largely) positive.

However, I found myself emotionally devastated by medical misfortune, avoidable error and a lack of compassion or care.

These things contrived to leave me with PTSD and anxiety. I struggled. I had placed my emotions in a box, not knowing what was wrong or how to access the positive love I felt for my new family without rage, anger and pain overwhelming me. I had a breakdown around 4 months postpartum and reached out for help from the GP.

It took a further 7 months to see a psychologist and start to reverse the damage. Lucky for us, my husband and mother-in-law were able to meet the emotional needs of my new baby in this time until I got better.

The medical issues I had, errors notwithstanding, weren't anyone's fault but the emotional damage and the source of my flashbacks and nightmares was a midwife being very unkind when I was incredibly emotionally vulnerable. Although I fedback to the hospital, I don't think she'll ever understand the impact of her words on my life.

She told me I would hurt my baby, to 'motivate' me, then I had a massive PPH and baby went to NICU. We were apart for 36 incredibly painful hours, where I thought my baby was dead and I had caused it. I convinced myself they weren't telling me as I was too poorly to hear it. I had other physical problems, sepsis, undiagnosed accreta, nerve damage in my back, etc. but the emotional pain was the worst. Health anxiety for my family, especially my birth trauma baby, is still a powerful fear.

It took 3 years (and more) of psychological therapy to unpick everything.

When I felt better enough to try for another baby, I had support for my medical issues and emotional help from the Perinatal Mental Health specialist midwife. Her kindness and reassurance was invaluable.

I'm not 100% today, PTSD is something I don't think really ever leaves you. We go into remission and have good times and bad.

Parenthood changed my emotional landscape fundamentally. I hope I am today the kind and gentle, emotionally connected mummy I wanted to be but I will always doubt my competence and fear for my daughters.

CASE STUDY 30.3   Pete's Story – PTSD

Six years ago my family went through unimaginable tragedy after Martha and Merlin's mum Mair died from cancer just 5 months after being diagnosed and just 10 weeks after Merlin was born.

The experience of diagnosis in pregnancy was so unreal, scary and confusing but thankfully we were well looked after in pregnancy and postpartum too.

I was a very active Dad anyway, and so quickly got used to juggling them both with Mair's needs in terms of care. Sadly, when Mair actually died my day-to-day logistically didn't change. It was the grief that was the tough part.

If I backtrack to before Mair died, I knew in my heart I was wasn't bonding with Merlin. I felt so torn between him and Mairs' health/needs. I felt like I was searching for how to prioritize when I didn't need to. I finally crashed one evening when chatting to Mair on the sofa and it became very apparent that I needed to seek some help. I had done what sadly many men do in situations like this. I was being tough and strong for my family and 'not wanting to seem weak'.

I started to talk and a monumental weight lifted.

In the years since, the kids grew, I grew emotionally and in 2016, my friend Nicola and I got together.

I had never had reason to consider what becoming a dad again would be like but the moment we got together I/we knew we would love to have a baby.

Nic got pregnant really quickly and we're just over the moon that we were going to grow our family.

Nic had a rough time of it for the first 20 weeks.

Seeing my loved one ill in a pregnancy setting again. It was horrible. Feeling useless and the deja vu was suffocating.

The even harder part was around the corner.

The magical pregnancy we were enjoying began to highlight the trauma I had actually experienced 5 years prior. I had complete black spots on my memory. I would rest my head on Nic's bump and then realize later that I have no visible memory of doing the same when Mair was pregnant with Merlin. I would chat away to bump at bedtime or sing ... but nothing in my head from Merlin. It was heartbreaking and scary at the same time. I went back to my counsellor in a panic wondering what on earth was wrong with me and that is when I heard the word trauma for the first time!

I cried uncontrollably that day at what I had lost. I'd lost so much of that previous birth experience.

Our baby boy Flynn was delivered safe and well in March '18 and that was a moment of pure and utter joy. The postpartum period saw a new series of things

raise their head. More evidence of birth trauma that just caught me so off guard.

A week after Flynn was born I was sat on the sofa just rocking back and forth. Nic offered to take Flynn from me so I could rest but I just refused to let go of him. My thoughts in that moment: I couldn't hear Nic.

How could there be someone else to share parenting with?

How am I not his everything as I was the last time I held a baby, i.e. Merlin?

I couldn't accept that this time was different!

And then to compound this, the more time I spent with Flynn playing, cuddling, soothing him, I realized how much I had lost with Merlin or more importantly, how little of that early time I remember with him. The little noises, the first cries, the snuggling.

This is my experience of birth trauma and it is just horrible, almost crippling at times.

Now please don't be confused into thinking I am envious of Flynn getting that time when Merlin didn't because in my mind I know that Merlin probably did. It's the fact that the memories are gone, which is the hardest thing to comprehend.

Delayed, unexpected and crippling at times. Perhaps not a typical depiction of birth trauma but one that will affect people nonetheless.

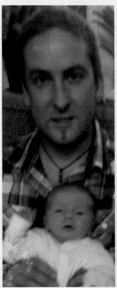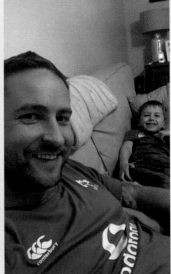

BOX 30.5 Summary of Key Points

- In the UK, pregnancy and the postnatal period are unparalleled periods when women engage with health care and have repeated contact with healthcare professionals.
- Women during pregnancy, labour and the puerperium are in a state of transition punctuated by heightened emotions and anxiety. Family life and daily routines become disrupted by the arrival of a new baby.
- Vulnerability factors such as domestic abuse, poverty and social isolation, can impact on the mother–baby relationship with consequences for child development.
- Risk identification of vulnerable groups of women antenatally presents a unique opportunity for multidisciplinary and multiagency collaboration in promoting mental health and wellbeing.

PART B: PERINATAL PSYCHIATRIC CONDITIONS

INTRODUCTION

Perinatal psychiatric disorder is now an accepted term used both nationally and internationally. It emphasizes the importance of psychiatric disorder in pregnancy as well as following childbirth and the variety of psychiatric disorders that can occur at this time, not just the ubiquitously known 'postnatal depression' (PND). It also places emphasis on the significance of psychiatric disorders that were present before conception, as well as those that arise during the perinatal period (Box 30.6).

BOX 30.6 What is Perinatal Psychiatric Disorder?

- Psychiatric disorders that complicate pregnancy, childbirth and the postnatal period
- Includes not only those illnesses that develop at this time but also pre-existing disorders such as schizophrenia, bipolar illness and depression
- Care involves consideration of the effects of the illness itself and of its treatment on the developing fetus and infant
- Care involves multidisciplinary and multiagency working, especially close relationships with Maternity Mental Health and Children's Services.

The emotional wellbeing of women is of primary importance to midwives. Not only can mental illness affect obstetric outcomes but also the transition to parenthood and emotional wellbeing and health problems in the infant. Perinatal psychiatric disorder is also a leading cause of both maternal morbidity and mortality. Worldwide, the WHO (2018) estimates that about 10% of pregnant women and 13% of women who have just given birth, experience a mental disorder, primarily depression. In developing countries this is even higher, i.e. 15.6% during pregnancy and 19.8% after child birth and in the worst case scenario, mothers' suffering might be so severe that they may even commit suicide (WHO 2018).

In the UK, Knight (2019) reported that maternal suicide is the second largest cause of direct maternal deaths and it remains a leading cause of direct deaths occurring within a year after the end of pregnancy. The report for the previous triennium 2014–2016 (Knight et al. 2018) found that many of the women who died from suicide had multiple adversities and other complexities such as alcohol or substance misuse or interpersonal violence. It was also reported that the most common diagnosis among women who died by suicide was of recurrent depressive disorder, and the majority of women had a prior history of mental health problems. However, unlike previous reports, very few women had previous psychotic disorder, whether bipolar, postpartum or non-affective.

Guidance to clinicians and practitioners from the UK's National Institute for Health and Care Excellence (NICE 2016) rightly emphasizes the importance of taking deliberate steps to identify any mental health problems in women presenting to maternity services, and recognizing that women who have, or have had, a psychiatric disorder may be fearful of volunteering this information because of the perceived risk of stigma. Any healthcare professional referring a woman with a history of current or past psychiatric disorder to maternity services has a responsibility to communicate this, but midwives should also make their own assessment. In addition to asking about any previous and current history of mental health problems and the care received, NICE (2016) recommends that midwives ask about any history of severe perinatal mental illness in a first-degree relative (mother, sister or daughter). It also recommends that midwives screen for depression and anxiety at booking, during the early postnatal period and following birth using the 'Whooley Questions' (see Part A of this chapter). Midwives should also screen for alcohol and drug misuse. Further details on how to recognize and screen for psychiatric disorders are set out in Section 1.5 of NICE (2014a): Antenatal and postnatal mental health: clinical management and service guidance, at: www.nice.org.uk/guidance/cg192/chapter/1-Recommendations#recognising-mental-health-problems-in-pregnancy-and-the-postnatal-period-and-referral-2.

Systems should be in place locally to ensure that women with mental health problems and those at risk of developing them receive the appropriate care.

It is therefore essential that all midwives have education and training to be familiar with common emotional changes women experience as they transition to motherhood, commonplace distress and adjustment reactions as well as the signs and symptoms of more serious psychiatric illnesses.

TYPES OF PSYCHIATRIC DISORDER

The term 'mental health problem' is commonly used to describe all types of emotional difficulties from transient and temporary states of distress, often understandable, to severe and uncommon mental illness. It is also used frequently to describe learning difficulties, substance misuse problems and difficulties coping with the stresses and strains of life. It is therefore too general and too nonspecific to be of use to the midwife. The term does not discriminate between severity and need and does not help the midwife distinguish between those conditions that she can manage and those that require specialist attention. For this reason, in this chapter, the term 'psychiatric disorder' is preferred, as it can be further categorized and the different types can be described aiding recognition and the planning of care.

Psychiatric disorders are conventionally categorized as in the list below.

Serious Mental Illnesses

These include schizophrenia, other psychotic conditions, bipolar illness and severe depressive illness. These conditions have in the past, and are sometimes still, referred to as psychotic disorders, because they can present with psychotic symptoms and loss of insight.

Mild to Moderate Psychiatric Disorders

These were previously known as 'neurotic disorders'. These include non-psychotic mild to moderate depressive illness, mixed anxiety and depression, anxiety disorders, including phobic anxiety states, panic disorder, obsessive–compulsive disorder and post-traumatic stress disorder.

Adjustment Reactions

These would include distressing reactions to life events, including death and adversity.

Substance Misuse

This includes those who misuse or who are dependent upon alcohol and other drugs of dependency, including both prescription and legal/illegal drugs.

Personality Disorders

This is a term that should be used only to describe people who have persistent severe problems throughout their adult life in dealing with the stresses and strains of normal life, maintaining satisfactory relationships, controlling their behaviour, foreseeing the consequences of their own actions and which persistently cause distress to themselves and other people.

Learning Disability

This is a term used to describe people who have a lifetime evidence of intellectual and cognitive impairment, developmental delay and consequent learning disabilities. This is usually graded as mild, moderate or severe. Overall psychiatric disorders are very common in the general population. The Adult Psychiatric Morbidity Survey (APMS) provides the UK's National Statistics for the monitoring of mental illness and treatment access in the household population. The most recent survey at the time of writing revealed that approximately 1 in 4 people in the UK will experience a mental health problem each year. In England, 1 in 6 people report experiencing a common mental health problem (such as anxiety and depression) in any given week (McManus et al. 2016). The survey is performed every 7 years, where a rigorous assessment of the nation's mental health is carried out. England has the longest running programme using consistent methods in the world (McManus et al. 2016). The APMS series provide data on the prevalence of both treated and untreated psychiatric disorder in the English adult population (aged 16 and over).

The data series capture statistical information relating to a range of mental disorders, substance disorders and self-harm behaviours. Surveys have been carried out in 1993, 2000, 2007 and 2014 using comparable methods so trends can be examined. The survey published in 2016 included interviews from a large representative sample of the household population – 7500 people aged 16 or more, including those who do not access services. Some of the key findings highlighted are:

- One in six adults (17%) surveyed in England met the criteria for a common mental disorder (e.g. anxiety/depression) in 2014.
- Women were more likely than men to have reported a common mental disorder (one in five women (19%) compared with one in eight men (12%)).
- Women were also more likely than men to report severe symptoms of common mental disorder (10% of women compared with 6% of men). Further information is available at: https://files.digital.nhs.uk/pdf/s/5/adult_psychiatric_study_executive_summary_web.pdf.

It is clear that anxiety and depression are commoner in women than in men, with the exception of substance misuse problems. Young women have become a key high-risk group with more self-harm being reported (McManus et al. 2016). However, the majority of psychiatric disorders in the community are mild to moderate conditions, particularly general anxiety and depression. As mentioned previously, mild to moderate depressive illness and anxiety disorders are at least twice more common in women than in men, and are particularly common in young women with children under the age of 5. The majority of these disorders are managed in primary care and do not require the attention of specialist psychiatric services. Mild to moderate depressive illness and anxiety states respond to psychological treatments. Despite this, perhaps because of shortage of such treatments, prescription of antidepressants is widespread in the community, particularly among women.

Serious mental illnesses are less common. Both schizophrenia and bipolar illness affect approximately 1% of the population. Bipolar illness affects men and women equally. However, schizophrenia, particularly the more severe chronic forms, is commoner among men. These conditions require the attention of specialist psychiatric services and require medical treatments as well as psychological care.

In the UK, psychiatric services are usually organized separately for adult mental health (serious mental illnesses), substance misuse (drug and alcohol treatment services) and learning disability. There are also, but not

TABLE 30.1 Incidence of Perinatal Psychiatric Disorders

Psychiatric Disorder	(%)
'Depression'	15–30
PND (postnatal depression)	10
Moderate/severe depressive illness	3–5
Referred psychiatry	2
Admitted to hospital	0.4
Admitted psychosis	0.2
Births to schizophrenic mothers	0.2

relevant to this chapter, separate services for psychiatric disorders in the elderly.

PSYCHIATRIC DISORDER IN PREGNANCY

In general, psychiatric disorder is not associated with a decrease in fertility. Therefore, all the previously described psychiatric disorders can and do complicate pregnancy and the postpartum period. The prevalence of psychiatric disorder in young women means that at least 20% of women will have current or previous psychiatric disorder in early pregnancy, many of whom will be taking psychiatric medication at the time of conception. However, it can be seen that only a small number will have a past history of a serious mental illness and an even smaller number will be currently suffering from such an illness. Pregnancy is not protective against a recurrence or relapse of a previous psychiatric disorder, particularly if the medication for these disorders is stopped when pregnancy is diagnosed. Women with a previous history of serious illness are at increased risk of a recurrence of that illness following birth. It is for these reasons that it is so important for midwives to enquire into women's current and previous mental health at early pregnancy assessment. Table 30.1 highlights the incidence of perinatal psychiatric disorders.

Mild–Moderate Conditions

The incidence (new onset) of psychiatric disorder in pregnancy is mostly accounted for by mild depressive illness, mixed anxiety and depression or anxiety states. They are probably predominantly of psychosocial aetiology, and for some women, they will represent a recurrence of a previous episode, of depression, anxiety, panic or obsessional disorders, particularly if they have suddenly stopped their antidepressant medication. Women may also be vulnerable at this time because of:

- previous fertility problems
- previous obstetric loss
- anxieties about the viability of their pregnancy
- social and relationship problems
- ambivalence towards the pregnancy
- other reasons for personal unhappiness.

Anxiety disorders overall appear to be no more common in the perinatal period compared with other points in a woman's lifecycle, (Vesga-López et al. 2008), but anxiety can be particularly debilitating in the perinatal period and may have adverse effects on the fetus. Anxiety can also be a presenting feature of depressive disorder, see below. Around two-thirds of women with a depressive disorder in pregnancy have a comorbid anxiety disorder. For these reasons, anxiety in pregnancy merits attention and where appropriate, treatment. In contrast, obsessive–compulsive disorder is up to twice as common in the perinatal period compared with other points in the lifecycle, and as a consequence, new cases frequently present in pregnancy.

In the past, it was often assumed that hyperemesis gravidarum (severe vomiting) was a psychosomatic manifestation of personal unhappiness and psychological disturbance. This condition is less common than in the past and usually resolves by 16 weeks of pregnancy. Psychological factors, anxiety and cognitive misattribution remain a significant factor in some women.

Prognosis and management

Most of the conditions are likely to improve as the pregnancy progresses. Psychological treatments and psychosocial interventions are effective for these conditions and caution needs to be exercised before pharmacological interventions are initiated during pregnancy, although medication may be necessary for the more severe illnesses.

For others, particularly those who develop a psychiatric illness in the later stages of pregnancy, their condition is likely to continue and worsen in the postpartum period.

Serious Conditions

This term refers to schizophrenia, other psychoses, bipolar illness (manic depressive illness) and severe depressive illness.

Incidence

Kendell et al.'s (1987) historical study revealed that women are at a lower risk of developing a serious mental illness for the first time during pregnancy than at other times in their lives. This is in marked contrast to the elevated risk of suffering from such a condition in the first few months following childbirth. While these conditions are uncommon, they require urgent and expert treatment, particularly as an acute psychosis in pregnancy can pose a risk to the mother and developing fetus, both directly because of the disturbed behaviour and indirectly because of the treatments. There is a possibility that such an illness can interfere with proper antenatal care.

Prevalence

While new onset psychosis in pregnancy is relatively rare, the prevalence of these illnesses (pre-existing) at the beginning of pregnancy will be the same as at other times. Women suffering from schizophrenia or bipolar illness are as likely to become pregnant as the rest of the general population. This means that approximately 2% of women in pregnancy will either have had such an illness in the past or be currently suffering from one. It is important to realize that these women may range from women who are well and stable, leading normal lives through to those who are disabled, chronically symptomatic and on medication. The management of these women in pregnancy therefore has to be individualized and plans made on a case-by-case basis. Nonetheless, there are three broad groups of women.

Group 1. The first group includes women who have had a previous episode of bipolar illness or a psychotic episode earlier in their lives. They are usually well, stable not on medication and may not be in contact with psychiatric services. These women, if their last episode of illness was >2 years ago, may not be at an increased risk of a recurrence of their condition during pregnancy but face at least a 50% risk of becoming psychotic in the early weeks postpartum. The most important aspect of their management is therefore a proactive management plan for the first few weeks following birth.

Group 2. The second broad group of women are those who have had a previous and/or recent episode of a serious mental illness, who are relatively well and stable but whose health is being maintained by taking medication. This may be antipsychotic medication or in the case of bipolar illness, a mood stabilizer (lithium or an anticonvulsant). These women are at risk of a relapse of their condition during pregnancy. This risk is particularly high if they stop their medication at the diagnosis of pregnancy. As some of these medications may have an adverse effect on the development of the fetus and yet an acute relapse of the illness is also hazardous, it is important that these women have access to expert advice on the risks and benefits of continuing the treatment or changing it as early as possible in pregnancy.

Group 3. The third broad category includes women who are chronically mentally ill with complex social needs, persisting symptoms and on medication. These women will usually be in contact with psychiatric services. Midwifery and obstetric care needs to be closely integrated into the case management of these women and there needs to be a close working relationship between maternity, psychiatric and social services.

Ideally, all women who have a current or previous history of serious mental illness should have advice and counselling before embarking upon a pregnancy. They should be able to discuss the risk to their mental health of becoming pregnant and becoming a parent as well as the risks to the developing fetus of continuing with their usual medication and perhaps the need to change it. However, in the general population, at least 50% of all pregnancies are unplanned at the point of conception. Midwives should therefore enquire at the early pregnancy assessment, about the women's previous and current psychiatric history and alert psychiatric services as soon as possible about the pregnancy, so that relapses of the psychiatric illness during pregnancy and recurrences postpartum can be avoided wherever possible.

PSYCHIATRIC DISORDER AFTER BIRTH

The majority of postpartum onset psychiatric disorders are affective (mood) disorders. However, symptoms other than those due to a disorder of mood are frequently present. Conventionally, three postpartum disorders are described:

- the 'blues'
- postpartum (puerperal) psychosis
- postnatal depression.

The 'blues' is a common dysphoric, self-limiting state, occurring in the first week postpartum (see Part A of this chapter).

Postpartum (Puerperal) Psychosis

Globally, postpartum psychosis, the most severe form of postpartum affective (mood) disorder has been recognized and described since antiquity. It leads to 2 in 1000 women being admitted to a psychiatric hospital following childbirth, mostly in the first few weeks postpartum. Although a relatively rare condition, there is a marked increase in the risk of suffering from a psychotic illness following childbirth (Kendell et al. 1987; Munk-Olsen et al. 2012). It is also remarkably constant across nations and cultures.

Risk factors

Most women who suffer from this condition will have been previously well, without obvious risk factors, and the illness comes as a shock to them and their families. However, some women will have suffered from a similar illness following the birth of a previous child, some may have suffered from a non-postpartum bipolar affective disorder from which they have long recovered or they may have a family history of bipolar illness. For others there may be marked psychosocial adversity. It is generally accepted that biological factors (neuroendocrine and genetic) are the most important aetiological factors for this condition. This implies that postpartum psychosis can and does strike without warning – women from all social and occupational backgrounds; those in stable marriages with much-wanted babies, as well as those living in less fortunate circumstances.

Clinical features

Postpartum psychosis is an acute, early onset condition. The overwhelming majority of cases present in the first 14 days postpartum. They most commonly develop suddenly between day 3 and day 7, at a time when most women will be experiencing the 'blues'. Differential diagnosis between the earliest phase of a developing psychosis and the 'blues' can be difficult. However, postpartum psychosis steadily deteriorates over the following 48 h, while the 'blues' tends to resolve spontaneously.

During the first 2–3 days of a developing postpartum psychosis, there is a fluctuating rapidly changing, undifferentiated psychotic state. The earliest signs are commonly of perplexity, fear – even terror – and restless agitation associated with insomnia. Other signs include: purposeless activity, uncharacteristic behaviour, disinhibition, irritation and fleeting anger, resistive behaviour and sometimes incontinence.

A woman may have fears for her own and her baby's health and safety, or even about its identity. Even at this early stage, there may be, variably throughout the day, elation and grandiosity, suspiciousness, depression or unspeakable ideas of horror.

Women suffering from postpartum psychosis are among the most profoundly disturbed and distressed found in psychiatric practice (Dean and Kendell 1981; VanderKruik et al. 2017). In addition to the familiar symptoms and signs of a manic or depressive psychosis, symptoms of schizophrenia (delusions and hallucinations) may occur. Depressive delusions about maternal and infant health are common. The behaviour and motives of others are frequently misinterpreted in a delusional fashion. A mood of perplexity and terror is often found, as are delusions about the passage of time and other bizarre delusions. Women can believe that they are still pregnant or that more than one child has been born or that the baby is older than it is.

Women often seem confused and disorientated. In the very common mixed affective psychosis, along with the familiar pressure of speech and flight of ideas, there is often a mixture of grandiosity, elation and certain conviction alternating with states of fearful tearfulness, guilt and a sense of foreboding. The sufferers are usually restless and agitated, resistive, seeking senselessly to escape and difficult to reassure. However, they are usually calmer in the presence of familiar relatives.

The woman may be unable to attend to her own personal hygiene and nutrition and be unable to care for her baby. Her concentration is usually grossly impaired and she is distractible and unable to initiate and complete tasks. Over the next few days, her condition deteriorates and the symptoms usually become more clearly those of an acute affective psychosis. Most women will have symptoms and signs suggestive of a depressive psychosis, a significant minority a manic psychosis and very commonly a mixture of both – a mixed affective psychosis.

Relationship with the baby

Some women are so disturbed, distractible and their concentration so impaired, that they do not seem to be aware of their recently born baby. Others are preoccupied with the baby, reluctant to let it out of their sight and forever checking on its presence and condition. Although delusional ideas frequently involve the baby and there may be delusional ideas of infant ill-health or changed identity, it is rare for women with postpartum psychosis to be overtly hostile to their baby and for their behaviour to be aggressive or punitive. The risk to their baby lies more from an inability to organize and complete tasks, and to inappropriate handling and tasks being impaired by their mental state. These problems, directly attributable to the maternal psychosis, tend to resolve as the mother recovers.

Management

Most women with psychotic illness following childbirth will require admission to hospital, which should be to a specialist mother and baby unit, the only setting in which the physical needs of the mother who has recently given birth can be met, and where specialist psychiatric nursing is available. This ensures that the physical and emotional needs of both mother and baby are met and the developing relationship with the baby promoted.

Prognosis

In spite of the severity of postpartum psychoses, they frequently resolve relatively quickly over 2–4 weeks. However, initial recovery is often fragile and relapses are common in the first few weeks. As the psychosis resolves, it is common for women to pass through a phase of depression and anxiety and preoccupation with their past experiences and the implications of these memories for their future mental health and their role as a mother. Sensitive and expert help is required to assist women through this phase, to help them understand what has happened and to acquire a 'working model' of their illness. The overwhelming majority of women will have completely recovered by 3–6 months postpartum. However, they face at least a 50% risk of a recurrence should they have another child and some may go on to have bipolar illness at other times in their lives (Robertson et al. 2005; Larsen and Saric 2017).

Postnatal Depressive Illness

Approximately 10% of all postnatal women will develop a depressive illness. The studies, from which this figure is derived, are usually community studies using the Edinburgh Postnatal Depression Scale (EPDS), either as a diagnostic tool or as a screen prior to the use of other research tools. It is often misused (Cox 2019), and NICE (2014a) recommendations suggest its use as an adjunct to asking the two Whooley screening questions for depression, as explained in part A of the chapter. Studies using a cut-off point of 14 usually give an incidence of 10%;

those using lower scores will give a higher incidence. A score on a screening instrument is not the same as a clinical diagnosis. Nonetheless, a score of 14 is said to correlate with a clinical diagnosis of major depression and the lower scores with that of major and minor depression (Cox 2019). The incidence of women who would meet the diagnostic criteria for moderate to severe depressive illness is lower, probably between 3% and 5% (Cox et al. 1993; Fisher et al. 2016; Munk-Olsen et al. 2016). Depression following childbirth has the same range of severity and subtypes as depression at other times. According to the symptomatology, duration and severity, they may be graded as mild to moderate or severe, and subtypes may have prominent anxiety and obsessional phenomena.

Postnatal depressive illness of all types and severities is therefore relatively common and represents a considerable burden of disability and distress in these women. Although postnatal depressive illness is popularly accepted, with the exception of the most severe forms, it is no more common than during pregnancy or in non-childbearing women of the same age (O'Hara and Swain 1996; Rasmussen et al. 2017). However, this does not detract from its importance. Depressive illness of any severity occurring at a time when the expectation is of happiness and fulfilment and when major psychological and social adjustments are being made together with caring for an infant, creates difficulties not found at other times in the human lifespan.

The term 'postnatal depression' is often used as a generic term for all forms of psychiatric disorder presenting following birth. While in the past this has undoubtedly been helpful in raising the profile of postpartum psychiatric disorders, improving their recognition and reducing stigma, it has also become problematic. Use of the term in this way can diminish the perceived seriousness of other illnesses, and has led to a 'one size fits all' view of diagnosis and treatments. Consequently, NICE (2014a) advises caution in the use of the term 'postnatal depression' as it can be misused to include any mental illness occurring postnatally, and may result in other serious illnesses failing to be identified.

The term 'postnatal depression' should only be used for a non-psychotic depressive illness of mild to moderate severity, which arises within 3 months of childbirth.

Severe Depressive Illness

Severe depressive illness affects at least 3% of all women who have given birth, with a seven-fold increase in risk in the first 3 months (Cox et al. 1993; Munk-Olsen et al. 2016). Again, the majority of women who suffer from this condition will have been previously well. However, women with a previous history of severe postnatal depressive illness or severe depression at other times or a family history of severe depressive illness or postnatal depression, are at increased risk. Psychosocial factors are more important in the aetiology of this condition than in puerperal psychosis, although biological factors play an important role in the most severe illnesses. Nonetheless, severe postnatal depression can affect women from all backgrounds not just those facing social adversity.

Like puerperal psychosis, severe depressive illness is an early onset condition in which the woman commonly does not regain her normal emotional state following birth. However, unlike puerperal psychosis, the onset tends not to be abrupt; rather, the illness develops over the next 2–4 weeks. The more severe illnesses tend to present early, by 4–6 weeks postpartum, but the majority present later, between 8 and 12 weeks postpartum. These later presentations may be missed. This is partly because some of the symptoms may be misattributed to the adjustment to a new baby and partly because the mother may 'put on a brave face', concealing how she feels from others.

Risk factors

A variety of risk factors for postnatal depressive illness have been identified and include those associated with depressive illness at other times. To these can be added ambivalence about the pregnancy, high levels of anxiety during pregnancy and adverse birth experiences, previous perinatal death to name but a few. Many of these risk factors, though statistically significant are so common as to have little positive predictive value. However, a clustering of these risk factors might lead to those caring for the woman to be extra vigilant. Of more use are those risk factors that have a higher positive predictive value. These include a family history of severe affective disorder, a family history of severe postnatal depressive illness, developing a depressive illness in the last trimester of pregnancy and the loss of the previous infant (including stillbirth). There might also be an increased risk in those women who have conceived through assisted means of reproduction such as IVF (Vikström et al. 2017).

Clinical features

The familiar symptoms of severe depressive illness are often modified by the context of early maternity and the relative youth of those suffering from the condition:

The *somatic syndrome* (*biological features*) of broken sleep and early morning wakening, diurnal variation of mood, loss of appetite and weight, slowing of mental functioning, impaired concentration, extreme tiredness and lack of vitality can easily be misattributed to a crying baby, understandable tiredness and the adjustment to new routines.

The all-pervasive *anhedonia* or *loss of pleasure* in ordinary everyday tasks, the lack of joy and fearfulness for the future may be misattributed by the woman herself to 'not loving the baby' or 'not being a proper mother' and all too easily described as 'bonding problems' by professionals. Anhedonia is a particularly painful symptom at a time when most women would expect to feel overwhelmed with joy and happiness and in turn contributes to feelings of *guilt, incompetence* and *unworthiness* that are very prominent in postnatal depressive illness. These overvalued ideas can verge on the delusional.

It is also common to find *overvalued morbid beliefs* and fears for the woman's own health and mortality and that of her baby. She may misattribute normal infant behaviour to mean that the baby is suffering or does not like her. A baby that settles in the arms of more experienced people may confirm the mother's belief that she is incompetent. Commonplace problems with establishing breastfeeding may become the subject of morbid rumination.

Some women with severe postnatal depressive illness may be slowed, withdrawn and retreat easily in the face of offers of help, avoid the tasks of motherhood and their relationship with the baby. Others may be agitated, restless and fiercely protective of their infant, resenting the contribution of others.

Anxiety and obsessive–compulsive symptoms

Anxiety symptoms, including obsessive-compulsive symptoms, can be the presenting features of an underlying depressive illness, and may even dominate the clinical picture. They frequently underpin mental health crises, calls for emergency attention and maternal fears for the infant. Repetitive intrusive, and often deeply repugnant, thoughts of harm coming to loved ones, particularly the infant, are commonplace, often leading to repetitive doubting and checking. The woman may doubt that she is safe as a mother and believe that she is capable of harming her infant. Crescendos of anxiety and panic attacks may result from the baby's crying or being difficult to settle and may lead the mother to be frightened to be alone with her child. This is easily misinterpreted by professionals who may fear that the child is at risk.

Obsessional, vacillating indecisiveness is also common and contributes to an overwhelming sense of being unable to cope with everyday tasks in marked contrast to premorbid levels of competence. While complex obsessive–compulsive behavioural rituals are relatively rare, obsessive cleaning, housework and checking are common. Intrusive obsessional thoughts and the typical catastrophic cognitions associated with panic attacks frequently lead to a fear of insanity and loss of control; see Sherry's story (Case Study 30.4).

CASE STUDY 30.4   Sherry's Story – OCD

After witnessing domestic abuse in the home and being raped repeatedly by the age of 6 years old, I developed OCD. The sexual abuse began again aged 11–14 and I was placed into foster care once I spoke out. I never received the psychological help I needed for the traumatic experiences that led to OCD.

As time went by, I had three children. Each time I had a child it would exacerbate my ruminations, which consisted of hurt, sick and dead children. I would see dead children laying under the Christmas tree, so I would have to put soft toys under the tree until it was taken down. I would check over and over again, check

that my baby as breathing, check the doors, check my calendar and diaries for tasks needed, to the point of exhaustion. I did not tell anyone through fear of them thinking I would hurt my children.

When my third baby was born my mum had died 3 months prior. My OCD began extremely troublesome and the ruminations were sometimes so violent that I would vomit. I would obsess about Baby P, researching about his case in great detail even though I would vomit but the urge to keep going was too powerful. If I didn't continue something bad would happen and I would lose my daughters. I would check all three diaries, my

CASE STUDY 30.4 Sherry's Story – OCD—cont'd

phone diary and the calendar numerous times a day. When my daughter got to 6, I was so poorly that I would not leave the house because seeing people tell their kids off in the street would make me shout out at them. This happened a few times. I would always be checking if my daughter was okay, if she was hungry or thirsty and told her how much I loved her in case she didn't know. I would also ask for reassurance so regularly that my family would become tired of me.

I do believe having children had an affect on my OCD, the fact they were female and when they were 6, made it unbearable. The hormones certainly played their part, making the devil louder and easier to manipulate me into thinking I was a horrible person.

I went on to pass a BSc in Adult Nursing and am currently studying BSc Psychology. Helping others

seems to help but I still ruminate that my daughter is going to die or that my loving husband is raping her. I also worried that if my ward manager knew about what went through my mind I would lose my job. This made me anxious even more, worrying about losing my job and my children.

I became brave, asked for help and had 11 months of Psychotherapy and with the help of an amazing Psychotherapist I now know I am the least dangerous person and that the devil on my shoulder who tells me how evil I am and who makes me believe I want to do the things he makes me see in my head is just a thought and that I am a good mother. It took a while but I know OCD takes the individual's worst fear and uses them. Pregnancy and birth made it more difficult, physically and mentally.

For further information, see: www.ocduk.org.

Relationship with the baby

Severe depressive symptomatology, particularly when combined with panic and obsessional phenomena, can have a profound effect on the relationship with the baby, in many, but by no means all, women. Most women who suffer from severe postnatal depressive illness maintain high standards of physical care for their infants. However, many are frightened of their own feelings and thoughts and few gain any pleasure or joy from their infant. They may find smiling and talking to their babies difficult. Most affected women feel a deep sense of guilt and incompetence and doubt whether they are caring for their infant properly. Normal infant behaviour is frequently misinterpreted as confirming their poor views of their own abilities. While a fear of harming the baby is commonplace, overt hostility and aggressive behaviour towards the infant is extremely uncommon. It should be remembered that the majority of mothers who harm small babies are not suffering from a serious mental illness. The speedy resolution of maternal illness usually results in a normal mother–infant relationship. However, prolonged chronic depressive illness can interfere with attachment, social and cognitive development in the longer term, particularly when combined with social and mental problems (Cooper and Murray 1997; Murray et al. 2015).

Management

These conditions need to be speedily identified and treated, preferably by a specialist perinatal mental health team. The value of early contact with professionals who recognize and validate the symptoms and distress, and can re-attribute the overvalued ideas of the mother and instil hope for the future cannot be underestimated. The treatment of the depressive illness is the same as the treatment of depressive illness at other times. The use of antidepressants together with good psychological care should result in an improvement of symptoms within 2 weeks and the resolution of the illness between 6 and 8 weeks (NICE 2014a).

Prognosis

With treatment, these women should fully recover. Without, spontaneous resolution may take many months and up to one-third of women can still be ill when their child is 1 year old.

Women who have had a severe depressive illness face a 1:2 to 1:3 risk of a recurrence of the illness following the birth of subsequent children (Cooper and Murray 1995). They are also at elevated risk from suffering from a depressive illness at other times in their lives. However, the long-term prognosis would appear to be better than when the first episode is in non-childbearing women, both in terms of the frequency of further episodes and in their overall functioning (Robling et al. 2000; Rutigliano et al. 2018).

Mild Postnatal Depressive Illness

This is the commonest condition following childbirth, affecting up to 10% of all women postpartum. It is in fact no commoner after childbirth than among other non-childbearing women of the same age.

Risk factors

Some women who suffer from this condition will be vulnerable by virtue of previous mental health problems or psychosocial adversity, unsatisfactory marital or other relationships or inadequate social support. Others may be older, educated and married for a long time, perhaps with problems conceiving, previous obstetric loss or high levels of anxiety during pregnancy. Unrealistically high expectations of themselves and motherhood and consequent disappointment are commonplace. Also common are stressful life events such as moving house, family bereavement, a sick baby, experience of special care baby units and other such events that detract from the expected pleasure and harmony of this stage of life.

Clinical features

The condition has an insidious onset in the days and weeks following childbirth but usually presents after the first 3 months postpartum. The symptoms are variable, but the mother is usually tearful, feels that she has difficulty coping and complains of irritability and a lack of satisfaction and pleasure with motherhood. Symptoms of anxiety, a sense of loneliness and isolation as well as dissatisfaction with the quality of important relationships are common. Affected mothers frequently have good days and bad days and are often better in company and anxious when alone. The full biological (somatic subtype) syndrome of the more severe depressive illness is usually absent. However, difficulty getting to sleep and appetite difficulties, both over-eating and under-eating, are common.

Relationship with the baby

Dissatisfaction with motherhood and a sense of the baby being problematic are often central to this condition, particularly when compounded by difficulty in meeting the needs of older children. Lack of pleasure in the baby, combined with anxiety and irritability, can lead to a vicious circle of a fractious and unsettled baby, misinterpreted by its mother as critical and resentful of her and thus a deteriorating relationship between them. However, it should also be remembered that the direction of causality is not always mother to infant. Some infants are very unsettled in the first few months of their life. A baby who is difficult to feed and cries constantly during the day or is difficult to settle at night can just as often

be the cause of a mild postnatal depressive illness as the result of it. Even mild illnesses, particularly when combined with socioeconomic deprivation and high levels of social adversity, can lead to longer-term problems with mother–infant relationships and subsequent social and cognitive development of the child (Cooper and Murray 1997; Murray et al. 2015). A very small minority of sufferers from this condition may experience such marked irritability and even overt hostility towards their baby that the infant is at risk of being harmed.

Management

Early detection and treatment is essential for both mother and baby. For the milder cases, a combination of psychological and social support and active listening from a health visitor will suffice. For others, specific psychological treatments, such as cognitive behavioural psychotherapy and interpersonal psychotherapy, are as effective, if not more than, antidepressants, as outlined in Antenatal and Postnatal Mental Health guidelines (NICE 2014a).

Prognosis

With appropriate management, postnatal depression should improve within weeks and recover by the time the infant is 6 months old. However, untreated there may be prolonged morbidity. This, particularly in the presence of continuing social adversity, has been demonstrated to have an adverse effect not only on the mother–infant relationship but also on the later social, emotional and cognitive development of the child.

Breastfeeding

There is no evidence that breastfeeding increases the risk of developing significant depressive illness, nor that its cessation improves depressive illness. Continuing breastfeeding may protect the infant from the effects of maternal depression and improve maternal self-esteem.

TREATMENT OF PERINATAL PSYCHIATRIC DISORDERS

The Role of the Midwife

Midwives need knowledge and understanding of the different management strategies for perinatal psychiatric disorders and of the use of psychiatric drugs in pregnancy and lactation. This knowledge is required because the women themselves may wish for advice, because the midwife may have to alert other professionals, for example GPs and psychiatrists, to ask for a review of the woman's medication and because in case of serious mental illness, the midwife will be part of a multiprofessional team caring for the women.

Midwives should routinely ask all women at the antenatal booking clinic whether they have had an episode of serious mental illness in the past and whether they are currently in contact with psychiatric services (NICE 2008). Those women who have a previous episode of serious mental illness (schizophrenia, other psychoses, bipolar illness and severe depressive illness) should be referred to a psychiatric team during pregnancy even if they have been well for many years. This is because they face at least a 50% risk of becoming ill following birth. The midwife should also urgently inform the psychiatric team if the woman is currently in contact with psychiatric services. The psychiatric team may not be aware of the pregnant woman who is taking psychiatric medication at the time when the midwife first sees her should be advised not to abruptly stop her medication. The midwife should urgently seek a review of the woman's medication from the GP, obstetrician or psychiatrist, as appropriate. This may result in the woman being advised to reduce, change or undertake a supervised withdrawal of her medication.

There are three components to the management of perinatal psychiatric disorder: psychological treatments and social interventions, pharmacological treatments and the skills, resources and services needed.

Those who are seriously mentally ill will require all three. Those with the mildest illnesses may benefit from facilitated self-help or psychological and social interventions delivered by primary care psychology services, like IAPT (Improving Access to Psychological Therapies) in the UK (NICE 2014a).

Psychological Treatments

All illnesses of all severities and indeed those who are not ill but experiencing commonplace episodes of distress and adjustment need good psychological care. This can only be based upon an understanding of the normal emotional and cognitive changes and common concerns of pregnancy and the puerperium. It also requires a familiarity with the symptoms and clinical features of postpartum illnesses.

For most women with mild depressive illness or emotional distress and difficulties adjusting, extra time given by the midwife or health visitor, 'the listening visit',

will be effective (NICE 2014a). For others, particularly those with more persistent states associated with high levels of anxiety, brief cognitive therapy treatments and brief interpersonal psychotherapy, are as effective as antidepressants and may confer additional benefits in terms of improving the mother–infant relationships and satisfaction (NICE 2014a). Similar claims have been made for infant massage and other therapies that focus the mother's attention on enjoying her baby. It is particularly important during pregnancy to use psychological treatments wherever possible and avoid the unnecessary prescription of antidepressants (NICE 2014a).

Social Support

Lack of social support, particularly when combined with adversity and life events, has long been implicated in the aetiology of mild to moderate depressive illness in young women (McManus et al. 2016). Social support not only includes practical assistance and advice but also having an emotional confidante, female friends and people who improve self-esteem. There is evidence that services that are underpinned by social support theory, such as 'Home Start', can have a beneficial effect on maternal and infant wellbeing and perhaps on mild postnatal depression (Barlow et al. 2011).

Pharmacological Treatment

In general, psychiatric illnesses occurring during the perinatal period respond to the same treatments as at other times. There are no specific treatments for perinatal psychiatric disorder. Moderate to severe depressive illnesses respond to antidepressants, psychotic illnesses to antipsychotics and mood stabilizers may be needed for those with bipolar illnesses. However, the possibility of adverse consequences on the embryo and developing fetus and via breastmilk on the infant makes the choice and dose of the drug important.

The evidence base for the safety or adverse consequences of psychotropic medication is constantly changing both in the direction of increased concern and of reassurance. Any text detailing specific advice is in danger of being quickly out of date and the reader is directed to the regularly updated information published by: the UK Teratology Information Service at www.uktis.org/; the US Toxicology Data Network at https://toxnet.nlm.nih.gov; and to the latest National Institute for Health and Care Excellence Guidelines on Antenatal and Postnatal Mental Health (NICE 2014a).

Chapter 8 of the NICE (2014a) full guidelines provide in-depth information and the evidence base for both pharmacological treatment and physical interventions, this is accessible at: www.nice.org.uk/guidance/cg192/evidence/full-guideline-pdf-4840896925.

However, it is worth noting that no matter what the changing evidence is, some general principles apply:

- The absence of evidence of harm is not the same as evidence of safety.
- It may take 20–30 years after the introduction of a drug for its adverse consequences to be fully realized. An example of this is sodium valproate in pregnancy.
- In general, there is more evidence on older than on newer drugs, although this does not necessarily mean they are safer.
- All psychotropic medication passes across the placenta and into the breastmilk.
- Both the architecture and function of the fetal central nervous system continues to develop throughout pregnancy and in early infancy. Concern should not be confined to the adverse effects in the first 3 months of pregnancy.
- The threshold for initiating medication in pregnancy and breastfeeding should be high. If there is an alternative, non-pharmacological treatment of equal efficacy, then that should be the treatment of choice.
- Serious mental illness requires robust treatment. In all cases of illness, occurring in a pregnant or breastfeeding mother, the clinician must endeavour to balance the risk of not treating the mother on both mother and baby against the risk to the fetus or infant of treating the mother. The more serious the illness is, the more likely it is that the risks of not treating outweigh the risks of treating.
- The risks to both mother and baby of a serious maternal mental illness may be greater than the risks of medication.
- The fetus and baby is no less likely to suffer from the side-effects of psychotropic medication than an adult. Fetal and infant elimination of psychotropic medication is slower and less than in adults and their central nervous systems more sensitive to the effects of these drugs.
- Adverse consequences of medication on the fetus and infant are dose-related. If medication is used it should be used in the lowest effective dose and if necessary given in divided dosages throughout the day.

> ### BOX 30.7   Perinatal Mental Health: National Documents (Regularly Updated)
>
> - Royal College of Psychiatrists: CR88
> - SIGN Guidelines – postnatal and puerperal psychosis
> - National Screening Committee
> - NICE guidelines on antenatal care: routine care for the healthy pregnant woman
> - NICE guidelines on antenatal and postnatal mental health
> - NICE guidelines on postnatal care: routine postnatal care of women and their babies
> - MBRRACE–UK: Saving Lives, Improving Mothers' Care triennial reports.

- The exposure of the baby to psychotropic medication in breastmilk will depend on the volume of milk, the frequency of feeding, weight and age. A totally breastfed baby under 6 weeks old will receive relatively more psychotropic medication than an older baby who is partially weaned.

The midwife should note that use of psychiatric medication during pregnancy and breastfeeding is an area of specialist medical expertise. Advice of the benefits and potential deleterious effects of medication should be sought from a mental health service, preferably a specialist perinatal mental health service. Detailed guidance on this, and other aspects of perinatal mental health care, are set out in the NICE clinical management and service guidance (NICE 2014a; Cantwell et al. 2018; Knight et al. 2019).

SERVICE PROVISION

There are a number of national recommendations for the needs of women with perinatal psychiatric disorders (see Box 30.7). The distinctive clinical features of the conditions, their physical needs and the professional liaison with maternity services all require specialist skills and knowledge. The frequency of the serious conditions at locality level makes it difficult for general adult psychiatric services to manage the critical mass of patients required to develop and maintain their experience and skills. It is difficult for maternity services to relate to multiple psychiatric teams. However, at supra-locality (regional) level, the frequency of serious perinatal psychiatric disorder is sufficient to justify the joint commissioning and provision of specialist services. Mothers, who require admission to a psychiatric hospital in the early months postpartum should, unless it is positively contraindicated, be admitted to a mother and baby unit. This is not only humane but also in the best interests of the infant and cost-effective, as it shortens inpatient stay and prevents re-admission. There should be specialist perinatal community outreach services available to every maternity service, to deal with psychiatric problems that arise postpartum but also to see women in pregnancy who are at high risk of developing a postnatal illness.

The majority of women suffering from postnatal mental illness will not require to be seen by specialist psychiatric services. However, there is a need for integrated care pathways to ensure that women are effectively identified and managed in primary care and, if necessary, referred on to specialist services. There is a need to enhance the skills and competencies of health visitors, midwives, obstetricians and GPs to deal with the less severe illnesses themselves.

PREVENTION AND PROPHYLAXIS

Prevention

NICE (2014a) guidelines do not promote routine screening using the EPDS and other 'paper and pen' scales in the antenatal period for those at risk of postnatal depression. They also find that there is a lack of evidence to support antenatal interventions to reduce the risk of non-psychotic postnatal illness. In contrast, these and other bodies (NICE 2008; Knight et al. 2019 for MBRRACE) all recommend that women should be screened at early pregnancy assessment for a previous or family history of serious mental illness, particularly bipolar illness, because they face at least a 50% risk of recurrence of that condition following birth. Those who undertake early pregnancy assessment will need training to refresh their knowledge of psychiatric disorder.

There is little point in screening for women at high risk of developing severe postnatal illness if systems for the proactive peripartum management of these conditions are not in place and if appropriate resources are not available. It is recommended that all women who are at high risk of developing a severe postpartum illness by virtue of a previous history are seen by a specialist psychiatric team during the pregnancy and a written management plan placed in the maternity records in late pregnancy and shared with the woman, her partner, her GP, midwife, obstetrician and psychiatrist.

Prophylaxis

If a woman has a previous history of bipolar illness or postpartum psychosis, consideration should be given to starting medication on day 1 postnatally, following guidance from a specialist mental health team.

The most important aspect of preventative management and one that will promote early identification and the avoidance of a life-threatening emergency is close surveillance, contact and support in the early weeks, the period of maximum risk. A specialist community perinatal psychiatric nurse, together with the midwife, should visit on a daily basis for the first 2 weeks and remain in close contact for the first 6 weeks. The local perinatal mental health mother and baby unit should be aware of the woman's expected date of birth and systems put in place for direct admission if necessary.

CONCLUSION

The full range of psychiatric disorders can complicate pregnancy and the postpartum year. The incidence of affective disorder, particularly at the most severe end of the spectrum, increases following birth. The familiar signs and symptoms of psychiatric disorder are all present in postpartum disorders as well, but the early maternity context and the dominance of infant care and mother–infant relationships exert a powerful effect on the content, if not the form, of the symptomatology. Early maternity is a time when there is an expectation of joy, pleasure and fulfilment. The presence of psychiatric disorder at this time, however mild, is disproportionately distressing. No matter how ill the woman feels, there is still a baby and often other children to be cared for. She cannot rest and is reminded on a daily basis of her symptoms and disability. Compassionate care and understanding and skilled care aimed at speedy symptom relief and re-establishing maternal confidence are thus essential. See Amy's story (Case Study 30.5).

CASE STUDY 30.5 Amy's Story – Postpartum Depressive Illness

In my first pregnancy, I was taken off my antidepressants by my GP and became very depressed before and after birth. I was seen by the perinatal mental health team and put back on antidepressants but I felt really sad that it affected me bonding with my daughter and kind of ruined much of my first year with her.

When I got pregnant again, I was very scared of it happening again but did lots of research into the actual evidence of antidepressant use in pregnancy and decided the risk of postnatal depression was greater, so decided to stay on them. I think there's a real stigma around this and I wish GPs were better informed. Again my GP tried to encourage me to come off them, despite me having written evidence from a perinatal psychiatrist.

Because of what happened before, I put in place a plan for my pregnancy and birth, with the support of the perinatal psych team. This included my husband getting as much paternity leave as he could, making sure my medication was right, trying to protect my sleep

both in and out of hospital, and getting additional practical help (we were lucky enough to afford a cleaner!). This plan helped so much and I haven't had PND with this child.

I have noticed less assertive friends go untreated and I do think more could be done for women by health professionals. There's so much stigma around PND many women may struggle to share their true feelings and I think by recognizing signs that women seem low and addressing this, many women could be helped … perhaps giving them written depression scoring sheets so they don't have to say the words out loud? Also reassuring them that it happens to lots of people and that their children won't be taken away. Big triggers seem to be birth trauma and people who have set themselves up for 'ideal' labours and breastfeeding and feel they've failed if they can't achieve these things. PND can look so different for different people but the more I share my story the more I realize how common it really is and that practical help can make all the difference.

REFLECTIVE ACTIVITY FOR SELF-ASSESSMENT

1. Discuss the range of emotions (positive and negative) a couple may experience during pregnancy, labour and postpartum as they transition to parenthood.
2. During a woman's pregnancy how should midwives and other key health professionals that the woman may have contact with, screen for:

   a. domestic abuse/violence
   b. mental illness?

3. Identify strategies the midwife could have in her toolkit to promote emotional wellbeing and mental health for mothers and fathers.

REFERENCES

Baldwin, S., Malone, M., Sandall, J., et al. (2018). Mental health and wellbeing during the transition to fatherhood: A systematic review of first time fathers' experiences. *JBI Database of Systematic Reviews and Implementation Reports*, 16(11), 2118–2191.

Barlow, J., Smailagic, N., Bennett, C., et al. (2011). Individual and group based parenting programmes for improving psychosocial outcomes for teenage parents and their children. *Cochrane Database of Systematic Reviews* (3), CD002964.

Beck, C. T. (2009). Birth trauma and its sequelae. *Journal of Trauma Dissociation*, 10(2), 189–203.

Beck, C. T. (2001). Predictors of postpartum depression: an update. *Nursing Research*, 50(5), 275–285.

Biaggi, A., Conroy, S., Pawlby, S., et al. (2015). Identifying the women at risk of antenatal anxiety and depression:

A systematic review. *Journal of Affective Disorders*, 191, 62–77 2016.

Bowden, S. J., Dooley, W., Hanrahan, J., et al. (2019). Fast-track pathway for elective caesarean section: A quality improvement initiative to promote day 1 discharge. *BMJ Open Quality*, 8, e000465.

Cantwell, R., Youd, E., Knight, M.; on behalf of the MBRRACE-UK mental health chapter-writing group. (2018). Messages for mental health. In M. Knight, K. Bunch, D. Tuffnell, et al. (Eds.), on behalf of MBRRACE-UK. *Saving Lives, Improving Mothers' Care – Lessons learned to inform maternity care from the UK and Ireland confidential enquiries into maternal deaths and morbidity 2014–16.* (pp. 41–60). Oxford: NPEU.

Choi, P., Henshaw, C., Baker, S., et al. (2005). Supermum, superwife, super everything: Performing femininity in the transition to motherhood. *Journal of Reproduction and Infant Psychology*, 23(2), 167–180.

Cook, K., & Loomis, C. (2012). The impact of choice and control on women's childbirth experiences. *Journal of Perinatal Education, 21*(3), 158–168.

Cook, N., Ayers, S., & Horsch, A. (2018). Maternal posttraumatic stress disorder during the perinatal period and child outcomes: A systematic review. *Journal of Affective Disorders, 225*, 18–31.

Cooper, P. J., & Murray, L. (1995). The course and recurrence of postnatal depression. *British Journal of Psychiatry, 166*, 191–195.

Cooper, P. J., & Murray, L. (1997). Effects of postnatal depression on infant development. *Archives of Disease in Childhood, 77*, 97–101.

Cox, J. (2019). Thirty years with the edinburgh postnatal depression scale: Voices from the past and recommendations for the future. *British Journal of Psychiatry, 214*(3), 127–129.

Cox, J. L., Murray, D., & Chapman, G. (1993). A controlled study of the onset, duration and prevalence of postnatal depression. *British Journal of Psychiatry, 163*, 27–31.

CQC (Care Quality Commission). (2018). survey of women's experiences of maternity care. Available at: www.cqc.org .uk/sites/default/files/20190424_mat18_statisticalrelease.pdf.

Crespi, I., & Ruspini, E. (2015). Transition to fatherhood: New perspectives in the global context of changing men's identities. *International Review of Sociology, 25*(3), 353–358.

de Graaff, L. F., Honig, A., van Pampus, M. G., & Stramrood, C. A. I. (2018). Preventing post-traumatic stress disorder following childbirth and traumatic birth experiences: A systematic review. *Acta Obstetricia et Gynecologica Scandinavica, 97*, 648–656.

Dean, C., & Kendell, R. E. (1981). The symptomatology of puerperal illnesses. *British Journal of Psychiatry, 139*, 128–133.

DHSC (Department of Health and Social Care). (2011). *Preparation for birth and beyond: A resource pack for leaders of community groups and activities*. London: DHSC.

Doss, B. D., Rhoades, G. K., Stanley, S. M., et al. (2009). The effect of the transition to parenthood on relationship quality: An 8-year prospective study. *Journal of Personality and Social Psychology, 96*(3), 601–619.

Dunkel Schetter, C., & Tanner, L. (2012). Anxiety, depression and stress in pregnancy: Implications for mothers, children, research and practice. *Current Opinion in Psychiatry, 25*(2), 141–148.

East, C. E., Biro, M. A., Fredericks, S., et al. (2019). Support during pregnancy for women at increased risk of low birthweight babies. *Cochrane Database of Systematic Reviews,* (4), CD000198.

Ferrari, G., Agnew-Davies, R., Bailey, J., et al. (2016). Domestic violence and mental health: A cross-sectional survey of women seeking help from domestic violence support services. *Global Health Action, 9*, 29890.

Fisher, A. D., Wisner, K. L., Clark, C. T., et al. (2016). Factors associated with onset timing, symptoms, and severity of depression identified in the postpartum period. *Journal of Affective Disorders, 203*, 111–120.

Furuta, M., Sandall, J., & Bick, D. (2012). A systematic review of the relationship between severe maternal morbidity and post-traumatic stress disorder. *BMC Pregnancy Childbirth, 12*(125), 1–26.

Genesoni, L., & Tallandini, M. A. (2009). Men's psychological transition to fatherhood: An analysis of the literature. *Birth, 36*(4), 305–318 1989–2008.

Giallo, R., Seymour, M., Dunning, M., et al. (2015). Factors associated with the course of maternal fatigue across the early postpartum period. *Journal of Reproductive and Infant Psychology, 335*, 528–544.

Glover, V., & Barlow, J. (2014). Psychological adversity in pregnancy: What works to improve outcomes? *Journal Children's Services, 9*(2), 96–108.

Glover, V., O'Connor, T. G., & O'Donnell, K. (2010). Prenatal stress and the programming of the HPA axis. *Neuroscience & Biobehavioral Reviews, 35*(1), 17–22.

Grabowska, C. (2017). Unhappiness after childbirth. In C. Squire (Ed.), *The social context of birth* (3rd ed.). Oxon: CRC, Ch. 14.

Harris, B., Lovett, L., Newcombe, R. G., et al. (1994). Maternity blues and major endocrine changes: Cardiff puerperal mood and hormone study 2. *British Medical Journal, 308*, 949–953.

Howard, L. M., Oram, S., Galley, H., et al. (2013). Domestic violence and perinatal mental disorders: A systematic review and meta-analysis. *PLoS Medical, 10*(5), e1001452.

Jones, F., Taylor, B., MacArthur, C., et al. (2016). The effect of early postnatal discharge from hospital for women and infants: A systematic review protocol. *Systematic Reviews, 5*(24), 1–7.

Kaźmierczak, M., & Karasiewicz, K. (2018). Making space for a new role – gender differences in identity changes in couples transitioning to parenthood. *Journal of Gender Studies, 28*(3), 271–287.

Kendell, R. E., Chalmers, J. C., & Platz, C. (1987). Epidemiology of puerperal psychoses. *British Journal of Psychiatry, 150*, 662–673.

Knight, M. (2019). MBRRACE-UK Update: Key messages from the UK and Ireland confidential enquiries into maternal death and morbidity 2018. *The Obstetrician & Gynaecologist, 21*, 69–71.

Knight, M., Bunch, K., Tuffnell, D., et al. (Eds.), on behalf of MBRRACE-UK. (2018). *Saving Lives, Improving Mothers' Care – Lessons learned to inform maternity care from the UK and Ireland Confidential Enquiries into Maternal Deaths and Morbidity 2014–16*. Oxford: NPEU.

Knight, M., Bunch, K., Tuffnell, D., et al. (Eds.), on behalf of MBRRACE-UK. (2019). *Saving Lives, Improving Moth-*

ers' Care – Lessons learned to inform maternity care from the UK and Ireland Confidential Enquiries into Maternal Deaths and Morbidity 2015–17. Oxford: National Perinatal Epidemiology Unit, University of Oxford.

Larsen, E., & Saric, K. (2017). Pregnancy and bipolar disorder: The risk of recurrence when discontinuing treatment with mood stabilisers: a systematic review. *Acta Neuropsychiatrica*, 29(5), 259–266.

McManus, S., Bebbington, P., Jenkins, R., & Brugha, T. (Eds.). (2016). *Mental health and wellbeing in England: Adult psychiatric morbidity survey 2014*. Leeds: NHS digital.

Mihelic, M., Morawska, A., & Filus, A. (2018). Preparing parents for parenthood: Protocol for a randomized controlled trial of a preventative parenting intervention for expectant parents. *BMC Pregnancy Childbirth*, 18(1), 311.

Miller, M., Kroska, E. B., & Grekin, R. (2017). Immediate postpartum mood assessment and postpartum depressive symptoms. *Journal of Affective Disorders*, 207, 69–75.

Munk-Olsen, T., Maegbaek, M. L., Johannsen, B. M., et al. (2016). Perinatal psychiatric episodes: A population-based study on treatment incidence and prevalence. *Translational Psychiatry*, 6, e919.

Munk-Olsen, T., Munk-Laursen, T., Meltzer-Brody, S., et al. (2012). Psychiatric disorders with postpartum onset: Possible early manifestations of bipolar affective disorders. *Archives of General Psychiatry*, 69(4), 428–434.

Murray, L., Fearon, P., & Cooper, P. (2015). Postnatal depression, mother-infant interactions, and child development. In J. Milgrom, & A. W. Gemmill (Eds.), *Identifying perinatal depression and anxiety: evidence-based practice in screening, psychosocial assessment and management*. Chichester: Wiley-Blackwell.

NHS England. (2016). The National Maternity Review: Better Births – improving outcomes of maternity services in England a five year forward view for maternity care. Available at: www.england.nhs.uk/wp-content/uploads/2016/02/national-maternity-review-report.pdf.

NICE (National Institute for Health and Clinical Excellence). (2006). *Postnatal care up to 8 weeks after birth: CG 37*. London: NICE (updated 2018).

NICE (National Institute for Health and Care Excellence). (2008). *Antenatal care: Routine care for the healthy pregnant woman: CG. 62*. London: NICE (updated 2019).

NICE (National Institute for Health and Clinical Excellence). (2014a). *Antenatal and postnatal mental health: The NICE Guideline on Clinical Management and Service Guidance*. London: NICE (updated 2018).

NICE (National Institute for Health and Care Excellence). (2014b). *Domestic violence and abuse: How health services, social care and the organisations they work with can respond effectively (PH50)*. London: NICE.

NICE (National Institute for Health and Care Excellence). (2016). Antenatal and postnatal mental health Quality standard. Available at: www.nice.org.uk/guidance/qs115.

Nicholson, P. (2010). What is "psychological" about "normal" pregnancy? *Psychologist*, 23(3), 190–193.

NRCN (National Rural Crime Network). (2019). *Captive and controlled domestic abuse in rural areas*. Available at: www.nationalruralcrimenetwork.net.

O'Hara, M. W., & Swain, A. M. (1996). Rates and risk of postpartum depression – a meta-analysis. *International Review of Psychiatry*, 8, 87–98.

O'Keane, V., Lightman, S., Patrick, K., et al. (2011). Changes in the maternal hypothalamic–pituitary–adrenal axis during the early puerperium may be related to the postpartum 'blues'. *Journal of Neuroendocrinology*, 23(11), 1149–1155.

O'Doherty, L., Hegarty, K., Ramsay, J., et al. (2015). Screening women for intimate partner violence in healthcare settings. *Cochrane Database of Systematic Reviews*, (7), CD007007.

O'Donnell, K., O'Connor, T. G., & Glover, V. (2009). Prenatal stress and neuro-development of the child: focus on the HPA axis and the role of the placenta. *Development Neuroscience*, 31(4), 285–292.

Philpott, L. F., Leahy-Warren, P., FitzGerald, S., et al. (2017). Stress in fathers in the perinatal period: A systematic review. *Midwifery*, 55, 113.

Rasmussen, M. H., Strøm, M., Wohlfahrt, J., et al. (2017). Risk, treatment duration, and recurrence risk of postpartum affective disorder in women with no prior psychiatric history: A population-based cohort study. *PLoS Medical*, 14(9), e1002392.

RCM Royal College of Midwives. (2012). *Maternal emotional wellbeing and infant development: A good practice guide for midwives*. Available at: www.maternalmental-health.org.uk/wp-content/uploads/2015/09/RCM-Maternal-Emotional-Wellbeing-and-Infant-Development.pdf.

Regier, D. A., Kuhl, E. A., & Kupfer, D. J. (2013). The DSM-5: classification and criteria changes. *World Psychiatry*, 12, 92–98.

Robertson, E., Jones, I., Hague, S., et al. (2005). Risk of puerperal and non-puerperal recurrence of illness following bipolar affective puerperal (postpartum) psychosis. *British Journal of Psychiatry*, 186(6), 258–259.

Robling, S. A., Paykel, E. S., Dunn, V. J., et al. (2000). Long-term outcome of severe puerperal psychiatric illness: A 23 year follow-up study. *Psychological Medicine*, 30, 1263–1271.

Rutigliano, G., Merlino, S., Minichino, A., et al. (2018). Long term outcomes of acute and transient psychotic disorders: The missed opportunity of preventive interventions. *European Psychiatry*, 52, 126–133.

Singley, D. B., & Edwards, L. M. (2015). Men's perinatal mental health in the transition to fatherhood. *Professional Psychology: Research and Practice*, 46(5), 309–316.

Strickland, P., & Allen, G. (2018). House of Commons Library Domestic Violence in England and Wales, Briefing Paper Number 6337 Available at: https://research-briefings.parliament.uk/ResearchBriefing/Summary/SN06337.

Talge, N. M., Neal, C., & Glover, V. (2007). Antenatal maternal stress and long-term effects on child neuro-development: How and why? *Journal of Child Psychology and Psychiatry, 48*, 245–261.

Teixeira, C., Figueiredo, B., Conde, A., et al. (2009). Anxiety and depression during pregnancy in women and men. *Journal of Affective Disorders, 119*(1–3), 142–148.

VanderKruik R, Barreix M, Chou D, et al. On behalf of the Maternal Morbidity Working Group. (2017) The global prevalence of postpartum psychosis: a systematic review. *BMC Psychiatry,* 17(272):1–9.

Vesga-López, O., Blanco, C., Keyes, K., et al. (2008). Psychiatric disorders in pregnant and postpartum women in the United States. *Archives of General Psychiatry, 65*(7), 805–815.

Vikström, J., Sydsjö, G., Hammar, M., et al. (2017). Risk of postnatal depression or suicide after in vitro fertilisation treatment: A nationwide case–control study. *BJOG, 124*(3), 435–442.

Werner-Bierwisch, T., Pinkert, C., Niessen, K., et al. (2018). Mothers' and fathers' sense of security in the context of pregnancy, childbirth and the postnatal period: an integrative literature review. *BMC pregnancy and childbirth, 18*(1), 473.

WHO (World Health Organization). (2014). *Who Recommendations on Postnatal Care of the Mother and Newborn.* Geneva: WHO.

WHO (World Health Organization). (2017). Violence against women factsheet. Available at: www.who.int/news-room/fact-sheets/detail/violence-against-women.

WHO (World Health Organization). (2018). *Maternal Mental Health.* Geneva: WHO.

Zhanga, S., Wanga, L., Yanga, T., et al. (2019). Maternal violence experiences and risk of postpartum depression: A meta-analysis of cohort studies. *European Psychiatry, 55*, 90–101.

ANNOTATED FURTHER READING

Crown Prosecution Service. (2018). Violence against women and girls report. Available at: www.cps.gov.uk/sites/default/files/documents/publications/cps-vawg-report-2018.pdf.

Lerardi, E., Ferro, V., Trovato, A., et al. (2019). Maternal and paternal depression and anxiety: Their relationship with mother-infant interactions at 3 months. *Archives of Women's Mental Health, 22*(4), 527–533.

An original study that examines the joint effects of maternal and paternal depression and anxiety on mother–baby interactions.

Lysell, H., Dahlin, M., Viktorin, A., et al. (2018). Maternal suicide – register based study of all suicides occurring after delivery in Sweden 1974–2009. *PLOS ONE, 13*(1) e0190133.

An interesting national cohort study of maternal suicide in the postpartum period. Addresses the key prosecution issues in tackling violence against women and girls.

Okun, M. L., Mancuso, A., Hobel, C. J., et al. (2018). Poor sleep quality increases symptoms of depression and anxiety in postpartum women. *Journal of Behavioral Medicine, 41*(5), 703–710.

In terms of risk identification this study evaluated the relationship between the quality of sleep and features of anxiety and depression in women during pregnancy and postpartum.

United Nations Office on Drugs and Crime. (2018). Global study on homicide: Gender-related killing of women and girls. Available at: www.unodc.org/documents/data-and-analysis/GSH2018/GSH18_Gender-related_killing_of_women_and_girls.pdf.

This sobering report provides evidence that globally gender-related killings of women and girls remain a grave problem for contemporary society. It highlights that while the vast majority of homicide victims are men, killed by strangers, women are far more likely to die at the hands of someone they know. Women killed by intimate partners or family members account for 58% of all female homicide victims reported globally in 2017, and little progress has been made in preventing such murders – concluding that this is an area that needs more targeted response.

USEFUL WEBSITES

Department of Health and Social Care (UK): www.gov.uk

e-Learning for Healthcare. An e-learning programme on perinatal mental health consists of three modules primarily aimed at Health Visitors but has some useful information/video clips. This is accessible at: www.e-lfh.org.uk/programmes/perinatal-mental-health/

Fathers Institute: www.fatherhoodinstitute.org

MIND: www.mind.org.uk

National Institute for Health and Care Excellence (UK): www.nice.org.uk

NHS Digital: www.digital.nhs.uk

MacMillan Cancer: https://www.macmillan.org.uk

Mothers and Babies: Reducing Risk Through Audits and Confidential Enquiries across the UK: www.mbrrace.ox.ac.uk

Mummy's Star: http://www.mummysstar.org

National Institute for Health and Care Excellence: www.nice.org.uk

Perinatal Illness UK: www.chimat.org.uk

Perinatal Mental Health Toolkit by the Royal College of General Practitioners: www.rcgp.org.uk/clinical-and-research/resources/toolkits/perinatal-mental-health-toolkit.aspx

Royal College of Psychiatrists (UK): www.rcpsych.ac.uk

Scottish Intercollegiate Guideline Network: www.sign.ac.uk

The International Marcé Society for Perinatal Mental Health: https://marcesociety.com

The US Toxicology Data Network: https://toxnet.nlm.nih.gov

UK Teratology Information Service: www.uktis.org

World Health Organization: www.who.int

31

Perinatal Loss and Bereavement in Maternity Care

Joanne Dickens, Jayne E. Marshall

CHAPTER CONTENTS

This chapter introduces the reader to the principal aspects of perinatal loss and bereavement within the maternity setting. Emphasis is placed on the reader gaining understanding and confidence in order to provide compassionate, proficient individualized care to bereaved parents and the wider family.

THE CHAPTER AIMS TO

- explore the terminology, national statistics and risk factors pertaining to perinatal loss
- discuss the nature of grief in perinatal settings and consider how personal choices and memory-making for bereaved families can be facilitated by the healthcare professional

- explain the types of investigations that are offered following pregnancy loss, stillbirth or neonatal death
- draw on research evidence and other knowledge to review the care of those affected by perinatal loss
- discuss the importance of signposting towards the support available for bereaved parents and for the healthcare professional caring for them.

INTRODUCTION

When choosing a career in midwifery the anticipation is one of sharing the joy of bringing new life into the world by using a high level of social and clinical skills to ensure a safe and healthy outcome for the baby, parents and the wider family. Sadly, for some families the trauma of pregnancy or perinatal loss is very real, and the care and support demanded of healthcare professionals, including midwives, will make a profound difference to the ability of the family to cope with the event of loss and its impact on their enduring psycho-social wellbeing, as well as face possible future pregnancies. Despite the UK being globally recognized as an economically high-income country, the rates of perinatal death do not compare very favourably with other such countries (Lawn et al. 2016) and have therefore become a driver of both public and political interest (Royal College of Midwives, RCM 2017).

Perinatal loss, or the loss of a baby due to miscarriage, stillbirth or neonatal death, in the maternity setting may be perceived as a relatively uncommon occurrence compared with the incidence of live healthy babies. In 2016, the stillbirth and neonatal death rates for pregnancies >24 weeks' gestation were 3.93 and 1.72 per 1000 births, respectively (Draper et al. 2018). Therefore, as an individual, the midwife may not be providing care to bereaved families on a very regular basis. This, combined with the uniqueness of a death that occurs simultaneously with birth (Mander 2014), can leave healthcare professionals feeling unprepared for caring for families affected by the often long-term and devastating consequences of what is essentially an unanticipated bereavement.

In recent years, there has been increased awareness around issues of pregnancy loss, stillbirth and the death of a baby, which is actively advocated by parents and stakeholders alike (Barbar et al. 2016) and reflected in the culture and social media that surrounds everyone

(Stillbirth and Neonatal Death Society, Sands 2015a). Accordingly, healthcare professionals need to be knowledgeable and feel confident in providing compassionate and proficient care to women and their families who are bereaved through pregnancy and perinatal loss. This chapter offers the reader insight into the types of pregnancy and perinatal loss experienced by families, associated risk factors and how clinical investigations and good quality and sensitive bereavement care can be facilitated by the caring midwife.

GRIEF AND LOSS

Grief, like death and other fundamentally important matters, is a fact of life. All human beings invariably face grief in some form, possibly when young. Despite its universality, a woman in a high-income country experiencing childbearing loss may have not encountered the grief of death previously. This is a further reason for the uniqueness of childbearing loss. When an adult or child dies, family members and friends will have memories to reflect on, and a life to remember, but when a baby dies, parents grieve for the future they had hoped for with their child. Consequently, there will be no tangible memories. Once a pregnancy is confirmed, parents tend to visualize their baby as a full-term healthy baby. Some will begin planning their future with the baby, including their hopes and dreams as parents and for the larger family. Such aspirations can be lost at the point of diagnosis of fetal anomaly, miscarriage, stillbirth or neonatal death. There is no right or wrong way to grieve or to experience a pregnancy loss or the death of a baby; each parent is individual, as are their circumstances and needs, and consequently, the death of their baby will be unique. Robinson et al. (1999) asserts that perinatal loss may be best understood through the framework of attachment theory.

Attachment

Limited understanding of mother–baby attachment, or *bonding,* long prevented the recognition of the significance of perinatal loss. The strength of the growing relationship between the woman and her fetus develops with feeling movement and experiencing her changing shape as pregnancy progresses, as well as various investigations that are undertaken. Continued advances in medical technology, including prenatal diagnostic procedures, such as ultrasound and 3D presentations (that mean the fetus is more likely to be perceived as a baby than a fetus) and any resulting decisions have influenced issues of both perinatal attachment and loss and continue to provide challenges for health professionals. Ordinarily, attachment continues to develop beyond the birth (Bowlby 1997). Attachment during pregnancy means that, should the relationship not continue, it will have to end as with any parting. Thus, the reality of the mother–baby relationship needs to be recognized before the loss can be accepted. These processes are crucial for the initiation of healthy grieving.

Grief

Through grieving an individual adjusts to more serious, and lesser, losses throughout life. Healthy grief means that they can move forward, although probably not directly, from the initial distraught hopelessness. Eventually, some degree of resolution, or perhaps integration, is achieved, which permits ordinary functioning much of the time. Through grief, an individual can learn something about both themselves and their resilience.

Grief has been viewed historically as apathetic passivity, but it is really a time when the bereaved person actively struggles with the emotional tasks facing them. The stages of grief through which the person moves have been described in various ways: one notable model being that attributed to Kübler-Ross (2014). The five stages of grief, as outlined in Box 31.1, are not necessarily negotiated in sequence; individual variations in the grieving process, can cause the individual to move back and forth between them before reaching a degree of resolution.

The initial response to loss comprises a defence mechanism protecting the individual from the full impact of the news or realization. This reaction comprises *shock or denial,* which shields the bereaved individual from the unbearably unthinkable reality. Facilitating coping with impending realization, this initial response allows some

---

BOX 31.1 The Five Stages of Grief

1. **Denial**
   - Shock
   - Isolation

2. **Anger**

3. **Bargaining**

4. **Depression**
   - Apathy
   - Bodily changes

5. **Acceptance**
   - Equanimity
   - Anniversary reactions

---

breathing space, during which time the individual gathers together their emotional resources.

Denial soon becomes ineffective and awareness of the reality of loss emerges. *Awareness* brings out powerful emotional reactions, together with physical manifestations. Sorrowful feelings surface but, other emotions simultaneously overwhelm the bereaved individual. These include *guilt, self-blame* and *dissatisfaction,* as well as *compulsive searching* and *anger.* Realization dawns in waves as the bereaved person tries coping strategies to *bargain* with themselves to delay accepting the grim reality.

When such fruitless strategies are exhausted, the despair of full *realization* materializes, bringing apathy and poor concentration, together with bodily changes. At this point, the bereaved individual may display *anxiety* and *physical symptoms,* such as *depression.*

When the loss is eventually accepted, it begins to become integrated into the individual's life, but this by no means is straightforward and may be slow to progress due to many setbacks, with oscillation and hesitation. Although the individual may never get over the loss, it should eventually become integrated into their life experiences. This ultimate degree of *acceptance* or *resolution* is recognizable in the bereaved individual's composure whenever contemplating the strengths, and weaknesses, of the lost person and their relationship.

The sadness of losing a baby never goes away completely, but it should not remain at the centre of the woman's/parents' life. If the pain of the loss is so constant and severe, it would suggest the individual is experiencing ***complicated grief:*** an intense state of mourning. The individual has difficulty accepting the death long after it has occurred or otherwise be so preoccupied with the baby who died that it disrupts their daily routine and undermines other relationships.

Symptoms of complicated grief include:

- intense longing and yearning for the baby
- intrusive thoughts or images of the baby
- denial of the death/sense of disbelief
- imagining the baby is still alive
- searching for the baby in familiar places
- avoiding things that remind them of their baby
- extreme anger or bitterness over the loss
- feeling that life is empty or meaningless.

Distinguishing between grief and clinical depression is not always easy, as they share many symptoms. Midwives need to be aware that grief can be unpredictable and involves a wide variety of emotions with a mix of good and bad days. There will be moments of pleasure and happiness, but with depression, the feelings of emptiness and despair are constant (see Chapter 30). Support and guidance for these women and their partners is discussed later in this chapter.

Significance

Healthy grieving is vital as it contributes to the balance or homeostasis in the bereaved individual's life. Grief helps people to deal with the hurt inflicted by the greater and lesser losses of life. The hazards of being unable to grieve healthily have long been recognized in emotional terms, but there may be an association between perinatal loss and physical illness such as fatigue, nausea, lowered immunity, weight loss/weight gain, pain and insomnia (Boyce et al. 2002). This research suggested the woman's need for support by society regardless of the nature of the loss or the extent to which it is recognized, or her grief approved. Furthermore, studies have revealed that women and men show different patterns of grief, potentially exacerbating decline in a relationship (Kersting and Wagner 2012).

Culture

A general picture of healthy grieving, and individual variation, common to people of different ethnic backgrounds, has been described (Katbamna 2000). The manifestations of grief, and accompanying mourning rituals, vary hugely. These variations are influenced by many factors (Tseng et al. 2018; Shaw 2014; Kelley and Trinidad 2012) and reflect massive differences between ethnic groups in attitudes towards childbearing loss. A midwife may encounter difficulty understanding the different attitudes to loss in cultures other than her own (Mander 2006). Whether the midwife is able to work through such feelings, to support the woman with different attitudes, is uncertain. Closely bound up with culture, and influencing mourning, are the grieving person's religious beliefs, or lack thereof. These aspects, however, are difficult to separate from social class and prevalent societal attitudes.

Despite huge variations in its manifestation, mourning has a universal underlying purpose. It establishes support for those closely affected, by strengthening links between the people who remain. In perinatal loss, the midwife initially provides this support. The midwife's role is to be with the woman when she begins to realize the extent of her loss and to prevent interference in the woman's healthy initiation of grieving.

FORMS OF LOSS AND BEREAVEMENT DURING CHILDBIRTH

Defining types of loss will be significant to the midwife from both a medical and legal perspective. Table 31.1 details the terminology and legal requirements for the types of pregnancy loss most commonly encountered by the midwife. It is important to recognize that the significance of a pregnancy or perinatal loss, and consequently, the terminology adopted by individual parents, will vary significantly and that gestation or type of loss is not reflective of the duration and intensity of grief experienced (Brier 2008; Sands 2016; Miscarriage Association 2017). It is therefore helpful for the midwife to respond sensitively and appropriately to how the parents talk about their loss, rather than strictly adhering to the impersonal medical or legal terminology during such interactions, e.g. a bereaved mother who has experienced a fetal loss before 24 weeks' gestation as being stillborn, but there would be no stillbirth certificate issued in this case (see below).

Perinatal Loss

Babies who are still stillborn or who die within the first week are associated with perinatal loss. Attempts have been made to compare the severity of grief of loss at different stages of pregnancy and childbirth in order to demonstrate that certain women deserve more understanding and supportive care. However, to date there is no evidence to signify specific differences in the grief responses

TABLE 31.1   Perinatal Loss: Definitions and Legal Requirements

Term	Definition	Legal Requirements
Early miscarriage	Spontaneous loss of pregnancy before 14 weeks' gestation, including *'missed or silent'* miscarriage and ectopic pregnancy	• No requirement to register the birth • No legal requirement to bury or cremate. However, robust guidance provided by the HTA (2015)
Late miscarriage/fetal loss (LFL)	A baby born with no signs of life after 14 weeks' and before 24 weeks' gestation	• No current requirement to register the birth • No legal requirement to bury or cremate. However, robust guidance provided by the HTA (2015)
Termination of pregnancy (TOP) (prior to 24 weeks)	The elective discontinuation of a pregnancy	• Legislation for the provision of a termination of pregnancy is covered by the Abortion Act (1967) in the UK and the Health (Regulation of Termination of Pregnancy) Act (2018) in the Republic of Ireland • A feticide is recommended for TOPs after 21+[6] (RCOG 2010) so that the baby is not live born • No requirement to register the birth • No legal requirement to bury or cremate. However, robust guidance provided by the HTA (2015)
Termination of pregnancy for fetal anomaly (ToPFA)	The elective discontinuation of a pregnancy with a fetal anomaly diagnosed through antenatal screening methods	• Legislation for the provision of a termination of pregnancy is covered by the Abortion Act (1967) in the UK and the Health (Regulation of Termination of Pregnancy) Act (2018) in the Republic of Ireland • A feticide is recommended for TOPs after 21+[6] (RCOG 2010) so that the baby is not live born • Where the ToPFA has taken place before 24 weeks gestation, there is no requirement to register the birth and no legal requirement to bury or cremate. However, robust guidance provided by the HTA (2015) • Where the ToPFA has taken place after 24 weeks' gestation, a stillbirth certificate must be issued by a qualified midwife or clinician, the stillbirth must be registered, and the baby must be buried or cremated
Stillbirth	Where a baby is born with no signs of life after 24 weeks' gestation	• A stillbirth certificate must be issued by a qualified midwife or clinician and the stillbirth must be registered • The baby must be buried or cremated
Neonatal death	Where a baby is born at *any gestation* with signs of life and subsequently dies before 28 days	• A Medical Certificate of Cause of Death must be completed by a qualified clinician and the birth and neonatal death must be registered • The baby must be buried or cremated

between mothers losing a baby by miscarriage, termination of a baby, stillbirth or neonatal death. Fundamental to facilitating changes in care is for health professionals to understand the uniqueness of the developing mother–baby relationship, regardless of the gestational age.

Miscarriage

The term *miscarriage* is given to early pregnancy loss that occurs before 24 weeks (at which time the fetus reaches viability) and may be attributed to various pathological processes such as spontaneous miscarriage or ectopic pregnancy (see Chapter 14). The grief of miscarriage has long been ignored because of its frequency and common occurrence outside the hospital setting. In the UK, there is variation regarding the gestation from which women who have experienced a miscarriage and are admitted to hospital, are cared for by midwives on a maternity ward, as the majority tend to be admitted to a gynaecology ward. This is likely to have implications for the type of bereavement care offered at these earlier and mid-trimester gestations. There is an increasing level of understanding in relation to a section of bereaved parents who feel that the term *miscarriage* does not faithfully reflect their experience of loss at, or before, the limits of viability (Smith and Hinton 2018). A recent development in this area has been the *Pregnancy Loss Review*, which has been established to consider whether it would be beneficial to adapt existing legislation, so that parents can register a birth that occurs prior to 24 weeks' gestation (Department of Health and Social Care, DHSS 2018).

Stillbirth

Stillbirth is defined as a baby born without any signs of life after 24 completed weeks' gestation. Stillbirth is most commonly associated with an antepartum event, however, in rarer circumstances, the baby dies during labour and the loss is unexpected (Draper et al. 2017). When a diagnosis of intrauterine fetal death (IUFD) has been made before labour, there may be disparities in parents' and healthcare professionals' perception of the nature of the ongoing care. Parents may continue to perceive clinical management of the situation as being urgent and healthcare professionals can misapprehend the rationale for mothers requesting a caesarean section (such as avoiding contraction pain and regaining a sense of control) over a recommended induction of labour (Siassakos et al. 2018). The midwife should be mindful of the challenges of stillbirth in terms of those mothers who are already aware their baby has died before it is born, which bears particular emotional burdens, particularly the changing appearance of the baby by the time it is born.

Maternity care can be implicated when an intrapartum-related stillbirth occurs (Draper et al. 2017) and women may express higher levels of criticism relating to their care or their role in the decision-making when their baby has died in such circumstances (Redshaw et al. 2014). Regardless of timing, the impact of stillbirth is usually devastating, multifaceted and encompasses wide-ranging implications for the psychosocial and economic circumstances of parents and the wider family (Heazell et al. 2016). An understanding of these issues, improved bereavement care education and training, and a national pathway for management around stillbirth has been recommended (Siassakos et al. 2018) and may be addressed by the National Bereavement Care Pathway developed by Sands (2018a).

A stillbirth is a registerable birth, which means a doctor or midwife must complete a stillbirth certificate following the birth and the baby's birth will need to be registered in the same manner as a live birth. In England and Wales, registration is required to take place within 42 days of the birth; in Scotland within 21 days; and in Northern Ireland, parents have up to 1 year to register the stillbirth. In 2019, the UK government launched a consultation paper to consider whether all term stillbirths should be subject to coronial investigation in-keeping with the principles described in the neonatal death section below (HM Government 2019). The rationale being to help provide all parents experiencing stillbirth at term with vital details as to the circumstances leading to their baby's death, while ensuring any issues regarding management and care are identified to prevent future deaths.

When a baby is stillborn (or a termination for fetal anomaly is performed after 24 completed weeks' gestation), parents can still access financial benefits and entitlements commensurate with when a baby is live born, such as maternity and paternity leave, statutory or maternity benefits and free National Health Service (NHS) prescriptions (Money Advice Service 2018).

Neonatal Death

A neonatal death is defined as a baby born (at any gestation) with signs of life and who subsequently dies before 28 completed days. While signs of life may appear obvious in the baby deemed to be of a viable gestation, this may prove a more challenging assessment for extremely preterm babies (i.e. those below 24 weeks' gestation) (Macfarlane et al. 2003). The mother has seen and held her baby in this situation and will have memories, however limited.

A neonatal death, like a stillbirth, is a registerable birth and both the birth **and** the death are required to be registered. It is imperative that a medical doctor witnesses any signs of life present at birth, as a Medical Certificate of Cause of Death can only be completed by the doctor who saw the baby alive (with the exception of Scotland, where a clinician can certify based on the documented evidence of signs of life), and that they are satisfied the death does not need to be considered by the Coroner (England, Wales and Northern Ireland) or Procurator Fiscal (Scotland). Although Coroners' preferences for reporting neonatal deaths (and stillbirths in Northern Ireland) can vary from region to region, all unexplained or unexpected deaths (or where a medical doctor did not see the baby alive) should be reported to the Coroner/Procurator Fiscal. A decision is then made as to whether or not to proceed to a post mortem, depending on whether the Coroner/Procurator Fiscal is satisfied with the cause of death recorded by the clinician. A Coronial/Procurator Fiscal requested postmortem does **not** require parental consent and adequate information and support should be offered to parents regarding this in order to try to mitigate for the additional distress this may cause for them. Where the Coroner/Procurator Fiscal remains undecided following a postmortem or where the parents request it, an inquest may be held to determine the cause of death. An inquest should take place within 6 months of the death but may be considerably longer depending on the circumstances (Ministry of Justice 2014), and parents should be advised of this. All deaths of a child, including neonatal and infant deaths, are subject to the child death review process and in the case of sudden unexpected death in infancy, parents should be assigned a key worker to provide information and ongoing support (HM Government 2018; NHS England 2018).

Infertility

Grief associated with involuntary infertility is less focused than when grieving for a particular person, as the couple grieve for the hopes and expectations integral to the conception of a baby. Realization of their infertility, and the associated grief, is aggravated by the widespread assumption that conception is easy, which is sufficiently prevalent for the emphasis, in society and healthcare, to be on preventing conception. Complex investigations and prolonged infertility treatment result in a roller-coaster of hope and despair.

As with any grief, the couple who are in an infertile relationship grieve differently from each other, engendering tensions. Being told the diagnosis or cause of their infertility resolves some uncertainty, but raises other difficulties. These include one partner being assigned the *label of infertile* and, hence, *blamed* for the difficulty in conceiving. A complex spiral of blame and recrimination may escalate to damage an already vulnerable relationship (Allen 2009). Clearly, counselling an infertile couple differs markedly from counselling those bereaved through death, but requires sensitivity and compassion, just the same.

Loss Within a Multiple Pregnancy

Advances in assisted reproductive technology (ART) in the past three decades have resulted in substantially increased multiple birth rates (National Institute for Clinical Excellence, NICE 2011). The increased risks to mothers and babies associated with multiple pregnancy, particularly regarding prematurity, means that multiples have a two and a half times greater chance of resulting in a stillbirth and a five times greater chance of resulting in a neonatal death (Antoniou et al. 2017). Limitations have been placed on the number of embryos that can be transferred during in vitro fertilization (IVF) treatment (NICE 2013) in order to lower the rates of multiple births resulting from assisted reproduction and mitigate for their increased risk.

Cox and Wainwright's (2015) review of the literature pertaining to the experiences of parents who lose a baby from a multiple birth highlighted the complexity of the issues they face, including the theme of *disenfranchised grief*, relating to a lack of acknowledgement of the deceased baby in the presence of its live sibling(s). This can be felt not only in relation to encounters with family members or friends outside of the healthcare setting, but when the surviving baby is cared for on the neonatal unit. Such grief can be alleviated in part by continuity of a carer who knows the history and uses both the live and deceased babies' names (Richards et al. 2015).

Some maternity and neonatal units have now adopted a system for acknowledging that a baby is one of a multiple birth such as a sticker (e.g. a butterfly sticker) placed on the live baby's incubator or cot. Healthcare professionals can cause additional distress to parents when their insensitive comments suggest that the positive experience of having a surviving baby negates the grief felt for the baby that has died (Richards et al. 2015). Parents can also find it difficult when their surviving baby is cared for on the neonatal or maternity unit in proximity to multiples, where both or all babies have survived and an understanding of this can result in sensitive management of cot spaces by the unit. In the immediate aftermath of the death, a shifting focus to the surviving baby/ies can result in the sense that grief is delayed and may potentially manifest strongly at a time sometimes significantly further into the future (Richards et al. 2015). Striving to preserve the position of the deceased baby within the family as they also observe the living baby's milestones is a challenge faced by bereaved parents in the longer term (Jordan et al. 2018). Support that is specific to the parents' experience of losing one or more babies in a multiple birth may be beneficial to the long-term grieving process and the Twins Trust (formerly the Twins and Multiple Births Association, TAMBA) can provide befriending and written information to facilitate this (Fraser 2017).

TERMINATION OF PREGNANCY

It is known that grief associated with termination (TOP) of an uncomplicated pregnancy is problematic and consequently, it tends not to be included in the literature on grief. In comparison, the grief following termination for fetal anomaly and of guilt following TOP are recognized and accepted. In view of the frequency of TOP and the grief experienced, this deserves more attention.

Termination of Pregnancy for Fetal Anomaly

Choosing to end or continue a pregnancy when a fetal anomaly (ToPFA) is diagnosed, at any gestation of pregnancy, is a complex and challenging decision for parents to navigate. Parents often feel utterly unprepared for the routine screening test or ultrasound scan resulting in the identification of a chromosomal or significant structural problem (Hodgson et al. 2016). Screening in pregnancy is discussed in more depth in Chapter 13, however, it is vital that healthcare professionals give sufficient, balanced information about screening to prepare parents for potential outcomes, although it cannot be assumed that this will avoid the impact of a difficult diagnosis (Fisher 2012). Indeed the *agonizing wait* for confirmation of diagnosis can increase parents' distress, with them finding the actual decision to end a pregnancy extremely difficult to navigate (Hodgson et al. 2016). Adequate staffing levels of midwives working in fetal medicine who have had bereavement training and provide continuity of care, may improve the quality of information and counselling that parents going through ToPFA receive (Lotto et al. 2016). As with all forms of pregnancy and perinatal loss, grief responses can vary between individuals, and it may be assumed that the mother's reaction is solely one of relief at avoiding giving birth to a baby with a disability. However, Lafarge et al. (2013) have demonstrated that grief can be extreme and variations may be seen dependant on the time since the ToPFA, the age of the mother, the presence of subsequent live births and whether the parents would choose the same course of action if faced with a future pregnancy affected by anomaly.

Termination of Pregnancy for Reasons Other than Fetal Anomaly

Although termination of pregnancy for reasons other than fetal anomaly usually fall outside the scope of the midwife and is routinely managed in the gynaecology or private healthcare setting, all healthcare professionals should understand the need for best practice care for these women. Such care should be delivered in a considerate, compassionate manner with the women as the agents of their own decision-making process (RCOG 2015). Consideration also needs to be made for the potential effects that may be felt by women, particularly those who may be experiencing difficulty in reaching a decision to discontinue the pregnancy, and signposting towards emotional support services may be beneficial at this time (Rocca et al. 2015).

RELINQUISHING A BABY

It is assumed that relinquishment of a baby is voluntary and that grief is unlikely. However, Mander (1995) found that mothers in her study who gave up their babies for adoption had no alternative to do so and considered it to be an *involuntary* act. These women felt bereaved in the sense of the term's original meaning, which implies, *robbing, plundering, snatching and removing traumatically without consent.*

The grief of relinquishing a baby differs crucially from grief following death. First, after giving up a baby for adoption, the grief is delayed due in part to the woman's lifestyle and because of the secrecy imposed on her, as she does not mother her baby as would be usual. Second, the grief of relinquishment is not resolved in the short or medium term. This is because, ordinarily, acceptance of loss is crucial to resolving grief. After giving up a baby for adoption, such acceptance is impossible due to the likelihood that the one who was relinquished will make contact when legally able. Mander (1995) found that being reunited with the baby they had given up for adoption was fundamentally important to the mothers she interviewed.

Surrogacy involves a couple commissioning a woman to act as a host for their own genetic embryo and provides a solution for those women who do not have a uterus or for whom a pregnancy may be contraindicated. This can also be a means for a same sex male couple to become parents to their own baby who may share the genetic origin of one of their male parents. It is illegal in the UK to pay a surrogate for such a service, but any expenses incurred to attend appointments, etc., may be reimbursed by the adoptive couple. In English law, the woman who gives birth to the baby is the legal mother of the child, irrespective of the genetic origin of the child. The genetic parents therefore have to apply to adopt the baby from the birth mother who would be expected to voluntarily relinquish the baby. It is wise to clarify at the outset the exact role of the surrogate and the expectations beyond her giving birth and handing over the baby to the adoptive parents. This would then help prepare the woman to deal with her emotions and the grief of finally relinquishing the baby. However, in this case, there would be no secrecy as to who the adoptive parents are or where the baby is likely to be, so the woman is more inclined to accept the loss and consequently resolve her grief.

THE BABY WITH A DISABILITY

For various reasons a baby may be born with a disability, which may or may not be anticipated. Disabilities vary hugely in severity and their implications for the baby, the parents and the family, with adjustment to the possibility of the baby dying (see Chapter 38). However, many conditions permit the continuation of a healthy life.

The mother's reaction to a baby with a disability will involve some grief. This is particularly true if the condition was unexpected, as the mother must grieve for her *expected* baby before relating to the realities of the baby she has given birth to. The mother may be shocked to find herself thinking that her baby might be better off not surviving (Lewis and Bourne 1989). Although the mother may be reassured that such thoughts are not unique, she may still find it difficult to begin her grieving.

If a baby is born with an unexpected disability, the problem of breaking the news emerges. There are no easy answers to how this can be done to reduce the trauma, but clear, effective and honest communication is crucial (Wright 2008; Farrell et al. 2001).

LOSS IN HEALTHY CHILDBEARING

It can be hard to appreciate that even in uncomplicated healthy childbearing, grief may still present as a feature.

The 'Inside Baby'

During pregnancy, a woman will begin to develop a picture in her mind of what she perceives her perfect baby will look like when it is born: notably the *inside baby* (Lewis 1979). Most women will have seen an image of their baby before birth via ultrasound scan, but those who have not, may experience a degree of grief. Inevitably the live baby, the *outside baby*, will differ from the one with whom the woman came to love during pregnancy and who may have some minor imperfections, such as the amount or colour of the baby's hair or their crying behaviour. The mother may have moments of regret and disappointment, during which she grieves the loss of her fantasy *inside* baby, before being able to begin her relationship with her live *outside* baby.

The Mother's Birth Experience

A further form of loss, over which the mother may need to grieve, is her loss of her anticipated birth experience. If she hoped for an uncomplicated birth, even some of the more common interventions may leave her feeling like a failure with low self-esteem (Kjerulff and Brubaker 2018). Thus, in the same way as the woman may need to grieve her *inside baby,* even though all appears satisfactory, this disappointed mother has some grief work to complete.

Sudden Unexpected Death in Infancy

The incidence of Sudden Unexpected Death in Infancy (SUDI) up to 12 months in an apparently otherwise healthy baby has decreased sharply since the *back to sleep* campaign of the 1990s, when evidence overwhelmingly pointed to an association of SUDI with placing babies in the prone position to sleep. Healthcare messages designed to counter associations with co-sleeping, particularly with additional harmful practices such as parental alcohol/drug use or sleeping on sofas, have served to further reduce SUDI rates. However, this reduction has occurred to a lesser extent among the most economically deprived groups (Fleming et al. 2015).

The rarity of SUDI means that healthcare professionals are often inexperienced in offering care in circumstances which are particularly traumatic for parents, especially as they are usually the first to discover the death, raise the alarm and may witness or be involved in resuscitation attempts. In the case of SUDI, the police are always notified and will attend, and this can be shocking for parents (Sands 2018b). Memory-making opportunities such as hand and footprints, photographs or a lock of hair should always be offered to the bereaved parents. However, these must not be undertaken without the permission of the local Coroner/Procurator Fiscal and once samples have been taken for clinical investigation. The Coroner/Procurator Fiscal will always instigate a postmortem and the death may be subject to an inquest if the Coroner/Procurator Fiscal deems necessary. In most circumstances, parents will be issued with an interim death certificate while awaiting the outcome of the Coroner/Procurator Fiscal investigation (Sands 2018b), in order to be able to arrange the baby's funeral.

PERINATAL MORTALITY – THE CONTEMPORARY PICTURE

Failures in maternity care (Kirkup 2015) and recognition that, despite the UK's status as a high-income nation, rates of perinatal death compare less favourably with other comparable countries (Lawn et al. 2016); this has underpinned an increase in research and initiatives related to perinatal bereavement (Table. 31.2).

Risk Factors in Perinatal Loss

Understanding why pregnancies end in adverse outcomes or why babies die is a complex and important part of current research and clinical advancement. To this end, surveillance data on stillbirths and neonatal deaths is collected and reported annually by *Mothers and Babies: Reducing Risk through Audits and Confidential Enquiries across the UK (MBRRACE–UK)* for the UK and by the *National Perinatal Epidemiology Centre (NPEC)* for Ireland. Rates of stillbirth and neonatal deaths are higher in mothers <20 and >40 years of age, mothers affected by socioeconomic deprivation, mothers from Black or Asian ethnic backgrounds and babies who are one of a multiple pregnancy (Manktelow et al. 2016). Targeted interventions to ameliorate for these factors would therefore seem pertinent.

A history of previous stillbirth is associated with reoccurrence in a subsequent pregnancy (Lamont et al. 2015) and research has shown that there is an increased risk of stillbirth after 28 weeks' gestation in women who fall asleep in the supine position (Platts et al. 2014; Heazell et al. 2018). A pre-conceptual management plan for recognized risk factors such as smoking, obesity and pre-existing diabetes can be beneficial for improving outcomes

(Ladhani et al. 2018). Fetal growth restriction may be associated with the majority of unexplained stillbirths (Gardosi et al. 2013) and the widespread implementation across the UK of customized growth charts has been presented as being associated with the subsequent reduction in stillbirth rates (Gardosi et al. 2018). Emphasis is routinely placed on mothers monitoring their fetal movements as a way of perceiving fetal wellbeing during pregnancy (RCOG 2011) and raising awareness of reduced fetal movements is an element of the *'Saving Babies Lives Care Bundle'* (Table 31.2), which has demonstrated improved outcomes for babies (Widdows et al. 2018). However, Norman et al. (2018) reported there was no substantiation of any reduction in stillbirths following a randomized controlled trial of a care package to educate women regarding fetal movements.

MANAGING PERINATAL LOSS

Communication Considerations

It is important that every bereaved parent is given the opportunity to be involved with decisions about their care and the care of their baby. Making sense of the information and care choices that are being proposed by healthcare professionals can be unachievable for parents in their grief (Downe et al. 2013) and while the provision of written information is essential, this needs to be supported by sensitive discussion taken at the parents' own pace. The difficulty for grieving parents in assimilating complex information and performing decision-making is likely to be further compounded where there are additional language or communication requirements and reasonable steps must be taken to meet such parents' needs (Nursing and Midwifery Council, NMC 2018). Where the parent has limited English or other communication challenges such as a hearing impairment, the use of other family members should be avoided (Sands 2017) and a trained interpreter or advocate is the most appropriate way to provide information. As with all aspects of the woman's clinical care, documentation of discussions and plans for care should be accurate and written contemporaneously (NMC 2018).

Clinical Investigations for Pregnancy Loss or when a Baby Dies

The scope of investigations offered will vary depending on the clinical circumstances and type of pregnancy or perinatal loss. The RCOG outline the range

TABLE 31.2 Contemporary Initiatives Relating to Stillbirth and Neonatal Death

The RCOG *Each Baby Counts* programme (Robertson et al. 2017)	Commenced in 2014, with the aim to halve the number of preventable deaths and severe disabilities from intrapartum care issues (RCOG 2017). The aim was to achieve this by examining how hospital Trusts review their deaths and looking at the modifiable factors that contributed towards the death to find recommendations for improved clinical care.
The Government's *Halve It Campaign* (DHSS 2015, NHS England 2016)	Originally aimed to halve stillbirths and neonatal deaths (along with brain injuries related to birth and maternal deaths) by 2030. In November 2017, the Secretary of State for Health brought forward this ambition to halve them by 2025, as well as initiating a review to look at whether Coroners should have jurisdiction over term intrapartum stillbirths and announcing that all term intrapartum stillbirths and neonatal deaths within the first 6 days of life (or death) would be subject to an independent review via the Healthcare Safety Investigation Branch (HSIB) (DH 2017).
The National Maternity Review – *Better Births* (NHS England 2016)	A 5-year plan for improving safety outcomes of maternity services in England, which mandates the need for compassionate and good quality bereavement care, duty of candour when things go wrong, the offer of a postmortem to all parents experiencing a stillbirth, timely follow-up with a Consultant and consistency in the standard of local perinatal mortality investigations.
The Saving Babies Lives Care Bundle (O'Connor 2016; NHS England 2019)	Aims to reduce stillbirths by introducing the four aspects of reducing smoking in pregnancy, risk assessment and surveillance for fetal growth restriction, raising awareness of reduced fetal movements, and effective fetal monitoring in labour and has demonstrated improved outcomes for babies and mothers within the Trusts that piloted the project (Widdows et al. 2018).
The National Bereavement Care Pathway	The NBCP is led by Sands in collaboration with other pregnancy and baby loss charities and aims to improve quality of care for all types of loss across the five pathways of miscarriage, termination of pregnancy for fetal anomaly (ToPFA), stillbirth, neonatal death and sudden unexpected death in infancy (SUDI). The NBCP is supported by the All-Party Parliamentary Group on Baby Loss and the Department of Health and Social Care has recently undergone a final evaluation report (Donaldson 2019).

of investigations that should be offered in the case of late intrauterine fetal death or stillbirth (Siassakos et al. 2010) and hospitals are likely to base their local guidelines and checklists for the completion of such investigations on this. However, the knowledge and confidence of individual healthcare professionals in offering and carrying out such investigations can be lacking and the need for improved training in order to offer parents the opportunity to understand why their baby died and help prevent future perinatal loss is essential (Gardiner et al. 2016). In the case of ToPFA, the cause of fetal death would already be established, therefore the full range of maternal investigations associated with an intrauterine fetal death would not be appropriate however, a postmortem (supplemented by cytogenetic and microarray testing where appropriate) can be useful to confirm the antenatal findings or give additional information regarding the diagnosis. With

parental consent, a top-to-toe external examination of the baby should be undertaken by a clinician and documented in the maternal case notes.

Postmortem

The postmortem examination can establish critical information for parents about why their baby/babies died and how this may impact on the planning of future pregnancies. A complete postmortem is an invasive procedure, whereby an external examination, usually including photographs and X-ray imaging, is carried out along with internal examination of the organs on a macro- and microscopic level. Parents may request that their baby undergoes an external examination only, that the examination is limited to certain parts of the body or may decline an examination entirely. In some situations, the Coroner/Procurator Fiscal's jurisdiction allows for postmortem examination without parental consent. Postmortem consent must be completed by a healthcare professional who has adequate experience, undertaken the appropriate training and has ideally witnessed a postmortem (Human Tissue Authority, HTA 2017) Parents should be offered written information and although it is imperative that the mother has given written consent, it is best practice, if applicable, to have both parents' consent (Sands 2013a). Parents may choose to see their baby again once the postmortem has been completed and while the incision made during an internal examination is generally not visible if the baby is clothed and a hat placed on; it is important to prepare the parents for the baby's potential appearance.

It is essential that all parents are offered a postmortem, regardless of whether the healthcare professional feels a clinical diagnosis has already been established or a ToPFA has taken place, as the postmortem findings may reveal an alternative cause of death or offer additional information. The healthcare professional may feel worried that raising the subject of postmortem examination will add to the parents' distress (Downe et al. 2012; Heazell et al. 2012). There is evidence that some parents regretted declining the examination having made their decision based on inadequate information and would have appreciated healthcare professionals describing how respectfully their baby's examination would be carried out (Siassakos et al. 2018). Recent findings show that almost all parents who experience a stillbirth are offered a postmortem (Draper et al. 2018; Henderson and Redshaw 2017), however this offer is less common in the case of a neonatal death (Draper et al. 2018). Furthermore, Henderson and Redshaw (2017) found that healthcare professionals were inconsistent when seeking consent from women from different ethnic backgrounds. There are also variations in the acceptance of postmortem as Draper et al. (2018) found that around half the parents of stillborn babies and only one-third of parents of babies who die after birth, consented to a postmortem. Henderson and Redshaw (2017) discovered that there were differences in acceptability of a postmortem according to the mother's marital status and educational level. Reasons for declining a postmortem predominantly relate to the parents' wish for their baby's body not to undergo an invasive examination. However, Henderson and Redshaw (2017) found that a significant proportion of parents perceive that they already know the diagnosis or do not feel confident that a postmortem will show a cause of death. For parents who decline a postmortem due to

religious or other reasons, the development of non-invasive or minimally-invasive techniques such as magnetic resonance imaging (MRI) or laparoscopic methods may offer an acceptable alternative (Lewis et al. 2018).

Placental Histology

The placenta has been described as the *black box* of pregnancy (Kulkarni et al. 2017) and can provide significant clinical information, often including evidence of placental insufficiency leading to stillbirth (Ptacek et al. 2014), when undergoing histological examination alone. When undertaken as part of the baby's postmortem examination, placental histology significantly improves the likelihood of finding a cause of death, but for some parents, placental histology alone may be more acceptable than a postmortem (Kulkarni et al. 2017). It is therefore essential that placental examination is offered to **all** parents who experience perinatal death at any gestation.

BEREAVEMENT CARE

Time after Birth

Parents may be unsure whether they would like to see or hold their baby after birth and may fear their baby's appearance (Kingdon et al. 2015). While evidence remains inconclusive as to the implications on maternal and paternal mental health of either seeing or holding their stillborn baby (Redshaw et al. 2016; Hennegan et al. 2018), parents can be supported to arrive at the decision that is right for them. The midwife can guide them by gentle explanations of the baby's appearance and the way they handle the baby in a sensitive and respectful manner (Kingdon et al. 2015). It is considerate to refer to the baby by its name if the parents have chosen one or the terms *'he' or 'she'* if they are still to be given a name. The midwife/healthcare professional should take their cues from the language the parents use to describe their loss. For earlier gestation losses, it may be difficult to determine the gender of the baby easily (Siassakos et al. 2010) and such assertions should be avoided in the absence of definitive cytogenetic or postmortem conclusions. Use of a cold cot or cooling mattress can allow parents to spend more time with their baby, by potentially slowing down the rate at which the baby's appearance deteriorates. Parents should have the benefits of access to a cold cot or mattress gently explained to them; as well as how the baby may feel. A cooling system should not be used unless the parents' permission is obtained.

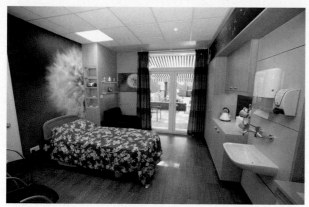

Fig. 31.1 Bereavement suite at Leicester General Hospital.

Environment

Findings from Redshaw et al. (2014) and Kingdon et al. (2015) explicated the distress felt by mothers where care was not provided in appropriate surroundings and the sound of another baby crying was apparent. Most maternity units now have a dedicated bereavement room or suite (Sands 2017), where care can be provided to bereaved parents in a private and comfortable environment (Dickens et al. 2016). However, the provision of equivalent facilities is less prevalent within neonatal units (Sands and Bliss 2018). It is helpful for such rooms (such as the one shown in Fig. 31.1), to be self-contained spaces with kitchen and washing facilities and a co-located private nursery area to attend to the baby if the parents wish for the baby to be outside the room for any given time. Consideration should also be given to the environment outside of the bereavement room when:

- parents require counselling for a difficult diagnosis
- a mother requires transfer from one clinical area to another
- care continues in the postnatal period.

Creating Memories and Offering Choices

All bereaved parents should benefit from memories of their baby being created with them. The study by O'Connell et al. (2016) found that most parents were facilitated to spend time undertaking memory-making and parenting activities with their baby. However, Downe et al. (2013) warn that such studies have mainly been small-scale qualitative analyses of self-selected parents who may not be reflective of the wider population). Therefore, when approaching memory-making with bereaved parents, it is important to understand that choices will be highly

individual and healthcare professionals should not make any assumptions or equally place any limitations on what parents will or will not want. It is also important to revisit the choices parents have made and re-offer memory-making activities in a sensitive way, as they may change their mind but not feel able to express this. The Sands *Creating Memories – Offering Choices* table is a suitable tool for ensuring that memory-making activities are re-offered in a timely manner (Sands 2016). Box 31.2 details potential memory-making activities based on current guidance and the author's experience as a bereavement support midwife. However, it is essential to note that these suggestions are not exhaustive, and that parental consent should be sought for all activities relating to their baby.

Funerals

Babies who are stillborn or die after birth must be cremated or buried and the legal responsibility for this remains with the parents. Parents may wish to maintain complete oversight of the arrangements and opt for a private funeral or may choose to allow the hospital to arrange the proceedings on their behalf (Institute of Cemetery and Crematorium Management 2015). As with all aspects of bereavement care, it is important to approach discussions regarding funeral options with no assumptions about what parents will require. Discussions should be based on their personal, cultural or religious background and the midwife must be mindful of the pathways for the management of distinct circumstances. This may include the request for urgent release of the baby's body in the case of Muslim or Jewish funerals. Input and support for bereaved parents from hospital chaplains can be invaluable where questions arise over the requirements for the funeral practices of a specific religion. Midwives should be knowledgeable about local funeral practices, such as the location of burial plots or the arrangements for the returning or scattering of their baby's ashes. It is also important to be aware of the funeral costs, including the burden this may have for some families (Heazell et al. 2016) and how parents on low income can access additional financial support.

There is no legal requirement for a baby born with no signs of life before 24 weeks' gestation to be buried or cremated. However, there are robust guidelines stating how the remains of such babies or pregnancy remains should be handled (HTA 2015). It is important to understand that women's approaches and choices in relation to what happens to the

BOX 31.2   Creating Memories

Spending Time and Parenting Activities with their Baby

Parents can spend time with their baby and include the wider family. Activities such as reading a book or talking to their baby can be comforting.

Clothing: The choice of clothing and blanket is highly personal. If parents are not able to bring appropriately-sized clothing for their baby, most hospitals will have a supply from which parents can choose, usually donated by the public. These should be available to keep should they not choose alternatives for a funeral and a sealable bag can be provided should they wish to retain the items to preserve their temporary olfactory memory of the baby.

Bathing and dressing: While some parents prefer the support of a healthcare professional, bathing and dressing their baby themselves can help demonstrate and validate their parental role. Care should be given to preparing parents with a sensitive and honest description of their baby's state of appearance, including anomalies.

Chaplaincy: Parents may wish to access support from a hospital Chaplain or non-religious pastoral carer. Parents may decide they wish for prayers to be said for their baby, a blessing or other religious observance to take place or to pray with other members of the family or a faith leader from their own community. Again, it is important not to make any assumptions about what parents will feel about their personal beliefs around the loss of their baby and grief, but to offer choices and support.

The Memory Box

These can be used to safely keep memory-making items from parents' time with their baby including items added later. Many charities now supply these free of charge to hospitals and they are often perceived as very precious (Sands 2016).

Teddy bears: Memory boxes are often supplied with two small teddy bears so that one teddy can remain with the baby and one teddy can be kept by the parents once the two are separated.

Measuring the baby: Marking a paper tape measure serves the purpose of both the memory of their baby's size and keeping an item that has touched their baby.

Hand- and footprints/impressions: Inkless kits to take hand and footprints without the need to place ink on the baby are now widely available. Hand and footprints can often be taken at relatively early gestations, but parents' expectations may need to be sensitively managed where requests are made for clay impressions or prints in a very small or macerated baby.

Acknowledgement of birth certificate: Offering an acknowledgement of the birth certificate can be particularly significant in the case of a non-registerable birth.

The suggestions above are not exhaustive and parents should be encouraged to place any items that are personal to them and their baby in the Memory Box.

Photographs

Offering photographs to bereaved parents is a significant part of a midwife's role and a collaborative aspect of the parent/healthcare professional relationship (Martel and Ives-Baine 2018). There may be personal, cultural or religious reasons why parents decline photographs and they should never be taken without the consent of parents; however, assumptions should not be made about which parents are likely to accept photographs and their offer should be universal. Photographs can capture evidence of the care that parents give to their baby (Martel and Ives-Baine 2014); memory-making activities such as bathing, dressing their baby or having a religious ceremony provide opportunities to record this parental care. Photographs can also offer a process for allowing other family members and friends to comprehend the parents' grief; in lieu of having met the baby themselves. As well as photographs that tell a story of the time parents have spent with their baby (Martel and Ives-Baine 2014), parents may wish to have more posed shots or photographs that evidence the baby's form or individual features. Examples of the types of photographs that may be taken are seen in Figs 31.2 and 31.3. Digital technology has removed the limitations on the number of photographs that can be taken, and parents can also be encouraged to take photographs themselves. Healthcare professionals should not delete or edit any photographs they believe to be of poor quality.

---

remains of her baby/pregnancy will vary considerably. While some families may opt for the hospital to carry out sensitive disposal, others choose to take the remains home or arrange a funeral themselves. Provision is also made for parents who decline any information or involvement at all (HTA 2015).

Fathers and Partners

Mander (2006) reflects on the contemporary attention to the needs of bereaved fathers that began to emerge in the latter half of the last century. The literature of that time is characterized by consideration of the gender

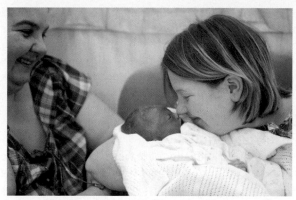

Fig. 31.2 'Nose Kiss' – Samuel and Mummy.

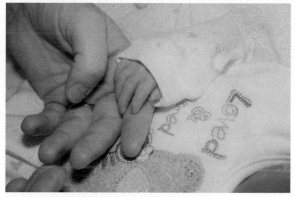

Fig. 31.3 Holding hands.

differences in bereavement and how these impact on the differing manifestations of grief, mechanisms for coping and the subsequent strain on a couple's relationship, as they seek to relate to each other's expressions of loss (Wing et al. 2001; Samuelsson et al. 2001). A recent systematic review of the literature also found differences between the intensity and duration of psychological consequences between men and women; demonstrating a higher frequency of the use of compensatory behaviours among men, e.g. use of alcohol (Due et al. 2017). Only one of the studies included has been published since 2010 and Due et al. (2017) comment on the lack of attention within the literature to issues of cultural and ethnic diversity or insight into single or gay fathers.

Fathers can feel a sense of needing to stay strong for their partner, taking on the role of arranging a funeral and informing family and friends of the baby's death (McCreight 2004). Their grief may be impeded by a reduced social awareness of a man's status as the father

to his deceased baby and a lack of opportunity for him to express his feelings. The provision of person-centred care towards fathers and respectful treatment of the deceased baby commensurate to that offered to a live baby, may serve to validate the bereaved father's role (Cacciatore et al. 2013).

There is currently an increasing appreciation of the potential fluidity of gender roles and the awareness of the increase in same sex partners exposes the lack of research around the experience of bereavement for the female parent who has not given birth to her baby. Recognition and validation of the distinctiveness of the experience of same-sex couples and appropriate compassionate support mechanisms are essential (Cacciatore and Raffo 2011).

Siblings

The death of a baby can have profound effects on other children within the family, which are not necessarily influenced by whether the baby died before birth or the length of time the baby lived and was known to the older sibling(s). Furthermore, Jonas-Simpson et al. (2015) found that the way a child related to their deceased sibling, developed over subsequent years even where the deceased baby's birth had preceded theirs. Parents can be reassured they are best placed to make decisions regarding how much detail they discuss about the baby's death with their surviving child(ren), based on their age and level of understanding. However, it is important to note that even very young children will have an awareness of the grief exhibited by parents and can be confused and distressed by a lack of explanation for it (Sands 2013b). Adolescent siblings have an increased understanding and therefore a unique perspective on the grief within the family, which may be characterized by feelings of isolation and the notion that their grief is not legitimate, particularly in relation to their parents' (Avelin et al. 2013). Therefore, supporting parents to find information to offer their surviving child(ren) that is appropriate to their developmental age is essential (O'Leary 2015) and can be facilitated through resources produced by the Child Bereavement UK (CBUK) organization (CBUK 2018). Encouraging parents to consider involving children with memory-making activities and family rituals, if their personal and cultural beliefs permit, may also be beneficial (O'Leary 2015). There is evidence from Avelin et al. (2013) that older children also find meeting their deceased baby sibling *enriching and natural*.

Grandparents

The death of a baby has been described as a double bereavement for the grandparent; as they grieve for the grandchild that has died and bear witness to their own child's grief (Sands 2016). However, there is a dearth of research pertaining to the effects of the death of an unborn or infant grandchild (Murphy and Jones 2014). Offering signposting for grandparents to bereavement support is an integral part of the healthcare professional's role in supporting the wider family. Supporting grandparents to be involved in memory-making activities can be beneficial where the parents have indicated that they welcome their participation (Sands 2016). Ultimately, the relationship established within the parents' and grandparents' shared grief can have profound effects on healing and a revalidation of the parents' role. Grandparents who are deemed *emotionally present* and who share the pain of loss have a more positive effect, in contrast to those grandparents who demonstrate a lack of understanding or who minimize the time spent openly grieving with the parents (O'Leary et al. 2011).

THE POSTNATAL PERIOD

Postnatal care on the maternity ward will depend, in part, upon the individual clinical needs of the bereaved mother. However, there are number of aspects of care specific to the area of bereavement that the midwife should be proficient in providing. Rapidly changing hormone levels following birth, uterine involution with associated afterpains and lochia as well the potential presence of perineal injury or caesarean wound, can be perceptibly more difficult to bear in the absence of a living baby. Adequate analgesia and information about what to expect is critical.

Mothers may find the production of breastmilk following the miscarriage, stillbirth or death of her baby distressing, particularly if they were unaware of this happening (Bakhbakhi et al. 2017). The midwife should provide adequate information to the bereaved mother, so she can make an informed decision about how she would like to manage her lactation. Most women will wish for support in preventing or discontinuing breastmilk production and advice should be competently supplied regarding lactation suppression: both natural and by pharmacological means such as the administration of *Cabergoline,* that may entirely suppress lactation

in over 90% of women (Siassakos et al. 2018). A small number of women will consider continuing to lactate following the birth either for personal reasons or with the intention to donate their breastmilk and they can be supported to do this through signposting to a local milk bank where available.

Going Home and Ongoing Care in the Postnatal Period

The emotional difficulty of leaving the hospital where they have received ongoing clinical care and leaving their baby behind can be particularly distressing for the mother (Lindgren et al. 2013). Sensitive discussion about how parents wish this to be managed, such as handing their baby to a trusted healthcare professional who has provided ongoing care or facilitating parents' individual wishes for transfer of the baby to the mortuary, can be helpful. There may be arrangements with a local children's hospice for families of babies whose care is being reoriented to palliation (Sands and Bliss 2018), but also sometimes for families of stillborn babies to spend further time together. It is therefore useful for the midwife to understand local pathways for this.

Another alternative to leaving the deceased baby in the hospital is taking the baby home (Lindgren et al. 2013), which can allow for more memory-making opportunities and the prospect of parents being able to care for their baby in their private environment alongside siblings and the wider family (Sands 2015b). Currently, there is limited evidence regarding the number of parents who would opt to take their baby home if all healthcare professionals felt confident to offer this, or how families experience time away from the clinical environment with their deceased baby. However, a recent small-scale local evaluation noted that nearly one-tenth of parents chose to take their baby home and advocated the importance of all maternity units providing cold cots to families to facilitate their time at home with the baby (Jones et al. 2017). Parents should be reassured that there is no legal reason that they cannot take their baby home, other than when the death has been referred to the Coroner/Procurator Fiscal; however, if they are wishing for a postmortem, it is advised that they return the baby to the hospital after around 24 hours (Sands 2015b). The parents retain legal responsibility for the burial or cremation of a baby who is stillborn or dies after birth once the baby has been taken home (Sands 2015b).

Whether the parents opt to take their baby home or not, communication with their General Practitioner (GP), community midwife, specialist community public health nurse (SCPHN)/health visitor and other specialist services, where appropriate, is vital; however adequate handover to postnatal care in the community can be lacking (Siassakos et al. 2018). Inconsistencies regarding the number of visits by the community midwife in the postnatal period have been evidenced (Redshaw et al. 2014; Redshaw et al. 2017), which seems inconceivable given the requirement for the provision of safe routine postnatal clinical care as well as the potential of the need for specialist bereavement and emotional support. The role of the bereavement midwife or specialist for bereavement care is endorsed by Sands (2015c) and is now common to many maternity units.

Bereavement midwives can assume a critical link between care in the hospital and in the community and provide specialist bereavement advice to both parents and healthcare professionals alike. Box 31.3 describes a typical day in the life of a bereavement midwife. Emphasizing the benefits of attending an appointment with the GP for a routine postnatal appointment, as well as signposting to local and national bereavement support groups, is important for the provision of ongoing support for bereaved women and the wider family. It is also essential that all future antenatal clinic appointments are cancelled and any pregnancy/baby-related mailing is suppressed to avoid the potential of future distressing communications for bereaved parents.

CONSIDERATIONS FOLLOWING PERINATAL LOSS

Follow-Up and Review

A consultant follow-up appointment should be offered to parents in a timely manner, once the results of all investigations are reported (NHS England 2016). Identifying an appropriate location for the follow-up, which is sensitive to the parents' recent loss is essential. Expectation that the appointment will provide a definitive answer to why their baby or babies died can be of paramount concern for parents (Sands 2016) and requires sensitive management when a clear cause has not been identified. Timing of the follow-up appointment may vary based on the timing of results with between one-quarter and one-third of postmortem results taking more than 12 weeks (Redshaw et al. 2017; Henderson and Redshaw

2017); although a recent interview study found that follow-up timing was not affected by awaiting postmortem results (Siassakos et al. 2018). The follow-up appointment is an opportunity for parents to have their questions about care and results explored, the risk factors for reoccurrence outlined (supplemented by referral to specialist services such as genetics where appropriate) and to discuss a plan for any future pregnancies if the parents feel ready.

Where the baby was live born or was an intrapartum stillbirth with attempted resuscitation, a joint follow-up with the Consultant Obstetrician and Consultant Neonatologist avoids the need for parents to attend multiple appointments and allows for a joined-up understanding of often interrelated clinical considerations. A sensitive and personalized letter detailing the follow-up discussion should be sent to the parents, with a copy sent to the GP.

The understanding of why a baby has died is enhanced by the undertaking of a review (RCOG 2017); however, there are inconsistencies across the UK in the prevalence and quality of perinatal mortality reviews (Kenyon et al. 2017). These inconsistencies may be addressed by the recent development and UK-wide implementation of a web-based tool developed to standardize the quality of a review (National Perinatal Epidemiology Unit 2018), underpinned by national guidance and with an emphasis on a multidisciplinary review and the seeking of parental views and feedback (Bakhbakhi et al. 2018). The Department of Health (DH 2017) issued a mandate that all term intrapartum stillbirths and neonatal deaths within the first 6 days of life (or the death) would be subject to an independent review via the Healthcare Safety Investigation Branch (HSIB).

Future Pregnancies

It is common for couples to plan another pregnancy relatively quickly after a stillbirth (Wojcieszek et al. 2018) or other types of perinatal loss. Embarking on a subsequent pregnancy is related to increased anxiety in women who have experienced perinatal loss, which may not be associated with the number of live children she already has. Concerns regarding the ability to sustain a pregnancy, a heightened anxiety of pregnancy signs and symptoms, particularly related to significant time-points in the pregnancy or labour, as well as attempts to create emotional distance from the developing fetus, may be apparent (Meredith et al. 2017). A request for more frequent antenatal appointments may be common among

BOX 31.3 A Day in the Life of a Bereavement Midwife (with personal reflections)

Monday 08.30

Check work mobile for messages left over the weekend – *always with a sense of trepidation but only three messages to respond to, often many more.*

Local Coroner's office asks me to facilitate a family viewing in our mortuary now the postmortem is complete on a 4-day old baby who died at an out of area A&E Department. Contact the family who have decided they would like me to help them with hand and footprint memories and suggest other memory-making activities. Call the mortuary to arrange the viewing for today – *always a delicate balance of pragmatic organization with the need for sensitive support to the family.*

Respond to a GP enquiry about local bereavement counselling for a family who had a miscarriage 3 months ago – *a bereavement midwife can be an expert source of such support, which can stretch over many months, even years beyond a bereavement.*

Organize in-house training for the multidisciplinary team with the help of Sands – *community support from voluntary organizations is vital to bridging the gap between the clinical and social care required.*

Respond to numerous e-mails including request to review clinical guidelines for stillbirth – *it is important that expertise of a specialist is reflected in such guidelines.*

10.30

Visit the birthing unit to check stocks of memory boxes, teddies, inkless hand- and foot-print as well as the paperwork needed by the midwives and doctors – *dealing with a death is always difficult for staff in birthing units, not having the practical things they need to enable that initial support makes the task even harder.*

While there, a recently qualified midwife asks for help in taking photographs of a baby (termination of pregnancy for complex cardiac anomalies) – *despite her correctly obtaining consent, the new midwife is naturally concerned about doing her best job for the family; demonstrating the importance of the bereavement photography training available to hospitals.*

Now that I have been introduced to the family, I spend more time discussing more memory-making activities and use this intimate time to establish what further information they want and their wishes for the baby's funeral – *finding the right moment, environment and opportunity to discuss some of the more sensitive, pragmatic and legal requirements is often a challenge, which affects the perceived level of care being offered.*

12.30

Meet with mortuary staff ahead of the at 13.00 viewing organized earlier today to ensure everything is prepared – *a viewing can be a most emotional time for parents and all the staff involved need to be prepared to ensure the visit with their baby is as smooth and sensitive as possible.*

Meet the parents at the bereavement office to discuss what they can expect to see when they visit their baby for the first time since A&E. They are overwhelmed by grief and anger but have come prepared for some of the memory-making activities such as dressing the baby and taking the hand and footprints, which I help with. I ensure the clothing and teddy the parents have brought are carefully logged to ensure they remain safely with the baby ready for the funeral – *the importance of being well organized and paying attention to the detail is vital to ensure the emotional expectations of the parents are met.*

Before they leave, the parents accept my offer of contacting their local bereavement midwife to ensure they can get access to local support services and counselling should they feel it helpful – *it is important to localize care available as much as possible, even when it falls outside of one Trust's catchment area.*

14.30

Several calls and e-mails regarding bereavement support have been received during the morning, so I begin to address these, including a call from a family contacted that have been discharged over the weekend. I offer a bereavement support visit, which is accepted and scheduled for later in the week. The mother has some questions about funerals and follow-up with the Consultant and has not felt able to read the leaflets that were provided when she was in the hospital – *while it is important to get information to the parents and families in a timely manner, it is often difficult to process when they are grieving. Print publications need to be supplemented by clear and sensitive verbal advice.*

16.30

Finish preparing notes for the perinatal mortality review meeting next week and chase-up paperwork for a cremation of a stillborn baby, without which a funeral cannot go ahead – *there are many administration actions that must be in place that bereaved parents are often not aware of. These processes need to be efficient to ensure the greatest level of care is given.*

Scan through the Bereavement Care Network (RCM 2018) for new threads on improving completion of bereavement care paperwork – *it is important to maintain and develop one's own knowledge and skills by looking for shared best practice.*

women with the highest anxiety, underlying their need for additional emotional support. Such raised anxiety levels are particularly distressing for parents. The communication of evidence that a nulliparous woman who experiences stillbirth has an almost five-fold chance of reoccurrence in a subsequent pregnancy (Lamont et al. 2015) or other difficult pregnancy outcomes, requires delicate management (Ladhani et al. 2018).

While Wojcieszek et al. (2018) found that the majority of parents received enhanced antenatal surveillance during a subsequent pregnancy to assess the chance of reoccurrence, the provision of specialist psychosocial support was lacking and there may be inequitable access to sensitive and appropriate care. This may be addressed by the provision of customized antenatal classes (O'Leary 2015), access to peer support (Ladhani et al. 2018), continuity of experienced carer and contact with a named professional between antenatal appointments (Mills et al. 2014). The concept of a specialist clinic for pregnancy following loss, which may combine the provision of services that improves outcomes with improved emotional support in subsequent pregnancies, has also gained some interest in recent years (Meredith et al. 2017; Abiola et al. 2016).

Placing a sticker on the maternal medical records has been recommended to highlight the history of perinatal loss and avoid bereaved mothers having to repeatedly relate their history to healthcare professionals (Sands 2016), although Aiyelaagbe et al. (2017) claims that in one-tenth of women, this initiative did not improve communication. Creating opportunities to remember and incorporate the bereaved parents' relationship with the deceased baby into the experience of being pregnant with the subsequent baby is a potentially useful aim of the healthcare professionals' care (O'Leary 2015).

THE DEATH OF A MOTHER

A form of loss that happens even less frequently than the death of a baby is when the mother dies; this is usually known as maternal death, which occurs during pregnancy and up to 6 weeks following childbirth or the end of pregnancy. In the UK, the rate of maternal deaths in the triennium 2015–17 was 9.2 women per 100,000 (Knight et al. 2019). This means that in a medium-sized maternity unit, the chance of midwives experiencing a maternal death is approximately once in every 3 years.

Although the obstetric and epidemiological aspects of maternal death have been well addressed through the *Confidential Enquiry into Maternal Deaths* triennial reporting in the UK since 1952, the more personal aspects have tended to be avoided. There is, however, little understanding of the family's experience, or the life of the motherless child. Palliative care principles may be appropriately applied to the care of the childbearing woman with or dying from an incurable condition (Mander 2011). The care of this woman and the implications for her baby and the other family members are becoming more important as women are choosing to delay childbearing into their mature years and consequently, has yet to be subjected to serious research attention.

Cauldwell et al. (2015) reported the devastating effects of a maternal death on maternity healthcare that included midwives, and doctors including consultant obstetricians. Maternal death was seen to have a major impact on the professionals' feeling of grief, guilt, stigma and shame, which they were reluctant to talk about to others; it was seen as a blemish on their career. There appeared to be a professional culture of silence around maternal death that did not encourage openness and reflection. Similar to Mander's (2001, 2004) research, Cauldwell et al. (2015) highlighted the health professionals' desperate need for support and debriefing by colleagues who had either shared the experience or have been through a similar one, as well as further education and training. The midwife's family also plays a fundamentally important role in supporting her (Mander 1999).

SUPPORT FOR THE HEALTHCARE PROFESSIONAL

Providing care during traumatic clinical and emotionally distressing events is associated with the incidence of symptoms related to post-traumatic stress disorder in the midwife, especially where a history of personal trauma pre-exists (Sheen et al. 2015). Feelings of upset may extend to all areas of the midwife's life and incorporate features of self-blame and fear of professional scrutinization. Peer support and discussion can be beneficial, however a lack of appropriate support from senior colleagues has been reported (Sheen et al. 2016). Therefore, opportunities for accessing support and non-judgemental reflection on the provision of care during perinatal loss events to help build resilience, should be made available through clinical supervisors/

Professional Midwife Advocates (PMA) and incorporated into the midwife's annual appraisal and professional revalidation.

Improved bereavement education and training has been espoused as a method of improving confidence in providing care to bereaved parents which in turn supports healthcare professionals (Sands 2016), however formal training may not mitigate the effects of distress. External support may be offered via the *Sands helpline*, which is available to all healthcare professionals as well as bereaved parents. The *Royal College of Midwives' Bereavement Care Network* (see Useful websites) are further sources of information and support.

CONCLUSION

Pregnancy loss or the death of a baby is arguably one of the most emotionally devastating life events for families and can also have significant effects on the healthcare professionals involved, including the midwife. It is important to recognize the wide range of possible impacts on not just the mother but the father, same-sex partner, siblings and wider family; these can be economic and practical as well as emotional. It is necessary to understand the complex, clinical, legal, ethical and psychological issues that have an impact, often contemporaneously and at a pace that can be difficult to manage. It is imperative for midwives to gain a quick and a thorough understanding of all the circumstances to be able to communicate effectively with families and the wider multidisciplinary team both within and outside of the maternity or neonatal unit. It is also important to be able manage families' expectations of the timeframe for the results of clinical investigations following pregnancy loss. Above all, midwives should be aware of the recognized care pathways after such an event to be able to signpost families to them; in order to support them beyond the clinical setting in the months and years ahead that will be impacted by such an event.

The management of bereavement and loss in maternity care continues to be an area of emphasis and study. There is a growing body of literature concerning both clinical and social impacts and research projects and initiatives continue to receive funding in a highly competitive environment and against the backdrop of a wider maternity safety agenda. Some of the new approaches outlined in this chapter have demonstrated a positive improvement in lowering the rates of pregnancy loss; adherence to a national care pathway for bereavement and a standardized method for reviewing the death of a baby is likely to improve outcomes further.

■ REFLECTIVE ACTIVITY FOR SELF-ASSESSMENT

1. How has your understanding of the *uniqueness* of grief pertaining to pregnancy loss or the death of a baby changed since reading this chapter?

2. What have you learnt about the legal definitions relating to perinatal loss and how would you relate your understanding of this to how you would communicate with parents regarding their bereavement?

3. How has your knowledge of the investigations that take place after a baby is stillborn or dies shortly after birth changed since reading this chapter?

4. Thinking about a situation when you have been involved with the care of bereaved parents in the hospital or community setting; what do you feel was helpful about the care that was provided and where do you think the care could have been improved based on your knowledge since reading this chapter?

5. How might you access support for yourself and colleagues following a baby or maternal death?

REFERENCES

Abiola, J., Warrander, L., Stephens, L., et al. (2016). *The Manchester Rainbow Clinic, a dedicated clinical services for parents who have experienced a previous stillbirth improves outcomes in subsequent pregnancies*. Manchester: Central Manchester University Hospitals NHS Foundation Trust. Available at: www.npeu.ox.ac.uk/downloads/files/m-brrace-uk/sharing-practice/pms-may-2016/prevention-management-of-risk-factors/The%20Manchester%20Rainbow%20Clinic%20-%20For%20parents%20of%20previous%20stillbirth.pdf.

Abortion Act. (1967). *England, Wales and Scotland*. Available at: www.legislation.gov.uk/ukpga/1967/87/pdfs/ukpga_19670087_en.pdf.

Aiyelaagbe, E., Scott, R. E., Holmes, V., et al. (2017). Assessing the quality of bereavement care after perinatal death: Development and piloting of a questionnaire to assess parents' experiences. *Journal of Obstetrics and Gynaecology, 37*(7), 931–936.

Allen, H. T. (2009). Managing intimacy and emotions. In *Advanced fertility care*. Keswick: M and K Publishing.

Antoniou, E., McCarthy, A., Turier, H., et al. (2017). *Twin pregnancy and neonatal care in England: A TAMBA Report – November 2017*. London: Twins and Multiple Births Association (TAMBA). Available at: www.tamba.org.uk/document.doc?id=903.

Avelin, P., Gyllens881wärd, G., Erlandsson, K., & Rådestad, I. (2013). Adolescents' experiences of having a stillborn half-sibling. *Death Studies, 38*(9), 557–562.

Bakhbakhi, D., Burden, C., Storey, C., & Siassakos, D. (2017). Care following stillbirth in high-resource settings: Latest evidence, guidelines, and best practice points. *Seminars in Fetal and Neonatal Medicine, 22*(3), 161–166.

Bakhbakhi, D., Burden, C., Storey, C., et al. (2018). PARENTS 2 Study: A qualitative study of the views of healthcare professionals and stakeholders on parental engagement in the perinatal mortality review – from "bottom of the pile" to joint learning. *BMJ Open, 8*, e023792.

Barbar, S., Pratt, A., & Sutherland, N. (2016). *Debate Pack Number CPD 2016/1075*. Available at: https://researchbriefings.parliament.uk/ResearchBriefing/Summary/CDP-2016-0175.

Bowlby J. (1997). *Attachment and loss* (Vol. 1). *Attachment*. London: Pimlico.

Boyce, P. M., Condon, J. T., & Ellwood, D. A. (2002). Pregnancy loss: A major life event affecting emotional health and well-being. *Medical Journal of Australia, 176*(6), 250–251.

Brier, N. (2008). Grief following miscarriage: A comprehensive review of the literature. *Journal of Women's Health, 17*(3), 451–464.

Cacciatore, J., & Raffo, Z. (2011). An exploration of lesbian maternal bereavement. *Social Work, 56*(2), 169–177.

Cacciatore, J., Erlandsson, K., & Rådestad, I. (2013). Fatherhood and suffering: A qualitative exploration of Swedish men's experiences of care after the death of a baby. *International Journal of Nursing Studies, 50*(5), 664–670.

Cauldwell, M., Chappell, L. C., Murtagh, G., & Bewley, S. (2015). Learning about maternal death and grief in the profession: A pilot qualitative study. *ACTA Obstetrica and Gynecologica, 94*, 1346–1353.

CBUK (Child Bereavement UK). (2018). *Death of a baby or child*. London: CBUK. Available at: https://childbereavementuk.org/for-families/death-of-a-baby-or-child/.

Cox, A., & Wainwright, L. (2015). The experience of parents who lose a baby of a multiple birth during the neonatal period – A literature review. *Journal of Neonatal Nursing, 21*(3), 104–113.

DH (Department of Health). (2017). *Safer Maternity Care: The national maternity safety strategy – progress and next steps*. Available at: https://assets.publishing.service.gov.uk/government/uploads/system/uploads/attachment_data/file/662969/Safer_maternity_care_-_progress_and_next_steps.pdf.

DHSS (Department of Health and Social Care). (2018). *The pregnancy loss review: Care and support when baby loss occurs before 24 weeks gestation. Terms of Reference*. Available at: https://assets.publishing.service.gov.uk/government/uploads/system/uploads/attachment_data/file/693820/Pregnancy_Loss_Review_ToR_gov.uk.pdf.

DHSS (Department of Health and Social Care). (2015). *News story: New ambition to halve rate of stillbirths and infant deaths gov.uk*. Available at: www.gov.uk/government/news/new-ambition-to-halve-rate-of-stillbirths-and-infant-deaths.

Dickens, J., Morrissey, J., & Adlerstein, D. (2016). *Developing the bereavement suite "Bubble". Leicester: University Hospitals of Leicester NHS Trust*. Available at: www.npeu.ox.ac.uk/downloads/files/mbrrace-uk/sharing-practice/pms-may-2016/bereavement-care/Support%20for%20bereaved%20parents-%20Developing%20the%20Beareavement%20Suite%20Bubble.pdf.

Donaldson, R. (2019). *Evaluation of the National Bereavement Care Pathway (NBCP): Final report (Wave two), May 2019*. London: Fiveways NP Ltd. Available at: https://nbcpathway.org.uk/sites/default/files/2019-05/N-BCP%20wave%20two%20evaluation%20report%207%20May%202019_0.pdf.

Downe, S., Kingdon, C., Kennedy, R., et al. (2012). Post mortem examination after stillbirth: Views of UK-based practitioners. *European Journal of Obstetrics and Gynecology, 162*(1), 33–37.

Downe, S., Schmidt, E., Kingdon, C., & Heazell, A. E. (2013). Bereaved parents' experience of stillbirth in UK hospitals: A qualitative interview study. *BMJ Open, 3*(2).

Draper ES Kurinczuk, JJ., Kenyon, S., (Eds); on behalf of the MBRRACE-UK Collaboration. (2017). *MBRRACE-UK 2017 Perinatal Confidential Enquiry: Term, singleton, intrapartum stillbirth and intrapartum-related neonatal death*. Leicester: The Infant Mortality and Morbidity Studies, Department of Health Sciences, University of Leicester. Available at: www.npeu.ox.ac.uk/downloads/files/mbrrace-uk/reports/MBRRACE-UK%20Intrapartum%20Confidential%20Enquiry%20Report%-202017%20-%20final%20version.pdf.

Draper, E. S., Gallimore, I. D., Kurinczuk, J. J., et al. (2018). *Perinatal mortality surveillance report. UK perinatal deaths for births from January to December 2016. The infant mortality and morbidity studies*. Department of Health Sciences, University of Leicester. Available at: www.npeu-

.ox.ac.uk/downloads/files/mbrrace-uk/reports/M-BRRACE-UK%20Perinatal%20Surveillance%-20Full%20Report%20for%202016%20-%20June%202018.pdf.

Due, C., Chiarolli, S., & Riggs, D. (2017). The impact of pregnancy loss on men's health and wellbeing: A systematic review. *BMC Pregnancy and Childbirth*, 17(1), 1–13.

Farrell, M., Ryan S., & Langrick, B. (2001). 'Breaking bad news' within a paediatric setting: An evaluation report of a collaborative education workshop to support health professionals. *Journal of Advanced Nursing*, 36(6), 765–775.

Fisher, J. (2012). Supporting patients after disclosure of abnormal first trimester screening results. *Current Opinion in Obstetrics and Gynecology*, 24(2), 109–113.

Fleming, P. J., Blair, P. S., & Pease, A. (2015). Sudden unexpected death in infancy: Aetiology, pathophysiology, epidemiology and prevention in 2015. *Archives of Disease in Childhood*, 100(10), 984.

Fraser, E. (2017). *Bereavement support group booklet: For parents who have lost one or more babies from a multiple birth*. London: Twins and Multiple Births Association (TAMBA). Available at: https://twinstrust.org/uploads/assets/1a37eb18-be5d-4b6b-83ee8af6bf19bf45/bereavement-booklet.pdf.

Gardiner, P. A., Kent, A. L., Rodriguez, V., et al. (2016). Evaluation of an international educational programme for health care professionals on best practice in the management of a perinatal death: IMproving Perinatal mortality Review and Outcomes Via Education (IMPROVE). *BMC Pregnancy Childbirth*, 16(1), 376.

Gardosi, J., Madurasinghe, V., Williams, M., et al. (2013). Maternal and fetal risk factors for stillbirth: Population based study. *British Medical Journal*, 346, 7893.

Gardosi, J., Francis, A., Turner, S., & Williams, M. (2018). Customized growth charts: Rationale, validation and clinical benefits. *American Journal of Obstetrics and Gynecology*, 218(2S), S609.

Health (Regulation of Termination of Pregnancy) Act. (2018). Republic of Ireland. Available at: https://data.oireachtas.ie/ie/oireachtas/act/2018/31/eng/enacted/a3118.pdf.

Heazell, A., McLaughlin, M. J., Schmidt, E., et al. (2012). A difficult conversation? The views and experiences of parents and professionals on the consent process for perinatal postmortem after stillbirth. *BJOG: An International Journal of Obstetrics and Gynaecology*, 119(8), 987–997.

Heazell, A. E. P., Siassakos, D., Blencowe, H., et al. (2016). Stillbirths: Economic and psychosocial consequences. *Lancet*, 387(10018), 604–616.

Heazell, A. E. P., Li, M., Budd, J., et al. (2018). Association between maternal sleep practices and late stillbirth – findings from a stillbirth case-control study. *BJOG: An*

International Journal of Obstetrics and Gynaecology, 125(2), 254.

Henderson, J., & Redshaw, M. (2017). Parents' experience of perinatal post-mortem following stillbirth: A mixed methods study. (Research Article) (Survey). *PLoS ONE*, 12(6), e0178475.

Hennegan, J. M., Henderson, J., & Redshaw, M. (2018). Is partners' mental health and well-being affected by holding the baby after stillbirth? Mothers' accounts from a national survey. *Journal of Reproductive and Infant Psychology*, 36(2), 120–131.

HM Government. (2018). *Working Together to Safeguard Children: A guide to inter-agency working to safeguard and promote the welfare of children*. London: HM Government. Available at: https://assets.publishing.service.gov.uk/government/uploads/system/uploads/attachment_data/file/729914/Working_Together_to_Safeguard_Children-2018.pdf.

HM Government. (2019). *Consultation on coronial investigations of stillbirths: HM Government*. Available at: https://consult.justice.gov.uk/digital-communications/coronial-investigations-of-stillbirths/supporting_documents/Consultation%20on%20coronial%20investigations%20of%20stillbirths%20web.pdf.

Hodgson, J., Pitt, P., Metcalfe, S., et al. (2016). Experiences of prenatal diagnosis and decision–making about termination of pregnancy: A qualitative study. *Australian and New Zealand Journal of Obstetrics and Gynaecology*, 56(6), 605–613.

HTA (Human Tissue Authority). (2015). *Guidance on the disposal of pregnancy remains following pregnancy loss or termination*. London: Human Tissue Authority. Available at: www.hta.gov.uk/sites/default/files/Guidance_on_the_disposal_of_pregnancy_remains.pdf.

HTA Human Tissue Authority. (2017). *Code of practice and standards code B: Post-mortem examination*. London: Human Tissue Authority. Available at: www.hta.gov.uk/sites/default/files/code%20b.pdf.

Institute of Cemetery, & Management, Crematorium (2015). *Policy and Guidance for Baby and Infant Funerals*. London: ICCM. Available at: www.iccm-uk.com/iccm/library/baby%20and%20infant%20funerals%20september%202015.pdf.

Jonas-Simpson, C., Steele, R., Granek, L., et al. (2015). Always with me: Understanding experiences of bereaved children whose baby sibling died. *Death Studies*, 39(1–5), 242–251.

Jones, E. R., Holmes, V., & Heazell, A. E. (2017). The use of cold cots following perinatal death. *European Journal of Obstetrics and Gynecology*, 217, 179–180.

Jordan, A., Smith, P., & Rodham, K. (2018). Bittersweet: A qualitative exploration of mothers' experiences of raising a single surviving twin, Psychology. *Health and Medicine*, 23(8), 891–898.

Katbamna, S. (2000). *Race and childbirth*. Buckingham: Open University Press.

Kelley, M. C., & Trinidad, S. B. (2012). Silent loss and the clinical encounter: Parents' and physicians' experiences of stillbirth: A qualitative analysis. *BMC Pregnancy and Childbirth*, 12, 137.

Kenyon S, Cross-Sudworth F, Keegan C, Johnston T; on behalf of MBRRACE-UK. (2017) Local review of intrapartum-related death. In: ES Draper, JJ Kurinczuk, S Kenyon (Eds); on behalf of MBRRACE-UK. *Perinatal confidential enquiry: Term, singleton, intrapartum stillbirth and intrapartum-related neonatal death,* (pp. 79–88) Leicester: The Infant Mortality and Morbidity Studies, Department of Health Sciences, University of Leicester.

Kersting, A., & Wagner, B. (2012). Complicated grief after perinatal loss. *Dialogues in Clinical Neuroscience*, 14(2), 187–194.

Kingdon, C., O'Donnell, E., Givens, J., & Turner, M. (2015). The role of healthcare professionals in encouraging parents to see and hold their stillborn baby: A meta-synthesis of qualitative studies. *PLoS ONE*, 10(7).

Kirkup, B. (2015). *The report of the Morecambe Bay investigation*. London: The Stationery Office.

Kjerulff, K. H., & Brubaker, L. H. (2018). New mothers' feelings of disappointment and failure after cesarean section. *Birth*, 45(1), 19–27.

Knight, M., Bunch, K., Tuffnell, D., et al. (Eds.). (2019). On behalf of MBRRACE-UK. *Saving Lives, Improving Mothers' Care - Lessons learned to inform maternity care from the UK and Ireland confidential enquiries into maternal deaths and morbidity 2015–2017.* Oxford: National Perinatal Epidemiology Unit, University of Oxford. Available at: www.npeu.ox.ac.uk/downloads/files/mbrrace-uk/reports/MBRRACE-UK%20Maternal%20Report%202018%20-%20Web%20Version.pdf.

Kübler-Ross, E. (2014). *On death and dying: What the dying have to teach doctors, clergy and their own families*. New York: Scribner.

Kulkarni, A., Palaniappan, N., & Evans, M. (2017). Placental pathology and stillbirth: A review of the literature and guidelines for the less experienced. *Journal of Fetal Medicine*, 4(4), 177–185.

Ladhani, N., Fockler, M., Stephens, L., et al. (2018). No. 369 – Management of Pregnancy Subsequent to Stillbirth: SOGC Clinical Practice Guideline. *Journal of Obstetrics and Gynaecology, Canada*, 40(12), 1669–1683.

Lafarge, C., Mitchell, K., & Fox, P. (2013). Perinatal grief following a termination of pregnancy for foetal abnormality: The impact of coping strategies. *Prenatal Diagnosis*, 33(12), 1173–1182.

Lamont, K., Scott, N. W., Jones, G. T., & Bhattacharya, S. (2015). Risk of recurrent stillbirth: Systematic review and meta-analysis. *British Medical Journal*, 350, h3080.

Lawn, J. E., Blencowe, H., Waiswa, P., et al. (2016). Stillbirths: Rates, risk factors, and acceleration towards 2030. *Lancet*, 387(10018), 587–603.

Lewis, E. (1979). Mourning by the family after a stillbirth or neonatal death. *Archives in Disease and Childhood*, 54, 303–306.

Lewis, E., & Bourne, S. (1989). Perinatal death. In M. Oates (Ed.), *Psychological aspects of obstetrics and gynaecology* (pp. 935–954). London: Baillière Tindall.

Lewis, C., Latif, Z., Hill, M., et al. (2018). We might get a lot more families who will agree: Muslim and Jewish perspectives on less invasive perinatal and paediatric autopsy. *PLoS ONE*, 13(8), e0202023.

Lindgren, H., Malm, M. C., & Radestad, I. (2013). You don't leave your baby–mother's experiences after a stillbirth. *Omega – The Journal of Death and Dying (Farmindale)*, 68(4), 337–346.

Lotto, R., Armstrong, N., & Smith, L. K. (2016). Care provision during termination of pregnancy following diagnosis of a severe congenital anomaly: A qualitative study of what is important to parents. *Midwifery*, 43, 14–20.

Macfarlane, P. I., Wood, S., & Bennett, J. (2003). Non-viable delivery at 20–3 weeks gestation: Observations and signs of life after birth. *Archives of Disease in Childhood – Fetal and Neonatal Edition*, 88(3), F199.

Mander, R. (1995). *The care of the mother grieving a baby relinquished for adoption*. Aldershot: Avebury.

Mander, R. (1999). Preliminary report: A study of the midwife's experience of the death of a mother. *RCM Midwives Journal*, 2(11), 346–349.

Mander, R. (2001). The midwife's ultimate paradox: A UK-based study of the death of a mother. *Midwifery*, 17(4), 248–259.

Mander, R. (2004). When the professional gets personal – the midwife's experience of the death of a mother. *Evidence Based Midwifery*, 2(2), 40–45.

Mander, R. (2006). *Loss and bereavement in childbearing* (2nd ed.). London: Routledge.

Mander, R. (2011). 'Being with woman': The care of the childbearing woman with cancer. In T. F. Fawcett, & A. McQueen (Eds.), *Perspectives on cancer care* (pp. 48–62). London: Wiley–Blackwell.

Mander, R. (2014). Bereavement and loss in maternity care. In J. Marshall, & M. Raynor (Eds.), *Myles textbook for midwives* (16th edn.) (pp. 555–567). Edinburgh: Churchill Livingstone.

Manktelow, B., Smith, L., Seaton, S., et al. (2016). *MBRRACE-UK Perinatal Mortality Surveillance Report, UK perinatal deaths for births from January to December 2014. Leicester: The infant mortality and morbidity studies*. Department of

Health Sciences, University of Leicester. Available at: www.npeu.ox.ac.uk/downloads/files/mbrrace-uk/reports/MBRRACE-UK-PMS-Report-2014.pdf.

Martel, S., & Ives-Baine, L. (2018). Nurses' experiences of end-of-life photography in NICU bereavement support. *Journal of Pediatric Nursing, 42*, e38–44.

Martel, S. L., & Ives-Baine, L. (2014). 'Most prized possessions': Photography as living relationships within the end-of-life care of newborns. *Illness, Crisis & Loss, 22*(4), 311–332.

McCreight, B. S. (2004). A grief ignored: Narratives of pregnancy loss from a male perspective. *Sociology of Health and Illness, 26*(3), 326–350.

Meredith, P., Wilson, T., Branjerdporn, G., et al. (2017). "Not just a normal mum": A qualitative investigation of a support service for women who are pregnant subsequent to perinatal loss. *BMC Pregnancy and Childbirth, 17*(1), 6.

Mills, T., Ricklesford, C., Cooke, A., et al. (2014). Parents' experiences and expectations of care in pregnancy after stillbirth or neonatal death: A metasynthesis. *BJOG, 121*(8), 943–950.

Ministry of Justice. (2014). *Guide to coroners services.* London: Ministry of Justice.

Miscarriage Association. (2017). *Your feelings after miscarriage.* Wakefield: The Miscarriage Association. Available at: www.miscarriageassociation.org.uk/wp-content/uploads/2016/10/Your-feelings-after-miscarriage-June-2014.pdf.

Money Advice Service. (2018). *If your baby is stillborn.* London: The Money Advice Service. Available at: www.moneyadviceservice.org.uk/en/articles/if-your-baby-is-stillborn.

Murphy, S., & Jones, K. S. (2014). By the way knowledge: Grandparents, stillbirth and neonatal death. *Human Fertility, 17*(3), 210–213.

NHS England. (2016). *Better Births – Improving outcomes of maternity services in England – A five year forward view for maternity care.* Available at: www.england.nhs.uk/wp-content/uploads/2016/02/national-maternity-review-report.pdf.

NHS England. (2018). *When a child dies: A guide for parents and carers.* London: NHS England.

NHS England. (2019). *Saving Babies' Lives, Version Two: A care bundle for reducing perinatal mortality NHS England.* Available at: www.england.nhs.uk/wp-content/uploads/2019/03/Saving-Babies-Lives-Care-Bundle-Version-Two-Final-Version2.pdf.

NICE (National Institute for Health and Clinical Excellence). (2011). *Multiple pregnancy: Antenatal care for twin and triplet pregnancies.* London: NICE. Available at: www.nice.org.uk/guidance/cg129/resources/multiple-pregnancy-antenatal-care-for-twin-and-triplet-pregnancies-pdf-35109458300869.

NICE (National Institute for Health and Clinical Excellence). (2013). *Fertility problems: Assessment and treatment.* London: NICE. Available at: www.nice.org.uk/guidance/cg156/chapter/Recommendations.

National Perinatal Epidemiology Unit. (2018). *Perinatal mortality review tool.* Oxford: NPEU. Available at: www.npeu.ox.ac.uk/pmrt.

Norman, J. E., Heazell, A. E. P., Rodriguez, A., et al. (2018). Awareness of fetal movements and care package to reduce fetal mortality (AFFIRM): A stepped wedge, cluster-randomised trial. *Lancet, 392*(3), 1629–1638.

NMC (Nursing and Midwifery Council). (2018). *The code: Professional standards of practice and behaviour for nurses, midwives and nursing associates.* London: NMC. Available at: www.nmc.org.uk/globalassets/sitedocuments/nmc-publications/nmc-code.pdf.

O'Connell, O., Meaney, S., & O'Donoghue, K. (2016). Caring for parents at the time of stillbirth: How can we do better? *Women and Birth, 29*(4), 345–349.

O'Connor, D. (2016). Saving Babies' Lives: A care bundle for reducing stillbirth: NHS England. Available at: www.england.nhs.uk/wp-content/uploads/2016/03/saving-babies-lives-car-bundl.pdf.

O'Leary, J. (2015). Subsequent pregnancy: Healing to attach after perinatal loss. *BMC Pregnancy and Childbirth, 15*(S1) 2393–15.

O'Leary, J., Warland, J., & Parker, L. (2011). Bereaved parents' perception of the grandparents' reactions to perinatal loss and the pregnancy that follows. *Journal of Family Nursing, 17*(3), 330–356.

Platts, J., Mitchell, E. A., Stacey, T., et al. (2014). The Midland and North of England Stillbirth Study (MiNESS). *BMC Pregnancy and Childbirth, 14*(1), 171.

Ptacek, I., Sebire, N. J., Man, J. A., et al. (2014). Systematic review of placental pathology reported in association with stillbirth. *Placenta, 35*(8), 552–562.

Redshaw, M., Dickens, J., Kenyon, S., et al. On behalf of the MBRRACE UK Collaboration. (2017). `Care after birth'. In: E. S. Draper, J. J. Kurinczuk, S. Kenyon (Eds.); on behalf of MBRRACE-UK. *Perinatal confidential enquiry: Term, singleton, intrapartum stillbirth and intrapartum-related neonatal death.* (pp. 67–72) Leicester: The Infant Mortality and Morbidity Studies, Department of Health Sciences, University of Leicester.

Redshaw, M., Rowe, R., & Henderson, J. (2014). *Listening to parents after stillbirth or the death of their baby after birth.* Oxford: National Perinatal Epidemiology Unit. Available at: www.npeu.ox.ac.uk/downloads/files/listeningtoparents/Listening%20to%20Parents%20Report%20-%20March%202014%20-%20FINAL%20-%20PROTECTED.pdf.

Redshaw, M., Hennegan, J. M., & Henderson, J. (2016). Impact of holding the baby following stillbirth on maternal mental health and well-being: Findings from a national survey. *BMJ Open, 6*(8), e010996.

Richards, J., Graham, R., Embleton, N. D., et al. (2015). Mothers' perspectives on the perinatal loss of a co-twin: A qualitative study. *BMC Pregnancy and Childbirth, 15*, 143.

Robertson, L., Knight, H., Prosser Snelling, E., et al. (2017). Each baby counts: National quality improvement programme to reduce intrapartum-related deaths and brain injuries in term babies. *Seminars in Fetal and Neonatal Medicine, 22*(3), 193–198.

Robinson, M., Baker, L., & Nackerud, L. (1999). The relationship of attachment theory and perinatal loss. *Journal of Death Studies, 23*(3), 257–270.

Rocca, C. H., Kimport, K., Roberts, S. C. M., et al. (2015). Decision rightness and emotional responses to abortion in the United States: A longitudinal study. *PLoS ONE, 10*(7), e0128832.

RCM (Royal College of Midwives). (2017). *Government drive to cut stillbirths.* London: RCM. Available at: www.rcm.org.uk/news-views-and-analysis/news/government-drive-to-cut-stillbirths.

RCM (Royal College of Midwives). (2018). Bereavement Care Network: RCM. Available at: https://bereavement-network.rcm.org.uk/.

RCOG (Royal College of Obstetricians and Gynaecologists). (2010). *Termination of pregnancy for fetal abnormality in England, Scotland and Wales: Report of a Working Party.* London: RCOG. Available at: www.rcog.org.uk/globalassets/documents/guidelines/terminationpregnancyreport-18may2010.pdf.

RCOG (Royal College of Obstetricians and Gynaecologists). (2011). *Reduced fetal movements: Green-top guideline No 57.* London: RCOG. Available at: www.rcog.org.uk/globalassets/documents/guidelines/gtg_57.pdf.

RCOG (Royal College of Obstetricians and Gynaecologists). (2015). *Best practice in comprehensive abortion care. Best Practice Paper No 2.* London: RCOG.

RCOG (Royal College of Obstetricians and Gynaecologists). (2017). *Each baby counts 2015 full report.* London: RCOG. Available at: www.rcog.org.uk/globalassets/documents/guidelines/research–audit/each-baby-counts-2015-full-report.pdf.

Samuelsson, M., Rådestad, I., & Segesten, K. (2001). A waste of life: Fathers' experience of losing a child before birth. *Birth, 28*(2), 124–130.

Sands (Stillbirth and Neonatal Death Society). (2013a). Guide for consent takers. *Seeking consent/authorisation for the post mortem examination of a baby.* London: Sands. Available at: www.hta.gov.uk/sites/default/files/5._Sands__Guide_for_consent_takers_Jan_2013.pd_.2017.pdf.

Sands (Stillbirth and Neonatal Death Society). (2013b). *Supporting children when a baby has died.* London: Sands. Available at: www.sands.org.uk/sites/default/files/%E2%80%A2AW%20SUPPORTING%20CHILDREN%20211113%20LR%20SP%20LINKED.pdf.

Sands (Stillbirth and Neonatal Death Society). (2015a). *EastEnders storyline media coverage.* London: Sands. Available at: www.sands.org.uk/about-sands/media-centre/news/2015/08/eastenders-stillbirth-storyline-media-coverage.

Sands (Stillbirth and Neonatal Death Society). (2015b). *Sands position statement: Taking the baby home.* London: Sands. Available at: www.sands.org.uk/sites/default/files/Position%20statement%20Taking%20the%20baby%20home_2.pdf.

Sands (Stillbirth and Neonatal Death Society). (2015c). *Sands Position Statement: Bereavement Midwives.* London: Sands. Available at: www.sands.org.uk/sites/default/files/Position%20statement%20Bereavement%20midwives_0.pdf.

Sands (Stillbirth and Neonatal Death Society). (2016). *Pregnancy loss and the death of a baby: Guidelines for professionals* (4th ed.). London: Sands.

Sands (Stillbirth and Neonatal Death Society). (2017). *Audit of bereavement care provision in UK maternity units 2016.* London: Sands. Available at: www.sands.org.uk/sites/default/files/Bereavement%20Care%20Audit%20Report%202016%20DIGITAL%20-%2010.01.17.pdf.

Sands (Stillbirth and Neonatal Death Society). (2018a). *Stillbirth Bereavement Care Pathway.* London: Sands. Available at: www.nbcpathway.org.uk/file/aw_5844_nbcp_stillbirth_pathway.pdf.

Sands (Stillbirth and Neonatal Death Society). (2018b). *Sudden Unexpected Death in Infancy (SUDI) up to 12 months: Bereavement care pathway.* London: Sands. Available at: www.nbcpathway.org.uk/file/aw_5844_nbcp_sudi_pathway.pdf.

Sands (Stillbirth and Neonatal Death Society) and Bliss (for babies born premature or sick). (2018). *Audit of bereavement care provision in UK Neonatal Units 2018.* London: Sands/Bliss. Available at: www.sands.org.uk/sites/default/files/27151%20Sands%20Neonatal%20Audit%20Report%20-%20updated%20Dec%202018.pdf.

Shaw, A. (2014). Rituals of infant death: Defining life and Islamic personhood. *Bioethics, 28*(2), 84–85.

Sheen, K., Spiby, H., & Slade, P. (2015). Exposure to traumatic perinatal experiences and post traumatic stress symptoms in midwives: Prevalence and association with burnout. *International Journal of Nursing Studies, 52*(2), 578–587.

Sheen, K., Spiby, H., & Slade, P. (2016). The experience and impact of traumatic perinatal event experiences in midwives: A qualitative investigation. *International Journal of Nursing Studies, 53*(C), 61–72.

Siassakos, D., Fox, R., Dracott, T., & Winter, C. (2010). *Late intrauterine fetal death and stillbirth. Green-top Guideline No 55.* London: RCOG. Available at: www.rcog.org.uk/globalassets/documents/guidelines/gtg_55.pdf.

Siassakos, D., Jackson, S., Gleeson, K., et al. (2018). All bereaved parents are entitled to good care after stillbirth: A mixed–methods multicentre study (INSIGHT). *BJOG: An International Journal of Obstetrics and Gynaecology, 125*(2), 160–170.

Smith, L. K., & Hinton, L. (2018). *This isn't a miscarriage: Losing a baby at 20 to 24 weeks of pregnancy.* Healthtalk. org. Available at: www.healthtalk.org/peoples-experiences/pregnancy-children/losing-baby-20-4-weeks-pregnancy-late-miscarriage-neonatal-death-stillbirth/isnt-miscarriage-losing-baby-20-4-weeks-pregnancy.

Tseng, Y. F., Hsu, M. T., Hsieh, Y. T., & Cheng, H. R. (2018). The meaning of rituals after a stillbirth: A qualitative study of mothers with a stillborn baby. *Journal of Clinical Nursing, 27*(5), 1134–1142.

Widdows, K., Reid, H. E., Roberts, S. A., et al. (2018). Saving babies' lives project impact and results evaluation (SPiRE): A mixed methodology study. *BMC Pregnancy and Childbirth, 18*(1), 43.

Wing, D. G., Clance, P. R., Burge-Callaway, K., & Armistead, L. (2001). Understanding gender differences in bereavement following the death of an infant: Implications for treatment. *Psychotherapy: Theory, Research, Practice, Training, 38*(1), 60–73.

Wojcieszek, A., Boyle, F., Belizán, J., et al. (2018). Care in subsequent pregnancies following stillbirth: An international survey of parents. *BJOG: An International Journal of Obstetrics and Gynaecology, 125*(2), 193–201.

Wright, J. (2008). Prenatal and postnatal diagnosis of infant disability: Breaking the news to mothers. *Journal of Perinatal Education, 17*(3), 27–35.

ANNOTATED FURTHER READING

Chute, A. (2017). Expecting sunshine: A journey of grief, healing and pregnancy after loss. Berkeley: She Writes Press.
A memoir of the author's subsequent pregnancy and the challenges she faced after the death of her child.

Kenworthy, D., & Kirkham, M. (2011). Midwives coping with loss and grief: Stillbirth, professional and personal losses. London: Radcliffe.
This book utilizes a phenomenological approach to portraying midwives' experiences of pregnancy loss and bereavement, which encourages midwives to reflect upon the effect of others' grief on themselves and improve support and understanding for all.

Pearson, G. (2013). The burden of choice: Collected stories from parents facing a diagnosis of abnormalities during pregnancy. Derby: Dormouse Press.
The stories of 25 mothers whose babies have died following the diagnosis of an abnormality, have been collected in this book to support anyone facing this impossible decision in pregnancy and subsequent devastating loss.

USEFUL WEBSITES

Registration and Statutory Documentation

England and Wales: General Register Office www.gro.gov-.uk/gro/content/

Northern Ireland: General Register Office Northern Ireland (GRONI) www.nidirect.gov.uk/gro

Scotland: National Records for Scotland www.nrscotland.gov-.uk/registration

Support Groups and Services for Bereaved Parents and Their Families

Antenatal Results and Choices (ARC): www.arc-uk.org/

Baby Mailing Preference Service (MPS): www.mpsonline.org.uk/bmpsr/

Bliss – for sick or premature babies: www.bliss.org.uk/

British Pregnancy Advisory Service (BPAS): www.bpas.org/

Child Bereavement UK (CBUK): www.childbereavementuk.org/

Cruse Bereavement Care Offers: www.cruse.org.uk/

Funeral Payments – Northern Ireland: www.nidirect.gov.uk/funeral-payments

Funeral Payments – United Kingdom: www.gov.uk/funeral-payments

Gifts of Remembrance Bereavement Photography: http://giftsofremembrance.co.uk/

Hearts Milk Bank: http://heartsmilkbank.org/

Human Tissue Authority (HTA): www.hta.gov.uk

Lullaby Trust: www.lullabytrust.org.uk/

MBRRACE-UK (Mothers and Babies: Reducing Risk through Audits and Confidential Enquiries across the UK): www.npeu.ox.ac.uk/mbrrace-uk

Miscarriage Association: www.miscarriageassociation.org.uk/

Money Advice Service: www.moneyadviceservice.org.uk

Muslim Bereavement Support Service: http://mbss.org.uk/

Remember My Baby Remembrance Photography: www.remembermybaby.org.uk/

Sands: The Stillbirth and Neonatal Death Society: www.uk-sands.org/

Together for Short Lives: www.togetherfor-
shortlives.org.uk/

Tommy's charity – funding research into miscarriage, stillbirth and premature birth: www.tommys.org/

The United Synagogue Burial Society – advice on Jewish
Burial www.theus.org.uk/article/about-us-burial-soci-
ety-0

Twins Trust Bereavement Support Group (Part of Twins
Trust, formerly TAMBA: Twins and Multiple Births Association): https://twinstrust.org/bereavement.html

Support for the Midwife

Association for Improvements in Maternity Services (AIMS):
www.aims.org.uk/

Bereavement Care Network Online: http://bereavement-net-
work.rcm.org.uk/

Nursing and Midwifery Council (NMC): www.nmc.org.uk/

Royal College of Midwives (RCM): www.rcm.org.uk/

The Neonate

32

Recognizing the Healthy Baby at Term Through Examination of the Newborn Screening

Hazel Ransome, Jayne E. Marshall

CHAPTER CONTENTS

The focus of this chapter is based on the characteristics of the healthy term baby and the role of the midwife in performing the ongoing systematic screening assessment of the baby's health and wellbeing from the point of birth until discharge from midwifery care. This includes the first top-to-toe assessment shortly after birth, the ongoing daily examination and the Full systematic physical examination of the newborn/Newborn and Infant Physical Examination (NIPE*) that is performed by healthcare professionals who have undergone specialist training, within 3 days (72 h) of birth. These examinations assess the baby's transition and adaptation to extrauterine life. Each examination undertaken should not be viewed in isolation but considered holistically, to build a picture of neonatal health and produce an individualized plan of care. The role of the midwife undertaking

*NIPE is not a UK-wide term, but is what Public Health England (PHE) use to describe the full systematic physical examination of the newborn within 72 h of birth and once again between 6 and 8 weeks of birth.

these examinations is not to make any diagnosis, but is to identify any subtle changes or abnormalities from that of the healthy baby and to escalate these appropriately and in a timely manner to appropriately trained healthcare professionals. It is therefore important that the midwife has a comprehensive knowledge of neonatal physiology and the skills to effectively examine the healthy term neonate. For the purpose of this chapter, the definitions of 'newborn' being immediately after birth and 'neonate' being within the first 28 days of life will be adopted, respectively (Nursing and Midwifery Council, NMC 2018; Resuscitation Council United Kingdom, RCUK 2015).

THE CHAPTER AIMS TO

- highlight the characteristics of a healthy term baby in order to recognize those babies that require referral
- emphasize the importance of gathering a comprehensive history from the woman's antenatal and labour records in conjunction with discussions with the parents prior to any examination of the baby
- identify the processes which should be followed when carrying out any examination of the neonate, such as obtaining informed consent from the parents
- understand the rationale for and the differing elements of the first examination of the newborn following birth, the daily examination of the baby

- and the full systematic physical examination of the newborn/NIPE assessment
- recognize that the outcomes of all examinations of the neonate provide a holistic indicator of the baby's health
- discuss how each screening examination provides an opportunity for the midwife to provide health education/promotion advice to parents on the health and wellbeing of their baby
- highlight the importance of clear, concise documentation of the findings of each examination and the communications that have taken place, including those with the parents.

THE FIRST EXAMINATION OF THE NEWBORN FOLLOWING BIRTH

It is essential that any examination that is performed on the neonate is not in isolation but is supported by the holistic picture, as shown in Fig. 32.1. In order for this to happen, the midwife is required to have an understanding of the mother's general health during the antenatal period, as well as the labour and birth outcome. This history should not only be taken from written records, but should also be clarified and confirmed by the parents, which in turn, assists in building a trusting relationship. It is often the case that something that may seem trivial to a mother may be significant in the view of the midwife/healthcare professional. Any conversations with parents need to be in a private environment where they feel comfortable and able to disclose information. Prior to any examination being undertaken, the parents should be fully informed regarding the process of the examination, its purpose and potential outcomes, so that informed consent can be gained (NMC 2018). Table 32.1 provides an overview of all the elements that should be assessed when any neonatal examination is undertaken, following a step-by-step process, as identified in Fig. 32.2.

The purpose of the first systematic examination of the newborn that encompasses all elements as detailed in Table 32.1, is to begin building a picture of the neonate's health and to identify any deviations that may compromise their health and wellbeing, which may require further investigation or monitoring (Perinatal Institute for Maternal and Child Health 2018). The midwife should first obtain informed consent from the mother/parents before undertaking the examination in their presence and within 24 h of the baby's birth. This examination should not be confused with the initial birth assessment, which is performed *at 1, 5 and 10 minutes following birth*, where Apgar scores are assigned (see Chapter 33). If the midwife has no concerns regarding the newborn's initial condition, it is recommended that the first systematic examination does not take place until at least 1 hour following the birth. This protected *'golden-hour'* enhances attachment between mother and baby and facilitates uninterrupted skin-to-skin contact and the initiation of breastfeeding (should this be the mother's preferred choice of infant feeding). Furthermore, the promotion of uninterrupted skin-to-skin contact within this first hour helps to regulate the newborn's temperature and cardiorespiratory response,

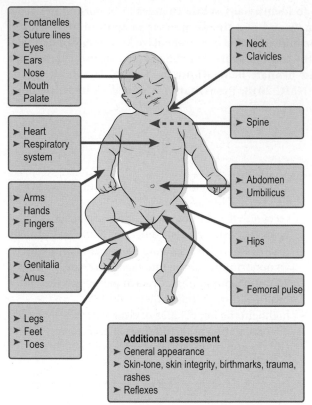

- Fontanelles
- Suture lines
- Eyes
- Ears
- Nose
- Mouth
- Palate

- Heart
- Respiratory system

- Arms
- Hands
- Fingers

- Genitalia
- Anus

- Legs
- Feet
- Toes

- Neck
- Clavicles

- Spine

- Abdomen
- Umbilicus

- Hips

- Femoral pulse

Additional assessment
- General appearance
- Skin-tone, skin integrity, birthmarks, trauma, rashes
- Reflexes

Fig. 32.1 Principles of holistic neonatal examinations. (Adapted from: www.niddk.nih.gov/health-information/urologic-diseases/urine-blockage-newborns.)

as well as stimulate the baby to self-attach to the mother's breast that is more likely to result in enhancing prolonged breastfeeding (UNICEF 2013).

The environment should be warm and draught-free with equipment ready for use if required. Thorough hand-washing is essential before the midwife commences the examination which should be undertaken in close proximity to the parents. The newborn should be lying at rest on a flat surface and the skills of observation, palpation and auscultation should be utilized. Box 32.1 identifies the guiding principles that should be communicated when screening is undertaken.

Visual Assessment

A generalized assessment of the newborn's overall appearance should be undertaken in the first instance, with the midwife observing for a newborn that appears well perfused, with good muscle tone, is responsive to touch and is easily roused if sleeping.

Skin Colour

The newborn baby's adaptation to extrauterine life can be directly observed through their skin colour. As the newborn transitions and establishes independent breathing, well-perfused skin should be observed. One of the first indications of potential problems related to this transition may be cyanosis: a blue tinge to the skin that is due to an accumulation of carbon dioxide and deprivation of oxygen. Therefore, skin colour may be used as an indicator of newborn health, although not the most reliable in isolation as cyanosis may present in cases of congenital heart disease, respiratory disease, hypothermia, hypoxia and infection (Baston and Durward 2017) (see Chapter 37). To assess cyanosis can be difficult in white ethnic groups and even more so in babies from black ethnic groups who have pigmented skin (Dawson and Morley 2010). The newborn's oral mucus membranes and tongue are not pigmented and will provide the midwife with reliable evidence of central cyanosis. The examination of the mouth, in particular the gums, can provide a more accurate indication of central cyanosis by appearing very pale or blue tinged.

A dull blue skin may indicate poor perfusion and can be assessed by measuring capillary refill time (CRT) by blanching the newborn's chest skin with a finger and on release, seeing how long it takes for the capillaries to refill. Any time over 2 seconds (s) indicates poor peripheral perfusion. Pallor of the skin is a result of peripheral shutdown and is always a serious sign, indicating acute blood loss, anaemia, the processes involved in cooling or/and the presence of infection. Jaundice that develops from birth in the first 24 hours (h) is considered pathological, is usually as a result of haemolysis (excessive breakdown of red blood cells) and the midwife should refer the baby immediately to the neonatal team (see Chapter 37).

Most newborns will have some degree of peripheral shutdown known as *acrocyanosis* in the hands and feet, as blood is diverted to the major organs. Parents often report the baby as having cold hands and feet accompanied by some discolouration and the midwife should reassure them that in isolation, this is a normal finding (Baston and Durward 2017). Occasionally, the newborn may present with a blue face as a result of *petechiae*, which are pinpoint haemorrhage spots on the skin, usually as a result of a tightening cord around the neck constricting the jugular veins during the descent of the fetus in the second stage of labour. The venous blood is trapped in the sinuses of the brain and finds an exit

TABLE 32.1   Comparison: The Elements Comprising the Systematic Neonatal Examinations

The First Examination of the Newborn	The Daily Examination of the Neonate	The Full Systematic Physical Examination of the Newborn/Neonatal and Infant Physical Examination (NIPE)

• General appearance
• Colour
• Visual inspection of:
  • the head including sutures and fontanelles
  • the face including eyes, ears, nose and mouth for palate and ankyloglossia
  • the neck
  • the chest and abdomen
  • the spine
  • the genitalia
  • the anus
  • the limbs including hands and feet
• Identification of any birthmarks or birth injuries
	• General appearance
	• Colour
	• Activity and tone
	• Eyes
	• Mouth
	• Cord
	• Skin/jaundice
	• Feeding
	• Urinary output
	• Stools
	• Sleeping pattern
		• General appearance
		• Colour
		• Visual inspection of:
		  • the head including sutures and fontanelles
		  • the face including eyes (red reflex), ears, nose and mouth for palate and ankyloglossia
		  • facial symmetry
		  • the neck
		  • the clavicles
		  • the chest and abdomen
		  • the spine
		  • the genitalia
		  • the anus
		  • the limbs including symmetry
		  • the hands: creases and digits
		  • the feet: digits, presence of talipes
		• Auscultation of:
		  • the heart
		  • the chest
		  • the abdomen
		• Palpation of:
		  • the palate
		  • the clavicles
		  • the abdomen
		  • the femoral arteries
		• Testes

Adapted from: https://evolve.elsevier.com/objects/apply/RN/HealthyNewborn/RN_HealthyNewborn_04.html.

point into the skin, causing the facial tissues to become bruised. Pulse oximetry can be used as a numerical reassurance that the newborn has successfully adapted to extrauterine life. This measures the oxygen saturation of the blood and a measurement of ≥95% is a normal finding for a baby in the first day of life (RCUK 2015).

The Head

The shape, size and symmetry of the head in relation to the face and rest of the body should be assessed. The head circumference measurement of the occipitofrontal diameter should be in the range of 32–36 cm for a term newborn baby. A head that is disproportionate to body size may indicate intrauterine growth restriction, where the head has been saved from any disruption to its growth (see Chapter 34). However, it is worth noting that a standalone head measurement may appear

perfectly normal, but its relationship with the body may render it large. Macrocephaly (a head circumference >97th centile) is also associated with hydrocephaly and congenital syndromes whereas microcephaly (a head circumference <2nd centile) is associated with poor brain development, significant with fetal alcohol spectrum disorders (FASD) and transplacental infections, respectively (England 2014).

As described in Chapter 7, the structure of the fetal skull is unique so that it can *mould* in order to reduce the presenting diameters to facilitate the process of birth. This reduction can be as significant as 1 cm. Moulding is perfectly normal and safe unless it happens rapidly or in an adverse direction, which can cause a shearing of the membranes and intracranial trauma (Campbell and Dolby 2018). Observation and palpation of the scalp will therefore indicate the presence and degree of *caput*

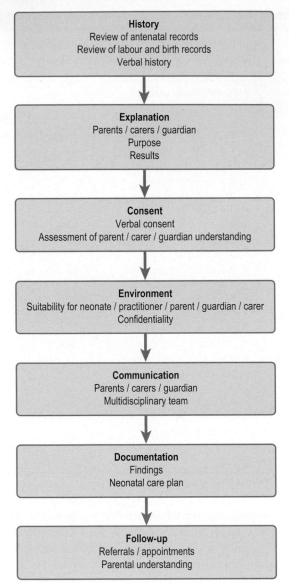

History
Review of antenatal records
Review of labour and birth records
Verbal history

Explanation
Parents / carers / guardian
Purpose
Results

Consent
Verbal consent
Assessment of parent / carer / guardian understanding

Environment
Suitability for neonate / practitioner / parent / guardian / carer
Confidentiality

Communication
Parents / carers / guardian
Multidisciplinary team

Documentation
Findings
Neonatal care plan

Follow-up
Referrals / appointments
Parental understanding

Fig. 32.2 Stages of the neonatal examination process.

United Kingdom National Screening Committee (2018) Newborn and Infant Physical Examination Screening Programme Handbook. Available at: www.gov.uk/government/publications/newborn-and-infant-physical-examination-programme-handbook/newborn-and-infant-physical-examination-screening-programme-handbook#maintaining-competency-in-undertaking-nipe-examinations.

succedaneum (the collection of fluid under the scalp resulting from the presenting part being subjected to excessive cervical pressure during labour following rupture of the membranes), which usually resolves within 2–3 days. Parents should be reassured that this is not a cause for concern but a normal mechanical process and the head will regain its normal shape. The direction and degree of moulding can indicate the engaging diameter of the fetal skull involved in the process of labour. The bones, fontanelles and sutures are then inspected to ensure that they are present and *craniosynostosis* (fusion of the bones) has not occurred. The anterior fontanelle (bregma) remains present and palpable for up to 18 months, while the posterior fontanelle (lambda) closes by 6 weeks after birth. Examination of the fontanelles should be performed when the newborn is at rest, as crying can affect their appearance and presentation during palpation. At rest, the fontanelles should be neither raised nor sunken. A raised, bulging bregma can be indicative of intracranial haemorrhage, infection such as meningitis and congenital or metabolic conditions, such as hydrocephaly, while a sunken bregma can be related to dehydration (Campbell and Dolby 2018). More than one lambda along the lamboidal suture lines often alongside a flat occiput, can indicate trisomy 21 as can abnormal patterns of hair growth (low hair lines and extra crowns) which are characteristics in a variety of syndromes.

The presence of any trauma on the newborn's head in the form of abrasions or bruising resulting from intrapartum processes such as artificial rupture of membranes, the application of fetal scalp electrodes, fetal blood sampling or instrumental births needs to be clearly documented. Any trauma needs to be discussed with parents and an explanation given as to the

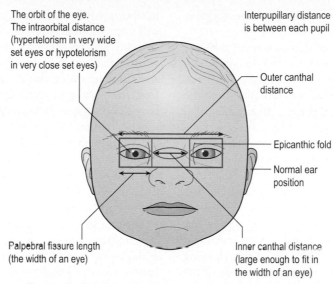

The orbit of the eye.
The intraorbital distance
(hypertelorism in very wide
set eyes or hypotelorism
in very close set eyes)

Interpupillary distance
is between each pupil

Outer canthal
distance

Epicanthic fold

Normal ear
position

Palpebral fissure length
(the width of an eye)

Inner canthal distance
(large enough to fit in
the width of an eye)

Fig. 32.3 Features of the baby's eyes in relation to the face.

potential causes and reasons why it may have occurred. It is also important to explain to parents that bruising increases the risk of the newborn developing physiological jaundice due to the presence of excessive blood collection in the bruised area and the subsequent need for breakdown and excretion (Podsiadly 2018). Trauma to the head should be escalated to the neonatal team, if it appears extensive or overlaps delicate structures such as the eyes to enable further investigation and monitoring and potentially reduce long-term complications (see Chapter 35).

The Face and its Features

It is essential that the midwife observes the facial features of both biological parents wherever possible before making assumptions and expressing concerns on an unusual looking face. Furthermore, it cannot be assumed that the male partner is the biological father of the baby.

Visual inspection of the face should take place in two parts. First, the face should be analysed as a whole and then each of the component parts should be examined independently. Dysmorphic features may be indicative of congenital abnormalities (Noonan et al. 2015), when they are combined with other features. The newborn's facial expression may indicate an underlying condition such as pain, irritability, distress and is important to note. The presence of two eyes, two ears, a nose and mouth are observed and that they are aligned symmetrically. Should one side of the face appear to droop, particularly

around the eye and mouth when the newborn is crying, would indicate birth trauma in the form of facial paralysis (see Chapter 35). This is a result of damage to the 7th cranial nerve (facial), known as Bell's palsy, during the application of forceps or from head compression against the sacral promontory during birth and requires referral to the neonatal medical team (Noonan et al. 2015). The extent of recovery will depend on the amount of damage to the myelin sheath that covers and nourishes the nerve.

The eyes should be visualized when they are open to ensure that they are both present and patent. Absence of one or both eyes may have an environmental or chromosomal cause and consequently warrants referral to the ophthalmologist. The symmetry is assessed in relation to the other facial features such as eyelids, eyebrows and the slant of the palpebral fissures as shown in Fig. 32.3. The outer canthal distance can be equally divided into thirds, with one eye-width fitting into the inner canthal space. Extremely wide (hypertelorism) or narrowly spaced (hypotelorism) eyes are abnormal and may indicate a syndrome as may epicanthic folds, however the latter finding can be a normal feature of some ethnic groups and so caution is required. The sclera should be white in colour, however conjunctival haemorrhages may be present both around the iris and in other parts of the sclera. These are often due to the pressure of the birth, especially in those that are rapid/precipitate. It is important that their appearance, size and position is documented, as they can be interpreted as non-accidental injury (Griffith 2009).

Parents should be reassured that conjunctival haemorrhages will not affect the newborn and do not require treatment but may take weeks to resolve fully. The iris of the newborn is navy blue with fibres radiating from the centre. It should be circular in shape with a round pupil in the centre. White specks on the iris called *Bushfield spots* are associated with Down syndrome. Opacity of the lens could indicate congenital cataract and clouding of the cornea may be significant of glaucoma. Small eyes can occur as a result of transplacental infection such as rubella and cytomegalovirus. Any profuse or purulent discharge from the eyes should be noted with swabs taken for culture and sensitivity, and conversations had with parents providing information regarding cleaning the eyes and monitoring the amount and colour of the discharge. The incidence of neonatal conjunctivitis is around 8% and is often caused by *Staphylococcus aureus*, which can be easily treatable (Grayson and Wylie 2011). Other causes of conjunctivitis may be the *herpes simplex virus*, *gonorrhoea* or *chlamydia*, which the newborn can acquire from the mother during the birth process and if left untreated, can lead to long-term sight complications. A more detailed examination of the eyes takes place around 72 h and includes a 'red-reflex' examination, which is discussed later in this chapter.

The position of the ears should be similar on both sides with the upper pinna in alignment with the inner to outer canthus of the eye. However, a finding of low-set ears alone may be a normal variation. Malformed and/or low-set ears are associated with chromosomal or urogenital anomalies and require referral (Campbell and Dolby 2018). Periauricular skin tags and dimples should also be documented and discussed with the parents as, although normally aesthetic, in some instances may indicate hearing impairment. The incidence of significant permanent congenital hearing impairment (PCHI) is 1:1000 births in high-to middle-income countries.

The shape of the nose will vary, but the two nares should be centrally placed on the face and patent. The neonate is an obligatory nose-breather and patency can be observed when the baby is breathing normally at rest (or via the mouth when crying). Nasal flaring may be indicative of respiratory distress and should not be ignored. Choanal atresia is a condition where one or both posterior nasal passages are blocked by either bone or tissue. If this is apparent in both nasal passages, the newborn will be centrally cyanosed at rest but perfusion will improve when they cry. Urgent referral to an ENT surgeon will be required. The neonate often sneezes, which may cause some parental concerns. Parents should be reassured that clear nasal secretions resulting from the clearing of excess amniotic fluid from the newborn's body system following birth, are common.

The mouth should appear symmetrical, with the lips being complete. At the midline of the mouth, two frenula should be visible; an upper frenulum labiisuperioris and a lower frenulum labiiinferioris. The frenulum linguae is found beneath the tongue and if this structure is short and thick it can restrict the normal movement of the tongue. This condition is commonly known as a 'tongue-tie' or 'ankyloglossia'. The extent and impact of a tongue-tie varies with a small percentage having little consequence to a high percentage, which severely limits the movement of the tongue. In those cases where feeding is affected, a frenotomy is offered, which involves dividing the frenulum linguae and freeing the tongue. Evidence supports frenotomy to improve breastfeeding as detailed in Chapter 27 and subsequent maternal comfort but is limited when considering speech development (Brookes and Bowley 2014). The tongue should also be examined for cysts and dimples.

Cleft lip and/or palate may be hereditary or as a consequence of maternal medication such as phenytoin or chromosomal anomalies such as Down or Patau syndrome and affects 1:700 babies in the UK (Cleft Lip and Palate Association, CLAPA 2019). Of these babies, 31% are cleft palates associated with a cleft lip, but approximately 45% of cleft palates will present independently and are often missed, resulting in a negative impact on feeding. When a cleft lip is detected by antenatal screening, automatic referral is made to the local cleft lip and palate (CLP) team that includes a plastic surgeon, ENT surgeon, audiologist, orthodontist surgeon and speech therapist, before the baby is born. For those newborns where the cleft lip is detected at birth, the midwife should in the first instance, refer to the neonatal team, who will then make referral to the cleft lip and palate team. Cleft lip can be either unilateral or bilateral and can extend into the hard and soft palate. A cleft palate is not always obvious and requires thorough assessment to confirm its presence. This is undertaken with a gloved finger inserted into the mouth to elicit the suck reflex. By palpating the hard palate, it should be possible to feel if a cleft is present. To detect clefts in the soft palate, visual inspection using a pen torch and tongue depressor should be used. The palate should be high-arched, intact with a central uvula. Detecting a cleft at birth will be a time of great anxiety for the parents, so additional support and information from the midwife and CLP team will be necessary. A small jaw (micrognathia) may be hereditary or part of a syndrome such as Pierre Robin, which comprises a midline cleft palate and protruding tongue (glossoptosis). The midwife must be aware of the tongue falling back and obstructing the oropharynx as well as potential feeding difficulties. Referral to the ENT and orthodontic surgeons will be made alongside the speech therapist.

A cluster of several white spots (Epstein's pearls) may be found in the mouth at the junction of the soft and hard palate in the midline. They are similar to milia and are of no significance and disappear simultaneously. The gums should be inspected for the presence of natal teeth, which may present as white ridges on the lower gums. They have no roots and may risk ulceration of the tongue and if they become loose, inhalation into the trachea. Referral to the orthodontic team for elective removal would be required in these situations.

The Neck

The neck is assessed in terms of its length and mobility as well as observed for any webbing with extra skin, any swelling, tumours or dimples. The neck should exhibit a good range of mobility, including flexion, extension, rotation and bending without any indication of discomfort to the neonate (Lewis 2014a). Any excess or folds of skin should be examined to ensure that they are not obscuring sinuses, tumours, cysts, birthmarks or birth injuries. It is also important to observe under the baby's chin, as this area is in the closest proximity to the airway so any inconsistencies or abnormalities in this area could affect successful respiration.

The Clavicles

The clavicles should be examined for any trauma such as fractures, particularly if there is any history of shoulder dystocia during the birth or suggestion of Erb's palsy (see Chapter 35). Although bruising is easily diagnosed, fractures and brachial plexus nerve damage can be challenging to identify and may be easily overlooked, particularly if the newborn is at rest. However, the midwife should observe for limited usage and movement of the affected arm as well as the absence of the moro (startle) reflex on the affected side (Lewis 2014b). This is often noticed initially by parents and as such, the midwife should always consider any parental concerns and respond accordingly.

The Chest and Abdomen

A visual examination of the chest should reveal symmetry with two nipples, equidistant and lateral to the mid-clavicular line. The nipples should be normal in shape and form and the presence of abnormal or supernumerary (extra) nipples should be recorded as a line drawing on a body map with referral to the neonatal team. This additional nipple has no known function and can be situated anywhere on the chest. Occasionally, the midwife may encounter a newborn baby with prominent, swollen breasts where the nipples leak fluid (galactorrhoea): referred to as 'witch's milk' and can occur in both male and female babies. The parents should be reassured that this is normal and is as a result of an excess of maternal hormones in the newborn's system and will eventually resolve itself (Madlon-Kay 1986).

Observation of respiratory movement should be equal on both sides of the chest, with a respiratory rate for the newborn ranging from 30 to 40 bpm, but should not exceed 60 bpm and will vary in rhythm with small periods of apnoea (absence of breathing for ≥20 s). Although this appears a broad range, it must be remembered that breathing can be affected by a number of factors such as periods of sleep, activity, feeding and crying. Not only can the rate of breathing be observed, but also the type of breathing. There should be no sternal or costal recession. Chest and abdominal movement are synchronous, as the diaphragm is the major muscle of respiration. Asymmetrical chest movement may be caused by either a unilateral pneumothorax or phrenic nerve damage on the side that is not moving. The presence of a diaphragmatic hernia would be indicative of a relatively large chest in comparison to a scaphoid (sunken) abdomen. Auscultation of ectopic bowel sounds in the chest may support this supposition (see Chapter 37). An auditory assessment of breathing should also take place as noisy breathing or 'grunting' is an indication of respiratory distress and should therefore be escalated to the neonatal team immediately (Bedford and Lomax 2015). The noise/grunt originates from the force of exhalation against the glottis, which is partially closed, in order to prevent complete lung collapse.

The abdomen should look symmetrical, with no swelling or distension and feel soft and rounded. The skin should be well perfused. Where the abdomen appears distended, the midwife should be aware that the bowel may be obstructed and that the presence of hernias may also alter the shape of the abdomen (Gordon 2015). Any concerns require further investigation. Gastroschisis is caused by a defect on the abdominal wall, which allows the bowel to protrude through it and is usually found on antenatal ultrasonography. At birth, the protruding bowel is covered by filmwrap to prevent fluid and heat loss prior to surgical repair.

The Umbilicus

The umbilicus should be firmly clamped and cut short enough to ensure that it does not get caught on the newborn's nappy or clothing. It should not be bleeding or actively excreting fluid and on examination, should contain two umbilical arteries and one larger umbilical vein. A single umbilical artery increases the chances of congenital anomalies, but further investigations are not justified on this finding alone. The size of the cord is often associated with the size of the newborn, with larger babies having a thicker cord containing more Wharton's jelly compared with the thinner cord of the low birth weight/growth restricted baby (Baston and Durward 2017).

The umbilicus should also be observed for any signs of herniation which present in 10–20% of newborns (Snyder 2007) and often cause parents concern. Although there appears to be no difference in the incidence of umbilical hernias among male and female babies, Ireland et al. (2014) affirm that they are more common in newborns of African or Afro-Caribbean descent. An umbilical hernia occurs when there is a defect in the anterior abdominal wall directly behind the umbilicus, meaning that adipose tissue or in some instances part of the small intestine covered by a transparent sac composed of amnion and peritoneum, protrudes through (known as 'exomphalos'). In the majority of cases, umbilical hernias are not associated with adverse health outcomes and are classified as uncomplicated, but in some instances the protruding small intestine may become strangulated, warranting immediate medical attention. Uncomplicated umbilical hernias are conservatively managed as in many cases they will resolve spontaneously. However, surgical repair would be warranted in cases of exomphalos or if there any complications associated with the hernia or if it has not closed spontaneously by the time the child reaches school age (Barreto et al. 2013).

The Spine

During the examination, the newborn should be held so that the spine can be visualized in its entirety. A good position to accomplish this is to rest the baby face-down along the forearm, while continuing to support the head and neck and running the other hand down the spinal processes. The spine should appear straight and central with no curvature. Particular attention needs to be paid to any swelling, fat pads, sacral dimples, dense areas of hair or birthmarks as *spina bifida occulta* (characterized by a missing vertebral process) may lie beneath them. Although the majority of spina bifida cases are diagnosed using ultrasonography screening in the antenatal period, some mild forms of this condition may be missed, demonstrating the importance of the first newborn examination. A sacral dimple should be carefully examined to ensure it is skin-lined with no sinus to the cerebrospinal fluid (CSF) pathway. If CSF is leaking, it presents a portal for infection, so referral to the plastic surgery and neurosurgical teams will be made. In the interim, an X-ray of the lumbosacral spine and an ultrasound scan of the lower spinal cord, kidneys and bladder will be arranged.

The Genitalia

At this first examination, the midwife should undertake a thorough assessment of the newborn's genitalia. In healthy term male newborns, there should be evidence of a penis about 3 cm in length, that is straight with no *chordee* (a bend in the shaft) and a scrotal sac containing two palpable distinct testicles. A small penis is more common, usually buried in suprapubic fat, but may cause some concern to parents. True *micropenis* is rare and associated with hypopituitarism and referral to the paediatric endocrinologist may be warranted (Hatipoğlu and Kurtoğlu 2013). *The midwife should never attempt to withdraw the foreskin.*

The urethral meatus should be situated at the tip of the penis. Observing the baby pass urine is helpful to detect a hypospadias, where the urethral meatus opens on the ventral (under) side of the penis and an epispadias, where the urethral meatus opens on the dorsal (upper) side. Parents should be advised not to have their baby circumcised for religious or cultural reasons, as the foreskin will be used to surgically repair the defect.

The testes originate in the abdomen then start to descend towards the scrotum through the internal inguinal ring, inguinal canal and external inguinal ring. It is thought that the descent of the testes occurs in two phases: 8–15 weeks' and 25–35 weeks' gestation, so that by term, they are located in the scrotal sac. Each testis is 1–1.5 cm in size and palpable along the route from the posterior abdomen to the scrotum, often found in the groin. Disruption at one or both of these hormonally controlled episodes of descent results in *cryptorchidism* (Gurney et al. 2017), which occurs in 2–4% of term newborns and is the most common testicular anomaly. The risk factors for cryptorchidism are:

- prematurity
- small for gestational age
- low birth weight
- family history: first-degree relative (Public Health England, PHE 2018a).

A number of theories regarding maternal risk factors for cryptorchidism including maternal age, smoking status, maternal diet and assisted conception have been proposed, however there is very limited evidence to support this claim (Yeap et al. 2019).

Undescended testes can be classified as palpable or impalpable, depending on their position. An impalpable testis may be absent or abdominal and a palpable testis can be positioned just above the scrotum (suprascrotal) in the inguinal canal (inguinal) or in another area of the groin (ectopic). If the testes are impalpable on examination, an urgent referral is required to confirm their presence and rule out gender ambiguity (Sumit 2016). Cryptorchidism is associated with increased risks of infertility and testicular cancers if left untreated (Cobellis et al. 2014).

Conservative management is sufficient for the majority of cases. However, if testes have still not descended by 6 months, surgery is planned to manually place the testes in the scrotal sac (orchidopexy). The optimum timing for this surgery is before the baby's first birthday, as the germ cells, which become spermatogenic stem cells, are affected by the higher temperatures in the abdomen, potentially affecting fertility (Yeap et al. 2019). By performing the orchidopexy, it also enables self-examination of the testes, which can prove vital for early detection of testicular tumours (Cobellis et al. 2014). Hormonal treatment has been attempted with neonates being prescribed gonadotropin-releasing hormone and human chorionic gonadotropin. These hormones were thought to assist the descent of the testes by promoting the release of the male sex hormones, however, there is limited evidence regarding their effectiveness (Yeap et al. 2019).

TABLE 32.2 Testicular Anomalies (Excluding Cryptorchidism)

Condition	Description
Hydrocele	• Scrotum is filled with fluid • Confirmed by ultrasound examination • Conservative management followed by surgical draining if it does not resolve spontaneously
Bifid scrotum	• Scrotal sack separated into two • Requires surgical treatment
Testicular torsion	• Testes become twisted • Presents as painful, swollen, discoloured scrotum • Requires surgical treatment
Bruising and oedema	• May be due to trauma or breech birth • Conservative management and pain relief if required

From: Campbell D, Dolby L. (2018) Physical examination of the newborn at a glance. Oxford: Wiley Blackwell.

To undertake the examination of the testes, the neonate should be in a warm environment, with the nappy removed, as the temperature can affect their position: a cold environment may cause them to ascend from the scrotum to maintain optimum temperature. A visual inspection should be carried out first to assess the size and symmetry of the scrotum and the presence of rugae as well as other anomalies such as those identified in Table 32.2. The scrotum should then be gently palpated from the top in a downward fashion with the thumb and a finger. If present, the testis will feel mobile within the scrotum. If the testes are not palpable in the scrotum, an examination of the inguinal canal needs to be carried out by using two fingers and gently palpating the groin again from the top in a downwards motion. If both of these examinations do not reveal the position of the testes they may be abdominal and an immediate referral is required (Gordon 2015).

Asymmetry of the scrotum may indicate a persistent connection between the abdominal cavity and scrotum so that fluid (hydrocele) or loops of bowel (inguinal hernia) can escape and occupy the scrotal sac on the affected side. A dark discoloration of the scrotum with or without swelling, is abnormal and may indicate testicular torsion. The testis twists on itself, reduces its own blood supply and the testis dies from ischaemia. Torsion can occur at any age and requires immediate surgical review.

The genitalia of newborn females comprise of the labia majora covering the two labia minora, a clitoris and a vaginal orifice. There should be no swelling or fusion of structures. Some female newborns may present with a mucus discharge from the vagina, which can be white in colour or be blood stained (pseudomenstruation). Parents should be reassured that this is a response to the newborn's withdrawal of maternal hormones following their birth and will resolve within days. However, if there appears to be any fresh bleeding, this must be escalated if in hospital or parents advised to seek medical advice as soon as possible, as this is an abnormal finding.

If there is any ambiguity regarding the genitalia of the newborn it is vital the midwife is positive, honest and does **not** assign a gender to the baby. The practice of placing the newborn into the mother's arms or on to her abdomen at the birth, enables the parents to examine their baby and make their own discoveries often before the midwife has had chance to see for themselves. Further investigations must be undertaken that require a multidisciplinary approach involving paediatricians, urologists, geneticists and endocrinologists **prior** to the gender being assigned (Lewis 2014b) (see Chapters 36 and 37).

The Anus

It is imperative that the midwife inspects for the presence, patency and appearance of the anus. The surrounding area should be examined and any dimples should be thoroughly assessed to rule out additional openings. The presence of meconium does not always exclude imperforate anus (anal atresia) (England 2014). In a perforate anus, the rectum and anal sphincter connect so that substantial amounts of meconium can be passed at any one time. If there is an underlying defect referred to as a high imperforate obstruction, there could be a rectal-vaginal fistula or a rectal-urethral fistula that may allow small amounts of meconium. A low anomaly may simply consist of a membrane covering the anal sphincter, which while in place will impede the passage of all meconium. Anal anomalies can indicate that other gastrointestinal defects may be present, so caution with feeding should be heeded. The passage of a nasogastric tube and withdrawal of hydrochloric acid may exclude oesophageal atresia, but does not necessarily exclude tracheo-oesophageal fistula.

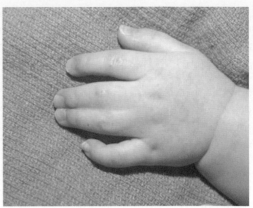

Fig. 32.4 Syndactyly. (With permission from James Chang (2019) Global reconstructive surgery. London: Elsevier)

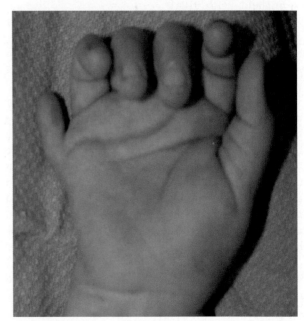

Fig. 32.5 Polydactyly. (With permission from Karen G. Duderstadt (2018) Pediatric physical examination: an illustrated handbook. London: Elsevier/Mosby.)

The Limbs, Hands and Feet

The term newborn will lie in a flexed position with the head in the midline or turned slightly to one side. The hands are flexed with the thumb lying beneath the fingers in a fist. The limbs and joints should be examined in terms of their length, symmetry and movement to exclude any hereditary conditions or birth injury. It is essential that the digits are counted and separated to ensure that webbing/fusion (syndactyly) as shown in Fig. 32.4 is not present on the hands and/or feet. Syndactyly may be inherited or occur sporadically. Each hand should be opened fully as any extra digits (polydactyly) shown in Fig. 32.5 may be concealed in the clenched fist and is often seen as a heredity trait. X-ray assessment will determine whether the defect requires referral to either the plastic surgeon (skin only) or orthopaedic surgeon (bone and skin). A single palmar (Simian) crease is associated with Down syndrome, however this is not an indication in isolation as 10% of the general population have single palmar crease on one hand and 5% have one on both hands.

The most common foot deformity occurring in 1:1000 births in the UK is congenital talipes equinovarusor club foot (talipes meaning ankle and foot) (Cooper and Jones 2014). In this condition, the foot is plantar-flexed (turned downwards like a horse's foot and inwards towards the midline of the baby). Newborn males are twice more likely to have this condition than females and in 50% of cases both feet are affected. The cause is unknown but is associated with Down syndrome and spina bifida and so swift referral to an orthopaedic surgeon is essential to favour effective long-term management and outcomes. First-line treatment would be gentle manipulation (Porseti method), serial plaster casting, which allows the foot to be gradually corrected over a period of about 6–8 weeks, and in most cases, surgery. Evidence suggests that treatment should be intensive and commence as soon as possible to improve outcomes (Ng et al. 2015).

Positional talipes equinovarus is caused by constricted uterine space. When gently manipulated, the position of the feet will easily correct. The newborn's foot can be turned outwards by 50–70° and upwards by 20°. If this can be achieved, a physiotherapist can advise the parents on gentle foot massage. It is not uncommon for a baby to have a structural talipes on one side and a positional one on the other, with no clear view if they are of the same entity. This means the midwife should always examine each foot individually and not automatically assume that both feet are affected in the same way.

Talipes calcaneo-valgus is characterized by dorsiflexion where the foot is turned upwards and outwards and is associated with the breech position and developmental dysplasia of the hip (DDH). Referral is to an orthopaedic surgeon. Gentle manipulation conducted by the parents will often bring about correct alignment with occasional need for a plaster cast.

Once the midwife has completed the first examination, the mother is able to resume skin-to-skin contact with her baby.

This first examination following birth is extremely important and needs to be undertaken thoroughly.

THE DAILY EXAMINATION OF THE BABY SCREENING

The frequency and number of subsequent examinations of the baby will depend on a number of factors, including place of birth and the midwife's judgement of the neonate's health and early development. Where the birth has taken place in hospital, the neonate will receive a daily examination by the midwife until they are transferred home to the care of the community midwife, where the examinations continue more intermittently until discharge to the care of the specialist community public health nurse (SCPHN)/health visitor, which usually occurs around the 10th to 14th day following birth in healthy neonates.

Although a large proportion of the same elements from the first systematic examination of the newborn following birth are included in the daily examination, it should not just be a duplication of this initial assessment. The daily examination should be used to assess the neonate's transition from fetal to extrauterine life, relating to the body systems and their impact on the baby's continued wellbeing. While performing the examination, the midwife should observe the neonate's behaviour. A term, healthy neonate would be well perfused, display good muscle tone and be responsive to touch. The midwife should also assess the neonate for any signs of jaundice and discuss with the mother the baby's feeding pattern and the frequency of urination and defaecation including the appearance of the stools. This examination also provides an opportunity to provide health education to the parents based on the neonate's general appearance and behaviour, discuss any parental concerns that may necessitate referral to other healthcare professionals and plan subsequent care with the parents as appropriate (Tappero and Honeyfield 2018). It is useful to begin the conversation by asking the mother how her baby is, as careful listening to her response is a crucial part of the examination and should determine the order in which the midwife undertakes the examination, beginning with any area of concern. Recording what the mother has said (and how she said it) is helpful to other healthcare professionals who may see the neonate at subsequent examinations.

In some areas of the UK, a Maternity Support Worker (MSW) may undertake postnatal visits to healthy women and their babies at home to support parents with infant feeding and discuss general health and wellbeing. However, the training of the MSW does **not** extend to perform the daily examination of either the neonate or the postnatal examination of the mother. Legally, only practising midwives or medical practitioners and their respective students under supervision are permitted to undertake such examinations as part of their role (NMC 2018). Any concerns identified during a visit by a MSW, or raised by the parents, should be escalated to the community midwifery team and documented in the health records.

Adaptations to Extrauterine Life and Body Systems Affected

The changes to the fetal circulation that occur at birth are described in Chapter 7; all being essential to enable the newborn to survive in the extrauterine environment, independent of the placenta that has provided the fetus with oxygen, nutrients and protection as well as remove waste products. Some of these changes occur at birth while others occur within the following few hours. When performing the daily examination, the neonate

TABLE 32.3 **Elements of the Daily Examination of the Baby and Related Body Systems**	
Questions Assessing	**Body System**
Activity, behaviour, cry and tone	• Respiratory • Cardiovascular • Skeletomuscular • Neurological
Colour and temperature	• Respiratory • Cardiovascular and blood physiology • Metabolic • Immunological
Urinary output	• Renal • Immunological
Feeding and stools	• Gastrointestinal • Immunological
Skin integrity/ rashes and spots	• Immunological

should be carefully assessed to identify any subtle deviations which may indicate abnormalities. Table 32.3 shows the links between the elements of the daily examination of the neonate to the body systems, which have undergone adaptation to support extrauterine life.

Respiratory, Circulatory and Cardiovascular Systems

The midwife should observe the neonate's respiratory rate that includes the diaphragm, chest and abdomen synchronously rising and falling. Neonates have a periodic breathing pattern that is erratic, with respirations being shallow and irregular, interspersed with brief 10–15 s periods of apnoea, which should be explained to the parents. As babies are either obligatory (required) or preferential nose-breathers, it is important to assess whether their nostrils are clear of any dried secretions. Tickling the edge of the nostril with cotton wool can induce sneezing, which aids some clearance. The midwife must consider that respiratory difficulties can occur because of neurological, metabolic, circulatory or thermoregulation dysfunction, as well as infection, airway obstruction or anomalies of the respiratory tract itself. Furthermore, an irritable neonate with excessive sniffling and sneezing could indicate opiate withdrawal.

The National Institute for Health and Care Excellence (NICE 2017) recommend that clamping of the umbilical cord at birth should be delayed between 1 and 5 min, unless the heart rate of the baby is <60 beats per min, and is not increasing or there is some concern about the integrity of the cord. Consequently, the total circulating blood volume at birth may exceed 80–90 mL/kg and assist in preventing neonatal iron-deficiency anaemia. The haemoglobin level may also be in excess of 18–22 g/L. The red cell count ($5–7 \times 10^{12}$/L) may contribute to the development of physiological jaundice (see Chapter 37). The conversion from fetal to adult haemoglobin commences around 36 weeks' gestation and is completed in the first 1–2 years of life. The white cell count is high initially (18.0×10^9/L), but then rapidly decreases. As there is no transplacental passage of coagulation proteins from the mother, the neonate's blood clotting system is immature and as a result, all levels of blood clotting reflect fetal synthesis, which is completed before the 30th week of pregnancy. Vitamin K is poorly transferred across the placenta and due to the low amount in breastmilk, the incidence of classic haemorrhagic disease of the newborn (HDN; also known as Vitamin K deficiency bleeding [VKDB]) occurring within the first week is enhanced in neonates who are exclusively breastfed until the bowel becomes colonized with *E. coli* and the Vitamin K-dependent clotting factors II (prothrombin), VII, IX and X can be synthesized in the presence of bile salts. In the UK, Vitamin K (intramuscular or oral suspension) is available to all newborns as a prophylactic precaution against HDN/VKDB. Early onset HDN/VKDB (within the first 24 h) is exclusively caused by transplacental transfer of anticoagulant medication that inhibits Vitamin K activity. The neonate would be prescribed a therapeutic dose of Vitamin K via intramuscular injection in such a situation.

Should the neonate appear cyanosed, on examination, it may be indicative of the failure of the foramen ovale or ductus arteriosus to completely close and warrants timely referral to the neonatal/paediatric team. The timing for these temporary structures to close range from the foramen ovale closing within minutes, compared with the ductus arteriosus sometimes taking hours. These timeframes guide practitioners in undertaking the full systematic physical examination of the newborn/ Newborn and Infant Physical Examination (NIPE), which is discussed below. However, as many heart anomalies do not always present in the first few days of life, PHE (2018a) state that early examination, with the potential for false-positives, proves less of a risk than not undertaking screening prior to the baby being transferred home. Some maternity service providers therefore implement a minimum age of 6 h before the NIPE is undertaken, which often corresponds with the timing of an early transfer home.

Renal System

Urine is produced *in utero* from between 9 and 10 weeks' gestation, with the amount increasing with gestational age. The urine produced forms part of the amniotic fluid. Evidence suggests that renal development *in utero* directly impacts on renal function as an adult (Blackburn 2013). *In utero*, the placenta is responsible for removing waste products and this function, along with fluid and electrolyte balance, must be taken over by the renal system at birth. Catecholamines are released when the placenta detaches and it is thought that these chemicals, among others, may stimulate the renin-angiotensin system. There is no specific examination that the midwife would perform in the neonatal period to assess that the renal system is functioning effectively.

About 20% of newborns will pass urine in the birthing room, with 90% voiding by 24 h and 99% by 48 h. The rate of urine formation varies from 0.05 to 5.0 mL/kg per hour at all gestational ages with a range of 15–60 mL/kg per day for a term baby, which increases with age (Blackburn 2013). The commonest cause of initial delay or decreased urine production is inadequate perfusion of the kidney. In addition, the kidneys are immature and the glomerular filtration rate is low, but mature within the first month of life. Tubular reabsorption capabilities are also limited, which renders the neonate unable to concentrate or dilute urine adequately, as well as to compensate for high or low levels of sodium, potassium and chloride in the blood. As a result, this creates a narrow margin between under- and over-hydration and restricts the neonate's ability to excrete medicines.

The midwife is responsible for asking the mother about the character of the baby's wet nappies and their frequency, in order to assess whether the neonate's urine output is within acceptable parameters: around four to six wet nappies in a 24-h period. The newborn's urine is dilute, straw coloured and odourless. Urate crystals may cause red brick staining in the nappy, which is often a sign of under-hydration and is usually insignificant, albeit be a cause of parental anxiety (Paul 2011). Any delay in urine production/passage of urine may be due to physiological stress, intrinsic renal anomalies or obstruction of the urinary tract. Examination of the antenatal records is important to ascertain if the results of any ultrasound scan identified the presence of oligohydramnios, which may indicate fetal difficulties with passing urine. A number of syndromes involve kidney function, especially those neonates with low-set ears, abnormal genitalia, anal atresia and low spine anomalies. The neonate should be assessed for dehydration, infection and a palpable abdominal bladder with referral to the neonatologist/paediatrician for further investigations as necessary.

Gastrointestinal System

The gastrointestinal (GI) system of the newborn is structurally complete, although functionally immature in comparison with that of an adult. The mucus membrane of the mouth is pink and moist, the teeth are buried in the gums and ptyalin secretion is low. Sucking and swallowing reflexes are coordinated. The tongue may be coated with milk plaques, which should be distinguished from the fungus *candida albicans*, which requires treatment. The stomach has a small capacity (15–30 mL), which increases rapidly in the first weeks of life. The cardiac sphincter is weak, predisposing to regurgitation of milk or posseting. Gastric acidity equal to that of the adult within a few hours after birth, diminishes rapidly within the first few days and by the 10th day, the neonate is virtually achlorhydric (without acid) and as a consequence from birth and for the first 6 months of life, the intestine is susceptible to infection across the mucosal layer (Blackburn 2013). Gastric emptying time is normally 2–3 h. Enzymes are present in the GI system, although there is a deficiency of amylase and lipase, which diminishes the neonate's ability to digest compound carbohydrates and fat. When milk enters the newborn's stomach, a gastrocolic reflex occurs and results in the opening of the ileocaecal valve. The contents of the ileum pass into the large intestine and rapid peristalsis means that *feeding is often accompanied by reflex emptying of the bowel.*

Bowel sounds can be heard on auscultation with a stethoscope within an hour of birth. This will provide some reassurance to the parents that the intestines are functioning. If there is an absence of these sounds, the midwife should ensure further investigations are initiated. Sterile meconium present in the large intestine from 16 weeks' gestation is passed within the first 24 h of life and should be totally excreted within 48–72 h. As a result of air entering the GI system, *E. coli* colonizes the bowel and the stools become brownish-yellow in colour and odorous. Regardless of the method, the timing of feeding is important as early feeding stimulates the gut and intestines to start functioning. Once feeding is established, the faeces become yellow. The consistency and frequency of stools reflect the type of feeding. Digested breastmilk produces loose bright yellow and inoffensive acid stools. The baby may pass 8–10 stools a day. The stools of the formula-fed baby are pale in colour, less acidic and have a more offensive odour. The midwife should therefore seek information from the mother regarding the baby's passing of stools and the frequency, informing her how the stools should change over time. A melaena stool contains digested blood from high in the GI system, has a tar-like appearance and may be caused by blood swallowed at birth, bleeding maternal nipples or damage to the neonate's GI system itself. Low GI system bleeding may result in frank blood, which is blood that can be seen in the stools with the naked eye and may be related to HDN/VKDB.

Glycogen stores are rapidly depleted in the newborn, so early feeding is required to maintain normal blood glucose levels (2.5–4.4 mmol/L) (British Association of Perinatal Medicine, BAPM 2017). Weight loss is usual in the first few days of life, but more than 10% body weight loss is abnormal and requires investigation. Most neonates regain their birth weight within 7–10 days, thereafter gaining weight at a rate of 150–200 g/week.

Thermoregulation

Newborns and neonates are unable to control their temperature in the same way as adults. They have a larger surface area-to-body mass ratio and less subcutaneous fat, which makes them more prone to heat loss (Blackburn 2013). According to Brown and Landers (2011) *a neutral thermal environment is one that is neither too hot nor too cold and enables the baby to use the minimal amount of energy to keep warm.* Babies are individuals and each have their own metabolic rate and thus, the clinical acceptable temperature range of 36.5–37.5°C is wide. In the first week of life, core temperature can be unstable as the heat-regulating centre in the hypothalamus and medulla oblongata is attempting to adapt from a **hot water intrauterine environment** to a **cooler extrauterine air environment** with concurrent threats of heat loss via:

- *evaporation:* heat loss through wet skin and towels
- *conduction:* coming into contact with cold items, scales, resuscitaires, clothes
- *convection:* draughts from open windows and doors
- *radiation:* heat being drawn to colder objects, windows, walls (Fig. 32.6).

Cooling babies are unable to shiver and instead attempt to maintain body heat by a means of non-shivering thermogenesis, whereby they utilize brown adipose tissue (BAT) and simultaneously increase their metabolic rate by increasing glucose and oxygen consumption to make more energy, carbon dioxide and heat. BAT is believed to constitute 2–7% of the baby's weight depending on gestation and weight and is deposited from 28 weeks' gestation. Unlike white adipose tissue, brown fat is capable of rapid metabolism, heat production and heat transfer to the peripheral circulation and is activated only after birth. The largest mass of BAT surrounds the kidneys and adrenal glands; smaller masses are around the blood vessels and muscles in the neck with extensions of these deposits under the clavicles and into the axillae (Fig. 32.7). The proximity of BAT to major organs and

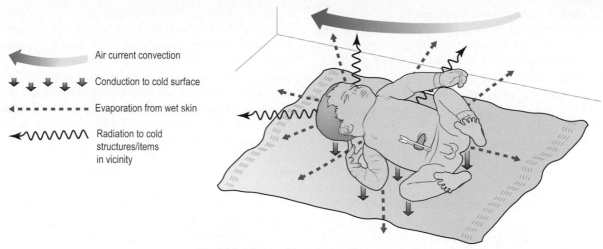

Air current convection

Conduction to cold surface

Evaporation from wet skin

Radiation to cold structures/items in vicinity

Fig. 32.6 Modes of heat loss in the neonate.

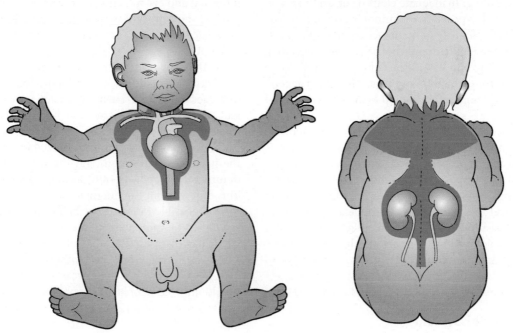

Fig. 32.7 Distribution of brown adipose tissue. (With permission from Brendan Ellis, medical illustrator, Royal Group of Hospitals, Belfast.)

large blood vessels provides the ability for rapid transfer of heat to the circulation when required.

For this process of *aerobic glycolysis* to function effectively, the neonate requires available oxygen and glucose. As oxygen is consumed, energy can be made in the absence of, or with minimal amounts of oxygen, which is referred to as *anaerobic glycolysis*, however the amounts of glucose to maintain this form of energy

production is >20 times greater to make the same amount of energy as in aerobic glycolysis. Hence, the baby becomes hypoxic and may begin to show signs of respiratory distress. In parallel, as the demands for glucose increase to generate heat, glycogen stores are utilized which, if prolonged, will lead to hypoglycaemia. This cascade effect is known as the *neonatal energy triangle* (Aylott 2006).

A transient respiratory grunt may be one of the first respiratory signs of cooling. Nasal flaring, tachypnoea, sternal or subcostal recession, are all signs of respiratory distress that may follow. It is vital the midwife listens to how the parents describe their baby in respect of the strange noise they make on each breath. Accompanying these fleeting episodes, may be subtle colour changes.

The midwife should observe the neonate overall and feel the head and chest to get a general sense of how warm they are. This is then followed by assessing the neonate's temperature using a thermometer via the axilla, tympanic membrane (ear) or in the groin. A clothed term neonate should maintain its body temperature satisfactorily, providing the environmental temperature is draught-free, sustained between 18°C and 21°C, nutrition is adequate and movements are not restricted by tight swaddling. Inadequate clothing or/and inadvertently being left exposed is a common cause of heat loss in the neonate. Skin-to-skin contact is one of the most efficient ways to regulate a newborn's temperature, along with the wearing of a hat, as the baby's head has a large surface area from which to lose heat. The baby's general condition and temperature should be reassessed after 30 min.

A term neonate with a pyrexia (≥37.7°C) may indicate infection, however hyperthermia can occur if the baby is exposed to an inappropriate heat source (by a sunny window) or dressed inappropriately for the ambient temperature. Placing the baby in the cot in the supine position with their feet to the foot, has contributed to the reduction in overheating and associated sudden infant death syndrome. Overheating increases the baby's metabolic rate and can draw upon supplies of glucose and oxygen to maintain the required energy level. Respiratory distress may follow unless the neonate is allowed to cool slowly.

Immunological System

The newborn has a marked susceptibility to infection, especially those gaining entry through the mucosa of the respiratory and gastrointestinal systems. Localization of infection is poor, with minor infections having the potential to rapidly become generalized. The newborn has some immunoglobulins at birth but the protective intrauterine existence limits the need for learned immune responses to specific antigens (Blackburn 2013). There are three main immunoglobulins: *IgG*, *IgA* and *IgM* that contribute to the neonate's developing immunological system.

Immunoglobulin G is small enough to cross the placental barrier. It affords immunity to specific viral infections and at birth, the newborn's level of IgG is equal to or slightly higher than those of the mother. This provides *passive immunity* during the first few months of life and by 2 months, the baby is able to produce a good response to protein vaccines, hence the timing for the commencement of routine childhood immunization programmes (Paterson 2010).

Immunoglobulin M and *immunoglobulin A* can be manufactured by the fetus and raised levels of IgM at birth are suggestive of infection. The relatively low level of IgM is considered to render the baby more susceptible to gastroenteritis. Levels of IgA are also low and increase slowly. Secretory salivary levels reach adult levels by 2 months and protect the baby against respiratory, gastrointestinal and eye infections. Colostrum and breastmilk provide the baby with passive immunity in the form of *Lactobacillus bifidus*, lactoferrin, lysozyme and secretory IgA.

As the baby passes through the birth canal in a vaginal birth, it is colonized by friendly maternal vaginal and faecal bacteria such as *Lactobacillus*, *Prevotella* and *Sneathia*, which assist the neonatal microbiome to develop (Mueller et al. 2015). In contrast, a neonate born by caesarean section is colonized by bacteria from the hospital environment and the maternal skin: predominantly *Staphylococcus* and *Clostridium difficile*. This difference in the microbiome *seeding* is thought to form a possible rationale for babies born by caesarean section to be more susceptible to an increased risk of particular diseases. There is some evidence to suggest that swabs taken from the mother's vagina and swept over the newborn post-caesarean section may assist in developing the neonatal microbiome and provide the baby with similar benefits as those who were born vaginally (Mueller et al. 2015). However, some pathogens can be particularly dangerous to an immature immune system such as *Herpes simplex virus*, *Chlamydia* and *Group B Streptococcus*, which emphasizes the importance of any antenatal infections being promptly diagnosed and treated during pregnancy or labour, with the newborn being monitored carefully for the first 24 h following birth. Midwives should always provide parents with information that supports them to recognize signs and symptoms of infection in their baby and where to seek prompt advice if they become concerned about their health (NICE 2015).

Skin Care

Although sterile at birth, the skin when exposed to air is quickly colonized by microorganisms which produce a pH of 4.9, creating an acid cover to protect the skin from infection. *Vernix caseosa* should be left to absorb into the skin because it is a highly sophisticated mixture of proteins and fatty acid that produce an antibacterial and antifungal skin barrier. If the baby is post-term it is likely the skin may be dry and cracked. The midwife should not be tempted to apply anything to the skin, because within a few days of peeling, perfect skin will be revealed underneath. Skin-to-skin contact just after birth and during subsequent feeding is an excellent way to colonize the baby's skin with friendly bacteria, which can still occur if the baby is being formula-fed. Great care must be provided to maintain the integrity of the lipids (fats) that seal each skin cell. Chemicals used in the manufacture of baby skin products can irreversibly damage epidermal lipids and lead to transepidermal water loss. There is no defined timeframe regarding when the baby should have their first bath, but only water should be used initially, with no products. However, should a cleansing agent be required this should be a mild soap and preferably non-perfumed (NICE 2015). Water as a sole cleaning agent is challenged by some and in a review of current evidence and products available, it was concluded that further research is required in this area (Kuller 2016).

The midwife should inspect the skin for rashes, septic spots, excoriation or abrasions. *Seborrhoeic dermatitis* (cradle cap) is commonly seen on the neonate's scalp, but can also occur in the axillae, groin and nappy area. It presents with scaly lesions that are greasy to the touch and is thought to be a response to irritants. Neonatal skin rashes such as *erythema toxicum* that occur within 72 h of birth as a red blotchy area usually over the face and trunk, may be a sign of the baby over-heating. Removing some of the baby's clothing or bedding is likely to resolve this. This is in comparison to septic spots that will need swabbing for culture and sensitivity, followed by topical or systemic antibiotic therapy as necessary. Similarly *paronychia* (infection of the nail cuticle caused by ragged nails) will be treated in the same way. Parents should be advised to file their baby's nails and *not use scissors or bite them off to keep them short*. The umbilical stump becomes colonized by non-pathogenic bacteria within hours of birth as a result of skin-to-skin contact with the mother. The cord quickly begins to necrose and separates by a process of dry gangrene, which usually takes between 7 and 15 days following the baby's birth. The cord is an ideal portal of entry for infection, especially *E. coli* as result of contamination from stools, and must be observed for any signs of redness in the surrounding abdominal skin: referred to as an *umbilical flare*. If the flare begins to spread and extend up the abdomen, this **must** be reported immediately as antibiotic therapy will be required.

Skin Conditions

There are a number of common benign newborn skin conditions, which are detailed in Table 32.4. If these skin conditions present in isolation, parental reassurance should be given. However, if they present with other symptoms such as fever, irritability, lethargy or reduced feeding, they should be investigated further immediately as this holistic picture may indicate infection.

There are numerous different types of birthmarks that can be present on the newborn skin and, depending on type, these will either become more prominent or disappear over time. It is essential that all birthmarks are shown to parents, discussed and clearly documented so that all those involved with the neonate's care are aware of their origin and they are not mistaken for injury. As a general rule, any birthmark that is raised or extends over the face and eyes in particular needs to be monitored and investigated, to ensure that they are not interfering with any other body function or negatively impacting on neonatal health and well-being. Chapter 36 details some of the most common birthmarks encountered.

FULL SYSTEMATIC PHYSICAL EXAMINATION OF THE NEWBORN/ NEWBORN AND INFANT PHYSICAL EXAMINATION

The Newborn and Infant Physical Examination (NIPE) is a screening programme, which aims to reduce morbidity and mortality. The full systematic examination is offered to parents and initially completed by 72 h after birth and then again at 6–8 weeks of age, with the aim of reducing morbidity and mortality (PHE 2018a). *It is important that this is not confused with the routine first top-to-toe examination at birth or the daily examination of the baby, previously discussed.*

TABLE 32.4 **Newborn Skin Conditions**

Milia

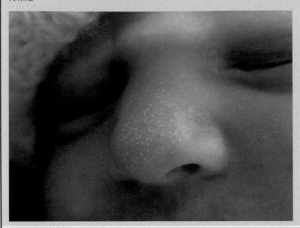

- Also known as 'milk spots'
- Very common
- Cysts filled with sebum and keratin
- Cysts erupt in 50% of newborns
- Can also be seen on gums
- Commonly clear by 4 weeks of age

Newborn acne

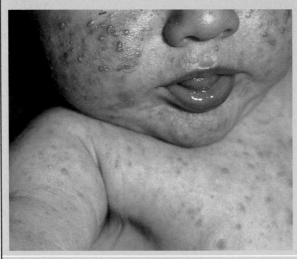

- Pimply appearance
- Caused by build-up of sebum
- Concentrated around the nose and forehead
- Normally presents between days 14–21
- Resolves spontaneously within months

Erythema toxicum

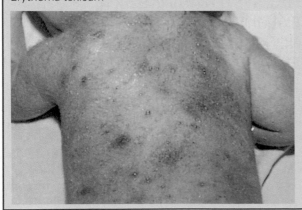

- Affects 40–70% of newborns
- Concentrated on face, chest, back and arms
- Usually occurs within first 3–5 days
- Resolves spontaneously within weeks

TABLE 32.4 Newborn Skin Conditions—cont'd

Transient pustular melanosis 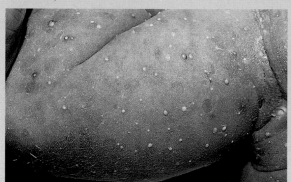	• Small white bumps on neck, chest, back and buttocks • Similar in appearance to erythema toxicum. • Common on pigmented skin • Can leave an area of darker pigment on the skin when resolves • Resolves spontaneously in weeks
Desquamation 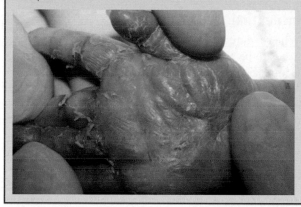	• Known as dry skin • Often associated with babies who are born post-dates

Milia: with permission from Marshall J and Raynor, M. (Eds). (2014) Myles textbook for midwives. Oxford: Elsevier, Fig. 28.2.
Newborn acne: with permission from Paller A, Mancini A. (2016) Hurwitz clinical pediatric dermatology: A textbook of skin disorders of childhood and adolescence. New York: Elsevier, Fig. 8.17.
Desquamation: with permission from Kliegman R. (2019) Nelson textbook of pediatrics, 2-Vol. Set, Fig. 245.4C.
Erythema toxicum: with permission from Kliegman R. (2019) Nelson textbook of pediatrics, 2-Vol. Set, Fig. 666.4.
Transient pustular melanosis: with permission from Kliegman R. (2019) Nelson textbook of pediatrics, 2-Vol. Set, Fig. 666.5.
See also: Templet and Lemoine (2017) and McLaughlin et al. (2008).

The Newborn and Infant Physical Examination relates to four screening elements: heart, hips, genitalia and eyes (PHE 2018a). The results of the screening are recorded in hospital notes, the baby's personal child health record and on the Nationwide Database (Royal College of Paediatrics and Child Health). This examination is generally carried out by a member of the neonatal team: a trained Advanced Nurse Practitioner or a Midwife, who has undertaken an accredited training programme (PHE 2018b). The examination does not necessarily have to take place in the hospital setting and can be undertaken at home with the use of a good light source, paediatric stethoscope, ophthalmoscope and depending on local Trust policy, a pulse oximeter.

Training

For healthy term babies born to mothers with no family history of congenital conditions and an uneventful pregnancy, the NIPE examination can be completed by a midwife who has undertaken an accredited training programme. In most instances, these training programmes are completed at postgraduate level and involve theoretical and practical assessment. Course participants have to undertake a predetermined number of assessments under the supervision and guidance of a suitably trained practitioner; a senior member of the neonatal team, a qualified nurse practitioner or a qualified NIPE trained midwife. A number of these assessments are usually observed by a neonatal consultant, or a neonatal Registrar assigned by the consultant, to ensure that the trainee has reached the adequate standard to be able to complete the examination independently.

Some Higher Education Institutes (HEIs) in England have integrated the NIPE skills into their undergraduate programmes, either as core or optional modules. However, from 2021 it will be a requirement that ALL HEIs in the UK have incorporated the essential theory and undertaken the assessment of every student midwife as being proficient at the point of registration in conducting the full systematic physical examination of the newborn (NMC 2019). The benefits of this include a greater skills base for students and an enhanced student experience, but more importantly, improved continuity for maternity service users (NHS England 2016).

Examination of the Heart

Congenital heart diseases (CHD) are the most common abnormalities occurring in the neonate, with an incidence of 4–10 in 1000 (PHE 2018a). Despite advances in routine antenatal ultrasonography, <50% of CHDs are diagnosed in the antenatal period or in the early neonatal period and before transfer home, if the baby was born in hospital. Hoffman and Kaplan (2002) suggest this is because often genetic abnormalities associated with CHD, although genetically present at birth, do not physically present and become symptomatic until later. Public Health England (PHE 2018a) indicate that there is no optimum time for the examination to take place, however, the risks of going home without screening outweighs completing the screening before a potential problem has presented. There are numerous CHDs, some of the more common along with the main causes are detailed in Table 32.5.

Zuppa et al. (2015) uses a mild, moderate and critical grading system for CHDs (Table 32.6) and the overriding themes that emerge when screening for heart conditions is that early intervention is key if any subtle abnormalities are detected or suspected.

Prior to the physical examination, a full history should be reviewed and discussed with parents. Sinha et al. (2018) identify a number of risk factors for CHD, which include: family history; antenatal maternal infection; the presence of maternal conditions such as diabetes mellitus; exposure to alcohol and drugs while *in utero* and the presence of syndromes such as Trisomy 21 (Down syndrome) and Turner syndrome. If on inspection of the notes, or when in discussion with parents, any of these risk factors become apparent or are disclosed, a heightened awareness of the potential for CHD is required. In order to ascertain whether the heart is functioning as expected, a visual inspection of the neonate should be carried out in conjunction with palpation of the heart and related pulses and auscultation of the heart. While it is recommended that the heart should technically be left until last with auscultation as the final step, if the baby starts to cry at any stage, it will make auscultation difficult, so many examiners listen to the heart much earlier.

Inspection

When conducting the visual examination, the neonate needs to be assessed holistically, as general dysmorphic features can be an indication to syndromes, which often have associated cardiac abnormalities (Carr and Foster 2014). The chest should be bare to enable the practitioner to assess skin colour, tone and respiratory rate and effort. The neonate should be well perfused and show no signs of respiratory distress such as recessional breathing or tachypnoea. There should be no signs of cyanosis, peripheral or central, observed, although Zuppa et al. (2015) states that cyanosis is not necessarily a good indication of CHD as some critical CHDs lead to hypoxaemia, which does not present as cyanosis. Pulse oximetry is being adopted as a screening tool for CHD, with an oxygen saturation of <95% being classified as a screen positive. When pulse oximetry is performed, pre- and post-ductal measurements are taken to evaluate cardiac function and efficiency, with probes positioned on the right hand and the left or right foot. If these oxygen saturation readings are too discordant, repeat measurements should be taken and if still different by >3%, appropriate referrals made to the neonatal team. Zuppa et al. (2015) affirms that of the cases where the oxygen saturation screened positive, over 80% showed some cardiac abnormality, however, over 80% of those abnormalities were subsequently transient.

If an abnormality is suspected, the neonate will be examined by a member of the medical team and if required, electrocardiography and ultrasound examinations would be performed. While these tests are more sensitive they are also resource intensive making them unsuitable for

TABLE 32.5   Types of Congenital Heart Disease

Defect/Condition	Cause and Effects
Atrial septal defects (ASDs)	• Cause due to developmental abnormalities of the atrial septum • More severe if it involves the mitral valve • Requires medical management including surgery
Ventricular septal defects (VSDs)	• Most common CHD • Different types and multiple defects may be present • Treatment depends on the severity and ranges from conservative management to surgery • Some neonates will be completely asymptomatic
Patent ductus arteriosus (PDA)	• Failure of the ductus arteriosus to close after birth • Relatively common • Treatment, if any, is dependent on size of duct
Coarctation of the aorta (COA)	• Constriction in the aorta in close proximity to the ductus arteriosus and distal left subclavian artery • Physical indications vary depending on the severity of the constriction • Should be considered when femoral pulses are weaker than brachial pulses or absent. • Requires medical intervention

Tetralogy of Fallot	• Multifaceted
	  • VSD
	  • Overriding aorta
	  • Narrowing of the pulmonary valve
	  • Right ventricular hypertrophy
	• Does not always present in the early neonatal period
	• Requires surgical treatment

Adapted from: Baston, H., & Durward, H. (2017). Examination of the Newborn. A Practical Guide, 3rd ed. London: Routledge; Lomax, A. and Appleton, J. (2015). Examination of the Newborn: An Evidence-based Guide, 2nd ed. Chichester: Wiley-Blackwell; Sinah, S., Miall, L. and Jardine, L. (2018) Essential Neonatal Medicine, 6th ed. Hoboken: Wiley, 2012.

TABLE 32.6   Grading of Congenital Heart Disease

Grade	Features	Examples
Mild	• Most common CHD • Often asymptomatic • Resolve spontaneously without intervention	Small ASDs Small PDA Small VSDs
Moderate	• Often asymptomatic • Depending on severity may require treatment	Large ASDs Complex VSDs
Critical	• Severe cardiac abnormalities • Requiring treatment • Treatment often necessary within the first year of life	Large VSD Large PDA COA Tetralogy of Fallot

ASD, Atrial septal defect; *VSD*, ventricular septal defects; *PDA*, Patent ductus arteriosus; *COA*, coarctation of the aorta.
From: Zuppa A, Riccardi R, Catenazzi P, et al. (2015) Clinical examination and pulse oximetry as screening for congenital heart disease in low-risk newborn. Journal of Maternal-Fetal and Neonatal Medicine 28(1):7–11.

routine screening. The benefits of using pulse oximetry for screening are that it provides a rapid indication of potential abnormalities while being non-invasive, easy to perform and without any risk to the neonate.

Palpation

Palpation of the heart and peripheral pulses for rhythm, strength, volume and character should form the next stage of the examination. The practitioner should gently place the hand onto the precordium, which is the area over the sternum and ribs to the left side of the chest. A palpable precordium murmur is referred to as a *'thrill'*: a vibration, which can be felt through the wall of the chest and can sometimes be also observed. It is diagnostic of CHD with a high volume overload such as a left-to-right shunt through the ductus arteriosus. Right ventricular enlargement is best sought with the fingertips placed between the 2nd, 3rd and 4th ribs along the left sternal edge. The apex beat is found in the 4th intercostal space along the mid-clavicular or nipple line. A diffuse, forceful and displaced apex beat, usually caused by hypertrophied heart muscle is relatively rare and is described as a *heave*. Palpation of the upper abdomen that reveals an enlarged liver (>1 cm below the costal margin) may indicate heart failure as the liver acts as a reservoir of blood because the heart cannot cope with the required workload. Complementing the clinical picture, is usually an enlarged spleen, palpable in the left upper quadrant of the abdomen.

Brachial and femoral pulses should be palpated simultaneously to assess heart rate and rhythm and to identify any divergence between the two pulse sites. The easiest pulse to feel is the brachial situated at the antecubital fossa. The rate should be counted over a period of 10 s. Coarctation of the aorta (COA) is suspected if the femoral pulses are weaker than the brachial pulse or absent altogether. Caution should be taken when palpating femoral pulses as they can easily be occluded by the pressure applied when attempting to palpate. From experience the femoral pulses are those which cause the most anxiety due to the difficulties in palpation. Equal, but bounding brachial pulses are found in PDA with a wide but diminishing pulse pressure in the lower limbs. A weak thread pulse is found in congestive heart failure (CHF) and in circulatory shock.

Rhythms originating in the sinoatrial node are called *sinus rhythms*. In a regular sinus rhythm, the rhythm and rate of the heartbeat are normal for the age of the baby.

In sinus tachycardia, with over 160 beats/min, it is wise to initially consider pyrexia as the cause. Hypoxia, circulatory shock, CHF and thyrotoxicosis are other possible causes. Sinus bradycardia is defined as below 80 beats/min and the causes may be attributed to hypothermia, hypoxia, increased intercranial pressure and hypothyroidism.

Auscultation

The final step of the heart examination is auscultation, which should be performed in five areas, namely: the four positions where the heart valves are located and mid-scapular. By auscultating these areas, the potential auscultation of murmurs and COA if present is improved. A paediatric stethoscope should be used and its diaphragm (the flat side) positioned over the aortic, pulmonary, tricuspid and mitral valves, respectively (Fig. 32.8) followed by the mid-scapular area to hear the high-pitched sounds of a systolic murmur. Landmarks are used on the neonate's chest to locate the four approximate valve areas (Carr and Foster 2014) for auscultation as shown below:

- *Aortic valve* – second intercostal space on the right side of the sternal edge. Also referred to as the upper right sternal border (**URSB**)
- *Pulmonary valve* – second intercostal space on the left side of the sternal edge. Also referred to as the upper left sternal border (**ULSB**)
- *Tricuspid valve* – fourth intercostal space on the left side of the sternal edge. Also referred to as the lower left sternal border (**LLSB**)

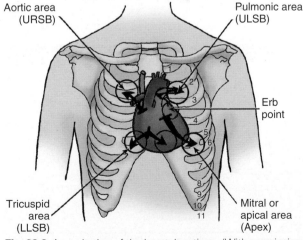

Fig. 32.8 Auscultation of the heart: locations. (With permission from Marilyn J. Hockenberry (2015) Wong's Nursing Care of Infants and Children, Elsevier/Mosby, Fig. 4.34.)

- *Mitral valve* – below the nipple on the mid-clavicular line in the 4th or 5th intercostal spaces (**the apex**).

Each cardiac cycle has two heart sounds that can be heard through a stethoscope when applied to the chest wall. The first heart sound (*S1*) is known as '*lub*' and is described as long and booming and occurs when the atrioventricular (AV) valves, the tricuspid and bicuspid (mitral) valves are closing at the beginning of ventricular contraction (systole). The second heart sound (*S2*) is known as '*dub*' and is short and sharp, reflecting the closure of the semi lunar valves of the aorta and pulmonary artery at the beginning of ventricular relaxation (dystole).

The best place to hear the first heart sound (S1) is at the apex or the LLSB. The second heart sound (S2) is heard in the ULSB (Lumsden 2010). Splitting of closure of the aortic and pulmonary artery valves is easily heard with a stethoscope and the degree of splitting normally varies with respiration, increasing on inspiration and decreasing (or becoming a single sound) on expiration. The third and fourth heart sounds are not usually heard, but can be best auscultated at the apex or LLSB. The third heart sound (S3) represents ventricular filling that begins as soon as the mitral and tricuspid valves open. The fourth heart sound (S4) represents ventricular filling that occurs in response to contraction of the atria. If S4 is heard at the apex, it is pathological and is associated with conditions of decreased ventricular compliance or CHF. Where there is a combination of a loud S3 or S4 with a tachycardia, common in CHF, this is referred to as a gallop rhythm. This information can only complement a clinical picture of a deteriorating neonate that is experiencing respiratory distress and is not feeding.

The heart should be auscultated for a full minute in each of the five areas, each with the examiner expecting to hear two clear sounds, '*lub dub*'/'*S1 and S2*'. The two audible heart sounds (S1 and S2) should be very clear and the presence of any muffling, whistling or background noise is referred to as a '*murmur*', the severity of which often depends on the volume of noise or level of interference heard. A murmur is caused by unstable and changeable blood flow moving through the heart. Bedford and Lomax (2015) use the analogy of slow and fast flowing rivers to describe the differences in sound from a heart without a murmur, to the presence of a murmur, respectively. Depending on where the murmur can be heard in relation to the normal heart sound, murmurs are described as either systolic or diastolic. A systolic murmur of VSD has a uniform high-pitched quality

often described as blowing, whereas an ejection systolic where stenosis is featured, has a harsh grating quality. Systolic murmurs occur between sounds S1 and S2 and diastolic murmurs occur after S2 and before the next S1 sound (Lumsden 2010). Murmurs are also classified according to their severity from Grades I to Grade VI: a Grade I murmur being barely audible to a Grade VI, which would be clearly audible even without the use of a stethoscope (Table 32.7). If a cardiac murmur is present, *details of location, timing in the cycle, grade, character* and *an illustration* should be provided and referral made for further review by the neonatal team.

Examination of the Hips

Developmental dysplasia of the hips (DDH) is the terminology used to describe a vast range of hip anomalies from a minor anomaly requiring conservative management, to irreducible hip dislocation (Pollet et al. 2017). Developmental problems may be associated with the formation of the acetabulum (joint socket) or the femoral head (the ball that fits into the socket). Such problems can occur at any time from fetal development up to early childhood. If the anomaly is not structural but presents as laxity of the joints, these problems can resolve spontaneously in the early postnatal period as the neonate matures and develops (Campbell and Dolby 2018). It is thought that the incidence of DDH is approximately 1–2 in 1000 (PHE 2018a), making it the most common lower limb congenital abnormality (McAllister et al. 2018). If DDH goes undetected and is not treated in a timely manner, it can have significant long-term

TABLE 32.7 Classification of Heart Murmurs

Grade	Description of Sound
I	Just audible
II	Comfortably audible
III	Loud
IV	Loud with a *thrill*
V	Audible with the stethoscope edge on the chest
VI	Audible without a stethoscope or with the stethoscope not touching the chest wall

From: Bedford CD, Lomax A. (2015) Cardiovascular and respiration assessment of the baby. In: A Lomax (Ed.) Examination of the newborn: an evidence-based guide (2nd ed.). Oxford: Wiley Blackwell, pp. 32–70.

debilitating effects, including osteoarthritis, pain and back problems. Terjesen (2011) states that one in six of those who are treated late for DDH will start to present with symptoms of osteoarthritis between the ages of 45 and 50 years old. The key to improving outcomes is therefore early detection and treatment in the form of physiotherapy and harnessing to reduce the risk of subsequent surgery. However, a study by Mace and Paton (2015) questions the effectiveness of the Pavlik harness and suggests that some hip abnormalities will not respond to early treatment, therefore inevitably requiring surgery. The risk factors for DDH identified in the NIPE Screening Handbook published by PHE (2018a) are:

- Family history presenting early in childhood – any member of the family with hip problems requiring physiotherapy, harnessing or surgery. This relates to both parents and siblings
- Breech presentation – any breech presentation, which persists or occurs after 36 weeks' gestation, regardless of the final mode of birth
- Breech birth prior to 36 weeks' gestation.

Multiple pregnancies are also highlighted as a risk factor, where one or more of the neonates fall into the above categories. This means that with twins, if one fetus is in the breech position after 36 weeks, both resulting neonates should be deemed high risk for DDH (PHE 2018a). Mace and Paton (2015) also recognize that female infants appear to be at higher risk for DDH than male infants and Pollet et al. (2017) include being first born as a risk factor. However, these two characteristics are not currently included in the screening pathway as a positive risk factor. All infants undergo a physical assessment for DDH during the NIPE examination. If a DDH is suspected following a positive physical screen, the NIPE screening programme Newborn Pathway (PHE 2018b) identifies that an ultrasound examination should be undertaken within 2 weeks. However, if the physical screen is negative but there are risk factors, as discussed above, follow-up with an ultrasound examination is still required at 6 weeks.

The neonate should be warm and comfortable, lying in the supine position, without a nappy, on a firm flat surface. It is essential that the midwife discusses the manoeuvres with the parents prior to performing them, as often the neonate will become agitated, due to the fact that the legs are being restrained. Parents require reassurance that this examination is not painful to their baby.

Before the physical examination takes place, a visual examination should be conducted. This should consist of first observing for symmetry and normal movement in both legs and then stretching the legs out to assess them for equal length. Any discordance in these visual elements may indicate DDH. The next stage of the examination is to undertake the physical manoeuvres; the *Ortalani* test and the *Barlow* test. Together these two manoeuvres are referred to as the *combined stress test*. The Ortalani manoeuvre is carried out to reduce a dislocated hip, if present, and the Barlow manoeuvre, if performed correctly, will dislocate an unstable hip (Jackson et al. 2014). The range of abduction in flexion is also a useful sign to indicate the degree of abnormality, if indeed there is any. The process for performing each of the manoeuvres is detailed below and shown in Fig. 32.9.

Ortalani Manoeuvre

The Ortalani manoeuvre (described here for the examination of the *left* hip using the practitioner's *right* hand). The practitioner steadies the pelvis between the thumb of the left hand on the baby's symphysis pubis and fingers under the sacrum. With the baby's left leg flexed in the palm of the right hand, the head of the femur is held between the practitioner's right thumb on the inner side of the thigh opposite the lesser trochanter and the middle longest finger over the greater trochanter. In an attempt to relocate a posteriorly displaced head of the femur forwards into the acetabulum, the middle finger applies gentle pressure upon the greater trochanter. The baby's thighs are flexed forward (to the head of the baby) onto the abdomen and rotated and **abducted** through an angle of 70–90° **towards** the examining surface. If the hip is dislocated, a clunk will be felt and sometimes heard as the head of the femur slips into the acetabulum. A high pitch-click is probably a product of soft tissue structures moving over bone prominences. The examination is then repeated with the right hip.

Remember Ortolani: Out to In

Barlow Manoeuvre

The Barlow manoeuvre (described here for the examination of the *left* hip using the practitioner's *right* hand). The neonate is in the same position as for the Ortalani and the practitioners hand position is the same. However, from a position of abduction, the hip is **adducted** to 70 degrees and gentle pressure is exerted by the practitioner's right thumb on the lesser trochanter in a **backwards** and lateral direction. If the thumb is felt to move

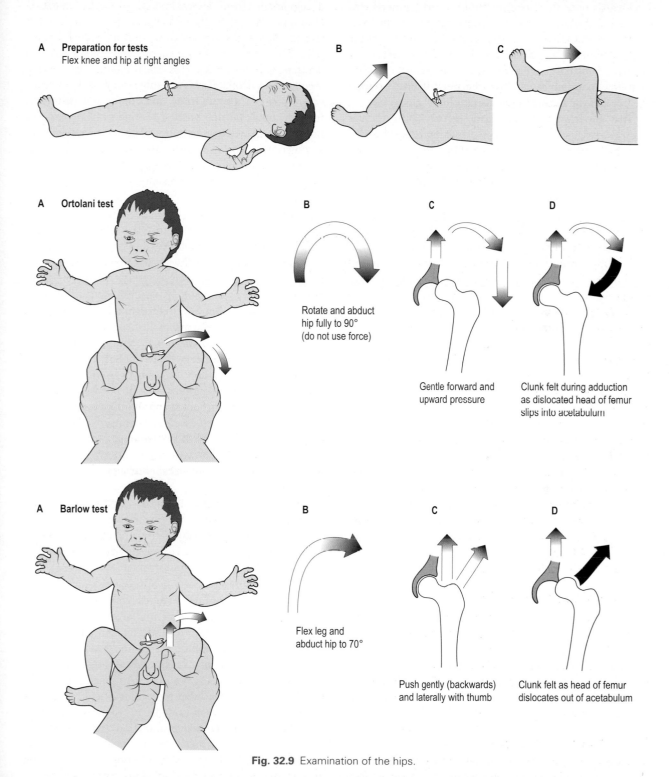

A **Preparation for tests**
Flex knee and hip at right angles

B

C

A **Ortolani test**

B

Rotate and abduct hip fully to 90° (do not use force)

C

Gentle forward and upward pressure

D

Clunk felt during adduction as dislocated head of femur slips into acetabulum

A **Barlow test**

B

Flex leg and abduct hip to 70°

C

Push gently (backwards) and laterally with thumb

D

Clunk felt as head of femur dislocates out of acetabulum

Fig. 32.9 Examination of the hips.

backwards over the labrum (the fibrocartilaginous rim of the acetabulum) onto the posterior aspect of the joint capsule, a clunk may be heard as the head of the femur dislocates out of the acetabulum. The dislocatable hip can feel unusually soft with little or no resistance. The Ortolani manoeuvre can then be performed to return the head of the femur to the acetabulum.

The Barlow and Ortolani tests require gentle manoeuvres, as very little pressure is required to dislocate the head of femur as the acetabulum is so shallow. The softer the touch the more information is elicited. A heavy-handed approach will often make the baby stiffen and resist being touched. In this situation, the practitioner will need to abandon the examination, talk to the baby to try and relax them (as well as the parents) and then attempt a further examination. Documentation of the findings should be made in the neonatal records and the parents informed of the outcome: notably that on **this occasion,** their baby's hips appear healthy.

As DDH is developmental it is possible that a screen negative during the earlier NIPE examination may become a screen positive at the 6–8 week examination. If this is the case, the baby should be referred for specialist follow-up before 10 weeks of age (PHE 2018a). Hip screening is still a contentious subject, as there is much conversation regarding practitioner expertise in relation to the effectiveness and interpretation of the manoeuvre findings and consistency of screening in different locations. McAllister et al. (2018) reported on a Scottish study, whereby the incidence of surgery halved in areas where early diagnosis had occurred due to the presence of specialist practitioners trained to undertake the neonatal hip examination. Hall and Sowden (2018) concur that practitioner expertise could impact on the effectiveness of screening and this needs to be addressed in order to reduce unnecessary surgery and long-term health problems.

Examination of the Genitalia

The examination of the genitalia forms part of the first examination of the newborn baby following birth and thus a detailed account has already been provided. However, further examination of the testes in particular is one of the four screening elements included in the full systematic physical examination/NIPE, allowing additional time for testes to descend.

Examination of the Eyes

The eyes are particularly vulnerable to teratogens, as the related ocular structures are present early in fetal development, from approximately 6 weeks' gestation (Noonan et al. 2015). The neonatal eye is 75% of the adult size but the visual system is immature and neural connections from eye to brain are incomplete. Babies have no depth perception because this relies on both eyes working together and neonatal eyes resemble those of chameleons where one eye appears to be functioning independently from the other. During the first 3 months of life, there is a need for both eyes to function well because reduced light stimulation to the eye causes the condition *amblyopia,* where the brain fails to pay enough attention to the messages from each eye and as a result, the neural connections for each eye are not created. By 6 months of age, the eyes and brain become locked on to each other and this then sets the stage for the baby's future visual acuity. Amblyopia can occur in one or both eyes and is usually caused by disruption of the light pathways to the retina when there is *corneal clouding* or *scarring, congenital cataract* or *clouding of the vitreous humour.* It is vital to screen for these media opacities within 72 h of birth and later at 6 weeks.

The incidence of eye anomalies requiring treatment is 2–3 in 10,000, with the most common abnormality being congenital cataracts (PHE 2018a). Although the incidence could arguably be seen to be quite low, the impact of eye abnormalities should not be underestimated, with the potential to cause blindness, early detection and intervention is essential for improved outcomes (Wan and VanderVeen 2015). There are a number of risk factors associated with eye abnormalities:
- family history of congenital cataracts
- premature birth
- the presence or suspicion of certain syndromes, including Trisomy 21
- a history of maternal infections or exposure during pregnancy, including cytomegalovirus, rubella, herpes simplex virus and gonorrhoea (PHE 2018a).

Although the presence of any of these risk factors does not evoke an automatic referral they provide additional information to highlight potential areas of concern for the practitioner. In order to undertake an effective, systematic, examination of the eye an understanding of eye development and structure is essential (Fig. 32.10).

Prior to commencing the examination, a review of the notes and a discussion with the parents should take place to ascertain the potential presence of risk factors and gain informed consent. A visual examination of the eyes should be carried out in the first instance. Positioning, patency and symmetry should all be considered along with observation of any external anomalies including discharge from the eye.

After the initial external examination is complete the *red-reflex* examination is performed to test for reflections from the pupil. This examination requires a darkened room and the use of an ophthalmoscope. The ophthalmoscope should be set to '0' on the illuminated lens and held approximately 30 cm from the eye. Both eyes should be examined individually when the baby opens them, but the responses should be compared for equal presence, size, colour and brightness (International Centre for Eye Health 2014). Prising eyelids open may add to any oedema and a ptosis (drooping of the eyelid) may go unnoticed, it may also increase the incidence of eye infection. Reducing the room lighting, sitting the baby up or asking the mother to hold the baby over her shoulder with the examiner approaching from behind the mother, often works well in the baby opening their eyes.

The *red-reflex* examination is used as a screen for abnormalities in the cornea, lens and vitreous humour and the expected result is an equal clear red fluorescence in each eye (Fig. 32.11). The shade of the opacity may vary according to the level of pigmentation in the eye and ethnicity. Neonates from Black and Asian backgrounds may have a reflex, which is a paler-red or pink in colour. One way of assessing this is to look at the reflexes in the parents eyes (International Centre for Eye Health 2014). However, if there is any ambiguity regarding the deviation from the red colouration of the reflex, this should be escalated for referral immediately along with any clear deviations, as they could be indications of a potential abnormality.

The *red-reflex* examination is quick, non-invasive, does not pose any risks and has been shown to be an efficient screening tool with greater sensitivity for ocular abnormalities in the anterior of the eye (Sun et al. 2016). There are limitations to the examination however, including practitioner experience and subjectivity, and there may also be some physical limitations in particular the presence of eyelid swelling, which prevents a clear visualization and examination of the eye (Russell et al. 2011). In some instances, parents may become aware of potential problems when they observe unequal or absent red-eye in photographs. This demonstrates the importance of communication with parents

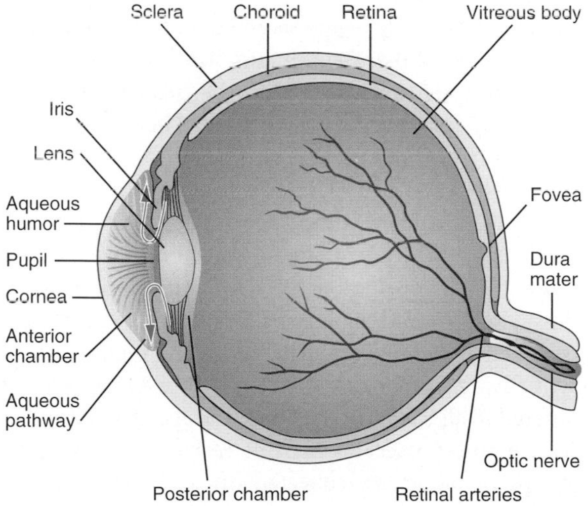

Fig. 32.10 Structure of the eye. (With permission from McCuistion et al. Pharmacology: A Patient-Centered Nursing Process Approach, fig 44.1, Elsevier 2020.)

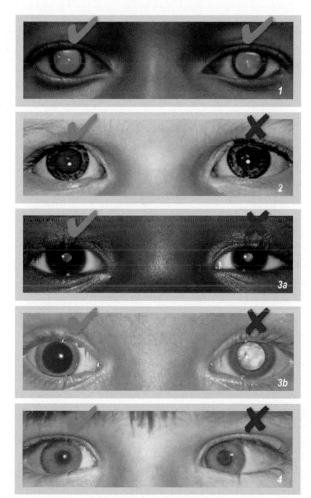

Fig. 32.11 Red-reflex. (With permission from: www.cehjournal.org/article/how-to-test-for-the-red-reflex-in-a-child.)

TABLE 32.8   Conditions Screened for with the 'Red-Reflex' Examination

Condition	Features
Congenital cataract	• most common congenital eye condition • presents as a white opacity (leucocoria) or absent red-reflex • can be unilateral or bilateral • requires immediate referral and should be assessed by an ophthalmologist within 2 weeks • early surgery, prior to 6–8 weeks normally yields the best results
Glaucoma	• often presents as a watery eye • on examination the eye appears cloudy but not always present at birth • can result in pressure on the optic nerve and subsequent blindness • requires prompt referral to an ophthalmologist
Retinoblastoma	• cancerous tumour in the retina • genetic – autosomal dominant • presents as a white reflex (leucocoria) or strabismus • requires immediate referral to an ophthalmologist • can be life-threatening

See: Rajavi and Sabbaghi H (2016); Ortiz and Dunkel (2016); Wan and VanderVeen (2015); Dimaras et al. (2012).

regarding the examination and what is being looked for, as this knowledge may empower them to seek medical advice if they suspect any abnormalities. The three main sight-threatening eye conditions, which the *red-reflex* is used to screen for are detailed in Table 32.8.

Due to the time-sensitive nature of the abnormalities associated with the eye and the very real potential for visual impairment, blindness and in the case of retinoblastomas, fatality, any suspected abnormalities should be referred to the ophthalmology team promptly.

NEUROLOGICAL EXAMINATION

Neurological responses can be continually assessed throughout any of the neonatal examinations, noting how the baby handles and behaviourly tolerates the examination. The healthy term neonate will make eye contact and follow a face when held about 30 cm away from the practitioner. There should be natural facial movements with blinking of the eyes. When lying supine, the baby will be flexed at the knees with hips abducted and the head turned to one side. Movements are smooth, symmetric and varied. The neonate should be able to demonstrate a rooting reflex and coordinated movements of lip, tongue, palate and pharynx are required to suck and swallow successfully. Failure to suck when the stomach is empty is indicative of abnormal function and an important sign of brain stem damage.

During the NIPE screen, the involuntary (primitive) reflexes detailed in Box 32.2 are assessed. These primitive reflexes are essential for survival and provide information about lower motor neuron activity and muscle tone. Primitive reflexes are best assessed at the end of the NIPE screen, as they are likely to unsettle or even distress the baby.

Controlled movements will replace these reflexes after a few months with the only exception being the suck reflex. Abnormalities, which can be seen when performing the neurological assessment include repetitive movements, which could be representative of convulsions, extreme lack of tone or conversely continual extension of the back (*opisthotonus*). The presence of any of these abnormal characteristics, as well as the absence of any of the primitive reflexes, always require immediate referral to the neonatal team and further investigation.

NEWBORN SCREENING TESTS

Various tests and examinations may be carried out in the early neonatal period in order to detect the presence of specific conditions. Early diagnosis and treatment may ameliorate the effects of many conditions. This means that some inborn errors of metabolism may be managed with diet and/or drugs, as described in more detail in Chapter 37.

Blood Spot Screening Test

The UK National Screening Committee recommend that all babies in the UK are offered screening for sickle-cell disease (SCD), cystic fibrosis (CF), congenital hypothyroidism (CHT) and a range of inherited metabolic diseases such as phenylketonuria (PKU) and medium-chain acyl-CoA dehydrogenase deficiency (MCADD). The test is offered to all babies in the UK at the age of 5–8 days and is via a blood spot test taken from the baby's heel, whereby 4 drops of blood are collected on a special absorbent card (Fig. 32.12). The parents must give their consent in advance of their baby undergoing the test. To minimize

BOX 32.2 Neurological Reflexes in the Newborn

- **Placing reflex.** While the baby is being held upright, the top of the foot is touched by the edge of a surface and the baby will lift and place its foot on the surface. Presents from 36 weeks' gestation and disappears at 3 months of age.
- **Palmar and plantar grasps.** Flexion of fingers/toes when an object is placed in the palm of the hand/on the ball of the foot. Presents at 28 weeks' gestation and disappears by 2–3 months.
- **Asymmetric tonic neck reflex** (the fencing sign). When the head is turned to one side, the arm and leg on that side extend, while the arm and leg on the other side remain flexed. Established from 36 weeks' gestation and disappears at 6 months.
- **Moro (startle) reflex.** On sudden head extension, symmetrical abduction and extension followed by flexion and adduction of the arms, with accompanying cry. Present at 37 weeks' gestation and disappears around 4 months of age. Absent in heavy sedation or hypoxic, ischaemic encephalopathy. Unilateral presentation implies fractured clavicle, hemiplegia, brachial plexus palsy.
- **Rooting reflex.** Stroking the baby's cheek with a finger causes the head to turn towards the stimulation and the mouth will open. Established at 34 weeks' gestation and disappears at 4 months of age, when visual cues take over.
- **Sucking reflex.** Elicited to assess the strength and coordination of the sucking reflex by placing a clean finger in the mouth. Disappears by age of 12 months. For visual display of reflexes, go to www.youtube.com/watch?v=Sv5SsLH70mY.

the distress to the neonate and optimize the collection of blood, it is good practice for the mother to cuddle or feed her baby to ensure they are comfortable and warm.

Sickle-cell disease (SCD) affects 1 in 2000 babies in the UK and is a debilitating inherited blood disease. The aim of screening is to identify those neonates who are affected with SCD to commence penicillin prophylaxis. These neonates are at risk of infections and severe acute anaemia in the first few years of life if left untreated.

Cystic fibrosis (CF) affects one in 2500 babies across the UK. It is an autosomal recessive inherited condition that affects the neonate's digestion and lung function. Early diagnosis improves nutrition and growth and reduces chest infection.

Congenital hypothyroidism (CHT) affects 1 in 3000 babies in the UK. Screening is undertaken by measuring the levels of thyroxine or thyroid-stimulating hormone (TSH) in the blood sample. If the condition is confirmed, early treatment with levothyroxine (thyroxine) sodium by the age of 21 days will prevent mental impairment and promote normal growth.

Phenylketonuria (PKU) is an autosomal recessive genetic condition and affects about 1 in 10,000 babies born in the UK. It is an inborn error of metabolism, where the baby is unable to metabolize phenylalanine, an amino acid found in protein, which if left untreated can lead to mental impairment. Treatment is via a phenylalanine free/limited diet with regular blood tests.

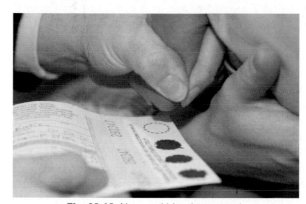

Fig. 32.12 Neonatal blood spot card.

Medium-chain acyl-CoA dehydrogenase deficiency (MCADD) affects 1 in 10,000 babies born in the UK, and is a condition that causes the accumulation of medium-chain fatty acids and impairs ketone production. This means that the baby with MCADD can become ill very quickly if their body's energy demands exceed their energy intake, such as during infections or vomiting, when they are less able to feed. As fat is only partially metabolized, this leads to a lack of energy and a build-up of fatty acids in the body.

Hearing Tests

The National Health Service (NHS) Newborn Hearing Screening programme (PHE 2016) offers hearing screening to all babies within the first week of life and aims to provide high quality detection, care and support for babies and their families in a timely fashion. Any abnormalities associated with the screening will prompt a re-test with further investigations by Ear, Nose and Throat (ENT) specialists if necessary. Recent technological advances have led to improved screening methods that can identify the majority of children with impaired hearing. The test is non-invasive and involves the measurement of *otoacoustic emissions* (OAE), which are low-level inaudible sounds produced by the inner ear. The value of this test is that children with hearing impairment can be given extra help at an early age to develop speech as the critical period for language and speech development is generally regarded as the first 2 years of life.

Vaccinations

The neonate is known to be susceptible to infections in the first 2 months of life, as the immune system of the newborn is immature and takes some time to develop.

The UK Joint Committee for Vaccination and Immunisation (UKJCVI) recommends that with parental consent, babies should be vaccinated against two of the most serious infections: tuberculosis (BCG) and hepatitis B, where necessary (PHE 2018c). If parents have immigrated to the UK from a country where there is high prevalence of tuberculosis or whose family members have previously been infected, the neonate should be vaccinated to reduce their risk of acquiring the infection. Hepatitis B is given within the first 12 h after birth to newborns whose mothers are chronic carries of hepatitis B virus or have had acute hepatitis B during pregnancy.

COMMUNICATION AND DOCUMENTATION

At the outset, the midwife is required to seek the permission from the mother/parents to undertake the examination before proceeding. It is important the midwife explains **in detail** to the parents, the purpose of the examination and its importance in screening the newborn for any anomalies that may subsequently affect their baby's health and may require a second opinion. As England and Morgan (2012) affirm, parents are often surprised by the course of events that unfolds if a problem or malformation is identified in their baby as a consequence of not being effectively prepared for the screening intervention. Some of this can be alleviated if the correct conversation content is used when gaining consent to perform an examination. England and Morgan (2012) highlight the importance of the words used when gaining consent and the impact on the parents' expectations of the examination process and potential outcomes. Parental understanding should be sought and the opportunity given for questions to be asked (Campbell and Dolby 2018). It is important to remember that communication can also be non-verbal and practitioners should be aware of facial expressions and body positioning throughout the examination. The midwife should subsequently document her dialogue with the parents, alongside details of the findings from the examination, parental reaction, referral details and support provided in the birth records (England and Morgan 2012; NMC 2018).

REFLECTIVE ACTIVITY FOR SELF-ASSESSMENT

1. Prior to commencement of any systematic physical examination of the newborn, what considerations should you give to the preparation, the environment, informed consent and the examination itself?
2. Why is it that the inclusion of the full systematic physical examination of the newborn/Newborn Infant Physical Examination should be considered as a natural extension of the role of the midwife? What benefits are there to the midwife performing these examinations within 72 h of birth and what are the incidences when this may not be appropriate?
3. Identify the different elements incorporated in the full systematic physical examination of a newborn

infant. Consider the value of each element and whether any one is more valuable than the others?
4. If, while performing a routine newborn examination, you discover an unexpected finding, what steps should you take and what information would you provide to the parents/carers?
5. During a routine newborn examination, you hear a heart murmur. What could be the possible causes for this heart murmur? What would be your next steps in relation to the subsequent management of this case? What information should you provide to the parents/carers with regards to the future health of the infant?

REFERENCES

Aylott, M. (2006). The neonatal energy triangle. Part 2: Thermoregulatory and respiratory adaption. *Paediatric Nursing*, 18(7), 38–42.

Barreto, L., Khan, A., Khanbhai, M., & Brain, J. (2013). Umbilical hernia. *British Medical Journal*, 347(7923), F4252.

Baston, H., & Durward, H. (2017). *Examination of the newborn A practical guide* (3rd edn.). London: Routledge.

Bedford, C. D., & Lomax, A. (2015). Cardiovascular and respiration assessment of the baby. In A. Lomax (Ed.), *Examination of the newborn: An evidence-based guide* (2nd edn.) (pp. 32–70). Oxford: Wiley Blackwell.

Blackburn, S. T. (2013). *Maternal, fetal, and neonatal physiology: A clinical perspective* (4th edn.). Amsterdam: Elsevier Saunders.

BAPM (British Association of Perinatal Medicine). (2017). *Identification and management of neonatal hypoglycaemia in the full term infant: A Framework for Neonatal Transitional Care*. London: BAPM. Available at: www.bapm.org/sites/default/files/files/Identification%20and%20Management%20of%20Neonatal%20Hypoglycaemia%20in%20the%20%20full%20term%20infant%20-%20A%20Framework%20for%20Practice%20revised%20Oct%202017.pdf.

Brookes, A., & Bowley, D. M. (2014). Tongue tie: The evidence for frenotomy. *Early Human Development*, 90(11), 765–768.

Brown, V. D., & Landers, S. (2011). Heat balance. In S. L. Gardner, B. S. Carter, M. Enzman-Hines, et al. (Eds.), *Neonatal intensive care.* (pp. 113–133). St Louis: Mosby.

Campbell, D., & Dolby, L. (2018). *Physical examination of the newborn at a glance.* Oxford: Wiley Blackwell.

Carr, N., & Foster, P. (2014). Examination of the newborn: The key skills, Part 2: The cardiovascular system and congenital heart disease. *Practising Midwife*, 17(2), 30–33.

CLAPA (Cleft Lip and Palate Association). (2019). *Dealing with diagnosis.* Available at: www.clapa.com/what-is-cleft-lip-palate/dealing-with-diagnosis.

Cobellis, G., Noviello, C., Nino, F., et al. (2014). Spermatogenesis and cryptorchidism. *Frontiers in Endocrinology Experimental Endocrinology*, 5, 63, 1–4.

Cooper, A., & Jones, S. (2014). Foot disorders in childhood. *Surgery (Oxford)*, 32(1), 46–49.

Dawson, J. A., & Morley, C. J. (2010). Monitoring oxygen saturation and heart rate in the early neonatal period. *Seminars in Fetal and Neonatal Medicine*, 15, 203–207.

Dimaras, H., Kimani, K., Dimba, E. A., et al. (2012). Retinoblastoma. *Lancet*, 379(9824), 1436–1446.

England, C. (2014). Recognizing the healthy baby at term through examination of the newborn screening. In J. E. Marshall, & M. D. Raynor (Eds.), *Myles textbook for midwives* (16th ed.) (pp. 591–609). Edinburgh: Elsevier.

England, C., & Morgan, R. (2012). *Communication skills for midwives. Challenges in everyday practice.* Maidenhead: Open University Press/McGraw-Hill Education.

Gordon, M. (2015). Examination of the newborn abdomen and genitalia. In A. Lomax (Ed.), *Examination of the newborn: An evidence-based guide* (2nd ed.) (pp. 124–141). Oxford: Wiley Blackwell.

Grayson, A., & Wylie, K. (2011). Towards evidence-based emergency medicine: Best BETs from the Manchester Royal Infirmary. BET 3: Fucidic acid or chloramphenicol for neonates with sticky eyes. *Emergency Medicine Journal*, 28(7), 634.

Griffith, R. (2009). Safeguarding children from significant harm. *British Journal of Midwifery*, 17(1), 58–59.

Gurney, J. K., McGlynn, K. A., Stanley, J., et al. (2017). Risk factors for cryptorchidism. *Nature Reviews Urology*, 14, 534–548.

Hall, D., & Sowden, D. (2018). Hip hip: no hurray. *Archives of Disease in Childhood*, 103(11), 1006–1007.

Hatipoğlu, N., & Kurtoğlu, S. (2013). Micropenis: etiology, diagnosis and treatment approaches. *Journal of Clinical Research in Pediatric Endocrinology*, 5(4), 217–223.

Hoffman, J. I., & Kaplan, S. (2002). The incidence of congenital heart disease. *Journal of the American College of Cardiology*, 39(12), 1890–1900.

International Centre for Eye Health. (2014). How to test for the red reflex in a child. *Community Eye Health Journal*, 27(86), 36.

Ireland, A., Gollow, I., & Gera, P. (2014). Low risk, but not no risk, of umbilical hernia complications requiring acute surgery in childhood. *Journal of Paediatrics and Child Health*, 50(4), 291–293.

Jackson, J. C., Runge, M. M., & Nye, N. S. (2014). Common questions about developmental dysplasia of the hip. *American Family Physician*, 90(12), 843–850.

Kuller, J. M. (2016). Infant skin care products: What are the issues? *Advances in Neonatal Care*, 16(5S), 3–12.

Lewis, M. L. (2014a). A comprehensive newborn examination: Part I. General, head and neck, cardiopulmonary. *American Family Physician*, 90(5), 289–296.

Lewis, M. L. (2014b). A comprehensive newborn examination: Part II. Skin, trunk, extremities, neurologic. *American Family Physician*, 90(5), 297–302.

Lomax, A. and Appleton, J. (2015). *Examination of the Newborn: An Evidence-based Guide,* 2nd ed. Chichester: Wiley-Blackwell.

Lumsden, H. (2010). Examination of the newborn. In H. Lumsden, & D. Holmes (Eds.), *Care of the Newborn by Ten Teachers* (pp. 34–50). London: Hodder Arnold.

Mace, J., & Paton, R. (2015). Neonatal clinical screening of the hip in the diagnosis of developmental dysplasia of the hip: A 15-year prospective longitudinal observational study. *Bone and Joint Journal*, 97-B(2), 265–269.

Madlon-Kay, D. J. (1986). 'Witch's milk'. Galactorrhea in the newborn. *American Journal of Diseases of Children, 140*(3), 252–253.

McAllister, D. A., Morling, J. R., Fischbacher, C. M., et al. (2018). Enhanced detection services for developmental dysplasia of the hip in Scottish children 1997–2013. *Archives of Disease in Childhood, 103*(11), 1021–1026.

McLaughlin, M. R., O'Connor, N. R., & Ham, P. (2008). Newborn skin: Part II. Birthmarks. *American Family Physician, 77*(1), 56–60.

Mueller, N. T., Bakacs, E., Combellick, J., et al. (2015). The infant microbiome development: Mom matters. *Trends in Molecular Medicine, 21*(2), 109–117.

NHS England. (2016). *National Maternity Review: Better Births, Improving outcomes of maternity services in England. A five year forward view for maternity care.* Available at: www.england.nhs.uk/wp-content/uploads/2016/02/national-maternity-review-report.pdf.

NICE (National Institute for Health and Care Excellence). (2015). *Postnatal care up to eight weeks after birth. Clinical guideline No 37.* London: NICE. Available at: www.nice.org.uk/guidance/cg37/resources/postnatal-care-up-to-8-weeks-after-birth-pdf-975391596997.

NICE (National Institute for Health and Care Excellence). (2017). *Quality Statement 6: Delayed cord clamping in intrapartum care: QS 105.* London: NICE. Available at: www.nice.org.uk/guidance/qs105/chapter/Quality-statement-6-Delayed-cord-clamping.

Ng, K. P., Chan, N. C., Chan, K. F., et al. (2015). New impact of physiotherapy management on children with congenital talipes equinovarus (CTEV): Preliminary results. *Hong Kong Physiotherapy Journal, 33*(2), 99.

Noonan, C., Rowe, F. J., & Lomax, A. (2015). Examination of the head, neck and eyes. In A. Lomax (Ed.), *Examination of the newborn: An evidence-based guide* (2nd ed.) (pp. 104–123). Oxford: Wiley Blackwell.

NMC (Nursing and Midwifery Council). (2018). *The Code: Standards of practice and behaviour for nurses, midwives and nursing associates.* London: NMC. Available at: www.nmc.org.uk/globalassets/sitedocuments/nmc-publications/nmc-code.pdf.

NMC (Nursing and Midwifery Council). (2019). *Standards of proficiency for midwives.* London: NMC. Available at: https://www.nmc.org.uk/globalassets/sitedocuments/standards/standards-of-proficiency-for-midwives.pdf.

Ortiz, M., & Dunkel, I. (2016). Retinoblastoma. *Journal of Child Neurology, 31*(2), 227–236.

Paterson, L. (2010). Infections in the newborn period. In H. Lumsden, & D. Holmes (Eds.), *Care of the newborn by ten teachers.* (pp. 113–145). London: Hodder Arnold.

Paul, S. (2011). An infant with a red-stained nappy. *Practice Nursing, 22*(8), 441–442.

Perinatal Institute for Maternal and Child Health. (2018). *Postnatal notes for baby: View the pages.* Available at: www.preg.info/PostnatalNotes/ViewThePagesBaby.aspx.

Podsiadly, E. (2018). Neonatal jaundice. In P. Lindsay, C. Bagness, & I. Peate (Eds.), *Midwifery skills at a glance* (pp. 132–133). Oxford: Wiley Blackwell.

Pollet, V., Percy, V., & Prior, H. J. (2017). Relative risk and incidence for developmental dysplasia of the hip. *Journal of Pediatrics, 181*, 202–207.

PHE (Public Health England). (2016). *Newborn hearing screening: programme overview.* Available at: www.gov.uk/guidance/newborn-hearing-screening-programme-overview.

PHE (Public Health England). (2018a). *Newborn and infant physical examination screening programme handbook.* Available at: www.gov.uk/government/publications/newborn-and-infant-physical-examination-programme-handbook/newborn-and-infant-physical-examination-screening-programme-handbook.

PHE (Public Health England). (2018b). *NIPE Screening Programme: Newborn Pathway.* Available at: https://assets.publishing.service.gov.uk/government/uploads/system/uploads/attachment_data/file/702100/NIPE_Screening_Programme_Newborn_Pathway.pdf.

PHE (Public Health England). (2018c). *Routine childhood immunisations from Autumn 2018.* Available at: https://assets.publishing.service.gov.uk/government/uploads/system/uploads/attachment_data/file/741528/Routine_childhood_immunisation_schedule_September2018.pdf.

Rajavi, Z., & Sabbaghi, H. (2016). Congenital cataract screening. *Journal of Ophthalmic and Vision Research, 11*(3), 310–312.

RCUK (Resuscitation Council UK). (2015). *Resuscitation and support of transition of babies at birth.* Available at: www.resus.org.uk/resuscitation-guidelines/resuscitation-and-support-of-transition-of-babies-at-birth.

Russell, H., Mcdougall, V., & Dutton, G. (2011). Congenital cataract. *British Medical Journal, 342*(1), D3075.

Sinha, S., Miall, L., & Jardine, L. (2018). *Essential neonatal medicine* (6th ed.). Oxford: Wiley-Blackwell.

Snyder, C. L. (2007). Current management of umbilical abnormalities and related anomalies. *Seminars in Pediatric Surgery, 16*(1), 41–49.

Sumit, D. (2016). A four-month-old boy with bilateral undescended testes. *Canadian Medical Association Journal, 188*(15), 1098–1099.

Sun, M., Ma, A., Li, F., et al. (2016). Sensitivity and specificity of red reflex test in newborn eye screening. *Journal of Pediatrics, 179* 192–6.e4.

Tappero, E. P., & Honeyfield, M. E. (2018). *Physical assessment of the newborn: A comprehensive approach to the art of physical examination* (6th ed.). New York: Springer Publishing Company.

Templet, T., & Lemoine, J. (2017). Benign neonatal skin conditions. *Journal for Nurse Practitioners, 13*(4), E199–E202.

Terjesen, T. (2011). Residual hip dysplasia as a risk factor for osteoarthritis in 45 years follow-up of late detected hip dislocation. *Journal of Child Orthopedics, 5*, 425–431.

UNICEF. (2013). *The evidence and rationale for the UNICEF UK Baby Friendly Initiative standards.* Available at: www.unicef.org.uk/wp-content/uploads/sites/2/2013/09/baby_friendly_evidence_rationale.pdf.

United Kingdom National Screening Committee. (2018). *Newborn and Infant Physical Examination Screening Programme Handbook.* Available at: www.gov.uk/government/publications/newborn-and-infant-physical-examination-programme-handbook/newborn-and-infant-physical-examination-screening-programme-handbook#maintaining-competency-in-undertaking-nipe-examinations.

Wan, M., & VanderVeen, D. (2015). Eye disorders in newborn infants (excluding retinopathy of prematurity). *Archives of Disease in Childhood – Fetal and Neonatal Edition, 100*(3), F264–F269.

Yeap, E., Nataraja, R., & Pacilli, M. (2019). Undescended testes. *Australian Journal of General Practice, 48*(1/2), 33–36.

Zuppa, A., Riccardi, R., Catenazzi, P., et al. (2015). Clinical examination and pulse oximetry as screening for congenital heart disease in low-risk newborn. *Journal of Maternal-Fetal and Neonatal Medicine, 28*(1), 7–11.

ANNOTATED FURTHER READING

Baston, H., & Durward, H. (2017). Examination of the newborn: where are we now? In H. Baston, & H. Durward (Eds.), *Examination of the newborn: A practical guide* (3rd edn.) (pp. 1–7). London: Routledge.

This chapter provides a comprehensive summary of the examination of the newborn and its effectiveness as a screening tool. It discusses elements of the Newborn and Infant Physical Examination and examines the relevant Key Performance Indicators along with suitability of practitioner and training.

Campbell, D., & Dolby, L. (2018). Part 5. Top to toe physical examination. In D. Campbell, & L. Dolby (Eds.), *Physical examination of the newborn at a glance* (pp. 63–103). Oxford: Wiley Blackwell.

This chapter provides the details of a top-to-toe examination and can be used as a revision guide for the practical elements of the examination.

England, C., & Morgan, R. (2012). Communication challenges in maintaining professional behaviour. In C. England, & R. Morgan (Eds.), *Communication skills for midwives: challenges in everyday practice* (pp. 6–20). Maidenhead: Open University Press/McGraw-Hill Education.

Communication skills are fundamental to all newborn examinations, but according to parents, this is an area where improvements can be made. This chapter explores communication and the professional responsibilities and expectations placed on midwives when dealing with colleagues, families and students. The authors examine the skills required to ensure information is imparted effectively and efficiently in an appropriate manner, which is often dependent on the target audience.

PHE (Public Health England). (2018). *Newborn and infant physical examination screening programme handbook.* Available at: www.gov.uk/government/publications/newborn-and-infant-physical-examination-programme-handbook/newborn-and-infant-physical-examination-screening-programme-handbook.

This is a comprehensive guide to the Newborn and Infant Physical Examination detailing the relevant care pathways in place. It also provides information regarding practitioner competencies and missed examinations.

USEFUL WEBSITES

Cleft Lip and Palate Association (CLAPA): www.clapa.com/

Joint Committee on Vaccination and Immunisation: www.gov.uk/government/groups/joint-committee-on-vaccination-and-immunisation

Perinatal Institute for Maternal and Child Health: https://perinatal.org.uk/

Public Health England: NIPE Screening Standards. www.gov.uk/government/publications/newborn-and-infant-physical-examination-screening-standards

Public Health England: NIPE Newborn Screening Pathway: https://assets.publishing.service.gov.uk/government/uploads/system/uploads/attachment_data/file/702100/NIPE_Screening_Programme_Newborn_Pathway.pdf

Resuscitation Council UK (RCUK): www.resus.org.uk/

The Auscultation Assistant: www.wilkes.med.ucla.edu/inex.html (a useful website that differentiates the various heart sounds and murmurs.

United Kingdom National Screening Committee: www.gov.uk/government/groups/uk-national-screening-committee-uk-nsc

33

Resuscitation of the Healthy Baby at Birth: The Importance of Drying, Airway Management and Establishment of Breathing

Michelle Knight

CHAPTER CONTENTS

Midwives are the experts and the lead practitioners in normal physiological birth. They attend and facilitate most births within a hospital and home setting. It is important therefore that midwives have applicable knowledge and skills in supporting the transition and resuscitation of babies at birth. Caring for the newborn baby and the parents is an essential component and must be done in an effective and supportive manner. The aim of this chapter is to uphold the standards of care offered by the Resuscitation Council United Kingdom (RCUK) and explore the specific role of the midwife in drying, assessing the baby and airway management. Resuscitation or support with this transition is more likely to be required by babies with intrapartum evidence of significant fetal compromise. Noting the time of birth and starting the clock on the Resuscitaire (when applicable) is always deemed the point of initiation of care for the baby and documentation requirements. Requesting assistance from the multiprofessional team at any stage during the process is fundamental to the ongoing care of the newborn (RCUK 2015).

THE CHAPTER AIMS TO

- emphasize the importance of thoroughly drying the baby at birth to prevent heat loss
- support the principle of transition and enabling the baby to resuscitate itself by placing its head in the neutral position
- detail how to open the airway by giving inflation breaths in order to clear the lung fluid
- reiterate the importance of starting and maintaining a documented record of events of the resuscitation process
- emphasize the requirement to escalate and seek appropriate assistance from the multiprofessional team at any stage of the resuscitation process.

DRYING THE BABY

At birth, the small size of the baby and the fact that they are born wet, means that they are liable to cool very quickly, losing heat by evaporation and convection (RCUK 2015). Thorough effective drying of the baby is always the first step to the management of their transition and any resuscitation required at birth. Taking the time to dry the baby's head, to include the face alongside the arm and leg creases, is sometimes not performed as thoroughly as it should be. According to Connolly (2010), heat loss and cooling of the baby is inevitable but failure to spend time doing this task meticulously can result in the baby using unnecessary oxygen and glucose to maintain or raise its metabolic rate. Therefore drying and covering the newborn and maintaining a normal body temperature between 36.5°C and 37.5°C will stabilize oxygen and glucose levels accordingly. Placing the baby in skin-to-skin contact with their mother or the father helps the baby in maintaining their body heat, but *the baby needs to be thoroughly dry*. Furthermore, the mother (parent providing the skin-to-skin contact) also needs to be dry so that the baby can benefit from *conductive heat* gains.

When drying the newborn, which can take up to a minute, this process will provide stimulation and gives time for the midwife to assess the baby's breathing and heart rate while observing their colour and muscle tone. The Apgar score developed by Virginia Apgar in 1952, albeit criticized for its simplicity and limited prognostic relevance, is a universal communication tool, which is used to inform other team members of the baby's condition if necessary (Apgar 1952; American College of Obstetricians and Gynecologists, ACOG 2015; National Institute for Health and Care Excellence, NICE 2017a). Assessment is made at 1, 5 and 10 min intervals of five indicators of the baby's condition as shown in Table 33.1, which are numerically scored and subsequently documented into the birth record (Nursing and Midwifery Council, NMC 2018). The most important elements within this scoring system, notably heart rate, respiratory rate and tone, will determine the nature and timing of active resuscitation. A score of **8+** indicates the newborn is in good condition however, a healthy baby's skin will be **blue** at birth, which indicates that there is an accumulation of carbon dioxide (CO_2) in the blood and tissues. It is important to remember that CO_2 is a stimulant to the respiratory centre in the medulla oblongata,

so therefore is a *normal physiological* sign and most babies will not require resuscitating. However, an excess of CO_2 will depress respiration and this may account for why the baby may be showing little or no respiratory effort. *White or mottled grey skin* is an indication of peripheral shut down as the baby is responding to low oxygen levels and is conserving the available oxygen for their heart and brain by diverting blood away from the skin and other non-essential organs (Leone and Finer 2012). Babies born in this poor condition will utilize their reserves of oxygen, therefore thoroughly drying this particular baby and maintaining their warmth is essential in order to help reduce further oxygen consumption. The midwife should ensure their own anxiety or that of others does not inhibit this drying process. All wet towels should be discarded, and the baby covered in warmed dry ones. Identification name bands should be placed on the baby in the hospital setting, should the baby require separation from their mother at any time and/or transferring to a neonatal intensive care unit or special care baby unit.

At birth, the healthy term baby will be blue, but will have good tone, will cry within a few seconds, and within a few minutes of birth, will have established a good heart rate (RCUK 2015). According to Rennie and Kendall (2013), the assessment of muscle tone indicates to what degree the nerves are stimulating the skeletal muscles. When a baby is well toned for its gestational

TABLE 33.1 The Apgar Score

Sign	SCORE		
	0	1	2
Appearance (colour)	Pale or blue	Body pink, extremities blue	Completely pink
Pulse (heart rate)	Absent	Slow <100 bpm	Fast >100 bpm
Grimace (reflex irritability)	No response	Grimace	Cry, cough
Attitude (muscle tone)	Limp, floppy	Some flexion of extremities	Active
Respiratory effort	Absent	Slow, irregular	Good/crying

age, i.e. adopting an attitude of flexion, this signifies that the baby is in good condition, even though they may not be breathing. An unwell baby that is both white and hypotonic (*floppy*), reflects the possibility of long-term hypoxia and severe acidaemia as a result of the labour and birth process or some other co-existing factor, such as infection. The midwife should simultaneously assess whether the baby is breathing by assessing the presence or absence of chest movement and any other signs, such as gasping. *If the baby is crying, the baby has an open airway.* This assessment is followed by auscultation of the chest using a stethoscope to assess the heart rate. Pulse oximetry will allow for accurate assessment of the heart rate and oxygen saturations within 2 min. A midwife should establish if there is a heart rate and whether it is above or below 60 beats/min (bpm). In the first minute of life, the average heart rate of a healthy term baby is around 100 bpm, however by the second minute, it has usually risen to around 140 bpm and by 5 min to 160 bpm. A less healthy infant may have a slow heart rate <100 bpm while an unwell baby may have a very slow or an unrecordable heart rate (RCUK 2015). Assessment of the baby's heart rate is considered to be a reliable indicator of wellbeing and it is crucially important to make a regular assessment, hence the 1 and 5 min timeframe of the Apgar score (Apgar 1952). During this time of assessment, the umbilical cord can remain uncut to allow for placental transfusion so that extra red blood cells are transported to the baby to enhance the baby's oxygen-carrying capacity, even if the heart rate is really slow. For healthy uncompromised term babies, delay in cord clamping for at least 1 min or until the cord stops pulsating and turns white, improves iron status through infancy (RCUK 2015; NICE 2017b). Box 33.1 highlights the benefits of delayed cord clamping.

The requirement for active resuscitation is not always predictable and all midwives should have skills in the resuscitation of the newborn baby that follow the Newborn Life Support (NLS) guidelines from RCUK (2015) and always ensure that the birth environment has the appropriate equipment for *every* birth, as outlined in Box 33.2. A useful algorithm is shown in Fig. 33.1 and outlines the steps that the midwife should take to support the baby's physiological transition.

Even if the baby's heart rate is really slow, opening and managing the airway must be the first task to achieve. Without an open airway, the baby is unable to breathe effectively and has no way of being oxygenated,

---

BOX 33.1   Benefits of Optimal Cord Clamping

(leaving up to 5 min before clamping and cutting the umbilical cord)

- Baby receives 30% more of its circulating blood from the cord and placenta
- Decreased risk of anaemia with increased iron stores
- Increased iron stores may increase infant neurological development
- More oxygen to vital organs through increased haematocrit
- More stem cells, which function as the building blocks for the immune system, prolonging long-term health
- In preterm babies, decreases the risk of intraventricular haemorrhage, late onset sepsis, necrotizing enterocolitis and blood transfusions
- For the mother, less intervention promotes the natural physiology of birth and may prevent complications with the birth of the placenta.

Adapted from: www.bloodtobaby.com based on Mercer and Erickson-Owens (2012) and Anderson et al. (2015).

BOX 33.2   Neonatal Resuscitation Equipment

- Pre-warmed towels/blankets
- Umbilical cord clamp
- Flat, stable surface
- Clock with second hand
- Light
- Warmth/heat source
- Oxygen supply
- Stethoscope
- Suction equipment, tubing and suction catheters
- A 500 mL self-inflating bag with a pressure limiting device (Laerdal)
- Oxygen reservoir attachment for self-inflating bags
- Size 00 and 01 masks conformable to the baby's face
- T-piece connector and tubing
- Guedel airway sizes 000/ISO 3.5 (pink); 00/ISO 5.0 (blue); 0/ISO 5.5 (grey)
- Laryngoscope (suction under direct vision)
- Endotracheal tubes sizes 2.5, 3.0 and 3.5
- Nasogastric tubes fine gauge sizes 8 and 10
- Syringes: 2 mL, 5 mL and 10 mL
- Needles: 21 and 25 fine gauge
- Blood gas syringes.

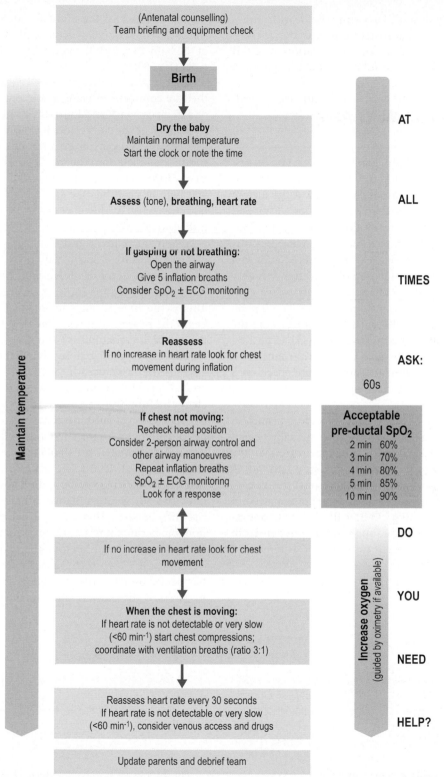

Fig. 33.1 Newborn life support algorithm. (From Resuscitation Council UK. 2015 Newborn life support. London: RCUK. (With permission from S Macdonald, G Johnson (Eds) (2017) Mayes' Midwifery. London: Elsevier.)

as this is the only means of assisting the heart to function. The midwife should therefore note the **A**irway, **B**reathing and **C**irculation of resuscitation when **B** *must* follow **A** and **C** *must* follow **B**: *there is no room for any short cuts.*

AIRWAY MANAGEMENT AND BREATHING

If the baby is not breathing, emphasis should be on initiating lung inflation within the first minute of life and *opening the airway is* **always the first step.** A flat surface is needed so the umbilical cord can be clamped, cut and secured as appropriate. In the home setting, the floor may be a tempting location to place the baby, but it is not an ideal place because it can be cluttered and even in the summer it may often be cold and too draughty and therefore likely to cool the baby. *Furthermore, in any resuscitation situation, the first consideration is practitioner safety.* The midwife must always make sure the environment is safe for her to function, and bad posture in particular can contribute to poor performance and awkward communications. Creating a safe space on a table or the seat of a firm chair can be a better option to place the baby on.

The prominence of the neonatal occipital protuberance can affect the natural position of the baby's head, when lying on its back, with the result of either the chin falling down to the chest in flexion or extending into the *chin-up* position. Both these postures consequently close the airway. The head should be placed in the *neutral* position (Fig. 33.2) with the nose uppermost. Assistance should be sought where possible from another member of the multiprofessional team to hold the baby's head for the midwife. Alternatively, a small sheet/towel or equivalent can be placed under the neck of the baby to secure the neutral position (*sniffing position*) (Fig. 33.3).

Intermittent positive pressure ventilation (IPPV) will then be commenced using a bag and mask if available or a T-piece, mask and Resuscitaire in the hospital. The mask must be the correct size for the baby to prevent any leaks of air to occur on inflation of the bag. The mask should be rolled onto the face from the chin, using the stem of the mask (like the stem of a champagne glass) and held in position. The soft part of the mask should not be touched as this may distort its shape and lead to leakage of air (Fig. 33.4).

When manually compressed, the bag will deliver positive pressure of air at 30 cmH_2O. Given that the alveoli in the lungs are filled with fluid, this pressure should be applied for 2–3 s: these are *inflation breaths*. This is the time it takes to steadily count '*1-2-3*', to begin the process of forcing the lung fluid out and into the lymphatic channels of the lungs. The bag should be allowed to refill before giving the second breath, '*2-2-3*', the third breath, '*3-2-3*', '*4-2-3*' and finally '*5-2-3*'. **Five inflation breaths should be sufficient to clear the lung fluid to make room for the air.** While these inflation breaths are being given, the baby should be covered but with the chest exposed so that any chest movement (which is the sign of an open airway) can be seen and noted. It must be acknowledged that, while there is an exchange of lung fluid with air, it can take until the 4th or 5th inflation breath before full chest rise may be seen. This can be an anxious time for the midwife because it is natural to think that the chest will rise on the first inflation and it is easy for midwives to question their own technique. Once chest movement has been observed, the face mask should be removed to assess if the baby is spontaneously breathing. The

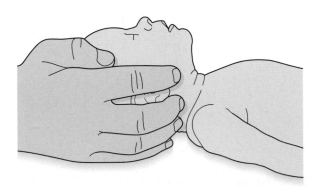

Fig. 33.2 Neutral position.

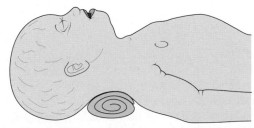

Fig. 33.3 Small towel under the neck (sniffing position).

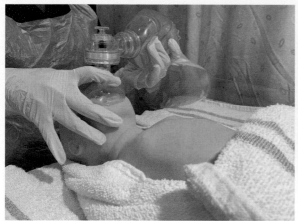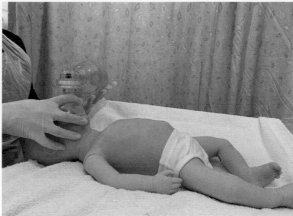

Fig. 33.4 Bagging demonstration.

heart rate should also be assessed at this time to establish whether the rate has increased. If the heart rate has increased, then the midwife can be assured the lungs have been successfully aerated.

Babies that are blue with good muscle tone and a heart rate above 60 bpm often do not need any further assistance. As soon as normal respiratory effort is established, and their heart rate is over 100 bpm, they can be given to their mother for skin-to-skin contact. However, some babies in this category may not be breathing spontaneously because there remains too much CO_2 in their blood and tissues (*hypercapnia*) that is depressing their respiratory effort. Repeating five more inflation breaths as per RCUK (2015) guidance may be considered at this point. Alternatively, *ventilatory breaths* should be commenced to provide oxygen (21% in air) and blow off the excess CO_2. Ventilation breaths are performed at a rate of 30 breaths per minute: these breaths are therefore 2 s in duration. It is important to assess the baby every 30 s to see if they are making spontaneous efforts to breathe. It is vital that the midwife does not over-aerate the baby and reduce their CO_2 too much and cause apnoea. Babies should be allowed to resuscitate themselves, noting the time when the baby is breathing spontaneously.

The time spent **not** undertaking IPPV is wasted time, as the baby is not receiving any benefit from the midwife/health professional. If a baby is not breathing it is **NOT** acceptable to simply blow oxygen onto the baby's face rather than using IPPV with a bag and mask. This is because resuscitation gas now consists of air, instead of oxygen. Air is a cold gas and if this is blown onto the face

of the baby, the baby will quickly cool. The main aim is to inflate the lungs within a minute of birth in order to aid spontaneous breathing.

Difficulties in Establishing an Open Airway

If there is no chest movement after giving five inflation breaths, this indicates that the airway is **not** open, so the alveoli will remain filled with lung fluid. This will be a good time to escalate and call for medical assistance, because failure to aerate the lungs may require further interventions and the need for tracheal intubation (RCUK 2015). In the home, paramedic support will take longer to arrive so early anticipation of problems is considered good practice. If the baby has a poor colour and muscle tone, this may indicate that the position of their head has not been maintained in the neutral position. This indicates the definite need for a second person to assist, both to hold the baby's head and apply jaw thrust to enable better management of the airway as shown in Fig. 33.5. The jaw of a floppy baby can fall backwards and as the tongue is attached to the jaw, the tongue falls back into the airway, blocking the airway. A second person, with their fingers on each side of the jaw, can push the jaw forwards and hold it in that position. This is an easily performed manoeuvre because the baby does not offer any muscle tone resistance. Five inflation breaths should be given, lasting 2–3 s in duration. If there is still no chest movement, suction to the oropharynx under direct vision using the light of a laryngoscope may be considered should there be an obstruction. This task is performed in the main by neonatal practitioners, unless midwives have been trained

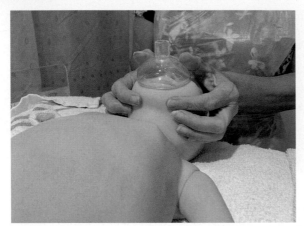

Fig. 33.5 Two-person jaw thrust. (With permission from S Macdonald, G Johnson (Eds) (2017) Mayes' Midwifery. London: Elsevier.)

and assessed as competent in performing oropharyngeal suction (NMC 2018). However, midwives may utilize simple suction to remove the contents from the baby's mouth and cheeks: recognizing this would be the limit of their scope of practice. Occasionally, if there is maternal bleeding at the birth, some blood may have entered the baby's mouth, initially as fluid but then over time may have clotted. (*Note: The management of meconium is not considered in this context, as the resuscitation would be approached in a different way;* see Chapters 36 and 37).

Following suction to the oropharynx, five inflation breaths are given and if not successful, an oropharyngeal (*Guedel*) airway can be inserted to open the airway mechanically, especially in babies who may have congenital anomalies such as *choanal atresia* and/or *micrognathia*. The correct sizing of the airway is vital. When held along the line of the lower jaw with the flange at the level of the middle of the lips, the end of the airway should reach the angle of the jaw. The airway is slipped over the tongue in the same attitude that it will finally lie. The midwife should make sure that the tongue is not pushed back into the back of the mouth. Once *in situ* the mask can be placed over the airway (*both* the *mouth* and *nose*) and a further five inflation breaths should be given. If the chest fails to rise after these interventions, intubation of the trachea will be required and an experienced neonatologist will be required to assist. Chest compressions may help to trigger the heart using either two fingers or by gripping the chest in both hands in such a way that the two thumbs press on the lower third

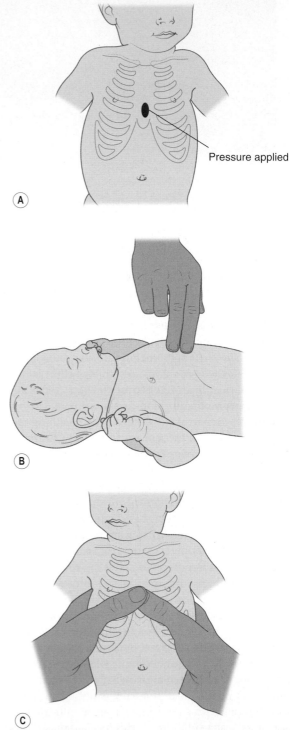

Pressure applied

(A)

(B)

(C)

Fig. 33.6 Cardiac compression A, B, C. (With permission from S Macdonald, G Johnson (Eds) (2017) Mayes' Midwifery. London: Elsevier.)

of the sternum, just below an imaginary line joining the nipples with the fingers over the spine at the back as shown in Fig. 33.6. The chest should be compressed quickly and firmly reducing the anteroposterior diameter of the chest by about one-third. These are coordinated with ventilation breaths at the ratio of 3:1. The heart rate should be assessed after 30 s and once the heart rate is above 60 bpm, cardiac compressions can end.

In rare cases, should the heart rate fail to respond, despite effective ventilation breaths and cardiac compressions being delivered, the attending neonatologist may decide that it is essential to administer drugs such as adrenaline, sodium bicarbonate, sodium chloride and dextrose to the baby. These drugs are best administered via an umbilical venous catheter directly into the inferior vena cava via the ductus venosus. If this is not possible, the route of drug administration may be either intra-tracheal or intra-osseous (into the bone marrow). Following resuscitation, the temperature and glucose levels of the baby should always be checked and the results used to inform the subsequent care management decisions of the baby.

PARENTAL SUPPORT THROUGH EFFECTIVE COMMUNICATION

According to England and Morgan (2012), as resuscitation of the baby will occur in the presence of the parents, a clear, simple explanation in a calm tone should be given to inform and support them during the process. Without a doubt, this will be a stressful and anxious time for the parents, which will affect how they receive and respond to information about their baby's condition (RCUK 2015). Clear concise documentation should always reflect obtained consent and specific aspects of the resuscitation, including any interactions and discussions between the parents and the multiprofessional team (NMC 2018). It is important to realize that any medical records could be requested for inquest and lawyers and therefore should always be sequentially detailed. These records will support the midwife's care and actions given at the time and may be used at a later date and read out in court or at the NMC, should there ultimately be an adverse outcome.

REFLECTIVE ACTIVITY FOR SELF-ASSESSMENT

1. When assessing a newborn baby, what fundamental elements reassure the midwife that the baby is well?
2. What is meant by transition of the newborn?
3. Outline the steps that should be taken in the process of neonatal resuscitation?
4. What support should the midwife provide to parents whose baby has undergone resuscitation?

REFERENCES

Anderson, O., Lindquist, B., Lindgren, et al. (2015). Effect of delayed cord clamping on neurodevelopment at 4 years of age: A randomized clinical trial. *JAMA Pediatrics, 169*(7), 631–638.

Apgar, V. (1952). Proposal for a new method of evaluation of newborn infants. *Anaesthesia and Analgesia, 32,* 260–267.

ACOG (American College of Obstetricians and Gynecologists). (2015). The Apgar Score, Committee Opinion, No 644. *Obstetrics and Gynecology, 126,* e52–5.

Connolly, G. (2010). Resuscitation of the newborn. In G. Boxwell (Ed.), *Neonatal intensive care nursing* (pp. 65–86). London: Routledge.

England, C., & Morgan, R. (2012). *Communication skills for midwives: Challenges in everyday practice.* Maidenhead: McGraw-Hill/Open University Press.

Leone, T. A., & Finer, N. N. (2012). Resuscitation in the delivery room. In C. A. Gleason, & Devaskar SU (Eds.), *Avery's diseases of the newborn* (pp. 328–340). Philadelphia: Elsevier.

Mercer, J. S., & Erickson-Owens, D. A. (2012). Rethinking placental transfusion and cord clamping issues. *Journal of Perinatal and Neonatal Nursing, 26*(3), 202–207.

NICE (National Institute for Health and Care Excellence). (2017a). *Intrapartum care of healthy women and babies: Clinical Guideline No 190.* London: NICE.

NICE (National Institute for Health and Care Excellence). (2017b). *Quality Statement 6: Delayed cord clamping in intrapartum care: QS 105.* London: NICE. Available at: www.nice.org.uk/guidance/qs105/chapter/Quality-statement-6-Delayed-cord-clamping.

NMC (Nursing and Midwifery Council). (2018). *The Code: Standards of practice, and behaviour for nurses, midwives and nursing associates.* London: NMC.

Rennie, J. M., & Kendall, G. S. (2013). *A manual of neonatal intensive care.* London: Taylor and Francis.

RCUK (Resuscitation Council UK). (2015). *Newborn life support.* London: RCUK.

ANNOTATED FURTHER READING

England, C., & Morgan, R. (2012). *Communication skills for midwives: Challenges in everyday practice.* Maidenhead: McGraw-Hill/Open University Press.

Chapter 7 provides details regarding personal interactions in acute clinical situations and explores in-depth how the midwife should communicate with parents and members of the multiprofessional team in the neonatal resuscitation situation.

Laptok, A. R. (2014). Neonatal and infant death: The Apgar score reassessed. *Lancet, 384*(9956), 1727–1728.

This article critically reviews the Apgar score and its impact on neonatal resuscitation. This systematic, rapid assessment of infants after birth has proven to be an effective way of communicating details of the baby's health among the multiprofessional team. It is also used widely within multidisciplinary simulation training.

Medical Aid Films: How to resuscitate a newborn baby. Available at: www.youtube.com/watch?v=lRjWSAutses.

This is a useful visual resource that clearly illustrates the stages of neonatal resuscitation: keeping the baby warm, assessing the baby, opening the airway and breathing and chest compressions that are based on the Resuscitation–UK guidelines. A summary is provided that acts as a valuable revision aid for students and practitioners alike.

Mosley, C. M. J., & Shaw, B. N. J. (2013). A longitudinal cohort study to investigate the retention of knowledge and skills following attendance on the Newborn Life Support course. *Archives of Disease in Childhood, 98*(8), 582–586.

This article reports that practitioners following specialist training, over time experience deterioration in neonatal resuscitation ability and technique, especially if they are not exposed to clinical resuscitation situations on a regular basis. Practitioners failed on simple but essential interventions such as not removing the wet towel from the baby and not assessing the baby's heart beat. It is suggested that practitioners should attend resuscitation updates on a regular basis to maintain and hone their skills, which should improve confidence.

USEFUL WEBSITES

Advances in Neonatal Care: https://journals.lww.com/advancesinneonatalcare/pages/default.aspx

Blood to Baby: www.bloodtobaby.com

British Association of Perinatal Medicine: www.bapm.org

National Institute for Health and Care Excellence: www.nice.org.uk

National Institute for Health Research (NHIR): www.nihr.ac.uk

Nursing and Midwifery Council: www.nmc.org.uk

Resuscitation Council UK (RCUK): www.resus.org.uk

Royal College of Paediatrics and Child Health: www.rcpch.ac.uk

34

The Healthy Low Birth Weight Baby

Michelle Knight, Jayne E. Marshall

CHAPTER CONTENTS

Low birth weight (LBW) is the international term used to identify babies who are born weighing <2500 grams (g). In the UK, approximately 7% of all babies fall into this category. Preterm babies including those born in multiples, contribute around two-thirds of this figure with the other one-third being small for gestational age (SGA), some of which will be born at term. Small for gestational age (SGA) refers to an infant born with a birth weight less than the 10th centile. Midwives need to be mindful that ethnicity can play a part in these statistics, as data from the Office of National Statistics (ONS) confirms that the percentage of babies born to Bangladeshi women who are of LBW is more than double that of the white British childbearing population (5.6% compared with 2.4%, respectively). Keeping mothers and babies together should be the cornerstone of newborn care. Healthy LBW babies are eligible for neonatal transitional care (NTC), which is provided by midwives as the lead practitioner on a postnatal ward or in the home setting. Babies with a gestational age of >33 weeks, a birth weight of >1600 g and who are able to maintain their body temperature, will be stepped down from neonatal care and managed under the NTC framework on a postnatal ward with the main care-giver being the mother. The majority of these babies will remain well and have minimal or no illness in the neonatal period. This chapter will examine the role of the midwife in supporting parents to care for their *healthy* LBW baby and the specific knowledge and skills the midwife requires to fulfil this effectively (RCOG 2014; ONS 2017; British Association of Perinatal Medicine, BAPM 2017).

THE CHAPTER AIMS TO

- examine the terminology and classifications of babies in relation to gestational age and birth weight
- critically discuss the importance of skin-to-skin contact and early responsive feeding in the prevention of cold stress and neonatal hypoglycaemia
- discuss measures that help to stimulate the LBW baby who is reluctant to feed
- discuss the provision of an accommodating environment that supports the developing needs of the LBW baby on the postnatal ward.

CLASSIFICATION OF BABIES BY GESTATION AND WEIGHT

Definitions of gestational age disregard any considerations of birth weight and, similarly, definitions of low birth weight (LBW) are based upon weight alone and do not consider the gestational age of the baby.

Gestational Age

According to Smith (2012), babies should preferably be classified by gestational age, as this is a better physiological measure compared with birth weight. A preterm baby is born before completion of the 37th gestational week (259 days), which is calculated from the first day of the mother's last menstrual period (LMP) and has no relevance to the baby's weight, length, head circumference, or indeed any other measurement of fetal or neonatal size. Smith (2012) states that gestational age estimates by first-trimester ultrasonography are accurate within 4 days, so the combination of fetal crown–rump length and menstrual history are now considered more accurate indices for estimating gestational age.

Birth Weight

The (United Nations Children's Fund/World Health Organization, UNICEF/WHO 2004) definition of low birth weight babies is internationally adopted and as babies are surviving at earlier gestations due to advances in fetal and neonatal medicine and subsequent neonatal care, further LBW categories are recognized, as follows:

- Low birth weight (LBW): lower than 2500 g at birth
- Very low birth weight (VLBW): lower than 1500 g at birth
- Extremely low birth weight (ELBW): lower than 1000 g at birth
- Small for gestational age (SFA): less than 10th centile
- Appropriate for gestational age (AGA): between the 10th and 90th centile.

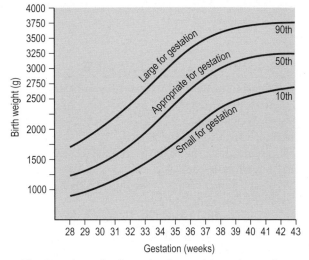

Fig. 34.1 A centile chart, showing weight and gestation.

It is the *relationship* between weight (for assessment of *growth*) and gestational age (for assessment of *maturity*) that is of great importance. This relationship can be seen plotted on centile charts (Fig. 34.1) to visually demonstrate that growth is appropriate, excessive or diminished for gestational age and that the baby is either preterm, term or post-term. Growth charts, should be derived from studies of local populations, because genetically derived growth differences exist between countries, cultures and lifestyles. The growth charts produced by the Royal College of Paediatrics and Child Health (RCPCH 2013) are based on measurements collected by the WHO from six different countries to provide a more representative guide. However, some maternity units are using customized growth charts to plot a baby's growth deriving information from the maternal ethnicity, height, weight and previous birth weights of their existing children.

Various presentations of LBW babies can be described as follows:

1. *Babies whose assessment of intrauterine growth is normal at birth, but are small because labour began* **before**

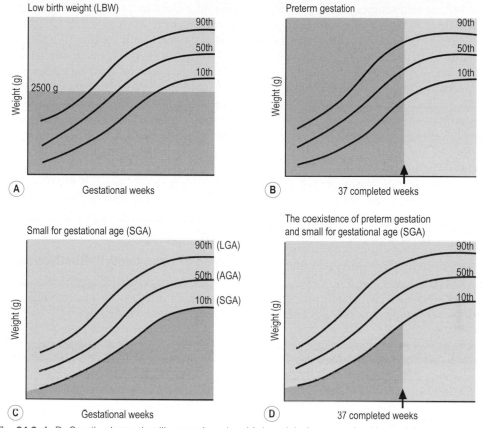

Fig. 34.2 A–D: Centile charts that illustrate how low birth weight is categorized by weight and gestation.

the end of the 37th gestational week. These babies are 'appropriately grown' for their gestational age (**AGA**) but are technically preterm. Their weight is between the 10th and 90th centiles for their gestational age.

2. *Babies whose assessment of intrauterine growth has slowed down, and who are born at, or post-term.* These term or post-term babies are 'under-grown' for gestational age and are consequently small for their gestational age (**SGA**). Their weight is measured **below** the 10th centile for their gestational age.

3. *Babies whose assessment of intrauterine growth has slowed down and who are also born* **before** *term.* These preterm babies are small by virtue of both their early birth and impaired intrauterine growth. They are both **pre-term** and **SGA** babies because their weight will be **below** the 10th centile for their reduced gestational age.

Babies are considered **large** for their gestational age (**LGA**) when their weight exceeds the 90th centile. Consequently, it should be recognized that both term and preterm babies can fall into the category of AGA, SGA or LGA (Fig. 34.2).

SMALL FOR GESTATIONAL AGE

Babies that are small for their gestational age (SGA) are of a size that is smaller when compared with other babies. If a baby is 'under-grown' and below the 10th centile for weight, historically for some, there has been an *automatic assumption* that as a fetus, the baby has experienced growth restriction *in utero* (now known as *fetal growth restriction*, FGR). Wilkins-Haug and Heffner (2012) define FGR as a rate of fetal growth that is less than the normal growth potential for a specific baby. This does not however, indicate that all SGA babies are small as a result of FGR. Some small babies are genetically small because they have small parents or grandparents and this familial factor determines their comparative size. They are otherwise healthy, well babies who need to be cared for accordingly.

Customized charts delineate the Gestation Related Optimal Weight (GROW) for each baby by adjusting for characteristics such as maternal height, weight, parity and ethnic origin and predicting the growth potential by excluding pathological factors such as smoking and diabetes. The rationale, validation and clinical benefits for using GROW charts have been articulated by Gardosi et al. (2018). As a consequence, GROW charts aim to:

- improve the antenatal detection of fetal growth problems
- avoid unnecessary investigations
- reduce anxiety by reassuring mothers when growth is normal.

In the UK, GROW is provided as part of the comprehensive Growth Assessment Protocol (GAP), and training programmes have been shown to significantly reduce stillbirth rates (Gardosi et al. 2013). However, although GAP and GROW centile charts provide advice and direction for clinicians, they can only act as guides. Trotter (2018) states that maternal characteristics, obstetric history and birth details in addition to the appearance and behaviour of the baby should determine what care is required. For example,

should a baby be born at 36 weeks' gestation with a birth weight of 2100 g, which according to weight, is well below the 50th centile, this baby would not fall below the 10th centile line for weight, so should **not** be identified as SGA but may be under-grown. Similarly, it should not be assumed that all infants of diabetic mothers (IDM) (either insulin-dependent or gestationally-acquired) are macrosomic and only fall into the LGA category. Diabetes and obesity are conditions that deleteriously affect maternal circulation and perfusion, so some babies may become growth restricted (FGR) and could be *small* for their gestational age. Increased prevalence of diabetes within Asian women populations correlates more to a higher rate of LBW babies.

Types of Fetal Growth Restriction

There are two recognized types of fetal growth restriction (FGR). The causes and predisposing factors are viewed as multifactorial (Box 34.1).

BOX 34.1   Causes of Small for Gestational Age (SGA)

Fetal growth restriction (FGR) is not synonymous with SGA (RCOG 2014), 50–70% of SGA babies are physically and naturally small with fetal growth proportional for maternal size and ethnicity. Fetal growth restriction is regulated by maternal, placental and fetal factors and represents a mix of genetic mechanisms and environmental influences through which growth potential is expressed. The mechanisms that appear to limit fetal growth are multifactorial.

Maternal Factors
- Pregnancy-induced hypertension, pre-eclampsia, to include HELLP syndrome
- Congenital and acquired heart disease, to include chronic hypertension
- Diabetes mellitus
- Undernutrition, BMI <20 underweight mother/small stature. Eating disorders
- Raised BMI >30 obesity
- Smoking, significant increase with women smoking >11 cigarettes per day
- Alcohol misuse
- Drugs: therapeutic (anticancer, thyroid medication), recreational (narcotic, prescription)
- Renal disease, collagen disorders, anaemia, thyroid disorders and epilepsy
- Genetic diseases such as maternal phenylketonuria and cystic fibrosis

- APLS (antiphospholipid syndrome)
- Maternal age >35 years with increased risk in women >40 years of age
- Maternal SGA
- IVF
- Poor obstetric history that includes preterm labour, previous stillbirth
- Respiratory disorders, to include asthma
- Daily vigorous exercise
- Diet.

Fetal Factors
- Multiple gestation
- Chromosomal/genetic abnormality (particularly trisomy conditions), including inborn errors of metabolism, achondroplasia
- Intrauterine infection: toxoplasmosis, rubella, cytomegalovirus, herpes simplex (ToRCH) and syphilis. Malaria, significant worldwide and should be considered in women travelling to and from high prevalent areas.

Placental Factors
- Abruptio placenta
- Placenta praevia
- Chorioamnionitis
- Abnormal cord insertion
- Oligohydramnios.

(RCOG 2014; Smith 2012).

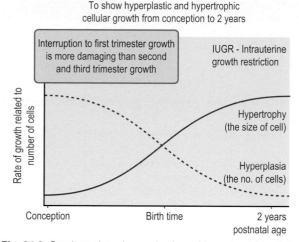

Fig. 34.3 Graph to show hyperplastic and hypertrophic cellular growth from conception to 2 years.

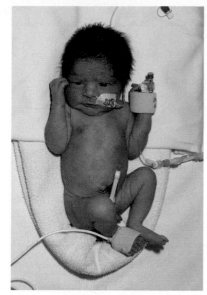

Fig. 34.4 Baby with asymmetrical growth restriction.

Fetal Growth Restriction that Begins Early in the First Trimester Caused by a Combination of Intrinsic and Extrinsic Factors, Results in *Symmetrical* Fetal Growth

In this situation, the fetus suffers significant interruption to *hyperplastic* (new cell) division (Fig. 34.3). As a result, the head circumference, length and weight are all proportionately reduced for gestational age. The main causes are referred to as *intrinsic factors* that operate from *within* the fetus and cause *symmetrical* growth restriction, often as a result of early intrauterine or transplacental infections such as cytomegalovirus, rubella and toxoplasmosis or chromosomal/genetic defects. In addition, the deleterious effects of maternal lifestyle where a poor quality diet may be in combination with smoking, drug and/or alcohol misuse, can impact on fetal growth and development. These examples are referred to as *extrinsic factors* that can act upon the fetal environment and contribute to congenital malformations that culminate in conditions such as fetal alcohol syndrome (FAS) or chronic hypoxia associated with maternal smoking. Affected babies suffer interruption in the process of hyperplasia and as a consequence, appear small with reduced potential for normal growth. It is worth noting that a small head equates to a small brain. Such babies make up 10–30% of all SGA babies in Western societies (Sinha et al. 2012).

Fetal Growth Restriction that Begins in the Last Trimester, Caused by Extrinsic Factors, Results in *Asymmetrical* Fetal Growth

This type of fetus has been growing normally, then starts to experience interruption to hypertrophic cell growth

(Fig. 34.3). This is influenced by *extrinsic* factors in its *intrauterine environment* that cause disruption to placental perfusion of oxygen and nutrients. When serial ultrasound scans of head and abdominal circumference in addition to umbilical artery Doppler measurements indicate poor and disproportionate growth, the birth of many affected fetuses are expedited early, usually by elective caesarean section or induction of labour dependent on the gestational age. For those women where an early birth is not possible (in multiples, the smaller twin or triplet; a concealed pregnancy or through failing to access antenatal care), their baby will to varying degrees have a characteristic brain-sparing appearance. The baby's head appears relatively large compared with the body (Fig. 34.4); however, the head circumference is usually within normal parameters and brain growth is usually spared. The skull bones are within gestational norms for length and density but the anterior fontanelle may be larger than expected, owing to diminished bone formation. The abdomen appears sunken owing to shrinkage of the liver and spleen, which surrender their stores of glycogen and red blood cell mass, respectively, as the fetus adapts to the adverse conditions of the uterus and the ribs are clearly visible. As subcutaneous fat is used as a source of glucose and ketones, the skin becomes loose, giving the baby a wizened, old appearance. Vernix caseosa is frequently reduced or absent as a result of diminished skin perfusion. In the absence of this protective

---

BOX 34.2   Causes of Preterm Labour and Preterm Birth

Preterm birth is the single biggest cause of neonatal mortality in the UK and around 7.3% of live births in England and Wales in 2012 were born preterm <37 weeks (NICE 2019).

Spontaneous Causes
- 40% unknown
- Ethnicity
- Multiple gestation – the higher the multiple, the greater the chance
- Mid-trimester loss
- Sepsis viral or bacterial infection – urinary tract infections
- Preterm prelabour rupture of the membranes (P-PROM) can be caused by maternal infection, especially chorioamnionitis; also polyhydramnios
- Maternal age (<17 or >40 years) and parity
- Maternal uterine malformation – bicornuate uterus or significant fibroids
- Obstetric history of preterm labour
- Cervical length ≤25 mm – history of cone biopsy, large loop excision of the transformation zone (LLETZ) and cervical surgery or trauma
- Maternal substance abuse – particularly recreational drugs, alcohol and cigarette smoking
- Domestic abuse, including physical, emotional or sexual

Elective Causes
- Pregnancy-induced hypertension, pre-eclampsia, chronic hypertension
- Maternal disease: renal, heart
- Placenta praevia, abruptio placenta
- Rhesus incompatibility
- Congenital abnormality of the baby
- IUGR
- Stress at home or in the workplace.

---

covering, the skin is continuously exposed to amniotic fluid and its cells will begin to desquamate (shed) so that the skin appears pale, dry and coarse. If the baby is of a mature gestation and has passed meconium *in utero*, the skin may be stained with meconium. The umbilical cord is thin and may also be meconium-stained. Fetal distress in labour and hypoglycaemia are more likely to be seen in this group of babies. Unless severely affected, these babies appear hyperactive with a good muscle tone, hungry, tending to suck a fist and have a lusty cry. The neurological responses usually correlate to the gestation age of the baby.

THE PRETERM BABY

The preterm baby is born before the completion of 37 weeks of pregnancy, regardless of birth weight. Most of these babies are 'appropriately grown', some are 'SGA' and a small number are 'LGA'. The factors that play a role in the initiation of preterm labour are largely unknown

and mainly overlay with factors that impair fetal growth. They are divided into those labours that commence spontaneously and those where a decision is made to terminate a viable pregnancy before term: referred to as *elective causes* (Box 34.2).

Typical Characteristics of the Preterm Baby (e.g. 32 Weeks' Gestation)

The appearance of the preterm baby at birth will depend upon the gestational age. Preterm babies rarely grow large enough *in utero* to develop muscular flexion and fully adopt the fetal position. As a result, their posture appears flattened, with hips abducted, knees and ankles flexed. Lissauer and Fanaroff (2011) describe a generally hypotonic baby with a weak and feeble cry. The size of the head is in proportion to the body size and the skull bones are soft with large fontanelles and wide sutures due to lack of ossification. The chest is small and narrow and appears underdeveloped. The abdomen is prominent because the liver and spleen are large and abdominal muscle tone

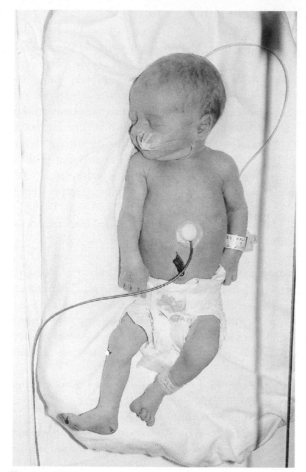

Fig. 34.5 Healthy preterm baby born at 32 weeks' gestation.

is poor (Fig. 34.5). The liver is large because it receives a good supply of oxygenated blood and is active in the production of red blood cells. The umbilicus appears low in the abdomen because linear growth is cephalo-caudal, being more apparent nearer to the head than rump, by virtue of fetal circulation oxygenation. Subcutaneous fat is laid down from 28 weeks' gestation, therefore its presence and amount will affect the redness and transparency of the skin. Vernix caseosa is abundant in the last trimester and tends to accumulate at sites of dense lanugo growth, such as the face, ears, shoulders and sacral region, protecting the skin from amniotic fluid maceration. The ear pinna is flat with little curve, the eyes bulge and the orbital ridges are prominent. The nipple areola is poorly developed and barely visible. The umbilical cord is white, fleshy and glistening. The plantar creases are absent before 36 weeks' gestation but soon begin to appear, as fluid loss

occurs through the skin. In girls, the labia majora fail to cover the labia minora and in boys, the testes descend into the scrotal sac at about the 37th gestational week. Suck and swallow reflexes tend to be uncoordinated

CARE OF THE HEALTHY LOW BIRTH WEIGHT BABY

Many of the care issues relevant to the LBW baby apply to both the preterm and the SGA infant. Where differences do exist, these will be highlighted.

Management at Birth

Given the unpredictability of the birth process on growth and maturity, the role of the midwife in the birthing room is to prepare the environment, staff and parents for certain eventualities, be this in the hospital or home setting. This takes the form of informing members of the multiprofessional team such as a second midwife, neonatal practitioner and neonatal nurse, to be on standby for the birth. The incidence of perinatal asphyxia and congenital malformation is greater in SGA babies and the baby with a scaphoid abdomen could be physically normal, albeit thin, but may also deteriorate quickly if presenting with a diaphragmatic hernia. The midwife should be fully aware of the availability of cots in the neonatal intensive care unit (NICU), transitional care unit or postnatal ward according to the condition of the baby and their potential care demands following birth. The birthing room ambient temperature should ideally be between 23°C and 26°C and the neonatal Resuscitaire and accompanying equipment should be ready for use.

It is particularly important that the midwife attaches the correct labels to the baby at birth in case separation from the mother should occur at any time if the baby's condition becomes unstable. Current National Institute for Health and Care Excellence (NICE 2017) guidance recommend that clamping of the umbilical cord should be delayed between 1 and 5 min, unless the heart rate of the baby is <60 beats/min and is not increasing or there is concern about the integrity of the cord. When the cord is clamped, the midwife should cut the cord leaving extra length to allow for easy access to the umbilical vessels in case they are needed at a later time. At birth, the midwife should ensure that the baby is thoroughly dried before skin-to-skin contact is attempted in order to prevent evaporative heat losses. Skin-to-skin contact for a period of up to 60 min is recommended to secure the baby's conductive heat transfer gains and help the baby to become physically stabilized to feed. If the mother chooses not to engage in skin-to-skin contact, the father may wish to do so (Huang et al. 2019) but if not, the baby can be dressed, wrapped and held by the parents. The baby's axilla temperature should be maintained between 36.5°C and 37.5°C. Early attempts at breastfeeding should be encouraged (UNICEF/WHO 2018).

Assessment of Gestational Age

With developments of more accurate dating by antenatal ultrasound techniques, it is argued by Smith (2012) that there is less justification for a full assessment of gestational age in healthy LBW babies. The exception is applied when the mother has concealed her pregnancy (see Chapter 12) or has difficulty/is unable to communicate. The neonatal practitioner, with the view that no harm is caused as a result of the process, should carefully conduct any assessments that need to be carried out using a tool such as the Ballard Maturation Score (Ballard et al. 1991) (Fig. 34.6). Sasidharan et al. (2009) considers that this tool can give an accurate assessment of gestational age until 7 days of life and consequently it continues to be the most effective and widely used assessment tool.

The RCPCH (2013) growth charts internationally developed by the WHO, describe *optimal* rather than average growth based on *exclusively* breastfeeding: highlighting how all healthy children are expected to grow. Appropriate centile charts are used to plot the weight, head circumference and length of the baby to make an assessment of the baby's growth. This initiates a dynamic growth record that guides subsequent neonatal management. There is a *preterm chart* to record the measurements of babies born before 37 completed weeks of pregnancy until 2 weeks after the expected date of birth (42 weeks). From 42 weeks, the baby's measurements should then be plotted on the 0–1 year chart with *gestational correction*: i.e. at the **actual age** with a line being drawn back to the number of weeks the baby was preterm, marking the spot with an arrow to show the *gestationally corrected percentile* (Fig. 34.7). It is important that midwives are educated to use these specialized charts efficiently, so that the baby's subsequent growth and development can be monitored effectively (DH 2009). Accurate charting will reflect the natural weight losses and gains of this category of baby as similar to term babies, LBW babies will also lose some weight in the first few days of life.

Thermoregulation

Thermoregulation is the balance between heat production and heat loss. The prevention of cold stress, which may lead to hypothermia – which is a body temperature below 35°C is critical for the entire survival of the LBW baby. Newborn babies are unable to shiver, move very much or seek extra warmth for themselves and therefore rely upon physical adaptations that generate heat by raising basal metabolic rate and utilize brown fat deposits. Thus, exposure to cool environments can result in multisystem changes. As body temperature falls, tissue oxygen consumption rises as the baby attempts to burn brown fat, which generates energy and heat. Diversion of blood away from the gastrointestinal tract reduces all forms of digestion. *Attempting to warm a cold baby by feeding is ineffectual and carries the danger of milk inhalation.* Care measures should aim to provide an environment that supports the *neutral thermal environment.* This environment constitutes: a range of ambient temperatures within which the metabolic rate is minimal; the baby is neither gaining nor losing heat; oxygen consumption is negligible; and the core-to-skin temperature gradient is small (Blackburn 2013).

In the baby, the head accounts for at least one-fifth of the total body surface area and brain heat production is thought to be 55% of the total metabolic heat production. Rapid heat loss due to the large head-to-body ratio and large surface area is exaggerated. Wide sutures and large fontanelles add to the heat-losing tendency. Once the baby is thoroughly dried (which includes the face) and their axilla temperature is taken, they are wrapped in pre-warmed blankets and a hat (the latter being to minimize heat loss from the baby's head). Asymmetric SGA babies have increased skin maturity but often depleted stores of subcutaneous fat, which are used for insulation. Their raised basal metabolic rate helps them to produce heat, but their high energy demands in the presence of poor glycogen stores and minimal fat deposition can soon lead to *hypoglycaemia* (<2.5 mmol/L followed by physiological cooling (<36°C) to reach a state of *hypothermia* (<35°C) (Bedford and Lomax 2011).

All preterm babies are prone to heat loss because their ability to produce heat is compromised by their immaturity, so factors such as their large ratio of surface area to weight, their varying amounts of subcutaneous fat and their ability to mobilize brown fat stores will be affected by their gestational age (Blackburn 2013). During cooling, immaturity of the heat-regulating centre in the

Neuromuscular maturity

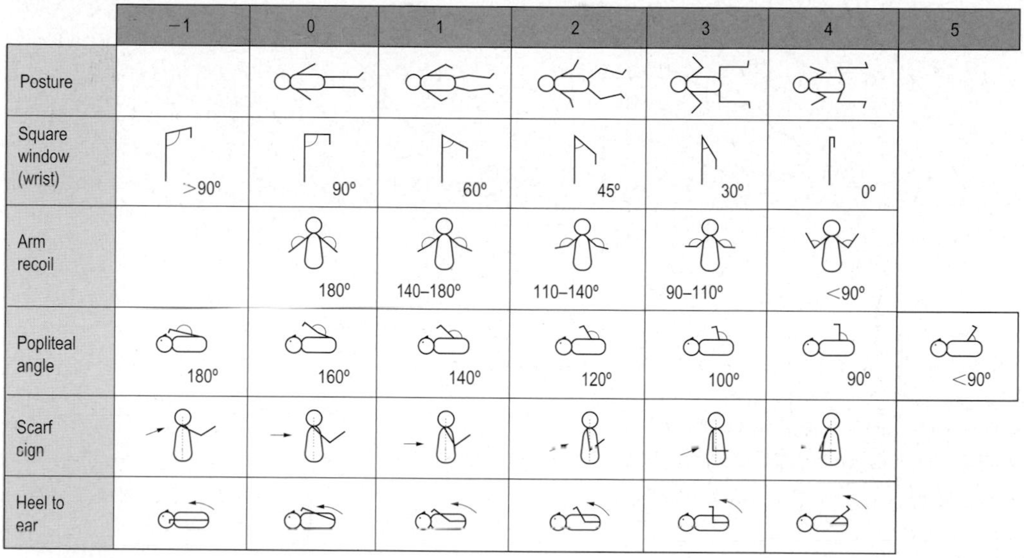

	−1	0	1	2	3	4	5
Posture							
Square window (wrist)	>90°	90°	60°	45°	30°	0°	
Arm recoil		180°	140–180°	110–140°	90–110°	<90°	
Popliteal angle	180°	160°	140°	120°	100°	90°	<90°
Scarf sign							
Heel to ear							

Physical maturity

Skin	Sticky, friable, transparent	Gelatinous, red, translucent	Smooth pink, visible veins	Superficial peeling and/or rash, few veins	Cracking, pale areas, rare veins	Parchment, deep cracking, no vessels	Leathery, cracked, wrinkled
Lanugo	None	Sparse	Abundant	Thinning	Bald areas	Mostly bald	
Plantar surface	Heel-toe 40–50 mm: −1 <40 mm: −2	>50 mm, no crease	Faint red marks	Anterior transverse crease only	Creases over anterior 2/3	Creases over entire sole	
Breast	Imperceptible	Barely perceptible	Flat areola; no bud	Stippled areola, 1- to 2-mm bud	Raised areola; 3- to 4-mm bud	Full areola; 5- to 10-mm bud	
Eye/ ear	Lids fused loosely: −1 tightly: −2	Lids open; pinna flat and stays folded	Slightly curved pinna; soft; slow recoil	Well-curved pinna; soft but ready recoil	Formed and firm; instant recoil	Thick cartilage; ear stiff	
Genitals (male)	Scrotum flat, smooth	Scrotum empty; faint rugae	Testes in upper canal; rare rugae	Testes descending; few rugae	Testes down; good rugae	Testes pendulous; deep rugae	
Genitals (female)	Clitoris prominent; labia flat	Prominent clitoris; small labia minora	Prominent clitoris; enlarging labia minora	Labia majora and minora equally prominent	Labia majora large; labia minora small	Labia majora cover clitoris and labia minora	

Maturity rating

Score	Weeks
−10	20
−5	22
0	24
5	26
10	28
15	30
20	32
25	34
30	36
35	38
40	40
45	42
50	44

Fig. 34.6 The Ballard score. (With permission from Johnston PGB, Flood K, Spinks K. (2003) The newborn child (9th ed.). Edinburgh: Churchill Livingstone.)

hypothalamus and medulla oblongata causes *failure to recognize the need to act*. In addition, preterm babies are unable to increase their oxygen consumption effectively through normal respiratory function and their calorific intake is often inadequate to meet increasing metabolic requirements. Furthermore, their open resting postures increase their surface area and, along with insensible water losses, these factors render the preterm baby more susceptible to evaporative heat losses. Fellows (2011) affirms that when the baby is not receiving skin-to-skin

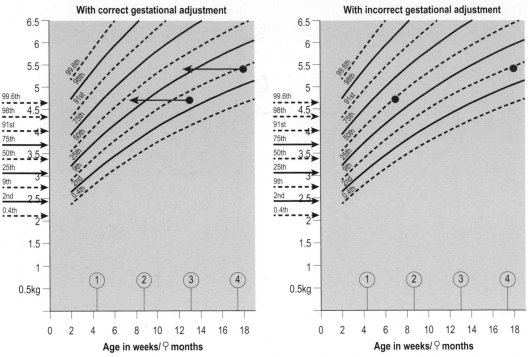

Fig. 34.7 Correct gestational age adjustment and incorrect gestational adjustment (baby born at 34 weeks).

contact with either parent and weighs under 2 kg, they should be placed in a warm incubator, where the temperature can be maintained by either heating the air to 30–32°C (*air mode*) or by *servo-mode*: controlling the baby's body temperature at a desired set point (36°C). In servo-mode, a *thermocouple* is taped to the upper abdomen and the incubator heater maintains the skin at that site at a pre-set constant temperature (Fig. 34.5). Most preterm babies between 2.0 kg and 2.5 kg will be cared for in a cot, in a room temperature of 24–26°C.

Hypoglycaemia

The term *hypoglycaemia* refers to a low blood glucose concentration and is usually a feature of failure to adapt from the fetal state of continuous transplacental glucose consumption to the extrauterine pattern of intermittent milk supply (WHO 1997). Within the first hour of life, the blood glucose levels fall, which triggers the pancreas to stimulate the alpha cells of the Islets of Langerhans to produce glucagon, with the consequential effect of releasing glucose from glycogen stores in the liver to maintain the blood glucose levels within *safe* limits. For the majority of babies, a physiological fall in blood

glucose is not a problem if their brains have the normal substrate stores to utilize. In rare circumstances, neonatal hypoglycaemia is sufficiently severe to cause brain injury and long-term neurodevelopmental impairment. It is therefore questioned whether LBW babies are as effective in this metabolic process compared with appropriately grown term babies and consequently, some caution is recommended when caring for these babies in the initial days following birth (WHO 1997). Asymmetrical SGA babies may have greater brain-to-body mass with a tendency towards *polycythaemia* (an increase in red blood cells defined as a venous haematocrit >65%), which increases their energy demands, and since both the brain and the red blood cells are obligatory glucose users, these factors can increase glucose requirements. Glycogen storage is initiated at the beginning of the third trimester of pregnancy but may be incomplete as a result of preterm birth or, in the asymmetrical SGA baby, may have been drawn upon before birth.

Hypoglycaemia in healthy LBW babies is more likely to occur in conditions where they become cold or where the initiation of early feeding (within the first *golden* hour) is delayed. However, hypoglycaemia is associated with mild to moderate perinatal asphyxia and maternal history of beta-blocker use (e.g. labetalol) as it causes *hyperinsulinism* and interferes with glycogenolysis. The midwife should consider that there may be some underlying medical condition that may call for more thorough investigation (see Chapter 37).

The signs of hypoglycaemia are varied and the BAPM (2017) acknowledges that hypoglycaemia can present with no or few clinical signs. The clinical picture of tremor and irritability may occasionally lead to convulsion and decreased consciousness. A high-pitched cry, hypotonia, unexplained apnoea and bradycardia with central cyanosis are also recognized as serious signs of deterioration in the baby's health and prompt escalation and referral to a neonatal practitioner is vital. Pre-term, SGA, FGR babies are at risk of hypoglycaemia. Jitteriness is not a sign of hypoglycaemia (UNICEF 2013). The aim of management is to maintain the true blood glucose level above 2.5 mmol/l, which is considered to be the lowest level of normal in the first few days of life (BAPM 2017).

Healthy LBW babies who show no clinical signs of hypoglycaemia, are often demanding and taking nutritive feeds on a regular basis. They can maintain their body temperature, and therefore do not need assessing for hypoglycaemia. The emphasis of care is placed upon the concept of *adequate feeding* and the key to the success lies in the midwife's regular assessment of whether the baby is feeding sufficiently well to meet energy requirements. The preterm baby may be sleepy and attempts to take the first feed may reflect its gestational age. Midwives should be guided by the local policies within their employing organization regarding the assessment of hypoglycaemia, but prior to the baby's second feed is the best time to ascertain whether the first feed was effective in maintaining the capillary blood glucose level above 2 mmol/dL. If a baby, despite regular feeds presents with *clinical signs of hypoglycaemia*, a venous blood sample should be taken by the skilled proficient practitioner to assess the *true* blood glucose level, which can be measured locally using a glucose monitor or dispatched to the laboratory. A true blood glucose level that remains <2.5 mmol/dL, despite the baby's further attempts to feed by breast or take colostrum by cup, may warrant transfer to the NICU, because glucose by intravenous bolus may be necessary to correct the metabolic disturbance. Healthy mature SGA babies with an asymmetrical growth pattern will usually breastfeed within the first 30–60 min of birth and demand feeds every 2–3 h thereafter. For the majority of LBW babies, hypoglycaemia is relatively short-lived and limited to the first 48 h following birth.

Responsive Feeding

Midwives and healthcare professionals should always consider best practice when supporting parents to feed their babies, regardless of their choice. Responsive feeding involves a mother responding to her own baby's cues as well as her own desire to feed her baby. This means that feeding responsively recognizes that feeds are not just for nutrition, but also for love, comfort and reassurance between baby and mother (UNICEF-UK 2016) (see also Chapter 27). Both preterm and SGA babies benefit from human milk because it contains long chain polyunsaturated omega-3 fatty acids, which are thought to be essential for the myelination of neural membranes and for retinal development. Preterm breast milk has a higher concentration of lipids, protein, sodium, calcium and immunoglobulins, alongside lipases and enzymes that improve digestion and absorption. The uniqueness of the mother's milk for her own baby cannot be overstated but she needs to understand what her baby may be able to achieve related to the stage of their development, which is based upon the combined influences of their gestational age at birth and their neonatal age.

For a baby to feed for nutritive purposes, the coordination of breathing with suck and swallow reflexes reflects neuro behavioural maturation and organization, which is thought to occur between 32 and 36 weeks' gestation. Blackburn (2013) argues that preterm babies are limited in their ability to suck because they lack *cheek pads*, which leads to a weaker suck, coupled with weak musculature and flexor control; both being vital for firm lip and jaw closure.

Parents should provide physical support for the head, trunk and shoulders, as sucking is part of the flexor pattern of development and may be enhanced by giving the baby something to grasp. The preterm baby's head is very heavy for the weak musculature of the neck and would, if not supported, result in considerable head lag, so correct positioning and attachment to the breast may be more challenging to achieve. Poor head alignment can result in airway collapse, which may lead to apnoea and bradycardia, therefore support from the midwife is essential when initiating breastfeeding.

Pollard (2017) reports that certain behaviours, such as licking and lapping, are well established *before* sucking and swallowing, and when babies are given the opportunity, it is not unusual to see them as early as 28 and 29 weeks licking milk that has been expressed onto the nipple by their mother. Babies born between 30 and 32 weeks' gestation can be given expressed breast milk (EBM) by cup. Pollard (2017) makes a further point that tongue movement is vital in the efficient stripping of the milk ducts, so cup-feeding is considered to be developmental preparation for breastfeeding. Between 32 and 34 weeks' gestation, cup-feeding can act as the main method of feeding, with the baby taking occasional complete breastfeeds. The baby uses less energy to take its feed by cup compared with a bottle, which supports their general wellbeing and homeostasis.

A preterm baby of <35 weeks' gestation can be gently wrapped/swaddled prior to a feed and this is thought to provide reassurance and comfort, not unlike the unique close-fitting tactile stimulation of the uterus. McGrath (2004) argues that this approach supports development of flexion as well as decreasing disorganized behaviours that could detract from feeding success.

The Reluctant Feeder

A preterm baby may easily become tired and show reluctance to feed. Long pauses between sucks are to be expected. This *burst–pause* pattern is a signal of normal development and seems to occur earlier with breastfeeding. The baby may appear to be asleep and a change in position may remind them of the task in hand, but it is considered to be unwise to force a reluctant pre-term baby to feed. The mother can be taught to start the flow of milk by hand expressing, before attempting to attach her baby to the breast. If it is obvious that the baby is more interested in sleeping, the mother can complete the feed by nasogastric tube.

If the baby requires feeding via a nasogastric tube, parents should always be supported to feed their own baby to help in developing their parenting relationship. The advantage with tube feeding is that the tube can be left *in situ* during a breast or cup feed and has been shown to eliminate the need to introduce bottles into a breastfeeding regimen. However, babies are preferential nose breathers and the presence of a nasogastric tube will inevitably take up part of their available airway. Flint et al. (2007) argue that the prolonged use of nasogastric tubes has been associated with delay in the development of a baby's sucking and swallowing reflexes simply because the mouth is bypassed. For these reasons, cup-feeding has been used in addition or as an alternative to tube-feeding, in order to provide the baby with a positive oral experience, to stimulate saliva and lingual lipases to aid digestion and to accelerate the transition from naso/orogastric feeding to breastfeeding. Oral gastric tubes have been associated with vagal stimulation and have resulted in bradycardia and apnoea.

Should an LBW baby be showing signs of reluctance to feed, it is good practice for the midwife to undertake a thorough clinical assessment of the LBW and SGA baby within 6 h of birth to differentiate between a healthy baby who is reluctant to feed and a baby whose feeding pattern may be affected by some deviation in their clinical state, in order to expedite care as appropriate. The healthy LBW baby should be left to establish their own volume requirements and feeding pattern and frequency of feeds can vary between 8 and 10 feeds per day. If necessary, the mother should use a breast pump to maintain her lactation in order to reflect her baby's feeding style.

OPTIMIZING THE CARE ENVIRONMENT FOR THE HEALTHY LOW BIRTH WEIGHT BABY

The normal sensory requirements of the developing neonatal brain depend upon subtle influences, first from the uterus and then from the breast (Reid and Freer 2010). Any disruption to this natural arrangement renders the LBW baby vulnerable to influences in the care environment, which can contribute to poor coordination as a result of delays in the development of different subsystems (autonomic, motor, sensory, etc.). Reid and Freer (2010) believe maternal role development depends upon the mother's self-esteem and her perception of mothering. By attempting to adapt the care environment to be more like the intrauterine environment, the midwife can help parents with responsive parenting and become aware of their baby's behavioural and autonomic cues and utilize them in organizing care according to their baby's individual tolerance.

Responsive Parenting

Responsive parenting supports the ethos of care and encouraging parents to listen and learn from their baby, to come to know and see them as an individual, competent for their stage of development and not merely *a baby born too early*, or a *dysfunctional term baby*. Parents should be supported in taking a major role in their baby's emerging developmental needs enabling them to understand the situation in which they find themselves, so they are further able to re-set their expectations and therefore provide more baby-led support (Teti et al. 2005; Reid and Freer 2010).

According to McGrath (2004), the emerging task of the term newborn baby is increasing alertness, with growing responsiveness to the *outside* world. By comparison, a preterm baby is at a stage of development that is more concerned with their *internal* world. Term babies have stable function of the autonomic and motor systems, whereas preterm babies will be at different stages of this development, depending on their gestational age and health status. They will spend more time in rapid eye movement (REM) sleep or drowsy states and have difficulty in achieving deep sleep. They are unable to shut out stimulation that prevents them from sleeping and resting, and sudden noise hazards provoke stress reactions, which can adversely affect respiratory, cardiovascular and digestive stability. The term baby can adapt to their environment shutting out stimuli for rest and sleep purposes. The degree to which SGA term babies have been affected by their unique intrauterine experience is difficult to assess in the short term, but hyperactivity is seen as a feature of an adaptive stress reaction. These babies, like their preterm counterparts, need an environment that supports their level of robustness. Should the baby wish to initiate or continue an interaction, they tend to demonstrate *approach signals* such as *raised eyebrows*, *head raising* and *engagement in different degrees of eye contact with their social partners*. The midwife can reassure parents that by being responsive to their baby's behaviour, they can work *with* their baby's capabilities, which is fundamental for maintaining their baby's healthy status.

Handling, Touch and Skin-to-Skin Care

Environmental disturbances, excessive or prolonged handling and even activities like feeding may add extra physiological burden to an already compromised state in the LBW baby. Social contact is considered a vital element for the development of parent–baby interaction, yet stereotypical notions of social contact that revolve around practical care-giving and feeding may not be suitable for some babies and when these activities are pooled together, may draw too heavily on the baby's physical resources. When the baby is over-stimulated and wishes to terminate the interaction, certain cues known as *coping signals* become apparent in the form of *fist clenching*, *furrowing of the brow*, *gaze aversion*, *splayed fingers* and *yawning*.

'Kangaroo care' is used to promote closeness between a baby and mother/father and involves placing the nappy-clad baby upright between the breasts for skin-to-skin contact (Fig. 34.8). The LBW baby can remain beneath the mother's clothing for varying periods of time that suit the mother (as well as the father) and contact may be repeated throughout the day, or planned for. Others may prefer to undertake kangaroo care at specific periods around which they can plan their daily activities. There are no rules or time limitations applied, but contact should be reviewed if there are any clinical signs of neonatal distress. Hake-Brooks and Anderson (2008) found that preterm babies of between 32 and 36 weeks' gestation who had unlimited skin-to-skin contact, breastfed for longer compared with those who had traditional nursery care. Conde-Agudelo and Belizan (2009) and Jeffries et al. (2013) also support this view, and consider that the baby remains more physiologically stable, with less reported incidence of infection.

Noise and Light Hazards

The time spent in a postnatal/transitional care ward should be a time of rest and recuperation for both the mother and her LBW baby. Careful consideration to extraneous noises should be eliminated from clinical area: harsh clattering footwear, telephones, radios, intercom systems and raised voices. Clinicians should be aware of noise hazards, such as the closing of incubator portholes, use of pedal bins, ward doors and general equipment. Ward areas have often polished floors and *quiet signs* can be posted on the wards and in patient areas to remind visitors not to disrupt the peace. In dimmed lighting conditions, preterm babies are more able to improve their quality of sleep and alert status. Reduced light levels during the day and night will help to promote the development of circadian rhythms and diurnal cycles. Light levels can be adjusted during the day with curtains or blinds to shade windows and protect the room from direct sunlight. Screens to shield adjacent babies from phototherapy lights are also essential. Restricted non-essential foot traffic through ward areas and the NICU can enhance the environment further.

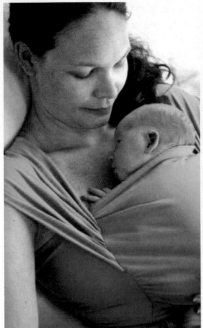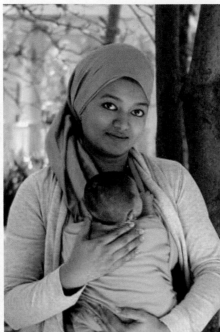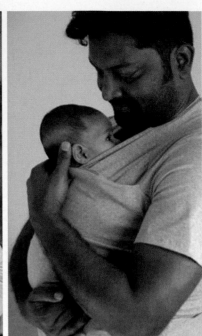

Fig. 34.8 Kangaroo care.

Sleeping Position

Hunter (2004) reports that preterm babies have reduced muscle power and bulk, with flaccid muscle tone, therefore their movements are erratic, weak or flailing. They exert energy to maintain their body position against the pull of gravity. Nesting preterm babies into soft bedding, in addition to the use of close flexible boundaries, helps to keep their limbs in midline flexion, however it is vital that they are nursed in a supine position to prevent asphyxia. The supine position is also thought to be effective in promoting engagement in self-regulatory behaviours such as exploration of the face and mouth, hand and foot clasping, boundary searching, flexion and extension of the limbs. Pressure on the occiput should, over time, ensure a more rounded head.

Placing healthy LBW babies to sleep in the prone position has been theoretically eradicated from neonatal practice and Warwood (2010) reiterates that all babies should be placed in the supine position. Midwives need to accustom the baby and educate the parents in adopting this approach. Teaching resuscitation to parents is part of routine preparation for transfer home, although according to Younger et al. (2007) this degree of preparedness can empower some parents but frighten others. The decision to receive training should be the parent's choice (Resuscitation Council United Kingdom, RCUK 2015).

The importance of providing an appropriate environment for the healthy LBW baby cannot be overstressed and the ideal environment should be provided at home or at least resemble that of the home setting, which provides a cycle of day and night, regular nourishment, rest, stimulation and loving attention. The midwife's role is to create such an environment, primarily for the physical development of the baby but at the same time to provide psychological support for the parents. According to Fleury et al. (2010) the mother should be encouraged to rely upon her own instincts and common sense, so that the rhythm of total care she adopts in hospital will thoroughly prepare her for when she goes home. Timing of transfer home should be dependent on the preparedness of the parents and their positive attitude and skills as opposed to the baby's maturity and inherent abilities and should include appropriate ongoing support for the family by the midwife and neonatal team until the baby is finally discharged from care.

REFLECTIVE ACTIVITY FOR SELF-ASSESSMENT

1. Consider a baby that you have cared for who was small for gestational age.
   a. What may have been the contributory factors leading to the baby being low birth weight?
   b. Describe the characteristics and behaviour of this particular baby that would indicate whether the baby is preterm or growth restricted.
2. What would be the main issues you would need to consider in planning the immediate and subsequent care of this baby to optimize their health and wellbeing?
3. What do you think the impact is likely to be on the mother/parents/family of a baby who is:
   a. born before term (AGA)
   b. growth restricted (SGA)
   c. both preterm AND growth restricted?
4. In what ways are parents supported to care for their LBW baby in your maternity/neonatal units?
5. What facilities are available in your local community to support the mother and baby once they have transferred home?

REFERENCES

Ballard, J. L., Khoury, C., Wedig, K., et al. (1991). New Ballard Score expanded to include extremely premature infants. *Journal of Paediatrics, 119*, 417–423.

Bedford, C. D., & Lomax, A. (2011). Development of the heart and lungs and transition to extrauterine life. In A. Lomax (Ed.), *Examination of the newborn: An evidence-based guide* (pp. 47–58). Chichester: Wiley-Blackwell.

Blackburn, S. T. (2013). *Maternal, fetal and neonatal physiology: A clinical perspective* (4th ed.). Philadelphia: Mosby: Elsevier.

BAPM (British Association of Perinatal Medicine). (2017). *Identification and management of neonatal hypoglycaemia in the full term infant: A framework for neonatal transitional care*. London: BAPM. Available at: www.bapm.org/sites/default/files/files/identification%20and%20management%20of%20neonatal%20hypoglycaemia%20in%20the%20-%20full%20term%20infant%20-%20a%20framework%20for%20practice%20revised%20oct%202017.pdf.

Conde-Agudelo, A., & Belizan, J. (2009). Kangaroo mother care to reduce morbidity and mortality in low birthweight infants. *Cochrane Database of Systematic Reviews* (2), CD002771.

DH (Department of Health). (2009). *Using the new UK–World Health Organization 0–4 years growth charts*. London: DH. Available at: https://assets.publishing.service.gov.uk/government/uploads/system/uploads/attachment_data/file/215564/dh_127422.pdf.

Fellows, P. (2011). Management of thermal stability. In G. Boxwell (Ed.), *Neonatal intensive care nursing*. (pp. 87–120). London: Routledge.

Fleury, C., Parpinelly, M., & Makuch, M. Y. (2010). Development of the mother–child relationship following pre-eclampsia. *Journal of Reproductive and Infant Psychology, 28*(3), 297–306.

Flint, A., New, K., & Davies, M. (2007). Cup feeding versus other forms of supplemental enteral feeding for newborn infants unable to fully breastfeed. *Cochrane Database of Systematic Reviews* (2), CD005092.

Gardosi, J., Giddings, S., Clifford, S., et al. (2013). Association between reduced stillbirth rates in England and regional update of accreditation training in customized fetal growth assessment. *BMJ Open, 3*, 1–10.

Gardosi, J., Francis, A., Turner, S., & Williams, M. (2018). Customised growth charts and rationale, validation and clinical benefits. *American Journal of Obstetrics and Gynecology, 218*(2S), S609–S618.

Hake-Brooks, S., & Anderson, G. (2008). Kangaroo care and breastfeeding of mother–preterm infant dyads 0–18 months: A randomised controlled trial. *Neonatal Network, 27*, 151–159.

Huang, X., Chen, L., & Zhang, L. (2019). Effects of paternal skin-to-skin contact in newborns and fathers after cesarean delivery. *Journal of Perinatal and Neonatal Nursing, 33*(1), 68–73.

Hunter, J. (2004). Positioning. In C. Kenner, & J. M. McGrath (Eds.), *Developmental care of newborns and infants: A guide for health care professionals* (pp. 299–320). St Louis: Mosby.

Jeffries, A. L., & Canadian Paediatric Society, Fetus and Newborn Committee. (2013). Kangaroo care for the preterm infant and family. *Paediatrics and Child Care, 17*(3), 141–143.

Lissauer, T., & Fanaroff, A. A. (2011). *Neonatology at a glance*. Chichester: Wiley-Blackwell.

McGrath, J. M. (2004). Feeding. In C. Kenner, & J. M. McGrath (Eds.), *Developmental care of newborns and infants: A guide for health care professionals* (pp. 321–342). St Louis: Mosby.

NICE (National Institute for Health and Care Excellence). (2017). *Quality Statement 6: Delayed cord clamping in intrapartum care: QS 105*. London: NICE. Available at: www.nice.org.uk/guidance/qs105/chapter/quality-statement-6-delayed-cord-clamping.

NICE (National Institute for Health and Care Excellence). (2019). *Preterm labour and birth*. London: NICE. Available at: www.nice.org.uk/guidance/NG25.

ONS (Office of National Statistics). (2017). *Percentage term low birthweight live births by ethnic group, 2006 to 2012 and 2014 to 2015, England and Wales*. Available at: www.ons.gov.uk/peoplepopulationandcommuni-ty/birthsdeathsandmarriages/deaths/adhocs/006681per-centagetermlowbirthweightlivebirthsbyethnicgroup-2006to2012and2014to2015englandandwales.

Pollard, M. (2017). *Evidence-based care for breastfeeding mothers* (2nd ed.). Abingdon: Routledge.

Reid, T., & Freer, Y. (2010). Developmentally focused nursing care. In G. Boxwell (Ed.), *Neonatal intensive care nursing* (pp. 16–39). London: Routledge.

RCOG (Royal College of Obstetricians and Gynaecologists). (2014). *Green-top Guideline No 31: The Investigation and management of the small -for-gestational-age fetus* (2nd edn). February 2013; minor revisions January 2014.

RCUK (Resuscitation Council UK). (2015). *Newborn life support* (4th ed.). London: RCUK. Available at: www.re-sus.org.uk/publications/newborn-life-support-resuscita-tion-at-birth-manual.

RCPCH (Royal College of Paediatrics and Child Health). (2013). *UK-WHO Growth Charts 0–4 years* (2nd ed.). Available at: www.rcpch.ac.uk/resources/uk-who-growth-charts-0-4-years.

Sasidharan, K., Dutta, S., & Narang, A. (2009). Validity of new Ballard score until 7th day of postnatal life in moderately preterm infants. *Archives of Diseases in Childhood Fetal and Neonatal Edition*, *94*, 39–44.

Sinha, S., Miall, L., & Jardine, L. (2012). *Essential neonatal medicine* (5th ed.). Chichester: Wiley-Blackwell.

Smith, V. C. (2012). The high-risk newborn: Anticipation, evaluation, management and outcome. In J. P. Cloherty, E. C. Eichenwald, A. R. Hansen, et al. (Eds.), *Manual of neonatal care* (pp. 74–90). London: Wolters Kluwer – Lippincott Williams and Wilkins.

Teti, D. M., Hess, C. R., & O'Connell, M. (2005). Parental perceptions of infant vulnerability in a preterm sample: Prediction from maternal adaptation to parenthood during the neonatal period. *Journal of Development and Behavioral Paediatrics*, *26*, 283–292.

Trotter, C. W. (2018). Gestational age assessment. In E. P. Tappero, & M. E. Honeyfield (Eds.), *Physical assessment of the newborn. A comprehensive approach to the art of physical examination* (6th ed.). (pp. 23–44). New York: Springer.

UNICEF (United Nations Children's Fund). (2013). *Guidance on the development of policies and guidelines for the prevention and management of hypoglycaemia of the newborn.* Available at: www.unicef.org.uk/babyfriendly/wp-content/uploads/sites/2/2010/10/hypo_policy.pdf.

UNICEF/WHO. (2004). *Low birth weight: Country, regional and global estimates.* New York: UNICEF/WHO.

UNICEF/WHO. (2018). *Capture the moment. Early initiation of breastfeeding: the best start for every newborn.* New York: UNICEF. Available at: www.unicef.org/publications/files/unicef_who_capture_the_moment_eibf_2018.pdf.

UNICEF-UK. (2016). Baby Friendly Initiative Infosheet. *Responsive feeding: Supporting close and loving relationships.* Available at: www.unicef.org.uk/babyfriendly/wp-content/uploads/sites/2/2017/12/responsive-feeding-infosheet-unicef-uk-baby-friendly-initiative.pdf.

Warwood, G. (2010). Teaching resuscitation to parents. In H. Lumsden, & D. Holmes (Eds.), *Care of the newborn by ten teachers* (pp. 168–177). London: Hodder Arnold.

Wilkins-Haug, L. E., & Heffner, L. J. (2012). Fetal assessment and prenatal diagnosis. In J. P. Cloherty, E. C. Eichenwald, A. R. Hansen, et al. (Eds.), *Manual of neonatal care* (pp. 1–10). London: Wolters Kluwer – Lippincott Williams and Wilkins.

WHO (World Health Organization). (1997). *Hypoglycaemia of the newborn: Review of the literature.* Geneva: WHO.

Younger, J. B., Kendell, M. J., & Pickler, R. H. (2007). Mastery of stress in mothers of preterm infants. *Journal of Specialist Paediatric Nursing*, *2*, 29–35.

ANNOTATED FURTHER READING

Gardosi, J., Francis, A., Turner, S., & Williams, M. (2018). Customized growth charts: Rationale, validation and clinical benefits. *American Journal of Obstetrics and Gynecology*, *218*(2S), S609–S618.

This paper debates the rationale for the development of customized growth and birth weight charts adjusted for the characteristics of each mother, taking her ethnic origin and her height, weight and parity to set a growth and birth weight standard for each pregnancy, against which actual growth can be assessed. Since adopted in the UK as part of the Growth Assessment Protocol (GAP), there has been a steady increase in antenatal detection of babies who are at risk because of fetal growth restriction and a year-on-year fall in stillbirth rates to their lowest ever levels in England.

Jeffries, A. L., & Canadian Paediatric Society, Fetus and Newborn Committee. (2012). Kangaroo care for the preterm infant and family. *Paediatrics and Child Care*, *17*(3), 141–146.

An interesting systematic review that provides evidence of the positive benefits of skin-to-skin care for both babies and parents, with no reported detrimental effect on physiological stability for preterm infants as young as 26 weeks' gestation, including those on assisted ventilation. Furthermore, kangaroo care was found to enhance breastfeeding and contributed to improved neurodevelopmental outcome. The paper also provides guidance to assist nurseries in developing best-practice guidelines and protocols for implementation.

UNICEF-UK. (2016). Baby Friendly Initiative Infosheet. *Responsive feeding: Supporting close and loving relationships.* Available at: www.unicef.org.uk/babyfriendly/wp-content/uploads/sites/2/2017/12/responsive-feeding-infosheet-unicef-uk-baby-friendly-initiative.pdf.

This infosheet assists health professionals to support parents to feed their babies responsively, advising them of specific cues to observe that will help them to develop a close and loving relationship, regardless of gestational age. The Baby Friendly Initiative standards require that healthcare professionals explain a **responsive feeding** *style to mothers, helping them to respond appropriately to their baby.*

USEFUL WEBSITES

Ballard Score: www.ballardscore.com/Pages/ScoreSheetInteractive.aspx
British Association of Perinatal Medicine: www.bapm.org
National Institute for Health and Care Excellence: www.nice.org.uk
Resuscitation Council UK (RCUK): www.resus.org.uk
Royal College of Paediatrics and Child Health: www.rcpch.ac.uk
UNICEF-UK Baby Friendly Initiative: www.unicef.org.uk/babyfriendly
World Health Organization: www.who.int

35

Trauma During Birth, Haemorrhages and Convulsions

Shalini Ojha, Liana Tsilika, Aarti Mistry

CHAPTER CONTENTS

This chapter focuses on complications occurring in specifically vulnerable babies; the midwife's awareness of this vulnerability may prevent such complications. If a complication does occur, the midwife must report it to the paediatrician/neonatologist within the hospital setting or expedite referral should the baby be born at home. Subsequent care from the midwife will be dependent on the type of complication and the severity of the neonate's condition, but should be based on a multiprofessional approach in aiding diagnosis and implementing effective treatment. Parents may be distressed when their baby experiences a complication associated with the birth, so the midwife plays a vital role in helping them to understand the complication, facilitating their discussions with the multiprofessional team members, and assisting them to care for their baby.

THE CHAPTER AIMS TO

- identify the types of trauma a newborn may sustain to their skin, superficial tissues, muscle, nerves and bones during the birth process
- discuss the major types of neonatal haemorrhage that occur as a result of birth trauma, disruptions in blood flow, coagulopathies and other causes

- explore the causes and treatment of neonatal convulsions
- discuss the significance of specific neonatal interventions and the importance of informing parents about their baby's health and wellbeing.

TRAUMA DURING BIRTH

Despite skilled midwifery and obstetric care in developed, Western societies and a reduction in the incidence, birth trauma still occurs. Efforts continue to reduce the incidence even further.

Trauma to the baby during the birth process includes:
- trauma to skin and superficial tissues
- muscle trauma
- nerve trauma
- fractures.

Trauma to Skin and Superficial Tissues
Skin
Skin damage is often iatrogenic, resulting from forceps blades (Fig. 35.1), vacuum extractor cups, scalp electrodes and scalpels. Poorly applied forceps blades

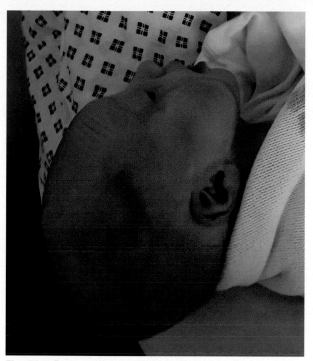

Fig. 35.1 Forceps abrasion on cheek.

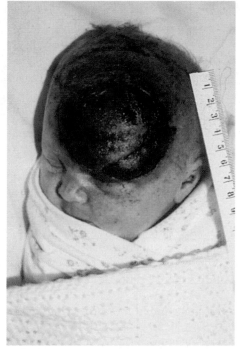

Fig. 35.2 Scalp abrasion during vacuum-assisted birth. Note the chignon. (Reproduced from Thomas R, Harvey D (1997) Colour guide: neonatology (2nd ed.). Edinburgh: Churchill Livingstone, with permission of Elsevier.)

or a vacuum extractor cup may result in scalp abrasions (Fig. 35.2), although less so with softer vacuum extractor cups. Forceps blades may cause bruising, scalp electrodes cause puncture wounds, as do fetal blood sampling techniques. Occasionally laceration of the baby's skin may occur during uterine incision at caesarean section. While rare, subcutaneous fat necrosis may result from the pressure of forceps blades, as well as following severe asphyxia/hypoxaemia, meconium aspiration syndrome and hypothermia (Grewal 2018).

While superficial fat necrosis usually presents between days 1 and 28 with well-defined areas of induration (Grewal 2018), all other skin injuries should be detected during the midwife's detailed examination of the baby immediately after birth (see Chapter 32). All trauma should be indicated to parents and reported to the paediatrician and General Practitioner (GP).

Abrasions and lacerations should be kept clean and dry. If there are signs of infection, further medical consultation should be sought by the midwife or parents. Antibiotics may be required. Deeper lacerations may

require closure with butterfly strips or sutures. Healing is usually rapid with no residual scarring (Sorantin et al. 2006). Pain relief should be considered if the infant appears to be in distress due to the injury. If related causes are successfully treated, fat necrosis should spontaneously resolve (Grewal 2018).

Superficial Tissues

This type of trauma involves oedematous swellings and/or bruising. During labour, the fetal part overlying the cervical os may be subjected to pressure, i.e. a *girdle of contact*, with reduced venous return and resultant congestion and oedema.

Caput Succedaneum

With cephalic presentation, there may be a diffuse oedematous swelling under the scalp but above the periosteum, called a *caput succedaneum* (Fig. 35.3). With an occipitoanterior position, one caput succedaneum may present. With an occipitoposterior position, a caput succedaneum may form, but if the occiput rotates anteriorly a second caput succedaneum may develop.

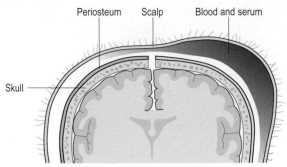

Fig. 35.3 Caput succedaneum.

If, during the second stage of labour, the birth of the head is delayed, the perineum may act as another *girdle of contact* with a further caput succedaneum forming. A *false* caput succedaneum can also occur if a vacuum extractor cup is used; because of its distinctive shape and position, the swelling is known as a *chignon* (Fig. 35.2).

A caput succedaneum is present at birth, thereafter decreasing in size. This swelling can *pit* on pressure, can cross a suture line, may be discoloured or bruised, may be associated with increased moulding, and the oedema may move to the dependent area of the scalp. The baby may appear to be in discomfort and, although care continues as normal, the baby should be handled gently. Abrasion of a chignon may occur.

The swelling is usually self-limiting and resolves within 36 h, with no long-term consequences (Sorantin et al. 2006). An abraded chignon usually heals rapidly if the area is kept clean, dry, and is not irritated.

Other Injuries

The cervical os may also restrict venous return when the fetal presentation is not cephalic. When the face presents, it becomes congested, bruised and the eyes and lips become oedematous. In a breech presentation, oedematous genitalia and buttocks may be bruised. In both instances, there may be discomfort and pain, therefore gentle handling of the newborn baby is essential and mild analgesia should be considered.

For babies with bruised or oedematous buttocks, maintaining nappy area hygiene with care to not cause further skin trauma is important. Barrier ointment or cream may be applied, particularly if nappies designed to limit the contact of urine and faecal fluid with the skin are not available. If skin excoriation occurs, the infection risk increases and consultation with a wound care specialist nurse may be required to ensure best skin care practice is undertaken.

Uncomplicated oedema and bruising usually resolve within days. However, if the baby suffers significant superficial trauma during birth, resulting serious complications requiring treatment could take longer to resolve. These complications include excessive haemolysis resulting in hyperbilirubinaemia; and rarely excessive blood loss resulting in anaemia, hypovolaemia, shock and disseminated intravascular coagulation (DIC). Sometimes, excessive damage to muscles can result in difficulties with micturition and defecation.

Muscle Trauma

Injuries to muscles can result from tearing or when the blood supply is disrupted.

Torticollis

The sternocleidomastoid (sternomastoid) muscles run from the side of the top of the sternum and the middle-third of the clavicle, alongside the neck, and are inserted into the mastoid process of the temporal bone. Torticollis is the result of tightness and shortening of one sternomastoid muscle. The aetiology of torticollis is not fully understood. It may occur if the muscle is torn due to excessive traction or twisting during the birth of the anterior shoulder of a fetus with a cephalic presentation, or during rotation of the shoulders when the fetus is being born by vaginal breech or caesarean section.

A 1–3 cm, apparently painless, hard lump of blood and fibrous tissue is felt on the affected sternomastoid muscle. The muscle length is shortened, therefore the neck is twisted to the affected side: a *torticollis* or *wry neck*. If the techniques for assisting at the above stages of birth are correctly applied, the incidence of torticollis can be prevented (Saxena 2019).

Torticollis management involves carers and parents performing passive muscle-stretching exercises, initially under the guidance of a physiotherapist, actively encouraging the baby to move the neck. The swelling usually resolves over several weeks to months with minimal sequelae. Surgical intervention may be required if there is no resolution by 1 year of age and therefore follow-up by the paediatric team to ensure achievement of normal movement, is recommended (Saxena 2019).

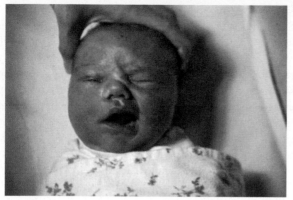

Fig. 35.4 Right-sided facial palsy. Note that the eye is open on the paralysed side and the mouth is drawn over to the non-paralysed side. (Reproduced from Thomas R, Harvey D (1997) Colour guide: neonatology (2nd ed.). Edinburgh: Churchill Livingstone, with permission of Elsevier.)

Nerve Trauma

The nerves most vulnerable to birth trauma are the facial nerve and the brachial plexus. Spinal cord injury is very rare and is not discussed here; an excellent explanation is given in Brand (2006).

Facial Nerve

The facial or seventh (VII) cranial nerve runs close to the skin surface and is vulnerable to compression, resulting in unilateral facial palsy. Compression may occur in the uterus but is more likely during birth by the maternal sacral promontory or by a misapplied forceps blade, especially when the baby is macrosomic. On the affected side, the baby appears to have no nasolabial fold, the eyelid remains open and the mouth is drawn over to the unaffected side (Fig. 35.4). The baby will drool excessively and may be unable to form an effective seal on the breast or teat, resulting in initial feeding difficulties, and may also have difficulty swallowing (Bruns 2019).

There is no specific treatment. If the eyelid remains open, regular instillation of eye drops lubricate the eyeball. Feeding difficulties are usually overcome by the baby's own adaptation, although alternative feeding positions may help. Spontaneous resolution is usually within weeks, with improvement appearing within 24–48 h. Recovery may be delayed but referral for appropriate plastic surgery must be made if recovery is delayed (Bruns 2019).

Brachial Plexus

Nerve roots exiting from the spine at the fifth to eighth cervical (C5–C8) and the first thoracic (T1) vertebrae form a matrix of nerves in the neck and shoulder: the brachial plexus. Brachial plexus birth palsy occurs due to traction on the brachial plexus at the time of birth. During vaginal or even caesarean section births, such injuries can happen due to forces of uterine contraction or assistance at the birth. Risk factors are difficult to determine but maternal diabetes, maternal obesity and prolonged second stage of labour may increase risk (British Medical Journal [BMJ] Evidence Centre 2012).

Nerve injury can be a stretch injury with a conduction block that resolves over a few months (*neuropraxia*). This is by far the most common. More severe injury, classified as *axonotmesis*, occurs when there is rupture of the axon but the nerve sheath is intact. Complete recovery can be expected; generally by 3–6 months. The most severe type of brachial plexus injury is *neurotmesis*, where there is complete division of the nerve. There is minimal recovery of function by 6 months and consequently, the baby will require surgical repair.

Narakas (1986) classification defines groups according to the potential areas of concern during recovery:
Group 1: paralysis of shoulder and biceps
Group 2: paralysis of shoulder, biceps, and wrist extensors
Group 3: paralysis of the entire limb
Group 4: paralysis of entire limb with temporary Horner's sign
Group 5: paralysis of entire limb with persistent Horner's sign and poor recovery.

Trauma to C5–C6 results in **Erb's palsy** (Erb–Duchenne/Duchenne–Erb), where there is paralysis of the shoulder muscles, biceps, elbow flexor and forearm supinator muscles. The baby's affected arm is limp, inwardly rotated, the elbow extended and the wrist pronated. When C7 is also traumatized, the baby presents with an extended Erb's palsy, in which the wrist and finger extensor muscles are affected, resulting in wrist and finger flexion – the 'waiter's tip position' (Fig. 35.5).

When there is trauma to C8–T1, **Klumpke's palsy** presents. The shoulder and upper arm are unaffected but the lower arm, wrist and hand are paralysed, resulting in wrist drop, no grasp reflex and a claw-like appearance of the hand. If there is associated trauma to the cervical sympathetic nerves, *Horner syndrome* may

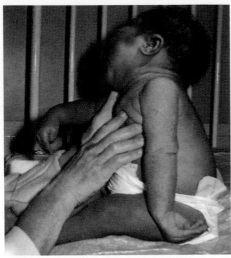

Fig. 35.5 Erb's palsy. (Reproduced from Thomas R, Harvey D (1997) Colour guide: neonatology (2nd ed.). Edinburgh: Churchill Livingstone, with permission of Elsevier.)

present with no sensation on the affected side, pupil constriction and eyelid ptosis.

If there is trauma to C5–T1, the result is **total brachial plexus palsy** (Erb–Klumpke), where there is complete paralysis of the shoulder, arm and hand, lack of sensation and circulatory problems. *Horner syndrome* may also occur. If there is bilateral paralysis, spinal injury should be suspected (Benjamin 2005; Foad et al. 2009; Semel-Concepcion 2018).

Investigations are not usually necessary in all cases. An X-ray may identify clavicle or humeral fractures if there are concerns, and an ultrasound scan may be used to investigate a dislocated shoulder or diaphragmatic paralysis.

Careful handling of the baby that avoids any extremes of motion, including the affected arm from dangling, is essential to enable the initial inflammation to subside. The baby should not be lifted by the arms or axilla, rather supported under the head and shoulders with one hand and the other hand placed under the buttocks. When changing clothes, the affected arm should be dressed first and undressed last.

After the initial phase, parents should receive physiotherapy advice on home-based exercise programmes with regular monitoring (Benjamin 2005, Foad et al. 2009, BMJ Evidence Centre 2012). Natural recovery still can occur post 3 months of age and surgical treatment has showed benefit in the recovery of regaining movement.

Fractures

Fractures are rare but the most commonly affected bones are the clavicle, humerus, femur and those of the skull. With all such fractures, a *crack* may be heard during the birth. With most fractures, distortion, deformity, swelling or bruising are usually evident on examination; crepitus may be felt; the baby appears to be in pain and is reluctant to move the affected area. The baby requires gentle handling to avoid further pain and an analgesic may be necessary. An X-ray examination may be undertaken to confirm the diagnosis.

Clavicle

Clavicular fractures are the most common fractures and may occur with shoulder dystocia, vaginal breech birth or if the baby is macrosomic. The affected clavicle is usually the one that was nearest the maternal symphysis pubis. Brachial plexus and phrenic nerve injuries should be excluded by careful examination in the affected baby (Laroia 2015; Mavrogenis et al. 2011). Fractures of the clavicle require no specific treatment and a stable union usually occurs within 7–10 days, while the humerus and femur can take between 2 and 4 weeks to repair (Laroia 2015).

Humerus

Midshaft humeral fractures can occur with shoulder dystocia or during a vaginal breech birth if the extended arm is forced down and born (Laroia 2015). To immobilize a fractured humerus, a pad should be placed in the baby's axilla and the arm firmly splinted with the elbow bent across the chest with a bandage, ensuring respirations are not embarrassed.

Femur

Midshaft femoral fractures can occur during vaginal breech birth if the extended legs are forced down and born (Laroia 2015). A fractured femur should be immobilized using a splint and bandage. Traction and plaster casting may be required.

Skull

Traumatic skull fractures from instrumental or difficult births are rare, with an incidence of around 4 per 100,000 births and a single parietal linear fracture is the most common form (Mohan et al. 2013). There may be no signs but an overlying swelling, cephalhaematoma or signs of associated complications such as intracranial haemorrhage or neurological disturbances, may suggest the presence of a fracture.

X-ray examination may confirm the fracture. However, if there are neurological concerns, a computerized tomography (CT) scan may be undertaken to detect intracranial haemorrhage that could require surgical intervention. A simple linear fracture usually requires no treatment and heals quickly with no sequelae. Treatment of a depressed fracture depends on the depth of the concavity. Shallow depressions in asymptomatic babies usually resolve spontaneously. With a deeper depression or where there are signs of complications, such as a basal skull fracture that can cause cerebrospinal fluid (CSF) leakage via the ear or nose, there is a requirement for surgical repair and antibiotic therapy to reduce the incidence of contamination and subsequent infection.

Babies may also present with a unique form of skull injury known as a *ping-pong* or *pond* skull fracture. This is a depressed skull fracture on the surface of the newborn skull caused by inner buckling of the calvarium due to the soft and resilient nature of the neonatal skull (Suneja et al. 2015). The fracture is called a *ping pong* fracture because it resembles a ping pong ball that has been indented inwards with a finger (Fig. 35.6). Such fractures can occur as a consequence of birth trauma or from the pressure caused by the

mother's pelvic bones against the soft fetal skull during labour. Most fractures of this nature are managed without any intervention but occasionally, surgical intervention is required, depending on the severity of the depression. Generally, these fractures do not cause any long-term damage but rarely, should complications occur, permanent neurological damage is possible (Qureshi 2018).

HAEMORRHAGES

Blood volume in the term baby is approximately 80–100 mL/kg and in the preterm baby 90–105 mL/kg, therefore even a small volume haemorrhage may be potentially fatal. In this section, haemorrhages are discussed according to their principal cause, or in relation to other factors. Haemorrhages may be due to:

- trauma
- disruption in blood flow

or can be related to:

- coagulopathies
- other causes.

Haemorrhages Due to Trauma

Cephalhaematoma

A cephalhaematoma (cephalohaematoma) is an effusion of blood under the periosteum that covers the skull bones (Fig. 35.7). During a vaginal birth, if there is friction between the fetal skull and maternal pelvic bones, such as in cephalopelvic disproportion or precipitate labour, the periosteum may be torn from the bone, causing bleeding underneath. Cephalhaematomas may also occur during vacuum-assisted births. Factors that increase pressure on the fetal head and the risk of developing a cephalhaematoma include a long labour, prolonged

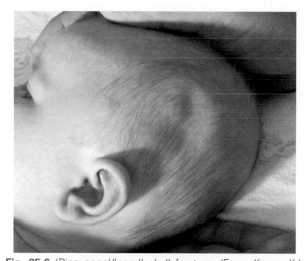

Fig. 35.6 'Ping pong'/'pond' skull fracture. (From Knoop KJ, Stack LB, Storrow AB, Thurman RJ. (2016) The atlas of emergency medicine (4th ed.). New York: McGraw-Hill Education. Copyright McGraw-Hill Education. All rights reserved.) Available at: www.accessemergencymedicine.

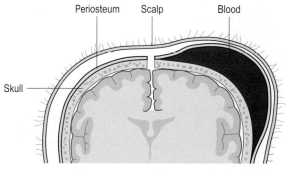

Fig. 35.7 Cephalhaematoma.

second stage of labour, macrosomia, weak or ineffective uterine contractions, abnormal fetal presentation, instrument-assisted birth with forceps or vacuum extractor and multiple gestations.

Due to the fact that the fetal or newborn skull bones are not fused, and as the periosteum is adherent to the edges of the skull bones, a cephalhaematoma is confined to one bone. However, more than one bone may be affected; therefore multiple cephalhaematomas can develop. A double cephalhaematoma is usually bilateral (Fig. 35.8). A caput succedaneum can also co-exist with a cephalhaematoma.

Unlike caput succedaneum, a cephalhaematoma is not always present at birth; the swelling appears after around 12 h of age, grows larger over subsequent days and can persist for weeks. The swelling is firm, does not pit on pressure, does not cross a suture and is fixed (Blackburn and Ditzenberger 2007). Factors that increase pressure on the fetal head and the risk of developing a cephalhaematoma include, long labour, prolonged second stage of labour, macrosomia, weak or ineffective uterine contractions, fetal malpresentation, instrumental assisted birth with forceps or vacuum extractor and multiple gestations (Raines and Jain 2019). No treatment is necessary and the swelling subsides when the blood is reabsorbed. Hyperbilirubinaemia may complicate recovery due to haemolysis of the extravasated blood. More rarely, complications such as sepsis, osteomyelitis and meningitis may occur. An underlying skull fracture may be associated with cephalhaematoma (Paul et al. 2009; Laroia 2015).

Subaponeurotic Haemorrhage

Subaponeurotic (subgaleal) haemorrhage is rare. Under the scalp, the *epicranial aponeurosis*, a sheet of fibrous tissue that covers the cranial vault allowing for muscles to attach to the bone, provides a potential space above the periosteum through which veins travel. Excessive traction on these veins results in haemorrhage, the epicranial aponeurosis is pulled away from the periosteum of the skull bones and swelling is evident (Fig. 35.9). Subaponeurotic haemorrhage may occur spontaneously with any type of birth but is more often associated with forceps and vacuum-assisted births, and severe dystocia (Reid 2007).

The swelling is present at birth, increases in size and is a firm, fluctuant mass. The scalp is moveable rather than fixed. The swelling can cross sutures and extend into the subcutaneous tissue of the neck and eyelids. Babies can lose large volumes of blood relatively quickly and may appear pale, be hypotonic, tachycardic and tachypnoeic (*hypovolaemic shock*). There can be discomfort or pain with head movement or handling of the swelling. A caput succedaneum and/or a cephalhaematoma may co-exist with a subaponeurotic haemorrhage. If the subaponeurotic haemorrhage is excessive, there is the potential for severe shock, disseminated intravascular coagulation (DIC) and death. This emergency situation requires immediate medical assistance, resuscitation, stabilization and full supportive care, including large volumes of blood transfusion and replacement of coagulation factors (Blackburn and Ditzenberger 2007).

With a smaller haemorrhage and in the babies who survive a larger haemorrhage, the blood is reabsorbed and the swelling and bruising resolve over 2–3 weeks.

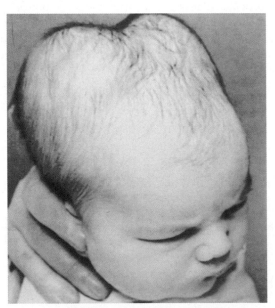

Fig. 35.8 Bilateral cephalhaematoma.

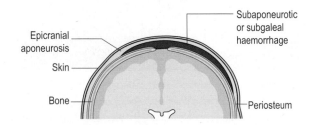

Fig. 35.9 Subaponeurotic haemorrhage.

Hyperbilirubinaemia complicates recovery (Reid 2007; Schierholz and Walker 2010).

Subdural Haemorrhage

A sickle-shaped, double fold of dura mater, the falx cerebri, dips into the fissure between the cerebral hemispheres. Attached at right angles to the falx cerebri, between the cerebrum and the cerebellum, is a horseshoe-shaped fold of dura mater – the tentorium cerebelli. In these folds of dura run large venous sinuses draining blood from the brain.

Normally, moulding of the skull bones and stretching of the underlying structures during birth are well tolerated. Trauma to the fetal head, such as excessive compression or abnormal stretching, may tear the dura, particularly the *tentorium cerebelli*, rupturing venous sinuses and resulting in a subdural haemorrhage. Predisposing factors include rapid, abnormal or excessive moulding, such as in precipitate labour or rapid birth, malpositions, malpresentations, cephalopelvic disproportion or undue compression during forceps manoeuvres (Barker 2007; Inder et al. 2018a).

A baby with a small haemorrhage may demonstrate no signs and resolution is spontaneous. Alternatively, the haemorrhage may initially be small but if blood continues to leak, signs develop over several days. As blood accumulates, there is cerebral irritation, cerebral oedema and raised intracranial pressure. The baby is likely to vomit, be unresponsive, have a bulging anterior fontanelle, be hypotonic, hyperthermic, apnoeic, bradycardic and experience convulsions.

With small lesions, close surveillance of the baby's condition is almost always followed by a favourable outcome. However, rapid detection and prompt surgical evacuation in the presence of progression of neurological signs is essential for large haemorrhages. Surgical referral should not be delayed if clear neurological deterioration becomes apparent.

The best imaging modality for those with suspected subdural haemorrhage are CT scans. Magnetic resonance imaging (MRI) may be more helpful if other brain pathologies are suspected. Supportive treatment focuses on replacing blood volume and controlling the consequences of asphyxia and raised intracranial pressure. Surgery to relieve pressure or subdural taps or shunt placement to drain large collections of blood may be required. A shunt is a drainage tube surgically inserted and connected to a one-way valve placed subcutaneously behind the ear. The valve's outflow tube is attached to a catheter allowing drainage into a large vein in the neck, or into the peritoneum, allowing reabsorption and elimination (Blackburn and Ditzenberger 2007). The prognosis for all affected babies, except those who experience massive haemorrhage, is usually good (Barker 2007; Inder et al. 2018a).

Haemorrhages Due to Disruptions in Blood Flow

Subarachnoid Haemorrhage

A primary subarachnoid haemorrhage involves bleeding directly into the subarachnoid space. Preterm babies who suffer perinatal hypoxia resulting in disruption of cerebral blood flow are most often affected. A secondary haemorrhage involves leakage of blood into the subarachnoid space from an intraventricular haemorrhage. Although classified here as a haemorrhage due to a disruption in blood flow, a subarachnoid haemorrhage may also occur due to birth trauma, particularly in term babies, similar to that which results in subdural haemorrhage (Inder et al. 2018a).

Depending on the extent of the haemorrhage, the affected baby may demonstrate no signs, while others may have generalized convulsions from the second day of life and have apnoeic episodes. Although rare, a massive subarachnoid haemorrhage may occur and is usually fatal despite emergency resuscitation and stabilization efforts. These babies have usually sustained severe perinatal asphyxia, sometimes with an element of trauma at the time of birth (Inder et al. 2018a).

Subarachnoid haemorrhage can be diagnosed with a CT scan or MRI. Supportive treatment focuses on replacing blood volume and controlling the consequences of asphyxia and raised intracranial pressure. Surgery to relieve pressure or subdural taps or shunt placement to drain large collections of blood may be required (Barker 2007).

Most subarachnoid haemorrhages are small, self-limiting and do not cause long-term damage. If post-haemorrhagic hydrocephalus occurs, drainage via a shunt may be required. The prognosis is usually very good for all affected babies, except those with related damage due to hypoxia (Barker 2007; Inder et al. 2018a).

Germinal Matrix Haemorrhage, Intraventricular Haemorrhage and Periventricular Haemorrhagic Infarction (Intraparenchymal Lesion)

Germinal matrix haemorrhage (GMH), *intraventricular haemorrhage* (IVH) and *periventricular haemorrhagic infarction* (PVHI) also known as *intraparenchymal lesion* (IPL), primarily affect babies born at <32 weeks' gestation and those weighing <1500 g at birth, although, rarely, more mature babies may be affected. The incidence and severity of these haemorrhages/lesions are inversely correlated with gestational age.

There are three grades of GMH and IVH:

1. A grade I haemorrhage that extends into the germinal matrix is a *germinal matrix, periventricular* or *subependymal haemorrhage*.
2. A grade II haemorrhage that extends into the lateral ventricle(s)without ventricular enlargement is known as an *intraventricular haemorrhage*.
3. A grade III haemorrhage is a grade 2 haemorrhage that is complicated by a blockage to the outflow of CSF (produced by the choroid plexus of the lateral ventricles) causing enlargement (i.e. dilatation) of the ventricles (Annibale and Hill 2018; Inder et al. 2018b).

Initially it was understood that a grade III haemorrhage may extend into the cerebral tissue, resulting in a *parenchymal haemorrhage*, known as a grade IV haemorrhage (Papile et al. 1978). Volpe (1997) proposed that the intraventricular clot in a grade III haemorrhage disrupts venous drainage, causing stasis and infarction. Reperfusion of the area causes haemorrhage into the infarcted area and necrotic damage of the white matter. Therefore, a grade IV haemorrhage was reclassified as a complication of a grade III IVH where the lesions persist and there is damage to the brain parenchyma, referred to as a PVHI with IPL used interchangeably (Annibale and Hill 2018; Inder et al. 2018b).

The stage of brain development is a crucial factor in the aetiology of GMH, IVH and PVHI/IPL. The two lateral ventricles are lined with ependymal tissue. Tissue lying immediately next to the ependyma is the germinal matrix, also known as the subependymal layer. From 8 to 32 weeks' gestation, neuroblasts and glioblasts are produced in the germinal matrix and migrate to the cerebral cortex. Neuronal migration is complete by 20 weeks' gestation but glial cell development and migration continues until approximately 32 weeks' gestation. During this period, a rich blood supply is provided to the germinal matrix through fragile immature capillaries that lack supporting muscle or collagen fibres. These vessels are particularly vulnerable to fluctuations in cerebral blood flow and pressure, rupturing easily causing haemorrhage. The ability of preterm babies to autoregulate cerebral blood flow and pressure is immature, resulting in an increased vulnerability to haemorrhage. After 32 weeks' gestation, the germinal matrix becomes less active and by term, has almost completely involuted: the capillaries become more stable and autoregulation becomes established; therefore GMH, IVH and PVHI/IPL in more mature babies are less common than in those babies born at <32 weeks' gestation (Annibale and Hill 2018).

The venous drainage from white matter and the deep areas of the brain, including the lateral ventricles, involves a peculiar U-turn route in the area of the germinal matrix. Disruptions to venous flow lead to congestion, with a risk of venous infarctions and ischaemia. With reperfusion of these ischaemic areas, there may be haemorrhage, demonstrated as PVHI (Volpe 2008a; Inder et al. 2018b).

Multiple factors may compromise cerebral haemodynamics resulting in GMH, IVH and PVHI/IPL. Early factors include obstetric haemorrhage, lack of antenatal steroids, maternal intrauterine infection, a low 1-min Apgar score and low umbilical artery pH. Later risk factors include acidosis, hypotension, hypertension, hypoglycaemia, hyperglycaemia, anaemia, mechanical ventilation, apnoea, rapid volume expansion, rapid administration of hyperosmolar solutions, pneumothorax and tracheal suctioning. Also implicated are excessive handling, exposure to light and noise, lateral flexion of the baby's head and crying (Blackburn 2018; Annibale and Hill 2018).

Most affected babies show no signs or signs that are nonspecific, therefore the haemorrhage/infarction/lesion is detectable only on ultrasound scan. If the haemorrhage is larger or extends, the clinical features may gradually appear and worsen, including apnoeic episodes that become more frequent and severe, bradycardia, hypotension, pallor, declining packed cell volume, tense anterior fontanelle, metabolic acidosis and convulsions. The baby may be limp or unresponsive. If the haemorrhage is large and sudden in onset, apnoea and circulatory collapse may present (Annibale and Hill 2018). At-risk babies should be screened by 7 days of life for IVH. Serial scanning may determine any increase, extension or complication (Inder et al. 2018a).

Care of at-risk babies is focused on prevention (Blackburn and Ditzenberger 2007). The birth of preterm babies should be in a regional obstetric unit with neonatal intensive care facilities. Prenatal maternal steroids and postnatal surfactant replacement therapy should be administered. Delayed cord clamping may also reduce the risk of IVH. Postnatally, haemodynamic stability is essential, as is prevention of complications. Prevention of hypoxic events and blood flow and pressure fluctuations may reduce the risk of IVH. Care is focused on maintaining normothermia, normoglycaemia, adequate oxygenation and ensuring the handling of the baby is restricted. The baby's developmental needs should be met, particularly in relation to supportive flexed positioning, reduction in bright lighting, maintaining a quiet, undisturbed environment and ensuring appropriate interaction with parents and others (Blackburn and Ditzenberger 2007; Inder et al. 2018b).

Despite preventative measures, babies do develop GMH, IVH and PVHI/IPL. The outcome depends on the nature of the haemorrhage/lesion and associated conditions/complications. The neurological prognosis for babies with a GMH or a small IVH is usually good. An IVH associated with ventricular dilatation may resolve spontaneously with no long-term consequences. However, with a large IVH and ventricular dilatation, the accumulating CSF may require temporary drainage using ventricular taps or external ventricular drainage. Some babies may require permanent CSF drainage via a shunt. Approximately 30–40% of these babies will have cognitive or motor disabilities. Although the incidence of major neurological sequelae (e.g. spastic motor deficits, major cognitive deficits) after minor degrees of haemorrhage is slightly higher than that in infants without haemorrhage and increases to approximately 50% in infants with severe haemorrhage, a *clearly higher* incidence occurs in babies with IVH complicated by periventricular haemorrhagic infarction or cystic periventricular leucomalacia (PVL), or both. For those babies who, in addition to severe IVH, also exhibit apparent periventricular haemorrhagic infarction, mortality rates approach 50% in the infants weighing <750 g at birth and are approximately 20% in those with a birth weight of 751–1500 g, with the incidences of

subsequent hydrocephalus being even higher; survival is usually complicated in the majority by significant cognitive and motor disabilities. Long-term follow-up is essential and parents need much support (Blackburn and Ditzenberger 2007; Annibale and Hill 2018; Inder et al. 2018b).

Periventricular Leucomalacia

Although not a haemorrhage, *periventricular leucomalacia* (PVL) is included here because of its association with GMH, IVH and PVHI/IPL. Between 27 and 30 weeks' gestation, the area of white matter around the lateral ventricles and within the watershed area of the deep cerebral arteries undergoes considerable development. It is sensitive to any insult that results in reduced cerebral perfusion, such as those associated with GMH, IVH, PVHI and chorioamnionitis. The cerebral blood flow autoregulation ability in preterm babies is limited, increasing their risk of developing PVL. Reduced perfusion results in areas of ischaemia and degeneration of the nerve fibre tracts that disrupts nerve pathways between areas of the brain and between the brain and spinal cord. This softening and necrosis of the white matter is PVL; it may be a classic focal necrotic cystic type or a diffuse non-cystic type. Only the former is seen on ultrasound scan but MRI may detect both types (Blackburn and Ditzenberger 2007; Volpe 2008a; Zach 2015).

Similar pathogenesis is seen in the older preterm and term baby, but the lesion occurs in the subcortical region rather than the periventricular region. This is because the watershed moves away from the ventricles to the cortex once the germinal matrix involutes. These lesions are known as subcortical leucomalacia (Volpe 1997).

Care instituted to reduce the incidence of GMH, IVH and PVHI/IPL may reduce the incidence of PVL or the severity of the related ischaemic damage. The prognosis is variable; some babies have little resulting impairment, others develop cognitive and neurodevelopmental impairment, while the most severely affected babies may develop spastic diplegic cerebral palsy (Blackburn and Ditzenberger 2007; Zach 2015; Inder et al. 2018a).

Haemorrhages Related to Coagulopathies

These haemorrhages occur due to disruption of the baby's blood-clotting abilities.

Vitamin K Deficiency Bleeding

Vitamin K deficiency bleeding (VKDB) may occur up to 6 months of age, although it more commonly occurs between birth and 8 weeks of life. It was previously known as haemorrhagic disease of the newborn (HDN). Several proteins, factor II (prothrombin), factor VII (proconvertin), factor IX (plasma thromboplastin component), factor X (thrombokinase) and proteins C and S, require vitamin K for their conversion to active clotting factors. A deficiency of vitamin K, as in VKDB, leads to a deficiency of these clotting factors and resultant bleeding.

Vitamin K_1 (phytomenadione/phytonadione/phylloquinone) is poorly transferred across the placenta and fetal liver stores are low. Stores are quickly depleted after birth and for normal clotting to occur, the baby must receive dietary vitamin K_1, the absorption of which requires fat and bile salts. Vitamin K_2 (menaquinone) is synthesized by bowel flora and may assist in the conversion of proteins to active clotting factors. Because the neonate's bowel is sterile, vitamin K_2 production is restricted until colonization has occurred. Therefore all newborns are deficient in vitamin K and vulnerable to VKDB.

There are three forms of VKDB that were first described by Lane and Hathaway (1985):

1. *early* (0–24 hours)
2. *classical* (1–7 days)
3. *late* (1–6 months, although the peak onset is before 8 weeks).

Early VKDB is rare, principally affecting babies born to women who, during pregnancy, have taken anticonvulsants, e.g. phenytoin, barbiturates or carbamazepine; antitubercular drugs, e.g. rifampin, isoniazid; or vitamin K antagonists, e.g. warfarin (contraindicated during pregnancy) for treatment of their medical conditions. As these drugs interfere with vitamin K metabolism, avoidance during pregnancy reduces the risk of early VKDB.

The babies most susceptible to developing classic VKDB are those with birth trauma, asphyxia, postnatal hypoxia and those who are preterm, or of low birth weight. They are more likely to spontaneously bleed or have invasive interventions resulting in bleeding that cannot be controlled. Disruptions to the colonization of the bowel due to antibiotic therapy, or lack of, or poor enteral feeding, may also result in *classic* VKDB.

The bowel of a breastfed baby colonizes with lactobacilli that do not synthesize menaquinone. The amount of vitamin K_1 in breastmilk is naturally low, although colostrum and hindmilk do contain higher levels than foremilk. The vitamin K_1 in breastmilk is considered insufficient for the exclusively breastfed baby's needs. Artificial infant formulae are fortified with vitamin K_1, offering some prophylaxis against VKDB (Blackburn 2018). Therefore *late* VKDB occurs almost exclusively in breastfed babies. However, babies who have liver disease or a condition that disrupts vitamin K_1's absorption from the bowel, for example cystic fibrosis, may develop *late* VKDB (Blackburn 2018).

The baby who has VKDB may have bruising; or bleeding from the umbilicus, puncture sites, the nose or the scalp; or severe jaundice for >1 week and/or persistent jaundice for >2 weeks. Gastrointestinal bleeding manifests as melaena and haematemesis. In early and late VKDB, there may be extracranial and intracranial bleeding. With severe haemorrhage, circulatory collapse occurs. Late VKDB is associated with higher mortality and morbidity. Blood tests reveal prolonged prothrombin time (PT) with a usually normal partial thromboplastin time (PTT) and a normal platelet count.

Babies diagnosed with VKDB require investigation and monitoring to assess their need for treatment. With all forms of VKDB, the baby will require administration of vitamin K_1, 1–2 mg intramuscularly. In severe cases, when coagulation is grossly abnormal and there is severe bleeding, replacement of deficient clotting factors is essential. If circulatory collapse and severe anaemia occur, blood transfusion or exchange transfusion may be required. Affected babies usually require other supportive therapy to assist in their recovery.

As VKDB is a potentially fatal condition, prophylactic administration of vitamin K is recommended for all babies and is administered to all preterm and ill babies as part of their treatment regime (Nimavat 2019; Blackburn 2018). For otherwise healthy term babies, the National Institute for Health and Clinical Excellence ([NICE] 2015) recommends that vitamin K_1 1 mg given intramuscularly after birth is the most effective prophylaxis for prevention of early onset VKDB. Some vitamin K_1 remains within the muscle and acts as a slow release depot, providing prophylaxis for classic and probably also for late VKDB (Hey 2003).

For healthy term babies, whose parents decline a single intramuscular injection of vitamin K_1, an oral prophylaxis regimen is recommended (NICE 2015), although there is no consensus on the most effective oral regime. It is suggested that whatever oral regime is used, multiple doses are required in the first week of life and if the baby is breastfed, a further dosing regime is required until at least 12 weeks of age, if not longer. Such prophylaxis should reduce the risk of all forms of VKDB, however this is dependent on the involvement, motivation and compliance of healthcare professionals and parents. Medical advice should be sought if the baby vomits within 1 h of oral administration or is too unwell to take the preparation orally.

All parents should be given the opportunity to discuss vitamin K_1 prophylaxis during pregnancy, understand the specific management of preterm, ill and *at-risk* babies, and agree on their choice of prophylaxis. They should also understand the signs and treatment of VKDB, especially if their baby has one or more of the risk factors (NICE 2015).

Thrombocytopaenia

Thrombocytopaenia results from a decreased rate of formation of platelets or an increased rate of consumption and is defined as a platelet count of $<150 \times 10^9/L$, and severe thrombocytopaenia is a platelet count of $<50 \times 10^9/L$ (Roberts and Murray 2008; Chakravorty and Roberts 2012; Bagwell 2013; Dror et al. 2016).

Thrombocytopaenia may be classified according to fetal, neonatal and late onset causes. Fetal causes include alloimmunity, congenital infection and trisomics. Early onset (<72 h) neonatal causes include placental insufficiency, perinatal asphyxia, perinatal infection, disseminated intravascular coagulation (DIC) and autoimmunity. Late onset (>72 h) neonatal causes include late onset sepsis, necrotizing enterocolitis (NEC), congenital infection and autoimmunity (Chakravorty and Roberts 2012).

The most at-risk babies are those with an older sibling who was diagnosed with thrombocytopaenia, babies born preterm who have had chronic intrauterine hypoxia such as with pregnancy-induced hypertension or diabetes and/or associated intrauterine growth restriction (Roberts and Murray 2008; Chakravorty and Roberts 2012).

Neonatal alloimmune thrombocytopaenia (NAIT) occurs when there is incompatibility between maternal and fetal platelets. Maternal antibodies cross the placenta destroying the fetal platelets – a mechanism similar to that of haemolytic disease of the newborn. If the fetus is severely affected, an intracranial haemorrhage and severe bleeding may result in fetal death. If a previous sibling has developed NAIT, in subsequent pregnancies, the fetus should be monitored using fetal blood sampling and/or ultrasound scan to determine the need for maternal immunoglobulin administration and/or steroids and/or intrauterine platelet transfusions, and possibly elective birth at 32–34 weeks' gestation (Roberts and Murray 2008). If diagnosed with NAIT postnatally, babies usually require specially treated platelet transfusions to achieve and maintain a platelet count within normal limits.

Neonatal autoimmune thrombocytopaenia may occur in babies whose mothers have autoimmune conditions such as idiopathic thrombocytopaenic purpura or systemic lupus erythematosus. The antibodies produced by the mother against her own platelets may cross the placenta, destroying the baby's platelets. The resultant thrombocytopaenia is usually mild, but in severe cases, immunoglobulin administration is effective (Roberts and Murray 2008; Chakravorty and Roberts 2012).

Thrombocytopaenia may appear as a petechial rash, presenting in a mild case with a few localized petechiae. In a severe case, there is widespread and serious haemorrhage from multiple sites. Intracranial haemorrhage may be fatal. Diagnosis is based on history, clinical examination and a reduced platelet count. It is differentiated from other haemorrhagic disorders because coagulation times, fibrin degradation products and red blood cell morphology are normal. Mild or moderate thrombocytopaenia is usually self-limiting and requires no treatment. In severe cases, the treatment usually includes platelet concentrate transfusion/s, although the optimum regime is yet to be determined (Roberts and Murray 2008).

Disseminated Intravascular Coagulation

Disseminated intravascular coagulation (DIC), also known as '*consumptive coagulopathy*', is an acquired coagulation disorder associated with the release of thromboplastin from damaged tissue, stimulating abnormal coagulation in the microcirculation as well as excess fibrinolysis. There is excessive consumption of clotting factors and platelets, predisposing the baby to haemorrhage. DIC is secondary to primary conditions. Maternal causes of neonatal DIC include pre-eclampsia,

eclampsia and placental abruption. Fetal causes include severe fetal compromise, the presence of a dead twin in the uterus and traumatic birth. Neonatal causes include conditions resulting in hypoxia and acidosis, severe infections, hypothermia, hypotension and thrombocytopaenia (Bagwell 2013; Levi 2013).

As clotting factors and platelets are depleted and fibrinolysis is stimulated, the baby will develop a generalized purpuric rash and bleed from multiple sites. With stimulation of the clotting cascade, multiple microthrombi may occlude vessels, with organ and tissue ischaemia, particularly affecting the kidneys, resulting in haematuria and reduced urine output. As the cycle of consumptive coagulopathy continues, multiorgan failure results (Bagwell 2013; Levi 2013). The diagnosis is made from clinical signs and laboratory findings that show a low platelet count, low fibrinogen level, distorted and fragmented red blood cells, low haemoglobin and raised fibrin degradation products (FDPs) with a prolonged PT and PTT (Bagwell 2013; Levi 2013).

Treatment must focus on correction of the underlying cause if possible and full supportive care will be required. Control of DIC requires transfusions of fresh frozen plasma, concentrated clotting factors and platelets. Cryoprecipitate is an excellent source of fibrinogen. If anaemia is diagnosed, transfusions of whole blood or red cell concentrate are required. Occasionally, an exchange transfusion of fresh heparinized blood may be performed, to remove FDPs, while replacing the clotting factors. If treatment of the primary disorder and/or replacement of clotting factors is ineffective, the administration of heparin may reduce fibrin deposition (Levi 2013). The prognosis depends on the severity of the primary condition, as well as of the DIC and the baby's response to treatment.

Haemorrhages Related to Other Causes
Umbilical Haemorrhage

This usually occurs as a result of a poorly applied cord ligature. The use of plastic cord clamps has almost eliminated this type of haemorrhage, although it is essential to avoid catching or pulling the clamp. Tampering with partially separated cords before they are ready to separate is discouraged. Umbilical haemorrhage is a potential cause of death. A purse-string suture should be inserted if bleeding continues after 15 or 20 min of manual pressure.

Vaginal Bleeding

A small temporary vaginal discharge of bloodstained mucus occurring in the first days of life: pseudo-menstruation, is due to the withdrawal of maternal oestrogen. This is a normal physiological phenomenon. Parents need to know that this is a possibility and is self-limiting. Continued or excessive vaginal bleeding warrants further investigation to exclude pathological causes (Grider and Hillard 1997).

Haematemesis and Melaena

These signs may present when the baby has swallowed maternal blood during birth, or from cracked nipples during breastfeeding. The diagnosis must be differentiated from VKDB, from other causes of haematemesis that include oesophageal, gastric or duodenal ulceration and from other causes of melaena, that include necrotizing enterocolitis and anal fissures. These causes need specific and usually urgent treatment (Wolfram 2018). If the cause is swallowed blood, the condition is self-limiting and requires no specific treatment. If the cause is cracked nipples, appropriate treatment for the mother must be implemented.

Haematuria

Haematuria may be associated with coagulopathies, vascular thrombosis, urinary tract infections and structural malformations of the urinary tract. Birth trauma may cause renal contusion and haematuria (Joseph and Gattineni 2016; Jernigan 2014). Occasionally, after suprapubic aspiration of urine, transient mild haematuria may be observed. Treatment of the primary cause should resolve the haematuria.

CONVULSIONS

A convulsion (seizure/fit) is a sign of neurological disturbance, not a disease, and the occurrence of a convulsion is a medical emergency. Because the newborn brain is still developing, its function is immature and there is an imbalance between stimulation and inhibition of neural networks. Convulsions present quite differently in the neonate and may be more difficult to recognize than those in later infancy, childhood or adulthood (Volpe 2008b).

Convulsive movements can be differentiated from jitteriness or tremors in that, with the latter two, the movements are rapid, rhythmic, equal and are often stimulated or made worse by disturbance and can be stopped by touching or flexing the affected limb. They are normal in an active, hungry baby and are of no consequence, although their occurrence should be documented. Convulsive movements in contrast, tend to be slower, less equal and are not necessarily stimulated by disturbance. They cannot be stopped by restraint, they may be accompanied by abnormal eye movements and cardiorespiratory changes and are always pathological. Convulsive movements should also be differentiated from the benign bilateral or localized jerking that occurs normally in neonatal sleep, particularly rapid eye movement sleep.

Abnormal, sudden or repetitive movements of any part of the body that are not controlled by repositioning or containment holds, require investigation. Volpe (2008b) suggests that the type of movement can help classify the convulsion as *subtle, tonic, clonic* or *myoclonic*:

- *Subtle* convulsions include movements such as blinking or fluttering of the eyelids, chewing and cycling movements of the legs and apnoea. There may or may not be associated abnormal electroencephalogram (EEG) activity.
- Focal *tonic* convulsions affect one extremity and abnormal brain electrical activity can be detected on EEG. With generalized tonic convulsions, which are more common than focal tonic convulsions, the baby sustains a rigid extended posture, similar to decerebrate posturing; not usually detected on EEG.
- Focal *clonic* convulsions are unilateral, affecting the face, neck or the trunk or upper or lower extremity, whereas multifocal clonic convulsions affect several areas of the body that jerk asynchronously and migrate. The movements are slow (one to three jerks per second), rhythmic and are most likely to be associated with EEG activity.
- *Myoclonic* convulsions differ from clonic convulsions, in that they are faster and are not associated with EEG activity. Focal myoclonic convulsions affect the upper body flexor muscles. Multifocal myoclonic convulsions affect several parts of the body with asynchronous jerks. Generalized myoclonic convulsions affect the upper and sometimes lower extremities with jerking flexion movements.

During a convulsion, the baby may have tachycardia, hypertension, raised cerebral blood flow and raised

TABLE 35.1 Selected Causes of Neonatal Convulsions

Category	Selected Causes
Central nervous system	Intracranial haemorrhage Intracerebral haemorrhage Hypoxic-ischaemic encephalopathy Kernicterus Congenital malformations
Metabolic	Acquired disorders of metabolism Hypoglycaemia and hyperglycaemia Hypocalcaemia and hypercalcaemia Hyponatraemia and hypernatraemia Inborn errors of metabolism
Other	Hypoxia Congenital infections Severe postnatally acquired infections Neonatal abstinence syndrome Hyperthermia
Idiopathic	Unknown

intracranial pressure, which predispose to serious complications.

As convulsions may be difficult to recognize, all at-risk babies must be continuously assessed. The underlying conditions that may result in a convulsion are classified as central nervous system, metabolic, other and idiopathic conditions (Table 35.1). Convulsions may be acute, recurrent or chronic (Blackburn and Ditzenberger 2007).

If a convulsion is suspected, a complete history and physical and laboratory investigations related to the possible cause should be undertaken. An EEG may help detect abnormal electrical brain activity and guide treatment. Immediate treatment necessitates obtaining assistance from a doctor while ensuring that the baby has a clear airway and adequate ventilation, either spontaneously or mechanically. The baby can be turned to the semi-prone position, with the head in a neutral position. Facial oxygen should be applied, and gentle oral and nasal suctioning may be required to remove any mucus or milk. In some cases active resuscitation maybe required (see Chapter 33). The need for intravenous access should be assessed. Any necessary handling must be gentle and the baby is usually nursed in an incubator to allow for observation and to monitor temperature regulation.

It is important that the nature of the convulsion is documented, noting the type of movements, the areas affected, the length of the convulsion, the baby's state of consciousness, colour change, alteration in heart rate, respiratory rate or blood pressure and immediate sequelae (Blackburn and Ditzenberger 2007).

The aims of care are to treat the primary cause/s and the pharmacological control of the convulsions. The latter is controversial due to the potential of incurring further damage from the drugs versus the potential damage from the convulsion on the developing brain (Rennie and Boylan 2007; Volpe 2008b). While there is little robust research evidence for the use of any anticonvulsants in neonates, there is consensus for the use of such drugs, particularly when the baby experiences prolonged or frequent convulsions (Volpe 2008b; Jensen 2009).

If pharmacological treatment is prescribed, the drugs most commonly used are phenobarbital and phenytoin; less frequently, benzodiazepines may be used. Over the past decade, additional anticonvulsants such as levetiracetam have been developed and are increasingly being used, but their effectiveness in neonatal seizures is still to be evaluated. Anticonvulsant therapy may be discontinued when convulsions cease, preferably before the baby is transferred home from hospital.

The outcome for babies who have convulsions is likely to depend on the cause, onset, type of convulsion and frequency, whether it was demonstrated on EEG and whether the tracing became normal following treatment, what type of treatment was used and how long it was before the baby showed signs of improvement. A good prognosis is usual if convulsions were due to hypocalcaemia, hyponatraemia or an uncomplicated subarachnoid haemorrhage. Much poorer prognoses are associated with severe hypoxic ischaemia, severe IVH, severe infections and central nervous system congenital anomalies (Blackburn and Ditzenberger 2007). Complications of neonatal seizures may include cerebral palsy, hydrocephaly, epilepsy and spasticity (Sheth 2017).

SUPPORT OF PARENTS

Trauma during birth, haemorrhages and convulsions are unexpected complications and parents may be shocked and anxious, and perhaps find themselves in a crisis situation. However, not all parents experience such feelings and some can adapt quickly to their baby's condition (Fowlie and McHaffie 2004; Carter et al. 2005; McGrath 2013).

BOX 35.1   Summary of Key Principles Related to the Baby, Parents and Family

The baby must be valued as an individual person by:
- using the baby's name
- not predicting the future
- always keeping the baby with the parents where possible when sharing information.

The parents and family must be respected by:
- facilitating parental support and empowerment
- acknowledging cultural and religious differences
- listening to their views and taking their concerns seriously
- giving information honestly and sensitively using uncomplicated language
- ensuring understanding and providing opportunities for them to ask questions
- facilitating follow-up and providing further information when required.

(Adapted from Scope (2003) Right from the start template: good practice in sharing the news. London: Scope/Department of Health. Available at: www.yumpu.com/en/document/read/6786226/right-from-the-start-audit-template-scope)

The extent of the midwife's and other healthcare professionals' contact with parents will depend on the circumstances but the experiences parents have at this time have longer-term implications for them, their response to the situation, their relationships with the multiprofessional care team as well as their interaction with, and care of, their baby (McGrath 2013).

One of the most important aspects of caring for the parents is in relation to **communication**. All parents should be fully informed about their baby's condition, treatment and care in ways that are considered best practice. The *Right from the Start template* (Scope 2003), although published some years ago, provides an excellent guide, and the principles related to the baby, parents and family are summarized in Box 35.1.

Parental involvement in their baby's care is essential and the family-centred care/partnership with parents approach should now pervade all midwifery and neonatal settings. Staniszewska et al.'s (2012) study reported the collaborative development of the first robust philosophy of set principles that underpin the POPPY (Parents of Premature babies Project) model of care and a set of indicators to guide the global implementation in neonatal units. Such a model of care can assist neonatal units to better meet parents' needs for information, communication and support. Midwives and neonatal nurses therefore have an important role in promoting adaptive coping mechanisms and guiding parents to appropriate resources and support services (POPPY Steering Group 2009). The baby charity BLISS offers helpful information for parents and its website includes a parent message board. Additional support and information is available from specialized outside agencies and the charity 'Contact a Family' is a useful resource in the longer term.

REFLECTIVE ACTIVITY FOR SELF-ASSESSMENT

1. What is the significance of examining the baby's head immediately following birth and during the neonatal period? How would you distinguish between a caput succedaneum and a cephalhaematoma?

2. Explain the difference between Vitamin K deficiency bleeding (VKDB; previously known as 'haemorrhagic disease of the newborn') and haemolytic disease of the newborn. How would you diagnose these conditions and what would be the subsequent management of the baby?

3. What would be your immediate action and the subsequent care of a baby who was demonstrating convulsive movements? What could be the possible causes?

4. How would you support parents to interact and care for their baby who has experienced birth trauma to the brachial plexus as a result of shoulder dystocia during birth?

REFERENCES

Annibale, D. J., & Hill, J. G. (2018). *Intraventricular hemorrhage in the preterm infant*. Available at: https://emedicine.medscape.com/article/976654-overview.

Bagwell, G. A. (2013). Haematologic system. In C. Kenner JW. Lott (Ed.), *Comprehensive neonatal nursing care* (5th ed.) (pp. 334–375). New York: Springer.

Barker, S. (2007). Subdural and primary subarachnoid haemorrhages: A case study. *Neonatal Network, 26*(3), 143–151.

Benjamin, K. (2005). Part 2: Distinguishing physical characteristics and management of brachial plexus injuries. *Advances in Neonatal Care, 5*(5), 240–251.

Blackburn, S. T. (2018). *Haematologic and hemostatic systems, maternal, fetal and neonatal physiology: A clinical perspective* (5th ed.). Philadelphia: Saunders/Elsevier.

Blackburn, S. T., & Ditzenberger, G. R. (2007). Neurologic system. In C. Kenner, & JW. Lott (Eds.), *Comprehensive neonatal care: An interdisciplinary approach* (4th ed.) (pp. 277–294). Philadelphia: Saunders/Elsevier.

Brand, M. C. (2006). Part 1: Recognizing neonatal spinal cord injury. *Advances in Neonatal Care, 6*(1), 15–24.

British Medical Journal (BMJ) Evidence Centre. (2012). *Erb's Palsy*. Available at: http://bestpractice.bmj.com/best-practice/monograph/746.

Bruns, A. D. (2019). *Congenital facial paralysis*. Available at: https://emedicine.medscape.com/article/878464-overview #showall.

Carter, J. D., Mulder, R. T., Bartram, A. F., et al. (2005). Infants in a neonatal intensive care unit: Parental response. *Archives of Disease in Childhood, Fetal and Neonatal Edition, 90*(2), F109–F113.

Chakravorty, S., & Roberts, I. (2012). How I manage neonatal thrombocytopenia. *British Journal of Haematology, 156*(2), 155–162.

Dror, Y., Chan, A. K. C., Baker, J. M., & Avila, M. L. (2016). Hematology. In M. G. MacDonald, & M. M. K. Seshia (Eds.), *Avery's neonatology: Pathophysiology and management of the newborn* (7th ed.) (pp. 872–929). Philadelphia: Wolters Kluwer.

Foad, S. L., Mehiman, C. T., Foad, M. B., et al. (2009). Prognosis following neonatal brachial plexus palsy: An evidence-based review. *Journal of Children's Orthopedics, 3*(6), 459–463.

Fowlie, P. W., & McHaffie, H. (2004). Supporting parents in the neonatal unit. *British Medical Journal, 329*, 1336–1338.

Grewal, S. K. (2018). *Subcutaneous fat necrosis of the newborn*. Available at: https://emedicine.medscape.com/article/1081910-overview.

Grider, A. R., & Hillard, P. A. (1997). Vaginal bleeding in pediatric patients. *Journal of Pediatric and Adolescent Gynecology, 10*(3), 173.

Hey, E. (2003). Vitamin K – what, why and when. *Archives of Disease in Childhood Fetal and Neonatal edition, 88*(2), F80–F83.

Inder, T. E., Perlman, J. M., & Volpe, J. J. (2018a). Intracranial hemorrhage: Subdural, subarachnoid, intraventricular (term infant), miscellaneous. In J. J.

Volpe, T. E. Inder, B. T. Darras, et al. (Eds.), *Volpe's neurology of the newborn* (6th ed.) (pp. 593–622). Philadelphia: Elsevier.

Inder, T. E., Perlman, J. M., & Volpe, J. J. (2018b). Preterm intraventricular haemorrhage/posthemorrhagic hydrocephalus. In J. J. Volpe, T. E. Inder, B. T. Darras, et al. (Eds.), *Volpe's neurology of the newborn* (6th ed.) (pp. 637–700). Philadelphia: Elsevier.

Jensen, F. E. (2009). Neonatal seizures: An update on mechanisms and management. *Clinics in Perinatology*, *36*(4), 881–900.

Jernigan, S. M. (2014). Hematuria in the newborn. *Clinics in Perinatology*, *41*(3), 591–603.

Joseph, C., & Gattineni, J. (2016). Proteinuria and hematuria in the neonate. *Current Opinion in Pediatrics*, *28*(2), 202–208.

Lane, P. A., & Hathaway, W. E. (1985). Vitamin K in infancy. *Journal of Pediatrics*, *106*, 351–359.

Laroia, N. (2015). *Birth trauma*. Available at: https://emedicine.medscape.com/article/980112-overview.

Levi, M. (2013). Disseminated intravascular coagulation. In R. Hoffman, E. J. Benz, LE Silberstein, et al. (Eds.), *Hematology: Basic principles and practice* (6th ed.) (pp. 2001–2012). Philadelphia: Saunders/Elsevier.

Mavrogenis, A. F., Mitsiokapa, E. A., Kanellopoulos, A. D., et al. (2011). Birth fractures of the clavicle. *Advances in Neonatal Care*, *11*(5), 328–331.

McGrath, J. M. (2013). Family: Essential partner in care. In C. Kenner, & J. W. Lott (Eds.), *Comprehensive neonatal nursing care* (5th ed.) (pp. 739–772). New York: Springer.

Mohan, S., Rogan, E. A., Batty, R., et al. (2013). CT of the neonatal head. *Clinical Radiology*, *69*, 1155–1166.

NICE (National Institute for Health and Care Excellence). (2015). *Postnatal care up to 8 weeks after birth: CG 37*. London: NICE. Available at: www.nice.org.uk/guidance/cg37/resources/postnatal-care-up-to-8-weeks-after-birth-pdf-975391596997.

Narakas, A. O. (1986). Injuries to the brachial plexus. In F. W. Bora (Ed.), *The pediatric upper extremity: Diagnosis and management* (pp. 247–258). Philadelphia: WB Saunders.

Nimavat, E. J. (2019). Vitamin K deficiency bleeding. Available at: https://emedicine.medscape.com/article/974489-overview.

Papile, L. A., Burnstein, J., Burnstein, R., et al. (1978). Incidence and evolution of subependymal and intraventricular hemorrhage: A study of infants with birth weights less than 1500 g. *Journal of Pediatrics*, *92*(4), 529–534.

Paul, S. P., Edate, S., & Taylor, T. M. (2009). Cephalhaematoma – a benign condition with serious complications: Case report and literature review. *Infant*, *5*(5), 146–148.

POPPY Steering Group. (2009). *Family-centred care in neonatal units. A summary of research results and recommendations from the POPPY project*. London: National Childbirth Trust. Available at: www.nna.org.uk/assets/poppy_family-centered-care.pdf.

Qureshi, N. H. (2018). *Skull fracture*. Available at: https://e-medicine.medscape.com/article/248108-overview.

Raines, D. A., & Jain, S. (2019). Cephalhaematoma, *StatPearls*,(Internet) Treasure Island (FL), *StatPearls* Publishing Available at: https://www.ncbi.nlm.nih.gov/books/NBK470192/.

Rewid, J. (2007). Neonatal subgaleal haemorrhage. *Neonatal Network*, *26*(4), 219–227.

Rennie, J. M., & Boylan, G. (2007). Treatment of neonatal seizures. *Archives of Disease in Childhood, Fetal and Neonatal Edition*, *92*(2), F148–F150.

Roberts, I., & Murray, N. A. (2008). Neonatal thrombocytopenia. *Seminars in Fetal and Neonatal Medicine*, *13*(4), 256–264.

Saxena, A. K. (2019). *Pediatric torticollis surgery*. Available at: https://emedicine.medscape.com/article/939858-overview.

Schierholz, E., & Walker, S. R. (2010). Responding to traumatic birth. *Advances in Neonatal Care*, *10*(6), 311–315.

Scope. (2003). *Right from the start template: Good practice in sharing the news*. London: Scope/Department of Health. Available at: www.yumpu.com/en/document/read/6786226/right-from-the-start-audit-template-scope.

Semel-Concepcion, J. (2018). *Neonatal brachial plexus palsies*. Available at: https://emedicine.medscape.com/article/317057-overview.

Sheth, R. D. (2017). *Neonatal seizures*. Available at: https://e-medicine.medscape.com/article/1177069-overview.

Sorantin, E., Brader, P., & Thimary, F. (2006). Neonatal trauma. *European Journal of Radiology*, *60*(2), 199–207.

Staniszewska, S., Brett, J., Redshaw, M., et al. (2012). The POPPY study: Developing a model of family-centred care. *Worldviews Evidence Based Nursing*, *9*(4), 243–255.

Suneja, U., Prokhorov, S., Kandi, S., & Rajegowda, B. (2015). Depressed skull fractures in a term newborn. *Pediatrics and Therapeutics*, *5*(4), 1000i109.

Volpe, J. J. (1997). Brain injury in the premature infant. *Clinics in Perinatology*, *24*(3), 567–587.

Volpe, J. J. (2008a). Intraventricular hemorrhage: Germinal matrix-intraventricular hemorrhage of the premature infant. In J. J. Volpe (Ed.), *Neurology of the newborn* (pp. 517–588). Philadelphia: WB Saunders.

Volpe, J. J. (2008b). Neonatal seizures. In J. J. Volpe (Ed.), *Neurology of the newborn* (pp. 203–244). Philadelphia: WB Saunders.

Wolfram, W. (2018). *Pediatric gastrointestinal bleeding*. Available at: https://emedicine.medscape.com/article/1955984-overview.

Zach, T. (2015). *Pediatric periventricular leukomalacia.* Available at: https://emedicine.medscape.com/article/975728-overview.

ANNOTATED FURTHER READING

Best Beginnings. Available at: www.bestbeginnings.org.uk/small-wonders and www.youtube.com/user/bestbeginnings

Best Beginnings has produced Small Wonders: 12 bite-size films following families and their journey in neonatal units throughout the UK.

Boxwell, G. (Ed.). (2010). *Neonatal intensive care nursing* (2nd ed.). London: Routledge.

This is a comprehensive, evidence-based text for neonatal nurses and midwives caring for ill newborn babies, focusing on the common problems occurring within the neonatal intensive care unit. It provides a useful resource to support healthcare professionals working in the field of newborn care, to recognize, rationalize and remedy such conditions using both a multisystems and an evidence-based approach.

Lissaueur, T., Fanaroff, A. A., Miall, L., & Fanaroff, J. (Eds.). (2019). *Neonatology at a glance.* Chichester: Wiley-Blackwell.

This text, written by leading international experts provides a concise, illustrated overview of neonatal medicine, including the normal newborn infant and neonatal problems encountered in neonatal intensive care units and their management. Each topic is supported by illustrations, diagrams and a range of video clips including neonatal resuscitation and the recognition of seizures.

Meeks, M., Hallsworth, M., & Yeo, H. (Eds.). (2010). *Nursing the neonate* (2nd ed.). Chichester: Wiley-Blackwell.

Written by a multidisciplinary team of medical and nursing experts, this 2nd edition provides evidence-based coverage of all frequently seen neonatal conditions in an accessible format and is highly illustrated with relevant diagrams and pictures. The text is divided into chapters based on body-systems and includes clear guidelines for procedure and discussion of best practice, including application to case studies.

Rennie, J. M. (Ed.). (2012). *Rennie and Roberton's textbook of neonatology* (5th ed.). Edinburgh: Churchill Livingstone.

A *classic textbook that provides the most contemporary methods of diagnosis, treatment and care of the neonate, alongside detailed pathophysiology of every significant neonatal condition, e.g. neonatal seizures, intracranial haemorrhage and hypoxic ischaemic brain injury, albeit from a medical perspective. Included in this edition are informative chapters on the psychological aspects of neonatology such as handling perinatal death.*

USEFUL WEBSITES

Best Beginnings: www.bestbeginnings.org.uk

BLISS – for sick or premature babies: www.bliss.org.uk

British Association of Perinatal Medicine: www.bapm.org

Child Bereavement UK (CBUK): www.childbereavementuk.org

Contact a Family: www.contact.org.uk

National Institute for Health and Care Excellence: www.nice.org.uk

Royal College of Paediatrics and Child Health: www.rcpch.ac.uk

Royal College of Obstetricians and Gynaecologists: www.rcog.org.uk

36

Congenital Malformations

Judith Simpson, Kathleen O'Reilly

CHAPTER CONTENTS

The incidence of major congenital malformations is 2–3% of all births, although this figure is subject to familial, cultural and geographic variations. It is therefore likely that every practising midwife will at some time in their career be confronted with the challenge of providing appropriate care and support for such babies and their families.

THE CHAPTER AIMS TO

- describe and explain specific congenital anomalies
- explore the role of the midwife in supporting parents who are faced with the diagnosis of a baby who has a congenital malformation

- discuss early management options including palliative care for life-limiting conditions.

COMMUNICATING THE NEWS

Improved prenatal screening and diagnostic techniques (see Chapter 13) have led to the increased recognition of malformations, particularly in early pregnancy. As a result, some women may make the decision to have their pregnancy terminated, while for others it provides time to adjust to and begin to come to terms with the news that their baby will be born with a particular problem. One advantage of prenatal diagnosis is that, if necessary, arrangements can be made for the woman to give birth in a unit where appropriate specialist neonatal services are available. The disadvantage of such a transfer is that the mother may then be separated from family, friends and the support of the midwives she knows best. This makes it even more important that the staff in these units are sensitive to the needs of such women.

Even with universal fetal screening, not all malformations will be identified prenatally and in this situation, it is often the midwife who first notices an anomaly either at birth or on routine newborn examination. While all anomalies should be notified to medical staff, there is sometimes uncertainty as to who should communicate the news to the parents. There is a strong argument for suggesting that this should be undertaken by the midwife present at the birth, with whom the parents will have formed a relationship. It is well recognized that one of the first questions a mother will ask the midwife after the birth is *'is the baby all right?'* It is preferable that the midwife informs the parents sensitively but honestly if they have any concerns and shows them any obvious anomaly in the baby.

Where there is doubt in the midwife's mind, for example in cases of suspected chromosomal disorders, it could be argued that the issue is less clear cut. Discretion could therefore be exercised in the precise form of words used, but the intention of inviting a second opinion should be made clear to the parents. It is advisable that both the parents and the midwife are present when an experienced paediatrician examines the baby and that the midwife is present during any dialogue between the parents and medical staff, so that they are aware of exactly what has been said. The midwife is then able to clarify or repeat any points that were not fully understood. Opportunities for follow-up consultation with the paediatrician should be offered as and when the parents desire. Patience, tact and understanding are prerequisites for midwives caring for these families.

Some malformations may appear minor to staff; however, it is important to appreciate that parental perceptions may be quite different and that the degree of distress can be unrelated to the apparent severity of the anomaly. The psychological impact on parents of being told and/or shown, that their baby has a congenital malformation has been likened to the grieving process discussed in Chapter 31. Great sensitivity is therefore required on the part of the midwife when communicating with the parents for the first time.

Whatever the anomaly, it is essential that families receive accurate, consistent and appropriate information about their baby's condition. It is preferable, where possible, for the baby to remain with its mother. Since a comprehensive discussion of every malformation is clearly not possible, selection has therefore been made of those that the midwife is most likely to encounter.

PALLIATIVE CARE

There are several severe congenital malformations, which are incompatible with sustained life, such as anencephaly. Many of these conditions are diagnosed antenatally and, whereas some parents opt for termination of the pregnancy, others choose palliative care after birth. It is important that parents feel supported in the choices they make. When parents opt to continue with the pregnancy, where possible, a plan for care of the baby when born should be made antenatally. This if often known as an *'Advance Care Plan'* or *'Anticipatory Care Plan'* and, with regard to previous discussions and parental wishes, is a valuable source of information for the attending health professionals at the time of the baby's birth.

Discussion with the parents should include information about the likely clinical course and explore any anxieties the parents may have, e.g. pain relief for the baby. It is important to be honest in cases where there is uncertainty. It may also be appropriate at this time to explore any specific wishes the parents may have, e.g. regarding religious ceremonies. Parents may find it helpful to meet with the palliative care team antenatally.

After birth, priority should be given to ensuring the comfort of the baby while at the same time, supporting the parents. The aim is to ensure that the baby's short life is as good as possible and to facilitate positive memory-making experiences for the family– this can take many forms, e.g. making hand and footprints, taking photographs, creating diaries and in caring for the baby through cuddling, bathing and dressing (see Chapter 38).

In cases where the baby survives for longer than expected, the specific aspects of the care plan may need to be reviewed and discussed with the parents (e.g. feeding). It is always important to treat the parents and the baby with kindness and dignity and to remember that the life of the baby is precious, no matter how short that life is.

Providing end-of-life care for infants with severe congenital malformations can be difficult and emotionally draining for staff. It is essential that staff caring for the baby feel comfortable with clinical decisions and are able to discuss any concerns they have. A formal debrief within the multiprofessional team may be useful.

DEFINITION AND CAUSES

By definition, a congenital malformation is any defect in form, structure or function. Identifiable defects can be categorized as follows (Fig. 36.1):
- chromosomal abnormalities
- single gene defects
- mitochondrial deoxyribonucleic acid (DNA) disorders

- teratogenic causes
- multifactorial causes
- unknown causes.

Chromosomal Malformations

Every human cell carries a blueprint for reproduction in the form of 44 chromosomes (autosomes) and two sex chromosomes. Each chromosome comprises a number of genes, which are specific sequences of DNA coding for particular proteins. The zygote should have 22 autosomes and one sex chromosome from each parent. Should a fault occur in either the formation of the gametes or following fertilization (see Chapter 5), variations in chromosome number (aneuploidies) or structure (deletions, duplications, inversions, translocations) may occur. Each abnormal chromosomal pattern has a characteristic clinical presentation, the most common of which will be discussed further, below.

Gene Defects (Mendelian Inheritance)

Genes are composed of DNA and each is concerned with the transmission of one specific hereditary factor. Genetically inherited factors may be *dominant* or *recessive*. A dominant gene will produce its effect even if present in only one chromosome of a pair. An autosomal dominant condition can usually be traced through several generations, although the severity of clinical expression may vary from generation to generation. *Congenital spherocytosis, achondroplasia, osteogenesis imperfecta, adult polycystic kidney disease* and *Huntington's chorea* are examples of dominant conditions.

A recessive gene needs to be present in both chromosomes before producing its effect. An individual who is carrying only one abnormal copy of the gene (a heterozygote) is unaffected. Examples of autosomal recessive conditions are *cystic fibrosis* or *phenylketonuria*.

Some congenital malformations are a consequence of single gene defects. In a dominantly inherited disorder the risk of an affected fetus is 1:2 (50%) for each pregnancy. In a recessive disorder, the risk is 1:4 (25%) for each pregnancy. In an X-linked recessive inheritance, the condition affects almost exclusively males, although females can be carriers. X-linked recessive inheritance is responsible for conditions such as *haemophilia A and B* and *Duchenne muscular dystrophy*. Spontaneous mutations commonly arise in X-linked recessive disorders. When a woman is a carrier of an X-linked condition, there is a 50% chance of each of her sons being affected

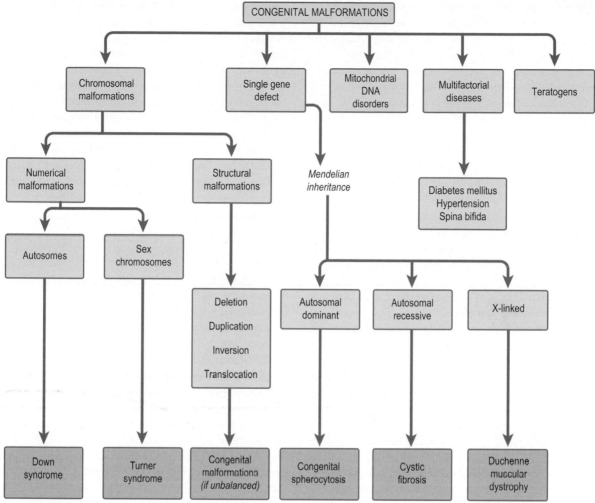

Fig. 36.1 Causes of congenital malformations. (Adapted from Beattie J, Carachi R (Eds.) (2005) Practical paediatric problems: a textbook for MRCPCH. London: Hodder Education.)

and an equal chance that each of her daughters will be carriers.

Chromosome microarray testing is a detailed genetic test that can detect extra or missing segments of DNA, known as duplications or deletions, respectively. Chromosome microarray testing is now widely available and may be useful for individuals whose clinical features do not fit with a specific syndrome but who demonstrate multiple congenital abnormalities. In such cases, discussion with or review by a clinical geneticist is often invaluable in aiding diagnosis given their expertise on dysmorphology and knowledge of appropriate genetic investigations.

Recent advancements in the understanding of inherited conditions have included increased awareness of the role of

epigenetic factors. Epigenetics is the study of factors other than the DNA structure, which can alter gene expression. Epigenetic regulation is important for tissue differentiation and normal embryonic development. Epigenetic factors influencing early development may be responsible for specific congenital syndromes. Continuing research may offer further diagnostic and treatment options in the future.

Mitochondrial Inheritance

Mitochondria are cellular structures responsible for energy production. Mitochondria are always inherited from the mother. Symptoms and signs of mitochondrial disorders can be diverse but tend to occur in tissues that have high energy requirements such as the brain and muscles.

Symptoms in the neonatal period may include hypotonia (which may be severe enough to necessitate respiratory support), cardiomyopathy, feeding difficulties, failure to thrive and vomiting and seizures. Mitochondrial disorders are very rare but include, *mitochondrial encephalomyopathy with lactic acidosis and stroke-like episodes* (MELAS) and *myoclonic epilepsy with ragged red fibres myopathy* (MERRF) (Chinnery et al. 1998).

Teratogenic Causes

A teratogen is any agent that raises the incidence of congenital malformation. The list of known and suspected teratogens is continually growing but includes:

- prescribed drugs (e.g. anticonvulsants, anticoagulants and preparations containing large concentrations of vitamin A such as those prescribed for the treatment of acne)
- drugs used in substance misuse (e.g. heroin, alcohol and nicotine)
- environmental factors such as radiation and chemicals (e.g. dioxins, pesticides)
- infective agents (e.g. rubella, cytomegalovirus, toxoplasmosis)
- maternal disease (e.g. diabetes).

It should be borne in mind that several factors influence the effect(s) produced by any one teratogen, such as gestational age of the embryo or fetus at the time of exposure, length of exposure and toxicity of the teratogen. Direct cause and effect are sometimes difficult to establish. Accurate recording of all congenital malformations on central registers, such as those included in the National Congenital Anomaly and Rare Disease Registration Service (NCAR-DRS), facilitates the early recognition of new teratogens.

Multifactorial Causes

These are due to interactions between specific genes (genetic susceptibility) and environmental influences (teratogens).

Unknown Causes

Despite a growing body of knowledge, the specific cause of many congenital anomalies remains unspecified and they occur sporadically in families.

CHROMOSOMAL MALFORMATIONS

Trisomy 21 (Down Syndrome)

Trisomy 21 or Down syndrome (commonly referred to as Down's syndrome) occurs when cells contain an extra copy of chromosome 21. The overall incidence of Trisomy 21 is around 1 in 700 live births. Trisomy 21 arising sporadically as a result of a non-disjunction process occurs in 95% of cases. Unbalanced translocation occurs in 2.5% of cases, usually between chromosomes 14 and 21. Mosaic forms (where not all cells have an extra copy of chromosome 21) may also occur. There is no difference between the types in clinical appearance. Parents who have a baby with Trisomy 21 should therefore be offered genetic counselling to establish the risk of recurrence.

The classic features of Trisomy 21 (Fig. 36.2) were first described in 1866 by physician John Langdon Down. He recognized a commonly occurring combination of facial features among individuals with low intelligence. Characteristic features include:

- up-slanting palpebral fissures
- a small head with flat occiput
- small nose
- small mouth with relatively large tongue
- short broad hands with an incurving little finger (clinodactyly), a single palmar (simian) crease
- a wide space between the great toe and second toe (sandal gap)
- Brushfield spots in the eyes
- generalized hypotonia.

Not all these manifestations need to be present and any of them can occur alone without implying chromosomal aberration. Babies born with Trisomy 21 also have a higher incidence of cardiac anomalies, cataracts, hearing loss, leukaemia and hypothyroidism. Although intelligence quotient is below average at 40–80, the degree of learning difficulty may vary considerably between individuals and while many are able to attend mainstream school and live semi-independent lives as adults, others require lifelong support for basic activities of daily living. Over the last 50 years, there has been a considerable change in both societal and medical attitudes towards people with Trisomy 21. As a consequence, the life expectancy of individuals with Trisomy 21 has increased over time. With appropriate medical care, the median life expectancy of people with Trisomy 21 is now almost 60 years, although there is a higher incidence of early onset Alzheimer's disease than in the general population (Bayen et al. 2018).

Although there may be little doubt in the midwife's mind that a baby has Trisomy 21 syndrome, they should be careful not to make any definitive statements. Family likeness alone may explain some babies' appearance. Parents themselves may voice their suspicions. If they do not, a sensitive but honest approach should be made by either

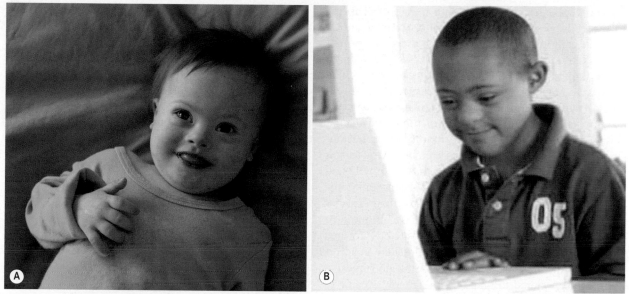

Fig. 36.2 (A) Baby with Down syndrome: note slant of eyes and incurving little finger. (B) With good parental involvement and stimulus these infants can reach maximum potential. (Photographs courtesy of A, iStock.com/ Tatiana Dyuvbanova (https://www.istockphoto.com/gb/photo/portrait-of-cute-baby-boy-with-down-syndrome -gm859395412-141970987); B, iStock.com/ Monkey Business Images (https://www.shutterstock.com/ image-photo/downs-syndrome-boy-laptop-202499914.)

the midwife or paediatrician to alert them to the possibility and to request permission to conduct further investigations. Investigations indicated include chromosome analysis and, following confirmation of a genetic diagnosis, echocardiography because of the increased risk of congenital heart disease. Rapid genetic testing is often available in the form of Quantitative Fluorescence-Polymerase Chain Reaction (QF-PCR) meaning that in cases where the diagnosis is suspected, this can be confirmed or refuted within 48 h (see Chapter 13). In confirmed cases, formal karyotype is required in order to identify possible inherited translocations. An individual baby's needs will vary depending on whether there are any co-existing anomalies. Although initial feeding problems are common owing to generalized hypotonia, breastfeeding should be encouraged and supported if that is what the mother had planned. The parents are likely to require a great deal of emotional support in the first few days following diagnosis. Providing audiovisual or reading material about Down syndrome for the parents may be helpful, or the address of the local branch of the Down Syndrome Association.

Ongoing paediatric follow-up is required both to manage any medical issues but also to monitor development and provide input from allied health services, e.g. physiotherapy and speech and language therapy to support the family and ensure that the child fulfils their developmental potential.

Trisomy 18 (Edwards Syndrome) and Trisomy 13 (Patau Syndrome)

Trisomy 18 (Edwards syndrome) occurs in approximately 1 in 5000 births. An extra 18th chromosome is responsible for the characteristic features. Facial features include a small head with a flattened forehead, a receding chin and frequently a cleft palate. The ears are low set and mal-developed. The sternum tends to be short, the fingers often overlap and the feet have a characteristic rocker-bottom appearance. Malformations of the cardiovascular and gastrointestinal systems, including exomphalos and oesophageal atresia are also common.

Trisomy 13 (Patau syndrome) occurs in around 1 in 5000–12,000 live births. An extra copy of the 13th chromosome leads to multiple abnormalities. Affected infants are small and microcephalic. Midline facial abnormalities such as cleft lip and palate are common and limb abnormalities are frequently seen. Brain, cardiac and renal abnormalities may co-exist with this trisomy.

The life expectancy for children born with Trisomy 13 and 18 is greatly reduced, with most affected children dying in early infancy. A small number do survive into early adulthood. This is more likely in cases of mosaicism where individuals are less severely affected. Those who do survive require long-term care because of significant physical and developmental needs. In many cases, the diagnosis may have been suspected or confirmed antenatally, which allows the opportunity for medical professionals and parents to make care plans even before the baby is born. Caring for families whose baby has Trisomy 13 and 18 requires kindness and sensitivity. It is important to be honest and help the parents to be realistic in their expectations, while remembering that each child is a unique individual. Management plans should therefore be informed by the clinical condition and needs of the child, in accordance with the wishes of the parents. Although surgery is not routinely offered to infants with Trisomy 13 and 18 (since it is unlikely to be beneficial in terms of improved survival) in some cases, it may be felt appropriate in order to alleviate symptoms or to facilitate discharge from hospital. Parents may find it useful to speak to other families where a child has Trisomy 13 or 18. SOFT UK may be a useful support and source of information for families.

Turner Syndrome (XO)

In this monosomal condition, affected females have only one normal X sex chromosome rather than the usual two. The absent chromosome is indicated by 'O'. Turner syndrome may be suspected on antenatal screening if there is increased nuchal translucency, aortic coarctation or a horseshoe kidney identified. Prenatal genetic testing may confirm the diagnosis. Physical characteristics at birth may include a short, webbed neck, widely spaced nipples and oedema of the hands and feet. In the absence of diagnostic clues antenatally or at the time of birth, the condition may not be identified until puberty, at which time short stature and delayed sexual development becomes apparent, because of underdeveloped ovaries.

GASTROINTESTINAL MALFORMATIONS

Prenatal ultrasound and increased access to fetal anomaly screening mean that many of these malformations are diagnosed before birth. This provides an opportunity for the parents to meet with the neonatal and surgical teams, and visit the specialist neonatal unit, in which their baby will be cared for, prior to the baby's birth.

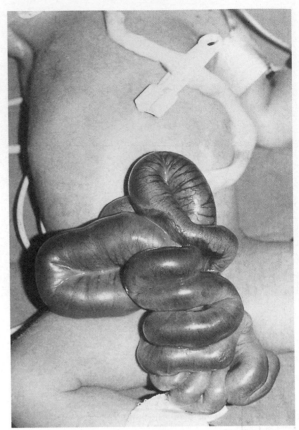

Fig. 36.3 Gastroschisis showing prolapsed intestine to the right of umbilical cord. (With permission from Rennie JM, Roberton NRC (Eds). (1999) Textbook of neonatology (3rd ed.). Edinburgh: Churchill Livingstone.)

Gastroschisis and Exomphalos

Gastroschisis and exomphalos are both referred to as defects of the anterior abdominal wall. They occur early in fetal development as a result of failure of the abdominal contents to return to within the abdominal cavity. They are almost always identified on prenatal ultrasound scanning, often within the first trimester (Prefumo and Izzi 2014). *Gastroschisis* (Fig. 36.3) is a paramedian defect of the abdominal wall with extrusion of bowel that is not covered by peritoneum. Closure of the defect is usually possible; the amount of extruded bowel will determine whether early primary closure is possible or whether a temporary silo (Fig. 36.4) made from synthetic materials (e.g. Silastic) is necessary until the abdominal cavity is able to accommodate all the abdominal organs (Prefumo and Izzi 2014).

Exomphalos or *omphalocele* (Fig. 36.5) is a defect in which the bowel or other viscera herniate into the

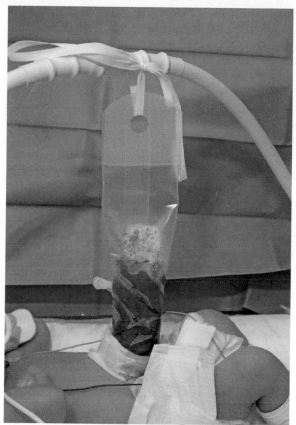

Fig. 36.4 Gastroschisis contained in a silo. (Reproduced with permission from the Medical Illustration Dept at the Royal Hospital for Sick Children, Glasgow.)

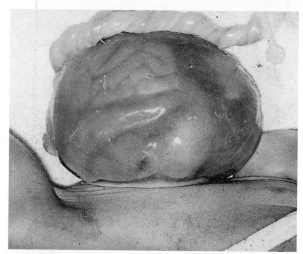

Fig. 36.5 Omphalocele defect with bowel visible through sac in the lower part and abnormally lobulated liver in the sac in the upper part. (With permission from Rennie JM, Roberton NRC (Eds). (1999) Textbook of neonatology (3rd ed.). Edinburgh: Churchill Livingstone.)

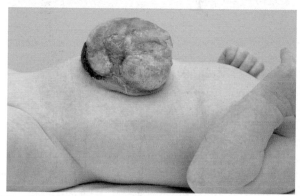

Fig. 36.6 Granulating omphalocele. (Reproduced with permission from the Medical Illustration Dept at the Royal Hospital for Sick Children, Glasgow (with approval of the parents.)

umbilical cord. Very often these babies have other problems, for example chromosomal or genetic defects, which require evaluation prior to surgery. The timing of surgical closure is determined by the size of the defect; small defects (exomphalos minor) undergo early primary closure, while a large defect (exomphalos major) is encouraged to granulate over (Fig. 36.6), prior to delayed closure at around 12 months (Prefumo and Izzi 2014).

The immediate management of both conditions is to cover the herniated abdominal contents with occlusive wrap (e.g. Clingfilm) to reduce fluid and heat loss and to give a degree of protection. An orogastric or nasogastric tube should be passed and stomach contents aspirated.

Atresias
Oesophageal Atresia
Oesophageal atresia occurs when there is incomplete canalization of the oesophagus in early intrauterine development. It is commonly combined with a tracheo-oesophageal fistula, which connects the trachea to the upper or lower oesophagus, or both. The commonest type of malformation is where the upper oesophagus terminates in a blind pouch and the lower oesophagus connects to the trachea. Around 50% of cases are associated with other malformations, often as part of a chromosomal or a genetic disorder such as the VACTERL spectrum (**V**ertebral anomalies, **A**nal anomalies, **C**ardiac, **T**racheo-**E**sophageal, **R**adial aplasia, renal and **L**imb anomalies). Further evaluation, particularly of the heart and great vessels, is required prior to surgery (Pedersen et al. 2012).

Oesophageal atresia may be suspected on prenatal ultrasound scan if the fetal stomach is not visualized but over half of cases are diagnosed after birth

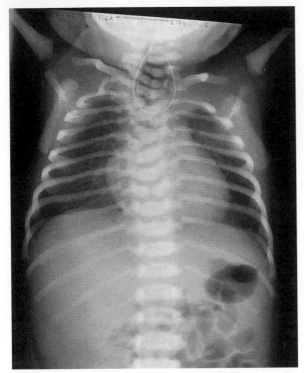

Fig. 36.7 Oesophageal atresia. Coiled feeding tube in proximal pouch. Note vertebral and rib abnormalities. Distal gas confirms a tracheo-oesophageal fistula. (With permission from Rennie JM, Roberton NRC (Eds). (1999) Textbook of neonatology (3rd ed.). Edinburgh: Churchill Livingstone.)

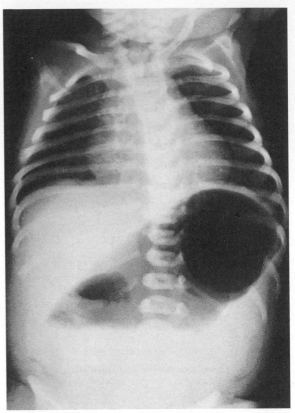

Fig. 36.8 Double bubble of duodenal atresia. The stomach is overlapping the duodenum with the second bubble being seen through the stomach. (With permission from Rennie JM, Roberton NRC (Eds). (1999) Textbook of neonatology (3rd ed.). Edinburgh: Churchill Livingstone.)

(Pedersen et al. 2012). The diagnosis should be considered in the presence of maternal polyhydramnios, especially if the baby appears 'mucousy' or noted to have 'colour changes' associated with copious oral secretions. The midwife should pass an orogastric tube but may feel resistance at <10–12 cm. Radiography will confirm the diagnosis (Fig. 36.7). The baby must be given no oral fluid and a wide bore oesophageal tube should be passed into the upper pouch and connected to gentle continuous suction apparatus to avoid build-up of secretions. Ideally, a double lumen (Replogle) tube is used. The baby should be transferred promptly to a neonatal surgical unit, ensuring that continuous suction is available throughout the transfer. It is usually possible to perform an early end-to-end anastomosis of the oesophagus and ligation of the fistula. Occasionally, if the gap in the oesophagus is too large, surgical repair is delayed. In this situation, a variety of techniques can be utilized to stretch the ends of the oesophagus, stimulate growth and eventually facilitate repair by end-to-end anastomosis.

Duodenal Atresia

Atresia can occur at any level of the bowel but the duodenum is the most common site. If this has not already been diagnosed in the prenatal period, the baby will present with persistent vomiting within 24–48 h of birth. The vomit may contain bile unless the obstruction is proximal to the entrance of the common bile duct, in which case it will be non-bilious. Abdominal distension is not necessarily present and the baby may pass meconium. A characteristic double bubble of gas is seen on radiological examination (Fig. 36.8). Treatment is by surgical repair. This anomaly is commonly associated with chromosomal disorders, in particular trisomy 21, which accounts for 30% of cases of duodenal atresia.

Anorectal Malformations

Careful examination of the perineum is an important aspect of the newborn examination. An imperforate anus

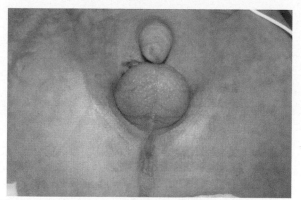

Fig. 36.9 Imperforate anus with rectovesical fistula (1). (Reproduced with permission from Donna Bain.)

should be obvious, but a rectal atresia might not become apparent until it is noted that the baby has not passed meconium. However, it is important to remember that a history of passing meconium does not exclude a diagnosis of an anorectal malformation. Occasionally, meconium is passed through a fistulous connection to the vagina, bladder or urethra and this may mask an imperforate anus (Figs 36.9–36.11). Whatever the anatomical arrangement, all babies should be referred for surgical assessment.

Malrotation/Volvulus

This is a developmental anomaly, whereby incomplete rotation (*malrotation*) of the small bowel has taken place. This predisposes the bowel to intermittent episodes of twisting (*volvulus*) and obstruction. A baby with malrotation may be entirely asymptomatic in the neonatal period; however episodes of obstruction can lead to bilious vomiting and abdominal distension. Due to the risk of severe, irreversible ischaemic bowel damage in unrecognized volvulus, any newborn infant with bile-stained vomiting requires urgent assessment. Surgical correction is necessary if a malrotation is confirmed.

Meconium Ileus (Cystic Fibrosis)

Around 15% of children with cystic fibrosis present with intestinal obstruction secondary to meconium ileus in the neonatal period. This occurs because their meconium is particularly viscous. Intravenous fluids and a contrast enema may relieve the obstruction but sometimes surgery is required. Histology of any resected bowel may suggest a diagnosis of cystic fibrosis, but genetic mutation analysis is required for confirmation. Subsequent treatment of cystic fibrosis is supportive

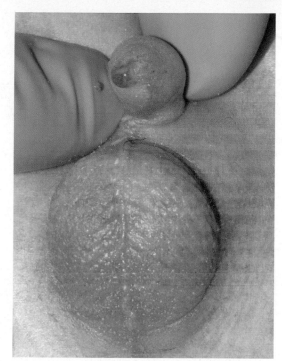

Fig. 36.10 Imperforate anus with rectovesical fistula (2). (Reproduced with permission from Donna Bain.)

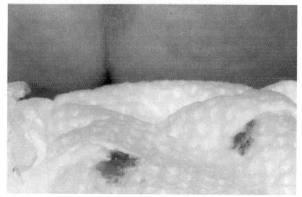

Fig. 36.11 Imperforate anus with rectovesical fistula and napkin containing meconium stained urine. (Reproduced with permission from Donna Bain.)

rather than curative and involves coordinated multi-disciplinary input including: optimized nutrition, chest physiotherapy and prophylactic antibiotics.

Hirschsprung Disease

In this disease, which has an incidence of 1 in 5000 live births, a segment of bowel does not contain the normal nerve supply and is referred to as aganglionic. This means

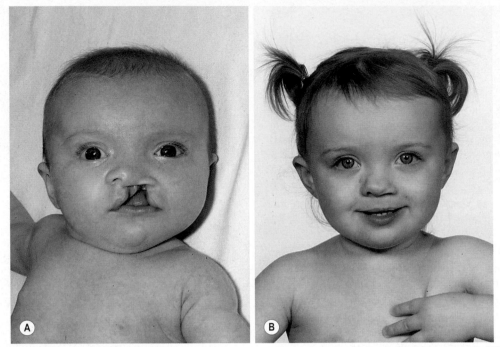

Fig. 36.12 (A) Pre-operative and (B) post-operative appearances of a left unilateral cleft lip and palate. (With permission from Paediatrics and Child Health Volume 22, Issue 4, April 2012, Pages 160-168, Figure 6.)

that bowel contraction (peristalsis) does not occur and it creates a functional bowel obstruction. The majority of babies present in the neonatal period with any combination of delayed passage of meconium (>24 h), abdominal distension and bile-stained vomiting. Hirschsprung disease is often suspected from radiography and contrast enema, however a rectal biopsy is required to confirm the diagnosis. Surgical resection of the aganglionic segment of bowel is indicated with a minority of babies requiring stoma formation (Bradnock et al. 2017).

Cleft Lip and Cleft Palate

The incidence of cleft lip occurring as a single malformation is 1.3 per 1000 live births. This anomaly may be unilateral or bilateral. Since cleft lip is very often accompanied by cleft palate, both will be considered together.

Clefts in the palate may affect the hard palate, soft palate or both. Some defects will include alveolar margins and some the uvula. The greatest problem for these babies initially is feeding. If the defect is limited to a unilateral cleft lip, mothers who had intended to breastfeed should be encouraged to do so. Where there is the additional problem of the cleft palate, establishing effective suck feeding can be more challenging, although a variety of specially shaped teats and bottles are available. Early referral to the local cleft lip and palate (CLAPA) multidisciplinary team including: specialist nursing staff, speech and language therapists, plastic surgeons, audiologists and orthodontists is recommended. Corrective surgery will be carried out at some stage, however agreement regarding optimal timing remains elusive (Shaye et al. 2015). To some extent, a compromise must always be made regarding the balance of risk from surgery, the psychological impact of the malformation, the effect on speech and language acquisition and future facial growth. In general, lips are repaired between 10 and 12 weeks and palates between 6 and 18 months. It can be helpful for the midwife to show families *'before and after'* photographs of babies for whom surgery has been a success (Fig. 36.12). In addition, ensuring that parents are aware of support groups such as the Cleft Lip and Palate Association is also important.

Pierre Robin Sequence

Pierre Robin sequence is characterized by micrognathia (underdevelopment of the lower jaw), posterior displacement of the tongue, which allows it to fall backward and occlude the airway, and a central cleft palate. This triad of anomalies presents challenges for neonatal care, notably airway obstruction and feeding difficulties. Minor airway obstruction can be managed with fairly straightforward interventions such as prone positioning or the use of a nasopharyngeal airway. However, in a minority of babies the anatomical anomaly is so severe that surgery, for example jaw distraction or tracheostomy, is required to create a safe airway (Bacher et al. 2010). Suck feeding can be problematic and supplemental tube feeding is sometimes required. A multidisciplinary team approach is essential for these babies and their parents will need considerable support during what may be a protracted period of hospitalization.

MALFORMATIONS RELATING TO RESPIRATION

Making a successful transition from fetus to neonate includes being able to establish regular respiration. Any malformation of the respiratory tract or accessory respiratory muscles is likely to hinder this process.

Congenital Diaphragmatic Hernia

This malformation occurs in 1 in 2000 live births and reflects failure of the development of the diaphragm, allowing herniation of abdominal contents into the thoracic cavity. It can occur as an isolated malformation but may be associated with other major anomalies. The extent to which lung development is compromised depends on the size of the diaphragmatic defect and the amount of herniated abdominal content. Around two-thirds of cases are diagnosed antenatally, although right-sided and/or small left-sided defects may not be identified before birth. Where there is a prenatal diagnosis, birth in a specialist neonatal surgical unit is advisable.

In the absence of a prenatal diagnosis, the condition may be suspected at birth if the resuscitation is unexpectedly difficult, especially if the heart sounds are displaced and the abdomen appears flat or scaphoid. A chest X-ray will confirm the diagnosis (Fig. 36.13).

Babies with this condition usually have significant respiratory distress and require intubation and mechanical ventilation. A large bore nasogastric tube on free drainage should be used to minimize gaseous distension of the displaced abdominal viscera. Surgical repair of the defect is necessary, but this is not urgent. It is more important to stabilize the baby's general condition before surgery. There is often co-existing pulmonary hypertension, requiring pulmonary vasodilators,

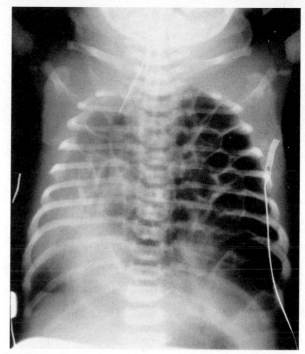

Fig. 36.13 Chest radiograph of a newborn at 1 h of life, showing left diaphragmatic hernia, displacement of air-filled viscera into the hemithorax and a marked shift of mediastinum and heart. (With permission from Rennie JM, Roberton NRC (Eds). (1999) Textbook of neonatology (3rd ed.). Edinburgh: Churchill Livingstone.)

inotropes and occasionally extracorporeal life support. Prognosis relates to the degree of pulmonary hypoplasia and reversibility of the accompanying pulmonary hypertension. A number of useful resources exist for health professionals and parents in relation to this condition, as detailed in the Useful websites section.

Congenital Pulmonary Airway Malformations

This group of malformations includes developmental lung anomalies previously known as *congenital cystic adenomatous malformation* (CCAM), *bronchopulmonary sequestration* (BPS) and *congenital lobar emphysema*. The incidence is thought to be around 1 in 2000 live births although with increased prenatal ultrasound scanning, more are being detected. Antenatal complications may include mediastinal shift and the development of *hydrops fetalis*, although many lesions seem to regress during the third trimester. Most lesions are asymptomatic in the early neonatal period but in certain situations, they can expand rapidly after birth, leading to air trapping, over-inflation and respiratory compromise.

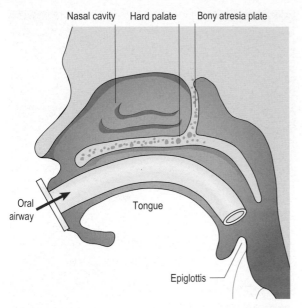

Fig. 36.14 Choanal atresia. A bony plate blocks the nose. (With permission from Rennie JM, Roberton NRC (Eds). (1999) Textbook of neonatology (3rd ed.). Edinburgh: Churchill Livingstone.)

In such cases, urgent surgical removal of the abnormal lung tissue is necessary. Babies known prenatally to have a CPAM should be monitored closely after birth for signs of respiratory distress.

Some CPAM have been reported to be associated with lung infection and malignant change in later life. The true incidence of such complications is unknown but is likely to be low. However, even in asymptomatic babies, surgical removal may be considered in childhood in order to prevent these long-term complications.

Choanal Atresia

Choanal atresia describes a unilateral or bilateral narrowing of the nasal passage(s) with a web of tissue or bone occluding the nasopharynx (Fig. 36.14). The incidence is 1 in 8000 live births. Respiratory compromise may be apparent from birth, particularly when a bilateral lesion is present or it may become obvious during feeding when the baby is unable to mouth breath. The diagnosis is confirmed if nasal catheters cannot be passed into the pharynx and if a mirror or cold metal spoon is held under the nose, no vapour will collect. Maintaining a clear airway is obviously essential and an oral airway may have to be used to achieve this. Surgery will be required to remove the obstructing tissue and nasal stents are generally left

in situ for a number of weeks postoperatively to prevent the obstruction from recurring.

Occasionally choanal atresia is associated with other genetic disorders such as CHARGE syndrome, a condition in which there are defects found in the eye (**C**oloboma), the **H**eart, occasionally oesophageal **A**tresia, usually growth **R**estriction, plus **G**enital and **E**ar abnormalities.

Laryngeal Stridor

This is a noise made by the baby, usually on inspiration and exacerbated by crying. The most common cause is laryngomalacia, where there is laxity of the laryngeal cartilage, which collapses inwards during inspiration. Laryngomalacia usually resolves over time and intervention is only required in the most severe cases.

There are a number of other rarer causes of stridor in the neonate, which should be considered, particularly if the stridor is accompanied by signs of respiratory distress or feeding problems. These include subglottic stenosis, laryngeal web, laryngeal cleft, vocal cord paralysis and extrinsic compression by a vascular ring. Investigations including laryngoscopy, bronchoscopy, computerized tomography (CT) angiography and barium swallow may be necessary in order to establish the diagnosis in these cases.

CONGENITAL CARDIAC DEFECTS

Babies with congenital heart defects comprise the second largest group of malformations. Approximately 8 per 1000 live births have some degree of congenital heart disease and about one-third of these babies will be symptomatic in early infancy.

Causes

Approximately 90% of cardiac anomalies cannot be attributed to a single cause. Chromosomal and genetic factors account for 8%, and a further 2% are thought to be caused by teratogens. The critical period of exposure to teratogens in respect of embryological development of cardiac tissue is from the **3rd to the 6th week of gestation**.

Prenatal Detection

An increasing number of cardiac anomalies are being identified by means of detailed prenatal ultrasound scanning (see Chapter 13). For babies with complex congenital heart disease, this enables a multidisciplinary plan for birth and immediate neonatal care, to be made well in advance of the baby's birth. However, the detection of many cardiac anomalies is still dependent upon accurate observation and examination during the early postnatal period.

Recognition Following Birth

Babies with congenital heart disease can present in a number of ways; a heart murmur, cyanosis, tachypnoea, weak or absent femoral pulses. Those babies in whom the pulmonary or systemic blood flow is dependent upon the arterial duct may present with severe cyanosis or shock when the duct closes, often around day 3–5 of life.

It is obviously important to try to identify those infants with life-threatening cardiac malformations as soon as possible and prior to transfer home, if born within a hospital or birthing centre setting. Additionally, early identification and referral of babies with significant cardiac malformations is desirable. While it must be remembered that not all babies with heart murmurs have an underlying cardiac malformation, it should also be noted that some babies with significant congenital heart disease may have no abnormal findings at the time of their routine newborn examination. As an adjunct to the routine newborn examination, most units also measure oxygen saturations. This has been shown to improve the detection of some duct-dependent heart lesions (Ewer et al. 2011).

Every baby should be examined by a competent practitioner within the first 72 h following birth. However, as some babies with significant congenital heart disease may have no clinical signs prior to transfer home, especially with shorter hospital stays or home birth, there is a need for community midwives to remain vigilant and to communicate effectively with parents. Parents who report any changes in the baby's behaviour such as breathlessness or cyanosis should be encouraged to seek prompt medical review.

Traditionally, babies with cardiac anomalies have been divided into two groups: those with central cyanosis and those without, i.e. *cyanotic* and *acyanotic* congenital heart disease.

Cardiac Defects Presenting with Cyanosis

Defects included in this group are:
- transposition of the great arteries
- pulmonary atresia
- tetralogy of Fallot
- tricuspid atresia
- total anomalous pulmonary venous drainage
- univentricular/complex heart.

Although cyanosis can be a presenting feature of a number of non-cardiac conditions (e.g. respiratory disease, persistent pulmonary hypertension of the newborn, sepsis), congenital heart disease should always be considered as a possible explanation. Administration of oxygen to babies with cyanotic heart disease may have little effect on their oxygen saturation levels. This observation, along with other routine investigations excluding other causes of cyanosis, may suggest a diagnosis of cyanotic heart disease. The definitive diagnostic investigation is echocardiography.

Cyanosis occurs when there is >5 g/dL of circulating deoxygenated haemoglobin. In congenital cyanotic heart disease, abnormal anatomy leads to mixing of oxygenated and deoxygenated blood ± inadequate pulmonary blood flow or, in the case of transposition of the great arteries, complete separation of the pulmonary and systemic circulations. In cases where there is severe obstruction to pulmonary blood flow, e.g. pulmonary atresia, there is often early presentation with marked cyanosis.

The most common cyanotic heart conditions are transposition of the great arteries and tetralogy of Fallot. Transposition of the great arteries is the most common cyanotic heart condition presenting in the neonatal period. This is a condition wherein the aorta arises from the right ventricle and the pulmonary artery from the left ventricle (Fig. 36.15). Consequently, oxygenated blood is circulated back through the lungs and deoxygenated blood back into the systemic circulation. It is apparent therefore that, unless there is an opportunity for oxygenated blood to access the systemic circulation, either by means of a patent arterial duct or through an accompanying septal defect, such a baby will die. In congenital cardiac defects such as this, where the patency of the arterial duct is essential for survival (*duct-dependent* lesions), a prostaglandin infusion should be commenced in order to maintain ductal patency pending more definitive management. For babies with transposition of the great arteries, a balloon septostomy is often performed to enlarge the foramen ovale and allow mixing of oxygenated and deoxygenated blood at the atrial level. Corrective surgery (arterial switch operation) is then carried out, usually within a few weeks of birth.

Tetralogy of Fallot has four anatomical components:
1. A pulmonary outflow tract obstruction
2. A ventricular septal defect
3. A right ventricular hypertrophy
4. An overriding aorta (Fig. 36.16).

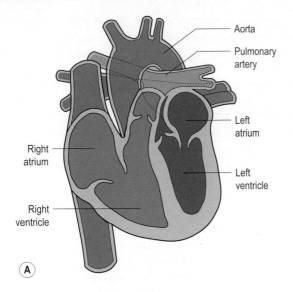

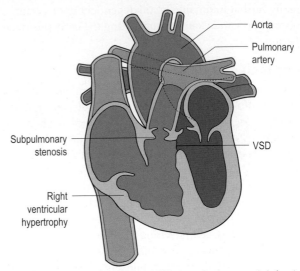

Fig. 36.16 Tetralogy of Fallot (VSD, ventricular septal defect).

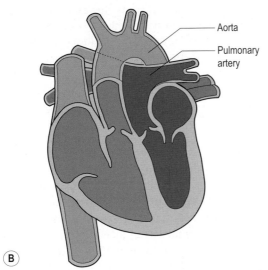

Fig. 36.15 Transposition of the great arteries. (A) Normal. (B) Transposition.

Tetralogy of Fallot seldom presents with cyanosis in the immediate newborn period, but this may become apparent within a few weeks of birth. Increasingly, the diagnosis is made prenatally. Most babies with this condition remain well in the neonatal period. Surgical treatment options include a *Blalock–Taussig shunt* for cases where it is necessary to increase pulmonary blood flow, and corrective repair, usually within the first year of life.

Although prostaglandin infusion is life-saving for duct-dependent heart conditions, it should be noted that it may lead to apnoea, particularly when higher doses are required. It is essential that there are facilities to provide respiratory support available for any baby on an infusion of prostaglandin.

Acyanotic Cardiac Defects

These congenital cardiac conditions include left-to-right shunt lesions and obstructive lesions.

> *Left-to-right shunts.*

- persistent arterial duct (also known as persistent ductus arteriosus)
- ventricular or atrial septal defects.

These lesions may present with a murmur or, if the shunt is large, with symptoms and signs of heart failure: tachypnoea, poor feeding, sweating, precordial heave, gallop rhythm or hepatomegaly.

A persistent arterial duct is more common in preterm babies and surgical closure is sometimes necessary if medical treatment with ibuprofen, indomethacin or paracetamol is ineffective. Term babies with a persistent arterial duct more commonly undergo cardiac catheterization with device closure in infancy or childhood.

Ventricular septal defects are a common cause of murmurs in the term neonate. Many of these defects are small, of no haemodynamic consequence and close spontaneously. Larger defects may lead to heart failure and surgical closure may be necessary, although not usually in the neonatal period (Fig. 36.17).

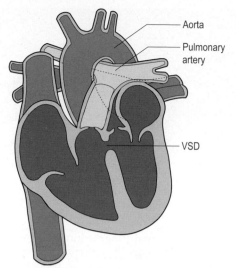

Fig. 36.17 Ventricular septal defect (VSD).

Obstructive lesions. These include:

- coarctation of the aorta
- pulmonary stenosis
- aortic stenosis
- hypoplastic left heart syndrome.

Some of these lesions may be difficult to identify clinically and a proportion of serious left heart obstructive lesions are not diagnosed before the baby is transferred home. Such lesions should always be considered in the baby with poor volume femoral pulses or unexplained tachypnoea, remembering that even severe lesions may have no associated murmur. If the obstruction is severe, e.g. critical aortic stenosis, then the systemic blood flow is often dependent upon the arterial duct and the baby will become very unwell when this closes. As in the duct-dependent cyanotic heart conditions, a prostaglandin infusion may be required while further investigations and discussions regarding the possibility of surgical correction take place.

Coarctation of the aorta and aortic stenosis are usually amenable to surgical correction. Hypoplastic left heart syndrome remains a major surgical challenge, requiring a number of surgical procedures in childhood, with a more guarded long-term outcome. Because of this, some parents opt for a palliative approach with no surgical intervention. Death usually occurs within a few days, although it may take substantially longer in some cases, particularly if the baby is preterm. If palliation is the chosen care path, then the priorities are to ensure the comfort of the baby and to support the family. Whatever treatment decisions they make, following confirmation of such a diagnosis there is a substantial psychological impact on the parents, which calls for particularly supportive management (see Chapter 38).

CENTRAL NERVOUS SYSTEM MALFORMATIONS

Neural tube defects are the most common malformations of the central nervous system. They arise from abnormalities during formation and closure of the neural tube, which is the embryonic precursor of the central nervous system.

Risk factors for neural tube defects include a family history of neural tube defects, maternal diabetes mellitus, maternal treatment with sodium valproate and carbamazepine and folic acid deficiency. Ingestion of folic acid supplements prior to conception and during the early stages of pregnancy has helped to reduce the incidence of such anomalies (Medical Research Council, MRC 1991). However, as the neural tube develops at a very early stage of pregnancy and, given that some pregnancies are not necessarily planned, women may not start taking folic acid until they realize they are pregnant, at which point it may already be too late to be of benefit. For this reason, many countries, supplement flour with folic acid, but this currently is ***not*** the case in the UK.

Prenatal screening is very effective at identifying central nervous system malformations (see Chapter 13). Some parents choose selective termination of pregnancies where severe neural tube defects are found but others elect to continue. Depending on the nature of the lesion and the prognosis, the neonatal care and management of the baby after birth may differ. Antenatal diagnosis enables health professionals to work with parents to formulate an individual plan for each baby even those with the most severe and life limiting malformations.

Anencephaly

This major anomaly describes the absence of the forebrain and vault of the skull. It is a condition that is incompatible with sustained extrauterine life, although babies who survive the birth process may breathe and live for a short period of time. Treatment in these situations is focused on ensuring the comfort of the baby and providing support for the family.

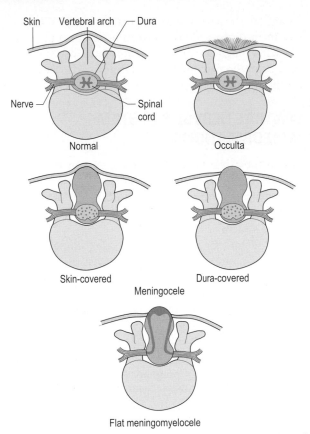

Fig. 36.18 Various forms of spina bifida. (With permission of the *Nursing Times*. From Wallis S, Harvey D. (1979) Disorders in the newborn. *Nursing Times* 75:1315–27.)

Spina Bifida

Spina bifida results from failure of fusion of the vertebral column. If there is no skin covering the defect, there is protrusion of the meninges, hence the term *meningocele* (Fig. 36.18). The meningeal membrane may be flat or appear as a membranous sac, with or without cerebrospinal fluid, but it does not contain neural tissue. A *meningomyelocele*, on the other hand, does involve the spinal cord (Fig. 36.19). This lesion may be enclosed, or the meningocele may rupture and expose the neural tissue. A meningomyelocele usually gives rise to neurological damage, producing paralysis or weakness distal to the defect, and impaired bladder and bowel function. The lumbosacral area is the most common site for these to present, but they may appear at any point in the vertebral column. When the defect is at base of skull level, it is known as an *encephalocele*. The added complication here is that the sac may contain varying amounts

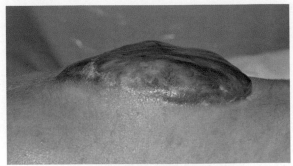

Fig. 36.19 Baby with meningomyelocele. (Reproduced with permission from Professor Robert Carachi.)

of brain tissue. Normal progression of labour may be impeded by a large lesion of this type.

Immediate management involves covering open lesions with a non-adherent dressing. Babies with enclosed lesions should be handled with the utmost care to preserve the integrity of the sac. This will limit the risk of meningitis occurring. If there is evidence of cerebrospinal fluid leak, then intravenous antibiotics should be given. Surgical closure is usually undertaken by a paediatric neurosurgeon. In cases where there is a large defect, a collaborative procedure with a plastic surgeon may be required in order to achieve skin closure. It is seldom necessary to close the back within 24 h of birth and priority should be given to stabilization of the baby and assessment of the defect (Jensen 2012). Surgical intervention for myelomeningocele carries a high rate of success of skin closure but has no impact on any damage already present in the cord or more distally. There is associated hydrocephalus (see below) in up to 90% of cases, with the majority requiring surgical shunting to prevent a rapid increase in the intracranial pressure.

Recent advances in the management of myelomeningocele include prenatal surgery performed at around 26 weeks' gestation. Compared with babies who have spina bifida surgery after birth, those who have prenatal surgery show improved neuromotor function by the age of 30 months and are less likely to require a shunt (Adzick et al. 2011). These benefits must be balanced against the potential risks of fetal surgery, which include the risk of oligohydramnios and preterm birth in addition to the requirement for caesarean section for all future pregnancies. Prenatal surgery for spina bifida was carried out in the UK for the first time in 2018 but is not currently considered the standard of care or is routinely available.

Spina Bifida Occulta

Spina bifida occulta (see Fig. 36.18) is the most minor type of defect where the vertebra is bifid. There is usually no spinal cord involvement. A tuft of hair or sinus at the base of the spine may be noted on first examination of the baby. Ultrasound investigation will confirm the diagnosis and rule out any associated spinal cord involvement.

Parents who have a baby with a neural tube defect should be offered genetic counselling, since there is a 50-fold increased risk of recurrence in future pregnancies (Saleem et al. 2009).

Hydrocephaly

This condition arises from a blockage in the circulation and absorption of cerebrospinal fluid, which is produced from the choroid plexuses within the lateral ventricles of the brain. The large lateral ventricles increase in size and eventually compress the surrounding brain tissue. It is a common accompaniment to the more severe spina bifida lesions because of a structural defect around the area of the foramen magnum known as the *Arnold–Chiari malformation*. In the absence of a myelomeningocele, congenital aqueduct stenosis is the commonest cause of hydrocephalus.

Signs of hydrocephalus include a large head, bulging fontanelle and widely spaced sutures. The condition may be identified antenatally on ultrasound scan or noted at routine examination of the newborn if the baby is found to have a large head. In severe cases detected antenatally, birth by caesarean section is usually planned. After birth, the risk of progressive cerebral damage may be minimized by the insertion of a ventriculo-peritoneal shunt to allow the excess cerebrospinal fluid to drain and to reduce the pressure on the brain. Signs of raised increased intracranial pressure include a tense, bulging fontanelle, vomiting and irritability, low heart rate and periods of apnoea. If the baby has signs of significant raised intracranial pressure, then an emergency ventricular tap to drain cerebrospinal fluid may be required prior to a planned ventriculo-peritoneal shunt insertion. Risks of shunt insertion include blockage, malfunction and infection leading to meningitis.

Microcephaly

This is where the occipitofrontal circumference is more than two standard deviations below normal for the gestational age of the baby. The disproportionately small head may reflect a familial pattern of head growth; however, it may also be a manifestation of abnormal brain development. Underlying aetiologies include conditions that adversely affect the early fetal brain, e.g. intrauterine infection, fetal alcohol exposure or chromosomal disorders. The longer-term neurodevelopmental sequelae are determined by the underlying cause but may include learning difficulties, cerebral palsy and seizures.

MUSCULOSKELETAL DEFORMITIES

These range from relatively minor anomalies, for example an extra digit, to major deficits such as absence of a limb.

Polydactyly and Syndactyly

Careful examination, including separation and counting of the baby's fingers and toes during the initial newborn examination is important, otherwise anomalies such as *syndactyly* (webbing) and *polydactyly* (extra digits) may go unnoticed.

Syndactyly more commonly affects the hands. It can appear as an isolated anomaly or as a feature of a syndrome such as *Apert syndrome*; this is a genetically inherited condition in which there is premature fusion of the sutures of the vault of the skull, cleft palate and complete syndactyly of both hands and feet. Whether or not any surgical division needs to be carried out depends on the degree of webbing or fusion.

In polydactyly the extra digit(s) may be fully formed or simply extra tissue attached by a pedicle. Even where there is only a rudimentary digit without bone involvement, better cosmetic results are obtained if the digit is surgically excised rather than 'tied off' to occlude its blood supply. Surgical excision is mandatory in more complex cases.

A family history of either of these defects is common, and in this situation, the parents will often have identified the anomaly before the baby is formally examined.

Limb Reduction Deficiencies

Limb reduction deficiencies describe the congenital absence or underdevelopment (hypoplasia) of a long bone and/or digits. The prevalence is around 0.7 per 1000 live births and the most common identifiable cause, present in a third of cases, is a developmental vascular disruption defect (Gold et al. 2011). An example of this is an amniotic band-related deficiency where the

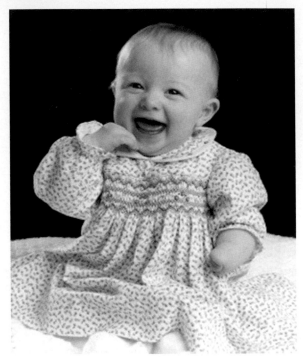

Fig. 36.20 A baby with a limb reduction defect quickly learns to adapt. (Photograph from Reach.)

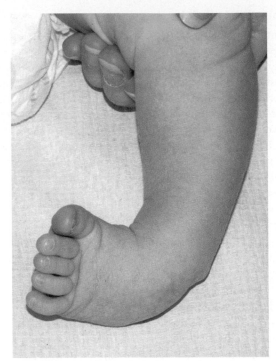

Fig. 36.21 Congenital talipes equinovarus.

amnion is believed to wrap itself around a developing limb causing strangulation and necrosis. Other identifiable causes include teratogens (such as thalidomide), genetic mutations, chromosomal disorders or as part of a syndrome such as the VACTERL spectrum described earlier in the chapter (McGuirk et al. 2001).

Limb reduction deficiencies may also be classified by site (upper versus lower limb), or by type (transverse versus longitudinal). In a transverse defect, the limb has developed normally to a particular level beyond which no skeletal elements exist (Fig. 36.20), while in a longitudinal defect, there is a reduction or absence of an element(s) within the long axis of the limb (Gold et al. 2011).

Specific management plans are often reached only after detailed assessment by an orthopaedic surgeon with a special interest in limb malformations. For those who require them, different types of prostheses are available and can be fitted as early as 3 months of age. Innovative surgical techniques such as limb lengthening or the transferring of toe(s) to hand to serve as substitute finger(s) are proving successful for some children. One of the most helpful things the midwife can do in these early days of parental adjustment, is to offer the address of a support group such as *Reach*. This appropriately-named support group for parents of children with upper limb deformities has branches throughout the UK.

Talipes

Talipes equinovarus (TEV, club foot) (Fig. 36.21) is the descriptive term for a deformity of the foot where the ankle is bent downwards (plantar flexed) and the front part of the foot is turned inwards (inverted). *Talipes calcaneovalgus* describes the opposite position where the foot is dorsiflexed and everted. TEV is a relatively common malformation, occurring in 1 in every 1000 live births. It is bilateral in 50% of cases and occurs in males more commonly than females, with a ratio of 2:1. Historically, it was thought that these deformities were more likely to occur when intrauterine space was restricted, for example in multiple pregnancy or oligohydramnios. It is now recognized that there is an important genetic element involved in their causation and parents who have had a baby with TEV have a 1 in 30 risk of recurrence in future pregnancies. TEV is also more likely to occur in conjunction with neuromuscular disorders such as spina bifida. In the mildest form, postural TEV, the foot may be easily returned to the correct position. The midwife should encourage the mother to exercise the baby's foot in this way several times a day. More severe, or *fixed* forms will require one or more of manipulation, splinting or surgical correction. In these cases, the advice of an orthopaedic surgeon should be sought as soon as possible after birth, as early treatment with manipulation or splinting may enhance results and minimize the need for surgery. Care should be taken to ensure that, for babies who have splints or casts applied, the strapping is not too tight and that the baby's toes are always well perfused.

Developmental Dysplasia of the Hip

Congenital hip dysplasia is an anomaly more commonly found when there is a family history in a first-degree relative or a breech presentation at term. It most often occurs in primigravida pregnancies and is commoner in females than males. The left hip is more often affected than the right. The dysplastic hip may present clinically in one of three ways:

1. Dislocated
2. Dislocatable
3. Subluxation of the joint.

Screening for hip dysplasia may prevent the need for later treatment and the options include: clinical examination, targeted hip ultrasound of high risk babies or universal hip ultrasound of all babies. Currently, there is insufficient evidence to support widespread hip ultrasound screening and babies should have their hips examined clinically after birth, with any abnormal findings prompting referral for a hip ultrasound, orthopaedic opinion or both (Shorter et al. 2013). Where the diagnosis is confirmed, it is usual for the baby to have a splint or harness such as the Pavlik harness applied (Fig. 36.22), which will keep the hips in a flexed and abducted position. The splint should **not** be removed for napkin changing or bathing and consequently, parents will require additional support in learning how to handle and care for their baby. Particular attention should be paid to skin care and examining the baby for signs of rubbing or excoriation.

Achondroplasia

Achondroplasia is an autosomal dominant condition where the baby is generally small with a disproportionately large head and short limbs. Some 80% of cases are due to new mutations of fibroblast growth factor

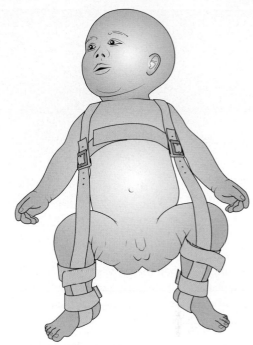

Fig. 36.22 Pavlik harness for congenital dislocation of the hip. (With permission from Barr DGD, Crofton PM, Goel KM. (1998) Disorders of bone, joints and connective tissue. In: AGM Campbell, N McIntosh (Eds) Forfar and Arneil's textbook of pediatrics. Edinburgh: Churchill Livingstone, Ch. 23, p. 1628.)

receptor genes and hence these families may have no anticipation of the disorder unless an antenatal diagnosis has been made.

Osteogenesis Imperfecta

Osteogenesis imperfecta (OI) is sometimes referred to as *brittle bone disease*. It is due to a disorder of collagen production that can result in multiple fractures either *in utero* or at birth. There are several different types and the severity of symptoms varies. Inheritance is usually autosomal dominant, but it is known that in a third of cases, the inheritance can be autosomal recessive, as new mutations arise (Basel and Steiner 2009). Recognition and genetic counselling are important for future pregnancies.

ANOMALIES OF THE SKIN
Vascular Naevi
Naevus Simplex

These are also known as *salmon patches* or *stork marks*. They are very common and often seen on the eyelids, bridge of the nose, upper lip and nape of the neck. They

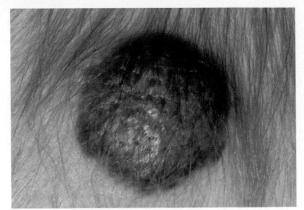

Fig. 36.23 Evolving capillary haemangioma. (Reproduced with permission from Sharon Murphy.)

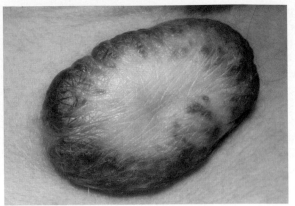

Fig. 36.24 Regressing capillary haemangioma with typical pallor. (Reproduced with permission from Sharon Murphy.)

are more obvious when the baby is crying. They are generally small and will fade during infancy although some, particularly those at the nape of the neck, may persist into adulthood. No treatment is necessary.

Capillary Vascular Malformation – Port-Wine Stain

This is a purple–blue capillary malformation. It can occur on any part of the body but most commonly affects the face and neck. It occurs in approximately 1 in 300 live births. It is generally fully formed at birth and does not regress with time. However, laser treatment and the skilful use of cosmetics may help to disguise the lesion if desired. In later life, the lesion may become raised or lumpy in appearance. If the malformation is in a visible area such as the face, the parents, and later the child, may benefit from psychological support.

Should the malformation mimic the distribution of the ophthalmic branch of the trigeminal nerve, further malformations in the eyes (glaucoma), meninges or brain (epilepsy) may be suspected. This is known as the *Sturge–Weber syndrome*.

Capillary Haemangiomata ('Strawberry Marks')

Capillary haemangiomata are not usually noticeable at birth but appear as red, raised lesions in the first few weeks of life (Fig. 36.23). These common lesions affect up to 10% of the population by the age of 1 year. They are five times more common in girls than boys and are also commoner in preterm babies. They can appear anywhere in the body but cause particular distress to the parents when they appear on the face. However, parents may be reassured that, although the lesion will grow bigger for the first few months, it will then regress with associated central pallor (Fig. 36.24) and usually disappears completely by the age of 5–6 years. In most cases, no treatment is required. Treatment may be considered in cases where the haemangioma is situated in an awkward area where it is likely to be subject to abrasion, such as on the lip, in the nappy area or around the eye, where it may interfere with vision. Treatment with topical timolol, oral propranolol, steroids or pulsed laser therapy is possible.

Pigmented (Melanocytic) Naevi

These are brown, sometimes hairy, marks on the skin that vary in size and may be flat or raised. A minority of this type of birthmark can become malignant. Surgical excision may be recommended to pre-empt this. It is unlikely that treatment for any of these birthmarks will be carried out in the immediate neonatal period, except in the case of larger pigmented naevi. The midwife's responsibilities are therefore to notify appropriate medical staff and offer parents general emotional support.

GENITOURINARY SYSTEM

Improved prenatal screening and diagnostic techniques (see Chapter 13) mean that information regarding urinary tract formation is often available at birth. In addition, knowledge of liquor volume provides reassurance that fetal renal function is adequate. If an anomaly has been prenatally identified, a plan regarding the timing of neonatal investigation(s) and subsequent management should be available at birth. Occasionally, renal tract malformations may be undiagnosed at birth, in which case the absence of urine for 24 h or a palpable kidney/bladder may indicate underlying problems.

Potter Syndrome

The impact of fetal renal agenesis or severe hypoplasia was first described in a series of stillborn infants, by Edith Potter, a perinatal pathologist, in 1946. A characteristic facial appearance due to the compressive effects of longstanding oligohydramnios is seen in association with limb contractures. The presence of adequate liquor volume is critical to the development of normal lungs and babies with renal agenesis will all die at or shortly after birth as a consequence of lung hypoplasia.

Posterior Urethral Valves

This is a malformation affecting male babies where the presence of valves in the posterior urethra obstructs the normal outflow of urine. As a result, the bladder distends, causing back pressure on the ureters and kidneys. This will ultimately cause bilateral hydronephrosis and renal parenchymal damage. Prenatal diagnosis is common and *in utero* intervention with the insertion of a shunt from the bladder to the amniotic fluid is possible, although not without risk (Morris et al. 2013). Improved long-term renal function following prenatal treatment is not guaranteed and postnatal valve ablation remains the mainstay of treatment (Morris et al. 2013). Unfortunately, even with early identification and management, many of these babies will have life-long renal impairment.

Cystic Kidneys

Cystic changes within the kidney(s) are often identified prenatally. Extensive bilateral changes are likely to be associated with impaired renal function and oligohydramnios. Unfortunately, the prognosis in this situation is poor, with some babies dying at birth and others developing renal failure. The severest forms of polycystic kidney disease are usually linked to an autosomal recessive inheritance, but an autosomal dominant variety also occurs with a better prognosis. Unilateral cystic changes, e.g. multicystic dysplastic kidney, have a good prognosis if the contralateral kidney is normal. Neonatal renal imaging and follow-up is required but the baby is usually well at birth and mother and baby do not have to be separated.

Hypospadias

Examination of a baby boy may reveal that the urethral meatus opens on to the under surface of the penis. The meatus can be placed at any point along the length of the penis and in some cases, will open onto the perineum. This anomaly often co-exists with *chordee*, in which the penis is short and bent and the foreskin is present only on the dorsal side of the penis. It is important that the parents are reassured that this can be corrected surgically but are made aware that circumcision should be deferred until consultation with the paediatric surgeon is completed.

Cryptorchidism

Undescended testes may be unilateral or bilateral and occur in 1–2% of male infants. If on examination of the baby after birth the scrotum is empty, the undescended testes may be found in the inguinal pouch. Sometimes the testis in this position can be manipulated into the scrotal pouch. If neither testis is palpable, further investigation to exclude endocrine or chromosomal causes is required. In unilateral undescended testis, parents should be advised to have their baby examined at regular intervals. If descent of the testis has not occurred by the time the child is 1 year old, arrangements for orchidopexy may be made.

DISORDERS OF SEX DEVELOPMENT

Disorders of sex development (DSD) are a diverse group of conditions in which the external genitalia and the reproductive organs do not develop normally. They may present at birth when the baby's external genitalia appear neither definitely male nor female. In this very challenging situation, it is vital that the midwife is positive, honest and does not assign a gender to the baby. Examination of the baby may reveal any of the following: a small hypoplastic penis, chordee, bifid scrotum, impalpable testes (careful examination should be made to detect undescended testes in the inguinal canal) or enlarged clitoris and incompletely separated or poorly-differentiated labia. It can be impossible to differentiate by clinical examination alone between female masculinization, male under-virilization or mixed gender and expert clarification is always required. The decision of gender attribution is made following chromosomal studies to determine genetic make-up, hormone assays and consideration of the potential surgical options (Ahmed and Rodie 2010). Specialist multidisciplinary input should be introduced from an early stage and families should be provided with psychological support and access to appropriate sources of information.

Congenital Adrenal Hyperplasia

Congenital adrenal hyperplasia is the commonest cause of female masculinization (i.e. genetically female with male-looking external genitalia). In this autosomal recessive inherited condition, the adrenal gland is stimulated to overproduce androgens because of a deficiency of an enzyme called 21-hydroxylase, which is necessary for normal production of steroid from cholesterol. If aldosterone production is also reduced, then these babies will rapidly lose salt and may present collapsed and dehydrated. Urea and electrolytes, blood glucose and 17-hydroxy progesterone levels should be measured and appropriate fluid replacement given. Prenatal diagnosis by genetic mutation analysis is possible and may allow consideration of prenatal steroid treatment to minimize virilization in affected females (Heland et al. 2016).

Androgen Insensitivity Syndrome

Androgen insensitivity syndrome is one of several causes of male under-virilization (i.e. genetically male with female-looking external genitalia). In this condition, cells are unresponsive to the effects of androgenic hormones. In the fetus, this prevents normal masculinization of the external genitalia, despite the presence of a Y chromosome.

TERATOGENIC CAUSES

Fetal Alcohol Syndrome/Spectrum

Fetal alcohol exposure remains a leading cause of intellectual impairment, despite Department of Health recommendations to abstain from drinking alcohol during pregnancy. This reflects the difficulties of translating health promotion objectives into successful outcomes, particularly in an environment where the alcohol consumption of young women is constantly increasing.

The teratogenic effects of alcohol include growth restriction, distortion of craniofacial features and brain damage (De Sanctis et al. 2011). The midwife may be alerted to the possibility of a baby being born with this syndrome if there have been concerns about *in utero* growth, particularly in the context of excess alcohol consumption. The following characteristics may be recognizable in the neonate: a small for gestational age baby with microcephaly, small palpebral fissures, a smooth philtrum and a thin upper lip. These facial features may become less pronounced as the child grows, however microcephaly, small stature and behavioural problems remain. The midwife will need to exercise excellent counselling skills to provide much-needed support for the mother. Collaboration with social services is usually called for to ensure that the care options decided are in the best interests of the baby and family.

Establishing such a direct link between a teratogen and a complex clinical pattern remains the exception rather than the rule although accurate recording of all congenital malformations on a central register can aid early recognition of potential new teratogens.

SUPPORT FOR THE MIDWIFE

Caring for a mother whose baby has a congenital malformation places extra demands on the midwife. This stress is compounded if the anomaly was not anticipated prior to birth or if the midwife has not previously encountered the particular problem. Good counselling and communication skills are invaluable in helping the family to adjust and in facilitating appropriate lines of support. The extra effort expended can be costly in terms not only of time but of the emotional stress the midwife may experience.

It is important that support is available for midwives in these situations and an opportunity to debrief with a senior colleague(s) or professional midwifery advocate (PMA)/clinical supervisor can be helpful. Preparatory courses on grief and bereavement counselling are also of some benefit, as many parents with affected babies will experience many of these emotions (see Chapter 31). Midwives who have acquired experience in this area should not, however, automatically be targeted as the experts and always be called upon to fulfil this role. Conversely, student midwives should not to be deliberately shielded from being involved in caring for such families. The provision of quality care for parents who have a baby with a congenital malformation is contingent upon meeting the needs of the carers.

Midwives may also find information available via the internet, however, they should be aware of the dubious quality of some of this information. They should therefore exercise caution in how they utilize it. It might also be wise to caution parents, who often search the internet for further information of this potential risk.

REFLECTIVE ACTIVITY FOR SELF-ASSESSMENT

1. What are the potential advantages and disadvantages of a woman whose fetus has a congenital anomaly, giving birth in a specialist centre rather than her local maternity unit?

2. What are the differences between the fetal and neonatal circulations? Why might a baby with significant congenital heart disease collapse at a few days of age, despite having no abnormality detected at routine examination of the newborn?

3. How might a baby with oesophageal atresia present after birth? What clues might there be on antenatal history/ultrasound scans, which may suggest the diagnosis?

REFERENCES

Ahmed, S. F., & Rodie, M. (2010). Investigation and initial management of ambiguous genitalia. *Best Practice and Research in Clinical Endocrinology and Metabolism*, 24(2), 197–218.

Adzick, N. S., Thom, E., Spong, C., et al. (2011). A randomized trial of prenatal versus postnatal repair of myelomeningocele. *New England Journal of Medicine*, 364(11), 993–1004.

Bacher, M., Linz, A., Buchenau, W., et al. (2010). Treatment of infants with Pierre Robin sequence. *Laryngorhinootologie*, 89(10), 621–629.

Basel, D., & Steiner, R. D. (2009). Osteogenesis imperfecta: recent findings shed new light on this once well understood condition. *Genetic Medicine*, 11(6), 375–385.

Bayen, E., Possin, K. L., Chen, Y., et al. (2018). Prevalence of aging, dementia and multimorbidity in older adults with Down syndrome. *Journal of the American Medical Association Neurology*, 75(11), 1399–1406.

Bradnock, T. J., Knight, M., Kenny, S., et al. (2017). Hirschsprung's disease in the UK and Ireland: incidence and anomalies. *Archives of Disease in Childhood*, 102(8), 722–727.

Chinnery, P. F., Howell, N., Lightowlers, R. N., et al. (1998). MELAS and MERRF: The relationship between maternal mutation load and the frequency of clinically affected offspring. *Brain*, 121, 1889–1894.

De Sanctis, L., Memo, L., Pichini, S., et al. (2011). Fetal alcohol syndrome: new perspectives for an ancient and underestimated problem. *Journal of Maternal Fetal and Neonatal Medicine*, 24(1), 34–37.

Ewer, A. K., Middleton, L. J., Furmston, A. T., et al. (2011). Pulse oximetry screening for congenital heart defects in newborn infants (Pulse Ox): a test accuracy study. *Lancet*, 378, 785–794.

Gold, N. B., Westgate, M. N., & Holmes, L. B. (2011). Anatomic and etiological classification of congenital limb deficiencies. *American Journal of Medical Genetics*, 155A(6), 1225–1235.

Heland, S., Hewitt, J. K., McGillivray, G., et al. (2016). Preventing female virilisation in congenital adrenal hyperplasia: The controversial role of antenatal dexamethasone. *Australian and New Zealand Journal of Obstetrics and Gynaecology*, 56(3), 225–232.

Jensen, A. (2012). Nursing care and surgical correction of neonatal myelomeningocele. *Infant*, 8(5), 142–146.

McGuirk, C. K., Westgate, M. N., & Holmes, L. B. (2001). Limb deficiencies in newborn infants. *Pediatrics*, 108(4), E64.

MRC (Medical Research Council) Vitamin Study Research Group. (1991). Prevention of neural tube defects: results of the Medical Research Council Vitamin Study. *Lancet*, 338, 131–137.

Morris, R. K., Malin, G. L., Quinlan-Jones, E., et al. (2013). Percutaneous vesicoamniotic shunting versus conservative management for fetal lower urinary tract obstruction (PLUTO): A randomized trial. *Lancet*, 382(9903), 1496–1506.

Pedersen, R. N., Calzolari, E., Husby, S., & EUROCAT Working Group, et al. (2012). Oesophageal atresia: prevalence, prenatal diagnosis and associated anomalies in 23 European regions. *Archives of Disease in Childhood*, 97(3), 227–232.

Prefumo, F., & Izzi, C. (2014). Fetal abdominal wall defects. *Best Practice and Research in Clinical Obstetrics and Gynaecology*, 28(3), 391–402.

Saleem, S. N., Said, A. H., Abdel-Raouf, M., et al. (2009). MRI in the evaluation of fetuses referred for sonographically suspected neural tube defects: impact on diagnosis and management decisions. *Neuroradiology*, 51(11), 761–762.

Shaye, D., Liu, C. C., & Tollefson, T. T. (2015). Cleft lip and palate: an evidence based review. *Facial Plastic Surgery Clinics of North America*, 23(3), 357–372.

Shorter, D., Hong, T., & Osborn, D. A. (2013). Cochrane review: screening programmes for developmental dysplasia of the hip in newborn infants. *Evidence Based Child Health*, 8(1), 11–54.

ANNOTATED FURTHER READING

Jones, K. L. (Ed.). (2013). *Smith's recognizable patterns of human malformation* (7th ed.) Philadelphia: Saunders/Elsevier.

This book provides a comprehensive and systematic approach to dysmorphic syndromes.

Rennie, J. M. (Ed.). (2014). *Rennie and Roberton's textbook of neonatology* (5th ed.) Edinburgh: Churchill Livingstone.

This definitive text explores the most contemporary methods of diagnosis, treatment and care of the neonate, alongside detailed pathophysiology of every significant neonatal condition of the neonate. Included in this edition are contributions from fetal medicine experts and obstetricians who provide valuable detail and insight, essential in the field of neonatology.

USEFUL WEBSITES

Antenatal Results and Choices (ARC): www.arc-uk.org

Children's Heart Federation: www.chfed.org.uk

Cleft Lip and Palate Association (CLAPA): www.clapa.com

Congenital Diaphragmatic Hernia (CDH) UK: https://cd-huk.org.uk

Contact a Family: www.contact.org.uk

Cystic Fibrosis Trust (CF): www.cysticfibrosis.org.uk

Down Syndrome Association: www.downs-syndrome.org.uk

Genetic Alliance UK: www.geneticalliance.org.uk

On-line Mendelian Inheritance in Man (OMIM): www.omim.org

Reach: The Association for Children with Upper Limb Deficiencies: https://reach.org.uk

Scottish Differences of Sex Development Network: www.sdsd.scot.nhs.uk

Scottish Down Syndrome Association (SDSA): www.dsscotland.org.uk

Shine (formerly Association for Spina Bifida and Hydrocephalus): www.shinecharity.org.uk

SOFT UK (Support Organization for Trisomy 13/18): http://soft.org.uk

STEPS (National Association for Children with Lower Limb Deficiencies): www.steps-charity.org.uk

Wolfson Institute of Preventative Medicine: www.qmul.ac.uk/wolfson/services/antenatal-screening

37

Significant Problems in the Newborn Baby

John McIntyre

CHAPTER CONTENTS

A wide variety of conditions may present in the newborn baby that require early referral to the neonatal multi-professional team. The midwife needs to be able to recognize and assess problems that distinguish healthy babies from those that are ill. Some problems will be life-threatening and require urgent assistance; others may be more subtle in their presentation but nevertheless important. Knowledge of the signs, characteristics and features of the conditions presented will enable the midwife to make well-informed and appropriate referrals and also provide valuable support for the parents.

THE CHAPTER AIMS TO

- assist the midwife in the assessment and identification of the ill newborn baby

- summarize possible problems that may be identified in a newborn baby and offer an approach to dealing with them.

INTRODUCTION

The majority of newborn babies are born in good condition and require no intervention after birth except to be dried with a warm towel and then to have skin-to-skin contact with their mother (see Chapter 33). Labour and birth may have been straightforward but the baby may still need to be observed at this time to ensure a healthy transition from uterine to neonatal life. Approximately 5–10% of babies are admitted to a neonatal intensive care unit (NICU). Many of these are preterm babies or those with antenatally detected problems but 6–9% of term babies are admitted to an NICU (Tracy et al. 2007). The length of time a mother spends in hospital with her newborn baby has decreased significantly in recent years and many babies may be born outside the hospital setting, at home or in a midwifery-led unit. Context may impact on early recognition and management of problems in the early newborn period. The focus of this chapter is to aid the early detection of problems, to enable the midwife to distinguish the ill from the well baby and to support decision-making of when to intervene and what that initial action should be. The aim is not to give detailed management about specific conditions that require ongoing specialist input, but to summarize those conditions that may first be recognized or come to the attention of midwives and require their involvement.

INITIAL EXAMINATION AND RECOGNITION OF PROBLEMS

Most of the information the midwife requires for the assessment of a baby's wellbeing comes from observation. The healthy term baby will lie with their limbs partially flexed and active and the skin colour reflecting warm and well perfused skin. After the initial observation, there should follow a more systematic examination to ensure the newborn baby is well (see Chapter 32). The following areas should be examined carefully.

The Skin

The skin of a neonate varies in its appearance and can often be the cause of unnecessary anxiety in the mother, midwife and medical staff. However, it can sometimes be the first clue to an underlying problem in the baby. The skin of all babies should be examined for pallor, plethora, cyanosis, jaundice and skin rashes.

Pallor

Pale, mottled skin may indicate poor peripheral perfusion. The hands and feet are often blue soon after birth (acrocyanosis) and this in isolation does not indicate an underlying problem. It is best practice to always examine the baby's face and chest when assessing colour. An anaemic baby will appear pale pink, white or, in severe cases where there is vascular collapse, grey. Accompanying signs of severe anaemia are tachycardia, tachypnoea and poor capillary refill (CR). A test is to press the skin briefly on the forehead or chest and observe how long it takes for the colour to return; this should be **<2 seconds**. The most likely causes of anaemia immediately after birth are:

- haemolytic disease of the newborn (HDN)
- twin-to-twin transfusions *in utero* (which can cause one baby to be anaemic and the other polycythaemic)
- fetomaternal haemorrhage
- fetal haemorrhage from vasa praevia or bleeding from the umbilical cord.

Pallor can also be observed in babies who are hypothermic or hypoglycaemic. Significant pallor can be associated with:

- anaemia and shock
- respiratory disorders
- cardiac anomalies
- sepsis.

Plethora

Babies who are very red in colour may be described as plethoric. Their colour may indicate a high level of circulating red blood cells (polycythaemia). Newborn babies can become polycythaemic if they are recipients of:

- twin-to-twin transfusion *in utero*
- a large placental transfusion.

Contributing factors may include delayed clamping of the umbilical cord or holding the baby below the level of the placenta, thereby allowing blood to flow into the baby and giving a greater circulating blood volume (can occur in unassisted births). Other babies at risk are:

- those that are small for their gestational age (SGA) as a means to increase oxygen carrying capacity in the hypoxic situation (see Chapter 34)
- infants of diabetic mothers (IDM) as a result of increased levels of growth hormone and an overactive metabolism.

The diagnosis of polycythaemia is based upon levels of haemoglobin and haematocrit (the relationship between red blood cells and plasma in the blood) and how they compare with normal values, based on gestational age. Some poor outcomes have been associated with polycythaemia, but there is a lack of evidence that a particular level of haematocrit requires treatment or that treatment is of any benefit (Özek et al. 2010).

Cyanosis

Peripheral cyanosis of the hands and feet is common during the first 24 h of life and is of no significance. However, *central* cyanosis should always be taken seriously and requires urgent attention. The tongue and mucous membranes are the most reliable indicators of central colour in all babies and if they appear blue, this indicates low oxygen saturation levels in the blood, usually of respiratory or cardiac origin. Episodic central cyanosis may be an indication that the baby is having convulsions. (See later sections on respiratory problems and assessment of the cyanosed baby).

Other factors that affect the appearance of the skin

Preterm babies have thinner skin that is redder in appearance than that of term infants. In post-term babies, the skin is often dry and cracked. The skin is a good indicator of the nutritional status of the baby. The small for gestational age (SGA) baby may look malnourished and have folds of loose skin over the joints, owing to the lack or loss of subcutaneous fat. This predisposes to hypothermia. The baby is also at increased risk of hypoglycaemia due to poor glycogen stores in the liver. If the baby is dehydrated, the skin looks dry and pale and is often cool to the touch. If gently pinched, the skin will be slow to retract. Other signs of dehydration are tachycardia, pallor or mottled skin, sunken eyes and anterior fontanelle. The best clinical indicator of dehydration is a change in the baby's weight.

Skin rashes

Skin rashes are quite common in newborn babies but most are benign and self-limiting. There are some rashes, however, which may indicate significant illness and should not be ignored:

- *Petechiae* (small red or purple spots of about 1–2 mm in diameter) or purpura (red or purple spots 3–10 mm in diameter) over the upper part of the body, particularly the face and chest, may occur due to venous obstruction after physiological or prolonged birth. However, petechiae can occur when there is a low platelet count (thrombocytopenia) and this may present with a petechial rash over the whole body with prolonged bleeding from puncture sites and/or the umbilicus and bleeding into the intestinal system.
- *Bruising* can occur following breech extractions, forceps and ventouse-assisted births. In a subaponeurotic haemorrhage (see Chapter 35), there is bleeding in the scalp tissues that can result in anaemia, a decrease in circulating blood volume and, if severe, hypotension.
- *A vesicular rash* is where there are small fluid-filled raised lumps on the skin. This can occur with some congenital viral infections, in particular herpes simplex or congenital chicken pox (Varicella). *These can be very serious infections in the newborn and should always be carefully assessed.* The midwife should enquire about a history of maternal genital herpes infection, although it can occur without any known history of infection. It is essential to refer the baby for further assessment.

- *A **blistering rash*** is where areas of skin are raised and are fluid-filled. The surface of the skin may also slough off, leaving red raw areas. This can occur in bacterial infections, particularly with *Staphylococcus aureus* (*S. aureus*). It presents as widespread tender erythema, followed by blisters, which break, leaving raw areas of skin or sometimes yellow-filled bullae. This is particularly noticeable around the napkin area but can also cause umbilical sepsis, breast abscesses, conjunctivitis and, in systemic infections, there may also be involvement of the bones and joints. Babies with this condition are likely to be very unwell and require admission to the NICU. A blistering skin rash should always be treated with broad spectrum intravenous (IV) antibiotics that cover *S. aureus*. It may be a sign of rare but important congenital skin diseases such as *epidermolysis bullosa* (EB), some of which are very serious and associated with significant morbidity and mortality; there may be a family history.

The Respiratory System

Healthy babies should establish normal regular breathing within minutes of birth. Many babies may display a slightly irregular breathing pattern for a few minutes after birth but then have regular breathing with a respiratory rate of 40–60 breaths/min by approximately 2 min. The baby's breathing pattern will alter depending on their level of activity but a respiratory rate consistently above 60 breaths/min is considered as tachypnoea.

Cardiorespiratory adaptations at birth

- Before birth, the lungs are fluid-filled. At birth, the newborn baby must clear this fluid in order to establish respiration. Some fluid is removed by physical means during physiological labour (Stephens et al. 1998) but most is absorbed into the pulmonary lymphatics and capillaries.
- Satisfactory lung inflation requires surfactant. In some preterm babies, infants of diabetic mothers (IDM) and ill term babies, surfactant production may be decreased, resulting in respiratory distress.
- Newborn babies are obligate nasal breathers. Obstruction to the nares (nostrils) results in respiratory distress.
- The shape of the newborn thorax and the rib orientation limit the potential for thorax expansion. The baby's soft and flexible ribs also make the chest wall subject to collapse during increased respiratory efforts.

This means that a baby with respiratory difficulty will have clinical signs of respiratory distress that are different from other patient groups. The following features may be seen:

- *Expiratory grunting*: a characteristic noise due to partial closure of the glottis during expiration. The baby is attempting to preserve some internal lung pressure and prevent the airways from collapsing completely at the end of the breath.
- *Intercostal recession*: using the intercostal muscles more effectively, but as a result, the spaces between the ribs and the sternum are sucked in during each breath.
- *Tachypnoea*: an increased respiratory rate as the baby attempts to compensate for an increased carbon dioxide concentration in the blood and extracellular fluids. A normal respiratory rate in the newborn is 40–60 breaths/min.
- *Nasal flaring*: an attempt to minimize the effect of the airways' resistance by maximizing the diameter of the upper airways. The nares are seen to flare open with each breath.
- *Apnoea*: an absence of breathing for >20 s that may occur as a result of increasing respiratory fatigue in the term baby. The preterm baby may also experience apnoea of prematurity due to immaturity of the respiratory centre and/or obstructive apnoea from occluded airways.

A baby with significant signs of respiratory distress should be reviewed by the neonatal team. The cause of respiratory distress may not always be clear on initial assessment. Occasionally in the first few minutes after birth, particularly following a caesarean section, a baby may have mild respiratory anomalies that settle quickly, but babies with abnormal signs should always remain under observation, as deterioration can occur rapidly in some cases. The initial assessment and treatment is described later in the chapter.

The importance of body temperature control

A neutral thermal environment is defined as the ambient air temperature at which oxygen consumption or heat production is minimal, with body temperature in the normal range (Lissauer and Faranoff 2006). The normal body temperature range for term babies is 36.5–37.3°C. Merenstein and Gardner (2011) assert the importance of the neutral thermal environment and how everyone caring for babies should understand the need for maintenance of normal body temperature. Mothers are often hot during labour and measures may be taken to produce a cooler environment for their comfort. It is important to always consider this effect and maintain a suitable environmental temperature for the newborn baby. In addition to skin-to-skin contact, this may require extra measures such as the use of a radiant heater or cot warmer, in some circumstances. When outside the neutral thermal environment, a baby can become too cold or too warm. As they attempt to regulate their temperature, they can become unstable especially more vulnerable babies such as those who are low birth weight (preterm or SGA). An abnormal temperature, either high or low, can be an early sign of an underlying problem such as an infection, a respiratory or cardiac problem, a metabolic abnormality or encephalopathy.

Hypothermia is defined as a core body temperature below 36°C (Jain 2012). When the body temperature is below this level, the baby is at risk from cold stress. This can cause complications such as increased oxygen consumption, lactic acid production, apnoea and hypoglycaemia. In preterm babies, cold stress may also cause a decrease in surfactant production, which is associated with increased mortality (Costeloe et al. 2000; Confidential Enquiries into Stillbirths and Deaths in Infancy, CESDI 2003). The hypothermic baby often looks pale or mottled and may be uninterested in feeding.

An abnormally high temperature is defined as a core temperature above 38.0°C (Jain 2012). A common cause is overheating due to environmental factors (hyperthermia). However, a high temperature can also be due to a fever and an important clinical sign of sepsis. A high temperature can result in an increased respiratory rate, increased fluid loss and hypernatraemia, and apnoea.

The Central Nervous System

Assessment of a baby's neurological status is usually carried out when they are awake but not crying. Important signs are the tone and quality of a baby's movements, level of activity, posture and presence of normal newborn reflexes. An abnormal posture (e.g. neck retraction, frog-like posture, hyperextension or hyperflexion of the limbs), abnormal involuntary movements and a high-pitched or weak cry, may indicate neurological impairment and a need for investigation (Lawn and Alton 2012).

Terms used to describe abnormal movements in babies (e.g. *fits, convulsions, seizures, twitching, jumpy, jittery*) are often used inconsistently. If an abnormal movement is seen, it is important to document a clear description to help understand its nature. A baby with poor muscle tone is described as *hypotonic* or *floppy*. It can be difficult to distinguish a seizure from jitteriness or irritability. Jitteriness is often used to describe a baby with tremors and rapid movement of the extremities or fingers that are stopped when the limb is held or flexed. Jitteriness is not a sign of a specific underlying illness and can be seen in otherwise healthy babies. However, it is important to consider if there are any other clinical findings that may point to a specific cause and distinguish it from a seizure that requires urgent assessment and investigation.

Hypotonia

Hypotonia describes reduced muscle tension and tone. On normal handling, the baby will feel floppy and at rest, often adopts an abnormal posture commonly referred to as '*frog like*'. If there has been prolonged lack of movement and hypotonia before birth, then limb contractures may also be seen. It is normal for preterm babies below 30 weeks' gestation to have a resting position that is hypotonic. The healthy term newborn baby has a position of total flexion with immediate recoil. Hypotonia in a term baby is *not* normal and requires investigation. It is also important to determine whether the hypotonia is associated with weakness and this distinction helps focus the search for a likely cause. It is important to observe for spontaneous movements and the quality and strength of these. There are several causes of hypotonia in the newborn.

- *Systemic causes:*
  - maternal sedation or drugs (in particular some antidepressants)
  - prematurity
  - infection
  - Down syndrome
  - endocrine (e.g. hypothyroidism)
  - metabolic problems (e.g. hypoglycaemia, hyponatraemia, inborn errors of metabolism).
- *Central (brain) causes:*
  - perinatal hypoxia-ischaemia or neonatal encephalopathy
  - traumatic brain injury

- structural brain abnormality, e.g. holoprosencephaly.
- *Peripheral nervous system causes:*
  - neurological problems (e.g. spinal cord injuries sustained during birth)
  - neuromuscular disorders (e.g. spinal muscular atrophy, myasthenia gravis related to maternal disease, myotonic dystrophy etc.).

The Renal and Genitourinary System

Passage of urine after birth is important to document, as it provides a record that may help if later concerns arise. The genitourinary tract is a common site for congenital or genetic abnormalities and many of these will have been detected by antenatal scans with an agreed plan made for early assessment and intervention. Urine that only dribbles out, rather than being passed with a good stream, may be an indication of a bladder outflow obstruction and in male infants is seen with posterior urethral valves. Other renal problems may present as a failure to pass urine. Urinalysis using reagent strips will give information that may be helpful in diagnosis. Urinary infections in the newborn period are uncommon. The signs of urinary tract infection are often vague and can be mistaken for other problems. The baby typically presents with lethargy, poor feeding, increasing jaundice and vomiting. Urine infections when present are important, however, because repeated untreated infections can lead to renal scarring. Reduced urine output is usually due to low fluid intake but other reasons should also be considered:

- increased fluid loss due to hyperthermia (e.g. with use of radiant heaters or phototherapy units)
- perinatal hypoxia-ischaemia
- congenital abnormalities
- infection.

The Gastrointestinal Tract

The baby's abdomen should be assessed, observing for signs of distension, discoloration or tenderness. Most babies should feed early and pass meconium within the first 8–12 h of birth. Healthy babies should be able to feed within 30 min of birth. Posseting small amounts of milk often with winding and over-handling after feeding, is common and normal. Vomiting can be a sign of a problem and babies with large vomits should be evaluated. The midwife needs to be alert to *red flag* symptoms that require urgent assessment, particularly a bile vomit (dark green in colour) or blood in the vomit.

Bile-stained vomiting

There should **never** be green bile in the vomit of a newborn baby and this always requires prompt evaluation. If bile-stained vomiting is seen or reported, the baby should be examined, observing for abdominal distension or tenderness. The anus should be observed for patency. It may indicate bowel obstruction from a variety of causes including infection, bowel atresias, meconium ileus, anorectal malformations or necrotizing enterocolitis (NEC). Of particular concern in the newborn is malrotation and volvulus. This can lead to the baby quickly becoming ill due to bowel ischaemia, if not promptly investigated. An X-ray and contrast study is usually required to rule out bowel obstruction and malrotation.

NEC is generally a problem in premature babies but may also occur in term babies, particularly those who have risk factors such as perinatal hypoxia, polycythaemia and hypothermia. It is an acquired disease of the small and large intestine caused by ischaemia of the intestinal mucosa. NEC may present with vomiting, which may be bile-stained. The abdomen becomes distended, stools may be loose and have blood in them or the baby may not open their bowels. In the early stages of NEC, the baby can display nonspecific signs of temperature instability, unstable glucose levels, lethargy and poor peripheral circulation. As the illness progresses, the baby may become apnoeic and bradycardic and may need respiratory support.

Passage of meconium

According to Metaj et al. (2003), 97% of babies will pass meconium by 24 h of age; an event that should be documented. If a baby has not passed meconium, the abdomen should be examined for signs of distension or tenderness and the anus checked for patency. Possible causes of delayed passage of meconium include bowel atresia, meconium ileus, meconium plug, imperforate anus and Hirschsprung disease. Passage of the first meconium occurs later with earlier gestational age (Kumar and Dhanireddy 1995).

The healthy term baby may pass about eight stools a day. Breastfed babies' stools are looser and more frequent than those of formula-milk fed babies, and the colour varies more and sometimes appears greenish. The baby who has a systemic infection can often display signs of gastrointestinal problems, usually poor feeding and vomiting. Diarrhoea may be a feature of this or may indicate a more serious gastrointestinal disorder such as NEC. Diarrhoea caused by gastroenteritis is unusual in the newborn, although it may be seen after the first week. Outbreaks of viral diarrhoea due to Rotavirus have been reported. Babies with this condition must be isolated and scrupulous hand-washing must be adhered to. Loose stools can also be a feature of babies receiving phototherapy.

RECOGNITION OF PROBLEMS AT THE TIME OF RESUSCITATION

Aspects of resuscitation of the newborn are covered in Chapter 33, but problems that might be encountered, or may present during or immediately after resuscitation, are addressed here. It is important to promptly recognize those babies who have adapted poorly to extrauterine life and are in poor condition at birth because of hypoxia-ischaemia, or have tolerated the birth process poorly as a result of pre-existing problems.

Neonatal Encephalopathy

Neonatal encephalopathy is a clinical syndrome of an altered level of consciousness, abnormalities in tone, primitive reflexes, autonomic function and sometimes seizures.

Which babies get encephalopathy?

The commonest cause is hypoxia-ischaemia, termed 'hypoxic ischaemic encephalopathy' (HIE). There may be a clear intrapartum sentinel event such as cord obstruction, placental abruption or uterine rupture. However, it is important to remember that not all encephalopathy is due to hypoxia-ischaemia; important other causes such as metabolic, infective, malformation or trauma should also be considered.

The term *neonatal HIE* should be used only when there is clear evidence of hypoxia and ischaemia. The incidence varies depending on the definition used but is approximately 1.5/1000 live births (Kurinczuk et al. 2010). Globally, neonatal HIE is a very large problem, with a high morbidity and mortality in low-income countries. In the past, management of babies with HIE was general supportive treatment. However, research evidence demonstrates that whole body cooling can improve outcomes (Shankaran et al. 2005; Azzopardi et al. 2009; Jacobs et al. 2013). Midwives play a vital role in recognizing the need for cooling and supporting the

> **BOX 37.1   Features Suggestive of Hypoxia-Ischaemia**
>
> **A. Before birth**
> - evidence of antenatal compromise
> - decreased fetal movements
> - abnormal fetal heart rate patterns
> - low fetal pH
> - meconium-stained amniotic fluid.
>
> **B. Poor condition at birth**
> - low heart rate
> - failure to establish normal respiration soon after birth (apnoea or gasping respiration)
> - acidotic cord pH
> - cyanosis or pallor.
>
> **C. Abnormal neonatal neurology**
> - decreased consciousness
> - decreased tone
> - poor suck and other primitive reflexes.

initiation of it. Neonatal encephalopathy is often classified according to a grading system that was originally described by Sarnat and Sarnat (1976). Features suggestive of hypoxia-ischaemia are detailed in Box 37.1.

Infants who are ≥36 weeks' gestation will require careful assessment for signs of encephalopathy and suitability for cooling if:
- Apgar score is ≤5 at 10 min after birth
- there is continued need for resuscitation including intubation or mask inflation at 10 min after birth
- acidosis within 60 min of birth (pH <7.00 in umbilical cord, arterial or capillary sample)
- base deficit ≥16 mmol/L in umbilical cord or any blood sample within 60 min of birth.

In these babies, who have moderate or severe encephalopathy (Table 37.1) whole body cooling should be considered. This treatment requires 72 h of cooling of core body temperature to 33–34°C. Evidence shows that this treatment reduces the risk of cerebral palsy and increases the likelihood of survival without significant disability, by 50% (Shankaran et al. 2005; Azzopardi et al. 2009; Jacobs et al. 2013). If cooling is being considered, the neonatal team may commence *passive* cooling before a firm decision is made. This means active warming of the baby is stopped and their body temperature is allowed to fall passively towards the levels required. Active cooling requires the use of a cooling jacket or mattress (Fig. 37.1) to cool the whole body. The treatment is started as

TABLE 37.1	Grading Criteria for Neonatal Encephalopathy		
	Grade 1 (Mild)	**Grade 2 (Moderate)**	**Grade 3 (Severe)**
Clinical features	• Hyper-alert, staring • May be normal or mild decreased tone/activity • Weak suck and may have poor feeding for up to 24 h	• Lethargy, hypotonia • Decreased activity • Seizures • Weak suck and poor feeding for >24 h	• Decreased consciousness/coma • Hypotonia/flaccid • Frequent prolonged seizures • Absent gag/sucking reflexes • Multi-organ involvement – breathing, kidneys, blood pressure affected
Management	May be able to stay with mother on postnatal ward but requires observation/feeding support	Will require admission to neonatal unit, cooling	Intensive care, cooling
Outcome (Jacobs et al. 2013)	Complete recovery, normal outcome	Most recover well but up to 25% may have long-term neurological problems. Cooling has significant benefits	• Generally poor • Death or significant neuro-disability likely, but with cooling, approximately 70% die or have major disability

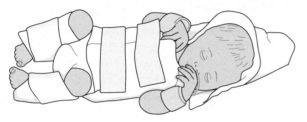

Fig. 37.1 Cooling jacket.

soon as possible after diagnosis and should be within the first 6 h after birth. It is continued for 72 h, after which the baby is gradually warmed. A systematic review of 10 randomized controlled trials (RCTs) (1320 babies in total) by Jacobs et al. (2013) reported a lower risk of death in cooled babies (whole body or head) in the first 18 months of life than in babies treated by standard care. In three of these studies, with 18-month follow-up (767 babies in total), the combined risk of death and severe disability was significantly lower in cooled babies compared with those treated by standard care, and cooling increased survival with normal neurological function compared with standard care at 18-month follow-up. In summary therefore, using cooling decreases the risks of death by >20% and increases the chance of survival without disability by 50%.

Babies with less severe problems

Babies with mild encephalopathy need careful observation and may need additional feeding support but they are often well enough to remain with their mother rather than being admitted to the NICU. These babies are expected to improve quickly and should not have any long-term consequences from their encephalopathy. Babies with mild encephalopathy have not been shown to benefit from whole body cooling.

Seizures and Abnormal Movements

Seizures in the newborn period are an important indicator of potentially serious problems. However, they can be subtle and are not always easy to recognize. The most common cause is neonatal encephalopathy, typically HIE, but readily treatable causes such as hypoglycaemia must not be missed. Different types of seizures may be seen and include *tonic seizures* (sustained posturing of the limbs or trunk or deviation of the head), *clonic* (usually involves one limb or one side of the body jerking rhythmically at 1–4 times/s) or *myoclonic* (rapid isolated jerking of muscles). Subtle seizures may include behaviours such as repetitive lip smacking, staring, blinking or repetitive movements of the limbs such as cycling movements.

Causes of seizures

Seizures in the newborn almost always have an identifiable cause. Examples include:

- HIE (49%)
- cerebral infarction (neonatal stroke) (12%)
- cerebral trauma (7%)

- infections (meningitis or encephalitis) (5%)
- metabolic abnormalities, including hypoglycaemia (3%).

It is important to distinguish seizures from jitteriness and neonatal sleep myoclonus: both of which are benign. Jitteriness is symmetrical rapid movements of the hands and feet. It is often stimulus-sensitive and may be initiated by sudden movement or noise and there are no associated eye movements. Benign sleep myoclonus involves bilateral or unilateral jerking during sleep. It occurs during active sleep, is not stimulus-sensitive and tends to be seen in the upper limbs more than the lower limbs. It is important to ensure that the baby is not at risk from the seizure, the airway is clear and they are breathing. The treatable causes should be identified. The blood glucose should be assessed to exclude hypoglycaemia and electrolytes, including calcium and sodium. Infection should also be considered.

INFECTION IN THE NEWBORN

Infection is one of the commonest reasons for newborn babies becoming unwell and requiring admission to a neonatal unit, consequently it remains an important cause of mortality and morbidity. Newborn babies may acquire infections antenatally (*transplacental infection*), during birth or after birth. They get some protection from the passive transfer of antibodies from their mother against infections they may come into contact with. The immune system is functional at birth and newborn babies can mount their own humeral (*antibody*) response to new infections. However, preterm babies are particularly vulnerable to infection, as placental transfer of IgG mainly occurs after 32 weeks' gestation and their own antibody response is immature.

Umbilical Cord

Until its separation, the umbilical cord can be a focus for infection by bacteria that colonize the skin of the newborn. The umbilical stump should be dry. If periumbilical redness occurs or a discharge is noted, it may be necessary to start antibiotic therapy to prevent ascending infection.

Bacterial Infection in the Newborn

Early signs of infection may be subtle and difficult to distinguish from other problems. The mother or midwife may simply feel the baby is *off colour or not right*. The physical signs that may be apparent are:

- *Temperature instability.* This may be a low temperature just as much as an increased temperature. Always carefully assess any appropriately grown baby who is unable to maintain a temperature of 37°C with a normal room temperature and normal wrapping/clothing.
- *Lethargy or poor feeding.* In general, babies, particularly those who are breastfeeding, will get only small volumes of colostrum in the first 24 h after birth, however, they should show an interest in feeding, be able to attach to the breast and have a sucking reflex.
- Unexplained bradycardia (heart rate <100/min) or tachycardia (heart rate >180/bpm) and any apnoea or episodes of cyanosis
- Increased respiratory rate or signs of respiratory distress
- Irritability, abnormal movements
- Skin mottling, rashes, prolonged capillary refill time.

If bacterial infection is suspected, then investigations are performed (often referred to by neonatologists as a *septic screen*) and antibiotics administered until blood and cerebrospinal fluid (CSF) cultures have confirmed no growth of pathogenic organisms (usually between 36–48 h). The usual investigations are:

- blood culture
- full blood cell count and blood film
- C-reactive protein measurement
- lumbar puncture for examination and culture of CSF.

Treatment of infection and management of babies with risk of infection

The overall aim is to reduce the risk of septicaemia and life-threatening septic shock in the vulnerable newborn baby. Bacterial infections are an important cause of neonatal morbidity and mortality. The two commonest organisms in the newborn are group *B streptococcus* (GBS; also known as *Streptococcus agalactiae*) and *Escherichia* (*E.*) *coli*, which are both organisms the baby may come into contact with via the maternal birth canal. Risk factors for early onset neonatal infection (Oddie and Embleton 2002; Ungerer et al. 2004; Hughes et al. 2017; National Institute for Health and Care Excellence, NICE 2012), include the following:

- maternal intrapartum fever (>38°C) or confirmed or suspected chorioamnionitis
- prolonged rupture of membranes >18 h

- prematurity <37 weeks
- maternal GBS colonization, bacteriuria or infection in the current pregnancy
- parenteral antibiotic treatment given to the woman for confirmed or suspected invasive infection during labour or in the 24 h before and after birth
- previous baby with GBS disease
- suspected or confirmed infection in another baby in the case of a multiple pregnancy.

These factors are used in the UK to decide which babies should receive antibiotics based on a risk-based approach (NICE 2012). In high-risk pregnancies, early onset neonatal GBS infection can be reduced with antibiotics during labour (Law et al. 2005). Similarly, antibiotic use for preterm rupture of membranes is associated with reduced neonatal morbidity (Kenyon et al. 2010). Generally therefore, risk factors should be identified before labour so that, if possible, intrapartum antibiotics should be given at least 4 h prior to birth to obtain maximal antibiotic concentration in the amniotic fluid (Pylipow et al. 1994). There is, however, also some evidence that suggests 2 h may be adequate (de Cueto et al. 1998). In babies with more than one risk factor, observation or treatment with antibiotics after birth is required.

The age of presentation of early onset GBS varies between studies. In a prospective UK study, when intrapartum antibiotics were not given, 50% of babies with early onset GBS presented by 1 h of age, 72% by 24 h and 92% by 48 h (Oddie and Embleton 2002). Bromberger et al. (2000), in a retrospective study, found that 95% of term babies with early onset GBS presented within the first 24 h of life. Additionally, intrapartum antibiotics did not alter the constellation and timing of onset of clinical signs of early onset GBS. Therefore, if babies are well by 12 h of age they are unlikely to develop early onset disease.

Group *B streptococcus* infection

GBS is recognized as the most frequent cause of sepsis in the newborn (Oddie and Embleton 2002; Heath et al. 2004). In England and Wales, there has been an increase in overall infection rates over the 20 years 1991–2010, with infant disease rates rising to around 0.7 per 1000 live births (Lamagni et al. 2013). One-third of the population carry GBS in the gut and over 20% of women have vaginal colonization (Barcaite et al. 2008). In the USA, Australia and several European countries, screening of pregnant women is used with antibiotic treatment during labour, which is effective in reducing the incidence of early onset

GBS. This approach, however, has not been shown in trials to reduce the risk of death or long-term harm from GBS; its introduction in the UK has been hotly debated but the introduction of screening has not been recommended. The current UK recommendations (Hughes et al. 2017;) are therefore based on a risk factor approach described above, whereby intrapartum antibiotic prophylaxis (IAP) is offered to all women with recognized risk factors for early onset GBS disease. Mathematical modelling in the USA suggests that this approach will result in approximately 25% of women being offered IAP with a decrease in the incidence of early onset GBS disease of 50.0–68.8%. UK data suggest that approximately 16% of pregnancies will have one or more risk factors for early onset GBS disease and approximately 60% of early onset GBS cases will have a risk factor (Oddie and Embleton 2002; Hughes et al. 2017).

Meningitis

Neonatal meningitis is an inflammation of the membranes covering the brain and spinal column caused by such organisms as GBS, *E. coli*, *Listeria monocytogenes* and, less often, *Candida* and herpes. In the UK, neonatal meningitis is most often caused by GBS (Law et al. 2005). Very early signs are often nonspecific, followed by those of meningeal irritation and raised intracranial pressure such as crying, irritability, bulging anterior fontanelle, increasing lethargy, seizures, severe vomiting, diminished muscle tone and alterations in consciousness. Babies may also present with abnormal neurological signs. Early diagnosis and treatment are critical to prevent collapse and death. Diagnosis may be confirmed by examination of CSF. Very ill babies require intensive support and antibiotic therapy. Although acute phase mortality has declined in recent years, long-term neurological complications still occur in many surviving babies. de Louvois et al. (2005) reported that in one group aged 5 years, 23% had a serious disability, with isolation of bacteria from CSF the best single predictor. For such babies, long-term comprehensive developmental assessment is essential, including audiometry and vision testing.

TORCH Infections

Infections may be acquired through the placenta, from amniotic fluid or the birth canal. The acronym **TORCH** is often used for congenital infections:

- **T**oxoplasmosis
- **O**ther (includes syphilis, varicella-zoster, parvovirus B19)

- **R**ubella
- **C**ytomegalovirus (CMV)
- **H**erpes.

All of these may cause significant illness in the newborn.

Toxoplasmosis

Toxoplasmosis is caused by *Toxoplasma gondii* (*T. gondii*), a protozoan parasite. It is found in uncooked meat, cat and dog faeces. Primary infection can be asymptomatic, or characterized by malaise, lymphadenopathy and ocular disease. Primary infection during pregnancy can cause severe damage to the fetus (Montoya and Liesenfeld 2004). Childhood-acquired infection also causes half of toxoplasma ocular disease in UK and Irish children (Gilbert et al. 2006).

Incidence and effects during pregnancy. Risks for the infected fetus can include intrauterine death, low birth weight, enlarged liver and spleen, jaundice, anaemia, intracranial calcifications, hydrocephalus, retinochoroidal and macular lesions. Infected neonates may be asymptomatic at birth, but can develop retinal and neurological disease. Those with subclinical disease at birth can develop seizures, cognitive and motor problems and reduced cognitive function over time (Gilbert et al. 2006; Schmidt et al. 2006; Systematic Review on Congenital Toxoplasmosis Group, SYROCOT 2007). In one group of 38 children with confirmed toxoplasma infection, 58% had congenital infection. Of these, 9% were stillborn while 32% of the live births had intracranial abnormalities and/or developmental delay, and 45% had retinochoroiditis with no other abnormalities. Of the 42% of children infected after birth, all had retinochoroiditis (Gilbert et al. 2006).

The effectiveness of antenatal treatment in reducing the congenital transmission of *T. gondii* is not proven. A meta-analysis of 1438 treated mothers (26 cohorts) also found no evidence that antenatal treatment significantly reduced the risk of clinical signs (SYROCOT 2007). Babies with congenital toxoplasmosis are usually treated with pyrimethamine, sulfadiazine and folinic acid for an extended period (Montoya and Liesenfeld 2004; Schmidt et al. 2006).

Prevention. Midwives have an essential role in prevention as health education can result in a 92% reduction in pregnancy seroconversion. In the UK, the National Health Service (NHS Choices 2017) website provides useful information, as well as the Toxoplasmosis Trust for women, their families and healthcare professionals. Appropriate information includes advising women about washing kitchen surfaces following contact with uncooked meats, stringent hand-washing and avoiding cat and dog faeces.

Varicella zoster

Varicella zoster virus (VZV) is a highly contagious virus of the herpes family that causes varicella (chickenpox). Transmitted by respiratory droplets and contact with vesicle fluid, it has an incubation period of 10–20 days and is infectious for 48 h before the rash appears and until vesicles crust over. After primary infection, the virus remains dormant in the sensory nerve root ganglia and with any recurrent infection can result in *herpes zoster* (shingles). Most childbearing women in the UK have had varicella and are immune. However, a primary infection during pregnancy can result in serious adverse outcomes (Meyberg-Solomayer et al. 2006).

Incidence and effects during pregnancy. Fetal effects vary with gestation at the time of maternal infection. During the first 20 weeks of pregnancy, the fetus has about a 2% risk of *fetal varicella syndrome* (FVS). Signs can include skin lesions and scarring, eye problems, such as chorioretinitis and cataracts. Skeletal anomalies include limb hypoplasia. Severe neurological problems may include encephalitis, microcephaly and significant developmental delay. About 30% of babies born with skin lesions die in the first months of life. From 20 weeks' gestation up to almost the time of birth, infection can result in milder forms of neonatal varicella that do not result in negative sequelae for the neonate. The child may have shingles during the first few years of life. Maternal infection after 36 weeks, and particularly in the week before the birth (when cord blood VZV IgG is low) to 2 days after, can result in infection rates of up to 50%. About 25% of those infected will develop neonatal clinical varicella. Most affected babies will develop a vesicular rash and about 30% will die. Other complications of neonatal varicella include pneumonia, pyoderma and hepatitis.

Diagnosis and treatment. Diagnosis can be made if there has been a recent history of maternal chickenpox, and polymerase chain reaction (PCR) to identify VZV in amniotic fluid. Antenatal ultrasound may confirm the effects of fetal varicella syndrome, e.g. limb contractures and malformations, cerebral anomalies, borderline ventriculomegaly, intracerebral, intrahepatic and myocardial calcifications, articular effusions and intrauterine growth restriction (IUGR) (Degani 2006; Meyberg-Solomayer et al. 2006).

Women infected during the first 20 weeks may request termination of pregnancy. Varicella zoster immunoglobulin (VZIG) can be offered to seronegative pregnant women who are exposed to chickenpox, within 72 h of contact, and always within 10 days. VZIG should also be administered to a baby whose mother develops chickenpox between 7 days before and 7 days after the birth, or whose siblings at home have chickenpox (if the mother is seronegative). Although no clinical trials have shown that antiviral chemotherapy prevents fetal infection, the antiviral drug *acyclovir* may reduce the mortality and risk of severe disease in some groups, particularly if VZIG is not available. These include pregnant women with severe complications, and newborns if they are unwell or have added risk factors such as prematurity or corticosteroid therapy (Sauerbrei and Wutzler 2000, 2001; Hayakawa et al. 2003).

Rubella

For most immune-competent children and adults (including pregnant women), the rubella virus, that is spread by droplet infection, causes a mild, insignificant illness. Congenital rubella syndrome (CRS) in the newborn however, remains a major cause of developmental anomalies that include blindness and deafness (Banatvala and Brown 2004). Maternal rubella is rare in many countries as a result of successful rubella vaccination programmes (Robinson et al. 2006). The measles, mumps and rubella (MMR) vaccine has significantly reduced the incidence of rubella (Wright and Polack 2006), albeit vaccination rates have declined in the UK and some other countries over recent years due to adverse press coverage. This potentially could result in an increase in the incidence of rubella. Countries without routine MMR programmes report rates similar to those of countries before vaccination became available (Banatvala and Brown 2004). As part of their public health role, midwives can encourage women who have not had the MMR vaccination to get protected before and after – but *not* during – pregnancy. They should also discuss the importance of vaccinating their children. Generally individuals will only be infected with rubella once during their lifetime, as they then develop an antibody response. Primary rubella infection is most likely to cause problems if it is acquired in the first 12 weeks of pregnancy when maternal–fetal transmission rates are as high as 85%. Intrauterine infection is unlikely when the mother's rash appears before, or within 11 days after

the last menstrual period; with infection later than the 16th week, the risk of severe fetal sequelae is much lower (Enders et al. 1988). First trimester infection can result in spontaneous miscarriage and in surviving babies, a number of serious and permanent consequences. These include cataracts, sensorineural deafness, congenital heart defects, microcephaly, meningoencephalitis, dermal erythropoiesis, thrombocytopenia and significant developmental delay (Banatvala and Brown 2004; Bedford and Tookey 2006).

Diagnosis and treatment. Congenital rubella can be recognized when there has been a maternal history of infection during pregnancy, or as a result of anomalies detected in the fetus or the newborn. All women have screening for rubella titres at booking in the UK and those not protected can be offered immunization **after** pregnancy. They should also avoid contact with anyone known to have the illness during pregnancy. If there is any contact, then rubella titres should be measured with increased surveillance of the fetus. Women with first trimester infection may request termination of pregnancy. Babies with CRS are highly infectious and should be isolated from other babies and pregnant women (but not their own mothers). Long-term follow-up is essential, as some problems may not become apparent until the baby is older.

Candida

Candida is a Gram-positive yeast fungus with a number of strains (see Chapter 15). *Candida (C.) albicans* is responsible for most fungal infections, including thrush in babies. Infection can affect the mouth (*oral candidiasis*), skin (*cutaneous candidiasis*) particularly the nappy area and internal organs (*systemic candidiasis*).

Oral candidiasis is a common mild illness that may present as white patches on the baby's gums, palate or tongue. It can be acquired during birth or from caregivers' hands or feeding equipment. Raw areas on the edge of the baby's tongue can assist diagnosis. Risk factors for thrush include bottle use during the first 2 weeks, the presence of siblings (Morrill et al. 2005) and antibiotic exposure (Dinsmoor et al. 2005). Women who breastfeed their babies may experience breast infection with flaky or shiny skin of the nipple/areola, sore, red nipples and persistent burning, itching or stabbing pain in the breasts (see Chapter 27). Accurate diagnosis and treatment of thrush is important for continued breastfeeding. Morrill et al. (2005) found only 43% of women with thrush 2 weeks after the birth, were breastfeeding at 9 weeks, compared with 69% of women without.

Cutaneous candidiasis often co-exists with oral thrush and presents as a moist papular or vesicular skin rash, usually in the axillae, neck, perineum or umbilicus. Although it is usually benign, recognition and treatment is important in preventing problems (Smolinski et al. 2005). Management includes keeping the area dry and applying topical antifungals. In preterm babies, the thin cutaneous barrier, invasive procedures and immune system immaturity may contribute to the early onset of *systemic Candida* infection. Antifungal prophylaxis may be used to prevent systemic *Candida* colonization. Systemic candidiasis in a preterm baby is a serious problem and requires a prolonged course of treatment with intravenous antifungal medication. It is associated with significant morbidity and mortality.

Significant Eye Infections

Eye infection caused by *Chlamydia* or *Gonococcus* will present with a red sore eye and a large amount of purulent discharge. *Ophthalmia neonatorum* refers to any purulent eye discharge in the baby within 28 days of birth. A swab must be taken for culture and sensitivity testing, with immediate medical referral. Identification of the organism responsible is essential as chlamydial and gonococcal infections can cause conjunctival scarring, corneal infiltration, blindness and systemic spread. Treatment includes local cleaning and care of the eyes with normal saline, and appropriate drug therapy for the baby and the mother if required.

RESPIRATORY PROBLEMS

There are several important causes of respiratory distress in the newborn such as infection, *transient tachypnoea of the newborn* (TTN) and *surfactant-deficient lung disease of prematurity*. The latter (previously known as *hyaline membrane disease*) is confusingly called respiratory distress syndrome (RDS). It is not always easy to be certain of the cause of respiratory distress at initial presentation.

Initial Management of Babies Presenting with Respiratory Distress

Typical signs of respiratory distress in the newborn period include tachypnoea (>60 breaths/min), intercostal and subcostal recession, 'grunting', and nasal flaring.

Babies should be assessed in a good light, ideally where oxygen and airway support can be given if necessary (e.g. a Resuscitaire). Signs of respiratory distress after birth require careful observation. A baby who has increased work of breathing and/or central cyanosis should be reviewed urgently. The history of the pregnancy and birth may give important clues as to the most likely cause of respiratory distress. Relevant factors are:

- gestation
- meconium in amniotic fluid
- mode of birth (caesarean section rather than vaginal)
- high vaginal swabs during pregnancy
- antenatal scans.

The baby should be observed for:

- the respiratory rate, heart rate, work of breathing
- the colour of the tongue and lips for central cyanosis
- skin colour and perfusion, e.g. pallor, mottled or white
- the baby's level of activity and tone
- feeding ability: babies with significant respiratory distress will not be able to feed safely
- apnoea.

The midwife will need to recognize the ill baby and liaise with the medical team. There may be need to proceed as for resuscitation at birth (see Chapter 33).

Possible Causes of Respiratory Distress in the Newborn

Infection

Respiratory distress can be a presenting feature of a serious infection (particularly GBS) and it can be very difficult to distinguish it from other causes of respiratory distress. It is usual practice to undertake an infection screen and treat with intravenous (IV) antibiotics until infection is excluded as the cause of the respiratory distress.

Meconium aspiration syndrome

Meconium in the amniotic fluid is common and usually does not require treatment or intervention if the baby is in good condition at birth and shows no signs of respiratory distress. Meconium aspiration occurs because hypoxia-ischaemia causes the fetus to pass meconium into the amniotic fluid. Gasping respiration may also occur as a result of hypoxia-ischaemia. *Consequently, it is the baby showing signs of fetal hypoxia, which develops meconium aspiration syndrome.* The incidence for meconium aspiration syndrome is known to vary from country to country with rates as low as 0.2/1000 live births in the UK compared with a higher incidence of 2–5/1000 in the USA (Greenough and Milner 2012). The initial respiratory distress may be mild, moderate or severe with a gradual deterioration over the first 12–24 h in more severe cases. The baby may present with cyanosis, increased work of breathing and a barrel-shaped chest. This is because of air trapping, leading to hyper-expansion of the lungs. The meconium can become trapped in the airways and cause a ball-valve effect: air can enter the lung during inhalation but the meconium then blocks the airway during expiration so that air accumulates behind the blockage. This accumulation can then lead to air leaks and the baby to develop a pneumothorax. Where the meconium has contact with the lung tissue a chemical pneumonitis occurs and there is a risk of super-added infection. Endogenous surfactant is also broken down in the presence of meconium.

These babies may need intensive care and ventilation. Specialized treatments such as nitric oxide (Finer et al. 2017) are of benefit in reducing death or the need for extracorporeal membrane oxygenation (ECMO) in some babies. ECMO has been shown to increase survival by 50% (UK Collaborative ECMO Trial Group 1996). Although the majority of infants make a full recovery, a number of the most severely affected babies will have signs of respiratory distress for some months, with ongoing residual respiratory problems during early childhood.

Transient tachypnoea of the newborn

The recorded incidence of transient tachypnoea of the newborn (TTN) varies widely, partly as a result of the variety of recording methods, differences in radiological interpretation and lack of clear diagnostic features. It is frequently seen as a diagnosis of exclusion of other possible respiratory causes. Babies may present with mild to moderate signs of respiratory distress and require admission to the NICU for further observation. Supplemental oxygen may be required initially but the condition gradually resolves during the 24 h following birth. The chest X-ray may show a streaky appearance with fluid in the horizontal fissure of the right lung. However, sometimes it is only the clinical course that distinguishes between TTN, respiratory distress syndrome (RDS) and infection. The lungs are completely fluid-filled before birth. This fluid is partly squeezed out through chest compression during vaginal birth, the rest being absorbed via the lymphatic system. When born by elective caesarean section, the baby's thorax has not been squeezed, which goes some way to explaining the increased risk of respiratory morbidity; birth at each week below 39 weeks approximately doubles the risk (Morrison et al. 1995). Although babies with TTN may require initial care on the NICU, their stay is usually of a short duration for observation and supplemental oxygen.

Respiratory distress syndrome

RDS is a condition that primarily affects preterm babies but can also occur in those born at term, when other disorders that can inhibit surfactant production are present. Approximately 50% of babies born before 30 weeks' gestation develop RDS, while 1% of all newborn babies may develop the condition (Greenough and Milner 2012). Surfactant is made up of phospholipids and proteins and is produced by the type II pneumocytes. It reduces the surface tension within the alveoli, preventing their collapse at the end of exhalation. When collapsed, alveoli require much greater pressures and exertion to re-inflate and the terminal airways become lined with *hyaline membranes*. The introduction of surfactant therapy into neonatal care during the 1980s and 1990s, combined with much wider use of antenatal steroids in the 1990s, significantly decreased the mortality and morbidity previously seen in RDS.

In preterm babies with RDS, the clinical picture is typically of a baby with progressive respiratory distress developing over the first hours. The X-ray shows a homogenous ground-glass appearance (indicating poorly aerated alveoli) with air bronchograms (black air-filled bronchi seen against white airless alveoli), although this may be less obvious if the baby has already received exogenous surfactant. Without administration of exogenous surfactant, babies with RDS experience increasing respiratory distress and work of breathing over the first 48–72 h followed by a slow improvement as endogenous surfactant is produced. In extremely preterm babies, surfactant is often given at the time of birth, usually in the context of the baby also requiring intubation and positive pressure ventilation. Alternative approaches using continuous positive airways pressure (CPAP) can also be used (Morley et al. 2008; SUPPORT 2010). Exogenous surfactant can be given as *rescue treatment* if the baby develops significant early signs of worsening respiratory distress. There is also increasing interest in the use of less invasive surfactant administration (LISA) in spontaneously breathing preterm infants with respiratory distress, although it has yet to become standard practice (Aldana-Aguirre et al. 2017).

Pneumothorax

Pneumothoraces may occur spontaneously in 1% of the newborn population either during or after birth; however, only one-tenth will be seen (Steele et al. 1971). A pneumothorax at birth may be caused by the large pressures generated by the baby's first breaths, often in the range of 40–80 cmH$_2$O. This can lead to alveoli distension and rupture that allows air to leak to a number of sites, most notably the potential space between the lung pleura. Babies receiving any assisted ventilation have an increased susceptibility to a pneumothorax. This could be due to either maldistribution of the ventilated gas in the lungs, high ventilation settings or baby-ventilator breathing interactions. Spontaneous pneumothorax can occur in otherwise healthy term babies. They may present with signs of respiratory distress on the postnatal ward. Although it is difficult to diagnose a pneumothorax in the absence of a chest X-ray, there may be reduced breath sounds on the affected side, displaced heart sounds and a distorted chest/diaphragm movement. A baby with a suspected pneumothorax will need closer observation and may need intervention with a chest drain. Many spontaneously breathing term babies who are stable can be managed without a chest drain, as long as they are closely observed, as most small pneumothoraces in this context will resolve spontaneously.

Congenital diaphragmatic hernia

CDH has an incidence of 3.5/1000 live births. It is an important condition because, despite improvements in neonatal care, reported mortality rates remain high (Wright et al. 2010). Most babies with a diaphragmatic hernia are diagnosed prenatally, usually made at the 20th week anomaly scan. However in some babies, the diagnosis is not made until after birth. Where there is an prenatal diagnosis, the usual care at birth is immediate intubation, insertion of a large bore nasogastric (NG) tube to decompress the stomach and bowel and early sedation/muscle relaxation. This allows optimal ventilation as early as possible to try to allow the underdeveloped lungs to expand and prevent significant problems with persistent

pulmonary hypertension and continual right-to-left shunting of blood through the foramen ovale and ductus arteriosus. Intensive care is difficult in these babies and the priorities are to maintain good ventilation and perfusion to avoid hypoxia. A surgical repair of the diaphragm will usually be performed at 2–7 days after birth if the underlying lung development is sufficient to enable stabilization of the baby. In all babies presenting with respiratory distress, a chest X-ray is important to discover the cause, one of which is a CDH. Babies with this condition typically have unilateral chest movement, heart sounds and an apex beat on the right side (in the case of left-sided CDH, which is more common) and a scaphoid abdomen. Babies with a postnatal diagnosis of CDH have a much better prognosis, with greater expected survival rates (van den Hout et al. 2010).

Upper airway obstruction and stridor

Upper airway obstruction in the newborn baby is uncommon but is characterized by noisy breathing on inspiration and is different to 'grunting', which is an expiratory noise. Obstruction to the upper airway significantly increases the work of breathing for a newborn baby and in the most severe cases, can quickly lead to exhaustion. Babies with stridor therefore always need medical assessment. It is important to evaluate the degree of respiratory distress and assess whether the baby is managing to breathe comfortably despite the stridor. There are many possible causes. One of the commonest is *laryngomalacia* and the baby may have mild respiratory distress but the work of breathing may increase when the baby is placed on their back. Although most babies do gradually improve with time, it is occasionally severe and the diagnosis needs to be confirmed with endoscopy. *Stridor* can be caused by external compression of the trachea, e.g. vascular anomalies, and requires specialist investigation.

CONGENITAL HEART DISEASE

The reported prevalence of CHD is influenced by the context of healthcare provision but recent estimates are of 9/1000 (Liu et al. 2019). Although many newborn infants may be asymptomatic, early diagnosis is extremely important for some conditions and it is vital that newborn babies are examined carefully to look for signs of

CHD (see Chapter 32). There are a number of ways that CHD may present in the newborn period and these give some clues as to the underlying anatomical diagnosis:

- prenatal diagnosis on antenatal scan
- associated with a syndrome or other congenital problems, e.g. Down syndrome
- asymptomatic murmur
- cyanosis
- sudden collapse
- heart failure.

Many countries and areas in the UK have also introduced the routine use of pulse oximetry measurement of oxygen saturation as part of the assessment of all newborn infants. There is evidence that it may help aid earlier diagnosis of serious congenital heart disease (Thangaratinam et al. 2012). There is however, ongoing debate in the UK as to whether it should be adopted as a part of the universal neonatal screening programme.

Management of a Baby with an Antenatal Diagnosis of Congenital Heart Disease

In a baby where an antenatal diagnosis of CHD has been made, there is usually a pre-agreed plan, which should be available to those providing the neonatal care. For some types of serious congenital malformations (e.g. transposition of the great arteries; pulmonary atresia (with or without VSD); coarctation of the aorta, hypoplastic left heart syndrome), a prostaglandin infusion to maintain patency of the ductus arteriosus is required immediately after birth, with stabilization and transfer to a cardiology centre. Some types of CHD do not require immediate intervention, but the baby will need follow-up with a cardiologist.

Care of a Baby with a Murmur

Babies found to have an asymptomatic heart murmur on their newborn examination (see Chapter 32) need careful assessment observing for other signs of cardiac disease. A pulse oximeter measurement of oxygen saturation is important with normal values being >96%. *It is worth noting that babies with a saturation of 85% often do not look cyanosed on visual inspection.* Measuring pre- and post-ductal saturations can be useful alongside measuring the blood pressure in all four limbs to look for signs of coarctation of the aorta (lower pressures in lower limbs). All babies with a cardiac murmur should be evaluated by a neonatologist and local guidelines are usually in place for appropriate cardiac referral.

JAUNDICE

Jaundice refers to the yellow colouration of the skin and the sclera caused by a raised level of bilirubin in the circulation *(hyperbilirubinaemia)*. Approximately 60% of term and 80% of preterm babies develop jaundice in the first week after birth, and about 10% of exclusively breastfed babies are still jaundiced at 1 month of age. In most babies, early jaundice is harmless. However, a few babies will develop very high levels of bilirubin, which can be harmful if not treated. Jaundice may also be an early sign of a more serious underlying condition and it is therefore important that the midwife is aware of this and refers appropriately for medical attention.

Clinical recognition and assessment of jaundice can be difficult, particularly in babies with dark skin tones. In the UK, the use a transcutaneous bilirubinometer (TCB) is recommended to measure the bilirubin level and if not available, to measure the serum bilirubin (NICE 2016). If a transcutaneous bilirubinometer measurement indicates a bilirubin level >250 μmol/L, the serum bilirubin should be assessed. Once the midwife recognizes jaundice in the baby, it is important to have a clear management plan. In the UK, there are national guidelines (NICE 2016) that have tried to standardize monitoring and treatment and similar guidelines exist in other countries (American Academy of Pediatrics, AAP 2004).

Bilirubin Physiology

It is important to understand bilirubin metabolism when planning the management of babies who present with jaundice. Bilirubin is produced as one of the breakdown products of haemoglobin (Fig. 37.2B). Ageing, immature or malformed red cells are removed from the circulation and broken down in the reticuloendothelial system (liver, spleen and macrophages). Haemoglobin from these cells is broken down into haem, globin and iron. *Haem* is converted to unconjugated bilirubin, a fat soluble product; *globin* is broken down into amino acids, which are used by the body to make proteins and *iron* is stored in the body or used for new red blood cells. The unconjugated bilirubin is transported to the liver bound to albumin from where detachment occurs and then it combines with glucose and glucuronic acid, resulting in *conjugation*, using the enzyme uridine diphosphoglucuronyl transferase (UDP-GT). The conjugated bilirubin is now water-soluble and can be excreted via the biliary

Physiological change in bilirubin concentration after birth

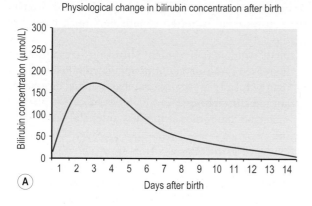

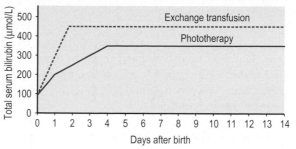

Fig. 37.3 Bilirubin chart.

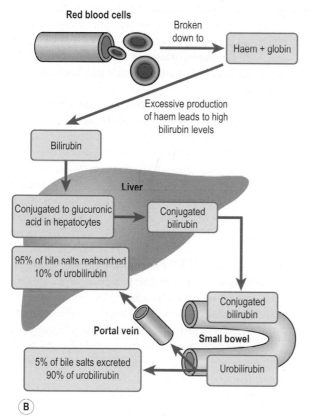

Fig. 37.2 Bilirubin pathway (A) Physiological change in bilirubin concentration after birth. (B) Production and circulation of bilirubin.

system into the small intestine, where normal bacteria change the conjugated bilirubin into urobilinogen. This is then oxidized into orange-coloured urobilin. Most is excreted in the faeces, with a small amount excreted in urine (Ahlfors and Wennberg 2004; Kaplan et al. 2005).

Physiological Jaundice

The turnover of haemoglobin is high before birth but the bilirubin is removed efficiently via the placenta. All newborn babies have a rise in unconjugated bilirubin during the first few days after birth for several reasons:

- At birth, as lungs increase blood oxygen levels, there is haemolysis of excess red blood cells (RBC) that are no longer required.
- At birth, the newborn liver enzymes systems may be immature and not as effective in conjugating and excreting bilirubin.

As a result of these factors, there is a rise in serum unconjugated bilirubin in healthy babies during the first few days after birth and this physiological jaundice follows a characteristic pattern (Fig. 37.2A). Typically, babies on the first day after birth will not appear jaundiced but most babies will have a yellow tinge by day 3–4. As unconjugated bilirubin levels rise, the serum albumin becomes saturated and then any excesses spill over into the blood plasma. Unconjugated bilirubin is fat-soluble and will deposit in subcutaneous fat, which makes the skin appear yellow. Once these sites are saturated, the brain is the next target, particularly the basal ganglia. High levels of unconjugated bilirubin can potentially be a serious problem because, when not bound to albumin, bilirubin can cross the blood–brain barrier and be deposited in the basal ganglia in the brain. This can cause a typical clinical picture of bilirubin encephalopathy and in the longer term, result in cerebral palsy, sensorineural hearing loss and learning difficulties. The cerebral palsy is typically an athetoid type due to the site of the damage in the brain. *Kernicterus* is the pathological finding at postmortem of the characteristic pattern of yellow staining in the brainstem seen after bilirubin encephalopathy. Bilirubin encephalopathy is serious but rarer now because of the decrease in incidence of Rhesus haemolytic disease since the introduction of anti-D pro-phylaxis (see Chapter 13) and the use of other interventions to control high unconjugated bilirubin levels in babies. However, there have been concerns that the incidence is starting to increase again (Manning et al. 2007) and midwives can play a pivotal role in trying to prevent this devastating complication.

Causes of Concern in Jaundice

There are several situations where a midwife should be concerned about jaundice in the newborn:

- jaundice in the first 24 h after birth
- history of antibodies (which may cause RBC haemolysis) identified on the maternal antibody screen
- any baby who is visibly jaundiced; this will require further evaluation with bilirubinometer and/or serum bilirubin (SBR) as the visual assessment of jaundice is not sufficiently accurate (NICE 2016)
- any baby who remains jaundiced beyond 14 days of age.

Early jaundice (within first 5 days after birth)

Possible causes include:

- physiological jaundice
- haemolysis (Rhesus isoimmunization, ABO incompatibility, other blood group antigen problems)
- infection
- bruising
- polycythaemia
- dehydration (unlikely in the first 48 h but must be considered in babies presenting between 2–7 days after birth).

This is not an exhaustive list but these are the causes that midwives will encounter on a regular basis. As a general rule, haemolysis must always be considered when a baby is jaundiced in the first 24 h after birth.

Assessment and Diagnosis of Physiological Jaundice

Two important areas to consider at the outset are:

- *Is the jaundice physiological due to the normal process of breakdown of bilirubin or is there a pathological process?*
- *Is the baby at risk of bilirubin encephalopathy?*

Individual risk factors

The initial assessment of a baby should include identifying risk factors for jaundice. These include any disease or disorder that increases bilirubin production, or alters the transport or excretion of bilirubin. Such examples being:

- birth trauma or evident bruising (resulting in increased production of unconjugated bilirubin)
- family history of significant haemolytic disease or jaundice in siblings
- maternal antibodies at the first antenatal visit/booking
- evidence of infection
- prematurity
- timing of jaundice; jaundice within the first 24 h should be regarded as pathological as it is commonly due to haemolysis. Jaundice at 3–6 days of age could be related to dehydration. At this age, it is good practice to take a feeding history, assess the baby's weight and evaluate the hydration status. Even with significant weight loss, the midwife should always consider other causes.

Physical assessment of the baby includes observation of the extent of changes in skin and sclera colour, skin bruising or cephalohaematoma (see Chapter 35) and other clinical signs such as lethargy, decreased eagerness to feed and accompanying dehydration. Signs of infection should be considered (e.g. temperature, vomiting, irritability or high-pitched cry) and the colour of the urine and stools observed: dark urine and light stools could indicate intrahepatic or extrahepatic obstructive disease.

Relevant laboratory investigations are determined by the clinical assessment. In the presence of an elevated SBR, the following are commonly undertaken:

- direct antiglobulin test (DAT; also referred to as Direct Coomb's test, DCT) to detect the presence of maternal antibodies on the baby's red blood cells
- blood groups (baby and mother) and Rh type for possible incompatibility
- haemoglobin concentration to assess anaemia/polycythaemia
- total bilirubin, including conjugated bilirubin if there are any factors to suggest conjugated hyperbilirubinaemia.

Management of Jaundice

If maternal antibodies were present on the first antenatal visit screen, the neonatal team should be informed and regular SBR concentrations should be assessed. These babies may need early phototherapy. In the case of Rh-D antibodies and some other blood group antigens with a high likelihood of causing haemolysis, other interventions such as the use of immunoglobulin or exchange transfusion may be needed that require admission to a NICU. Plotting the SBR concentration on a treatment threshold chart is always useful and deemed best practice by NICE to see how the level compares with phototherapy intervention and/or exchange transfusion interventions. In using such a chart, it is important to select the relevant chart for the gestation of the baby. (An example of a bilirubin chart is shown in Fig. 37.3.) The trend or change in bilirubin can also be assessed from the chart as a guide to whether the level is rising too quickly or is following the normal physiological pattern. Treatment strategies for jaundice include *phototherapy, immunoglobulin therapy* and occasionally *exchange transfusion.*

Phototherapy

It was observed in the 1950s at Rochford Hospital, Essex, that babies cared for in sunlight became less jaundiced (Dobbs and Cremer 1975). Light therapy is effective because ultraviolet blue light (wavelength 420–448 nm) catalyses the conversion of *transbilirubin* into the water-soluble *cis-bilirubin isomer* that can then be excreted via the kidneys. Thresholds for commencing phototherapy are based on SBR levels (NICE 2016). Commercially available phototherapy systems include those delivering light via fluorescent bulbs, halogen quartz lamps, light-emitting diodes and fibreoptic mattresses (Stokowski 2006). Conventional phototherapy systems use high intensity light from conventional white and/or blue, blue–green and turquoise fluorescent phototherapy lamps. Fibreoptic light systems use a woven fibreoptic pad that delivers high intensity light with no ultraviolet or infrared irradiation. They can be used as bilibeds in especially adapted cots or fitted around the chest and abdomen of the baby. These systems may be more comfortable for babies and allow easier accessibility and handling for parents.

Phototherapy is a safe and effective treatment. Any side-effects tend to be mild but can include hyperthermia, increased fluid loss and dehydration, damage to the retina from the high intensity light, lethargy or irritability, decreased eagerness to feed, loose stools, skin rashes and skin burns and alterations in a baby's state and neurobehavioural organization. Phototherapy may be intermittent or continuous (Lau and Fung 1984) with mild/moderate jaundice. It can be administered in the home setting (Snook 2017), although babies would need to be carefully selected for this approach. Babies receiving phototherapy should be nursed naked in an incubator or cot with lid: a minimum of 40 cm from the light. Phototherapy equipment should be routinely checked for safety. The baby's temperature should be measured and recorded at least 4-hourly, more frequently if unstable, and the baby should be turned regularly to maximize exposed areas of skin. For overhead fluorescent therapy, the baby's eyes should be shielded using eye shields. If eye shields are used, these should not be applied too tightly to avoid constriction to the scalp and excessive pressure over eyes. The eye shields should be removed regularly and the baby's eyes inspected for signs of infection. Application of topical creams or lotions should be avoided, as there is a risk of burns and blistering. Particular attention should be paid to careful cleaning and drying of the skin, especially if the stools are loose. The baby should be assessed regularly for signs of dehydration using as a measure urine output or frequency of wet nappies. It is wise not to nurse babies on a white sheet because of reflective glare. Parents should be informed of the requirement for phototherapy and their consent obtained prior to commencement. The parents should also be encouraged to maintain contact with the baby and continue being involved with their routine care. The baby may not require continuous phototherapy and the phototherapy unit can be removed/switched off when caring for and feeding the baby, for up to 30 min in every 3-h period being acceptable while on single phototherapy. However, if the baby is requiring multiple phototherapy, this should not be interrupted.

Discontinuing phototherapy. The SBR should be measured at least every 6–12 h while phototherapy continues. It should be monitored more frequently when the rate of rise is rapid. Phototherapy may be safely discontinued when the bilirubin is 50 µmol/L below the threshold. Repeat SBR measurement is necessary 12–18 h after phototherapy is discontinued to assess for rebound hyperbilirubinaemia.

Immunoglobulin

When there is isoimmune haemolysis, infusion of a set volume of pooled human immunoglobulin may help prevent the need for an exchange transfusion by mopping up excess antibodies (Gottstein and Cooke 2003). Although it reduces the need for exchange transfusions, immunoglobulin slightly increases the risk of requiring a later top-up transfusion but these are safer and less invasive.

Exchange transfusion

If the bilirubin level cannot be controlled with phototherapy and good hydration and the level exceeds the recommended limits (NICE 2016), an exchange transfusion is performed to prevent the bilirubin level reaching levels known to be linked to bilirubin encephalopathy. Exchange transfusion carries significant risks and should always be carried out in an NICU (refer to individual hospital guideline) with experienced operators. It involves transfusing a large volume of blood to the baby (double the baby's blood volume or 160 mL/kg) while removing blood from the baby, usually via an umbilical venous catheter. This process removes excess bilirubin and, if the cause is isoimmunization, antibodies that may be causing the RBC haemolysis. With haemolytic disease of the newborn, sensitized erythrocytes are replaced with blood that is compatible with both the mother's and the baby's serum.

Pathological Jaundice
Haemolytic jaundice

Jaundice within the first 24 h after birth is assumed to be due to haemolysis until proven otherwise. Haemolysis in the fetus or newborn has several causes, the most important being blood group incompatibility. This can occur due to various antibodies, but the most important is caused by Rhesus (Rh-D) isoimmunization/incompatibility. This occurs if blood cells from a Rhesus-positive baby enter a Rhesus-negative mother's bloodstream. Her blood treats the D antigen on positive blood cells as a foreign substance and produces antibodies. These antibodies can then cross the placenta and destroy fetal red blood cells (Figs 37.4–37.9). This condition is particularly relevant for midwives who have a critical role in the injection of anti-D immunoglobulin (anti-D Ig). Without this anti-D prophylaxis, Rh-D isoimmunization can

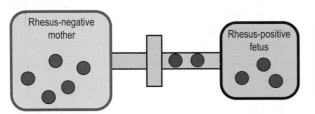

Fig. 37.4 Normal placenta with no communication between maternal and fetal blood.

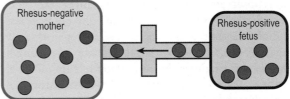

Fig. 37.5 Fetal cells enter maternal circulation through 'break' in 'placental barrier', e.g. at placental separation.

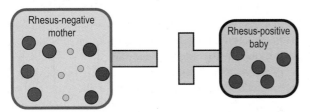

Fig. 37.6 Maternal production of Rhesus antibodies following introduction of Rhesus-positive blood.

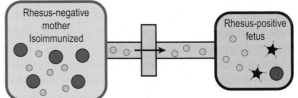

Fig. 37.7 In a subsequent pregnancy maternal Rhesus antibodies cross the placenta, resulting in haemolytic disease of the newborn.

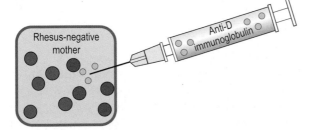

Fig. 37.8 Anti-D immunoglobulin administered within 72 h of birth or other sensitizing event.

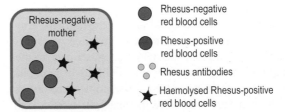

Fig. 37.9 Anti-D immunoglobulin has destroyed fetal Rhesus-positive red cells and prevented isoimmunization.

Figs 37.4–37.9 Isoimmunization and its prevention.

cause severe haemolytic disease of the newborn (HDN) with significant mortality and morbidity (NICE 2008). With the effectiveness of anti-D prophylaxis, antibodies against other blood groups are now more common than anti-D (e.g. anti-A, anti-B and anti-Kell). There are a few antibodies to blood group antigens other than those in the Rh system that cause severe haemolytic disease of the newborn. These include anti-E haemolytic disease of the fetus or newborn (Joy et al. 2005), and anti-Kell (van Dongen et al. 2005). ABO incompatibility can also occur and is the most frequent cause of mild to moderate haemolysis in the neonate.

Rh-D isoimmunization

Rh-D isoimmunization is commonest among Caucasians, about 15% of whom are Rh-negative, compared with 3–5% of African and about 1% of Asian populations (Bianchi et al. 2005). Before the introduction of anti-D Ig in 1969, Rh-D isoimmunization was a major cause of perinatal mortality and morbidity. In England and Wales, about 520 cases of Rh-D isoimmunization are estimated each year, requiring close monitoring. Between 10% and 12% of these babies would require intrauterine transfusions. It is estimated that fetal anaemia and HDN result in approximately 37 fetal/neonatal deaths, 21 children with minor developmental problems and eight with major developmental problems (NICE 2008).

Causes of Rh-D isoimmunization. The placenta usually acts as a barrier to fetal blood entering the maternal circulation (Fig. 37.4). However, during pregnancy or birth, fetomaternal haemorrhage (FMH) can occur, when small amounts of fetal Rh-positive blood can cross the placenta and enter the Rh-negative mother's blood (Fig. 37.5). The woman's immune system produces anti-D antibodies (Fig. 37.6). In subsequent pregnancies, these maternal antibodies can cross the placenta and destroy the red cells of any Rh-positive fetus (Fig. 37.7). Rh-D isoimmunization can result from a procedure or incident where positive Rh-positive blood leaks across the placenta, or from any other transfusion of Rh-positive blood (e.g. blood or platelet transfusion or drug use). Haemolytic disease of the fetus and newborn caused by Rh-D isoimmunization can occur during the first pregnancy. However, in most cases, sensitization during the first pregnancy or birth leads to extensive destruction of fetal red blood cells during subsequent pregnancies (Finning et al. 2004; Bianchi et al. 2005; Geifman-Holtzman et al. 2006; NICE 2008).

Prevention of Rh-D isoimmunization. Most cases of Rh-D isoimmunization can be prevented by injecting anti-D Ig within 72 h of birth or any other sensitizing event (Fig. 37.8). Anti-D Ig is a human plasma-based product that is used to prevent women producing anti-D antibodies. Anti-D Ig is of value to women with non-sensitized Rh-negative blood who have a baby with Rh-positive blood type (Fig. 37.9). *It is not used when anti-D antibodies are already present in maternal blood.* Furthermore, Anti-D Ig does not protect against the development of other antibodies that cause haemolytic disease of the newborn.

Routine prophylaxis. In the UK (and some other countries), since 2002, routine antenatal anti-D prophylaxis at 28 and 34 weeks' gestation is recommended for all non-sensitized Rh-negative women (NICE 2008). With postnatal anti-D Ig prophylaxis, about 1.5% of Rh-negative women still develop anti-D antibodies following a first Rh-positive pregnancy. A meta-analysis (Allaby et al. 1999) and Cochrane Review (Crowther et al. 2013) suggest the antenatal sensitization rate is further reduced by routine antenatal prophylaxis. Antenatal prophylaxis should always be given following possible sensitization events such as spontaneous miscarriage before 12 weeks, any threatened, complete, incomplete or missed abortion *after* 12 weeks of pregnancy, termination of pregnancy by surgical or medical methods regardless of gestational age, fetal death *in utero* or stillbirth, ectopic pregnancy or amniocentesis, cordocentesis, chorionic villus sampling, fetal blood sampling or other invasive intrauterine procedure such as shunt insertion. In addition, postnatal prophylaxis should be given. A systematic review of six eligible trials of more than 10,000 women found when given within 72 h of birth (and other antenatal sensitizing events), anti-D Ig lowered the incidence of Rh isoimmunization 6 months after birth and in a subsequent pregnancy, regardless of the ABO status of the mother and baby (Crowther et al. 2013)

Management of Rh-D isoimmunization. Destruction of fetal RBCs results in fetal anaemia and as less oxygen reaches fetal tissue, oedema and congestive cardiac failure can develop. Lesser degrees of red cell destruction may result in fetal anaemia only, while extensive haemolysis can cause *hydrops fetalis* and fetal death. Mortality rates are higher for those with hydrops fetalis (van Kamp et al. 2005). Early referral to specialist care for women with Rh-D antibodies detected at the first antenatal visit is essential in order to influence fetal outcome (Ghi et al. 2004; Craparo et al. 2005; van Kamp et al. 2005) and ongoing midwifery information and support are important. Treatment aims to reduce the effects of haemolysis. Intensive fetal monitoring and intervention are often required in the pregnancy. Monitoring and treatment can include the principles outlined in Box 37.2.

Postnatal treatment of isoimmunization. Management requires early monitoring of the SBR level. If levels are high or increasing rapidly, early intervention is required to try and prevent reaching potentially harmful levels. The following management principles should be considered:

- using phototherapy from birth helps to prevent a rapid rise in some babies
- regular SBR measurements from birth every 4 h
- a low haemoglobin concentration at birth may indicate the need for early intervention with an exchange transfusion
- If the SBR level is increasing too rapidly or is too high then intervention is required.

In mild to moderate haemolytic anaemia and hyperbilirubinaemia, careful monitoring may be sufficient. However, severely affected babies with hydrops fetalis are pale, oedematous and have ascites and require early admission to the NICU. While early phototherapy is helpful, exchange transfusion is often required, and later packed-cell transfusion may be needed if there is ongoing haemolytic anaemia, which can persist up to 6–8 weeks of age. Treatment with IVIG can be effective at blocking ongoing haemolysis, resulting in a shorter duration of phototherapy and fewer exchange transfusions although this may also increase the likelihood of a later 'top-up' blood transfusion (Gottstein and Cooke 2003).

ABO isoimmunization

ABO isoimmunization usually occurs when the mother is blood group O and the baby is group A, or sometimes group B. Individuals with type O blood develop antibodies throughout life from exposure to antigens in food, Gram-negative bacteria or blood transfusion and by the first pregnancy may already have high serum anti-A and anti-B antibody titres. Some women produce IgG antibodies that can cross the placenta and attack the fetal red cells and destroy them. ABO incompatibility is also thought to protect the fetus from Rh incompatibility as the mother's anti-A and anti-B antibodies destroy any fetal cells that leak into the maternal circulation. Although first and subsequent babies are at risk, destruction is usually much less severe than with Rh incompatibility. In most cases, haemolysis is fairly mild but occasionally be more severe. ABO isoimmunization can in rare cases cause severe fetal anaemia and hydrops fetalis.

Antibodies are not often detected in pregnancy and it is usually a diagnosis made in a baby with an unexpectedly high SBR level. Postnatal management depends on the severity of haemolysis and, as with isoimmunization, aims to prevent bilirubin levels that may be harmful. The Direct Coombs' Test (DAT) is positive and the maternal and baby's blood groups are consistent with ABO incompatibility (i.e. maternal group O and baby A or B or AB). Early phototherapy is usually sufficient but in rare cases, babies with high SBR levels require exchange transfusion. IVIG administered to newborns with significant hyperbilirubinaemia due to ABO haemolytic disease has reduced the need for exchange transfusion (Miqdad et al. 2004).

Late Neonatal Jaundice

This is generally defined as hyperbilirubinaemia beyond 14 days of age. Investigation is important because, while uncommon, some of the causes are conditions with significant long-term implications that require early diagnosis and treatment.

Causes of late neonatal jaundice

Any disease or disorder that increases bilirubin production or alters transport or metabolism of bilirubin is superimposed upon normal physiological jaundice. One approach is to divide the causes into those conditions that result in a raised unconjugated bilirubin (fat soluble) and those that cause a raised conjugated bilirubin (water soluble).

Late neonatal (>14 days) unconjugated hyperbilirubinaemia. Increased red cell destruction or haemolysis causes raised unconjugated SBR levels. This may be immune mediated blood type/group incompatibility, including Rhesus (Rh-D) and ABO incompatibility, anti-E and anti-Kell. Other factors include sepsis (e.g. urinary tract infection), hypothyroidism and galactosaemia. Non-immune haemolysis can occur with abnormally-shaped red cells such as spherocytosis or with certain enzyme deficiencies. Glucose-6-phosphate dehydrogenase (G6PD) is an enzyme that maintains the integrity of the cell membrane of RBCs and deficiency results in increased haemolysis. G6PD is an X-linked genetic disorder that is typically carried by females, affects male babies and is more common in African, Asian and Mediterranean ethnic groups.

Late neonatal (>14 days) conjugated hyperbilirubinaemia. Pale stools and dark urine are important *red flags*, which the midwife must be alert to and act urgently if they are present. They indicate underlying pathology and require urgent medical assessment. Important causes include:

- biliary atresia
- dehydration, starvation, hypoxia and sepsis (oxygen and glucose are required for conjugation)
- TORCH infections (toxoplasmosis, others, rubella, cytomegalovirus, herpes)
- other viral infections (e.g. neonatal viral hepatitis)
- other bacterial infections, particularly those caused by *E. coli*
- metabolic and endocrine disorders that alter uridine diphosphoglucuronyl transferase (UDPGT) enzyme activity (e.g. Crigler–Najjar disease and Gilbert syndrome)
- other metabolic disorders such as hypothyroidism and galactosaemia

HAEMATOLOGICAL PROBLEMS

Bleeding

Bleeding is generally rare in the newborn baby but there are a small number of significant conditions that the midwife should be aware of. Blood from the gastrointestinal tract (vomiting or passed per rectum as *malaena*) is sometimes seen and the commonest cause is swallowed maternal blood. This is supported if there is a clear history of maternal bleeding and bloodstained amniotic fluid. The baby should be carefully evaluated and the possibility of bleeding from the gastrointestinal tract considered. This could occur if there was a clotting or platelet abnormality, or occasionally with some serious gastrointestinal disorders such as necrotizing enterocolitis (NEC).

Possible Causes of Bleeding Abnormalities
Vitamin K-deficient bleeding

Early VKDB, occurring in the first 48 h is rare and usually occurs in babies born to mothers who have received medications that interfere with vitamin K metabolism. These include the anticonvulsants phenytoin, barbiturates or carbamazepine, the antitubercular drugs rifampicin or isoniazid and the vitamin K antagonists warfarin and phenprocoumarin. It is prevented by giving vitamin K to the mother (except those who require ongoing anticoagulation) in the last weeks of pregnancy and ensuring a dose of intramuscular (IM) vitamin K is given to the baby. In the UK, current guidance is that all parents should be offered vitamin K prophylaxis for their babies to prevent the rare but serious and sometimes fatal disorder of vitamin K deficiency bleeding; it is most effective when given as an IM injection (NICE 2006). The midwife needs to be well informed and has a crucial role in the consent process.

If there is unexplained bruising or bleeding, it is important to check that vitamin K has been given as some mothers may decline to consent. *Classic VKDB* occurs in the first week of life, often in ill babies or those slow to establish feeding. Gastrointestinal bleeding is common and may be severe; epistaxis or unexplained bruising or oozing from the umbilical cord are common features. Bleeding into the brain is uncommon. It is prevented by ensuring that an early first dose of vitamin K is given by any route.

Late VKDB occurs from the first week up to 6 months, usually between 4 and 12 weeks. This form is more commonly associated with intracranial bleeds (30–50%) than classic VKDB, and this can be fatal or leave permanent disability. It is almost completely confined to fully breastfed babies. About half will have an underlying liver disease or other malabsorptive state. Late VKDB can be optimally prevented by 1 mg vitamin K IM at birth or significantly reduced by repeated doses of oral vitamin K.

Thrombocytopenia

A low platelet count may present with bleeding or a petechial rash. The management will depend on the underlying cause, which may include:

- maternal idiopathic thrombocytopenic purpura (ITP), where autoimmune maternal antibodies destroy maternal and fetal platelets
- isoimmune thrombocytopenia, where maternal antiplatelet antibodies destroy fetal platelets of a different group
- congenital infections, both viral and bacterial
- drugs, administered to mother or baby
- severe Rhesus haemolytic disease.

Haemophilia and other inherited problems

Haemophilia A is an X-linked recessive disorder, which therefore affects only boys. Females may however be carriers. The diagnosis is often known or suspected antenatally because of a family history. In these cases investigation should occur after birth and IM injections

and invasive procedures should be avoided. The diagnosis can be made by checking a clotting profile and should always be considered in a male baby who has unexpected bleeding.

METABOLIC PROBLEMS

Many metabolic abnormalities can occur in the newborn, particularly in preterm or IUGR babies. By far the most common problem is hypoglycaemia.

Glucose Homeostasis

The fetus has a constant supply of glucose via the placenta. Following birth, this supply of nutrients ceases and there is a fall in glucose concentration (Srinivasan et al. 1986). At the same time, however, endocrine changes (decrease in insulin and a surge of catecholamines and release of glucagon) result in an increase in *glycogenolysis* (breakdown of glycogen stores to provide glucose), *gluconeogenesis* (glucose production from the liver), *ketogenesis* (producing ketones, an alternative fuel) and *lipolysis* (release of fatty acids from adipose) bringing about an increase in glucose and other metabolic fuel. Problems arise in the newborn when there is either a lack of glycogen stores to mobilize (preterm and IUGR babies) or excessive insulin production (infants of diabetic mothers) or when the babies are ill and have a poor supply of energy and increased requirements.

Low glucose concentrations are a potential problem in the newborn because if there is a lack of fuel or nutrients available for the brain, cerebral dysfunction and potentially brain injury may occur. The problem for those caring for newborn babies is not only to identify those who are at risk and treat them appropriately, but also to avoid excessive treatment and investigation in babies where intervention is not required.

Hypoglycaemia

The definition of hypoglycaemia is controversial and many different definitions can be found in the literature (Koh et al. 1988). It remains a confused and contentious issue (Cornblath et al. 2000). The reason that defining a specific level of blood glucose is unhelpful is because a baby's ability to compensate and use alternative fuels may be as important as the specific glucose concentration. However, guidelines will often use a specific level to aid management. In the literature a cut-off value in the newborn of 2.6 mmol/L is often cited although the evidence for the use of this level is not strong (Koh et al. 1988; Lucas et al. 1988). In the UK, operational thresholds in the British Association of Perinatal Medicine (BAPM 2017) guidance use those suggested by Cornblath et al. (2000), as follows:

- a value <1.0 mmol/L at anytime
- baby with abnormal clinical signs: single value <2.5 mmol/L
- baby at risk of impaired metabolic adaptation but without abnormal clinical signs: <2.0 mmol/L and remaining <2.0 mmol/L at the next measurement.

Signs of hypoglycaemia

A baby who has signs of hypoglycaemia has a glucose concentration that is too low and this should be treated whatever the exact glucose level. The signs of hypoglycaemia are lethargy, poor feeding, seizures and decreased consciousness level. Jitteriness is commonly ascribed to hypoglycaemia but is a common feature in the newborn and alone, should not be used as an indication for measuring blood glucose concentration.

Healthy term babies

It is likely that healthy term babies are able to tolerate low blood glucose concentrations using compensatory mechanisms and alternative fuels such as ketone bodies, lactate or fatty acids (Hawdon et al. 1992). These babies may have blood glucose concentrations as low as 2.0 mmol/L without any symptoms because, if responding normally, they are likely to have increased ketone body concentrations, so that fuel is available for the brain (Hawdon et al. 1992). Term babies who are breastfed are particularly likely to have low blood glucose concentrations, probably because of the low energy content of breastmilk in the first few postnatal days. However, these babies will have higher ketone body concentrations to compensate (Hawdon et al. 1992) and they are unlikely, therefore, to suffer any ill-effects. Unfortunately, however, routine measurements of ketone body concentrations are not readily available and when glucose measurements are made in these babies, some practitioners have found it difficult to resist giving treatment that may involve supplementary formula-feeding or even IV dextrose at the expense of breastfeeding. This should be avoided unless there are other clinical indications for intervention. Because of their ability to counter-regulate, clinically well, appropriately grown, full-term babies who are feeding do not require routine monitoring of

their glucose concentration. Doing so would result in many babies being inappropriately treated.

Babies at risk of neurological sequelae of hypoglycaemia

Babies where monitoring and treatment should be considered are those in whom counter-regulation may be impaired. Preterm babies (<37 completed weeks) and IUGR babies (<3rd centile for gestation) have lower glycogen stores and therefore cannot mobilize glucose as effectively during the immediate neonatal postnatal period. In addition, these babies have immature hormone and enzyme responses. They are also less likely to be enterally fed at an early stage. Infants of diabetic mothers (IDM) frequently have low blood glucose concentrations because of an excess of insulin production. This is produced by the fetal pancreatic gland as a result of stimulation by increased maternal glucose concentrations. This excess of insulin also acts as a growth factor and brings about excessive fat and glycogen deposition. This is why these babies have a characteristic appearance and are relatively macrosomic with increased adiposity, as shown in Fig. 37.10. Midwives have an important role in the management of IDM and can contribute timely support that enables mother and babies to stay together. In the UK, this is a focus of the ATAIN project (*'Avoiding Term Admissions Into Neonatal units'*) of NHS Improvement (2017). In ill babies following perinatal hypoxia-ischaemia or sepsis, there may be low substrate stores compounded by feeding difficulties that add to the problem and babies with an inborn error of metabolism (discussed later in this chapter) are also at risk of hypoglycaemia.

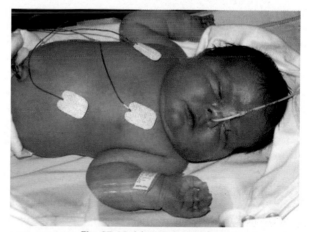

Fig. 37.10 Macrosomic infant.

Diagnosis, prevention and management of hypoglycaemia

Healthy term babies without identified risk factors for hypoglycaemia, who are admitted to the postnatal ward and are feeding, should not have blood glucose measured unless they are symptomatic. In particular, breastfeeding advice and intervention should not be based on blood glucose concentrations. Prevention is important in those babies susceptible to developing hypoglycaemia and therefore they should have:

- adequate temperature control with early skin-to-skin contact – *keep warm*
- *early breastfeeding* – within 1 h of birth
- *frequent feeding* (≤3-hourly)
- *a blood glucose assessment* immediately before the second feed and then 4–6-hourly thereafter.

There is no advantage in assessing the blood glucose concentration earlier than this, providing there are no clinical signs, as it is likely to be low and the appropriate treatment at this stage is to feed the baby. If there are signs of hypoglycaemia, the blood glucose should be assessed and treatment given immediately. In at-risk breastfed babies, it is desirable to avoid supplemental feeding with formula milk to promote successful breastfeeding; however the risks associated with significant hypoglycaemia do at times outweigh this advantage. If the blood glucose concentration is <2.5 mmol/L, then a feed should be given at an increased volume and decreased frequency. The midwife needs to be aware of options to support babies who are reluctant to feed.

If the blood glucose concentration remains low, despite these measures, then additional intervention is required such as glucose gel or admission to a NICU for IV dextrose. There is evidence to support the use of glucose gel in specific circumstances, in that it can reduce the need for admission to an NICU (Harris et al. 2013). For babies admitted for IV dextrose therapy, it is important that enteral feeding is continued, as colostrum/milk contains much more energy than 10% dextrose and promotes ketone body production and metabolic adaptation. It is essential in these situations to accurately measure the overall fluid balance to avoid electrolyte disturbance such as hyponatraemia.

Hyperglycaemia

Hyperglycaemia is much less of a clinical problem than hypoglycaemia and occurs predominantly in preterm and severely affected IUGR babies. It is also seen in term babies in response to stress, especially following perinatal hypoxia-ischaemia, surgery or drugs (especially corticosteroids). In general, no treatment is required. In preterm babies, it is usually a transient phenomenon related to the immature autoregulation or inability to deal with excessive glucose intakes. In general, treatment is not required unless there is significant loss of glucose in the urine that may cause an osmotic diuresis. If treatment is required, the rate of glucose infusion can be decreased, but there may be some advantages in this situation of giving an IV insulin infusion. This allows glucose input to continue and sufficient calories to continue to be given and may result in better weight gain (Collins et al. 1991).

ELECTROLYTE IMBALANCES IN THE NEWBORN

In the first few days after birth, all babies lose weight due to a loss of extracellular fluid. This diuresis and loss of weight is associated with cardiopulmonary adaptation; it occurs rapidly in healthy babies but may be delayed in those with respiratory distress syndrome (RDS). As extracellular fluid is lost, there is a net loss of both water and sodium over these first few days after birth, although the baby's serum sodium should remain within the normal range. The healthy baby should lose up to 10% of its birth weight. This weight loss is physiological and should be expected.

Sodium

Sodium is normally excreted via the kidney, and sodium balance controlled by the renin–angiotensin system. This control mechanism is functional in the preterm baby but loss of sodium may occur in these babies because of renal tubule unresponsiveness. Term breast milk has relatively little sodium (<1 mmol/kg per day) and the healthy newborn can conserve sodium via the kidney in order to maintain growth. Normal sodium requirements are 1–2 mmol/kg per day in term babies and 3–4 mmol/kg per day in preterm babies. Changes in serum sodium reflect changes in sodium and water balance. In order to assess changes in sodium concentration, it is important to know a baby's weight. *Hypernatraemia* in the presence of weight loss suggests dehydration, whereas when there is weight gain it is due to fluid and sodium overload. *Hyponatraemia* in the presence of weight gain represents fluid overload. When associated with appropriate weight loss, it usually represents sodium depletion. The normal serum sodium concentration is 133–146 mmol/L (Ayling and Bowron 2012).

Hyponatraemia

Hyponatraemia is due either to fluid overload or sodium depletion. The latter may be due to inadequate intake or excessive losses.

Fluid overload

In the first few days after birth this is the commonest cause of a low sodium concentration. It is commonly seen in babies receiving IV fluids or in babies with oliguric renal failure or those on medication, e.g. indomethacin or ibuprofen given to preterm babies. Appropriate treatment is to limit the fluid intake whilst maintaining normal sodium intake.

Sodium depletion

In preterm babies, there can be increased renal losses that require increasing sodium intake to compensate for this. Sodium loss can also occur into the bowel due to ileus (resulting from intestinal obstruction, sepsis or prematurity) or severe vomiting. Medications such as diuretics can increase renal losses. Rare, but important causes of sodium depletion are abnormalities of adrenocortical function such as congenital adrenal hyperplasia or hypoplasia, or adrenal haemorrhage in an ill baby.

Hypernatraemia

Increased sodium concentration is almost always due to water depletion and loss of extracellular fluid but can also rarely be due to an excessive sodium intake. These causes can be easily differentiated, by weighing the baby to assess the change since birth.

Water depletion

This is rare in term babies but does occur occasionally in babies with an inadequate intake of breastmilk.

It is more common in preterm babies and reasons include:

- transepidermal water loss in preterm babies – this occurs particularly in babies <28 weeks' gestation and can be prevented by adequate environmental humidity and regular weighing to gauge fluid loss to predict fluid requirements

- excessive urine output in preterm babies during recovery from RDS
- high rates of fluid loss during vomiting, diarrhoea or bowel obstruction.

Water depletion is perhaps the most important cause of hypernatraemia. The incidence has been estimated as 2.5/10,000 live births and it typically occurs in term babies of breastfeeding primiparous mothers (Oddie et al. 2001). It can be associated with significant morbidity and even mortality (Edmondson et al. 1997). With sufficient assistance and supervision of feeding, it is preventable. Babies typically present at 5–9 days of age with lethargy and poor feeding. They have lost >15% of their birth weight and are usually significantly jaundiced. The serum sodium concentration can be between 150 and 200 mmol/L.

In general, many babies are not weighed during this period. Too frequent weighing may undermine those mothers breastfeeding their babies, particularly early on when lactogenesis is only just starting at between 48 and 72 h; the volume of milk transferred to the baby is still rising sharply between 72 and 96 h of age. However, weighing babies can be very useful when a baby is unwell or if there are concerns about intake and fluid and electrolyte balance. It has been suggested that routine weighing of babies may be useful to prevent dehydration and hypernatraemia in breastfed babies with referral to hospital if weight loss exceeds 10% (van Dommelen et al. 2007). The baby's fluid deficit can be calculated from the loss in weight and this is then replaced by gradual rehydration over 24–48 h. Feeding can continue but careful IV treatment is often required. Assistance with lactation can be given to continue promoting breastfeeding.

Excessive sodium intake

Overall, an excessive sodium intake is rare in term babies, although it may be seen in ill preterm babies due to excessive bicarbonate and other sodium-containing fluids. Causes are:
- incorrect fluid prescription
- excessive administration of sodium bicarbonate
- incorrectly formulated powdered feeds
- fabricated or induced illness by carers (FII or sometimes referred to as Münchausen syndrome by proxy) – *intentional administration of salt to a baby*.

Potassium

Potassium is the major intracellular cation. A low serum concentration therefore implies significant potassium depletion. Abnormalities in serum potassium concentration are important because they can cause significant arrhythmias. Potassium concentrations can be severely affected by measurement technique, and haemolysis of the blood sample, especially from capillary sampling, can lead to a falsely high value.

Hyperkalaemia

Causes include:

- acidosis
- acute renal failure
- congenital adrenal hyperplasia.

The treatment is to remove all potassium supplements from IV fluids, and to consider giving: calcium gluconate IV; sodium bicarbonate to increase pH; IV glucose and insulin; and IV salbutamol. Calcium resonium given rectally can help remove potassium but can cause rectal plugs and obstruction. In general, these measures will be required only where there is a confirmed serum potassium that is very high (>8 mmol/L) and/or evidence of an abnormal electrocardiogram (ECG) or arrhythmia.

Hypokalaemia

Causes include:

- inadequate intake of potassium
- bowel losses (vomiting or diarrhoea)
- diuretic therapy
- hyperaldosteronism.

Hypokalaemia is treated by adding potassium to IV infusion fluids or given orally. The normal daily requirement of potassium is 2 mmol/kg per day.

Calcium

Calcium metabolism is closely linked to phosphate metabolism and these are very important minerals for bone development. Preterm infants require much higher concentrations of phosphate and calcium and this can be achieved with IV supplements, by supplementing breast milk with fortifier (Lucas et al. 1996) or by giving specific preterm milk formula milk rather than term formula. The normal serum concentration is 2.2–2.7 mmol/L; this must be interpreted with the serum albumin concentration as serum calcium is bound to albumin and a low albumin concentration will lead to a falsely low serum value. Calcium concentrations fall within 18–24 h of birth as the baby's supply of placental calcium ceases but accretion into bone continues. In the past, hypocalcaemia during the first week after birth

used to be caused by giving unmodified cow's milk. This has a high phosphate concentration and a relatively low calcium concentration that depresses the serum calcium concentration and causes seizures. This is now rare with contemporary formula-milk feeds.

Hypocalcaemia can cause seizures, tremors, jitteriness, lethargy, poor feeding and vomiting. Severe signs can be treated by IV replacement of calcium. Longer-term management depends on the cause. Hypocalcaemia can be caused by:

- prematurity
- significant hypoxia-ischaemia
- renal failure
- hypoparathyroidism including DiGeorge syndrome (discussed later)
- maternal diabetes mellitus.

Hypercalcaemia is uncommon in the newborn infant. Causes include excess Vitamin D and rare genetic conditions such as Williams syndrome.

INBORN ERRORS OF METABOLISM IN THE NEWBORN

Inborn errors of metabolism (IEM) are rare inherited disorders occurring in approximately 1 in 5000 births. They result mainly from enzyme deficiencies in metabolic pathways causing an accumulation of a toxic substrate, and/or important deficiencies in metabolites. *In utero*, the placenta generally provides an effective system for removing toxic metabolites. Most affected babies are usually born in good condition with normal birth weight and initially may appear well. A high index of suspicion is required when evaluating an acutely ill neonate, as many disorders are treatable and early diagnosis and treatment can reduce morbidity.

The mode of inheritance is usually autosomal recessive. In taking a family history, the following information should be sought from the woman:

- any affected siblings
- previous stillbirth/neonatal death
- parental consanguinity
- features associated with feeding, fasting or a surgical procedure
- improvement when feeds are stopped and relapse on restarting.

A clinical examination often reveals little specific evidence and the baby can appear healthy. The features in Box 37.3 may be seen in isolation with many diagnoses,

BOX 37.3 Clinical Features Associated with Many Diagnoses

A Combination of These Features Could be Indicative of an Inborn Error of Metabolism

- Septicaemia
- Hypoglycaemia
- Metabolic acidosis
- Convulsions
- Coma
- Cataracts
- Cardiomegaly
- Jaundice/liver disease
- Severe hypotonia
- Unusual body odour
- Dysmorphic features
- Abnormal hair
- Hydrops fetalis
- Diarrhoea.

however multiple features indicate that an underlying IEM should be seriously considered.

The following laboratory tests are a basic first step in the investigation process:

- full blood count
- septic screen
- creatinine, urea and electrolytes (including chloride)
- liver enzymes
- blood gas
- blood glucose and lactate concentration
- urine reducing substances (sugar)
- urine ketones (dipstick)
- plasma ammonia concentration
- coagulation tests.

Additional investigations are usually necessary and are planned with a consultant biochemist or paediatrician with an interest in metabolic disorders. Principles of emergency management are to reduce any abnormal load on affected pathways, removing toxic metabolites and stimulating residual enzyme activity. Hypoglycaemia is corrected, adequate ventilatory support and hydration are maintained, convulsions are treated and significant metabolic acidosis and electrolyte abnormalities are corrected. In general, antibiotics are frequently given as infection may have precipitated metabolic decompensation. Occasionally, renal dialysis may also be required.

In the UK, midwives have a crucial role in implementing the routine Newborn Blood Spot Screening Programme, which is ideally undertaken when the baby is 5 days old. As part of this programme, the following inherited metabolic disorders are screened for:

- phenylketonuria (PKU)
- medium-chain acyl-CoA dehydrogenase deficiency (MCADD)
- maple syrup urine disease (MSUD)
- isovaleric acidaemia (IVA)
- glutaric aciduria type 1 (GA1)
- homocystinuria (pyridoxine unresponsive) (HCU).

Providing detail about the various metabolic disorders is beyond the scope of this chapter but two conditions, PKU and galactosaemia, are discussed further to illustrate some relevant aspects and key principles of management and treatment.

Phenylketonuria

Phenylketonuria (PKU) was one of the first disorders to be part of mass screening. If detected during the first week of life and appropriate management initiated in the first 2–3 weeks, a good outcome can be anticipated.

PKU is an autosomal recessive disorder of protein metabolism that has an incidence of approximately 1 in 10,000 in the UK. Babies with PKU are born in good condition but begin to be affected by their condition during the first few weeks after birth. If PKU is left untreated, it will lead to irreversible brain damage and associated severe learning difficulties/disability (Intelligence Quotient, IQ <30). Early treatment is via a diet specifically restricted in phenylalanine. The common type of PKU is caused by the absence of, or reduction in an enzyme called 'phenylalanine hydroxylase' which, in the liver, converts the essential amino acid phenylalanine to another essential amino acid, tyrosine. The toxic accumulation of phenylalanine and lack of tyrosine leads to brain damage.

PKU is particularly suitable for mass screening because there is a simple widely available diagnostic test and subsequent treatment is effective. Midwives collect the blood sample for PKU screening in the UK ideally when the baby is around 5 days old with the knowledge that the baby has been taking milk feeds. The level of phenylalanine is analysed and babies with increased levels should be prescribed a low phenylalanine diet and have further assessment to determine whether they are affected by the 'classic' type of the disease or other variants. If it is treated early, a normal outcome can be expected. Affected people will have to stay on a low phenylalanine diet for life and women who wish to become pregnant require good pre-conception management to prevent congenital anomalies such as microcephaly in their developing fetus. This is because fetal brain injury may result from exposure to maternal high concentrations of phenylalanine and its metabolites.

Galactosaemia

Galactosaemia is a disorder of carbohydrate metabolism that is autosomal recessive in inheritance and has an incidence of 1 in 60,000. It is caused by an absence or severe deficiency of an enzyme for metabolizing galactose, most typically galactose-1-phosphate uridyl-transferase (often referred to as Gal-1-PUT). The main sugar in milk is lactose, a disaccharide containing glucose and galactose. Babies with this condition cannot metabolize galactose and rapidly become affected when fed either human breastmilk or cow's milk formulae. The metabolite that builds up and is harmful, is galactose-1-phosphate. Galactosaemia is not currently included in the UK national screening programme, although it is screened for in some other countries.

The clinical signs of the disorder are those of liver failure and renal impairment. Affected babies tend to present with vomiting, hypoglycaemia, jaundice, bleeding, acidosis, failure to gain weight and hypotonia during the first few days after birth. Another important clinical feature is congenital cataract. These babies may also present with septicaemia (particularly *E. coli*) due to damage to the intestinal mucosa by high levels of galactose in the bowel. Galactosaemia is an important differential diagnosis to consider when dealing with a baby with unresponsive hypoglycaemia and prolonged or severe jaundice. Babies with galactosaemia will have galactose but not glucose in their urine. The diagnosis therefore can be made by looking for urine-reducing substances (galactose) using a Clinitest, whereas a urine test for glucose will be negative. Confirmation of the diagnosis is by assay of the enzyme level (Gal-1-PUT) within red blood cells.

Treatment is with a lactose-free milk formula, commenced as soon as the diagnosis is suspected. This results in a rapid correction of the abnormalities. However, cataracts and mild brain injury have still occurred, even when galactosaemic babies have been fed lactose-free milk from birth. Screening for this disorder is possible but many babies will have presented clinically before the screening test is undertaken so calling into question whether screening can alter the long-term outcome.

ENDOCRINE PROBLEMS

Endocrine problems in the newborn are relatively rare and although they may be serious are nearly always treatable, so identification and diagnosis is important.

Thyroid Disorders

The thyroid gland produces hormones that have an effect on the metabolic rate in most tissues. They are also essential for normal neurological development. Thyroid stimulating hormone (TSH) is produced by the anterior pituitary gland and this stimulates production of T3 and T4 by the thyroid gland with a feedback mechanism to the anterior pituitary.

Hypothyroidism

The incidence of hypothyroidism in the newborn is 1 in 3500. There are several possible causes for hypothyroidism in the newborn, including abnormalities in gland formation (thyroid dysgenesis), defects in hormone synthesis (dyshormonogenesis) and rarely, secondary pituitary causes. The latter causes a decrease or lack of TSH, whereas *primary* (thyroid) causes result in very high TSH values and this has implications for screening. The clinical presentation however, is the same. Babies with hypothyroidism tend to be large, post-term and have a large posterior fontanelle. They may have coarse features and often have an umbilical hernia. These features are often missed, which is why screening for this disorder is so important. Untreated babies develop impaired motor development with growth failure, a low IQ, impaired hearing and language difficulties. It is essential to commence treatment as early as possible to avoid long-term problems. Screening for hypothyroidism involves measuring thyroid stimulating hormone (TSH) on a blood spot taken when the baby is 5 days old. This method detects almost all cases, however it cannot detect cases caused by *secondary* (pituitary) hypothyroidism that will have a low TSH. This condition is, however, much less common, with an incidence of 1 in 60,000 to 1 in 100,000 (Fisher et al. 1979).

Hyperthyroidism

Graves' disease is an autoimmune disorder that causes hyperthyroidism. Neonatal hyperthyroidism occurs relatively rarely but is possible when the mother has, or previously had, Graves' disease. It occurs as a result of maternal thyroid stimulating immunoglobulins transferring across the placenta. These are autoantibodies that are produced and act in the same way as TSH. This can occur when a mother has active, inactive or treated Graves' disease (Teng et al. 1980) and thyrotoxicosis in the fetus can lead to preterm labour, low birth weight, stillbirth and fetal death. Although uncommon, babies of mothers with Graves' disease may show signs of thyrotoxicosis. In the baby the signs are irritability, jitteriness, tachycardia, prominent eyes, sweating, excessive appetite and weight loss. These may be present immediately after birth or presentation may be delayed for as long as 4–6 weeks (Skuza et al. 1996). Therefore, even if well at birth, there needs to be a clear plan for regular clinical review and investigation. Severe neonatal hyperthyroidism has a high mortality. It requires treatment, usually with carbimazole and propranolol, until the effects of the maternal antibodies have resolved which can take several months.

Adrenal Disorders

The adrenal glands are vital for the normal function of many systems within the body. They are divided into a medulla and a cortex. The medulla produces catecholamines, which help to maintain blood pressure and are produced at times of stress. Abnormalities of function of the adrenal medulla are not described in the newborn. The adrenal cortex produces three groups of hormones – glucocorticoids, mineralocorticoids and sex hormones – that have distinct functions.

Glucocorticoids regulate the general metabolism of carbohydrates, proteins and fats on a long-term basis. They have a particular role in modifying the metabolism in times of stress.

Mineralocorticoids regulate sodium, potassium and water balance. The *sex hormones* are responsible for normal development of the genitalia and reproductive organs. Abnormalities in function of the glands represent the functions of these different groups of hormones.

Adrenocortical insufficiency

This is caused by congenital hypoplasia, adrenal haemorrhage, enzyme defects or can be secondary to pituitary problems. It can present with vomiting, poor feeding and weight loss and prolonged jaundice. The baby may become acutely unwell with hyponatraemia, hypoglycaemia, hyperkalaemia and acidosis. Treatment is by IV therapy with glucose and electrolytes followed by replacement of corticosteroid and mineralocorticoid hormones.

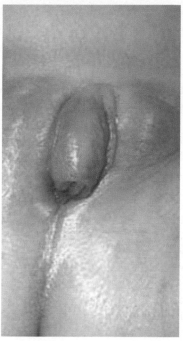

Fig. 37.11 Female infant with ambiguous genitalia due to congenital adrenal hyperplasia. (Adapted from: Chavhan GB, Parra, DA, Oudjhane K et al. 2008. Imaging of ambiguous genitalia: classification and diagnostic approach, Fig. 2. RSNA Education Exhibit.)

Adrenocortical hyperfunction

This most commonly results from congenital adrenal hyperplasia (CAH) and is the name given to a group of inherited disorders that are due to deficiency of enzymes responsible for hormone production within the adrenal gland. The most common enzyme deficiency results in an excess of androgenic hormones and a deficiency of glucocorticoid and mineralocorticoids.. These disorders can cause abnormalities in the formation of the genitalia leading to ambiguous genitalia (virilization of females or inadequate virilization of males) (Fig. 37.11) and features of adrenal insufficiency (vomiting, diarrhoea, vascular collapse, hypoglycaemia, hyponatraemia, hyperkalaemia). The classification of disorders of sexual differentiation and consensus statement on the management of inter-sex disorders has been reported by Hughes et al. (2006).

It is important to make a prompt diagnosis. The genetic sex must be determined (chromosome analysis) and it is important not to assign a sex until the diagnosis has been established (see Chapter 32). The biochemical diagnosis is made by analysing urine and plasma for steroid hormone metabolites. Treatment is as for adrenocortical insufficiency by replacement of glucocorticoid and mineralocorticoid hormones. Virilized girls may also require surgical intervention for the genital abnormalities.

Pituitary Disorders

Pituitary insufficiency is rare in the newborn. It may occur in association with other abnormalities, particularly midline developmental defects. Presentation is with signs of glucocorticoid deficiency such as hypoglycaemia, prolonged jaundice or signs of hypothyroidism. Growth hormone deficiency generally causes hypoglycaemia but no other signs in the newborn. When it is recognized, treatment is with replacement of the missing hormones.

Parathyroid Disorders

The parathyroid glands are responsible for control of calcium metabolism but abnormalities of the parathyroid glands are rare causes of hypocalcaemia and hypercalcaemia in the newborn. When hypoparathyroidism does occur it may be familial or may occur in association with deletions of chromosome 22 (22q11 deletion or DiGeorge syndrome). The signs associated with hypocalcaemia are detailed above.

EFFECTS ON THE NEWBORN OF MATERNAL DRUG ABUSE/USE DURING PREGNANCY

There is a large geographical variation in the incidence of drug withdrawal among babies, reflecting the variation of drug use within the UK population. Opiates and other drugs cross the placenta and the fetus is likely to be exposed to the same peaks and troughs of drug exposure as the mother. Withdrawal may be manifest before birth. The increased incidence of fetal distress may be related in part to drug withdrawal during labour. The effects of drugs and withdrawal on the fetus and newborn are related to the timing of drug doses. Babies born to mothers who have used illicit drugs during pregnancy are at risk of withdrawal effects. Other problems that are more common in these pregnancies are:

- obstetric complications of pregnancy including placental abruption, IUGR, signs of fetal compromise during labour, stillbirth
- poor attendance for antenatal care
- non-disclosure of information regarding drugs taken during pregnancy

- risk of infectious disease (hepatitis B and C, and HIV)
- social problems such as poor housing, chaotic lifestyle, care of other children
- poor attendance for neonatal follow-up.

Attendance for antenatal care and supervision during pregnancy may be improved by midwifery support and community liaison. It is important to identify these women during pregnancy in order to try to prevent some of the above problems and offer appropriate support. Identification during pregnancy also allows screening for infectious diseases and this is particularly important for hepatitis B and HIV, where treatments are available to decrease the chance of the newborn being affected.

Signs of Withdrawal

Many drugs have been reported to cause problems of withdrawal in the newborn. The most common seen in the UK are opiates in the form of heroin and methadone but barbiturates, benzodiazepines, cocaine and amphetamines are also frequently seen. Multidrug use is common and usually leads to prolonged difficult withdrawal. Each drug has a different half-life and this leads to different patterns of withdrawal behaviour. In general, methadone produces effects for longer periods than heroin (Herzlinger et al. 1977) but benzodiazepines may also contribute to this (Sutton and Hinderliter 1990).

The signs most frequently seen are jitteriness, irritability and constant high-pitched crying. Babies often fail to settle between feeds and are hyperactive. When feeds are offered, they often feed voraciously although some have a poor suck. Vomiting is common. Diarrhoea and an irritant nappy rash are also often seen. Sneezing and yawning may be seen, as well as episodes of high temperature in the absence of infection. In rare circumstances, babies may also have seizures.

Several scoring systems have been developed to help to guide when to give pharmacological treatment (Finnegan et al. 1975). These scoring systems aim to make the assessment more objective, however most of the features and their severity are difficult to quantify. Babies assessed for signs of drug withdrawal by a scoring system may have less inappropriate treatment and a shorter hospital stay. It is important not to over-treat with drugs as the long-term effects are not clear and the treatment may then be difficult to withdraw. Furthermore pharmacological treatment in many maternity hospitals means admitting the baby to the NICU therefore possibly separating mother and baby. Non-pharmacological management can be very effective and often sufficient as a standalone treatment or if necessary used in combination with pharmacological therapy (Ryan et al. 2019).

Treatment

Treatment can be divided into general care given to these babies and pharmacological treatment. It is important, if at all possible, to keep mother and baby together. Interaction and care of these babies by their mother should be positively encouraged. The mother is likely to be feeling upset and guilty because of the baby's appearance/behaviour and the co-existing social problems for these families can make for a challenging time for all involved. Breastfeeding can be encouraged as long as there is no evidence of HIV or ongoing drug use, such as heroin and cocaine that precludes this. A quiet environment with reduced light and noise is helpful in keeping stimuli to a minimum. Swaddling is useful and feeds may need to be given frequently. These babies will often take large volumes of milk, which is acceptable as long as vomiting is not a problem. Rocking or cradling are also useful interventions.

Pharmacological treatment

Several different treatments have been recommended in the past (AAP 1998). A number of randomized trials have been performed attempting to assess the use of various drugs in the treatment of neonatal abstinence syndrome (NAS) (Theis et al. 1997). It seems logical to treat opiate withdrawal with opiates and the two most commonly used treatments are oral methadone and oral morphine. These appear to control withdrawal symptoms much more effectively (Lawn and Alton 2012). Doses can be titrated as necessary until the features are controlled and then the dose gradually reduced. Other medication may sometimes be useful, e.g. clonazepam for benzodiazepine use or chloral hydrate as a general sedative.

Cocaine

Cocaine deserves special mention because its effects on the newborn are different. It is a larger problem in the USA than in the UK but the incidence of its use during pregnancy is unknown. It is only present in maternal urine for 24 h after exposure and therefore detection is difficult (Zuckerman et al. 1989). It can produce significant withdrawal signs, although these are often less severe and less troublesome than with other drugs, but it is associated with many other harmful effects on the fetus (Fulroth et al. 1989). These include significant fetal IUGR, brain injury due to haemorrhage or infarction (Hadeed and Siegel 1989), abnormalities of brain development, limb reduction defects and atresias of the gastrointestinal system. Correlation between cocaine exposure, small head size and developmental scores has also been reported (Chasnoff et al. 1992).

Discharge and Long-Term Effects

Discharge must be planned with the involvement of other support agencies. This may include a planning meeting involving all agencies concerned with the care of the mother and baby. Although it seems intuitive that exposure to drugs *in utero* would cause neurodevelopmental impairment, this is not borne out by carefully controlled studies (Lifschitz et al. 1985). This implies that impairment in intellectual outcome in these children relates to other adverse prenatal and postnatal factors. Babies born to these mothers are smaller and have smaller head circumferences (Kandall et al. 1976). However, it is difficult to be certain about the exact causes of any long-term harmful effects because so many factors are involved, all of which are interlinked. These include:

- the effects of the drugs themselves on the developing fetus
- the use of other harmful substances by mothers who use drugs (e.g. cigarettes and alcohol)
- the effect of pregnancy complications
- the effect of the withdrawal syndrome on the developing neonate
- the effect of treatment to prevent withdrawal behaviours
- the effect of the home environment of the chaotic drug-user for the developing child
- genetic effects
- reporting bias means that negative associations with drug-taking are more likely to be reported (Koren et al. 1989).

REFLECTIVE ACTIVITY FOR SELF-ASSESSMENT

1. In the immediate period after birth what will reassure you that the newborn baby is making a successful adaptation from uterine to neonatal life? What findings would prompt you to ask for urgent review from the paediatric team?

2. In what ways will the midwife be involved in the care of families whose baby is *'cooled'* as part of their management for hypoxic ischaemic encephalopathy?

3. When a newborn baby has visible jaundice, what circumstances and findings would be consistent with physiological jaundice and in what situations should it be regarded as pathological requiring further investigation/referral?

4. Midwives have an important role in reducing unnecessary admissions of term babies to a neonatal unit. In this context, consider your actions with particular reference to those admissions related to hypoglycaemia.

5. Midwives are involved in the full systematic physical examination of the newborn infant and NBS (newborn blood spot screening). Can you explain why these screening tests are undertaken and what conditions they might detect? What will be expected of you as a midwife in preparing families for these screening tests?

REFERENCES

Ahlfors, C. E., & Wennberg, R. P. (2004). Bilirubin-albumin binding and neonatal jaundice. *Seminars in Perinatology*, 28(5), 334–339.

Aldana-Aguirre, J. C., Pinto, M., Featherstone, R. M., & Kumar, M. (2017). Less invasive surfactant administration versus intubation for surfactant delivery in preterm infants with respiratory distress syndrome: A systematic review and meta-analysis. *Archives of Disease in Childhood Fetal and Neonatal Edition*, 102, F17–F23.

Allaby, M., Forman, K., Touch, S., & Chilcott, J. (1999). *The use of routine anti-D prophylaxis antenatally to Rhesus negative women*. Universities of Leicester. Nottingham and Sheffield: Trent Institute for Health Services Research.

AAP (American Academy of Pediatrics). (1998). Neonatal drug withdrawal. American Academy of Pediatrics Committee on Drugs. *Pediatrics*, 101(6), 1079–1088.

AAP (American Academy of Pediatrics). (2004). Clinical Practice guideline: Management of hyperbilirubinemia in the newborn infant >35 weeks of gestation. *Pediatrics*, 114(1), 297–316.

Ayling, R. M., & Bowron, A. (2012). Neonatal biochemical reference ranges. In J. M. Rennie (Ed.), *Rennie and Roberton's textbook of neonatology* (5th ed.) (pp. 1309–1318). Edinburgh: Churchill Livingstone.

Azzopardi, D. V., Strohm, B., Edwards, A. D., et al. (2009). Moderate hypothermia to treat perinatal asphyxial encephalopathy. *New England Journal of Medicine*, 361(14), 1349–1358.

Banatvala, J. E., & Brown, D. W. G. (2004). Rubella. *Lancet*, 363(9415), 1127–1137.

BAPM (British Association of Perinatal Medicine). (2017). *Identification and management of neonatal hypoglycaemia in the full term infant: A Framework for Neonatal Transitional Care*. London: BAPM. Available at: www.bapm.org/sites/default/files/files/Identification%20and%20Management%20of%20Neonatal%20Hypoglycaemia%20in%20the%20%20full%20term%20infant%20-%20A%20Framework%20for%20Practice%20revised%20Oct%202017.pdf.

Barcaite, E., Bartusevicius, A., Tameliene, R., et al. (2008). Prevalence of maternal group B streptococcal colonisation in European countries. *Acta Obstetrica et Gynecologica Scandinavica*, 87(3), 260–271.

Bedford, H., & Tookey, P. (2006). Rubella and the MMR vaccine. *Nursing Times*, 102(5), 55–57.

Bianchi, D. W., Avent, N. D., Costa, J. M., & van der Schoot, C. E. (2005). Noninvasive prenatal diagnosis of fetal rhesus D. Ready for prime(r) time. *Obstetrics and Gynecology*, 106(4), 841–844.

Bromberger, P., Lawrence, J. M., Braun, D., et al. (2000). The influence of intrapartum antibiotics on the clinical spectrum of early-onset group B streptococcal infection in term infants. *Pediatrics*, 106(Pt 1), 244–250.

CESDI (Confidential Enquiries into Stillbirths and Deaths in Infancy) Project 27/28. (2003). In M. Macintosh (Ed.), *An enquiry into quality of care and its effect on the survival of babies born at 27–28 weeks*. Norwich: TSO.

Chasnoff, I. J., Griffith, D. R., Freier, C., & Murray, J. (1992). Cocaine/polydrug use in pregnancy: two year follow-up. *Pediatrics*, 89(2), 284–289.

Collins, J. W., Hoppe, M., Brown, K., et al. (1991). A controlled trial of insulin infusion and parenteral nutrition in extremely low birth weight infants with glucose intolerance. *Journal of Pediatrics*, 118(6), 921–927.

Cornblath, M., Hawdon, J. M., Williams, A. F., et al. (2000). Controversies regarding definition of neonatal hypoglycaemia: suggested operational thresholds. *Pediatrics, 105*(5), 1141–1145.

Costeloe, K., Hennessy, E., Gibson, A. T., et al. (2000). The EPIcure study: Outcomes to discharge from hospital for infants born at the threshold of viability. *Pediatrics, 106*(4), 659–671.

Craparo, F. J., Bonati, F., Gementi, P., & Nicolini, U. (2005). The effects of serial intravascular transfusions in ascetic/hydropic-alloimmunized fetuses. *Ultrasound in Obstetrics and Gynecology, 25*(2), 144–148.

Crowther, C. A., Middleton, P., & McBain, R. D. (2013). Anti-D administration during pregnancy for preventing rhesus alloimmunization. *Cochrane Database of Systematic Reviews* (2), CD000020.

de Cueto, M., Sanchez, M. J., Sampedro, A., et al. (1998). Timing of intrapartum ampicillin and prevention of vertical transmission of group B streptococcus. *Obstetrics and Gynecology, 91*(1), 112–114.

de Louvois, J., Halket, S., & Harvey, D. (2005). Neonatal meningitis in England and Wales: Sequelae at 5 years of age. *European Journal of Pediatrics, 164*(12), 730–734.

Degani, S. (2006). Sonographic findings in fetal viral infections: a systematic review. *Obstetrical and Gynecological Survey, 61*(5), 329–336.

Dinsmoor, M. J., Viloria, R., Lief, L., & Elder, S. (2005). Use of intrapartum antibiotics and the incidence of postnatal maternal and neonatal yeast infections. *Obstetrics and Gynecology, 106*(1), 19–22.

Dobbs, R. H., & Cremer, R. J. (1975). Phototherapy. *Archives of Disease in Childhood, 50*(11), 833–836.

Edmondson, M. B., Stoddard, J. J., & Owens, L. M. (1997). Hospital readmission with feeding-related-problems after early postpartum discharge of normal newborns. *Journal of the American Medical Association, 278*(4), 299–303.

Enders, G., Pacher, U. N., Miller, E., & Cradock-Watson, J. E. (1988). Outcome of confirmed periconceptional maternal rubella. *Lancet, 1*(8600), 1445–1446.

Finer, N., Barrington, K. J., Pennaforte, T., & Altit, G. (2017). Nitric oxide for respiratory failure in infants born at or near term. *Cochrane Database of Systematic Reviews, 1*, CD000399.

Finnegan, L. P., Kron, R. E., Connaughton, J. F., & Emich, J. P. (1975). Assessment and treatment of abstinence in the infant of the drug dependent mother. *International Journal of Clinical Pharmacology and Biopharmacy, 12*(1–2), 19–32.

Finning, K., Martin, P., & Daniels, G. (2004). A clinical service in the UK to predict fetal Rh (Rhesus) D blood group using free fetal DNA in maternal plasma. *Annals of the New York Academy of Sciences, 1022*, 119–1123.

Fisher, D. A., Dussault, J. H., Foley, T. P., et al. (1979). Screening for congenital hypothyroidism: results of screening one million North American infants. *Journal of Pediatrics, 94*(5), 700–705.

Fulroth, R., Phillips, B., & Durand, D. (1989). Perinatal outcome of infants exposed to cocaine and/or heroin in utero. *American Journal of Diseases of Children, 143*(8), 905–910.

Geifman-Holtzman, O., Grotegut, C. A., & Gaughan, J. P. (2006). Diagnostic accuracy of noninvasive fetal Rh genotyping from maternal blood – a meta-analysis. *American Journal of Obstetrics and Gynecology, 195*(4), 1163–1173.

Ghi, T., Brondelli, L., Simonazzi, G., et al. (2004). Sonographic demonstration of brain injury in fetuses with severe red blood cell alloimmunization undergoing intrauterine transfusions. *Ultrasound in Obstetrics and Gynecology, 23*(5), 428–431.

Gilbert, R., Tan, H. K., Cliffe, S., et al. (2006). Symptomatic toxoplasma infection due to congenital and postnatally acquired infection. *Archives of Disease in Childhood, 91*(6), 495–498.

Gottstein, R., & Cooke, R. W. I. (2003). Systematic review of intravenous immunoglobulin in haemolytic disease of the newborn. *Archives of Disease in Childhood Fetal and Neonatal Edition, 88*(1), F6–F10.

Greenough, A., & Milner, A. D. (2012). Acute respiratory disease. In J. M. Rennie (Ed.), *Rennie and Roberton's textbook of neonatology* (5th ed.) (pp. 468–551). Edinburgh: Churchill Livingstone.

Hadeed, A. J., & Siegel, S. R. (1989). Maternal cocaine use during pregnancy: effect on the newborn infant. *Pediatrics, 84*(2), 205–210.

Harris, D. L., Weston, P. J., Signal, M., et al. (2013). Dextrose gel for neonatal hypoglycaemia (the Sugar Babies Study): a randomised, double-blind, placebo controlled trial. *Lancet, 382*(9910), 2077–2083.

Hawdon, J. M., Ward Platt, M. P., & Aynsley-Green, A. (1992). Patterns of metabolic adaptation for pre-term and term infants in the first neonatal week. *Archives of Disease in Childhood, 67*(4), 357–365.

Hayakawa, M., Kimura, H., Ohshiro, M., et al. (2003). Varicella exposure in a neonatal medical centre: successful prophylaxis with oral acyclovir. *Journal of Hospital Infection, 54*(3), 212–215.

Heath, P. T., Balfour, G., Weisner, A. M., & PHLS Group B Streptococcus Working Group., et al. (2004). Group B streptococcal disease in UK and Irish infants younger than 90 days. *Lancet, 363*(9405), 292–294.

Herzlinger, R. A., Kandall, S. R., & Vaughan, H. G. (1977). Neonatal seizures associated with narcotic withdrawal. *Journal of Pediatrics, 91*(4), 638–641.

Hughes, I. A., Houk, C., Ahmed, S. F., et al. (2006). Consensus statement on management of inter-sex disorders. *Archives of Disease in Childhood, 91*(7), 554–563.

Hughes, R. G., Brocklehurst, P., Steer, P. J., & on behalf of the Royal College of Obstetricians and Gynaecologists., et al. (2017). Prevention of early-onset neonatal group B streptococcal disease. Green-top Guideline No 36. *BJOG: An International Journal of Obstetrics and Gynaecology, 124*, e280–e305.

Jacobs, S. E., Berg, M., Hunt, R., et al. (2013). Cooling for newborns with hypoxic ischaemic encephalopathy. *Cochrane Database of Systematic Reviews, 1*, CD003311.

Jain, A. (2012). Temperature control and disorders. In J. M. Rennie (Ed.), *Rennie and Roberton's textbook of neonatology* (5th ed.) (pp. 263–276). Edinburgh: Churchill Livingstone.

Joy, S. D., Rossi, K. Q., Krugh, D., & O'Shaughnessy, R. W. (2005). Management of pregnancies complicated by anti-E alloimmunization. *Obstetrics and Gynecology, 105*(1), 24–28.

Kandall, S. R., Albin, S., Lowinson, J., et al. (1976). Differential effects of maternal heroin and methadone use on birthweight. *Pediatrics, 58*(5), 681–685.

Kaplan, M., Muraca, M., Vreman, H. J., et al. (2005). Neonatal bilirubin production-conjugation imbalance: effect of glucose-6-phosphate dehydrogenase deficiency and borderline prematurity. *Archives of Disease in Childhood: Fetal and Neonatal Edition, 90*(2), F123–F127.

Kenyon, S., Boulvain, M., & Neilson, J. (2010). Antibiotics for preterm rupture of membranes. *Cochrane Database of Systematic Reviews* (2), CD001058.

Koh, T. H., Eyre, J. A., & Aynsley-Green, A. (1988). Neonatal hypoglycaemia – the controversy regarding definition. *Archives of Disease in Childhood, 63*(11), 1386–1388.

Koren, G., Shear, H., Graham, K., & Einarson, T. (1989). Bias against the null hypothesis: The reproductive hazards of cocaine. *Lancet, 334*(8677), 1440–1442.

Kumar, S. L., & Dhanireddy, R. (1995). Time to first stool in premature infants: effect of gestational age and illness severity. *Journal of Pediatrics, 127*(6), 971–974.

Kurinczuk, J. J., White-Koning, M., & Badawi, N. (2010). Epidemiology of neonatal encephalopathy and hypoxic–ischaemic encephalopathy. *Early Human Development, 86*(6), 329–338.

Lamagni, T. L., Keshishian, C., Efstratiou, A., et al. (2013). Emerging trends in the epidemiology of invasive group B streptococcal disease in England and Wales, 1991–2010. *Clinical Infectious Diseases, 57*(5), 682–688.

Lau, S. P., & Fung, K. P. (1984). Serum bilirubin kinetics in intermittent phototherapy of physiological jaundice. *Archives of Disease in Childhood, 59*, 892–894.

Law, M. R., Palomaki, G., Alfirevic, Z., et al. (2005). The prevention of neonatal group B streptococcal disease: A report by a working group of the Medical Screening Society. *Journal of Medical Screening, 12*(2), 60–68.

Lawn, C., & Alton, N. (2012). The baby of the substance abusing mother. In J. M. Rennie (Ed.), *Rennie and Roberton's textbook of neonatology* (5th ed.) (pp. 431–442). Edinburgh: Churchill Livingstone.

Lifschitz, M. H., Wilson, G. S., Smith, E. O., & Desmond, M. M. (1985). Factors affecting head growth and intellectual function in children of drug addicts. *Pediatrics, 75*(2), 269–274.

Lissauer, T., & Faranoff, A. A. (2006). *Neonatology at a glance* (2nd ed.). London: Blackwell Science.

Lucas, A., Fewtrell, M. S., Morley, R., et al. (1996). Randomized outcome trial of human milk fortification and developmental outcome in preterm infants. *American Journal of Clinical Nutrition, 64*(2), 142–151.

Lucas, A., Morley, R., & Cole, T. J. (1988). Adverse neuro developmental outcome of moderate neonatal hypoglycaemia. *British Medical Journal, 297*(6659), 1304–1308.

Liu, Y., Chen, S., Zühlke, L., et al. (2019). Global birth prevalence of congenital heart defects 1970–2017: updated systematic review and meta-analysis of 260 studies. *International Journal of Epidemiology, 48*(2), 455–463.

Manning, D., Todd, P., Maxwell, M., & Platt, M. J. (2007). Prospective surveillance study of severe hyperbilirubinaemia in the newborn in the UK and Ireland. *Archives of Disease in Childhood Fetal and Neonatal Edition, 92*(5), 342–346.

Mari, G., Zimmermann, R., Moise, K. J., & Deter, R. L. (2005). Correlation between middle cerebral artery peak systolic velocity and fetal hemoglobin after 2 previous intrauterine transfusions. *American Journal of Obstetrics and Gynecology, 193*(3), 1117–1120.

Merenstein, G. V., & Gardner, S. L. (2011). *Merenstein and Gardner's handbook of neonatal intensive care* (7th ed.). St Louis: Mosby.

Metaj, M., Laroia, N., Lawrence, R. A., & Ryan, R. M. (2003). Comparison of breast- and formula-fed normal newborns in time to first stool and urine. *Journal of Perinatology, 23*, 624–628.

Meyberg-Solomayer, G. C., Fehm, T., Muller-Hansen, I., et al. (2006). Prenatal ultrasound diagnosis, follow-up, and outcome of congenital varicella syndrome. *Fetal Diagnosis and Therapy, 21*(3), 296–301.

Miqdad, A. M., Abdelbasit, O. B., Shaheed, M. M., et al. (2004). Intravenous immunoglobulin G (IVIG) therapy for significant hyperbilirubinemia in ABO hemolytic disease of the newborn. *Journal of Maternal-Fetal and Neonatal Medicine, 16*(3), 163–166.

Montoya, J. G., & Liesenfeld, O. (2004). Toxoplasmosis. *Lancet*, *363*(9425), 1965–1976.

Morley, C. J., Davis, P. G., Doyle, L. W., & COIN Trial Investigators., et al. (2008). Nasal CPAP or intubation at birth for very preterm infants. *New England Journal of Medicine*, *358*(7), 700–708.

Morrill, J. F., Heinig, M. J., Pappagianis, D., & Dewey, K. G. (2005). Risk factors for mammary candidosis among lactating women. *Journal of Obstetric, Gynecologic and Neonatal Nursing*, *34*(1), 37–45.

Morrison, J. J., Rennie, J. M., & Milton, P. J. (1995). Neonatal respiratory morbidity and mode of delivery at term: influence of timing of elective caesarean section. *British Journal of Obstetrics and Gynaecology*, *102*(2), 101–106.

NHS Choices. (2017). Toxoplasmosis. Available at: www.nhs.uk/conditions/toxoplasmosis.

NHS Improvement. (2017). *Reducing harm leading to avoidable admission of full-term babies into neonatal units: Findings and resources for improvement*. London: NHSI. Available at: https://improvement.nhs.uk/documents/764/Reducing_term_admissions_final.pdf.

NICE (National Institute for Health and Care Excellence). (2016). *Jaundice in newborn babies before 28 days: CG 98*. London: NICE. Available at: www.nice.org.uk/guidance/cg98/resources/jaundice-in-newborn-babies-under-28-days-pdf-975756073669.

NICE (National Institute for Health and Care Excellence). (2012). *Neonatal infection (early onset). Antibiotics for prevention and treatment: CG149*. London: NICE. Available at: www.nice.org.uk/guidance/cg149/resources/neonatal-infection-early-onset-antibiotics-for-prevention-and-treatment-pdf-35109579233221.

NICE (National Institute for Health and Care Excellence). (2008). *Routine antenatal anti-D prophylaxis for women who are rhesus D negative: TA156*. London: NICE. Available at: www.nice.org.uk/guidance/ta156/resources/routine-antenatal-antid-prophylaxis-for-women-who-are-rhesus-d-negative-pdf-82598318102725.

NICE (National Institute for Health and Care Excellence). (2006). *Postnatal care up to 8 weeks after birth: CG37*. London: NICE. Available at: www.nice.org.uk/guidance/cg37/resources/postnatal-care-up-to-8-weeks-after-birth-pdf-975391596997.

Oddie, S., & Embleton, N. D. (2002). On behalf of the Northern Neonatal Network. Risk factors for early onset neonatal group B streptococcal sepsis: Case-control study. *British Medical Journal*, *325*(7359), 308.

Oddie, S., Richmond, S., & Coulthard, M. (2001). Hypernatraemic dehydration and breast feeding: a population study. *Archives of Disease in Childhood*, *85*(4), 318–320.

Oepkes, D., Seaward, G., Vandenbussche, F. P., et al. (2006). Doppler ultrasonography versus amniocentesis to predict fetal anemia. *New England Journal of Medicine*, *355*(2), 156–164.

Özek, E., Soll, R., & Schimmel, M. S. (2010). Partial exchange transfusion to prevent neurodevelopmental disability in infants with polycythemia. *Cochrane Database of Systematic Reviews* (1), CD005089.

Pylipow, M., Gaddis, M., & Kinney, J. S. (1994). Selective intrapartum prophylaxis for group B streptococcus colonization: Management and outcome of newborns. *Pediatrics*, *93*(4), 631–635.

Robinson, J. L., Lee, B. E., Preiksaitis, J. K., et al. (2006). Prevention of congenital rubella syndrome – what makes sense in 2006? *Epidemiologic Reviews*, *28*(1), 81–87.

Ryan, G., Dooley, J., Gerber Finn, L., & Kelly, L. (2019). Nonpharmacological management of neonatal abstinence syndrome: A review of the literature. *Journal of Maternal-Fetal and Neonatal Medicine*, *32*(10), 1735–1740.

Sarnat, H. B., & Sarnat, M. S. (1976). Neonatal encephalopathy following fetal distress: A clinical and electroencephalographic study. *Archives of Neurology*, *33*(10), 696–705.

Sauerbrei, A., & Wutzler, P. (2000). The congenital varicella syndrome. *Journal of Perinatology*, *20*(8), 548–554.

Sauerbrei, A., & Wutzler, P. (2001). Neonatal Varicella. *Journal of Perinatology*, *21*, 545–549.

Schmidt, D. R., Hogh, B., Andersen, O., et al. (2006). The national neonatal screening programme for congenital toxoplasmosis in Denmark: results from the initial four years, 1999–2002. *Archives of Disease in Childhood*, *91*(8), 661–665.

Shankaran, S., Laptook, A. R., Ehrenkranz, R. A., et al. (2005). Whole-body hypothermia for neonates with hypoxic-ischemic encephalopathy. *New England Journal of Medicine*, *353*(15), 1574–1584.

Skuza, K. A., Sills, I. N., Stene, M., & Rapaport, R. (1996). Prediction of neonatal hyperthyroidism in infants born to mothers with Graves' disease. *Journal of Pediatrics*, *128*(2), 264–268.

Smolinski, K. N., Shah, S. S., Honig, P. J., & Yan, A. (2005). Neonatal cutaneous fungal infections. *Current Opinion in Pediatrics*, *17*(4), 486–493.

Snook, J. (2017). Is home phototherapy in the term neonate with physiological jaundice a feasible practice? A systematic literature review. *Journal of Neonatal Nursing*, *23*(1), 28–39.

Srinivasan, G., Pildes, R. S., Cattamanchi, G., et al. (1986). Plasma glucose values in normal neonates: A new look. *Journal of Pediatrics*, *109*, 114–117.

Steele, R. W., Metz, J. R., Bass, J. W., & DuBois, J. J. (1971). Pneumothorax and pneumomediastinum in the newborn. *Radiology*, *98*, 629–632.

Stephens, R. H., Benjamin, A. R., & Walters, D. V. (1998). The regulation of lung liquid absorption by endogenous cAMP in postnatal sheep lungs perfused in situ. *Journal of Physiology*, *511*, 587–597.

Stokowski, L. A. (2006). Fundamentals of phototherapy for neonatal jaundice. *Advances in Neonatal Care*, *6*(6), 303–312.

SUPPORT Study. (2010). Group of the Eunice Kennedy Shriver NICHD Neonatal Research Network. Early CPAP versus surfactant in extremely preterm infants. *New England Journal of Medicine*, 362(21), 1970–1979.

Sutton, L. R., & Hinderliter, S. A. (1990). Diazepam abuse in pregnant women on methadone maintenance. Implications for the neonate. *Clinical Pediatrics*, 29(2), 108–111.

SYROCOT (Systematic Review on Congenital Toxoplasmosis Study Group). (2007). Effectiveness of prenatal treatment for congenital toxoplasmosis: a meta-analysis of individual patients' data. *Lancet*, 369(9556), 115–122.

Teng, C. S., Tong, T. C., Hutchinson, J. H., & Yeung, R. T. (1980). Thyroid stimulating immunoglobulins in neonatal Graves' disease. *Archives of Disease in Childhood*, 55, 894–895.

Thangaratinam, S., Brown, K., Zamora, J., et al. (2012). Pulse oximetry screening for critical congenital heart defects in asymptomatic newborn babies: A systematic review and meta-analysis. *Lancet*, 379(9835), 2459–2464.

Theis, J. G., Selby, P., Ikizler, Y., & Koren, G. (1997). Current management of the neonatal abstinence syndrome: a critical analysis of the evidence. *Biology of the Neonate*, 71(6), 345–356.

Tracy, S. K., Tracy, M. B., & Sullivan, E. (2007). Admissions of term infants to neonatal intensive care: A population based study. *Birth*, 34(4), 301–307.

UK Collaborative ECMO Trial Group. (1996). UK collaborative randomized trial of neonatal extracorporeal membrane oxygenation. *Lancet*, 348(9020), 75–82.

Ungerer, R. L., Lincetto, O., McGuire, W., et al. (2004). Prophylactic versus selective antibiotics for term newborn infants of mothers with risk factors for neonatal infection. *Cochrane Database of Systematic Reviews* (2), CD003957.

van den Hout, L., Reiss, I., Felix, J. F., et al. (2010). Risk factors for chronic lung disease and mortality in newborns with congenital diaphragmatic hernia. *Neonatology*, 98(4), 370–380.

van Dommelen, P., van Wouwe, J. P., Breuning-Boers, J. M., et al. (2007). Reference chart for relative weight change to detect hypernatraemic dehydration. *Archives of Disease in Childhood*, 92(6), 490–494.

van Dongen, H., Klumper, F. J., Sikkel, E., et al. (2005). Non-invasive tests to predict fetal anemia in Kell-alloimmunized pregnancies. *Ultrasound in Obstetrics and Gynecology*, 25(4), 341–345.

van Kamp, I. L., Klumper, F. J., Oepkes, D., et al. (2005). Complications of intrauterine intravascular transfusion for fetal anemia due to maternal red-cell alloimmunization. *American Journal of Obstetrics and Gynecology*, 192(1), 165–170.

Wright, J. C., Budd, J. L., Field, D. J., & Draper, E. S. (2010). Epidemiology and outcome of congenital diaphragmatic hernia: A 9-year experience. *Paediatric and Perinatal Epidemiology*, 25(2), 144–149.

Wright, J. A., & Polack, C. (2006). Understanding variation in measles–mumps–rubella immunization coverage – a population-based study. *European Journal of Public Health*, 16(2), 137–142.

Zuckerman, B., Frank, D. A., Hingson, R., et al. (1989). Effects of maternal marijuana and cocaine use on fetal growth. *New England Journal of Medicine*, 320, 762–768.

ANNOTATED FURTHER READING

MacDonald, M. G., & Seshia, M. K. (2015). *Avery's neonatology: Pathophysiology and management of the newborn* (7th ed.). Philadelphia: Lippincott Williams and Wilkins.

This key international text comprehensively defines the pathophysiology and management of both term and preterm neonates. This edition is accompanied by a bundled interactive e-book edition offering tablet, smartphone or online access, with a highlighting tool for easier reference of key content throughout the text and the facility to take and share notes with friends and colleagues.

Rennie, J. M. (Ed.). (2012). *Rennie and Roberton's textbook of neonatology* (5th ed.) Edinburgh: Churchill Livingstone.

This definitive text explores the most contemporary methods of diagnosis, treatment and care of the neonate, alongside detailed pathophysiology of every significant condition of the neonate. Included in this edition are informative chapters on the psychological aspects of neonatology, such as legal and ethical aspects of neonatal care and perinatal death.

Wylie, L. (2010). Newborn screening and immunization. In H. Lumsden, & D. Holmes (Eds.), *Care of the newborn by ten teachers* (pp. 51–64). London: Hodder Arnold.

This chapter provides further information on all conditions that are currently screened by blood spot, to include medium-chain acyl CoA dehydrogenase deficiency (MCADD), cystic fibrosis and sickle cell disease.

USEFUL WEBSITES

British Association of Perinatal Medicine: www.bapm.org

Group B Strep Support: https://gbss.org.uk

National Institute for Health and Care Excellence: www.nice.org.uk

National Society for Phenylketonuria: www.nspku.org

RCOG (Royal College of Obstetricians and Gynaecologists): www.rcog.org.uk

Royal College of Paediatrics and Child Health: www.rcpch.ac.uk

UK National Screening Committee: www.gov.uk/government/groups/uk-national-screening-committee-uk-nsc

38

Care of the Dying Baby: End-of-Life Issues and Rights of the Fetus/Neonate

Alison Ledward, Jayne E. Marshall

CHAPTER CONTENTS

This chapter outlines the unique circumstances of the neonate, that is the *never competent* individual and introduces the midwife to the debates pertaining to who is best placed as principal decision-maker as well as the ethical theories that underpin the decision-making process at the end of life in the care of the dying baby. Central to the chapter is the midwife's role in the care of the dying baby, whose comfort is paramount. The intention is to capture the significance and impact of the parents' perspectives and in conjunction with the midwifery perspective, consider how the midwife can guide and support decisions that minimize parental distress and enhance memories of their baby. The best ways of training and supporting midwives providing care at a time of intense uncertainty and vulnerability are also taken into account. The chapter adopts an approach, which aims to provide a basis for understanding the values of all parties involved in the dying baby's care. In this respect, the value of inter-professional learning and working and finding common threads may be important and supportive.

INTRODUCTION

Medical advances in recent years have raised stark dilemmas relating to the resuscitation, care and treatment of extremely low birth weight babies, premature babies and those with congenital anomalies. Enhanced antenatal screening in particular has led to an increase in the numbers of families learning during pregnancy that their baby has a life-limiting condition and will die (Peacock et al. 2015). Further, the shifting relationships between healthcare professionals and parents/carers and the increasing availability of information on the internet have intensified clinical, ethical and professional issues relating to end-of-life care.

While neonatal intensive care is able to save the lives of many babies, some will still die after a long stay in intensive care and many painful and distressing interventions. The decision to end a baby's life is one of the most challenging situations encountered in neonatal intensive care.

Despite technological advances, what remains unchanged are the problems and complexities associated with the care of the sick neonate and it may be difficult to establish where the thresholds for decisions lie. Testing circumstances raise a wide spectrum of issues; clinical, ethical and professional. Care is frequently strongly underpinned by value judgements and beneath the technicalities, lie perceptions of hopes and fears, social and family values. These are independent of prognosis, predicted mortality or other clinical information based on facts or probabilities presented by healthcare professionals to parents.

End-of-life care is in complete contrast to the joyous anticipated outcome of pregnancy, labour and the birth of a healthy baby. In the United Kingdom (UK) around 105,000 babies require specialist neonatal care services (Royal College of Paediatrics and Child Health, RCPCH 2018). Further, during 2017, 1267 babies died during the first 28 days of life (Draper et al. 2019). The need for continued developments to ensure all babies and their families have access to equitable palliative care services has never been clearer or more opportune (Together for Short Lives, TfSL 2017). Midwives may be unaccustomed to providing end-of-life care. Nonetheless, it is part of their scope of practice. This chapter identifies likely sources of difficulty encountered by midwives caring for neonates at the end-of-life, including their families, and considers strategies that may help.

The chapter inevitably raises issues relating to parental bereavement and loss (see Chapter 31) however, such issues are not its main focus. Rather, central to this chapter, is the midwife's role in caring for the neonate and supporting the baby's parents. End-of-life care can mean caring for the pregnant woman who discovers her fetus(es) have a life-limiting condition, providing care during labour and birth associated with previously unanticipated events and (perhaps most frequently) providing end-of-life-care to babies in the Neonatal Intensive Care Unit (NICU), Special Care Baby Unit (SCBU) or in the home setting.

THE UNIQUE CIRCUMSTANCES OF THE BABY

The Never Competent Individual

In the UK, the fetus has no legal personality, but once it is born and shows signs of life, the baby becomes an individual in their own right. Midwives have a duty of care to the women, babies and families in their care and must act within the framework of the law and the Nursing and Midwifery Council (NMC) Code (NMC 2018a). Any act or omission on the part of the midwife that has the intent of causing death to a baby (infanticide) is deemed unlawful (Pattinson 2017). However, despite the neonate's status ratified in legal terms, they are a 'never competent individual', or if they are, then that competence has still to be located.

The Baby's Inability to Make Informed Decisions

The newborn baby does not have the ability or opportunity to express their views about life or death, therefore it is plausible to suggest they cannot wish to escape the fate of death since they have no concept about what it might entail. Concurrently, they have no real concept of living, nor do they have the ability to communicate their wishes in a coherent way. This contrasts markedly with competent individuals who have the opportunity to express their views.

The Validity of Proxy Decision-Making

The most appropriate and practical alternative is that adult decision-makers act on the baby's behalf as proxies. However, the validity of proxy decision-making is associated with risks (Boland et al. 2019). This is because it is virtually impossible for adult decision-makers to place themselves in the baby's position, thereby gauge their response, and view life and death decisions exclusively from the baby's perspective.

DECISION-MAKERS: THE ONGOING DEBATE

In this context, it should be stressed that a decision to withhold/withdraw treatment from a baby should always be based upon professional, ethical and legal guidance.

The Case for Doctors as Principal Decision-Makers

Arguably, medical practitioners have been clinically trained and have the appropriate professional experience specific to their sphere of practice; in this case neonatology and/or paediatrics. This enables them to be better placed than parents to judge the risks over benefits, the comparisons of treatments, the long-term significance of a poor clinical outcome and intolerability of some interventions. The care of premature and sick babies is highly specialized and the baby's condition can change on an hour-by-hour, if not minute-by-minute basis. The neonatologist/paediatrician should be able to interpret

outcome data (Shah et al. 2015; Pisani et al. 2016) and recommendations in clinical guidelines (National Institute for Health and Clinical Excellence, NICE 2016). Further attributes include doctors' experience with the clinical components of neonatal care and interpretation of test results (Gillam et al. 2017).

On the other hand, doctors frequently find themselves unable to reach a consensus about the evidence of effectiveness of some treatments for the individual baby and how they might respond. The doctors' focus should always be doing what is in the best interests of the baby, but professional authority might not always be used to good effect, for example when overriding the parents' views, which could be seen as unjustified paternalism. Further, some doctors may feel ill-prepared for conversations with parents about end-of-life care for their baby (Placencia and McCullough 2012; Pelentsov et al. 2016). This can limit the overall perceived benefits of discussions with parents.

The Case for Parents/Carers as Principal Decision-Makers

Parents/carers are those with parental responsibility for the child. Arguably, parents are usually involved in decision-making with regard to their children. It has been argued that parents should be the principal decision-makers in end-of-life care and as Miller (2004) claims, it is somehow contradictory that parents should be denied the opportunity to make decisions when they would be caring for the surviving child. Sullivan et al. (2014) argue that when the baby's prognosis is very bleak or when it is uncertain what lies ahead, parents should be allowed to decide, but their decisions should be based upon best available evidence.

Although parents and doctors share the same goal, that is, to reach a good clinical outcome, there is evidence to suggest that prognostic data are less important to parents than doctors (Kugelman et al. 2012). Parents tend to take a wider, more holistic view of their baby's situation, that is, other considerations, for example, hopes and fears, family values and religious beliefs to influence their judgement (Barth and Lannen 2011).

On the other hand, medical science can be complex and parents' judgements about the risks and benefits of treatment and clinical outcomes may be rudimentary. The high technology NICU environment can be intimidating and limit parents' opportunities to be involved in the care of their baby (Finlayson et al. 2014). There can also be a tendency for parents to request the continuation of their baby's treatment, despite the chances of success being slim (Moro et al. 2011).

Information-giving to parents in the NICU/SCBU setting is challenging. Doctors cannot legislate for all eventualities and if they did, they could run the risk of information overload and parents becoming overwhelmed in a maze of medical information, which may be confusing or even frightening. Events in neonatal intensive care can change rapidly, making the timely exchange of information difficult in a practical sense. Any decision parents make about their baby will affect them for the rest of their lives. Hence, there may be instances in practice when doctors should override parental autonomy by acting paternalistically. There may be instances in clinical practice when relieving parents of the burden of decision-making could however, be seen as a caring act.

Shared Responsibility for Decision-Making

Shared decision-making in health care is widely advocated as a way to support service users/patients in making decisions (Elwyn et al. 2012; Jefferies and Kirpalani 2012; Cummings 2015). Similarly, in neonatal care, there is recognized value in doctors and parents engaging in shared decision-making (Adams and Winslade 2011; Caeymaex et al. 2013).

Shared decision-making implies a discussion between parents/carers and doctors and the multi-professional team that explores their respective criteria for defining the baby's best interests. Although whatever information is disclosed by doctors (and other healthcare professionals) will frame the parents' decision and provide the basis for their informed consent, research has shown that doctors and parents use different criteria to make their decision. Doctors will use the *best interests* criteria that are determined by the best available medical evidence regarding the probabilities of the baby's survival and morbidity (Haward et al. 2011). Parents, moreover, are guided by their desired level of involvement in the decision-making process, their interpretation of medical information, support received from and trust in doctors (Birchley et al. 2017) and their hopes and spiritual values (Sadeghi et al. 2016). Hence, shared decision-making at the end-of-life should exceed best available evidence on the risks, benefits and comparisons of the interventions being proposed.

Shared decision-making means doctors and parents both engage in a communicative style that enhances parents' opportunity to participate, if that is their wish. Doctors can best facilitate this approach to promote parental engagement by providing balanced information, discussing options relating to parents' concerns and personal values and encouraging parents' questions in order to develop a sense of each other's perspectives, and in so doing, establish a trusting relationship.

Further measures consistent with good clinical practice include allowing parents adequate time to consider their options whenever appropriate and identifying further appropriate opportunities for shared decision-making (Daboval et al. 2016). The ways in which doctors and the healthcare team act to keep parents involved can help prevent parental disengagement from the process during a very tense and anxious time. Continued uncertainty about the right course of action may lead to the involvement of a Clinical Ethics Committee (CEC) (Kirkbride 2013; Jansen et al. 2018).

A final resort, when parents and their caring team cannot agree is involvement of the courts. External second opinion may be sought before pursuing mediation or referring to the courts for legal review on the course of the action to take.

THE MAIN ETHICAL DEBATES RELATING TO END-OF-LIFE CARE

This section outlines the main ethical debates relating to end-of-life care and how the reasoning process can help the midwife reach a position when there is rarely a single correct answer. This involves deciding which is the weightier ethical position in a given case. The systematic use of the principles outlined below (1–5) can help ensure that the midwife has reflected on the full range of considerations. It is not intended that these arguments will resolve conflict, but may help the midwife to better understand why some people weight each argument differently. It should be stressed that knowledge of these concepts is but one part of the care process and should be combined with evidence-based knowledge, clinical and interpersonal skills as well as ethical decision-making frameworks (see Chapter 2).

1. The Sanctity of Life

In religion and ethics, the sanctity of life (or inviolability) is a principle of implied protection regarding aspects of sentient life that are deemed holy, sacred or otherwise of such value that they are not to be violated. Supporters of the sanctity of life doctrine hold that it is always wrong to end a human life, including those with predicted poor quality. Inherent is that all human life is intrinsically valuable and should be preserved at all costs. An example is parents who want everything possible to be done for their baby. However, in practice, this principle may be difficult to uphold when certain choices have to be made. This is because, taken literally, it would mean disregarding all quality of life principles and indefinitely prolonging the lives of babies with life-limiting conditions, such as those babies who have anencephaly or are brain-dead.

2. The Quality of Life

The quality of life is elusive to assess (Green et al. 2017). In the care of the neonate, debate usually centres around what constitutes a poor outcome and the baby's likely future quality of life. Continued life support could be seen as imposing suffering without any foreseeable benefit other than prolonging the baby's life, but without improving their quality of life, thereby conflicting with the principle of *primum non nocere/non-maleficence* (above all, do no harm) (Beauchamp and Childress 2019). Healthcare professionals and parents should consider what constitutes a good quality of life and concurrently, how much burden and risk is it reasonable to impose on a baby in order to achieve this goal. A further point is that this principle is difficult to maintain in practice because neonatal interventions have become increasingly more sophisticated and outcomes are often difficult to predict. The dilemma professionals and parents face is whether treatment will help to promote a good outcome.

3. Best Interests

Best interests is a nebulous concept, as it is not clear as to whether this means a decision is made on *best medical interests* or the *best overall interests*. The principle of *best interests* involves value judgements and how different/competing interests should be compared against each other. It becomes more challenging with uncertainty of outcomes (Birchley et al. 2017; Racine et al. 2017). The interests of the baby should be seen as the principle on which to base decision-making. Although high value is placed on the baby's life, the approach recognizes that certain interventions may not always benefit the baby

and that there are situations in practice when the withholding/withdrawal of treatment may ultimately be in the baby's best interests.

4. Killing/Letting Die

Under English law, the intentional killing of a child under 12 months of age (usually by a parent) is known as *infanticide*, whereas *neonaticide* is the term given to the practice of killing newborn babies within 24 h of their birth (more often by the mother); both are criminal acts (Laurie et al. 2019). While the withdrawal of mechanical life support may be seen as acceptable in letting a baby die, active measures to end the baby's life would constitute euthanasia, which is illegal in the UK. However, if the cause of death is the doctor's omission to act (letting die), they may not necessarily be liable if the inaction was considered benevolent. In the case of, e.g. a severely compromised baby whose prognosis is extremely poor and who develops a chest infection, the decision may be made not to administer any antibiotics. The doctor's judgement not to treat the baby would be based on their knowledge that antibiotic therapy would only temporarily alleviate the baby's symptoms and that in the longer-term, might impose more suffering by extending the baby's life.

5. Theories of Personhood

Personhood theories are in direct opposition to the sanctity of life principle. Some theorists claim that only the possession of certain characteristics, such as a sense of the past and future; curiosity and the ability to reason (Fletcher 1979); self-consciousness (Tooley 1985); and rationality and autonomy (Singer 2011) confer personhood on an individual. Based on this theory, it could be argued that, as the neonate does not possess these features, they **cannot** be classified as a person and therefore it would not be wrong to kill them/let them die. It is, however, virtually certain that the various philosophical arguments for the attribution of personhood could not be coherently applied in a practical sense and have limited usefulness in neonatal intensive care.

SPECTRUM OF CARE

End-of-life care is not confined to the care of the baby and parents in an NICU or SCBU. It is imperative that the development of palliative care and professional support based on the needs of babies and their families should start as soon as the diagnosis or recognition of the life-limiting condition is made; that is antenatally (Wilkinson 2013). See Case Study 38.1: Anna's story. Hence, there needs to be an expansion of the goals of antenatal care to those associated with neonatology. Such support requires healthcare professionals working together to ensure that appropriate and timely palliative care/end-of-life care is provided by knowledgeable individuals who have an awareness and respect for baby/family needs and the role that each can play to address those needs. Evidence however, suggests that such care can be fragmented and not introduced in a timely manner (British Association of Perinatal Medicine, BAPM 2010; Peacock et al. 2015).

CASE STUDY 38.1 Anna's Story

Some things are a blur now, in that time near the end of my pregnancy. But I remember clearly the ultrasonographer spending a long time on the scan, the feel of the cool gel on my abdomen as my excitement ebbed away, until she finally said with sadness, 'I'm so sorry Anna, I don't know how to tell you this…'

Then came more scans, MRIs, obstetricians and neurosurgeons. A strong memory of the emotion in the voice of my obstetrician as she explained the extent of my baby's brain tumour. The words 'inoperable' and 'no chance of survival' managed to permeate through the dark fog that had surrounded me. I heard a groan of sorrow coming from somewhere, it took some time to realize it was coming from me.

Packing my hospital bag for birth was done in a daze, not much was needed. As I walked on to the labour suite, I hung my head low, not wanting to see the couples leaving with their new, beautiful babies. Not wanting them to see me; pale faced, red-eyed. I didn't want to ruin their moment.

Then in the birth room, gentle lighting, subtle scent of jasmine and bright loving eyes met mine with strength. My midwife, Helen, gave me the gift of listening to my grief, bearing witness to my loss without shying away, but also giving me courage to go on. Every time I felt I couldn't do it, she made me trust that I could. I believe all women should have their choice for birth respected and listened to, and I opted to birth my baby without any painkillers. For me, being fully present for the short time I had left with my child, was most important and Helen helped me birth in the way I had chosen.

Labour was hard; I didn't want to let go of my child knowing that we would have to say goodbye. My birth partner held my hand and midwife Helen encouraged me to the end, helping me birth safely with one-to-one care. I screamed and swore: Helen didn't flinch. But as I then held my baby, she gently soothed me and I had an hour skin-to-skin in calm, loving awe before my daughter, Fatima passed away. One of the most precious and beautiful times of my life.

After my baby's body was taken and wrapped, I descended back in to the dense fog of loss. My placenta failed to birth and had to be removed manually, but I barely registered it. Leaving the hospital with just a memory box were the hardest steps I've taken. I cherish the foot and hand prints done for me now, but at the time my arms ached for my baby and nothing could cushion that.

Other midwives also featured strongly in my emotional recovery. Those present through labour, plus a very special bereavement midwife who helped organize photos of my baby, registering her birth and death, and who even held my hand at the funeral. I don't remember everyone's names or faces, but I remember clearly how they made me feel; listened to.

Needless to say, the loss is still a journey I am on and probably always will be. However I remain grateful for all the help and strength the NHS maternity team gave to me – it's not an exaggeration to say the midwives saved my life. I now have a healthy 3-year-old, and having her was the best thing that ever happened to me, so we have a lot to look forward to and I am thankful for that chance.

In memory of: Baby Fatima: 25:10:15–25:10:15: age 1 hour. Midwife Helen: 28:09:83–06:12:18: age 35 years.

The midwife may have a key role in helping the woman compose a birth plan, supporting the parents and liaising with other healthcare professionals and the wider multiprofessional team. In order to establish confidence and a trusting relationship with the mother/parents, the midwife must be sensitive to the fact that they will be extremely anxious and therefore will need to build the necessary foundation to develop mutual understanding and empathy (von Hauff et al. 2016).

There are also occasions during labour and the birth of the baby when unforeseen events occur, such as birth asphyxia, where the midwife is a key role player in

---

BOX 38.1 Criteria for Admission to an NICU/SCBU

- Extremely low birth weight babies (ELBW): <1000 g and usually <28 weeks' gestation
- Very low birth weight babies (VLBW) <1500 g and usually <32 weeks' gestation
- Birth defects: malformations, chromosomal disorders, some of which may be incompatible with life (e.g. Potter syndrome), some inborn errors of metabolism
- Acquired diseases: generally healthy full-term fetuses, who become ill during or post-birth as a result of birth asphyxia, bacterial infections, etc.

From Rennie JM, Roberton NRC. (2012) Rennie and Roberton's textbook of neonatolgy (5th ed.) Edinburgh: Churchill Livingstone.

BOX 38.2 When to Withhold/Withdraw Treatment and Provide End-of-Life Neonatal Care

- Treatment falls short of success/cure
- Treatment is intolerable
- The baby's condition is incompatible with life, e.g. anencephaly
- Little hope of survival, e.g. severe spina bifida and hydrocephalus; Down syndrome (Trisomy 21) with multiple malformations
- The quality of life is extremely poor, e.g. babies who would survive with life-sustaining treatment, but with severe disability or chronic ill health
- Parents refuse clinically warranted treatment.

---

expediting appropriate action and subsequent care of the baby. Furthermore, there may be instances when a baby becomes ill on the postnatal ward and the midwife's clinical judgement, prompt actions and communicative skills are paramount.

BABIES WHO WARRANT ADMISSION TO THE NICU/SCBU

The criteria for a baby being admitted to a neonatal intensive care unit or special care baby unit as outlined by Rennie and Roberton (2012) can be seen in Box 38.1. However, some parents who have a baby with a life-limiting condition may wish to care for their baby in their own home environment with support from the multiprofessional team including the community midwife.

WITHHOLDING/WITHDRAWAL OF TREATMENT

There is no ethical difference between withholding (restricting) treatment or withdrawing (stopping) treatment (Larcher et al. 2015). Box 38.2 provides details of those situations where a decision is made to withhold/withdraw treatment is made and when end-of-life care of the baby may be appropriate. However, as Sacco and Virata (2017) affirm, there are instances in practice when establishing a clear prognosis may be difficult and fraught with uncertainties such as when a baby's fluctuating condition raises the

dilemma of restricted treatment on an ongoing basis and ultimately, the appropriateness of end-of-life care (Metselaar et al. 2017). The worst of all possible outcomes would be a slow and distressing death or the survival of a baby with severe disability.

THE MIDWIFE'S ROLE IN THE CARE OF THE DYING BABY/END-OF-LIFE CARE

The midwife should develop an understanding of the role and importance of recommendations in evidence- based clinical guidelines in shaping the end-of-life care of babies with life-limiting conditions in order to provide safe and effective care (NICE 2016). When treatment that has no overall benefit is withdrawn, following discussion of the redirection of care, end-of-life care should follow as a natural sequence. It is very important that the baby's care plan is revised appropriately in order to reflect both their changing physical needs and the parents' wellbeing at this fraught time. Care ceases to have a technical focus. The baby's life is short and every minute is extremely precious. Rather, care becomes focused upon the baby in their vulnerability and the goals of good care should be comfort, relief of suffering and minimizing parental distress.

Sensitive and effective communication by the midwife is an essential part of good practice. The midwife should remain constantly alert to the fact that many factors influence parents' decision-making, for example, social, educational, cultural and religious (Sacco and Virata 2017). It is crucial that appropriate choice of words by midwives reflects the fact that care is supportive and no longer curative (Fagerlin et al. 2011).

Throughout the entire process, documentation relating to end-of-life care should be contemporaneous, accurate and include records of all discussions with the mother/parents (NMC 2018a). Ideally, discussions about the baby's palliative care should be undertaken in the presence of **both** parents. Their valid consent should always be obtained for care and treatment offered to the baby as part of an ongoing process.

The Scope of Midwifery Practice in End-of-Life Care of the Baby

The midwife should develop a clear understanding of their scope of practice in end-of-life care of the baby. Midwives may have a key role in providing much of the baby's care and part of their duty of care includes their interactions with the baby's family. In this respect, care should be family-centred, meaning that the care provided is both respectful of, and responsive to, the needs of the individual family (Davidson et al. 2017). It is very important that healthcare professionals never assume that they know what the preferences of each family may be and thus, along with their colleagues, the role of the midwife is to gently explore families' priorities and goals to inform the baby's care plan. The focus of this care should be the baby's comfort, which would also consider appropriate pain management. Warmth, hygiene, food and fluids are considered to be part of basic care, whereas artificially supplied fluids or nutrition via an intravenous infusion or nasogastric tube are viewed by some as treatment and in a similar category as ventilation.

Information-Giving/Exchange

It is essential at the outset and throughout the process that parents have an understanding of their role in caring for their baby (Trajkovski et al. 2016). Similarly, in order to provide individualized care and support, the midwife needs to be able to recognize parental capacity to be involved in their baby's care. In these respects, the importance of good communication cannot be over emphasized.

Information-giving is multifaceted; it includes the need for the midwife to be constantly alert to the knowledge asymmetry between parents and the healthcare professionals providing the care in order to appropriately pace the dialogue. In this respect, the process involves sensitivity in actively listening to parents and willingness to learn from them. It is challenging to establish the right level of information and the appropriate choice of words for individuals. It may be the midwife who assists parents to better comprehend the doctors' explanation about their baby's care and treatment, and provides those elements which clarify certain points to enhance their understanding. This may be particularly important when information is complex, dense and difficult for parents to grasp and assimilate what has been said. The midwife should be mindful that parents will perceive every piece of information that they are presented with as being valuable, which may subsequently overshadow other equally important details. In this respect, it is helpful for consistency if one or two designated midwives are identified as 'leads' for keeping parents informed about what to expect so as to minimize confusion and misunderstanding. These measures would also help in improving continuation of care (NHS England 2016), reducing fragmentation of care and maintaining a relationship of respect, trust and understanding about the baby's best interests. This is especially important if the baby's death is very protracted, which can prove challenging for the midwife in respect of sustaining strong connections with other members of the caring team.

The parents of a baby with a life-limiting condition will be experiencing a range of emotions and while they may feel in need of care themselves, they may also wish to be viewed as a significant partner in the decision-making process. What parents require are assurances from the midwife that they have made the most appropriate decision and care is consistent with their understanding of the baby's condition and prognosis, which can provide some comfort. Midwives should be particularly careful about their choice of words and refrain from giving false assurances and non-verbal cues, which may be misinterpreted by parents. Bry et al. (2016) suggest that the use of gestures, for example, affirmation that the baby will not suffer, the physical use of touch and even silence, may be helpful measures.

There are instances in practice when one baby from a multiple pregnancy dies, which raises additional challenges for parents who are constantly reminded of their loss (Jordan et al. 2018) (see Chapter 31). In this respect, a thoughtful initiative by the midwife would be to take a photograph **all** the babies together as well as separately, clearly differentiating the babies from one another. This approach further acknowledges the specific grief borne by the parents (Richards et al. 2015), but can assist in their eventual acceptance of the loss as well. Furthermore, such photographs can help to place the dying baby in context with surviving babies/siblings and ultimately serve in a permanent memory of their short lives in years to come. The midwife should remain vigilant to the unique difficulties and dilemmas these parents face in caring for a surviving baby alongside the dying sibling. All interactions with the parents should be undertaken sensitively, taking into account the specific difficulties that are confronting them, including clarifying their part in end-of-life care provision alongside the care of their surviving baby/babies.

Appropriate Environment for the Dying Baby

The NICU/SCBU is a highly technical environment. The midwife should consider the impact of noise, lights, interruptions and the presence of other parents. These may be minimized by transferring the baby to a designated family room/quiet room as appropriate. In accordance with end-of-life care, alarms should be silenced and monitors removed. Discussions with the multiprofessional healthcare team may result in transferring the baby to another unit nearer to the family home (Kilcullen and Ireland 2017). Such discussions can help parents express their autonomy by making choices.

Where parents choose to care for their baby in the comfort of their own home, support from appropriate healthcare professionals that include outreach and palliative/comfort care services will be essential from diagnosis through to bereavement. Parents will need to be taught how to care for their baby's specific needs, e.g. tube feeding/applying suction, etc., to maintain their baby's comfort. There should be regular updates with the parents to discuss their baby's care, answer any questions and address any issues that may subsequently arise. Practical and emotional assistance for the family, including siblings and any close friends, should always be at hand, which can be provided by support workers with doctors being available 24 h/day. This is particularly vital when the baby's condition further deteriorates and/or the baby dies. In this situation, parents may also welcome spiritual support from their local faith organization or the hospital chaplain. The parents should also be reassured that they may choose to return their baby to the NICU/SCBU at any time if they feel the situation of the baby remaining at home, is becoming too stressful for them and the rest of their family.

Pain Management

Appropriate symptom management to include timely administration of analgesia should be an integral part of palliative care to maintain the baby's comfort (Mancini et al. 2014). The process of accurately identifying neonatal pain is challenging, as neonates can perceive pain but their sensory systems are immature (Vinall and Grunau 2014). A useful tool for the midwife may be to use a pain assessment scale as part of the baby's observations and care. This can help identify actual or potential sources of pain and thereby the frequency of pain assessment and appropriate treatment (Beatriz et al. 2015). The midwife should be cognisant with the fact that analgesia and sedatives may expedite the baby's death, but this is not the primary intention: rather, the *baby's comfort should always be paramount.*

Withdrawal of Nutrition and Fluids

A contentious area in clinical practice is the withdrawal of food and fluids. Feeding a baby is an integral part of care and seeing a baby dehydrated may be deemed unacceptable to some midwives. However, a baby with marked lung disease, heart failure or renal disease may become further distressed if fluids are continued. Babies with anomalies of the brain/airway may also be prone to choking episodes and should attempts be made to feed babies who have anomalies of the mouth/throat that inhibit their ability to suckle or swallow, their condition would be made worse with the likelihood of vomiting or choking if any feed is aspirated into the lungs (Fox et al. 2017). On this premise, it would be beneficent to withdraw feeds as a comfort measure, but not to give feeds by a nasogastric tube could be seen as starving the baby to death and morally unacceptable. It is therefore essential that each midwife or nurse examines the ethical issues involved in end-of-life care and determine their own position, as there is never any consensus of opinion in such situations. While doctors determine the course of action to withdraw/withhold feeds to a baby, legally the midwife or nurse can follow this instruction without compromising their professional position. However, it is the midwife or nurse who has to care for the baby day by day and support the parents' as they observe their baby become dehydrated and wasted, which can cause much distress and anxiety (Miller 2004).

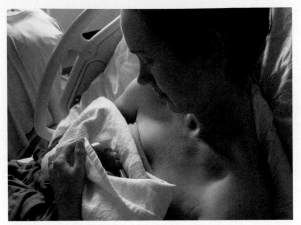

Fig. 38.1 Anna and Fatima.

Memory Making

The midwife's care should extend to exploring with the parents their goals and assisting them in creating distinctive memories of the short time they are likely to have with their baby. This could include preserving the precious moments where a mother caresses her baby following the withdrawal of life-support measures, as shown in Fig. 38.1. The research undertaken by Shelkowitz et al. (2015) found that parents greatly valued opportunities to preserve precious memories by bonding with and parenting their baby. In this respect, the midwife should consider and discuss with parents their perceptions of the best ways they can access and implement memory-making opportunities on a personal level (see Chapter 31).

Resources Available to Parents/Carers

The midwife's role is to always promote comprehensive family support in every situation. Where a baby has a life-limiting condition, the midwife's multifaceted role becomes even more vital and includes recognizing and responding to the baby's fluctuating condition as well as sensitively acknowledging the parents' varying needs. In some areas, this role may be undertaken by a Specialist Bereavement Midwife. In addition, the parents may appreciate the involvement of a minister of religion and/or social worker.

Following the baby's death, the parents should be supported by their midwife to spend as much time as they wish with their baby. Some parents may wish to take their baby home (if the death occurred in hospital) and arrange the funeral from there. This also assists other family members to acknowledge the baby's short life prior to saying their final farewells. Parents should be made aware of support groups such as Bliss, Child Bereavement UK, Stillbirth and Neonatal Death Society (Sands) and Together for Short Lives (TfSL). Such groups place the physical and psychosocial needs of the family, as well as the sharing of information between parents and their professional carers, at the heart of what they do, which in turn can help families to come to terms with their loss.

STRATEGIES TO SUPPORT MIDWIVES CARING FOR BABIES AT THE END-OF-LIFE

The experience of the death of a baby at any stage of pregnancy is not only devastating for the parents, but also those healthcare professionals, particularly the midwife, who have been involved in providing the maternity and any subsequent neonatal care. The following sections explore the strategies that may support midwives when providing care to babies with life-limiting conditions and their parents.

Midwifery Practice

In accordance with the Code (NMC 2018a), the midwife should act as the baby's advocate, which is a role-related responsibility of the healthcare professional. Some midwives may however, disagree with the medical decision to continue with or withdraw treatment, or with the parents' decision to withhold their permission for certain interventions or insist that everything possible is done to keep their baby alive. It is virtually certain that consensus will not be achievable in every case. The midwife should be mindful that parents' needs and wishes vary considerably and that they will not always make decisions based solely on the medical facts, but their unique set of personal values, their knowledge and cultural expectations and experiences relating to health care and disability (Haward et al. 2012). Hence, they may make decisions in a wider, relational sense and this is part of their autonomy. What becomes clear is that no parental decision to withdraw/withhold treatment and forego their dreams of including their baby in their life-plans is made easily (Enaudi et al. 2010; Gillam 2016; Weiss et al. 2016).

Midwives may need support to manage their own emotions as some may experience difficulty in *letting go*, whereas others may have difficulty expressing personal grief. In order to overcome these barriers, such emotions should be addressed. One way of doing this is to explore the lived experiences of those involved in caring for the baby within in a supportive environment (Widdershoven and Molewijk 2010). In this respect, *moral case deliberations* (ethical reflection meetings) based on a real case that has presented with challenging ethical issues to healthcare professionals, can be helpful (Daboval et al. 2014), assisting midwives to better understand the parents' position and remain open to their views (Metselaar et al. 2015). Further initiatives include staff referral for counselling and pastoral care (Green et al. 2016). Taken collectively, these measures should become a part of formal policy to support staff wellbeing at work.

For midwives working on the postnatal ward or in the community, it is essential that the lines of communication with their colleagues working in NICU/SCBU are clear and robust, so as to minimize misunderstandings between professional groups; the backdrop of which may compromise relationships with the baby's parents and diminish professional trust.

Education and Training

Less experienced and newly qualified midwives need to be prepared to deal with and offer the best possible care in difficult situations. It is imperative that education commences at the pre-registration stage and that student midwives are educated in moral and ethical decision-making theories to apply to challenging childbirth scenarios, including care of the dying baby and those with life-limiting conditions. However, previous studies have suggested significant omissions in the education of healthcare professionals in this area of care, notably NICU nurses who had received little in the way of palliative care education (Korzeniewska-Eksterowicz et al. 2013; Peng et al. 2013). Additional training and support should include developing communication skills and using ethical decision-making frameworks to deal with challenging and sensitive situations such as explaining the decision to withdraw/withhold treatment. Studies by Cavinder (2014) and Younge et al. (2015) found that educational interventions had a positive impact and helped in reducing moral distress among nurses providing end-of-life care to babies within the NICU.

Midwives are responsible to ensure their professional knowledge and skills remain contemporary, which is a requirement of their triennial professional revalidation (NMC 2019a). This can take the form of a variety of sources, including formal education and training sessions, online learning resources, debriefing and reflective case study discussions with colleagues and role play of typical challenging end-of-life scenarios.

Midwifery Research

In order to fully understand the role of healthcare professionals and appreciate the lived experiences of parents and in so doing, better accommodate the holistic needs of the dying baby and their family, it is essential research continues to be undertaken in this ethically challenging area of neonatal care. Undertaking a study to compare the experiences with those from Paediatric Intensive Care Units (PICU) would help in determining whether there are similarities or differences in how parents and healthcare professionals deal with situations where decisions to limit treatment are made. Furthermore, any lessons learned from similar clinical areas would serve in further improving ethical decision-making and subsequent care decisions affecting the dying neonate and their family.

THE VALUE OF INTER-PROFESSIONAL LEARNING AND WORKING

The report into the Bristol Inquiry (Kennedy 2001) identified the need to change the club culture found in the hospital setting to one in which collaborative teamwork is respected. Furthermore, the findings from the Francis (2013) Inquiry that investigated substandard care within Mid Staffordshire NHS Trust, attributed the failings in patient care to a constant lack of multidisciplinary team working. Similar findings were highlighted by Kirkup (2015) in the Inquiry into baby deaths at Morecambe Bay. The General Medical Council (GMC 2009) and the NMC (2018b, 2019b) endorse that doctors, midwives and nurses should understand the roles and expertise of health and social care professionals in the context of working and learning as a multiprofessional team, as well as appreciate the contribution this makes to the delivery of safe, effective and high quality care.

An inter-professional education initiative within the university setting that involved final year student midwives and children's nursing students exploring the challenges of perinatal and neonatal palliative care delivery, proved beneficial in improving their awareness of end-of-life care for babies in conjunction with the support of their families (Price et al. 2019). Both student groups reported that learning from and about each other's unique professional role in supporting babies diagnosed with life-limiting conditions and their families was important in developing their knowledge and future collaborative working practices, and welcomed more inter-professional education opportunities. This reaffirms the value of education relating to moral and ethical decision-making theories applied to challenging perinatal and neonatal palliative care commences at the pre-registration stage within an inter-professional context to optimize learning opportunities across professions.

CONCLUSION

Midwives can play a unique and pivotal role as a member of the multiprofessional healthcare team in providing high quality end-of-life care to the dying baby and developing a trusting and supportive relationship with the parents facing such a devastating and challenging situation. A knowledgeable and skilful midwife can help parents feel optimally supported and empowered following re-direction of care discussions with the caring team to end a baby's life.

In order to fulfil this deeply challenging role, and to adopt the most appropriate pathway/care plan, midwives need to familiarize themselves with ethical decision-making frameworks and to engage in inter-professional learning and working to ensure their knowledge and skills remain contemporary.

REFLECTIVE ACTIVITY FOR SELF-ASSESSMENT

1. As a midwife, how would you best support the mother/parents and the wider family in the following situations:
   a. During pregnancy when a life-limiting fetal anomaly is suspected/confirmed?
   b. During labour and birth in respect of (a) above and when a baby is unexpectedly stillborn?
   c. When a baby suddenly becomes unwell on the postnatal ward?
   d. Following withdrawal of a baby's treatment in a neonatal unit?

2. How might the application of ethical arguments/ethical decision-making frameworks assist you in handling difficult situations relating to the care of babies who have a life-limiting condition?
3. Following the medical decision to withdraw their baby's treatment, the parents have expressed they wish their baby to die at home. As a midwife, how would you and the multiprofessional team support this request, while also ensuring the interests of the dying baby remain central to your plan of action?

REFERENCES

Adams, D. M., & Winslade, W. J. (2011). Consensus, clinical decision making and unsettled cases. *Journal of Clinical Ethics, 22*, 310–313.

Barth, J., & Lannen, P. (2011). Efficacy of communication skills training courses in oncology: A systematic review and meta-analysis. *Annals of Oncology, 22*, 1030–1040.

Beatriz, V. O., Holsti, L., & Linhares, M. (2015). Neonatal pain and developmental outcomes in children born preterm: A systematic review. *Clinical Journal of Pain, 31*(4), 355–362.

Beauchamp, T. L., & Childress, J. E. (2019). *Principles of biomedical ethics* (8th ed.). Oxford: Oxford University Press.

Birchley, G., Gooberman-Hill, R., Deans, Z., et al. (2017). Best interests in paediatric intensive care: An empirical ethics study. *Archives of Disease in Childhood, 102*, 930–935.

Boland, L., Graham, I. D., Légaré, F., et al. (2019). Barriers and facilitators of pediatric shared decision-making: A systematic review. *BMC Implementation Science, 14*(7), 7.

BAPM (British Association of Perinatal Medicine). (2010). *Palliative care (supportive and end of life-care). A Framework for Clinical Practice in Perinatal Medicine.* Available at: www.bapm.org/resources/palliative-care-supportive-and-end-life-care-framework-clinical-practice-perinatal.

Bry, K., Bry, M., Hentz, E., et al. (2016). Communication skills training enhances nurses' ability to respond with empathy to parents' emotions in a neonatal intensive care unit. *Acta Pediatrica, 105*, 397–406.

Caeymaex, L., Jousselme, C., Vasilecu, C., et al. (2013). Perceived role in end–of–life decision making in the NICU affects long-term parental grief response. *Archives of Disease in Childhood-Fetal and Neonatal Edition, 98*, F26–31.

Cavinder, C. (2014). The relationship between providing neonatal palliative care and nurses' moral distress: An integrative review. *Advances in Neonatal Care, 14*(5), 322–328.

Cummings, J. (2015). Committee on fetus and newborn. Antenatal counselling regarding resuscitation and intensive care before 25 weeks of gestation. *Pediatrics, 136*(3), 588–595.

Daboval, T., Moore, G. P., Rhohde, K., et al. (2014). Teaching ethics in neonatal and perinatal medicine. What is happening in Canada? *Paediatrics and Child Health, 19*(1), e6–e10.

Daboval, T., Shidler, S., & Thomas, D. (2016). Shared decision-making at the limit of viability: A blueprint for physician action. *Plos One, 11*(11), e0166151.

Davidson, J. E., Aslakson, R. A., Long, A. C., et al. (2017). Guidelines for family-centred care in the neonatal, pediatric and adult ICU. *Critical Care Medicine, 45*, 103–128.

Draper, E. S., Gallimore, I. D., Smith, L. K., on behalf of the MBRRACE-UK Collaboration, et al. (2019). *MBRRACE-UK Perinatal Mortality Surveillance Report, UK Perinatal Deaths for Births from January to December 2017*. Leicester: The Infant Mortality and Morbidity Studies, Department of Health Sciences, University of Leicester.

Elwyn, G., Frosch, D., Thomson, R., et al. (2012). Shared decision-making: A model for clinical practice. *Journal of General Internal Medicine, 27*(10), 1361–1367.

Enaudi, M. A., Le Coz, P., Malzac, P., et al. (2010). Parental experience following perinatal death; Exploring the issues to make progress. *European Journal of Obstetrics, Gynecology and Reproductive Biology, 151*, 143–148.

Fagerlin, A., Zikmond-Fisher, B. J., & Ubel, P. A. (2011). Helping parents decide: Ten steps to better risk communication. *Journal of the National Cancer Institute, 103*, 1436–1443.

Finlayson, K., Dixon, A., Smith, C., et al. (2014). Mothers' perceptions of family centred care in neonatal intensive care units. *Sexual and Reproductive Healthcare, 5*, 119–124.

Fletcher, J. F. (1979). *Humanhood: Essays in biomedical ethics.* Buffalo: Prometheus Books.

Fox, G., Watts, T., & Hoque, N. (2017). *Oxford handbook of neonatology* (2nd ed.). Oxford: Oxford University Press.

Francis, R. (2013). *Mid Staffordshire NHS Foundation Trust public inquiry: Final report.* London: HMSO.

GMC (General Medical Council). (2009). *Tomorrow's doctors.* London: GMC.

Gillam, L. (2016). The zone of parental discretion: An ethical tool for dealing with disagreement between parents and doctors about medical treatment for a child. *Clinical Ethics, 11*, 1–8.

Gillam, L., Wilkinson, D., Xafis, V., & Isaacs, D. (2017). Decision-making at the borderline of viability: Who should decide and on what basis? *Journal of Paediatrics and Child Health, 53*, 105–111.

Green, J., Darbyshire, P., Adams, A., & Jackson, D. (2016). It's agony for us as well. Neonatal nurses reflect on iatrogenic pain. *Nursing Ethics, 23*(2), 176–190.

Green, J., Darbyshire, P., Adams, A., & Jackson, D. (2017). Quality versus quantity: The complexities of quality of life determinations for neonatal nurses. *Nursing Ethics, 24*(7), 802–820.

Haward, M. F., Kirshenbaum, N. W., & Campbell, D. E. (2011). Care at the edge of viability: Medical and ethical issues. *Clinics in Perinatology, 38*, 471–492.

Haward, M. F., John, L. K., Lorenz, J. M., & Fischhoff, B. (2012). Effects of description of options on perinatal decision-making. *Pediatrics, 129*, 891–902.

Jansen, M. A., Schlapbach, L. J., & Irving, H. (2018). Evaluation of a paediatric clinical ethics service. *Journal of Paediatrics and Child Health, 54*(11), 1199–1205.

Jefferies, A. L., & Kirpalani, H. M. (2012). Counselling and management for anticipated extremely preterm birth. *Paediatrics and Child Health, 17*(8), 443–446.

Jordan, A., Smith, P., & Rodham, K. (2018). Bittersweet: A qualitative exploration of mothers' experiences of raising a single surviving twin. *Psychology, Health and Medicine, 23*(8), 891–898.

Kennedy, I. (2001). *Bristol Royal Infirmary inquiry: Final report.* London: HMSO.

Kilcullen, M., & Ireland, S. (2017). Palliative care in the neonatal unit: Neonatal nursing staff perceptions of facilitators and barriers in a regional tertiary nursery. *BMC Palliative Care, 16*(1), 32.

Kirkbride, V. (2013). Managing complex ethical problems on the neonatal unit. *Medical Ethics, 9*(2), 66–70.

Kirkup, B. (2015). *The report of the Morecambe Bay investigation.* Preston: The Stationery Office.

Korzeniewska-Eksterowicz, A., Respondak-Liberska, M., Przyslo, L., et al. (2013). Perinatal palliative care: Barriers and attitudes of neonatologists and nurses in Poland. *Scientific World Journal, 2013*, 168060.

Kugelman, A., Bader, D., Lerner-Geva, L., et al. (2012). Poor outcomes at discharge among extremely premature infants: A national population-based study. *Archives of Pediatric and Adolescent Medicine, 166*, 543–550.

Larcher, V., Craig, F., Bhogal, K., et al. (2015). Making decisions to limit treatment in life-limiting and life–threatening conditions in children: A framework for practice. *Archives of Disease in Childhood, 100*, s1–s23.

Laurie, G. H., Harmon, S., & Dove, E. (2019). *Mason and McCall Smith's law and medical ethics* (11th ed.). Oxford: Oxford University Press.

Mancini, A., Uthaya, S., Beardsley, C., et al. (2014). *Practical guidance for the management of palliative care on neonatal units* (1st ed.). London: Chelsea and Westminster Hospital NHS Foundation Trust. Available at: www.chelwest.nhs.uk/services/childrens-services/neonatal-services/links/Practical-guidance-for-the-management-of-palliative-care-on-neonatal-units-Feb-2014.pdf.

Metselaar, S., Molewijk, B., & Widdershoven, G. (2015). Beyond recommendation and mediation: Moral case deliberation as moral learning in dialogue. *American Journal of Bioethics, 15*, 50–51.

Metselaar, S., Van Scherpenzeel, M., & Widdershoven, G. (2017). Dealing with moral dilemmas at the neonatology ward: The importance of joint case-by-case reflection. *American Journal of Bioethics, 17*(8), 21–23.

Miller, P. (2004). Ethical issues in neonatal intensive care. In L. Frith, & H. Draper (Eds.), *Ethics and midwifery* (2nd ed.) (pp. 127–142). Edinburgh: Books for Midwives.

Moro, T. T., Kavanaugh, K., Savage, T. A., et al. (2011). Parent decision-making for life support for extremely premature infants: From the prenatal through end-of-life period. *Journal of Perinatal and Neonatal Nursing, 25*(1), 52–60.

NHS England. (2016). *Better Births: Improving outcomes of maternity services in England: A five year forward view for maternity care*. London: NHS England.

NICE (National Institute for Health and Care Excellence). (2016). *End of life care for infants, children and young people with life- limiting conditions: Planning and management: NG 61*. London: NICE.

NMC (Nursing and Midwifery Council). (2018a). *The Code. Professional Standards of practice and behaviour for nurses, midwives and nursing associates*. London: NMC.

NMC (Nursing and Midwifery Council). (2018b). *Realising professionalism: Standards for education and training: Part 3: Standards for pre-registration nursing education*. London: NMC.

NMC (Nursing and Midwifery Council). (2019a). *Revalidation: How to revalidate with the NMC*. London: NMC.

NMC (Nursing and Midwifery Council). (2019b). *Realising professionalism: Standards for education and training: Part 3: Standards for pre-registration midwifery programmes*. London: NMC.

Pattinson, S. (2017). *Medical law and ethics* (5th ed.). London: Sweet and Maxwell.

Peacock, V., Price, J., & Nurse, S. (2015). Pregnancy to palliative care. *Practising Midwife, 18*(10), 18–25.

Pelentsov, L., Fielder, A., & Esterman, A. (2016). The supportive care needs of parents with a child with a rare disease: A qualitative descriptive study. *Journal of Pediatric Nursing, 31*(1), e207–e218.

Peng, N. H., Chen, N. H., Huang, L. C., et al. (2013). The educational needs of neonatal nurses regarding neonatal palliative care. *Nurse Education Today, 33*(12), 1506–1510.

Pisani, F., Facini, C., Pelos, A., et al. (2016). Neonatal seizures in preterm newborns: A predictive model for outcome. *European Journal of Paediatric Neurology, 20*(2), 243–251.

Placencia, F., & McCullough, L. (2012). Biopsychosocial risks of parental care for high-risk neonates: Implications for evidence-based parental counselling. *Journal of Perinatology, 32*(5), 381–386.

Price, J. E., Mendizabal-Espinosa, R. M., Podsiadly, E., et al. (2019). Perinatal/neonatal palliative care: Effecting improved knowledge and multi-professional practice of midwifery and children's nursing students through an inter-professional education initiative. *Nurse Education in Practice, 40*, 1–9.

Racine, E., Bell, E., Farlow, B., et al. (2017). The 'ouR-HOPE' approach for ethics and communication about neonatal neurological injury. *Developmental and Child Neurology, 59*, 125–135.

Rennie, J. M., & Roberton, N. R. C. (2012). *Rennie and Roberton's Textbook of Neonatology* (5th ed.). Edinburgh: Churchill Livingstone.

Richards, J., Graham, R., Embleton, N. D., et al. (2015). Mother's perceptions on the perinatal loss of a co twin: A qualitative study. *BMC Pregnancy and Childbirth, 15*, 143.

RCPCH (Royal College of Paediatrics and Child Health). (2018). *National Neonatal Audit Programme (NNAP) Annual 2018 Report on 2017 Data*. London: RCPCH.

Sacco, J., & Virata, R. (2017). Baby O and the withdrawal of life-sustaining medical treatment in the devastated neonate: A review of clinical, ethical and legal issues. *American Journal of Hospice and Palliative Medicine, 34*(10), 925–930.

Sadeghi, N., Hasaanpour, M., Heidarzadeh, M., et al. (2016). Spiritual needs of families with bereavement and loss of an infant in the neonatal intensive care unit: A qualitative study. *Journal of Pain and Symptom Management, 52*(1), 35–42.

Shah, P., Anvekar, A., McMichael, J., & Rao, S. (2015). Outcomes of infants with Apgar score of zero at 10 minutes: The West Australian experience. *Archives of Disease in Childhood: Fetal and Neonatal Edition, 100*(6), F492–F494.

Shelkowitz, E., Vessella, S. L., O'Reilly, P., et al. (2015). Counselling for personal care options at neonatal end of life: A quantitative and qualitative parent survey. *BMC Palliative Care, 14*, 70.

Singer, P. (2011). *Practical ethics* (3rd ed.). New York: Cambridge University Press.

Sullivan, J., Monagle, P., & Gillam, L. (2014). What parents want from doctors in end-of-life decision-making for children. *Archives of Disease in Childhood, 99*, 216–220.

TfSL (Together for Short Lives). (2017). *The perinatal pathway for babies with palliative care needs*. Bristol: TfSL. Available at: www.togetherforshortlives.org.uk/wp-content/uploads2018/01/ProRes-Perinatal-for-Babies-With-Palliative-Care-Needs.pdf.

Tooley, M. (1985). *Abortion and infanticide*. New York: Oxford University Press.

Trajkovski, S., Schmied, V., Vickers, M. H., & Jackson, D. (2016). Experiences of neonatal nurses and parents working collaboratively to enhance family centred care: The destiny phase of an appreciative inquiry project. *Collegian, 23,* 265–273.

Vinall, J., & Grunau, R. E. (2014). Impact of repeated procedural pain-related stress in infants born very preterm. *Pediatric Research, 75*(5), 584–587.

von Hauff, P., Long, K., Taylor, B., & van Manen, M. A. (2016). Antenatal consultation for parents whose children may require admission to neonatal intensive care: A focus group study for media design. *BMC Pregnancy and Childbirth, 16,* 103.

Weiss, E. M., Barg, F. K., Cook, N., et al. (2016). Parental decision-making preferences in neonatal intensive care. *Journal of Paediatrics, 179,* 36–41.

Widdershoven, G., & Molewijk, B. (2010). Philosophical foundations of clinical ethics: A hermeneutic perspective. In J. Schildmann, J. S. Gordon, & J. Vollman (Eds.), *Clinical ethics consultation: Theories and methods, implementation, evaluation* (pp. 37–51). Farnham: Ashgate.

Wilkinson, D. (2013). *We need palliative care for babies facing certain death. The Conversation.* Available at: https://theconversation.com/we-need-palliative-care-for-babies-facing-certain-death-15932.

Younge, N., Smith, P. B., Goldenberg, R. N., et al. (2015). Impact of a palliative care program on end-of-life care in a neonatal intensive care unit. *Journal of Perinatology, 35*(3), 218–222.

ANNOTATED FURTHER READING

Carter, B. S., & Jones, P. M. (2013). Evidence-based comfort care for neonates towards the end of life. *Seminars in Fetal and Neonatal Medicine, 18*(2), 88–92.

This paper focuses on the redirection of care from curative to supportive, with empathy and compassion at its core. Despite the lack of a firm evidence-base on this aspect of care, professional carers should apply their practical knowledge skilfully and sensitively.

Cortezzo, E. D., Sanders, M. R., Brownell, E., & Moss, K. (2015). End-of-life care in the neonatal intensive care unit: Experiences of staff and parents. *American Journal of Perinatology, 32,* 713–724

This paper explores the perceptions and experiences of healthcare professionals who cared for parents whose baby had died in the NICU. Most healthcare professionals' accounts suggested they were comfortable delivering end-of-life care, despite the fact that supportive measures such as debriefing and further education did not occur routinely. Parents' accounts suggested that consistency of care was sometimes lacking and emphasized the importance of memory-making and appropriate follow-up care.

Kirkbride, V. (2013). Managing complex ethical problems on the neonatal unit. *Medical Ethics, 9*(2), 66–70.

A useful paper that explores ways in which ethical dilemmas relating to neonatal care, may be managed through the discussion of authentic case studies.

McDougall, R., Delaney, C., & Gillam, L. (2016). *When doctors and parents disagree. Ethics, paediatrics and the zone of parental discretion.* Sydney: The Federation Press.

This text examines the vexed question of what happens when doctors and parents fail to reach an agreement about the care and treatment of a child. Written from a dominant medical discourse, it covers the doctor and parent relationship and the key ethical and social complexities of decision-making with families. It outlines a conceptual framework, namely the Zone of Parental Discretion (ZPD): an ethical tool that balances the child's welfare and the parent's rights of decision-making. The ZPD extends thinking from what is in the child's best interests to whether the parents' decision will cause the child harm.

Price, J. E., & McAlinden, O. (2017). *Essentials of nursing children and young people.* London: Sage.

This innovative and student-friendly text provides up-to-date information on the core content of child nursing courses and helps students understand how it applies to practice. Particularly useful to the focus of this chapter are Chapters 34 and 35 that explore the care of children and young people with life-limiting illness and the care of children and young people at the end-of-life, respectively. The text signposts the reader to consider critical aspects of practice throughout such as 'safeguarding stop points', 'what's the evidence?' boxes and links to critical thinking or reflection.

USEFUL WEBSITES

American Academy of Pediatrics: www.aap.org/en-us/Pages/Default.aspx

Bliss for babies born premature or sick: www.bliss.org.uk

British Association of Perinatal Medicine: www.bapm.org

Child Bereavement UK (CBUK): www.childbereavementuk.org

General Medical Council: www.gmc-uk.org

Mothers and babies reducing risk through audits and confidential enquiries across the UK (MBRRACE-UK): www.npeu.ox.ac.uk/mbrrace-uk

National Institute for Health and Clinical Excellence: www.nice.org.uk

Nuffield Council on Bioethics: http://nuffieldbioethics.org

Nursing and Midwifery Council: www.nmc.org.uk

Royal College of Paediatrics and Child Health: www.rcpch.ac.uk

Stillborn and Neonatal Death Society: www.uk-sands.org

Together for Short Lives: www.togetherforshortlives.org.uk

United Kingdom Clinical Ethics Network: http://ukcen.net

GLOSSARY OF TERMS AND ACRONYMS

Abruptio placenta   Premature separation of a normally situated placenta. This term is commonly used from viability (24 weeks).

Acridine orange   A stain used in fluorescence microscopy; it causes bacteria to fluoresce green to red.

Aetiology   The science of the cause of disease.

Affective awareness   An awareness of feelings and ability to express them.

Affective neutrality   Known as professional detachment.

Allantois   A sac-like structure or outpouching of the endodermic tissue.

Alveoli   Terminal sacs at the end of the bronchial tree where gaseous exchange takes place.

Anhedonia   The loss of pleasure.

Amenorrhoea   Absence of menstrual periods.

Amnion   The inner membrane of the placenta derived from the inner cell mass.

Amniotic fluid embolism   The escape of amniotic fluid through the wall of the uterus or placental site into the maternal circulation, triggering life-threatening anaphylactic shock in the mother. (*The word 'embolism', denoting a clot, is a misnomer.*)

Amniotomy   Artificial rupture of the amniotic sac.

Ankyloglossia   Tongue-tie, which is caused by a tight or short lingual frenulum that may affect the newborn breastfeeding.

Anteflexion   The uterus bends forwards upon itself.

Anterior obliquity of the uterus   Altered uterine axis. The uterus leans forward due to poor maternal abdominal muscles and a pendulous abdomen.

Anteversion   The uterus leans forward.

Antigen   A substance that stimulates the production of an antibody.

Anuria   Lack of urine production.

Apnoea   An absence of breathing for more than 20 seconds.

Asynclitism   The presentation of the fetal head at an oblique angle between the axis of the presenting part of the fetus and the pelvic planes during labour/childbirth (also known as obliquity).

Atresia   Closure or absence of a usual opening or canal.

Attitude   The degree of flexion or extension of the fetal head on the neck.

Augmentation of labour   Intervention to correct slow progress in labour.

Autonomy   Self-determination, independence and self-governing.

Bandl's ring   An exaggerated retraction ring seen as an oblique ridge above the symphysis pubis between the upper and lower uterine segments, which is a sign of obstructed labour.

Basal body temperature   The temperature of the body when at rest. In natural family planning, it is taken as soon as the woman wakes from sleep and before any activity occurs or after a period of at least 1 hour's rest.

Basal plate   The maternal side of the placenta.

Beneficence   To do good.

Bicornuate uterus   A structural congenital malformation of the uterus that results in two horns; commonly referred to as a 'heart-shaped' uterus.

Bioavailability   The degree to which, or rate at which, a drug or other substance becomes available to the target tissue after administration.

Bioequivalent   Acting on the body with the same strength and similar bioavailability as the same dosage of a sample of a given substance.

Bipolar disorder   A mental illness or mood disorder where the individual experiences periods of depression and elevated mood (mania). (*Previously known as manic depression*).

Birth centres   These may be freestanding (*away from hospital*) or in hospital grounds or in the hospital. The emphasis is on providing a less medical environment and supporting physiological birth.

Bishop Score   Rating system to assess suitability of the cervix for induction of labour.

Blastulation   The process from the development of the morula to the development of the blastocyst.

Bregma   Anterior fontanelle.

Bullying   Intimidating, malicious, offensive or insulting behaviour, or an abuse or misuse of power through means that undermine, humiliate, denigrate or injure the recipient.

Burns–Marshall manoeuvre   A method of breech birth involving traction to prevent the fetal neck from bending backwards.

Candour   Openness, honesty and frankness.

Caput succedaneum   A diffuse oedematous swelling under the scalp but above the periosteum.

Cardiotocogram/graphy   Measurement of the fetal heart rate and uterine contractions on a machine that is able to provide a paper printout of the information it records.

Carunculae myrtiformes   Hymenal tags/remnants.

Caseload practice   A personal caseload where named midwives care for individual women.

Cave of Retzius   Extraperitoneal space between the symphysis pubis and urinary bladder.

Central venous pressure line   An intravenous tube that measures the pressure in the right atrium or superior vena cava, indicating the volume of blood returning to the heart and by implication, hypovolaemia.

Cephalhaematoma (cephalohaematoma)   An effusion of blood under the periosteum that covers the skull bones.

Cephalopelvic disproportion   Disparity between the size of the woman's pelvis and the fetal head.

Cerclage   Non-absorbable suture inserted to keep the cervix closed.

Cervical eversion Physiological response by cervical cells to hormonal changes in pregnancy. Cells proliferate and cause the cervix to appear eroded.

Cervical intra-epithelial neoplasm Progressive and abnormal growth of cervical cells.

Cervical ripening Process by which the cervix changes and becomes more susceptible to the effect of uterine contractions. Can be physiological or artificially produced.

Cervicitis Inflammation of the cervix.

Chadwick's/Jacquemier's sign the increased vascularity within the cervical stroma that creates an ectocervical violet-blue tint.

Child sex exploitation (grooming) A child or young person coerced or manipulated into engaging in sexual activity in return for a reward, thus falsely feeling valued and in control.

Choanal atresia (Bilateral) membranous or bony obstruction of the nares; the baby appears blue when sleeping and pink when crying.

Chorion The outer placental membrane that is continuous with the edge of the placenta.

Chorionic plate The fetal side of the placenta.

Choroid plexus cyst Collection of cerebrospinal fluid within the choroid plexi, from where cerebrospinal fluid is derived.

Chromosome An organized structure of DNA and organized proteins that carries genes.

Clitoridectomy Partial or total removal of the clitoris and/or, in some cases, only the prepuce.

Coloboma A malformation characterized by the absence of, or a defect in, the tissue of the eye; the pupil can appear keyhole-shaped. It may be associated with other anomalies.

Colposcopy Visualization of the cervix using a colposcope.

Commensal Micro-organisms adapted to grow on the skin or mucous surfaces of the host, forming part of the normal flora.

Concealed pregnancy A complex, multidimensional and temporal process, where a woman is aware of her pregnancy and copes by keeping it secret and hidden.

Conjoined twins Identical twins, where separation is incomplete so their bodies are partly joined together and vital organs may be shared.

Coronal suture Membranous tissue separating the frontal bones from the parietal bones.

Couvelaire uterus (uterine apoplexy) Bruising and oedema of uterine tissue seen in placental abruption when leaking blood is forced between muscle fibres because the margins of the placenta are still attached to the uterus.

Cricoid pressure A technique whereby pressure is exerted on the cartilaginous ring below the larynx (the cricoid) to occlude the oesophagus and prevent reflux. Cricoid pressure is employed during the induction of a general anaesthetic to prevent acid aspiration syndrome.

Cryotherapy Use of cold or freezing to destroy or remove tissue.

Cryptorchidism Undescended testes, which may be unilateral or bilateral.

Decidualization The structural changes that occur in the endometrium in preparation for implantation.

De-infibulation Being opened.

Delusion A false fixed belief that is impenetrable to reason.

Deontology Duty-based theory.

Deoxyribonucleic acid The substance containing genes. DNA can store and transmit information, can copy itself accurately and can occasionally mutate.

Dextrorotation Rotation of the uterus to the right.

Diastasis symphysis pubis A painful condition in which there is an abnormal relaxation of the ligaments supporting the pubic joint; also referred to as pelvic girdle pain.

Dichorionic twins Two individuals who have developed in their own separate chorionic sacs.

Diploid Containing two sets of chromosomes.

Disseminated intravascular coagulation/coagulopathy A condition secondary to a primary complication where there is inappropriate blood clotting in the blood vessels, followed by an inability of the blood to clot appropriately when all the clotting factors have been used up.

Dizygotic (binovular) Formed from two separate zygotes.

Domestic abuse/violence Any incident or pattern of incidents of controlling, coercive or threatening behaviour between those aged 16 years and over who are, or have been, intimate partners or family members regardless of gender or sexuality. This may encompass psychological, physical, sexual, financial and emotional abuse.

Ductus arteriosus A temporary fetal structure, which leads from the bifurcation of the pulmonary artery to the descending aorta.

Ductus venosus A temporary shunt that connects the intrahepatic portion of the umbilical vein to the inferior vena cava.

Dysmenorrhoea Painful menses or menstrual cramps.

Dyspareunia Painful or difficult intercourse experienced by the woman.

Ectoderm The outermost layer of three primary germ cell layers present in the early embryo.

Ectopic pregnancy An abnormally situated pregnancy, most commonly in a uterine/fallopian tube.

Effacement Thinning out or taking up of the cervix.

Endocervical Relating to the internal canal of the cervix.

Endoderm The innermost layer of three primary germ cell layers present in the early embryo.

Engagement When the widest transverse diameter of the fetal head enters the pelvic brim.

Epicanthic folds A vertical fold of skin on either side of the nose, which covers the lacrimal caruncle. They may be common in Asian babies, but may indicate Down syndrome in other ethnic groups.

Episiotomy A surgical incision made to enlarge the vaginal orifice during childbirth.

Epulis Bleeding gums also known as *pyogenic granuloma*.

Erb's palsy Paralysis of the arm due to the damage to cervical nerve roots 5 and 6 of the brachial plexus.

Erythematous Reddening of the skin.

Erythropoiesis The process by which erythrocytes (red blood cells) are formed. After the 10th week of gestation, erythropoiesis production rises and seems to be involved in red cell production in the bone marrow during the third trimester.

Eumenorrhoea Denotes normal and regular menstruation.

Exomphalos (omphalocele) A defect in which the bowel or other viscera protrude through the umbilicus.

External cephalic version The use of external manipulation on the pregnant woman's abdomen to convert a breech to a cephalic presentation.

False-negative rate The proportion of affected pregnancies that would not be identified as high risk. Tests with a high false-negative rate have low sensitivity.

False-positive rate The proportion of unaffected pregnancies with a high-risk classification. Tests with a high false-positive rate have low specificity.

Fasciculus The predominant macroscopic structural element of the myometrium.

Female genital mutilation Also known as 'female circumcision' or 'genital cutting'. Any procedure that intentionally alters or causes injury to the external female genital organs for non-medical reasons. Four main types are reported.

Ferguson reflex Surge of oxytocin, resulting in increased contractions, due to stimulation of the cervix and upper portion of the vagina.

Fetal reduction The reduction in the number of viable fetuses/embryos in a multiple (usually higher multiple) pregnancy by medical intervention.

Feto-fetal transfusion syndrome Also known as 'twin-to-twin transfusion syndrome'. Condition in which blood from one monozygotic twin fetus transfuses into the other fetus via blood vessels in the placenta.

Fetus-in-fetu Parts of a fetus may be lodged within another fetus. This can only happen in monozygotic twins.

Fibroid (fibromyoma) Firm, benign tumour of muscular and fibrous tissue.

Fontanelles Soft areas on the fetal skull bones (cranium) where two or more sutures meet.

Foramen magnum A large opening in the occipital bone of the skull through which the spinal cord exits.

Foramen ovale A temporary structure of the fetal circulation allowing blood to be shunted from the right to left atrium *in utero*.

Fossa ovalis Oval-shaped depression in the intra-atrial septum. Formed following the closure of the foramen ovale at birth.

Framing effect A means of cognitive bias insofar that individuals react differently to a particular choice such as antenatal screening tests, based on the manner in which the information is presented, i.e. whether they perceive the risk of screening as a loss or a gain.

Fraternal twins Dizygotic *(non-identical)*.

Frenulum The membrane connecting the underside of the tongue to the floor of the mouth (see 'Ankyloglossia').

Fundal height The distance between the upper part of the uterus (*the fundus*) and the upper part of the symphysis pubis (*the junction between the pubic bones*). This assessment is undertaken to assess the increasing size of the uterus antenatally and decreasing size postnatally.

Funis The umbilical cord.

Gastroschisis A paramedian defect of the abdominal wall with extrusion of bowel that is not covered by peritoneum.

Gastrulation The beginning of morphogenesis.

Gingivitis Swelling/inflammation of the gingiva – the part of the gum that surrounds the base of the teeth.

Glabella The area between the eyebrows.

Globalization The increased interconnectedness and interdependence of people and countries.

Goodell's sign Cervical oedema that leads to softening of the anatomical structure.

Grande multipara A woman who has given birth five times or more.

Greater vestibular glands (Bartholin's glands) Two small glands that open on either side of the vaginal orifice, located in the posterior part of the labia majora.

Group practice A small group of midwives who provide care for a group of women.

Haematogenesis Formation of red blood cells.

Haematuria Blood in the urine.

Haemostasis The arrest of bleeding.

Hallucinations A sensory perception in the absence of any stimulus. Any of the five sensory modality can be affected.

Haploid Containing only one set of chromosomes.

Harassment Unwanted conduct related to a relevant protected characteristic, which has the purpose or effect of violating an individual's dignity or creating an environment for that individual that is not only hostile but is intimidating, degrading, humiliating or offensive.

Hegar's sign Softening of the isthmus between the cervix and uterus.

HELLP syndrome A condition of pregnancy characterized by Haemolysis, Elevated Liver enzymes and Low Platelets.

Herpes gestationis An autoimmune disease precipitated by pregnancy and characterized by an erythematous rash and blisters.

Hilum The point of entry for the renal artery and renal nerves plus the point of exit for the renal vein and the ureter.

Homan's sign Pain is felt in the calf when the foot is pulled upwards (*dorsiflexion*). This is indicative of a venous thrombosis and further investigations should be undertaken to exclude or confirm this.

Homeostasis The condition in which the body's internal environment remains relatively constant within physiological limits.

Human trafficking (modern slavery) The trade of humans (usually women and children) for the purposes of forced labour, sexual slavery or commercial exploitation for the trafficker or others.

Hydatidiform mole A gross malformation of the trophoblast in which the chorionic villi proliferate and become avascular.

Hydropic vesicles Fluid-filled sacs or blisters.

Hypercapnia An abnormal increase in the amount of carbon dioxide in the blood.

Hyperemesis gravidarum Protracted or excessive vomiting in pregnancy.

Hypertrophy Overgrowth of tissue.

Hypogastric arteries Temporary fetal structures that branch off from the internal iliac arteries and become the umbilical arteries when they enter the umbilical cord.

Hypospadias A condition where the urethral meatus opens on to the under-surface of the penis.

Hypothermia A core body temperature below 36°C.

Hypotonia The loss of muscle tension and tone.

Hypovolaemia Reduced circulating blood volume due to external loss of body fluids or to loss of fluid into the tissues.

Hypoxia Lack of oxygen.

Hypoxic ischaemic encephalopa-thy Condition where there is evidence of hypoxia and ischaemia.

Hysteroscope An instrument used to access the uterus via the vagina.

Immunoglobulins Antibodies.

Induction of labour Intervention to stimulate uterine contractions before the onset of spontaneous labour.

Infibulation Narrowing of the vaginal opening through the cutting of the labia minora and suturing or closing of the outer, labia majora, with or without removal of the clitoris.

Intermittent positive pressure ventilation Inflation breaths are given to clear lung fluid and ventilatory breaths are given to remove excess CO_2 and provide oxygen.

Internationalization Has no agreed definition but best describes the process of harmonizing relationships from a cross-cultural or international perspective.

Intervillous spaces The spaces between the chorionic villi that fill with maternal blood.

Intraepithelial Within the epithelium, or among epithelial cells.

Intrahepatic cholestasis of pregnancy An idiopathic condition of abnormal liver function.

Jaundice Yellow coloration of the skin and the sclera caused by a raised level of bilirubin in the circulation (*hyperbiliru-binaemia*).

Justice Being treated with fairness.

Kleihauer test A standard blood test used to quantitatively assess or measure the degree of feto-maternal haemorrhage.

Lacunae Hollowed out spaces or cavities.

LAM A method of contraception based upon an algorithm of lactation and amenorrhoea over a 6-month time period.

Lamda Posterior fontanelle.

Lamdoidal suture Membranous tissue separating the occipital bone from the two parietal bones of the fetal skull.

Lanugo Soft downy hair that covers the fetus *in utero* and occasionally the neonate. It appears at around 20 weeks' gestation and covers the face and most of the body. It disappears by 40 weeks' gestation.

Layer of Nitabusch A collagenous layer between the endometrium and myome-trium.

Ligamentum arteriosum Permanent lig-ament formed from the ductus arteriosus following birth.

Ligamentum teres Permanent ligament formed from the umbilical vein following birth.

Ligamentum venosum Permanent lig-ament formed from the ductus venosus following birth.

'Lightening' The feeling of relief a woman experiences when the presenting part of the fetus descends into the brim of the pelvis.

Linea alba A line that lies over the midline of the rectus muscles from the umbilicus to the symphysis pubis.

Linea nigra A common dark line of pigmentation running longitudinally in the centre of the abdomen below and sometimes above the umbilicus.

Lochia A Latin word traditionally used to describe the vaginal loss a woman experi-ences following the birth of a baby.

Løvset manoeuvre A manoeuvre for the birth of the fetal shoulders and extended arms in a breech presentation.

Macrosomia Large baby weighing 4–4.5 kg or greater.

Malposition A cephalic presentation other than a normal well-flexed anterior position of the fetal head, e.g. occipi-toposterior.

Malpresentation A presentation other than the vertex, i.e. face, brow, com-pound or shoulder.

Mauriceau–Smellie–Veit manoeuvre A manoeuvre to assist the birth of the fetal head in a breech presentation that in-volves jaw flexion and shoulder traction.

McRoberts manoeuvre A manoeuvre to rotate the angle of the symphysis pubis superiorly and release the impaction of the anterior shoulder of the fetus when there is shoulder dystocia. The woman brings her knees up to her chest.

Mendelson's syndrome A chemical pneumonitis caused by the reflux of gastric contents into the maternal lungs during a general anaesthetic.

Meningitis Inflammation of the mem-branes covering the brain and spinal column.

Menopause When the menstrual period does not occur for up to 12 months in a woman's reproductive cycle and the ovarian phase ceases.

Menorrhagia Heavy vaginal bleeding.

Menstrual cycle The name given to the physiological changes that occur in the endometrial layer of the uterus, which are essential to receive the fertilized oocyte.

Mentum Chin.

Mesenchyme A mesh of embryonic connective tissue.

Mesoderm The middle layer of three primary germ cell layers present in the early embryo.

Microchimerism The presence of a small number of cells in one individual that originated in a different individual.

Midwife-led care Midwives or a midwife take the lead role in care of a woman or group of women.

Miscarriage Spontaneous loss of pregnan-cy before viability.

Mittelschmerz   The pelvic and lower abdominal pain experience by some women during ovulation.

Modified Early Obstetric Warning Score (MEOWS/MEWS)   A chart or track and trigger system used to record maternal observations or physiological vital signs antenatally and postnatally for all mothers who are hospitalized in the maternity service.

Monoamniotic twins   Two individuals who have developed in the same amniotic sac.

Monochorionic twins   Two identical individuals who have developed in the same chorionic sac.

Monozygotic (monozygous)   Formed from one zygote (identical twins).

Morphogenesis   The process that controls the organized spatial distribution of cells during the embryonic period.

Moulding   The change in shape of the fetal head that takes place during its passage through the birth canal.

Morula   The spherical embryonic mass of cells/blastomeres resulting from cleavage of a fertilized ovum.

Multifetal reduction   see 'Fetal reduction'.

Myocytes   Elongated, spindle-shaped smooth muscle cells.

Naegele's rule   A method of calculating the expected date of birth.

Natural family planning   Methods of contraception based on observations of naturally occurring signs and symptoms of the fertile and infertile phases of the menstrual cycle.

Necrotizing enterocolitis   An acquired disease of the small and large intestine caused by ischaemia of the intestinal mucosa.

Neonatal encephalopathy   A clinical syndrome of abnormal levels of consciousness, tone, primitive reflexes, autonomic function and sometimes seizures in newborn babies.

Neoplasia   Growth of new tissue.

Neurulation   The formation of the neural plate and its transformation in to the neural tube.

Nerve innervation   Nerve supply.

Neutral thermal environment   The range of environmental temperature over which heat production, oxygen consumption and nutritional requirements for growth are minimal, provided the body temperature is normal.

Non-maleficence   Do no harm.

Oedema   The effusion of body fluid into the tissues.

Oligohydramnios   Abnormally small amount of amniotic fluid in pregnancy.

Oliguria   The production of an abnormally small amount of urine.

One-to-one midwifery   One midwife takes responsibility for individual women with a partner backing up the named midwife. Such a system integrates a high level of continuity of caregiver and midwifery-led care. It is geographically based and includes women regardless of their circumstances and health needs.

Oogenesis   Formation of oogonia in the germinal epithelium of the ovaries.

Operculum   Mucoid plug of the cervical canal that inhibits ascending infection.

Osiander's sign   The increased pulsation of the uterine artery felt in the lateral vaginal fornices from the 6th week of pregnancy.

Ovulation   The process whereby the dominant Graafian follicle ruptures and releases the secondary oocyte into the pelvic cavity.

PaCO$_2$ Carbon dioxide partial pressure. Measures the partial pressure of dissolved carbon dioxide. This dissolved CO$_2$ has moved out of the cell and into the bloodstream. The measure of a PaCO$_2$ accurately reflects the alveolar ventilation.

PaO$_2$ Arterial oxygen partial pressure. Measures the partial pressure of oxygen in the arterial blood. It reflects how the lung is functioning but does not measure tissue oxygenation.

Paronychia   An inflamed swelling of the nail folds; acute paronychia is usually caused by infection with *Staphylococcus aureus*.

Partnership   A relationship of trust and equity through which both partners are strengthened and power is diffused.

Peak mucus day   A retrospective assessment of the last day of highly fertile mucus, which is observed vaginally or felt around ovulation.

Pedunculated   Stem or stalk.

Pemphigoid gestationis   see 'Herpes gestationis'.

Perinatal   Events surrounding labour and the first 7 days of life.

Perinatal mental illness   A term used both nationally and internationally to emphasize the importance of psychiatric disorder in pregnancy as well as following childbirth and the variety of psychiatric disorders that can occur at this time, in addition to postnatal depression.

pH   A solution's acidity or alkalinity is expressed on the pH scale, which runs from 0 to 14. This scale is based on the concentration of hydronium (H+) ions in a solution expressed in chemical units called moles per litre (mol/L). Solutions with a pH less than 7 are said to be *acidic* and solutions with a pH greater than 7 are *basic* or *alkaline*. Pure water has a pH very close to 7. When the fetus is hypoxic, the increased acid produced raises the acidity of the blood and the pH falls.

Phenylketonuria   An autosomal recessive disorder of protein metabolism.

Pill-free interval   The 7 days when no pills are taken during the combined oral contraceptive regimen.

Placenta accreta   Abnormally adherent placenta into the muscle layer of the uterus.

Placenta increta   Abnormally adherent placenta into the perimetrium of the uterus.

Placenta percreta   Abnormally adherent placenta through the muscle layer of the uterus.

Placenta praevia   A condition in which some or all of the placenta is attached in the lower segment of the uterus.

Placental abruption   see 'Abruptio placenta'.

Placentation   The forming of the placenta.

Polyhydramnios   An excessive amount of amniotic fluid in pregnancy. Also referred to as *hydramnios*.

Polyp   Small growth.

Porphyria   An inherited condition of abnormal red blood cell formation.

Postnatal blues   A transitory emotional or mood state, experienced by 50–80% of women, depending on parity.

Postnatal period The period after the end of labour, during which the attendance of a midwife upon the woman and baby is required, being not less than 10 days, and for such longer period as the midwife considers necessary.

Postpartum After labour.

Precipitate labour The expulsion of the fetus within 3 hours of commencement of contractions.

Pre-eclampsia A condition peculiar to pregnancy, which is characterized by hypertension, proteinuria and systemic dysfunction.

Primary postpartum haemorrhage A blood loss in excess of 500 mL or any amount that adversely affects the condition of the mother within the first 24 hours of birth.

Progestogen Synthetic progesterone used in hormonal contraception.

Prostaglandins Locally acting chemical compounds derived from fatty acids within cells. They ripen the cervix and cause the uterus to contract.

Proteinuria Protein in the urine.

Proteolytic enzymes Enzymes that break down proteins.

Pruritus Itching.

Psychosis A disorder of the mental state that affects mood and cognitive processes, which may cause the individual to lose touch with reality (i.e. hallucinations and delusional thoughts are usually present).

Ptyalism Excessive salivation.

Pudendal block This is the procedure where local anaesthetic is infiltrated into the tissue around the pudendal nerve within the pelvis; employed for some operative procedures during vaginal births.

Puerperal psychosis Describes a rare but serious psychiatric emergency and the most severe form of postpartum affective (mood) disorder.

Puerperal sepsis Infection of the genital tract following childbirth; still a major cause of maternal death where it is undetected and/or untreated.

Puerperium A period after childbirth where the uterus and other organs and structures that have been affected by the pregnancy are physiologically returning to their non-gravid state, lactation is establishing and the woman is adjusting

socially and psychologically to motherhood. Usually described as a period of up to 6–8 weeks.

Quickening The first point at which the woman recognizes fetal movements in early pregnancy.

Reciprocity A mutual relationship between two individuals where there is an exchange of positive regard for each other.

Regional anaesthesia More commonly are epidural and intrathecal (spinal) anaesthetics.

Retraction The process by which the uterine muscle fibres shorten after a contraction. This is unique to uterine muscle.

Rubin's manoeuvre A rotational manoeuvre to relieve shoulder dystocia. Pressure is exerted over the fetal back to adduct and rotate the shoulders.

Sandal gap Exaggerated gap between the first and second toes.

Secondary postpartum haemorrhage Any abnormal or excessive bleeding from the genital tract occurring between 24 hours and 12 weeks postnatally.

Selective fetocide The medical destruction of a malformed twin fetus in a continuing pregnancy.

Sinciput The forehead.

Sheehan's syndrome A condition where sudden or prolonged shock leads to irreversible pituitary necrosis characterized by amenorrhoea, genital atrophy and premature senility.

Short femur Shorter than the average thigh bone, when compared with other fetal measurements.

Shoulder dystocia Failure of the shoulders to spontaneously traverse the pelvis after birth of the fetal head.

Show Discharge of the operculum.

Speculum (vaginal) An instrument used to open the vagina.

Striae gravidarum Stretch marks.

Subinvolution The uterine size appears larger than anticipated for the number of days postpartum, and may feel not well contracted. Uterine tenderness may be present.

Succenturiate lobe A small extra lobe of placenta separate from the main placenta.

Surfactant Complex mixture of phospholipids and lipoproteins produced by type 2 alveolar cells in the lungs that decreases surface tension and prevents alveolar collapse at end expiration.

Sulci Another word for furrows.

Sutures Junctions or joints between two adjacent cranial bones.

Symphysiotomy A surgical incision to separate the symphysis pubis and enlarge the pelvis to aid birth of the baby.

Symphysis pubis dysfunction see 'Diastasis symphysis pubis'.

Tachypnoea Increased respiratory rate that occurs as the baby attempts to compensate for an increased carbon dioxide concentration in the blood and extracellular fluids.

Talipes A complex foot deformity, affecting 1/1000 live births and more common in males. The affected foot is held in a fixed flexion (*equinus*) and in-turned (*varus*) position. It can be differentiated from positional talipes because the deformity in true talipes cannot be passively corrected.

Team midwifery Midwives are team-based rather than on a ward or within a community base. The team takes responsibility for a number of women. Teams may be restricted to hospital or community, or cover both areas.

Tentorium cerebelli An arched fold of the dura mater, covering the upper surface of the cerebellum.

Teratogen An agent believed to cause congenital malformations, e.g. thalidomide.

Tocophobia A morbid fear of childbirth.

Torsion Twisting.

Torticollis The result of tightness and shortening of one sternomastoid muscle.

Tregs Adapted T regulator cells that play a part in immunity.

Trigone base of the bladder.

Trizygotic Formed from three separate zygotes.

Trophoblasts Peripheral cells surrounding the blastocyst.

Twin-to-twin transfusion syndrome see 'Feto-fetal transfusion syndrome'.

Uniovular   Monozygotic.

Unstable lie   After 36 weeks' gestation, a lie that varies between longitudinal and oblique or transverse is said to be unstable.

Urachus   A fibrous band that extends from the apex of the bladder to the umbilicus.

Uterine involution   The physiological process that starts from the end of labour and results in a gradual reduction in the size of the uterus until it returns to its non-pregnant size and location in the pelvis.

Uterine souffle   Soft blowing sound heard using a stethoscope in the lower part of the uterus in the second trimester. It is synchronous with the maternal pulse.

Uterotonics   Also known as 'oxytocics' or 'ecbolics'. Pharmacological agents/drugs (e.g. syntometrine, syntocinon, ergometrine and prostaglandins) that are used in the active management of the third stage of labour to stimulate the smooth muscle of the uterus to contract.

Utilitarianism   Providing the greatest good for greatest number.

Vanishing twin syndrome   The reabsorption of one twin fetus early in pregnancy (usually before 12 weeks).

Vasa praevia   A rare occurrence in which umbilical cord vessels pass through the placental membranes and lie across the cervical os.

Vasculogenesis   The formation of new blood vessels.

Vernix caseosa   White creamy substance protecting the fetus from desiccation and is present from 18 weeks' gestation.

Wharton's jelly   Gelatinous substance surrounding the umbilical cord.

Withdrawal bleed   Vaginal bleeding due to withdrawal of hormones.

Wood's manoeuvre   A rotational or screw manoeuvre to relieve shoulder dystocia. Pressure is exerted on the fetal chest to rotate and abduct the shoulders.

Zavanelli manoeuvre   Last choice of manoeuvre for shoulder dystocia. The head is returned to its pre-restitution position, then the head is flexed back into the vagina. Birth is by caesarean section.

Zona pellucida   An extracellular glycoprotein matrix surrounding the plasma membrane of the oocyte, which aids with binding of the spermatozoa.

Zygote   A diploid cell resulting from the union of two haploid gametes, i.e. the ovum and the spermatozoon with the culmination of a fertilized ovum from which a fetus will develop.

Zygosity   Describing the genetic make-up of children in a multiple birth.

Acronyms

AA   arachidonic acid

ABM   Association of Breastfeeding Mothers

ABPM   ambulatory blood pressure monitoring

ACE   angiotensin converting enzyme

ACOG   American College of Obstetricians and Gynecologists

ACTH   adrenocorticotrophic hormone

ADH   antidiuretic hormone

AED   antiepileptic drug/automated external defibrillator

AEI   Approved Education Institution

A-EQUIP   Advocating for Education and Quality Improvement (England)

AFE   amniotic fluid embolism

AFLD   acute fatty liver disease

AGA   appropriate for gestational age

AIDS   acquired immunodeficiency syndrome

AIMS   Association for Improvements in Maternity Services

ALP   maternal alkaline phosphatase

ALT   alanine transaminase

AMROC   Academy of Medical Royal Colleges

AMTSL   active management of the third stage of labour

ANS   autonomic nervous system

ANP   atrial natriuretic peptide

Anti HBe   hepatitis B e-antibodies

APEC   Action on pre-eclampsia

APH   antepartum haemorrhage

APS   antiphospholipid syndrome

ARB   angiotensin receptor blocker

ARC   antenatal results and choices

ARM   artificial rupture of the membranes; Association of Radical Midwives

ART   antiretroviral therapy

ASD   atrial septal defect

AST   aspartate transaminase; aspartate aminotransferase

ATAIN   avoiding term admissions into neonatal units

ATP   adenosine triphosphate

BALT   bronchus-associated lymphoid tissue

BAME   black, Asian and minority ethnic

BAPM   British Association of Perinatal Medicine

BAT   brown adipose tissue

BF(H)I   Baby Friendly (Hospital) Initiative

BFLG   Baby Feeding Law Group

BHIVA   British HIV Association

BMI   body mass index

BMR   basal metabolic rate

BNF   British National Formulary

BNP   brain natriuretic peptide

BOC   British Oxygen Company

BP   blood pressure

BPA   bisphenol A

BPAS   British Pregnancy Advisory Service

BTS   British Thoracic Society

CAH   congenital adrenal hyperplasia

CBUK   Child Bereavement United Kingdom

CCA   clear-cell adenocarcinoma

CCG   Clinical Commissioning Group

CCT   controlled cord traction

CD   controlled drug

C. Diff   *Clostridium difficile*

CDH   congenital diaphragmatic hernia

CDOP   child death overview panel

CDR   child death review

CEMD   Confidential Enquiry into Maternal Deaths

CESDI   Confidential Enquiries into Stillbirths and Deaths in Infancy

CF   cystic fibrosis

C(E)FM   continuous (electronic) fetal monitoring

CHD   congenital heart disease

CHF   congenital heart failure

CHFed   Children's Heart Federation

CHRE   Council for Healthcare Regulatory Excellence (replaced by PSA)

CHT   congenital hypothyroidism

CIN cervical intraepithelial neoplasia

CLAPA Cleft Lip and Palate Association

CMACE Centre for Maternal and Child Enquiries

CMB Central Midwives Board

CMO Chief Midwifery Officer

CMS cervical membrane sweep

CMV cytomegalovirus

CNORIS Clinical Negligence and Other Risks Indemnity Scheme

CNR Clinical Research Network

CNS central nervous system

CNST Clinical Negligence Scheme for Trusts

CNO Chief Nursing Officer

CoA coarctation of the aorta

COC combined oral contraceptive

COMET Comparative Obstetric Mobile Epidural Trial

CONI care of the next infant

CPAM congenital pulmonary airway malformation

CPD cephalopelvic disproportion; continuing professional development

CPR cardiopulmonary resuscitation

CQC Care Quality Commission

CR capillary refill

CRH corticotrophin-releasing hormone

CRS congenital rubella syndrome

CRT capillary refill time

CS caesarean section

CSE child sex exploitation ('grooming')

CSF cerebral spinal fluid

CSfM Clinical Supervisor for Midwives (Wales, Scotland and Northern Ireland)

CSII continuous subcutaneous insulin infusion

CT computerized tomography

CTG cardiotograph(y)/cardiotocogram

CVA cerebral vascular accident

CVP central venous pressure

CVS chorionic villus sampling

CWS Cambridge Worry Scale

DAT direct antiglobulin test

DCT direct Coomb's test

DDH developmental dysplasia of the hip

DES Diethylstilboestrol

DfE Department for Education

DCDA Placenta with two chorions and two amnions

DH/DoH Department of Health (and social care) England

DHA docosahexaenoic acid

DIC disseminated intravascular coagulation

DNA deoxyribonucleic acid

DI donor insemination

DSD disorders of sex development

DVT deep vein thrombosis

DZ Dizygotic

EAS external anal sphincter

EB epidermolysis bullosa

EBM expressed breast milk

ECG electrocardiogram/graphy

E. coli *Escherichia coli*

ECM extracellular matrix

ECMO extracorporeal membrane oxygenation

ECV external cephalic version

EDB expected date of birth

EEG electroencephalogram

EFM electronic fetal monitoring (see also C(E)FM)

EFSA European Food Standards Agency

eGFR epidermal growth factor receptor

ELBW extremely low birth weight (below 1000 g)

EMC enhanced maternity care

EMTSL expectant management of the third stage of labour

ENT ear, nose and throat

EON examination of the newborn

EPDS Edinburgh Postnatal Depression Scale

ERPC evacuation of retained products of conception

EU European Union

FASD fetal alcohol spectrum disorders

FBC full blood count

FBS fetal blood sample/sampling

FDA Food and Drug Administration

FDP fibrin degradation product

FGM female genital mutilation (genital cutting/female circumcision)

FGMPO Female Genital Mutilation Protection Order

FGR fetal growth restriction

FHEQ Framework for Higher Education Qualifications

FHR fetal heart rate

FIGO International Federation of Gynecology and Obstetrics

FIL feedback inhibitor of lactation

FNP family nurse partnership/practitioner

FPA Family Planning Association

FSA Food Standards Agency

FSH follicle stimulating hormone

FSRH Faculty of Sexual and Reproductive Health

FVC forced vital capacity

FVS fetal varicella syndrome

GA1 glutaric aciduria type 1

GAD-2 generalized anxiety disorder 2

GALT gut-associated lymphoid tissue

Gal-1-PUT galactose-1-phosphate uridyl transferase

GAP growth assessment protocol

GAS Group A streptococcus

G6PD Glucose 6 phosphate dehydrogenase

GBS Group B streptococcus

GCS Glasgow Coma Score

GCP good clinical practice

GDM gestational diabetes mellitus

GF glomerular filtrate

GFR glomerular filtration rate

GGT γ-glutamyl transpeptidase

GI(T) gastrointestinal (tract)

GIFT gamete intrafallopian (intratubal) transfer

GLOSS Global Maternal Sepsis Study

GMH germinal matrix haemorrhage

GNC General Nursing Council

GnRH gonadotrophic-releasing hormone

GP General Practitioner

GROW gestation related optimal weight

GSL general sale list (medicines)

GTD gestational trophoblastic disease

GTI genital tract infection

GTN gestational trophoblastic neoplasia

GTT glucose tolerance test

HAART highly active antiretroviral therapy

HAMLET Human Alpha-lactalbumin Made LEthal to Tumour cells

Hb haemoglobin

HbA adult haemoglobin

HbAS sickle cell trait (heterozygous)

HbA1c glucated/glycosylated haemoglobin

HBeAg hepatitis B e-antigen

HbF fetal haemoglobin

HbH haemoglobin H disease

HbSS sickle cell anaemia/disease (homozygous)

HBV hepatitis B virus

HCAI healthcare-acquired infection

hCG human chorionic gonadotrophin

hCG-H hyperglycosylated human chorionic gonadotrophin

hCS human chorionic somatomammotropin hormone

HCU homocystinuria

HDCU high dependency care unit

HDL high-density lipoprotein

HDN haemolytic disease of the newborn

HEI higher education institution

HELLP haemolytic elevated liver enzymes low platelets

HFEA Human Fertilisation and Embryology Authority (UK)

HIE hypoxic ischaemic encephalopathy

HIS Healthcare Improvement Scotland

HIV Human Immunodeficiency Virus

HIW Healthcare Inspectorate Wales

HOOP hands-on hands-poised

HPA axis hypothalamic pituitary adrenal axis

hPGH human placental growth hormone

hPL human placental lactogen

HPT home pregnancy test

HPV human papilloma virus

HRA Health Research Authority

HSCIC Health and Social Care Information Centre (now NHS Digital)

HSE health survey for England; health, safety and environment

HSIB Healthcare Safety Investigation Branch

HSV herpes simplex virus

HTA human tissue authority

HVS high vaginal swab

IA intermittent auscultation

IAP intrapartum antibiotic prophylaxis

IAS internal anal sphincter

ICH International Confederation of Harmonization of Technical Requirements of Pharmaceuticals for Human Use

ICM International Confederation of Midwives

ICP intrahepatic cholestasis of pregnancy

ICU intensive care unit

ICS integrated care system

IDM infants of diabetic mothers

IEM inborn errors of metabolism

IFCC International Federation of Clinical Chemistry and Laboratory Medicine

IgA Immunoglobulin A

IGF-1 insulin-like growth factor

IHD ischaemic heart disease

IM intramuscular

IOL induction of labour

IOM Institute of Medicine (now the National Academy of Medicine in America)

IPL intraparenchymal lesion

IPPV intermittent positive pressure ventilation

IQ intelligence quotient

ITP idiopathic thrombocytopenic purpura

IUCD intrauterine contraceptive device

IUFD intrauterine fetal death

IUGR intrauterine growth restriction

IUI intrauterine insemination

IUS intrauterine system

IV/IVI intravenous/intravenous infusion

IVA isovaleric acidaemia

IVF *in vitro* fertilization

IVH intraventricular haemorrhage

JEC Joint Epilepsy Council

L3 third lumbar vertebra

LA Local Authority

LAM lactational amenorrhoea method; levator ani muscles

LBW low birth weight (below 2500 g)

LC-PUFA long chain polyunsaturated fatty acids

LFT liver function test

LGA large for gestational age

LGBTQ lesbian, gay, bisexual, transgender and queer (umbrella term for minority sexual orientations and gender identities)

LH luteinizing hormone

LLSB lower left sternal border

LME lead midwife for education (NMC UK)

LMP last menstrual period

LMWH low molecular weight heparin

LSA Local Supervising Authority

LSCB Local Safeguarding Children Board

LSCS lower segment caesarean section/CS

MA mento-anterior

MADGE IgM, IgA, IgD, IgG, IgE

MALT mucosa associated lymphoid tissue

MBF Multiple Birth Foundation

MBRRACE-UK Mothers and Babies: Reducing Risk through Audits and Confidential Enquiries across the UK

MCADD medium-chain acyl-CoA dehydrogenase deficiency

MCDA Placenta with one chorion and two amnions

MCH mean cell/corpuscular haemoglobin

MCMA Placenta with one chorion and one amnion

MCoC midwifery continuity of carer

MCV mean cell/corpuscular volume

MELAS mitochondrial encephalomyopathy with lactic acid and stroke-like episodes

MEOWS Modified Early Obstetric Warning Score

MERRF myoclonic epilepsy with ragged red fibres myopathy

MFPR Multifetal pregnancy reduction

MDT multidisciplinary team

MH(P)RA Medicines and Healthcare Products Regulatory Agency

MI myocardial infarction

MIDIRS Midwives Information and Resource Service

MMR measles, mumps and rubella

MODY mature onset diabetes of the young

MOH Medical Officer of Health

MPV mean platelet volume

MRI magnetic resonance imaging

MRSA methicillin-resistant *Staphylococcus aureus*

MSU/MSSU mid-stream specimen of urine

MSUD maple syrup urine disease

MSW Maternity Support Worker

MTP Maternity Transformation Programme

MV mento-vertical

MZ Monozygotic

NAIT neonatal alloimmune thrombocytopenia

NAS neonatal abstinence syndrome

NCT National Childbirth Trust

NEC necrotizing enterocolitis

NES NHS Education for Scotland

NET-EN norethisterone enanthate

NG nasogastric

NHS National Health Service

NHSLA National Health Service Litigation Authority (now NHS Resolution)

NICE National Institute for Health and Care Excellence

NICU/NNICU neonatal intensive care unit

NIHR National Institute for Health Research

NIPE newborn and infant physical examination (England)

NIPEC Northern Ireland Practice and Education Council for Nursing and Midwifery

NIPT non-invasive pregnancy test

NK natural killer

NLS newborn life support

NMC Nursing and Midwifery Council (UK)

NPEU/C National Perinatal Epidemiology Unit/Centre (Ireland)

NPSA National Patient Safety Agency (now NHS Improvement)

NSAID non-steroidal anti-inflammatory drug

NSPCC National Society for the Prevention of Cruelty to Children

NSPKU National Society for Phenylketonuria

NT nuchal translucency

NTC neonatal transitional care

NTD neural tube defect

NTE neutral thermal environment

OA occipitoanterior

OASI/OASIs obstetric anal sphincter injuries

OC obstetric cholestasis

OF occipitofrontal

ONS Office of National Statistics (UK)

OP occipitoposterior

OT occipitotransverse

PAP pulmonary artery pressure

PAP test Papanicolaou test/smear test

PCA patient-controlled analgesia

PCHI permanent congenital hearing impairment

PCR polymerase chain reaction

PCT Primary Care Trust (abolished in 2013 and their work taken over by CCGs)

PDA patent ductus arteriosus

PDS Personal Demographics Service

PE pulmonary embolism/embolus

PET pre-eclampsia toxaemia

PGD patient group direction; pre-implantation genetic diagnosis

(15-)PGDH (15-hydroxy)prostaglandin dehydrogenase

PGE2 prostaglandin E2

PGP pelvic girdle pain

PHE Public Health England

PHSO Parliamentary and Health Service Ombudsman

PID pelvic inflammatory disease

PIH pregnancy-induced hypertension

PKU phenylketonuria

PMA professional midwife advocate (England)

PND postnatal depression

POC point of care

POM prescription-only medicines

POP progesterone-only pill

PPH postpartum haemorrhage

PPI proton pump inhibitor

PPROM preterm prelabour rupture of the membranes

PROM prelabour rupture of the membranes (at term)

PSA Professional Standards Authority (formerly CHRE)

PSD patient specific directions

PSRB Professional Statutory Regulatory Body

PSTI pancreatic secretory trypsin inhibitor

PT prothrombin time

PTH parathyroid hormone

QF-PCR quantitative fluorescence-polymerase chain reaction

RAAS renin–angiotensin–aldosterone system

RBC red blood cells

RCoA Royal College of Anaesthetists

RCM Royal College of Midwives

RCOG Royal College of Obstetricians and Gynaecologists

RCPCH Royal College of Paediatrics and Child Health

RCPSG Royal College of Physicians and Surgeons of Glasgow

RCS restorative clinical supervision

RCT randomized controlled trial

RCUK Resuscitation Council of the United Kingdom

RDS respiratory distress syndrome

REM rapid eye movement

RNA ribonucleic acid

RPF renal plasma flow

RQIA Regulation and Quality Improvement Authority (Northern Ireland)

SACN Scientific Advisory Committee on Nutrition

SANDS Stillbirth and Neonatal Death Society

SBR serum bilirubin

SBAR situation, background, assessment and recommendation

SCBU Special Care Baby Unit

SCD sickle cell disease

SCPHN specialist community public health nurse (also known as health visitor)

SDGs Sustainable Development Goals

SDSD Scottish Differences of Sex Development Network

SFH symphysis fundal height

SFGA Small-for-gestational-age

SGA small for gestational age

sGR Selective growth restriction

SI statutory instrument

SIGN Scottish Intercollegiate Guidelines Network

SLE systemic lupus erythematosus

SMB submento bregmatic

SMV submento vertical

SOB suboccipito bregmatic; shortness of breath

SOF suboccipito frontal

SOFT Support Organization for Trisomy 13/18.

SoM Supervisor of Midwives

SPRM selective progesterone receptor modulator

SRY sex determining region on the Y gene

SSC skin-to-skin contact

STI sexually transmitted infection

STP sustainability and transformation partnership

SUDI sudden unexpected death in infancy

SUI stress urinary incontinence

T11 eleventh thoracic vertebra

TAMBA   Twins and Multiple Birth Association (now the Twins Trust Ltd)

TAPS   twin anaemia-polycythaemia sequence

TBG   thyroxine-binding globulin

TBV   total blood volume

TCB   transcutaneous bilirubinometer

TDF   testis determining factor

TED   thromboembolism deterrent

TENS   transcutaneous electrical nerve stimulation

TEV   talipes equinovarus

ToP(FA)   termination of pregnancy (for fetal anomaly)

TPR   temperature, pulse and respiration

ToRCH   Toxoplasmosis, other (e.g. syphilis, varicella zoster, parvovirus B19) Rubella, Cytomegalovirus, Herpes

TRAP   twin reversed arterial perfusion

TRH   Thyrotropin-releasing hormone

TSH   Thyroid-stimulating hormone

TTN   Transient tachypnoea of the newborn

TTTS   Twin-to-twin transfusion syndrome

UDP-GT   Uridine diphospho-glucuronyl transferase

UK   United Kingdom

UKAMB   United Kingdom Association for Milk Banking

UKCC   United Kingdom Central Council for Nursing, Midwifery and Health Visiting

UKCEN   United Kingdom Clinical Ethics Network

UK:JCVI   United Kingdom Joint Committee for Vaccination and Immunisation

UKOSS   United Kingdom Obstetric Surveillance System

ULSB   upper left sternal border

UN   United Nations

UNAIDS   United Nations Programme on HIV/AIDS

UNCRC   United Nations Convention on the Rights of the Child

UNFPA   United Nations Population Fund

UNICEF   United Nations International Children's Fund

UNOHCHR   United Nations Office of the High Commissioner for Human Rights

UPSI   unprotected sexual intercourse

URSB   upper right sternal border

USMERA   United States Midwifery Education, Regulation and Association collective

US(S)   ultrasound (scan)

UTI   urinary tract infection

VACTERL spectrum   vertebral anomalies, anal anomalies, cardiac, tracheoesophageal, radial aplasia, renal and limb anomalies

VE   vaginal examination

VEGF   vascular endothelial growth factor

VKDB   vitamin K deficiency bleeding

VLBW   very low birth weight (below 1500 g)

VSD   ventricular septal defect

VTE   venous thromboembolism

VZIG   varicella zoster immunoglobulin

VZV   varicella zoster virus

W-DEQ   Wijma Delivery Expectancy-Experience Questionnaire

WHO   World Health Organization

WMA   World Medical Association

ZIFT   zygote intrafallopian (intratubal) transfer

Note: Page numbers followed by "f" indicate figures, "t" indicate tables, and "b" indicate boxes.